Adult Health Nursing-II
(Medical Surgical Nursing)

Adult Health Nursing-II
(Medical Surgical Nursing)

As per the Revised Syllabus for BSc Nursing

Sukhpal Kaur PhD PGDS FNRSI
Professor-cum-Principal
National Institute of Nursing Education
Postgraduate Institute of Medical Education and Research
Chandigarh, India

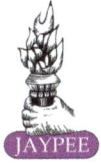

JAYPEE BROTHERS MEDICAL PUBLISHERS
The Health Sciences Publisher
New Delhi | London

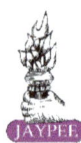

Jaypee Brothers Medical Publishers (P) Ltd

Headquarters
Jaypee Brothers Medical Publishers (P) Ltd
EMCA House
23/23-B, Ansari Road, Daryaganj
New Delhi - 110 002, India
Landline: +91-11-23272143, +91-11-23272703
+91-11-23282021, +91-11-23245672
Email: jaypee@jaypeebrothers.com

Overseas Office
J.P. Medical Ltd
83 Victoria Street, London
SW1H 0HW (UK)
Phone: +44 20 3170 8910
Email: info@jpmedpub.com

Website: www.jaypeebrothers.com
Website: www.jaypeedigital.com

Corporate Office
Jaypee Brothers Medical Publishers (P) Ltd
4838/24, Ansari Road, Daryaganj
New Delhi 110 002, India
Phone: +91-11-43574357
Fax: +91-11-43574314
Email: jaypee@jaypeebrothers.com

EU GPSR Authorised Representative
Logos Europe, 9 rue Nicolas Poussin
17000, La Rochelle, France
Phone: +33 (0) 6 67 93 73 78
E-mail: Contact@logoseurope.eu

© 2024, Jaypee Brothers Medical Publishers (P) Ltd

The views and opinions expressed in this book are solely those of the original contributor(s)/author(s) and do not necessarily represent those of editor(s) and publisher of the book.

All rights reserved. No part of this publication may be reproduced, stored or transmitted in any form or by any means, electronic, mechanical, photocopying, recording or otherwise, without the prior permission in writing of the publishers.

All brand names and product names used in this book are trade names, service marks, trademarks or registered trademarks of their respective owners. The publisher is not associated with any product or vendor mentioned in this book.

Medical knowledge and practice change constantly. This book is designed to provide accurate, authoritative information about the subject matter in question. However, readers are advised to check the most current information available on procedures included and check information from the manufacturer of each product to be administered, to verify the recommended dose, formula, method and duration of administration, adverse effects and contraindications. It is the responsibility of the practitioner to take all appropriate safety precautions. Neither the publisher nor the author(s)/editor(s) assume any liability for any injury and/or damage to persons or property arising from or related to use of material in this book.

This book is sold on the understanding that the publisher is not engaged in providing professional medical services. If such advice or services are required, the services of a competent medical professional should be sought.

Every effort has been made where necessary to contact holders of copyright to obtain permission to reproduce copyright material. If any have been inadvertently overlooked, the publisher will be pleased to make the necessary arrangements at the first opportunity.

Inquiries for bulk sales may be solicited at: jaypee@jaypeebrothers.com

Adult Health Nursing-II (Medical Surgical Nursing)

First Edition: **2024**

ISBN: 978-93-5465-919-5

Contributors

Abhishek Singh DNB (ENT)
Government Multi Specialty Hospital
Chandigarh, India

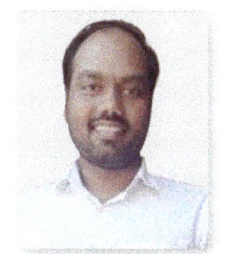

Aditi Mehta MD (Ophthalmology)
Consultant
Grewal Eye Institute
Chandigarh, India

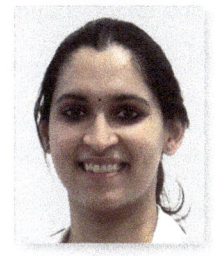

Alisha Talwar MSN
Team Lead–Nursing
Jaypee Brothers Medical Publishers
New Delhi, India

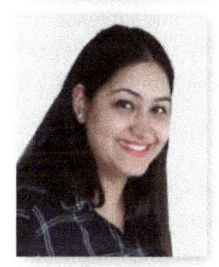

Anshul Chauhan BDS MPH PhD Scholar
Department of Ophthalmology
Postgraduate Institute of Medical
Education and Research
Chandigarh, India

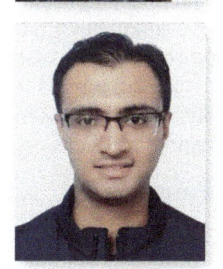

Anuradha Sharma PhD
Lecturer
Speech and Hearing Unit
Department of Otolaryngology
Postgraduate Institute of Medical
Education and Research
Chandigarh, India

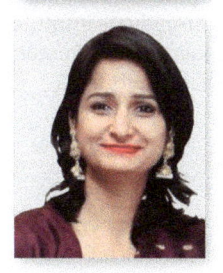

Arti Saini MSc
Nursing Officer
Postgraduate Institute of Medical
Education and Research
Chandigarh, India

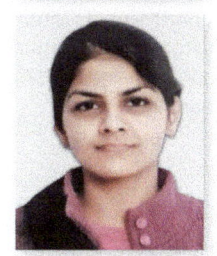

Ashok Kumar PhD
National Institute of Nursing
Education
Postgraduate Institute of Medical
Education and Research
Chandigarh, India

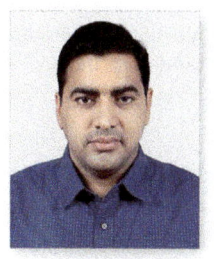

Atul Arora MBBS (Gold Medallist) MS
MCh (Vitreoretina)
Consultant (Ophthalmology)
Department of Telemedicine
Postgraduate Institute of Medical
Education and Research
Chandigarh, India

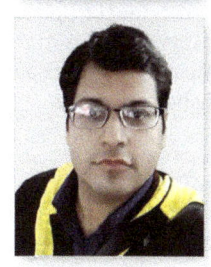

Daisy Sahni PhD
Former Professor and Head
Department of Anatomy
Postgraduate Institute of Medical
Education and Research
Chandigarh, India

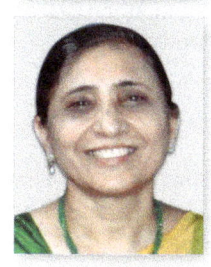

Deepak Goel MD DM (Neurology)
Professor and Head
Himalyan Institute of Medical Sciences
Dehradun, Uttarakhand, India

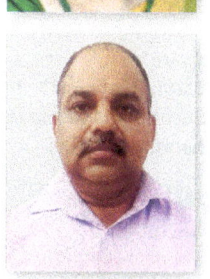

Dia Sharma DNB (ENT) Student
Government Multi Specialty Hospital
Chandigarh, India

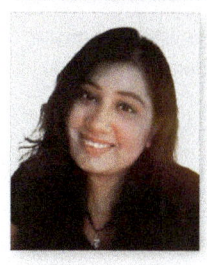

Divesh Kumar Munjal MSc
Stroke Nurse Coordinator
Department of Neurology
Postgraduate Institute of Medical
Education and Research
Chandigarh, India

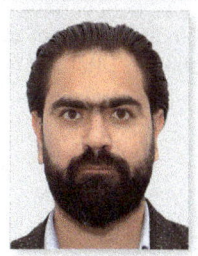

Contributors

Divya Dahiya MS
Professor
Department of General Surgery
Postgraduate Institute of Medical
Education and Research
Chandigarh, India

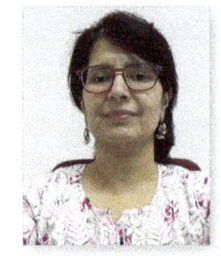

Faisal Thattaruthody MS (Ophthal)
Associate Professor
Advanced Eye Centre
Postgraduate Institute of Medical
Education and Research
Chandigarh, India

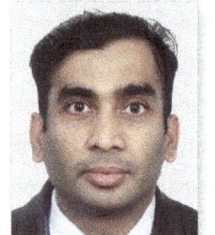

Gagandeep Kaur BSc
Bachelors of Optometry
Optometrist
Department of Ophthalmology
Postgraduate Institute of Medical
Education and Research
Chandigarh, India

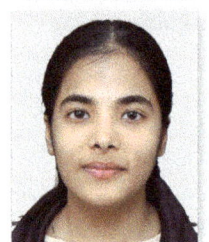

Gurpreet Kaur PhD
Public Health Nursing Officer
Postgraduate Institute of Medical
Education and Research
Chandigarh, India

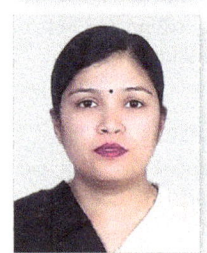

Himanshi Singh MS
Associate Consultant
Centre for Sight, Agra
Ex-Senior Resident
Advanced Eye Center
Postgraduate Institute of Medical
Education and Research
Chandigarh, India

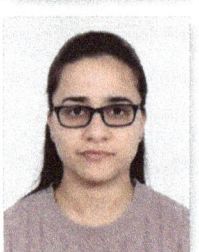

Jagat Ram MS FAMS
Director
Cataract and Refractive Surgery and
Cornea
Grewal Eye Institute
Chandigarh, India

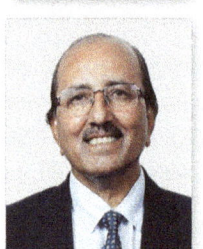

Jitender Chaturvedi MCh
(Neurosurgery)
Associate Professor
Department of Neurosurgery
All India Institute of Medical Sciences
Rishikesh, Uttarakhand, India

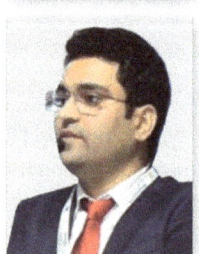

Jitendra Gairolla PhD
Senior Resident
Department of Microbiology
Nodal Officer
Drone Based Health Services
All India Institute of Medical Sciences
Rishikesh, Uttarakhand, India

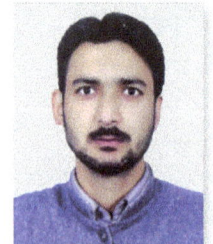

Jyoti Kathwal PhD
Assistant Professor
College of Nursing
Bilaspur, Himachal Pradesh, India

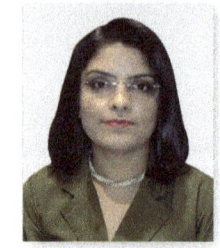

Jyoti Sharma MSc
Nursing Tutor
DMCH College of Nursing
Ludhiana, Punjab, India

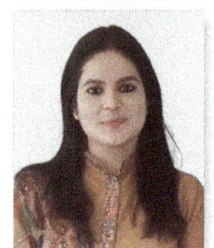

Kajree Gupta MS
Senior Resident
Advanced Eye Centre
Postgraduate Institute of Medical
Education and Research
Chandigarh, India

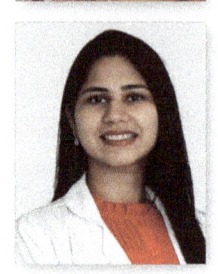

Kapil Goel MBBS MD (Community Medicine)
Assistant Professor of Epidemiology
Department of Community Medicine
and School of Public Health
Postgraduate Institute of Medical
Education and Research
Chandigarh, India

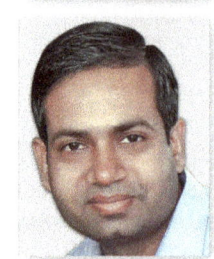

Kiran Kumari MS
Senior Resident
Advanced Eye Centre
Postgraduate Institute of Medical
Education and Research
Chandigarh, India

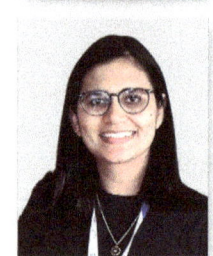

Lakshya Kumar BSc
Bachelors of Optometry
Optometrist
Department of Ophthalmology
Postgraduate Institute of Medical
Education and Research
Chandigarh, India

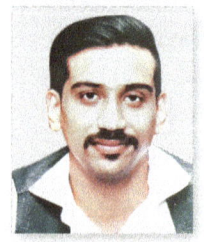

Latika Bajaj PhD
Assistant Professor
College of Nursing
All India Institute of Medical Sciences
Nagpur, Maharashtra, India

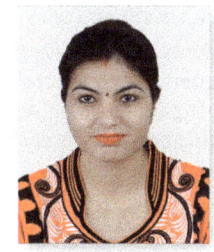

Manju Dhandapani PhD
Associate Professor
National Institute of Nursing
Education
Postgraduate Institute of Medical
Education and Research
Chandigarh, India

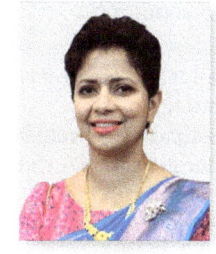

Latika Rohilla PhD
Public Health Nursing Officer
Postgraduate Institute of Medical
Education and Research
Chandigarh, India

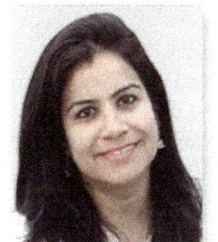

Manpreet Kaur MBBS MS FSEH
Consultant
Grewal Eye Institute
Chandigarh, India

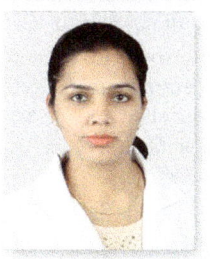

Lt Col Lata Mandal PhD
Head of Research Wing
Indigen Institute of Neuropsychology
Council
Kolkata, West Bengal, India

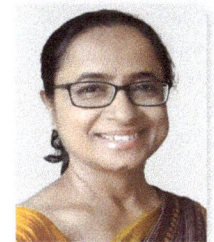

Manpreet Singh MS DNB FAICO FRCS
(GI) MNAMS
Associate Professor
Advanced Eye Centre
Department of Ophthalmology
Postgraduate Institute of Medical
Education and Research
Chandigarh, India

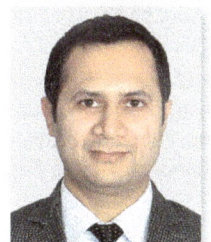

Madhuri Akella MS
Former Glaucoma Fellow
Advanced Eye Centre
Postgraduate Institute of Medical
Education and Research
Chandigarh, India

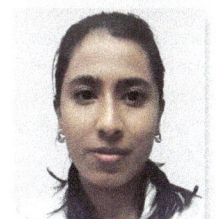

Manu Saini MS
Assistant Professor
Department of Ophthalmology
Postgraduate Institute of Medical
Education and Research
Chandigarh, India

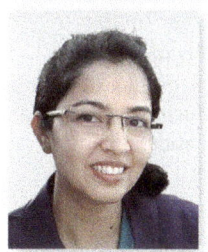

Maninderdeep Kaur PhD
Faculty
National Institute of Nursing
Education
Postgraduate Institute of Medical
Education and Research
Chandigarh, India

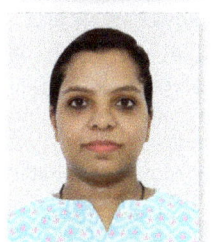

Manwinder Singh Walia MS
Head
Department of ENT
Government Multispecialty Hospital
Chandigarh, India

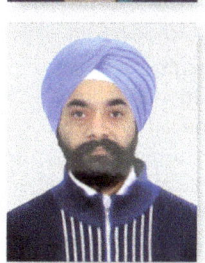

Manisha Nagi PhD
Faculty
National Institute of Nursing
Education
Postgraduate Institute of Medical
Education and Research
Chandigarh, India

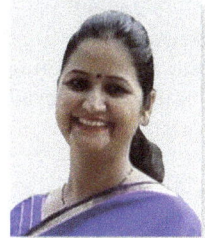

Md Noorain Alam PhD
Lecturer
Speech and Hearing Unit
Department of Otolaryngology
Postgraduate Institute of Medical
Education and Research
Chandigarh, India

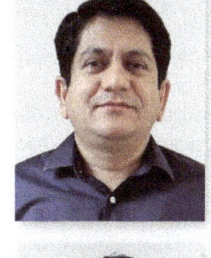

Manjeet Singh MD
Additional Director
Internal Medicine
Fortis Med Care
Chandigarh, India

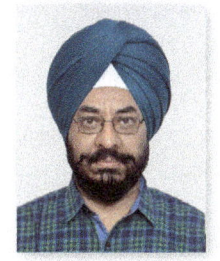

Mona Duggal MD MHS
Associate Professor Advanced
Eye Centre
Postgraduate Institute of Medical
Education and Research
Chandigarh, India

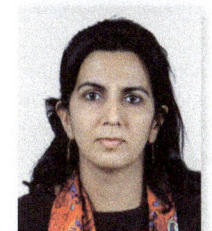

Contributors

Monaliza PhD
Associate Professor
National Institute of Nursing Education
Postgraduate Institute of Medical Education and Research
Chandigarh, India

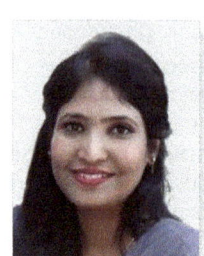

Navdeep Bansal PhD
Transplant Coordinator
Postgraduate Institute of Medical Education and Research
Chandigarh, India

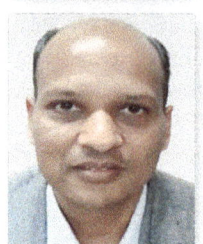

Neha Chauhan MS FICO FAICO
(Glaucoma)
Ex-Glaucoma Fellow
Postgraduate Institute of Medical Education and Research
Chandigarh, India

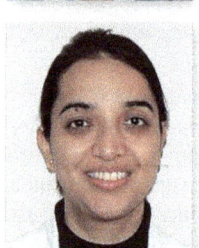

Neha Pundhir MSc
Nursing Officer
Postgraduate Institute of Medical Education and Research
Chandigarh, India

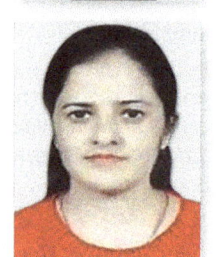

Nitasha Sharma MSc PhD
Faculty
National Institute of Nursing Education
Postgraduate Institute of Medical Education and Research
Chandigarh, India

Pankaj Arora MBBS MHA (AIIMS) DNB
Associate Professor
Department of Hospital Administration
Postgraduate Institute of Medical Education and Research
Chandigarh, India

Parul Chawla Gupta MS
Associate Professor
Advanced Eye Center
Postgraduate Institute of Medical Education and Research
Chandigarh, India

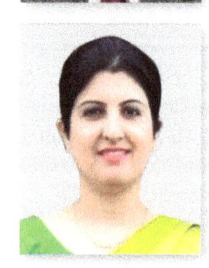

Pooja Nadholta PhD
Neuroscience Research Laboratory
Department of Neurology
Postgraduate Institute of Medical Education and Research
Chandigarh, India

Pooja Parihar MPH
Research Scholar
Department of Community Medicine and School of Public Health
Postgraduate Institute of Medical Education and Research
Chandigarh, India

Pooja Thakur PhD
Tutor
Adress-College of Nursing
All India Institute of Medical Sciences
Patna, Bihar, India

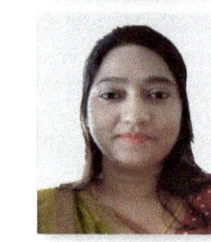

Pradeepti Nayak MS
Assistant Professor
Department of Otorhinolaryngology and HNS
School of Medical Sciences and Research
Sharda University
Greater Noida, Uttar Pradesh, India

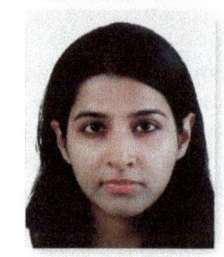

Pragya Pathak PhD
Professor-cum-Vice-Principal
College of Nursing
Dr Ram Manohar Lohia Institute of Medical Sciences
Lucknow, Uttar Pradesh, India

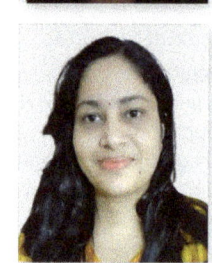

Pramod Kumar MSc
Nursing Officer
Postgraduate Institute of Medical Education and Research
Chandigarh, India

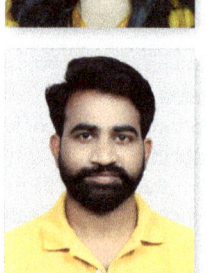

Priya Baby PhD
Lecturer, College of Nursing
National Institute of Mental Health and Neurosciences
Bengaluru, Karnataka, India

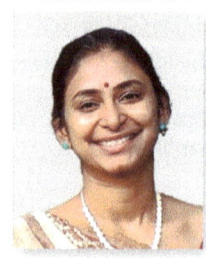

Priyanka Verma BDS MPH
Research Associate
Department of Ophthalmology
Postgraduate Institute of Medical
Education and Research
Chandigarh, India

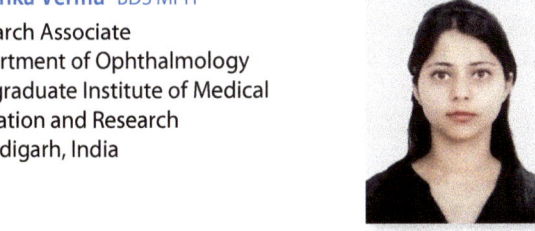

Puneet Kaur PhD Scholar MSc (Oncology Nursing)
Faculty
College of Nursing
Kasturba Hospital
Daryaganj, New Delhi, India

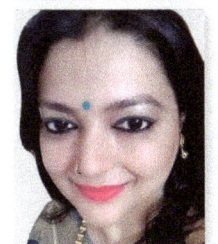

Rakesh Sharma PhD
Assistant Professor
College of Nursing
All India Institute of Medical Sciences
Rishikesh, Uttarakhand, India

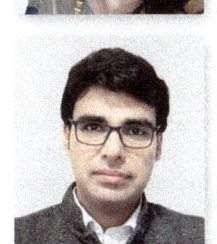

Ranjan Kumar Behera MS
Assistant Professor
Department of Ophthalmology
Maharishi Markandeshwar Institute of
Medical Sciences and Research
Mullana, Ambala, Haryana, India
Ex-Senior Resident
Advanced Eye Center
Postgraduate Institute of Medical
Education and Research
Chandigarh, India

Ravindra Khaiwal DSc
Professor of Environment Health
Department of Community Medicine
and School of Public Health
Postgraduate Institute of Medical
Education and Research
Chandigarh, India

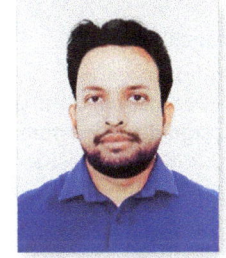

Reema Bansal MS
Professor
Department of Ophthalmology
Postgraduate Institute of Medical
Education and Research
Chandigarh, India

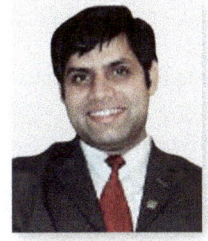

Richa Gupta MBBS MD (Anatomy)
Assistant Professor
Department of Anatomy
Postgraduate Institute of Medical
Education and Research
Chandigarh, India

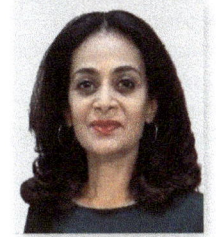

Rohan R Mahale MBBS DM (Neurology)
Postdoctoral Fellow (Movement Disorders) (SCTIMST)
Additional Professor
Department of Neurology
National Institute of Mental Health
and Neurosciences (NIMHANS)
Bengaluru, Karnataka, India

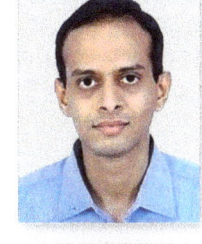

Ruchi Saini PhD
Faculty
National Institute of Nursing
Education
Postgraduate Institute of Medical
Education and Research
Chandigarh, India

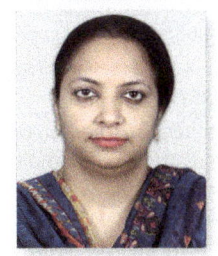

Sadhna Verma Masters in Yoga
Yoga Spok, CCRYN Collaborative
Centre for Mind Body Intervention
Through Yoga
Postgraduate Institute of Medical
Education and Research
Chandigarh, India

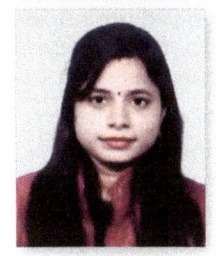

Sanjay Munjal PhD
Professor and In-Charge
Speech and Hearing Unit
Department of Otolaryngology
Postgraduate Institute of Medical
Education and Research
Chandigarh, India

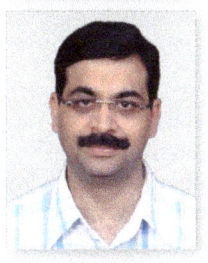

Santa De PhD
Professor-cum-Principal
NSHM Institute of Nursing
NSHM Knowledge Campus
Durgapur, West Bengal, India

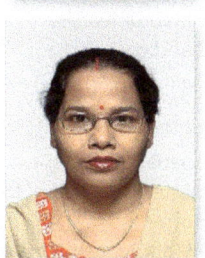

Saraswathi Nashi MBBS DM Post
Doctoral Fellow (Neuromuscular Disorders)
Associate Professor
Department of Neurology
National Institute of Mental Health
and Neurosciences (NIMHANS)
Bengaluru, Karnataka, India

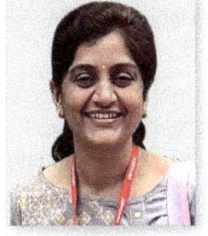

Shagun Korla MS
Senior Resident
Advanced Eye Centre
Postgraduate Institute of Medical
Education and Research
Chandigarh, India

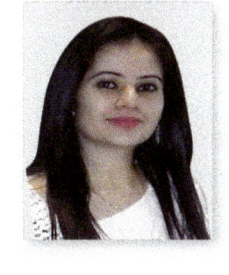

Contributors

Shivani Kalra MSc PhD Scholar
Professor
SKSS College of Nursing
Sarabha, Ludhiana, Punjab, India

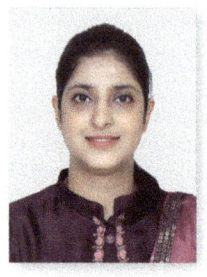

Shweta Chaurasia MS FICO FAICO (Pediatric Ophthalmology and Strabismus) DNB FRCS(I)
Associate Professor, Department of Pediatric Ophthalmology, Neuro-ophthalmology and Strabismus Services
Advanced Eye Centre
Postgraduate Institute of Medical Education and Research
Chandigarh, India

Sonali Banerjee PhD
Fertility Counsellor
Yoga and Wellness Mentor
Navi Mumbai, Maharashtra, India

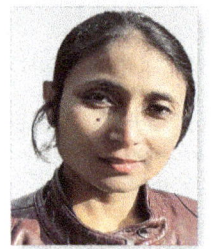
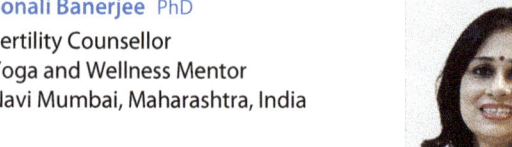

Suman Mor PhD
Professor
Department of Environment Studies
Former Coordinator
Centre for Public Health
Punjab University
Chandigarh, India

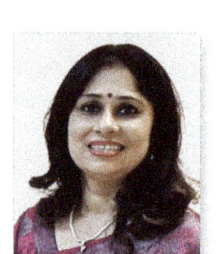

Sunita Sharma PhD
Associate Professor
National Institute of Nursing Education
Postgraduate Institute of Medical Education and Research
Chandigarh, India

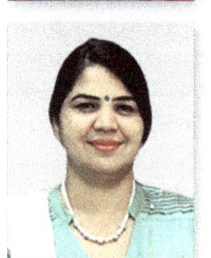

Surbhi Khurana MS
Ex-Senior Resident
Advanced Eye Center
Postgraduate Institute of Medical Education and Research
Chandigarh, India

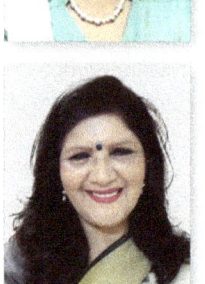

T Samuel Ravi Kumar RN MSc N (PhD Disaster Management)
Former Trauma Center Coordinator
Head
Department of Emergency Nursing
Christian Medical College
Vellore, Tamil Nadu, India

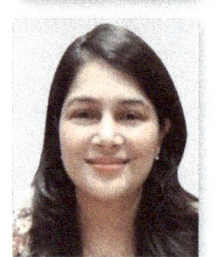

Tanmya Deswal BSc (Psychology)
Ashoka University
Sonipat, Haryana, India

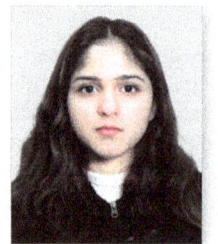

Tanvi Soni MS
Consultant
Cornea Services
CL Gupta Eye Institute
Moradabad, Gujarat, India

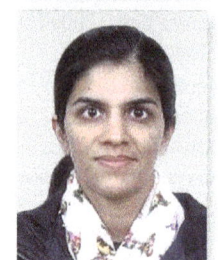

Tulika Gupta MD
Associate Professor
Department of Anatomy
Postgraduate Institute of Medical Education and Research
Chandigarh, India

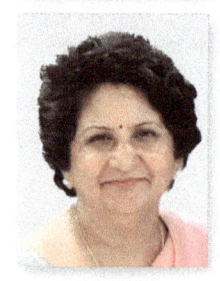

Vishali Gupta MD
Professor
Department of Ophthalmology
Postgraduate Institute of Medical Education and Research
Chandigarh, India

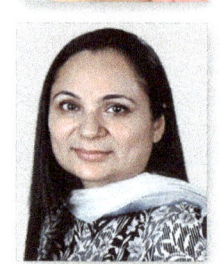

Vithal Malmande MBBS MS MCh (Plastic Surgery) DNB (Plastic Surgery)
Senior Consultant
Hosmat Hospitals
Bengaluru, Karnataka, India

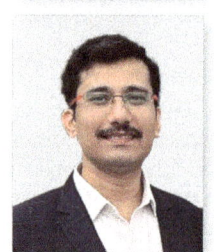

Vivek K Pathak MBBS MS (ENT)
Associate Professor
Department of ENT
School of Medical Sciences and Research
Sharda University
Greater Noida, Uttar Pradesh, India

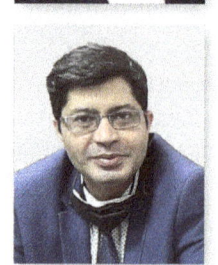

Vivek Kumar Garg PhD
Associate Professor
Department of Medical Laboratory Technology
Chandigarh University
Mohali, Punjab, India

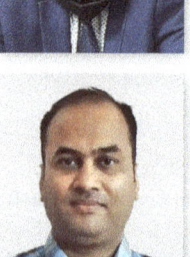

National Advisory

ANDHRA PRADESH

Suja Shamili
Principal
Dr Mallela Ramaiah College of Nursing
Nellore, Andhra Pradesh, India

J Roja Ramani
Professor
Medical Surgical Nursing
Government College of Nursing
Kadapa, Andhra Pradesh, India

M Ragha Sudha
Associate Professor
Medical Surgical Nursing, Cardiothoracic Nursing
LVTG College of Nursing
Kurnool, Andhra Pradesh, India

ASSAM

Manashi Sengupta
Dean Faculty of Nursing
Assam Downtown University
Guwahati, Assam, India

Mayengbam Benita Devi
Principal
Rahman Hospitals College of Nursing
(Under Rahman Institute of Nursing and Paramedical Sciences)
Guwahati, Assam, India

Mitali Barman
Associate Professor
Department of Medical Surgical Nursing
Asian Institute of Nursing Education
Guwahati, Assam, India

BIHAR

Usha Saldanha
Principal
Kurzi Holy Family Hospital College of Nursing
Patna, Bihar, India

CHHATTISGARH

Radhika Sahu
Associate Professor
Medical Surgical Nursing
Government College of Nursing
Rajnandgaon, Chhattisgarh, India

HARYANA

Abey Varughese
Principal
Sharbati College of Nursing
Mahendergarh, Haryana, India

Amrita Charlotte Kapoor
Principal
Himalayan Institute of Nursing
Ambala, Haryana, India

Baba Vajrala
Principal
Birender Singh College of Nursing
Uchana Jind, Haryana, India

Jyoti Sharma
Associate Professor
KVM College of Nursing
Rohtak, Haryana, India

Lalita Bhat
Principal
Maharaja Agrasen Nursing College
Bahadurgarh, Haryana, India

Lovejeet Kaur
Principal
Shaheed Baba Deep Singh College of Nursing
Ratia, Haryana, India

Loyd Melwyn Mendonca
Associate Professor
Maharaja Agrasen Nursing College
Bahadurgarh, Haryana, India

M Paul Dinagaran
Professor
Prem Institute of Medical Sciences
Panipat, Haryana, India

Mavitha VG
Assistant Professor
Maharaja Agrasen Nursing College
Bahadurgarh, Haryana, India

Subhasankari G
Principal
National College of Nursing
Hisar, Haryana, India

Rajkumari Ranjita Devi
Principal
Rural Nursing Training Institute
Sonipat, Haryana, India

Sunita Ahlawat
Principal
Government Nursing College
Safidon, Haryana, India

Sharda Rastogi
Principal and Director
Ved College of Nursing
Panipat, Haryana, India

HIMACHAL PRADESH

Anuja Sharma
Nursing Tutor
Medical Surgical Nursing
All India Institute of Medical Sciences
Bilaspur, Himachal Pradesh, India

Chanchal Sharma
Associate Professor
Medical Surgical Nursing
Shivalik Institute of Nursing
Shimla, Himachal Pradesh, India

Neha Patyal
Assistant Professor
Maharishi Markandeshwar University, MMCON
Solan, Himachal Pradesh, India

Suman Bharti
Principal
Maa Hateshwari College of Nursing
Himachal Pradesh, India

National Advisory

JAMMU AND KASHMIR

Ahrar Ahmed Dev
Tutor
Nursing Department
Government Medical College
Doda, Jammu and Kashmir, India

Frank JC
Principal
Bee Enn College of Nursing
Jammu, Jammu and Kashmir, India

Humaira Qadir Lone
Nursing Tutor
SMMCON and MT IUST
Awantipora, Jammu and Kashmir, India

Indra Devi Moza
Principal
Acharya Shri Chander College of
Nursing Education
Sidhra, Jammu and Kashmir, India

Insha
Nursing Officer
Government Nursing College
Srinagar, Jammu and Kashmir, India

Israel Jeba Prabu
Vice-Principal
Bee Enn College of Nursing
Jammu, Jammu and Kashmir, India

Poonam Paul
Associate Professor
Government Nursing College
Gandhinagar, Jammu and Kashmir, India

Pushpendra Kumar
Principal
College of Nursing, BGSB University
Rajouri, Jammu and Kashmir, India

Rajni Sharma
Principal
Government Nursing College
Gangyal, Jammu and Kashmir, India

Rehana Quasar
Tutor
Government College of Nursing
Srinagar, Jammu and Kashmir, India

Roohi Jan
Nursing Tutor
SMMCON and MT IUST
Awantipora, Jammu and Kashmir, India

Sameer Ahmad Dar
Assistant Professor
DIMS and T
Pulwama, Jammu and Kashmir, India

Shaila Nazir
Tutor
Dolphin Institute of Medical Sciences and Technology
Pulwama, Jammu and Kashmir, India

Dr Shailla Cannie
Principal and Dean
Shri Mata Vaishno Devi College of Nursing
Katra, Jammu and Kashmir, India

Shally Sharma
Nursing Tutor
Government Nursing College
Gangyal, Jammu and Kashmir, India

Shiekh Muneeb U Shaban
Nursing Tutor
Government College of Nursing
Srinagar, Jammu and Kashmir, India

Sufora Yaseen
Nursing Tutor
Government College of Nursing
Srinagar, Jammu and Kashmir, India

Titi Xavier
Associate Dean and Principal
Baba Ghulam Badshah University College of Nursing
Jammu and Kashmir, India

Ulfat Amin
Nursing Tutor
SMMCN and MT IUST
Awantipora, Jammu and Kashmir, India

Uzma Ashraf
Assistant Professor
College of Nursing GMC
Baramulla, Jammu and Kashmir, India

JHARKHAND

C Vasantha Kalyani
Principal
College of Nursing
All India Institute of Medical Sciences
Deoghar, Jharkhand, India

KARNATAKA

Dharam Singh Hajari
Assistant Professor
RIMS Government College of Nursing
Raichur, Karnataka, India

KERALA

Agnet Beena Mani
Professor/HOD and Coordinator
Medical Surgical
Baby Memorial College of Nursing
Kozhikode, Kerala, India

Alex John
Professor
Karuna College of Nursing
Palakkad, Kerala, India

Beena Koshy
Assistant Professor
Government College of Nursing
Thiruvananthapuram, Kerala, India

Betty P Kunjumon
Associate Professor (CAP)
Government College of Nursing
Kerala, India

Binutha VP
Associate Professor
Bishop Benziger College of Nursing
Kerala, India

KT Moly
Principal
Amrita College of Nursing
Kochi, Kerala, India

Priya Mary Stella
Professor-cum-Vice-Principal
Nehru College of Nursing
Palakkad, Kerala, India

Rani Jose
Professor and Head
Government College of Nursing
Kannur, Kerala, India

Reny Jose
Vice-Principal
Baby Memorial College of Nursing
Calicut, Kozhikode, Kerala, India

Shejila
Professor-cum-Vice-Principal
MIMS College of Nursing
Calicut, Kerala, India

Simple Rajagopal
Professor
Siddhi Sadan Lourde College of Nursing
Ernakulam, Kerala, India

Sindhu J Vayalil
Principal
Mercy College of Nursing
Kottayam, Kerala, India

Sindhu L
Associate Professor
Government College of Nursing
Thiruvananthapuram, Kerala, India

Sindhu R
Vice-Principal
PRS College of Nursing
Thiruvananthapuram, Kerala, India

MAHARASHTRA

Arundhati Karemore
Principal
Shashi Subhash Nursing College
Tumsar, Maharashtra, India

Avani Abhijit Bhanage
Principal
Namco College of Nursing and Research Institute
Nashik, Maharashtra, India

Hemlata Salve
Professor
Obstetrics and Gynecology
VSPM Madhuribai Deshmukh Institute of Nursing Education
Nagpur, Maharashtra, India

Kumari Nutan
Vice-Principal
MVP Samaj's Institute of Nursing Education
Nashik, Maharashtra, India

Mangesh Prakash Gawai
Professor
Medical Surgical Nursing
Sarswati Institute of Nursing Research and Sciences
Amaravati, Maharashtra, India

Mercy Aajore
Principal
Suretech College of Nursing
Nagpur, Maharashtra, India

Nutan Prakash Makasare
Assistant Professor and Head
Department of Medical Surgical Nursing
College of Nursing Government Medical College
Nagpur, Maharashtra, India

Rebecca Jadhav
Principal
Sumantai Wasnik Institute of Nursing
Nagpur, Maharashtra, India

Rupa Ashok Verma
Principal
MKSSS Sitabai Nargundkar College of Nursing for Women
Nagpur, Maharashtra, India

Samuel Fernandis
Vice-Principal
College of Nursing Wellness Hospital
Sangli, Maharashtra, India

Sharada Rakesh Chavan
Associate Professor
DES Smt Subhadra K Jindal College of Nursing
Pune, Maharashtra, India

Sheela Upendra
Deputy Director and Professor
Symbiosis College of Nursing
Symbiosis International (Deemed University)
Pune, Maharashtra, India

Shraddha Raut Meshram
Assistant Professor
Med Pro College of Nursing
Nagpur, Maharashtra, India

Sonam Methew
Principal
Central Institute of Nursing
Gondia, Maharashtra, India

Vaishali Tendolkar
Principal
Datta Meghe College of Nursing
Nagpur, Maharashtra, India

Veda Vivek
Principal
Panjabrao Deshmukh Nursing Institute
Amravati, Maharashtra, India

Veera Chandekar
Principal
Smt Sumitrabai Thakare Training College of Nursing
Yavatmal, Maharashtra, India

MADHYA PRADESH

Achamma Varghese
Principal
Shubhdeep College of Nursing
Indore, Madhya Pradesh, India

Keshkali Sharma
Principal
Vikrant College of Nursing
Indore, Madhya Pradesh, India

Maya Patila
Nursing Director
Malwanchal University
Indore, Madhya Pradesh, India

Prerna A Benson
Principal
SDPS College of Nursing
Indore, Madhya Pradesh, India

Prerna Pandey
Principal
Sri Aurobindo Institute of Medical Sciences
Indore, Madhya Pradesh, India

Rajan Joshi
Principal
Shreeji Institute of Nursing
Mandsaur, Madhya Pradesh, India

Rajni Udeniya
Principal
Renaissance University
Indore, Madhya Pradesh, India

Savita Vishwakarma
Principal
Shri Sadguru Sainath College of Nursing
Rewa, Madhya Pradesh, India

PUNJAB

Jasmine Kaur
Nursing Tutor
University College of Nursing
Faridkot, Punjab, India

Mercy Madan Lal
Assistant Professor
State Institute of Nursing and Paramedical Sciences
Sri Muktsar Sahib, Punjab, India

Navjot Kaur
Assistant Professor
Medical Surgical Nursing
(Cardiovascular and Thoracic Nursing)
Lala Lajpat Rai Institute of Nursing Education, Gulab Devi Hospital
Jalandhar, Punjab, India

Neelam Dass
Professor
Medical Surgical Nursing
(Critical Care Nursing)
College of Nursing Mohan Dai Oswal Hospital
Ludhiana, Punjab, India

Shridhar KV Iyengar
Principal
Adesh College of Nursing
Bathinda, Punjab, India

RAJASTHAN

Firoz Mansuri
Professor
Jaiswal College of Nursing
Kota, Rajasthan, India

Jagmohan Nagar
Professor
Jaiswal College of Nursing
Kota, Rajasthan, India

Pramendra Kumar Soni
Associate Professor
Jaiswal College of Nursing
Kota, Rajasthan, India

Sunil Kumar Dadheech
Principal
Mewar BSc Nursing College
Chittorgarh, Rajasthan, India

TELANGANA

Ammereddy Hemalatha
Assistant Professor
Medical Surgical Nursing Department
Deepthi College of Nursing
Nalgonda, Telangana, India

Aruna Kumari Gade
Principal
Aware College of Nursing
Hyderabad, Telangana, India

M Veguna Rani
Professor and Principal
Prathima College of Nursing
Karimnagar, Telangana, India

UTTARAKHAND

Akbar Nawaz
Vice-Principal
Graphic Era College of Nursing
Dehradun, Uttarakhand, India

Anil Kumar Purvia
Vice-Principal
Siddhartha Nursing Education and Research Institute
Dehradun, Uttarakhand, India

Bhaskar Bhatt
Professor
Government Medical College
Rudrapur, Uttarakhand, India

Govind Gaurav Pandey
Professor
Dr Susheela Tiwari Government Hospital and Medical College
Rudrapur, Uttarakhand, India

Manisha Dhyani
Principal
Government Nursing College
Dobh Srikot Pauri Garhwal
Uttarakhand, India

Manjeet Kaur
Assistant Professor
Medical Surgical Nursing
Shri Swami Bhumanand College of Nursing
Haridwar, Uttarakhand, India

Navneeta Khrist
Principal
Aarogyam Nursing College
Roorkee, Uttarakhand, India

Rosaline Lilly Mary
Professor
SGRR College of Nursing
Deharadun, Uttarakhand, India

Ruchi
Vice-Principal
Shri Swami Bhumanand College of Nursing
Haridwar, Uttarakhand, India

Rupali Verma
Assistant Professor
Punethi, Chhattar District
Champawat, Uttarakhand, India

Shabistan Ahmed
Principal
Government College of Nursing
New Tehri, Uttarakhand, India

UTTAR PRADESH

Amanjeet Kaur
Nursing Tutor
KGMU College of Nursing
Lucknow, Uttar Pradesh, India

Mrs Anjulika Yadav
Assistant Professor
Regency Institute of Nursing
Kanpur, Uttar Pradesh, India

Annu Kushwaha
Principal
Kamal Nehru Memorial Hospital School of Health Sciences
Prayagraj, Uttar Pradesh, India

Ashu
Registrar
Pushpanjali College of Nursing
Agra, Uttar Pradesh, India

Jayashree Ajith
Naraina Nursing College
Kanpur, Uttar Pradesh, India

Loveena Arpita Samuel
Nursing Tutor
KGMU College of Nursing
Lucknow, Uttar Pradesh, India

Ritu Tobit
Associate Professor
Sardar Patel College of Nursing
Lucknow, Uttar Pradesh, India

Savitha GR
Associate Professor
Abhishek Nursing and Paramedical Institute
Chandauli, Uttar Pradesh, India

Somesh Vashisth
Associate Professor
Ravi School of Nursing
Agra, Uttar Pradesh, India

Subin S
Assistant Professor
KGMU College of Nursing
King George's Medical University
Lucknow, Uttar Pradesh, India

WEST BENGAL

Aparna Saha Ghosh
Senior Lecturer
West Bengal Government College of Nursing, IPGME & R and SSKM Hospital Campus, Kolkata, West Bengal, India

Nabanita Sahu
Associate Professor
Shova Rani Nursing College
Kolkata, West Bengal, India

Shampa Gupta
Vice-Principal
Neotia Academy of Nursing
Kolkata, West Bengal, India

Preface

It gives me immense pleasure and satisfaction to bring out the first edition of *Adult Health Nursing-II: Medical Surgical Nursing*. Medical surgical nursing is the largest nursing specialty, worldwide. It is even known as the backbone of nursing practice. Registered nurses in this specialty practice primarily in hospitals and care for adult patients, having acute as well as chronic illnesses with a wide variety of medical and surgical problems. Today, the nurse practitioner is coming up as the new leading role in the nursing profession, even in the Indian settings. Irrespective of the role, the prime responsibility of a nurse is to provide high-quality evidence-based nursing care to the patients. The medical surgical nurses need a high level of critical thinking skills, vast knowledge of disease state and body systems, robust management skills, and the ability to stay calm under pressure.

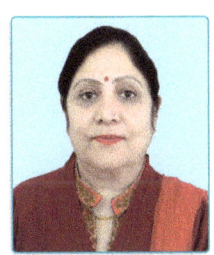

Audience

The current *Adult Health Nursing-II: Medical Surgical Nursing* has been authored and edited keeping in mind the needs of not only of various levels of students but the nursing educators and practitioners as well, to further refine their knowledge and skills regarding medical surgical nursing. An attempt has been made to explain the text clearly and succinctly.

Main Sections of the Text and the Sequencing of Chapters

The entire text as per the revised syllabus is being covered into two volumes. Each volume covers whole of the syllabus of the 3rd and 4th semester respectively. There are 101 chapters in volume I and 56 in volume II being covered under XXIV units. Unit I covering three chapters (1-3), introduces the readers to the foundations of medical surgical nursing. The basics of medical surgical nursing including its evolution, concept of health and illness, causation of disease, etc., are discussed in Chapter 1. The roles and feasibilities of a medical surgical nurse in OPD and IPD are highlighted in Chapter 2. The readers are introduced to the concept of quality improvement in Chapter 3. Unit II is about the introduction to medical surgical asepsis (Chapter 4). Unit III details perioperative nursing under three chapters preoperative, intraoperative, and postoperative nursing care (5-7). Unit IV provides information regarding common signs and symptoms and their management under five chapters (8-12) including fluid and electrolyte balance, acid-base balance, respiratory obstruction and other manifestations, pain, and shock. From unit V onwards various system-wise disorders are discussed very elaborately starting from Chapter 13 up to Chapter 97. Each system starts with a review of its anatomy and physiology followed by assessment and diagnostic evaluation and then a detailed description of the respective disorders. Unit V elaborates on disorders of the respiratory system; Unit VI highlights the disorders of the gastrointestinal system; Unit VII deliberates on the disorders of the cardiovascular system; Unit VIII is about hematological disorders; Unit IX discusses the disorders of the urinary system; Unit X is about male reproductive system; unit XI elaborates disorders of the endocrine system; unit XII highlights the disorders of the integumentary system; disorders of the musculoskeletal system are discussed in unit XIII; and unit XIV is about immunological disorders. Lastly, Unit XV in Volume I elaborates upon various communicable diseases under four chapters (98-101) including respiratory infections, surface and intestinal diseases, zoonoses and arthropod-borne infections, and sexually transmitted diseases.

Volume II starts with the disorders of ENT (Chapters 1-7), followed by disorders of the eye (Chapters 8-25), nervous system (Chapters 26-38), burns, reconstructive and cosmetic surgery (Chapter 39), and oncological disorders (Chapters 40-43). Emergency nursing and disaster are elaborated on in Chapters 44 and 45 respectively. Geriatric nursing has been discussed in detail over 5 chapters (46-50) under unit XXI. Critical care nursing has been discussed under unit XXII in Chapters 51 and 52. Chapter 53 is regarding occupational and industrial disorders. The second volume ends with unit XXIV having three special chapters (54-56) on patient safety, organ donation, and yoga in health care.

It is my sincere hope that the readers of this textbook will find it useful in understanding the concept of medical surgical nursing.

I wish to sincerely thank all the contributors to the book for taking time out of their busy schedules to write for me. Constructive comments and concrete suggestions to further improve this book are welcome and shall be gratefully acknowledged.

Sukhpal Kaur

Acknowledgments

It gives me immense pleasure to express my gratitude to various people who encouraged and supported me throughout my journey of completing this book.

First and foremost, I owe my deepest gratitude to the **Almighty**, the omnipresent **God**, for **His** grace and for giving me the strength, knowledge, ability, and abundant blessings to accomplish this enormous task. Thank you, so much dear Lord, for enabling me to take the daring stride into this expedition and helping me emerge as an achiever.

My wholehearted and sincere thanks to all the contributors for sparing their valuable time from their busy schedules and writing for me. I could never have dreamt of completing this endeavor without the support of each one of you.

I would like to thank my husband Dr Manjeet Singh, my good luck charm, who always is a strong pillar and a constant support for my academic work. Further, I extend my gratitude to my loving daughter Gunjeet and son Harshdeep, for bearing with me. I used to steal a lot of time from the time I was supposed to be giving to them to complete this work. The deepest affection and regard to my whole family, for their support, that kept me going enthusiastically.

I also appreciate the support of Shri Jitendar P Vij (Group Chairman), Mr Ankit Vij (Managing Director), Mr MS Mani (Group President), for their wholehearted support in publication of this book. I have no words to describe the role, efforts, inputs and initiatives undertaken by Dr Madhu Choudhary (Director-Educational Publishing), Ms Pooja Bhandari [Director-Production (Books and Journals)], Ms Sunita Katla (Executive Assistant to Group Chairman and Publishing Manager), Mr Ajay Kumar Sharma [Deputy General Manager (Books and Journals)], Mr Rishi Sharma (Regional Business Development Manager), Ms Samina Khan (Executive Assistant to Director-Educational Publishing), Ms Alisha Talwar (Team Lead-Nursing), Mr Rajesh Sharma (Production Coordinator), Ms Seema Dogra (Cover Visualizer), Mr Laxmidhar Padhiary (Proofreader), Mr Jagvir Singh Tomar (Typesetter), Mr Nitesh Jain (Graphic Designer) and all other staff members of M/s Jaypee Brothers Medical Publishers (P) Ltd,

I sincerely thank the entire JAYPEE team, for bringing out the book with utmost care and attractive presentation.

I welcome constructive comments and concrete suggestions for further improvement of this book. All the suggestions would be gracefully acknowledged.

Contents

UNIT I: Disorders of Ear, Nose and Throat

1. Review of Anatomy and Physiology: Ear, Nose and Throat 3
   Tulika Gupta, Daisy Sahni

2. Assessment and Diagnostic Evaluation of Ear, Nose and Throat 10
   Manwinder Singh, Abhishek Singh

3. Disorders of Ear 19
   Manwinder Singh, Dia Sharma, Sukhpal Kaur

4. Upper Airway Infections 33
   Vivek K Pathak, Pragya Pathak, Pradeepti Nayak

5. Obstruction and Trauma of the Upper Respiratory Airway 47
   Vivek K Pathak, Pragya Pathak, Pradeepti Nayak

6. Speech Defects and Speech Therapy 61
   Sanjay Munjal, Anuradha Sharma

7. Deafness and its Management 71
   Sanjay Munjal, Md Noorain Alam

UNIT II: Disorders of Eye

8. Review of Anatomy and Physiology: Eye 87
   Tulika Gupta, Tanvi Soni, Daisy Sahni

9. Assessment and Diagnostic Evaluation of Eye 93
   Anshul Chauhan, Gagandeep Kaur, Priyanka Verma, Lakshya Kumar, Mona Duggal

10. Ophthalmic Surgical Instruments 103
    Manpreet Singh, Manpreet Kaur, Aditi Mehta

11. Ocular Pharmacology and Lasers 108
    Himanshi Singh, Parul Chawla Gupta, Jagat Ram

12. Refractive Errors 111
    Himanshi Singh, Parul Chawla Gupta, Jagat Ram

13. Cataract 114
    Ranjan Kumar Behera, Parul Chawla Gupta, Jagat Ram

14. Disorders of Eyelid and Lacrimal System 120
    Manu Saini, Tanvi Soni

15. Orbital Disorders 126
    Manu Saini, Tanvi Soni

16. Disorders of Cornea 130
    Surbhi Khurana, Parul Chawla Gupta, Ranjan Kumar Behera, Jagat Ram

17. Glaucoma 136
    Faisal Thattaruthody, Neha Chauhan, Madhuri Akella

18. Disorders of Conjunctiva 145
    Surbhi Khurana, Parul Chawla Gupta, Ranjan Kumar Behera, Jagat Ram

19. Disorders of Retina and Vitreous 151
    Atul Arora, Reema Bansal, Vishali Gupta

20. Disorders of Sclera and Uvea 164
    Atul Arora, Reema Bansal, Vishali Gupta

21. Neuro-ophthalmology 170
    Shweta Chaurasia, Kajree Gupta

22. Strabismus 200
    Shweta Chaurasia, Shagun Korla, Kiran Kumari

23. Ocular Injuries 222
    Surbhi Khurana, Parul Chawla Gupta, Ranjan Kumar Behera, Jagat Ram

24. Eye Banking, Ocular Prosthesis and Rehabilitation 228
    Ranjan Kumar Behera, Parul Chawla Gupta, Jagat Ram

25. Community Ophthalmology 234
    Mona Duggal, Anshul Chauhan

UNIT III: Disorders of Nervous System

26. Review of Anatomy and Physiology: Nervous System 243
    Daisy Sahni, Richa Gupta

27. Assessment of Patients with Neurological Disorders 256
    Sonali Banerjee

28. Diagnostic Evaluation in Neurological Disorders 272
    Sonali Banerjee

29. Management of Common Problems in Neuroscience Patients 285
    Pooja Thakur

30. Traumatic Conditions 311
    Latika Bajaj

31. Cerebrovascular Disorders 327
    Manisha Nagi, Ashok Kumar, Vivek Kumar Garg, Divesh Kumar Munjal, Kapil Goel

32. Neoplasms of the Neurological System 344
    Manju Dhandapani
33. Chronic Neurological Problems 360
    Vivek Kumar Garg, Manisha Nagi, Ashok Kumar, Jitendra Gairolla, Kapil Goel
34. Neurological Infections 376
    Rakesh Sharma, Deepak Goel, Jitender Chaturvedi
35. Nerve and Muscle Disorders 387
    Priya Baby, Saraswathi Nashi
36. Movement Disorders 405
    Priya Baby, Rohan R Mahale
37. Cranial Nerve Disorders 414
    Rakesh Sharma, Deepak Goel, Jitender Chaturvedi
38. Neurodegenerative Diseases 423
    Monaliza

UNIT IV: Burns, Reconstructive and Cosmetic Surgery

39. Burns, Reconstructive and Cosmetic Surgery 447
    Latika Rohilla, Vithal Malmande

UNIT V: Oncological Disorders

40. Cancer 463
    Gurpreet Kaur, Latika Rohilla
41. Treatment Modalities of Cancer 473
    Maninderdeep Kaur, Divya Dahiya, Pramod Kumar
42. Oncological Emergencies 491
    Puneet Kaur, Sukhpal Kaur
43. Palliative Care 503
    Sukhpal Kaur, Jyoti Kathwal

UNIT VI: Emergency Nursing

44. Principles of Emergency Management 519
    Santa De
45. Disaster Management: Nursing Perspective 538
    T Samuel Ravi Kumar

UNIT VII: Geriatric Nursing

46. Ageing: Demography, Classification, Myths and Realities, and Theories 555
    Sukhpal Kaur, Manjeet Singh
47. Age-related Body System Changes and Common Health Problems in Elderly 566
    Manjeet Singh, Alisha Talwar, Sukhpal Kaur
48. Elderly Abuse, Legal and Ethical Issues of the Elderly 594
    Nitasha Sharma, Sunita Sharma
49. Provisions and Programs for Elderly 603
    Ruchi Saini, Nitasha Sharma, Sukhpal Kaur
50. Care of Elders 611
    Sukhpal Kaur, Alisha Talwar

UNIT VIII: Critical Care Nursing

51. Critical Care Nursing: General Concepts 631
    Lt Col Lata Mandal
52. Management of Patients in Critical Care Units 644
    Shivani Kalra, Jyoti Sharma

UNIT IX: Occupational and Industrial Disorders

53. Occupational and Industrial Disorders (Occupational Hazards Among Nurses) 667
    Ravindra Khaiwal, Pooja Parihar, Suman Mor

UNIT X: Special Topics

54. Patient Safety 677
    Arti Saini, Neha Pundir, Pankaj Arora
55. Organ Donation and Transplantation 689
    Navdeep Bansal, Sukhpal Kaur 689
56. Importance of Yoga for Nursing Professionals 699
    Tanmya Deswal, Pooja Nadholta, Sadhana Verma

Annexures
    Annexure 1: Important Clinical Signs 715
    Annexure 2: Clinical Triads 716
Appendix 717
Index 723

Syllabus

ADULT HEALTH NURSING-II

Placement: IV Semester
Theory: 7 Credits (140 hours)
Practicum: Laboratory/Skill Laboratory (SL) – 1 Credit (40 hours); Clinical – 6 Credits (480 hours)
Description: This course is designed to equip the students to review and apply their knowledge of anatomy, physiology, biochemistry and behavioral sciences in caring for adult patients with medical/surgical disorders using nursing process approach and critical thinking. It also intends to develop competencies required for assessment, diagnosis, treatment, nursing management, and supportive/palliative care to patients with various medical surgical disorders.
Competencies: On completion of the course the students will apply nursing process and critical thinking in delivering holistic nursing care with selected medical and surgical conditions.

At the completion of Adult Health Nursing-II course, students will:
1. Explain the etiology, pathophysiology, manifestations, diagnostic studies, treatments and complications of selected common medical and surgical disorders.
2. Perform complete health assessment to establish a data base for providing quality patient care and integrate the knowledge of diagnostic tests in the process of data collection.
3. Identify diagnoses, list them according to priority and formulate nursing care plan.
4. Perform nursing procedures skillfully and apply scientific principles while giving comprehensive nursing care to patients.
5. Integrate knowledge of anatomy, physiology, pathology, nutrition and pharmacology in caring for patients experiencing various medical and surgical disorders.
6. Identify common diagnostic measures related to the health problems with emphasis on nursing assessment and responsibilities.
7. Demonstrate skill in assisting/performing diagnostic and therapeutic procedures.
8. Demonstrate competencies/skills to patients undergoing treatment for medical surgical disorders.
9. Identify the drugs used in treating patients with selected medical surgical conditions.
10. Plan and provide relevant individual and group education on significant medical surgical topics.
11. Maintain safe environment for patients and the healthcare personnel in the hospital.

COURSE CONTENTS
T – Theory, L/SL – Laboratory/Skill Laboratory

Unit	Time (hours)	Learning outcomes	Content	Teaching/learning activities	Assessment methods

I	12 (T) 4 (SL)	Explain the etiology, pathophysiology, clinical manifestations, diagnostic measures and medical, surgical, nutritional and nursing management of patients with ENT disorders	**Nursing Management of Patient with Disorders of Ear, Nose and Throat** (Includes etiology, pathophysiology, clinical manifestations, diagnostic measures and medical, surgical, nutritional and nursing management)
			• Review of anatomy and physiology of the ear, nose and throat
			• History, physical assessment, and diagnostic tests
			• **Ear**
			  – *External ear:* Deformities otalgia, foreign bodies and tumors
			  – *Middle ear:* Impacted wax, tympanic, membrane perforation, otitis media, and tumors
			  – *Inner ear:* Meniere's disease, labyrinthitis, ototoxicity tumors
			• Upper respiratory airway infections: Rhinitis, sinusitis, tonsillitis, laryngitis
			• Epistaxis, nasal obstruction, laryngeal obstruction
			• Deafness and its management
				• Lecture and discussion
				• Demonstration of hearing aids, nasal packing, medication administration
				• Visit to audiology and speech clinic
					• MCQ
					• Short answer
					• Essay
					• OSCE
					• Assessment of skill (using checklist)
					• Quiz
					• Drug book

Unit	Time (hours)	Learning outcomes	Content	Teaching/learning activities	Assessment methods
II	12 (T) 4 (SL)	• Explain the etiology, pathophysiology, clinical manifestations, diagnostic measures and management of patients with disorders of eye • Describe eye donation, banking and transplantation	**Nursing Management of Patient with Disorder of Eye** • Review of anatomy and physiology of the eye • History, physical assessment, diagnostic assessment **Eye Disorders** • Refractive errors • **Eyelids:** Infection, deformities • **Conjunctiva:** Inflammation and infection bleeding • **Cornea:** Inflammation and infection • **Lens:** Cataract • Glaucoma • Retinal detachment • Blindness • Eye donation, banking and transplantation	• Lecture and discussion • Demonstration of visual aids, lens, medication administration • Visit to eye bank	• MCQ • Short essay • OSCE • Drug book
III	15 (T) 4 (L/SL)	• Explain the etiology, pathophysiology, clinical manifestations, diagnostic tests, and medical, surgical, nutritional, and nursing management of kidney and urinary system disorders • Demonstrate skill in genitourinary assessment • Prepare patient for genitourinary investigations • Prepare and provide health education on prevention of renal calculi	**Nursing Management of Patient with Kidney and Urinary Problems** • Review of anatomy and physiology of the genitourinary system • History, physical assessment, diagnostic tests • **Urinary tract infections:** Acute, chronic, lower, upper • Nephritis, nephrotic syndrome • Renal calculi • Acute and chronic renal failure • Disorders of ureter, urinary bladder and urethra • **Disorders of prostate:** Inflammation, infection, stricture, obstruction, and benign prostate hypertrophy	• Lecture cum Discussion • Demonstration • Case Discussion • Health education • Drug book • Field visit – Visits hemodialysis unit	• MCQ • Short note • Long essay • Case report • Submits health teaching on prevention of urinary calculi
IV	6 (T)	Explain the etiology, pathophysiology, clinical manifestations, diagnostic tests, and medical, surgical, nutritional, and nursing management of male reproductive disorders	**Nursing Management of Disorders of Male Reproductive System** • Review of anatomy and physiology of the male reproductive system • History, physical assessment, diagnostic tests • Infections of testis, penis and adjacent structures: Phimosis, epididymitis, and orchitis • Sexual dysfunction, infertility, contraception • **Male breast disorders:** Gynecomastia, tumor, climacteric changes	• Lecture, discussion • Case discussion • Health education	• Short essay
V	10 (T) 4 (SL)	Explain the etiology, pathophysiology, clinical manifestations, types, diagnostic measures and management of patients with disorders of burns/cosmetic surgeries and its significance	**Nursing Management of Patient with Burns, Reconstructive and Cosmetic Surgery** • Review of anatomy and physiology of the skin and connective tissues • History, physical assessment, assessment of burns and fluid and electrolyte loss • Burns • Reconstructive and cosmetic surgery for burns, congenital deformities, injuries and cosmetic purposes, gender reassignment • Legal and ethical aspects • **Special therapies:** LAD, vacuumed dressing. Laser, liposuction, skin health rejuvenation, use of derma filters	• Lecture and discussion • Demonstration of burn wound assessment, vacuum dressing and fluid calculations • Visit to burn rehabilitation centers	• OSCE • Short notes
VI	16 (T) 4 (L/SL)	Explain the etiology, pathophysiology, clinical manifestations, diagnostic measures and management of patients with neurological disorders	**Nursing Management of Patient with Neurological Disorders** • Review of anatomy and physiology of the neurological system • History, physical and neurological assessment, diagnostic tests • Headache, head injuries • **Spinal injuries:** Paraplegia, hemiplegia, quadriplegia • **Spinal cord compression:** herniation of in vertebral disc • Intra cranial and cerebral aneurysms	• Lecture and discussion • Demonstration of physiotherapy, neuroassessment, tracheostomy care • Visit to rehabilitation center, long-term care clinics, EEG, NCV study unit,	• OSCE • Short notes • Essay • Drug book

Unit	Time (hours)	Learning outcomes	Content	Teaching/learning activities	Assessment methods
			• Meningitis, encephalitis, brain, abscess, neuro-cysticercosis • **Movement disorders:** Chorea, seizures and epilepsies • **Cerebrovascular disorders:** Cerebrovascular accident (CVA) • **Cranial, spinal neuropathies:** Bell's palsy, trigeminal neuralgia • Peripheral neuropathies • **Degenerative diseases:** Alzheimer's disease, Parkinson's disease • Guillain-Barré syndrome, myasthenia gravis and multiple sclerosis • Rehabilitation of patient with neurological deficit		
VII	12 (T) 4 (L/SL)	• Explain the etiology, pathophysiology, clinical manifestations, diagnostic tests, and medical, surgical, nutritional, and nursing management of immunological disorders • Prepare and provides health education on prevention of HIV infection and rehabilitation • Describe the national infection control programs	**Nursing Management of Patients with Immunological Problems** • Review of immune system • **Nursing assessment:** History and physical assessment • **HIV and AIDS:** Epidemiology, transmission, prevention of transmission and management of HIV/AIDS • Role of nurse; Counseling, health education and home care consideration and rehabilitation • National AIDS Control Programme—NACO, various national and international agencies for infection control	• Lecture, discussion • Case discussion/seminar • Refer module on HIV/AIDS	
VIII	12 (T) 4 (L/SL)	Explain the etiology, pathophysiology, types, clinical manifestations, staging, diagnostic measures and management of patients with different cancer, treatment modalities including newer treatments	**Nursing Management of Patient with Oncological Conditions** • Structure and characteristics of normal and cancer cells • History, physically assessment, diagnostic tests • Prevention screening early detections warning sign of cancer • Epidemiology, etiology classification, pathophysiology, staging clinical manifestations, diagnosis, treatment modalities and medical and surgical nursing management of oncological condition • Common malignancies of various body system eye, ear, nose, larynx, breast, cervix, ovary, uterus, sarcoma, renal, bladder, kidney, prostate, brain, spinal cord • Oncological emergencies • Modalities of treatment: Chemotherapy, Radiotherapy: Radiation safety, AERB regulations, surgical intervention, stem cell and bone marrow transplant, immunotherapy, gene therapy • Psychological aspects of cancer: Anxiety, depression, insomnia, anger • Supportive care • Hospice care	• Lecture and discussion • Demonstration of chemotherapy preparation and administration • Visit to BMT, radiotherapy units (linear accelerator, brachytherapy, etc.), nuclear medicine unit • Completion of palliative care • module during clinical hours (20 hours)	• OSCE • Essay • Quiz • Drug book • Counseling, health teaching

Unit	Time (hours)	Learning outcomes	Content	Teaching/learning activities	Assessment methods
IX	15 (T) 4 (L/SL)	Explain the types, policies, guidelines, prevention and management of disaster and the etiology, pathophysiology, clinical manifestations, diagnostic measures and management of patients with acute emergencies	**Nursing Management of Patient in Emergency and Disaster Situations** **Disaster Nursing** • Concept and principles of disaster nursing, related policies • **Types of disaster:** Natural and manmade • **Disaster preparedness:** Team, guidelines, protocols, equipment, resources • Etiology, classification, pathophysiology, staging, clinical manifestation, diagnosis, treatment modalities and medical and surgical nursing management of patient with medical and surgical emergencies—polytrauma, bites, poisoning and thermal emergencies • Principles of emergency management • Medicolegal aspects	• Lecture and discussion • Demonstration of disaster preparedness (Mock drill) and triaging • Filed visit to local disaster management centers or demo by fire extinguishers • Group presentation (role play, skit, concept mapping) on different emergency care • **Refer trauma care management/ ATCN module** • Guided reading on National Disaster Management Authority (NDMA) guidelines	• OSCE • Case • presentations and case study
X	10 (T)	• Explain the concept, physiological changes, and psychosocial problems of ageing • Describe the nursing management of the elderly	**Nursing Care of the Elderly** • History and physical assessment • Aging process and age-related body changes and psychosocial aspects • Stress and coping in elder patient • Psychosocial and sexual abuse of elderly • Role of family and formal and non-formal caregivers • Use of aids and prosthesis (hearing aids, dentures) • Legal and ethical issues • National programs for elderly, privileges, community programs and health services • Home and institutional care	• Lecture and discussion • Demonstration of communication with visual and hearing impaired • Field visit to old age homes	• OSCE • Case presentations • Assignment on family systems of India focusing on geriatric population
XI	15 (T) 8 (L/SL)	Explain the etiology, pathophysiology, clinical manifestations, diagnostic measures and management of patients in critical care units	**Nursing Management of Patients in Critical Care Units** • Principles of critical care nursing • **Organization:** Physical set-up, policies, staffing norms • Protocols, equipment and supplies • **Use and application of critical care biomedical equipment:** Ventilators, cardiac monitors, defibrillators, infusion pump, resuscitation equipment and any other • Advanced cardiac life support • Nursing management of critically ill patient • Transitional care • Ethical and legal aspects • **Breaking bad news to patients and/or their families:** Communication with patient and family • End of life care	• Lecture and discussion • Demonstration on the use of mechanical ventilators, cardiac monitors, etc. • Clinical practice in different ICUs	• Objective type • Short notes • Case presentations • Assessment of skill on monitoring of patients in ICU. • Written assignment on ethical and legal issues in critical care
XII	5 (T)	Describe the etiology, pathophysiology, clinical manifestations, diagnostic measures and management of patients with occupational/ industrial health disorders	**Nursing Management of Patients Occupational and Industrial Disorders** • History, physical examination, diagnostic tests • Occupational diseases and management	• Lecture and discussion • Industrial visit	• Assignment on industrial health hazards

UNIT I

Disorders of Ear, Nose and Throat

OUTLINE

1. **Review of Anatomy and Physiology: Ear, Nose and Throat**
   Tulika Gupta, Daisy Sahni

2. **Assessment and Diagnostic Evaluation of Ear, Nose and Throat**
   Manwinder Singh, Abhishek Singh

3. **Disorders of Ear**
   Manwinder Singh, Dia Sharma, Sukhpal Kaur

4. **Upper Airway Infections**
   Vivek K Pathak, Pragya Pathak, Pradeepti Nayak

5. **Obstruction and Trauma of the Upper Respiratory Airway**
   Vivek K Pathak, Pragya Pathak, Pradeepti Nayak

6. **Speech Defects and Speech Therapy**
   Sanjay Munjal, Anuradha Sharma

7. **Deafness and its Management**
   Sanjay Munjal, Md Noorain Alam

CHAPTER 1
Review of Anatomy and Physiology: Ear, Nose and Throat

Tulika Gupta, Daisy Sahni

"Eyes are a deaf man's ears. Ears are a blind man's eyes."
—**Mokokoma Mokhonoana**

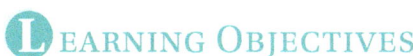 EARNING OBJECTIVES

After going through the chapter, the learner will be able to:
- Identify the parts of ear, nose and throat.
- Define parts of ear, nose and throat.
- Understand their relative position in the body.
- Comprehend their structure and functions.

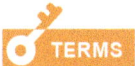 **TERMS**

- **Cochlea:** Spiral tubular structure which coils around the central core called modiolus.
- **Tympanic membrane:** Translucent partition between middle ear and external acoustic canal.
- **Vestibular folds:** False vocal cords formed by the vestibular ligament.
- **Vocal folds:** True vocal cords formed by vocal ligament and vocalis muscle.

INTRODUCTION

Anatomy of head and neck region, comprising ear, nose and throat is a very interesting and comprehensive topic. Ears not only receive and amplify sound, but also help in maintenance of balance. Nose is the part of the upper respiratory tract, responsible for humidification and filtration of air. Protection of the lower respiratory tract and phonation are major functions of larynx. It extends from the laryngeal inlet to the cricoid cartilage and continues distally with the trachea.

EAR

Ear is responsible for hearing and balance. It can be divided into external, middle and inner ear, lying lateral to medial side **(Fig. 1.1)**.

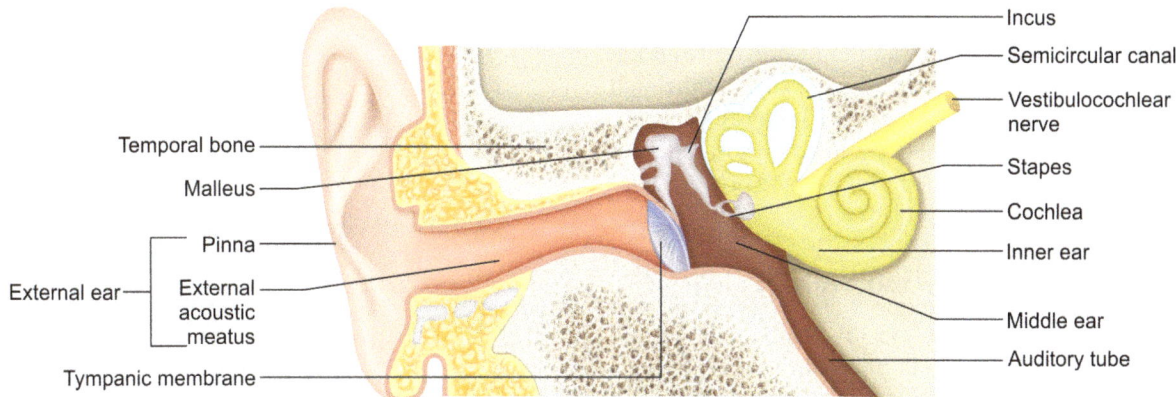

Fig. 1.1: External ear, middle ear and inner ear.

EXTERNAL EAR

It is made up of the auricle (pinna) and external acoustic meatus. The auricle is supported by elastic cartilage covered by skin, projecting from the side of the face with the purpose of catching the sound waves and directing them towards the eardrum via external acoustic meatus. Latter is an osteo-cartilaginous "S" shaped canal of about one inch, extending till the lateral surface of the tympanic membrane. It is an air-filled tubular space/canal, acts as resonator for speech waves. The canal can get blocked by wax, formed by collection of desquamated cells, cerumen and sebum; this might impede the sound wave transmission and hearing.

TYMPANIC MEMBRANE (EARDRUM)

It is a translucent partition between middle ear and external acoustic canal, directed laterally and downwards. Outer skin lined surface is concave while inner mucosae surface is convex and gives attachment to the handle of malleus. Point of maximum convexity is known as umbo. Myringotomy or incision of tympanic membrane is safely given at the posteroinferior quadrant. Sound waves cause vibrations in the tympanic cavity which are transmitted to the ear ossicles.

MIDDLE EAR

It lies in the temporal bone. It is a narrow biconcave space containing air. It has six sides, lateral wall is the tympanic membrane, medial wall separates it from the inner ear, roof separates it from the cranial cavity, floor is formed by the jugular fossa housing internal jugular bulb and the bony canal for the facial nerve is present in the posterior wall. The anterior wall has opening of the auditory tube which connects the middle ear to the nasopharynx and its lower part is related to the internal carotid artery. The medial wall of the middle ear has a rounded bulge, called promontory, two openings are present behind the promontory—the oval window and the round window. The oval window is closed by the foot plates of stapes which lie above, and the round window is closed by a membrane which lies below. The middle ear contains three ear ossicles (malleus, incus and stapes), ligaments and muscles related to the ossicles, vessels, nerves and air. Malleus (hammer) is the largest ossicle. The handle of malleolus attaches to the tympanic membrane while the upper end of the malleolus articulates with the incus, the lower end of incus forms joint with the head of stapes and the footplate of the stapes fits into the oval window present on the promontory. This ossicular chain amplifies and transmits the tympanic membrane vibrations to the internal ear through the oval window. Tensor tympani and stapedius are two muscles present in the middle ear, both contracts together to dampen the high-pitched sound waves for protection of the labyrinth or inner ear.

INTERNAL INNER EAR OR LABYRINTH

It lies in the temporal bone; it is formed by bony labyrinth, which suspends endolymph filled membranous labyrinth within it. The bony labyrinth has three parts oriented anterior to posterior—cochlea, vestibule and semicircular canals (Fig. 1.2).

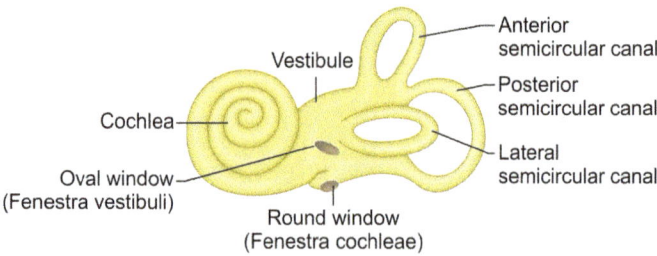

Fig. 1.2: The bony labyrinth.

It has two important functions—hearing and equilibrium—served by mechanoreceptors with directionally sensitive hairs.

ANATOMY AND PHYSIOLOGY OF HEARING

The cochlea is a spiral tubular structure which coils around the central core called modiolus taking two and half turns. Bony cochlear tube is divided into three chambers scala vestibule, scala media (membranous) and scala tympani. Scala media or cochlear duct contains spiral organ of Corti, which is made up of neuroepithelial hair cells (receptors for sound) and supporting hair cells present as a single cell layer lying on the basilar membrane. The apices of the hair cells are embedded in the acellular membrane tectoria.

Process of Hearing

Sound pressure waves are collected by funnel-shaped external ear which lead to vibrations in the taut tympanic membrane. These vibrations are transmitted to chain of ossicles through the handle of malleus. The footplate of stapes covering the oval window transmits the vibrations to the perilymph scala vestibule. The pressure waves travel to the endolymph of scala media and cause vibrations in the basilar membrane. This stimulates the hair cell receptors of organ of Corti. The basilar membrane is tonotopic—reaction by any sound is maximum at some particular area of the membrane; basal turn of cochlea (Fig. 1.3) responds to the high pitch (frequency) sounds and apex to the low pitch. The hair cell receptors transduce these vibrations into nerve impulse to be carried by the nerve fibers to the spiral ganglion (present in the modiolus) and on to the auditory area of cerebral cortex via the cochlear component of the vestibulocochlear cranial nerve.

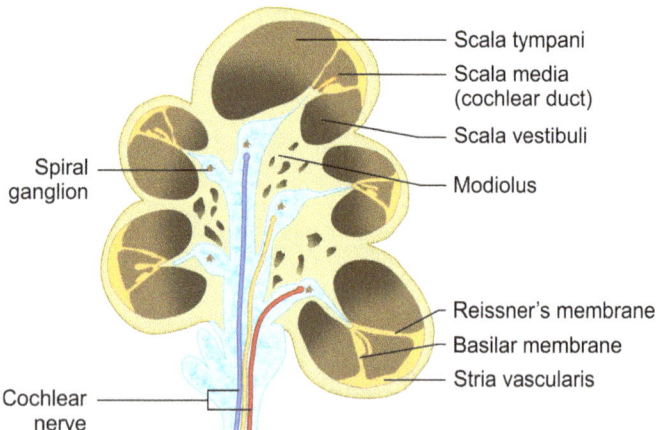

Fig. 1.3: A section of cochlea showing divisions of the cochlear canal, modiolus, and spiral ganglia.

ANATOMY AND PHYSIOLOGY OF EQUILIBRIUM

The vestibule lies medial to the middle ear cavity and is continuous with the cochlea adjacent to the oval window. It receives sound vibration waves via oval window and excessive pressure in the internal ear is relieved by the round window. The vestibule contains membranous saccule and utricle **(Fig. 1.4)**, which house receptors for static balance and linear acceleration, called macula. The macula consists of hair cells covered by otolithic gelatinous mass and sensitive to gravitational stimuli. The semicircular canals are three in number oriented at right angle to each other and they open anteriorly in the utricle by five openings. They contain membranous semicircular ducts which house organ of kinetic balance and angular acceleration known as crista ampullaris. The crista ampullaris consists of hair cell receptors covered by cone-shaped gelatinous cupula. Both macula and crista are supplied by vestibular part of vestibulocochlear nerve and provide important information about position, motion and gravity which is required to maintain equilibrium.

NOSE

Upper respiratory tract consists of nose, pharynx and larynx. Nose is the most proximal part of the upper respiratory tract. It modulates temperature and humidity of the inspired air and is an organ for olfaction. It can be divided into external nose and nasal cavity.

EXTERNAL NOSE

It is a surface projection on the face, consisting of root (part attached to the forehead), tip, dorsum (border present between the tip and the root). Nostrils or external nares are two piriform shaped openings seen at the lower end. These openings are bounded by ala nasi (wings of the nostrils) laterally and nasal septum medially. The skeletal framework of external nose is formed by bones (nasal bones and frontal processes of maxillae) and cartilages (superior and inferior nasal cartilages with minor alar cartilages). The overlying skin is thin and mobile except over alae. Sensory supply to the external nose is by branches of ophthalmic and maxillary nerves.

NASAL CAVITY

It is divided by the nasal septum into two halves. Each half extends from the anterior nare (nostrils) to the posterior nare (choana), latter opens in the pharynx. Nostrils lead to skin lined roomy area known as vestibule. The nasal cavity extends from palate to the cribriform plate vertically. Floor is concave and is formed by the palatine processes of the maxilla anteriorly and horizontal processes of the palatine bone posteriorly. The narrow roof is mainly formed by the cribriform plate of the ethmoid bone and is lined by the olfactory epithelium. Rest of the cavity is lined by the respiratory epithelium. Lateral wall of nasal cavity **(Fig. 1.5)** has three curved projections called conchae, directed

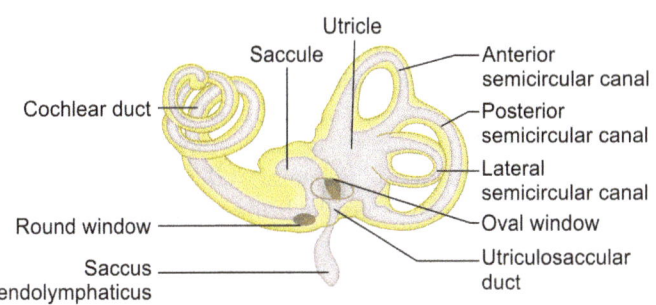

Fig. 1.4: The membranous labyrinth (blue) is seen within the bony labyrinth.

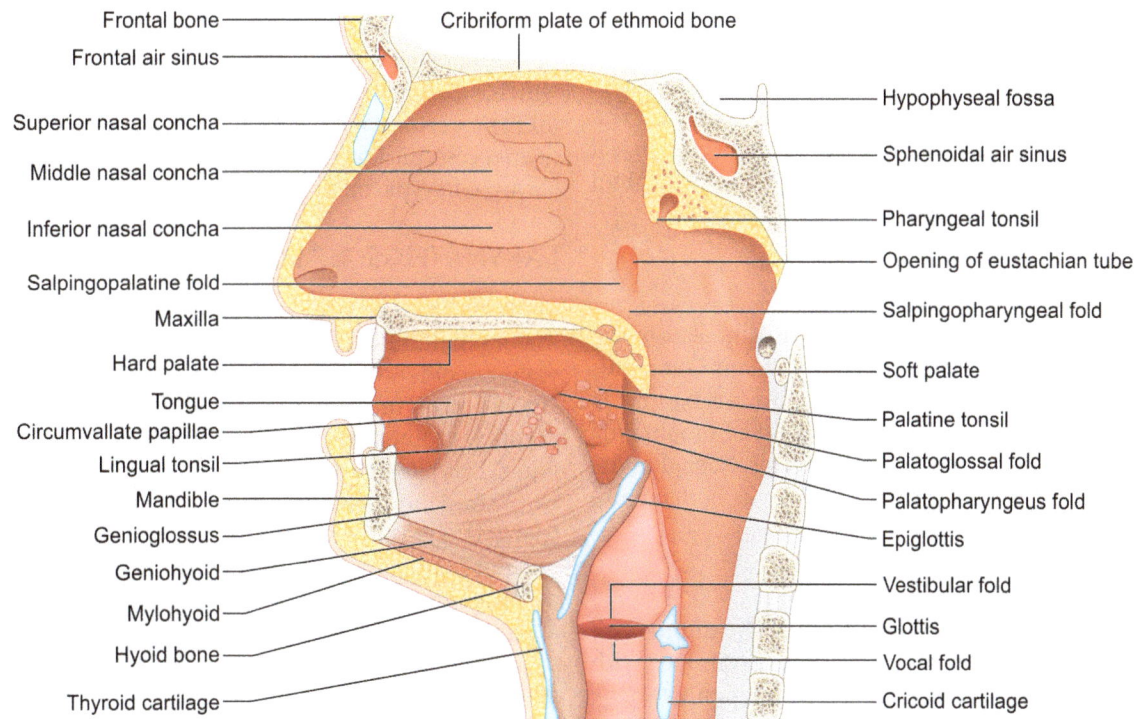

Fig.1.5: Sagittal section of pharynx.

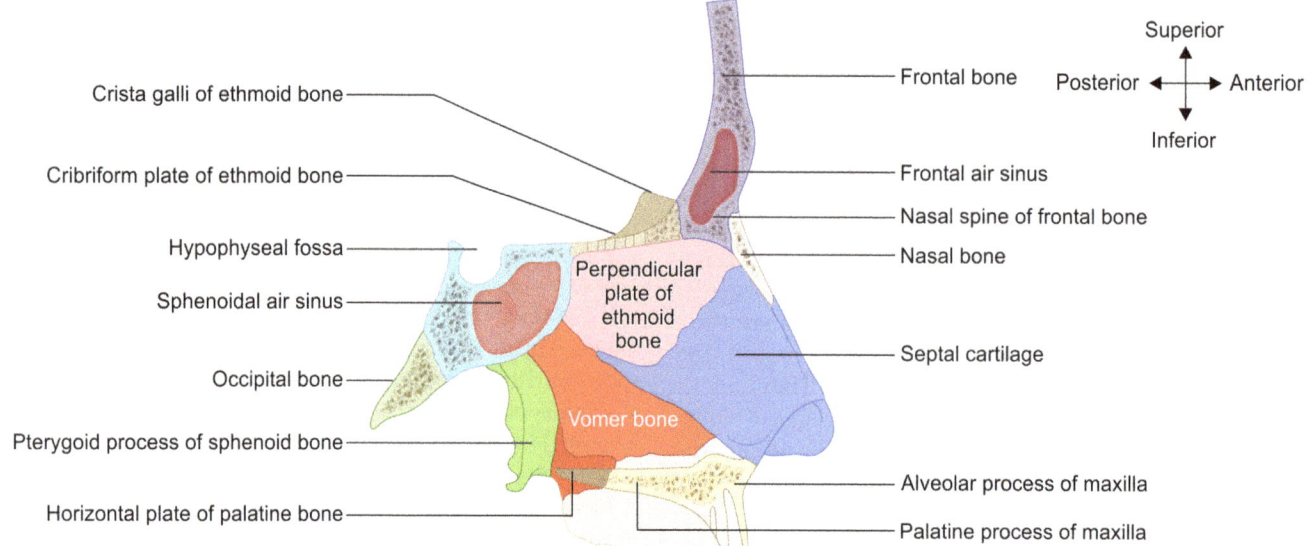

Fig. 1.6: Medial wall of nasal cavity showing the bones and cartilage forming the nasal septum.

downwards and medially. Meatuses are part of the nasal cavity present below overhanging conchae. Nasolacrimal duct opens in the inferior concha. Middle meatus has openings of frontal sinus, anterior and middle ethmoidal sinuses and maxillary sinuses. Posterior ethmoidal sinus opens at superior meatus. Area above the superior meatus is called sphenoethmoidal recess and it receives the opening of the sphenoidal sinus. The nasal septum is the osteo-cartilaginous medial wall formed by vomer and perpendicular plate of ethmoid bone, septal cartilages and cuticular part at lower end **(Fig. 1.6)**. Nasal septum is rarely in median plane; it is usually deflected to one side. Little's area, present in the anteroinferior part of the septum, is highly vascular and is the common site of nasal bleed.

PARANASAL SINUSES

These are the air-filled spaces present in the bones forming the nasal skeleton. These are frontal, maxillary, sphenoidal and ethmoidal (anterior, middle and posterior) sinuses. The sinuses are lined by respiratory mucosa and open in the nasal cavity. The sinuses lighten the skull, condition the inspired air and add resonance to voice.

PHARYNX

It is a muscular tube which starts at the base of the skull above and below it opens into the esophagus. It communicates anteriorly with the nose, oral cavity and larynx and is accordingly divided into three parts nasopharynx, oropharynx and laryngopharynx, from above downwards. Nasopharynx is a passage for air while oropharynx transmits both air and food.

Nasopharynx

It is present behind the nose, below the base of the skull and above the soft palate. Inferiorly, it is continuous with the oropharynx. The pharyngeal end of tympanic tube, a communication between the middle ear and nasopharynx, opens in its lateral wall. Adenoid or pharyngeal tonsils (aggregation of lymphoid tissue) are present on roof and adjoining posterior wall.

Oropharynx

It is a middle part of the pharynx located behind the oral cavity, and inferiorly it extends till the upper border of the epiglottis where it becomes continuous with laryngopharynx. Large mass of lymphoid tissue known as palatine tonsils or tonsils are present on the lateral wall of the oropharynx. Waldeyer's lymphatic (tonsillar) ring is located within the pharynx. The ring is formed by pharyngeal tonsil above, both palatine tonsils laterally and lingual tonsil posterior part of the tongue below (tubal tonsils).

Laryngopharynx

It lies behind the larynx and inferiorly continues as the esophagus at the level of 6th cervical vertebra. Anteriorly, it communicates with the larynx through the laryngeal inlet, which is bounded by epiglottis anteriorly, by inter-arytenoid folds posteriorly and laterally by two aryepiglottic folds. A deep recess, piriform fossa is present on the lateral wall of the laryngopharynx, on each side of the laryngeal inlet.

LARYNX (FIGS. 1.7 TO 1.9)

Protection of the lower respiratory tract and phonation are major functions of larynx. It extends from the laryngeal inlet to the cricoid cartilage and continues distally with the trachea. Hyoid bone is present above the larynx. Larynx is formed by cartilages joined by muscles, ligaments, membranes, and joints. Laryngeal cartilages are thyroid, cricoid and epiglottis (unpaired) and arytenoid, corniculate and cuneiform (paired). Thyroid cartilage is present anteriorly, this has two flat laminae which meet in the midline of the neck at an angle to make laryngeal prominence, which is more apparent in males and is called Adam's apple. Superior border of the thyroid cartilage is connected to the hyoid bone by thyrohyoid membrane and its inferior border is connected to the cricoid cartilage below. Cricoid is a ring-shaped cartilage with narrow anterior arch and broad posterior lamina.

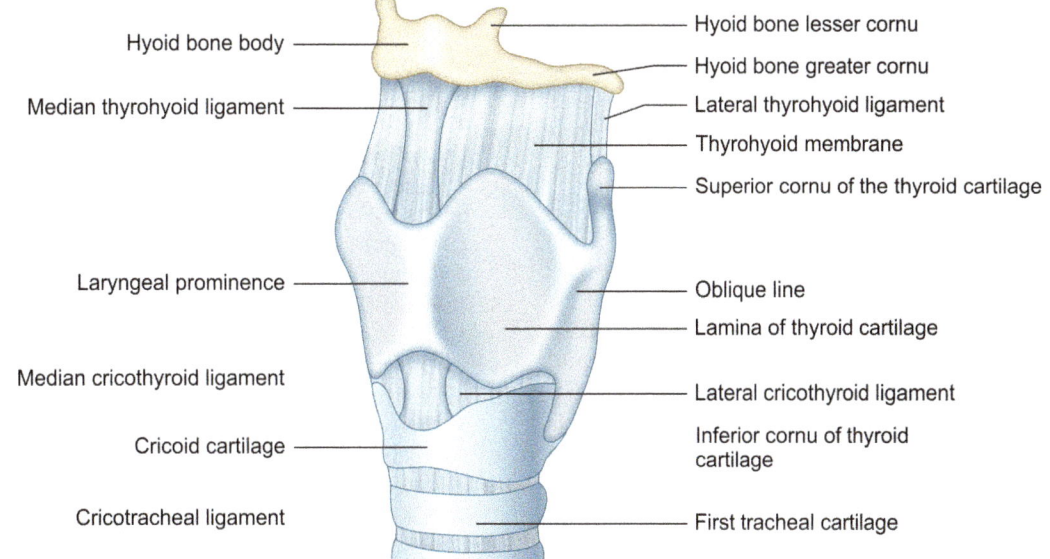

Fig. 1.7: Anterolateral view of laryngeal cartilages and ligaments.

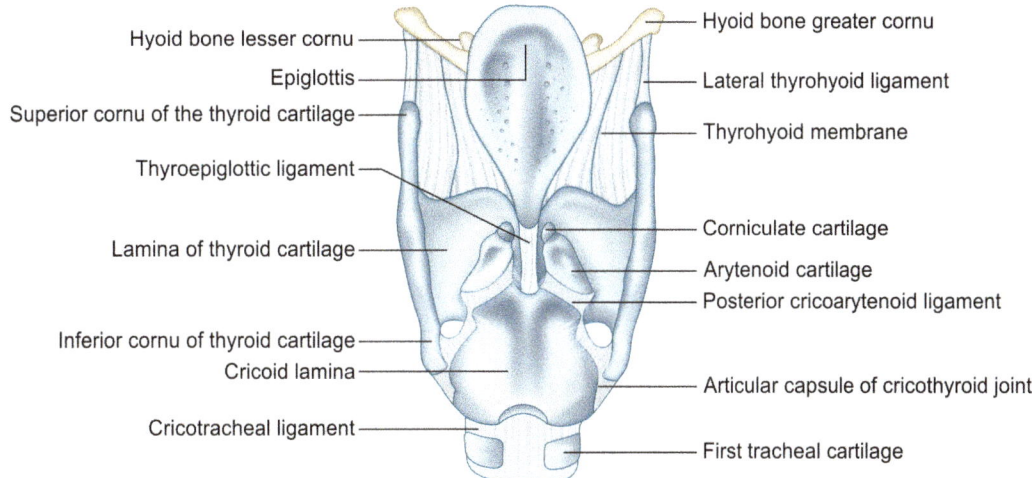

Fig. 1.8: Posterior view of laryngeal cartilages and ligaments.

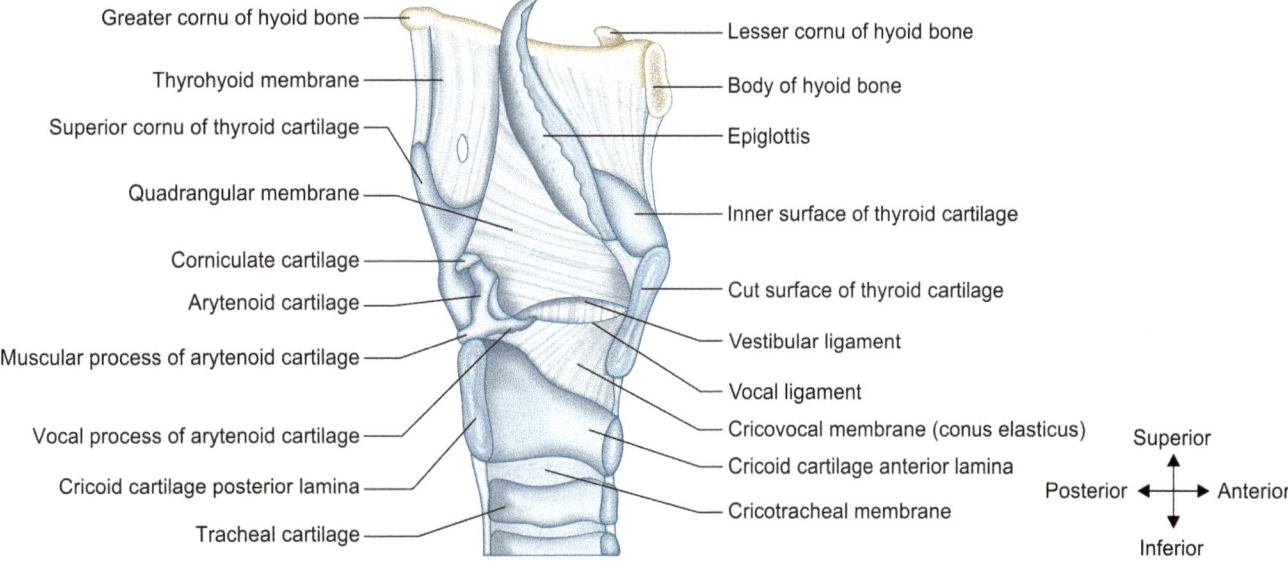

Fig. 1.9: Sagittal section of larynx showing the internal features.

Arytenoid cartilages are pyramidal in shape. Base of the arytenoid rests on the upper margin of the posterior cricoid lamina and the apex points upwards. Epiglottis is in the shape of droplet. Its wide rounded end is free and projects upwards behind tongue and hyoid bone, while lower narrow end is attached to the posterior aspect of thyroid cartilage, at the angle between the two thyroid laminae. Aryepiglottic fold is present between the sides of epiglottis to the apices of the arytenoid cartilage on both sides. Corniculate and cuneiform cartilages are very small in size and lie within the aryepiglottic folds.

The laryngeal cavity thus formed is lined by mucosa and it presents two pairs of folds, which lie between the thyroid and arytenoid cartilages. Superior fold is called vestibular folds or false vocal cords (by vestibular ligaments) and inferior pair is called vocal folds or true vocal cords (by vocal ligament and vocalis muscle). The laryngeal cavity is divided into three parts, vestibule or supraglottis (above the vestibular fold), glottis (between vestibular and vocal folds) and infraglottis (below the vocal folds) compartments. Space between the right and left vocal folds is known as rima glottides. Vibrations of the vocal cords lead to production of speech. Pitch of the sound depends on frequency of vibrations and loudness of sound depends upon the amplitude of vibrations. Longer vocal cords of males lead to lower pitch and louder voices. Muscles of the larynx and sensory supply below the vocal folds is by recurrent laryngeal nerve while sensory supply above the focal folds is by superior laryngeal nerve; all are branches of the vagus nerve.

SUMMARY

Ear can be divided into external, middle, and inner ear. External ear is made up of the auricle and external acoustic meatus. Tympanic membrane is a translucent partition between middle ear and external acoustic canal, directed laterally and downwards. Middle ear is a narrow biconcave space containing air cavity, lying in the temporal bone. Internal ear or labyrinth lies in the temporal bone, and it is formed by bony labyrinth and membranous labyrinth. Upper respiratory tract consists of nose, pharynx, and larynx. Nose is the proximal most part of the upper respiratory tract. It can be divided into external nose and nasal cavity. Nasal cavity is divided by the nasal septum into two halves and each half extends from palate to the cribriform plate vertically. Pharynx is a muscular tube which starts at the base of the skull above and opens into the esophagus below. It is divided into three parts nasopharynx, oropharynx, and laryngopharynx. Protection of the lower respiratory tract and phonation are major functions of larynx, which extends from the laryngeal inlet to the cricoid cartilage and continues distally with the trachea.

MULTIPLE CHOICE QUESTIONS

1. Which of the following structures open into the inferior meatus of nose?
    a. Maxillary sinus
    b. Sphenoid sinus
    c. Ethmoidal sinus
    d. Nasolacrimal duct
2. Identify the false statement regarding the nasopharynx.
    a. It communicates with the nose anteriorly
    b. It is a passage for air
    c. It transmits both air and food
    d. It continues inferiorly with oropharynx
3. The tubotympanic tube connects:
    a. Nasopharynx to the middle ear
    b. Oropharynx to the middle ear
    c. Nasopharynx to the external auditory meatus
    d. Oropharynx to the internal ear
4. Larynx extends from:
    a. Laryngeal inlet to cricoid cartilage
    b. Base of skull to esophagus
    c. Oblique line of thyroid cartilage to cricoids cartilage
    d. Laryngeal inlet to oblique line of thyroid cartilage
5. The membranous labyrinth contains:
    a. Cystolymph
    b. Otolymph
    c. Perilymph
    d. Endolymph
6. Footplate of stapes is attached to:
    a. Oval window
    b. Round window
    c. Tympanic membrane
    d. Cochlea
7. Which is the smallest bone of human body:
    a. Malleus
    b. Sphenoid
    c. Stapes
    d. Vomer
8. Study of ear, nose and throat diseases is known as:
    a. Cosmetology
    b. Otolaryngology
    c. Entomology
    d. Rheumatology
9. Vestibular folds are also known as:
    a. False vocal cords
    b. Vocal ligament
    c. Vocalis muscle
    d. True vocal cords
10. Protection of the lower respiratory tract and phonation are functions of:
    a. Nasopharynx
    b. Oropharynx
    c. Larynx
    d. Esophagus
11. All of the following are parts of bony labyrinth, *except*:
    a. Cochlea
    b. Semicircular canal
    c. Oval window
    d. Vestibule
12. Ossicles amplify and transmit tympanic membrane vibrations to:
    a. External ear
    b. Middle ear
    c. Both a and b
    d. Internal ear
13. Number of turns formed by cochlea around modiolus:
    a. One and half turns
    b. Two and half turns
    c. One turn
    d. Two turns
14. Paired laryngeal cartilages are all, *except*:
    a. Epiglottis
    b. Corniculate
    c. Arytenoid
    d. Cuneiform

15. Piriform fossa is present along:
    a. Lateral wall of larynx
    b. Posterior wall of larynx
    c. Lateral wall of laryngopharynx
    d. Posterior wall of laryngopharynx
16. Paranasal sinuses are examples of which type of bone:
    a. Flat bones
    b. Short bones
    c. Accessory bones
    d. Pneumatic bones
17. Waldeyer's ring is formed by one of the following:
    a. Celiac lymph nodes
    b. Deep inguinal lymph nodes
    c. Lingual tonsil
    d. Superficial inguinal lymph nodes
18. Roof of nasal cavity is formed by:
    a. Cribriform plate of ethmoid
    b. Middle cranial fossa
    c. Sphenoid sinus
    d. Vomer
19. All of the following statements about nasal septum are true, *except*:
    a. Nasal septum forms medial wall of nasal cavity
    b. It is a muscular structure
    c. It is formed by perpendicular plate of ethmoid bone
    d. The quadrangular cartilage makes up its front part
20. Supraglottic part of laryngeal cavity lies:
    a. Between vocal and vestibular folds
    b. Below vocal folds
    c. Above vestibular folds
    d. Behind sinus of larynx

ANSWERS

1. d	2. c	3. a	4. a
5. d	6. a	7. c	8. b
9. a	10. c	11. c	12. d
13. b	14. a	15. c	16. d
17. c	18. a	19. b	20. c

SUGGESTED READING

1. Barrett KE, Boitano S, Barman SM, Brooks HL. Ganong's review of medical physiology, 26th Edn; 2019.
2. Inderbir S. Textbook of human histology with color atlas. New Delhi: Jaypee Brothers Medical Publishers; 2006.
3. Kumar V, Abbas AK, Aster JC. Robbins basic pathology e-book. Elsevier Health Sciences; 2017.
4. LeMone PT, Burke KM, Gerene Bauldoff RN, Gubrud P. Medical-surgical nursing: Clinical reasoning in patient care. Pearson; 2014.
5. Ross MH, Pawlina W. Histology. Lippincott Williams & Wilkins; 2006.
6. Standring S, editor. Gray's anatomy E-Book: the anatomical basis of clinical practice. Elsevier Health Sciences; 2020.
7. Waugh A, Grant A. Ross & Wilson Anatomy and physiology in health and illness E-book. Elsevier Health Sciences; 2014.

CHAPTER 2

Assessment and Diagnostic Evaluation of Ear, Nose and Throat

Manwinder Singh, Abhishek Singh

"He who sees things grow from the beginning, will have the finest view of them".
—**Aristotle (384–322 BC)**

LEARNING OBJECTIVES

After going through the chapter, the learner will be able to:
- Define the terminology used in assessment and diagnostic evaluation of ENT disorders.
- Enumerate the complaints of patients related to the ear, nose and throat disorders.
- Discuss various diagnostic tests of ear, nose and throat disorders.

TERMS

- **Tuning fork test:** This is done to detect the type and extent of hearing loss.
- **Anterior rhinoscopy:** This is examining the anterior nasal cavity with the help of Thudichum speculum to visualize the septum, inferior and middle turbinates, floor of the nasal cavity, and nasal mucosa.
- **Foreshortened malleus:** The malleus appears shorter than it would appear in the normal tympanic membrane.
- **Posterior rhinoscopy:** This is examining the posterior choana and nasopharynx. Structures commonly seen are choana, posterior end of the turbinates and nasal septum, fossa of Rosenmüller, and eustachian tube.
- **Indirect laryngoscopy:** It is done for examination of the supraglottic and glottic region to visualize the base of tongue, vallecula, epiglottis, vestibule, true vocal folds, and pyriform sinuses.

INTRODUCTION

Assessment of any patient with ENT disorders begins with a complete and comprehensive history taking which is to be followed by the physical examination of ear, nose and throat depending on the patients' complaints. In the current chapter following the assessment of the patients, common diagnostic tests to rule out the ENT conditions are discussed.

EAR

Most common ear complaints with which the patients present to OPD are:

Otorrhea: Otorrhea means discharge from the ear. It can be either unilateral/bilateral. It may be—serous (watery), serosanguinous (blood stained), mucoid, mucopurulent (acute/chronic otitis media), purulent, watery, or bloody. It can be foul smelling, e.g., in squamous type of chronic otitis media.

Hearing loss: It can be unilateral/bilateral, sudden/gradual in onset and may be associated with discharge/pain/tinnitus/fullness.

Other symptoms can be:
- Earache
- Irritation and itching
- Tinnitus
- Vertigo
- Trauma
- Foreign body

EXAMINATION OF THE EAR

Ear should be examined in a systematic manner starting with external ear which consists of pinna **(Fig. 2.1)** and external auditory canal followed by the examination of tympanic membrane. Structures of the middle ear should be examined if there is a perforation of tympanic membrane.

External Ear

- **Preauricular region:** We should look for any anatomical defects or congenital lesions, e.g.:
  - *Skin tags:* There are some skin tags which may be present congenitally.
  - *Preauricular sinus or fistula/abscess:* These are the development defects which may be present at the opening in anterior aspect of the helix. It may also present as painful swelling in front of the pinna due to abscess formation. Treatment is excision of the complete sinus tract.
  - *Lymph node/vascular lesions:* Pre and Post auricular lymph nodes may be enlarged due to infection of pinna, or external auditory canal etc.
    Note should be made for the presence of any arteriovenous malformations in front of pinna which may present as red patches.
- **Pinna:** Both medial and lateral surface of the pinna should be examined. The skin over lateral surface of the pinna is adherent and on the medial surface is loose, hence any swelling on lateral surface will cause excruciating pain. The lateral surface has various landmarks like helix, antihelix, concha, tragus, etc., as has been shown in **Figure 2.1**. The pinna should be examined for the following:
  - *Position:* Low set – Down's syndrome
  - *Size:* Anotia, microtia, macrotia
  - *Shape:* Cauliflower ear, bat ear, contour, landmarks
  - *Color:* Red—perichondritis, hyperpigmentation
  - *Any swellings:* Pseudo cyst of pinna, abscess, keloid
- **Postauricular region:** This region consists of mastoid bone below and temporal region above. Any lesion in this area will present as follows. One should look for:
  - *Any swelling:* Mastoiditis, mastoid abscess
  - *Mastoid fistula*
  - *Scar:* suggestive of previous surgery.
  - *Lymph nodes:* Any infection can cause lymphadenopathy.
  - Any **cystic swelling** in this area may be dermoid, or a sebaceous cyst.

Examination of External Auditory Canal

Examination of external auditory canal can be performed without as well as with speculum.

Examination without Speculum

This should always be performed first before introducing a speculum. In order to visualize the external auditory canal, adult pinna is pulled upwards, backwards and laterally **(Fig. 2.2)**, however, infant's pinna is pulled backwards.

Look for

1. **Contents of the lumen:** wax, polyp, discharge, debris, etc.
2. Any swelling in the meatus, furuncle, abscess etc.

Examination with Speculum

The speculum should be of proper size, i.e., one should be able to introduced it easily into the canal. External auditory canal (EAC) is divided into two parts- inner two third is bony and outer one third is cartilaginous. The length of external auditory canal is approximately 2.5 cm. The following things need to be examined:

Look for

1. Walls of EAC: any sagging of posterosuperior wall.
2. Discharge, wax, polyp, or fungal debris etc.

Examination of Tympanic Membrane

The normal tympanic membrane **(Figs. 2.3A and B)** is semitransparent and pearly white in color. Examination is done using otoscope **(Fig. 2.4)**. An otoscope is gently introduced in the external auditory canal and after examining the external canal for any deformity the tympanic membrane is examined.

It should be examined for:
- **Color:** Red and congested—acute otitis media; if bluish- hemotympanum and if Chalky white—tympanosclerosis
- **Position:** Retraction or any bulges

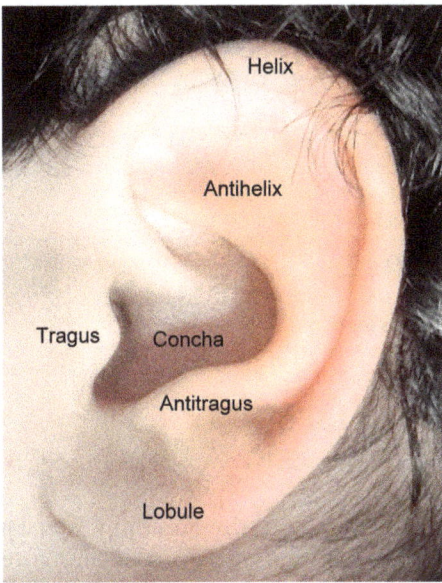

Fig. 2.1: Landmarks of pinna.

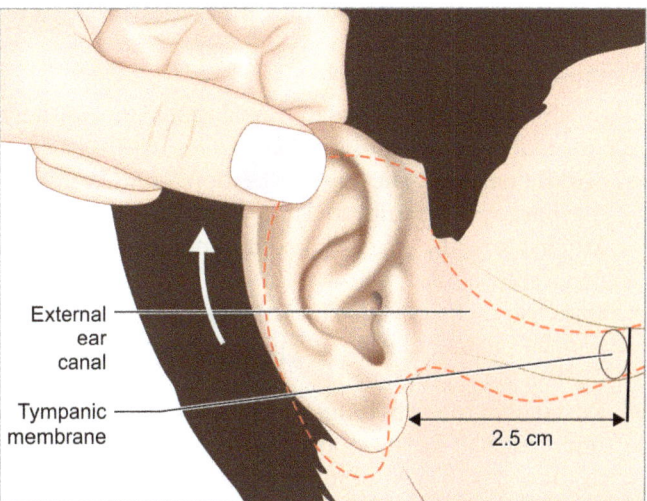

Fig. 2.2: External auditory canal.

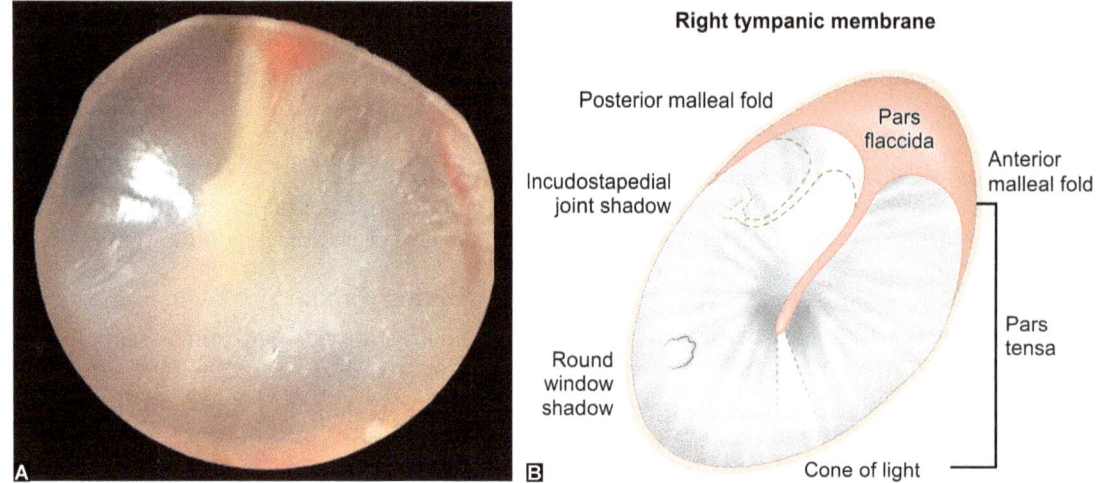

Figs. 2.3A and B: (A) Endoscopic view of tympanic membrane; (B) Right tympanic membrane.

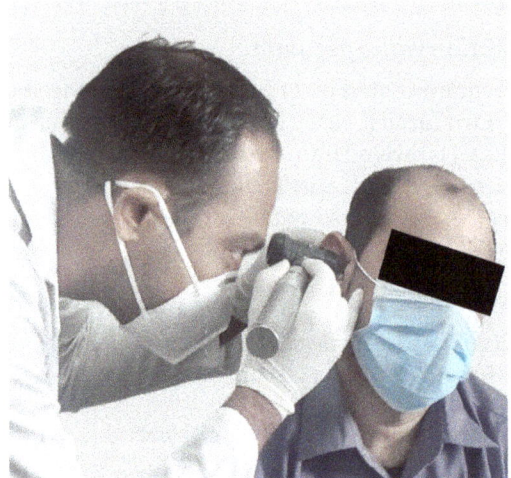

Fig. 2.4: Otoscopic examination.

- **Surface:** Any perforation in case of acute or chronic otitis media-shape, size, position and margins of perforation. Vesicles-Herpes zoster
- **Mobility:** The mobility of the tympanic membrane can be assessed by Valsalva maneuver or by Siegel's speculum. The conditions like eustachian tube dysfunction and tympanosclerosis of tympanic membrane affect the mobility. Mobility of tympanic membrane is important for conduction of sound to middle ear.

Examination of Middle Ear

Normally it cannot be examined directly but in the presence of perforation we can look for:
- **Middle ear mucosa:** Any congestion, granulations or discharge in the middle ear is sign of active disease. Mucosa may be pale/pink/red depending upon the congestion of the mucosa.
- **Ossicles:** In the posterosuperior region incudostapedial may be visible. In case of a perforation the handle of malleus is foreshortened.
- **Eustachian tube opening:** Eustachian tube connects the middle ear to the nasopharynx. Its opening is present in the anterior wall of middle ear and with tympanic membrane perforation its opening can be visualized.
- **Round window niche:** It is located in the posteroinferior region of medial wall of the middle ear. Round window niche can be visualized if there is any perforation in the posterior quadrant of tympanic membrane.

AUDIOLOGICAL EXAMINATION

Hearing starts with the outer ear. The sound wave travels down the external auditory canal and cause vibration of tympanic membrane. These vibrations are then passed through the auditory ossicles' malleus, incus and stapes in the middle ear, which send the sound to the inner ear. In the inner ear the sound waves are converted into electrical impulses. The auditory nerve sends these impulses to the brain and interprets them to sound. In case the patients are presenting with hearing difficulty the following audiological tests are done to establish the extent, type and site of hearing loss.

Tuning Fork Tests

It gives rough estimate of patient's hearing acuity. 512 Hz tuning fork is used for the examination. Various tuning fork tests are the Rinne's test, Weber's test, and Absolute Bone Conduction (ABC test) **(Table 2.1)**. Other audiological tests to establish the hearing loss are Pure tone audiometry and Impedance audiometry.

TABLE 2.1: Tuning fork tests.			
Test	Normal	Conductive deafness	SN deafness
Rinne	AC > BC (Rinne positive)	BC > AC (Rinne negative)	AC > BC
Weber	Not lateralized	Lateralized to diseased ear	Lateralized to better ear
ABC	Same as examiner's	Same as examiner's	Reduced

Rinne's Test (Fig. 2.5)

In this test air conduction is compared with bone conduction for each ear

It is done by first putting the vibrating tuning fork close to the ear canal and then putting the fork on the mastoid region, to determine if the sound is better heard in front of ear canal

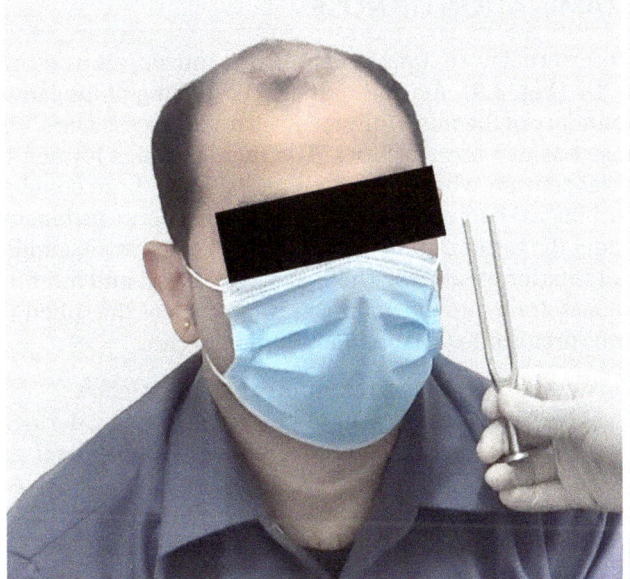

Fig. 2.5: Rinne's test.

(air conduction—AC) or when it was placed over the mastoid (bone conduction—BC). A patient with normal hearing and in sensorineural hearing loss cases, air conduction is better than bone conduction, i.e., **positive Rinne's test.** In cases of conductive hearing loss, bone conduction is better than air conduction, i.e., Rinne's negative.

Weber's Test (Fig. 2.6)

Bone conduction of both ears is compared in Weber's test. In this test the tuning fork is placed over the forehead in the midline and patient is asked in which ear he can hear well. If sound lateralized to normal side, then he may have sensorineural hearing loss. If lateralization is towards effected ear, then patient will have conductive hearing loss. Along with Rinne's test it is a great tool to diagnose both conductive and sensorineural hearing loss.

Absolute Bone Conduction (ABC) Test

In this test the hearing level of patient is compared with the examiner's hearing. The hearing status of the examiner is presumed to be within normal range. After occluding the ear canal, the vibrating tuning fork is placed over the mastoid process of the patient. When the patient is not able to hear the sound anymore, the tuning fork is placed at the mastoid process of the examiner after occluding his canal.

In case of normal hearing, the examiner will not hear any sound. However, in sensorineural hearing loss, the examiner will be able to hear the sound, interpreted as reduced ABC.

Pure Tone Audiometry (PTA)

This test is used to determine the degree and type of hearing loss. Patient is made to hear pure tones (sounds of a particular frequency) of 250 Hz, 500 Hz, 1000 Hz, 2000 Hz, 4000 Hz and 8000 Hz and his air conduction and bone conduction threshold for different frequencies are plotted on a graph and from there the degree **(Fig. 2.7)** and type of hearing loss is calculated.

Impedance Audiometry

It is an objective test to differentiate types of hearing loss, assess the middle ear status, and facial nerve status. This test is done by giving a sound stimulus through a sealed auditory canal and as per the impedance provided by the middle ear a graph is plotted. It helps in diagnosis of otosclerosis,

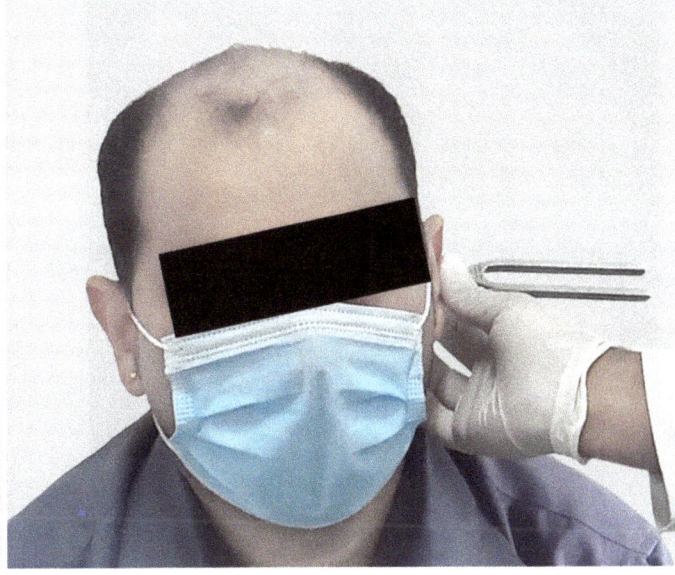

Fig. 2.6: Weber's test.

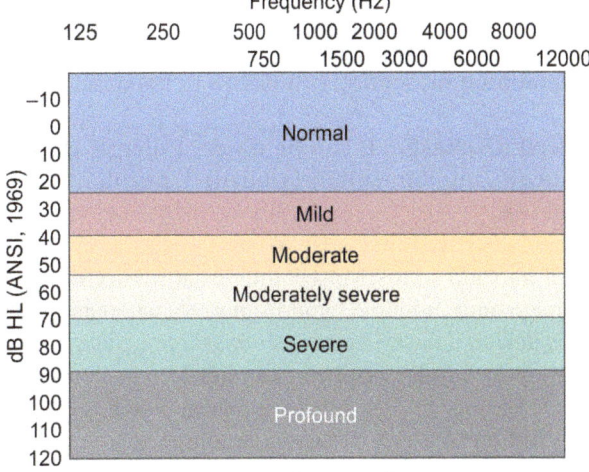

Fig. 2.7: Deafness grading.

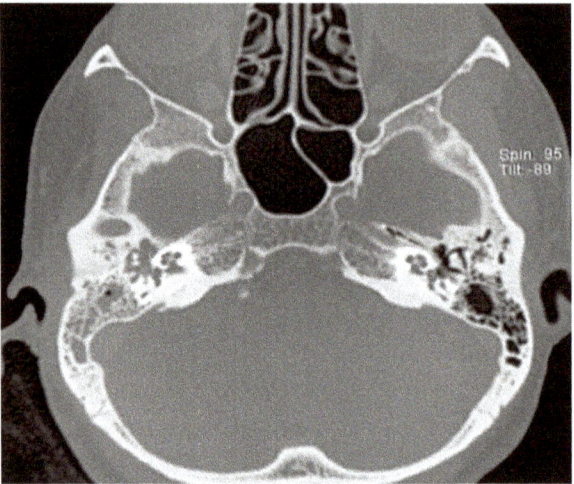

Fig. 2.8: HRCT temporal bone.

ossicular discontinuity and middle ear effusion. Stapedial reflex is also observed during the impedance audiometry. As the stapedius muscle is supplied by the facial nerve, it also helps in determining the status of facial nerve.

RADIOLOGICAL EXAMINATION

X-ray

Schuller's view is a lateral radiographic view of skull. It is primarily used to view the mastoid cells. Various structures seen are:
- Mastoid air cells
- External auditory canal
- Tympanic cavity
- Temporomandibular joint
- Dural plate
- Sinus plate
- Dense bone of labyrinth

High Resolution CT (HRCT)

It gives minute structural detail of both anatomy and pathology of temporal bone and gives a direct visual window into it.

It is the investigation of choice for ear diseases, e.g., Cholesteatoma and also helps to assess the bony landmarks and status of the ear ossicles and inner ear **(Fig. 2.8)**.

NOSE

Most common presenting complaints of the nasal diseases are:
- **Nasal discharge:** It can be watery (allergic rhinitis)/mucoid/mucopurulent (sinusitis)/purulent/blood-stained.
- **Nasal obstruction:** Cause of nasal obstruction varies in children and adults. Most common causes in children are foreign body, adenoid hypertrophy etc., whereas in adults it is deviated nasal septum, sinonasal polyposis, etc.
- **Other common symptoms can be:**
  - Sneezing
  - Epistaxis (Nasal bleeding)
  - Stuffiness
  - Mass or swelling
  - Headache
  - Loss of smell

EXAMINATION OF NOSE

The external nose consists of root, dorsum, tip, ala as shown in the **(Fig. 2.9)**. Ala is the tissue comprising of the lateral boundary of the nose, inferiorly, surrounding the naris. The nose has two nasal cavities. The medial wall is formed by nasal septum whereas the lateral wall has three conchae (turbinates) namely superior, middle, and inferior turbinates. Under the turbinates are the meatuses, i.e., superior, middle, and inferior meatuses. The maxillary, frontal and ethmoid sinuses drain into the middle meatus whereas the sphenoid sinus drains into the sphenoethmoidal recess.

The examination of various parts of nose is as follows:
- **Skin:** Signs of any inflammation, scar, swelling dermoid cyst, lipoma etc. Ulceration could be seen in basal cell carcinoma.
- **Dorsum:** Any deviation, deformity or bulge is looked for.
- **Vestibule:** It is examined by lifting the tip of the nose. The vestibular area is anterior hairy area of the nose. Look for any furuncle, crusting or deviated caudal end of septum.
- **Anterior rhinoscopy (Fig. 2.10):** It is an examination of nasal cavity using Thudichum speculum. It is placed into each nostril turn wise to widen it for better visualization. A headlight is worn by the doctor so that his hands are free for proper examination. This test helps to evaluate the condition of nasal cavity, nasal mucosa, any discharge, deviated nasal septum, hypertrophic turbinate, polyp, mass, foreign bodies, etc.
- **Septum:** Any deviation, hematoma, growth, perforation
- **Nasal floor:** Any foreign body, rhinolith, swelling
- **Roof:** Usually not visible except in cases of atrophic rhinitis.
- **Lateral wall:** Turbinates and the meatus

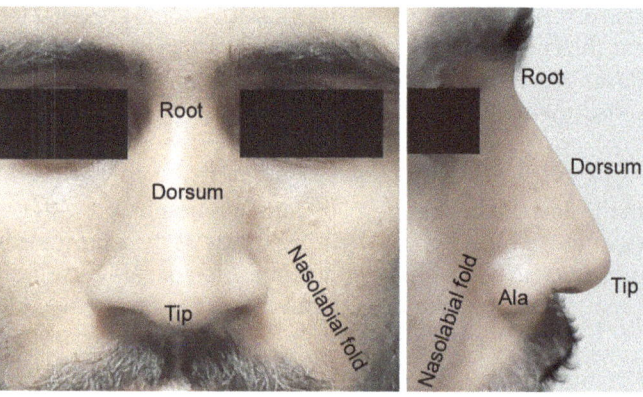

Fig. 2.9: External nose—anterior and lateral view.

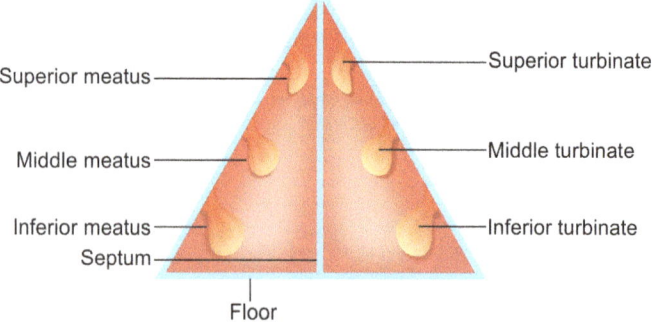

Fig. 2.10: Anterior rhinoscopy.

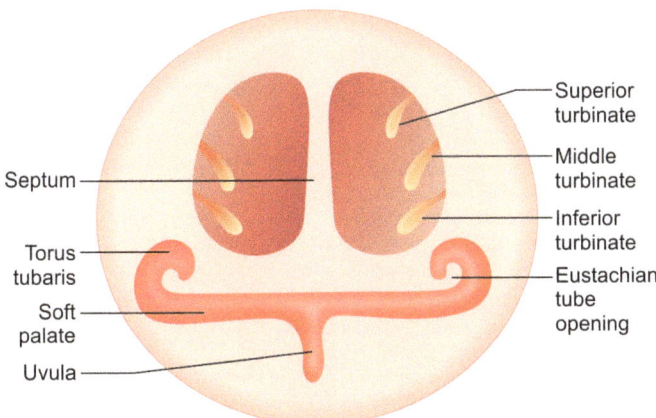

Fig. 2.11: Posterior rhinoscopy.

- **Posterior rhinoscopy (Fig. 2.11):** It is done for visualization of posterior end of nasal cavity and nasopharynx.

FUNCTIONAL TEST

Cold Spatula Test (Fig. 2.12)

This is a clinical method used to screen the nasal patency of the patient. Patient is asked to exhale on a cold tongue depressor or a metal spatula which is placed below the nostril. We look for the area of mist formation under the nostril and is compared on both the sides.

Cotton Wool Test

In this test a cotton fluff is held under each nostril and the degree of movement of the cotton fluff is compared on both the sides when the patient inhales and exhales.

Sense of Smell

To assess the sense of smell, the patient is asked to identify the smells while keeping the eyes closed. Each nostril is tested separately. Most commonly used substances are: Coffee powder, camphor, asafetida.

There are 7 primary odors:
1. Musky   – Perfumes
2. Putrid   – Rotten eggs
3. Pungent   – Vinegar
4. Camphoraceous – Mothballs
5. Ethereal   – Dry cleaning fluid
6. Floral   – Roses (floral scent)
7. Pepper minty – Mint gum

EXAMINATION OF PARANASAL SINUS

There are four groups of sinuses namely maxillary, frontal, ethmoidal and sphenoid. The presence of sinuses in the skull makes the skull light. The mucosa of sinuses is lined by ciliated pseudostratified columnar epithelium and the secretions of the sinuses are drained into the nasal cavity. Any obstruction of this drainage will lead to obstruction of drainage of secretions followed by sinusitis. These sinuses are examined as follows:

- **Maxillary sinus:** It is palpated over the canine fossa or anterolateral of maxilla.
- **Frontal** above the inner canthus of eye.
- **Anterior ethmoid** medial to inner canthus.
- **Posterior ethmoid** not able to palpate.
- **Sphenoid** not able to palpate.

  Each sinus should be palpated with moderate pressure.

RADIOLOGICAL EXAMINATION

X-ray

- **Water's view:** Preferred view for examination of maxillary sinuses, frontal sinus and sphenoid sinus.
- **Lateral view for nasal bones (Fig. 2.13):** Best view for fracture of nasal bone and always bilateral view should be obtained.

Computed Tomography (CT) of Nose and Paranasal Sinus (Fig. 2.14)

It is the imaging modality of choice.
CT scan helps in detailed examination of the bony landmarks of nose and paranasal sinuses and any anatomical anomalies like:

- **Concha bullosa:** Air in the middle turbinates
- **Haller cells:** Air cell in the floor of the orbit obstructing the opening of maxillary sinus
- **Onodi cell:** Air cell of posterior ethmoid extending posterior to the anterior wall of sphenoid above the sphenoid sinus.

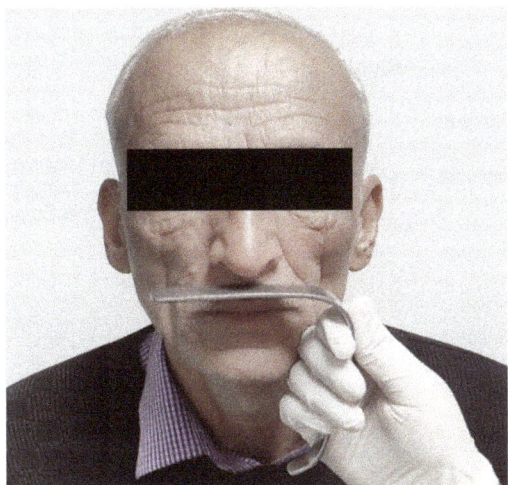

Fig. 2.12: Cold spatula test.

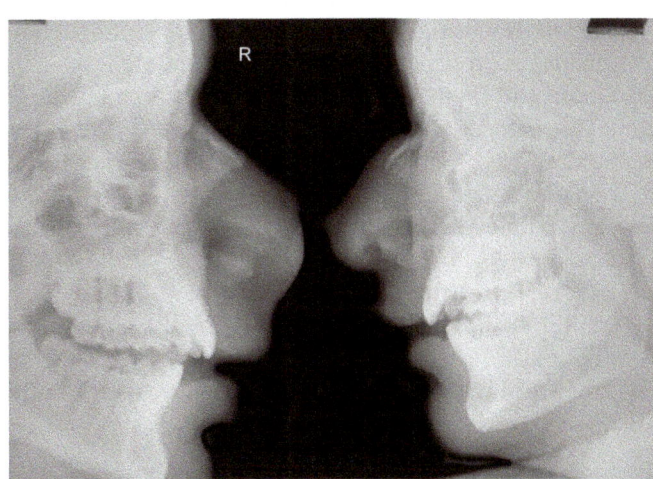

Fig. 2.13: X-ray lateral view.

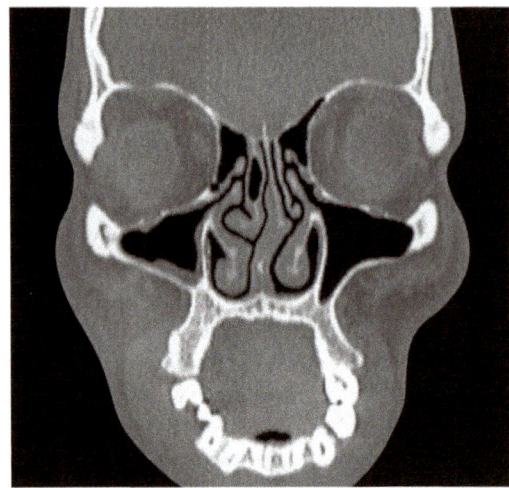

Fig. 2.14: CT PNS and nose.

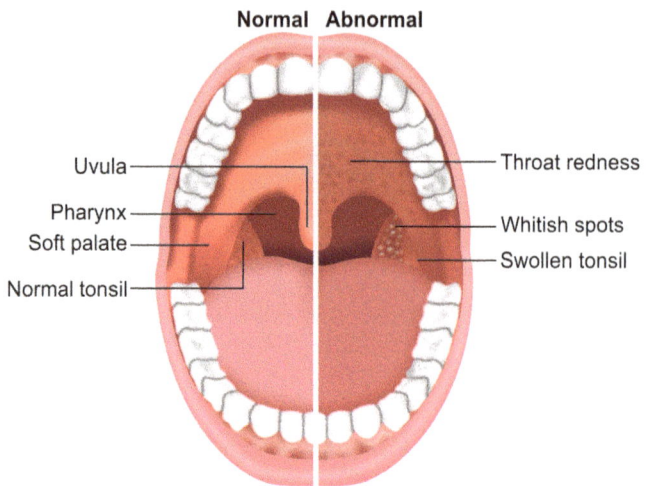

Fig. 2.15: Oral cavity.

It further helps in diagnosis of sinusitis or any tumor of nose and paranasal sinuses.

THROAT

Commonly seen complaints in throat disorders are:
- **Dysphagia:** It is difficulty in swallowing. Any disease involving the oropharynx or esophagus can result into dysphagia. We should inquire about the onset, duration, progression and if it is associated only for solids or for both solid and liquids.
- **Throat Pain:** Children most commonly present with throat pain. It is commonly seen in cases of acute tonsillitis, peritonsillar abscess, pharyngitis, etc.
- **Other symptoms can be:**
  - Pain while chewing
  - Swelling or growth
  - Ulceration or lesions in oral cavity
  - Throat pain
  - Difficulty in opening mouth

EXAMINATION OF ORAL CAVITY

Examination of oral cavity should be done by using some light source for better visualization. Examine each area of the oral cavity for any abnormal findings **(Fig. 2.15)**.
- **Lips:** Color change, ulceration, any tumor, cleft lip
- **Buccal mucosa:** Color, ulceration, white striae (lichen planus), submucosal fibrosis, leukoplakia, etc.
- **Gums and teeth:** Signs of caries, infection, pus, loose teeth, malocclusion.
- **Tongue:** Size, shape, color, surface, movement, any patch or plaque growth.
- **Hard palate:** Cleft palate, ulceration, any growth, oronasal fistula.
- **Floor of mouth:** Opening of submandibular duct, frenulum-tongue tie, any swelling, ranula, sublingual dermoid.
- **Retromolar trigone:** Submucosal fibrosis, growth, impacted last molar tooth.

Examination of Oropharynx

Examination of oropharynx involves the following:
- **Tonsils:** They are the lymphoid tissues present in the lateral wall of oropharynx between the anterior and posterior tonsillar pillars. We should look for any congestion, hypertrophy or membrane over tonsils. Any congestion of the anterior tonsillar pillars should also be noted. These are the signs of tonsillitis.
- **Soft palate:** It is the posterior part of palate with uvula hanging posteriorly. We should look for any congestion. Any swelling in the nasopharynx may cause bulge or swelling in soft palate which should be noted.
- **Posterior pharyngeal wall:** Any congestion or cobble stoning of pharyngeal wall due to inflammation of lymphoid tissue should be noted.
- **Base of tongue:** In the base of tongue, any bulge or growth in the base of tongue should be observed.
- **Indirect Laryngoscopy (Fig. 2.16):** It is done with the help of indirect laryngoscope mirror. It is done to visualize the vocal cords and also assess their mobility and for any growth in the vocal cords. Besides this, it is also done to visualize base of tongue, vallecula, epiglottis, aryepiglottic folds, false vocal cords and pyriform sinuses. Any growth or abnormalities are recorded.

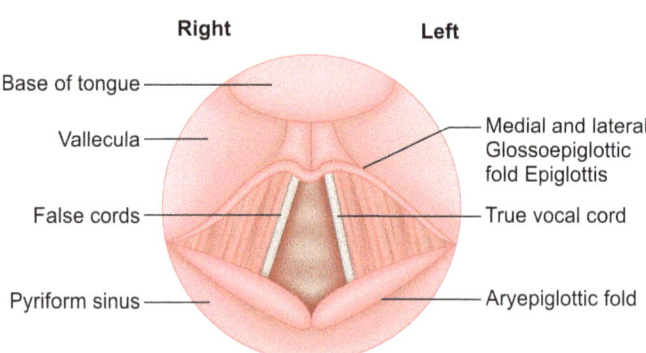

Fig. 2.16: Indirect laryngoscopy.

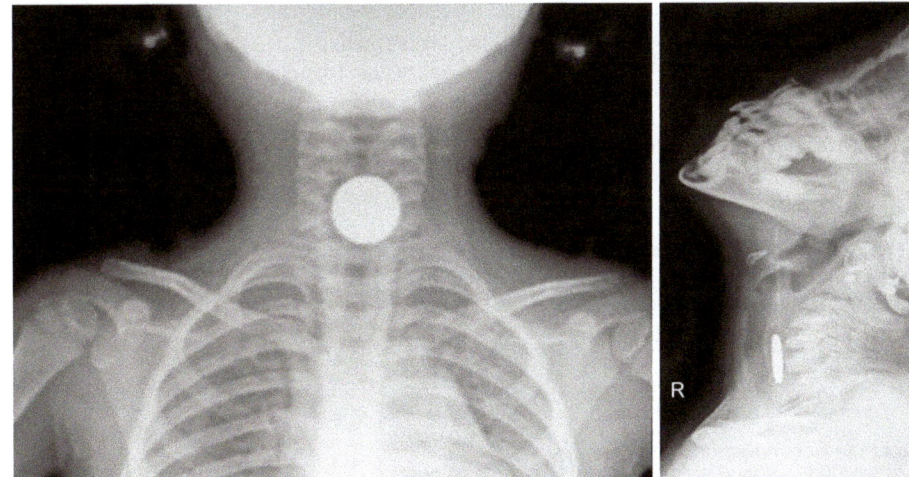

Fig. 2.17: X-ray neck AP and lateral view.

RADIOLOGICAL EXAMINATION

- **X-ray neck:** It helps in diagnosis of any foreign body in throat. X-ray AP and lateral view **(Fig. 2.17)** helps in diagnosing any foreign bodies, e.g., coin, fish bone, pin or dentures. Lateral view of neck also helps in knowing whether the foreign body is in the airway or esophagus. It also helps in diagnosing:
  - Acute epiglottitis
  - Retropharyngeal abscess
  - Fracture of laryngeal framework
  - Compression of trachea
- **Contrast-enhanced CT (CECT) neck:** It is the imaging modality of choice **(Fig. 2.18)** for lesions of neck spaces like retro pharyngeal space, parapharyngeal space, and submandibular space. Any abscess or growth will be very nicely delineated in contrast-enhanced CT. Besides this, it is very good diagnostic test to diagnose any condition of thyroid, larynx, lymph nodes, or any vascular conditions.

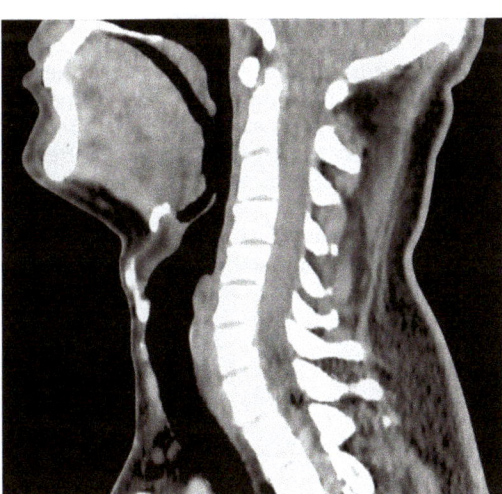

Fig. 2.18: CECT neck.

Case Scenario

1. A 15-year-old male patient comes to ENT OPD with severe pain in the throat and the left ear. The pain was increasing at the time of swallowing. It was of sudden onset with 3 days duration. Few days patient also had sore throat and fever. He also gives history of recurrent throat infection around 5-6 episodes/year. Patient was looking very ill. Temperature was 38.8°C and pulse 100/minute. The patient had malodor breath. He was unable to open his mouth. There was congestion of anterior pillars and bilateral tonsillar hypertrophy grade 3. There was painful lymphadenopathy of bilateral jugulodigastric nodes. The left tympanic membrane was normal. Routine blood investigations, i.e., complete blood count was done which showed leukocytosis. He was started on oral antibiotics, analgesics, antipyretics and betadine mouth gargles. With this his condition significantly improved. After a gap of 4–5 weeks, he underwent adenotonsillectomy and was discharged within 2 days with complete recovery.

2. A 45-year-female patient comes to ENT OPD with complaints of right ear discharge since last 10 years which has increased since last 2 weeks. It is associated with difficulty in hearing in the right ear since last 4 years. The discharge was mucopurulent, moderate in amount, non-foul smelling, non-blood tinged. It used to increase during episodes of cold and winter seasons. On examination, right external auditory canal was filled with yellowish mucopurulent discharge and after ear mopping, we could see a medium size central perforation and rest of the tympanic membrane was congested. Routine blood investigations showed leukocytosis. She was started on topical and oral antibiotics, antihistamines and decongestant nasal drops. She again visited OPD after 3 weeks with completely dry ear. At this time hearing was evaluated using pure tone audiometer (PTA) which showed moderate conductive hearing loss. She was diagnosed as right chronic otitis media mucosal type along with moderate conductive hearing loss and advised surgery. She underwent pre-op HRCT of temporal bone to look for the extent of disease and any anatomical variations. After 3 weeks, she underwent tympanoplasty and recovery was completely uneventful. On follow up there have been no new episodes of ear discharge. There was significant improvement in hearing.

SUMMARY

A meticulous history taking, local physical examination, audiological examination and radiology of ear, nose and throat will help us in proper anatomical, physiological and pathological assessment of ear, nose and throat. A thorough assessment will lead to correct diagnosis and ultimately the right treatment of the patient's problem.

MULTIPLE CHOICE QUESTIONS

1. Which of the following is true about Rinne's test?
   a. Air conduction is better than bone conduction in perceptive deafness
   b. Air conduction is better than bone conduction in conductive deafness
   c. Bone conduction is better than air conduction in conductive deafness
   d. Bone conduction is better than air conduction in perceptive deafness

2. Which of the following is true about Weber's test?
   a. Sound is heard better in diseased ear in conductive deafness
   b. Sound is heard better in healthy ear in conductive deafness
   c. Sound is heard in the center in perceptive deafness
   d. Sound is heard better in diseased ear in perceptive deafness

3. Identify the area marked 'X':

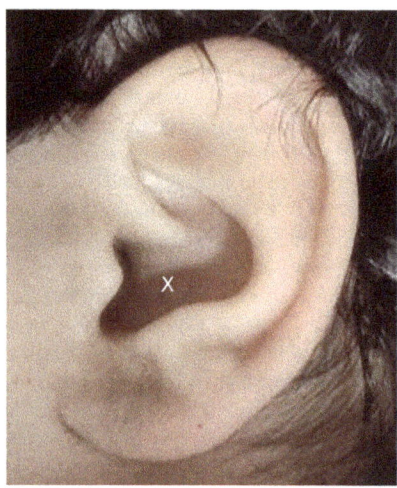

   a. Tragus   b. Concha
   c. Helix   d. Lobule

4. Thudichum speculum is used for visualizing:
   a. Posterior nasal cavity   b. Larynx
   c. Anterior nasal cavity   d. Posterior nares

5. Radiological finding of sinusitis includes all of the following, *except*:
   a. Bone destruction   b. Opacity of affected sinus
   c. Fluid level   d. Mucosal thickening

6. The most common site of nasal bleeding is:
   a. Little's area
   b. Mac Ewan triangle
   c. Pyriform fossa
   d. Sphenoethmoidal recess

7. The figure shows structure seen on posterior rhinoscopy - Identify the structure shown by 'X':

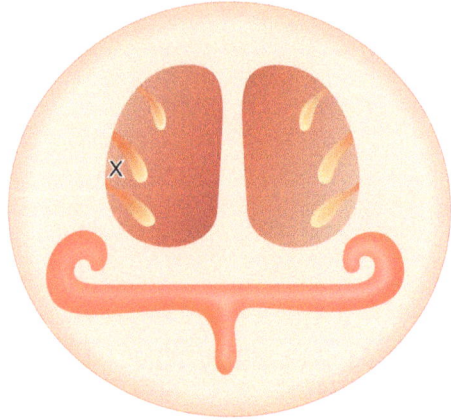

   a. Superior meatus   b. Middle meatus
   c. Inferior meatus   d. Eustachian tube opening

ANSWERS

| 1. c | 2. a | 3. b | 4. c |
| 5. a | 6. a | 7. b | |

SUGGESTED READING

1. Barnes ML, White PS. Outpatient Assessment. In: Watkinson JC, Clarke RW (Eds). Scott-Brown's Otorhinolaryngology Head and Neck Surgery, 8th edition. Florida, CRC Press Taylor and Francis Group; 2018. pp. 977-82.
2. Browning GG, Wormald PJ. Clinical Examination of The Ears and Hearing. In: Watkinson JC, Clarke RW (Eds). Scott-Brown's Otorhinolaryngology Head and Neck Surgery, 8th edition. Florida, CRC Press Taylor and Francis Group; 2018. pp. 919-29.
3. Francis HW. Anatomy of the Temporal Bone, External Ear, and Middle Ear. In: Flint PW, Francis HW, Haughey BH, Lesperance MM, Lund VJ, et al (Eds). Cummings Otolaryngology Head and Neck surgery, 7th edition. Pennsylvania: Elsevier; 2021. pp. 1928-37.
4. Nunez DA, Qi L. Tests for hearing. In: Hussain SM (Eds). Logan Turner's Diseases of the Nose, Throat and Ear Head and Neck Surgery, 11th edition. Florida, CRC Press Taylor and Francis Group; 2016. pp. 375-84.
5. Philpott C. Investigation of nasal diseases. In: Hussain SM (Eds). Logan Turner's Diseases of the Nose, Throat and Ear Head and Neck Surgery, 11th edition. Florida, CRC Press Taylor and Francis Group; 2016. pp. 13-22.

CHAPTER 3

Disorders of Ear

Manwinder Singh, Dia Sharma, Sukhpal Kaur

"Words might only be said once, but the hearing lasts forever."
—**Craig D Lounsbrough**

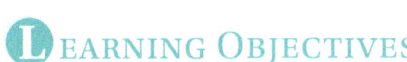

After going through the chapter, the learner will be able to:
- Identify the symptoms related to various disorders of ear.
- Make a diagnosis with key ENT findings in a patient.
- Learn treatment modalities for various ear disorders.
- Discuss the pre and postoperative nursing interventions for the patients undergoing ear surgery.
- Discuss the geriatric considerations related to disorders of ear.

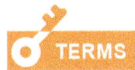

- **Acute otitis media:** It is infective disease of middle ear mucosa, more common in children but seen in adults also. It presents with excruciating pain, aural fullness, hearing loss and in later stages discharge from ear with relief from other symptoms.
- **Cerumen:** An excretory product of external auditory canal (EAC) which is produced by shedding of skin of EAC and other particulate substances that may have entered the EAC.
- **Chronic otitis media:** Chronic Infection of mucosa of middle ear which may or may not be accompanied with pars tensa perforation (mostly in mucosal type), pars flaccida and pars tensa retraction and cholesteatoma (in squamous type). Thus, patient will complaint of hearing loss and in active stage discharge.
- **Endolymph:** It is the fluid contained in the membranous labyrinth of the inner ear.
- **Otalgia:** It is the ear pain which can be due to various underlying ear disorders or referred pain due to dental disorders, oral cavity and oropharyngeal diseases.
- **Otitis externa:** Infection of EAC skin which will present with discharge from ear, pain, itching, and hearing loss.
- **Endolymphatic sac:** A non-sensory organ of the inner ear which is connected to the endolymphatic compartment that is filled with endolymph.
- **Tinnitus:** A symptom and not a disease which is defined by extra-abnormal sound heard by the patient.

INTRODUCTION

Disorders of ear include any pathological condition which hinders normal acoustic and vestibular functioning of ear. Various disorders of ear are discussed separately for external, middle and inner ear.

DISORDERS OF EXTERNAL EAR

The external ear includes the disease involving pinna and external auditory canal (EAC).

CERUMEN IMPACTION

Definition

Cerumen is naturally occurring extruded material in external ear which might get impacted in EAC. In layman terminology it is also called ear wax.

Epidemiology

Cerumen impaction presents in approximately 10% children, 5% normal healthy adults.

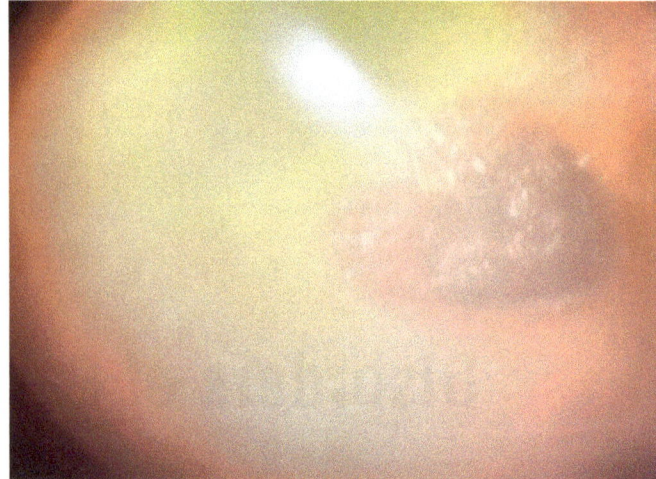

Fig. 3.1: Cerumen impaction.

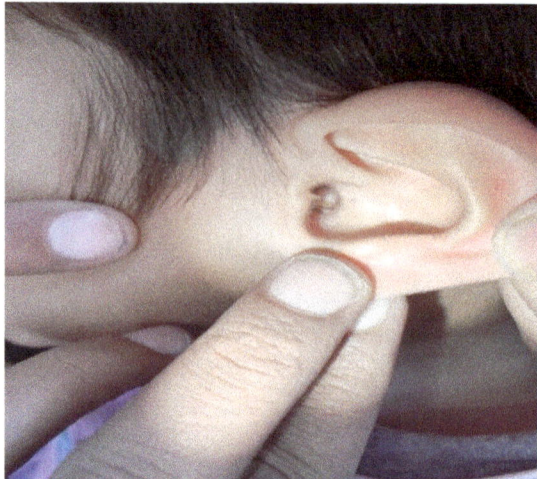

Fig. 3.2: Foreign body in EAC.

Etiology
An anatomically narrow EAC can predispose to impaction. Also, cerumen impaction is noted with attempted extrusion of cerumen by patient (e.g., ear swab, ear plugs).

Clinical Manifestation
Cerumen usually is asymptomatic. On impaction, patient can complaint of fullness of ear, decreased hearing, itching, discomfort and sometimes pain as well.

Diagnosis
Otoscopic examination of ear will show brown to black appearing cerumen collected in the EAC **(Fig. 3.1)**. Due to impaction, tympanic membrane might not be visible properly.

Treatment Modalities
It could be cleared by:
- **Ear drops:** Glycerine and paraffin ear drops can be prescribed. They make the cerumen loose and allow it to pass from EAC.
- **Aural syringing:** Using a 50cc syringe, lukewarm water (not cold or hot to trigger nystagmus) is pushed, mostly posterosuperiorly in EAC, with pressure to remove the cerumen.
- **Aural toileting:** Using Jobson's probe with cotton on the pointed end, doctor can clean the impacted cerumen.
- Precautions to be taken not to use ear swabs by patient to clean cerumen again. In case of narrow EAC, patients may require regular cleaning of ear.

FOREIGN BODY

Definition
Any unnaturally occurring particle ranging from organic material like lentil seed or insect to inorganic like pen cap in the EAC is defined as foreign body in ear. It can occur intentionally as well as unintentionally.

Epidemiology
It is more common in children. The incidence of 40% has been reported to be more in children within the age group of 7–12 years of age followed by children less than 6 years of age (32.4%) cases. The insertion was more in the right ear (66%) as compared to left ear (34%) (Awad AL et al).

Etiology
In patients with mental illness, patient is prone to insert various foreign bodies in the ear. Sometimes, EAC foreign body can be chance occurrence as well. And foreign body like insects can themselves get lodged in EAC.

Clinical Presentation
Patient generally presents with fullness of ear involved, pain in the ear. When foreign body is left undetected or untreated, patient may also present with ear discharge and edema of EAC.

Diagnosis
Using bull's lamp or head light, foreign body can be visualized in EAC when light is focused with or without ear speculum **(Fig. 3.2)**. If in doubt, otoscopic examination can confirm the presence of foreign body.

Treatment Modalities
Method of foreign body removal:
- Removal under bull's lamp: Any foreign body seen in EAC has to be removed under vision. Using bull's lamp with or without speculum, light is focused to visualize the foreign body and then removed using probe or crocodile forceps depending on size and type of foreign body.
- Syringing
- Suctioning
- Foreign body which is impacted and unable to remove by above mentioned method, removal under microscope can be tried. And if still no help, post aural approach to EAC should be tried.

For discharge from ear, local antibiotic ear drops are prescribed. Analgesics should be given for pain.

OTALGIA

Definition
Otalgia is defined as pain in ear due to local cause or referred pain.

Etiology

Various causes of pain may include:
- In external ear, conditions including impacted wax, foreign body, furuncle, herpes zoster, otitis externa, and otomycosis etc. Middle ear disorders may include acute otitis media, eustachian tube obstruction, mastoiditis also.
- The referred pain may be from dental disorders, temporomandibular joint (TMJ) disorders, acute tonsillitis, benign or malignant ulcers in oral cavity.

Clinical Manifestations

Patient will present with pain in ear along with symptoms according to the underlying cause for otalgia.

Treatment Modalities

Analgesics are given for pain. For resolution of pain, underlying cause must be treated.

EXOSTOSES

Definition

Exostosis is a hyperostotic benign outgrowth of periosteal bone in EAC. They are smooth, sessile, hemispherical swelling in EAC.

Epidemiology

Exostoses are more common in patients exposed to cold water. Prevalence is higher in surfer population to about 73.5%. The incidence of exostoses is correlated to length of exposure varying from 55.3% in patients who surfed 10 years or less to 90.9% in individuals who surfed for longer than 20 years (Graham MD).

Etiology

The commonly affected population as discussed earlier is individuals exposed to cold water as in case of water sports. It is anthropologically noted as evolutionary response to protect middle ear from immersion in cold water.

Pathology

Histopathological examination shows exostoses is seen as broad based, dense and composed of lamellated bone, covered with periosteum and its overlying squamous epithelium, lack fibrovascular channels.

Clinical Presentation

Exostoses are typically multiple and bilateral. Exostoses may be asymptomatic but if large and/or multiple, may occlude the EAC.

Diagnosis

The diagnosis is made clinically by otoscopic examination of EAC. Single or multiple sessile, bony swellings are seen in EAC near tympanic membrane. Under light, high-resolution CT scanning is used for defining the extent of pathology.

Treatment

Treatment is not required if the patient is asymptomatic.
Conservative treatment: Regular aural toilet is required to prevent complications and treatment of intercurrent otitis externa. Cold-water exposure in patients with exostoses should be avoided. If conservative management fails, surgical excision of both can be done.

OTITIS EXTERNA

Definition

Otitis externa is referred as generalized infection of external auditory canal skin characterized by itching, pain, discharge, and oedema of EAC.

Epidemiology

Otitis externa has a prevalence of approx. 0.4% per year and affects almost 10% of the population during their lifetime.

Etiology

Water and increased moisture can cause change of flora of the EAC skin from gram positive to gram negative. Bathing and exposure to water can predispose to otitis externa.

Bacteriology suggests of multiple bacterial strains in most cases, also including methicillin resistant *Staphylococcus aureus* (MRSA) and pseudomonas **(Table 3.1)**. Generally, exposure to water is enough to develop the condition and bacterial contamination is not required, although exposure to freshwater lakes containing pseudomonas contributed to a large outbreak in the Netherlands.

TABLE 3.1: Bacteriology of otitis externa.

Bacteria	Percentage
Pseudomonas spp.	50–65
Other gram-negative organisms	25–35
Staphylococcus aureus	15–30
Streptococcus spp.	9–15

Pathology

The course of disease can be divided into following stages:
- **Stage I (preinflammatory):** Edema of stratum corneum of EAC skin, blocking of sebaceous glands seen which cause aural fullness and itching.
- **Stage II (acute stage):** With disruption of epithelial layer, patient develop thickening exudate, further oedema, pain disproportionate to the disease progression and obliteration of EAC.
- **Stage III (chronic stage):** Continued infection of EAC for more than 6 months is referred to as chronic otitis externa and is characterized with thickening of EAC wall.

Clinical Features

Patients present with pain and tenderness (out of proportion to disease progression), ear discharge is seen serous and later thick and mucopurulent in acute stage and in chronic stage dried discharge debris. Meatus is edematous in early stage and scaling and fissuring seen in chronic stage.

Diagnosis

Diagnosis of otitis externa is made clinically. During ear examination, pressing over the tragus elicits tenderness. This is known as a tragal sign. Pain is also elicited when the pinna of patient is held during examination under bull's lamp and otoscopic examination.

On otoscopic examination, discharge is seen in EAC which is serous in pre inflammatory stage to mucopurulent in acute stage and discharge debris is seen in chronic stage. Edema is also seen of EAC skin with erythema noted. Acquired atresia of EAC can also be noted in few cases due to oedema of the skin.

Treatment

Treatment modalities include:
- **Aural toileting:** Most effective treatment. Using head light or bull's lamp, the EAC is visualized and thorough aural toileting is done regularly on OPD basis.
- Medicated ear wicks can also be used. Ichthammol and glycerol (90%: 10%) solution is commonly used as it causes dehydration and has anti-inflammatory and anti-bacterial properties against *Staphylococcus* and *Streptococcus*.
- Topical antibiotics are given to control the underlying bacterial infection.
- Systemic antibiotics are given in case of systemic infection is also present.
- Analgesia
- Prevention from predisposing factors. Ear wick coated with petroleum jelly (Vaseline) has proven to be effective in prevention of exposure to water.

DISORDERS OF MIDDLE EAR

Various disorders of middle ear include:
1. Tympanic membrane perforation
2. Acute otitis media
3. Serous otitis media
4. Chronic otitis media
5. Mastoiditis
6. Otosclerosis

TYMPANIC MEMBRANE PERFORATION

Definition

Perforation is any breach in the pars tensa of tympanic membrane through which middle ear can be visualized.

Etiology

Tympanic membrane perforation can be:
- **Traumatic:** Due to any external trauma to ear, noise induced trauma, barotrauma or iatrogenic trauma caused during aural syringing or aural toileting.
- **Pathological causes:** These include acute otitis media, chronic otitis, and sharp foreign body.

Pathology

Tympanic membrane consists of three layers. Most laterally lies epithelial layer, middle fibrous layer and medially the layer is continuous with mucosa of middle ear. Traumatic perforation due to barotrauma is due to change of pressure in the middle ear causing bulge and perforation of TM.

In acute otitis media, due to collection of mucopurulent discharge behind the perforation causes increase in middle ear pressure leading to perforation.

Clinical Presentation

Patient presents commonly with decreased hearing in the ear involved. According to underlying cause, symptoms vary. In case of trauma, patient might also present with aural fullness, pain and tinnitus in some cases. In middle ear pathologies and chronic cases of traumatic perforation, patient also can present with discharge too.

Depending on size, the perforation can be classified as: Small, Medium, Subtotal and Total perforation.

Depending on location, the perforation can be central or marginal involving one or more than one of the four quadrants.

Diagnosis

Diagnosis is made clinically. The tympanic membrane is visualized using bull's lamp or with otoscope. Traumatic perforation can be identified by:
- Irregular margins
- Congested margins, blood clot near the margins
- Everted margins

The location of perforation should be noted. In pathological condition, the margins of perforation are smooth due to epithelization, no congestion seen. Margins can be inverted too. Ear discharge can also be seen varying in quantity according to pathology, for example scanty discharge is seen in chronic otitis media squamous type whereas purulent in acute otitis media, foreign body, chronic otitis media mucosal type.

In case of chronic otitis media squamous type, pars flaccida dimpling and even cholesteatoma can be visualized.

Treatment

Depending on the size and cause of perforation, various treatment modalities are:
- In small traumatic perforations, we can wait and follow the patient as irregular margins of perforation without epithelization can heal.
- In case of perforation with inverted margins, the margins can be everted under local anesthesia using gel foam soaked in saline using straight pick.
- **Chemical cautery:** With application of 4% solution of Trichloroacetic acid to margins, the margins of the perforation can be made raw and patient is followed to see the closure of perforation.
- **Fat graft myringoplasty:** In small to medium sized perforations, fat graft can be tried. Under local anesthesia, the margins of perforation are made raw and fat harvested from ear lobule is used as graft to plug the perforation.

- ❖ **Myringoplasty/tympanoplasty:** It refers to surgical procedure for correction of tympanic perforation ranging from medium to total perforation. The graft is generally taken from temporalis fascia.

  Other graft materials that can be used are perichondrium and cartilage from tragus and cymba conchae, periosteum, subcutaneous tissue, fascia lata, skin graft.

  Depending on the ossicular status of the ear, the tympanoplasty can be further divided into:
- ❖ **Type I:** TM is repaired, no middle ear abnormality seen.
- ❖ **Type II:** Malleus is eroded. Thus, TM is repaired and grafting done to incus.
- ❖ **Type III:** Malleus and incus both are eroded. The graft to repair the TM is kept in relation to stapes head.
- ❖ **Type IV:** The suprastructure of stapes along with malleus and incus are eroded. Graft is placed in the relation with stapes footplate.
- ❖ **Type V:** The repair involves the stapes footplate, which is fixed. Fenestra in lateral semi-circular canal is created.

ACUTE OTITIS MEDIA (AOM)

Definition

Acute otitis media refers the infective pathology of mucosa of middle ear with short duration of symptoms. It could be due to bacterial or viral pathology.

Epidemiology

Acute otitis media is commonly a disease of childhood but can be seen in adults. According to a study, Acute otitis media affects up to 75% of children less than age 5 years.

Also, *Streptococcus pneumoniae* and *Haemophilus influenzae* are responsible for up to 80% of bacterial AOM.

Etiology

Bacterial AOM is more common in adults. Organisms commonly found include:
- ❖ *Haemophulis influenzae* (26%); *Streptococcus pneumoniae* (21%); *Moraxella catarrhalis*, and *Streptococcus aureus*.
- ❖ The routes of infection of middle ear are:
  - ➢ *Via eustachian tube:* Most common route. The infection travels along the lumen or subepithelial peritubal lymphatics.
  - ➢ *Via external ear:* In cases with traumatic perforation, the middle ear is exposed to infection.
  - ➢ Blood borne

The predisposing factors include recurrent episodes of cold or URTI, tonsillitis and adenoiditis, allergic rhinitis and sinusitis, tumors of nasopharynx.

Pathology

Acute otitis media has four stages of disease development:
- ❖ **Stage I:** Stage of tubal occlusion—there is edema and hyperemia of nasopharyngeal end of Eustachian tube causing negative pressure due to blockage of tube. Retraction of TM is seen.
- ❖ **Stage II:** Stage of presuppuration—in cases with prolonged tubal occlusion, the inflammatory exudate invades the tympanic cavity along with hyperemia. TM is congested.

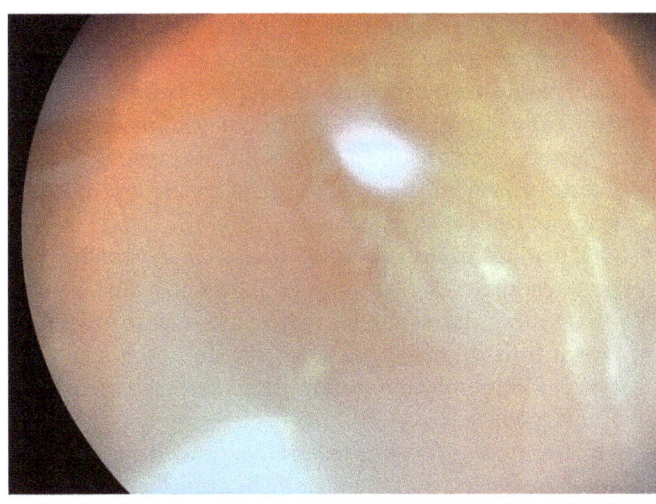

Fig. 3.3: Showing congested TM in suppurative phase of AOM.

- ❖ **Stage III:** Stage of suppuration—tympanic membrane is seen bulging due to pus formation in middle ear extending till mastoid air cells **(Fig. 3.3)**.
- ❖ **Stage IV:** Stage of resolution—tympanic membrane ruptures and pus are released which relieves pressure and inflammatory process resolves.
- ❖ **Stage V:** Stage of complications—in few cases where the virulence of organism is high or patient is immunodeficient, resolution does not occur. Disease progress to complications involving mastoiditis, labyrinthitis, subperiosteal abscess, facial paralysis, petrositis, brain abscess, meningitis, or lateral sinus thrombophlebitis.

Clinical Manifestations

Patient will present with short history of symptoms. The patient presents with deafness and aural fullness in initial stages of tubal occlusion and presuppuration.

In presuppurative stage and suppurative, the patient also complaints of marked earache. Few cases with AOM can also present with fever and vomiting episodes, more common in children.

In resolution stage, the patient complaints of muco-purulent ear discharge (otorrhea) along with resolution of previous symptoms.

Diagnosis

Using bull's lamp with or without speculum or using otoscope, the tympanic membrane is visualized.

In early stage, the tympanic membrane is seen retracted. Later, tympanic membrane is seen congested and bulged out.

During suppurative stage, the tympanic membrane is seen bulging and typical cartwheel appearance of congestion is seen. In few cases a dependent part is seen where the tympanic membrane will rupture in later stages.

In resolution stage, tympanic membrane perforation is seen along with mucopurulent discharge coming from middle ear.

Treatment

The treatment modalities include:
- ❖ **Antibiotic therapy:** The bacterial infection underlying the condition needs to be treated. For same, oral antibiotic

therapy is given. Broad spectrum antibiotics are used to cover gram positive as well as gram negative organisms. Commonly used antibiotics are cephalosporin.
- **Topical decongestant:** Nasal decongestants is used to relieve eustachian tube oedema and increase ventilation. Common nasal decongestant used are ephedrine, xylometazoline, oxymetazoline.
- Oral Antihistamines like fexofenadine, levocetirizine and oral decongestants are given for increasing ventilation.
- Analgesic and antipyretic for symptomatic treatment.
- Aural toileting is done to clear the discharge post tympanic membrane perforation cause release of pus from middle ear.
- **Myringotomy:** It refers to surgical procedure in which small passage is made, generally by grommet placement in Tympanic membrane. This provide passage for the discharge and negative pressure is released.

SEROUS OTITIS MEDIA/OTITIS MEDIA WITH EFFUSION (OME)

Definition
Otitis media with effusion is described as collection of fluid which extends in middle ear and till mastoid air cells.

Epidemiology
OME is generally a condition of children and can follow or precedes AOM. Adult cases are less commonly seen. According to a study, prevalence of OME is seen to 0.6% in population above the age of 15 (Robinson PM).

Etiology and Pathology
OME is an uncommon disease in adults with limited population affected.

The predisposing factors for the same include:
- **Infective pathology:** Population suffering from URTI or sinusitis will cause infective pathogen to travel via eustachian tube to the middle ear. Most commonly seen pathogens include *Staphylococcus aureus, Haemophilus influenzae* and in some cases *Moraxella catarrhalis*. Patient with HIV also show high incidence for middle ear pathologies including OME.
- **Allergic conditions:** Patient with genetic predisposition to allergic condition like allergic rhinitis will show symptoms including nasal obstruction, rhinorrhea, postnasal drip which in turn causes Eustachian tube dysfunction thus predisposing to OME.
- **Barotrauma:** Few cases of patients of OME also have shown association with travelling via air flights. This change in pressure of during the ascend and descend causes similar pressure changes in eustachian tube.
- Eustachian tube obstruction as seen in adenoid hypertrophy in children and skull base tumors, nasopharyngeal carcinoma, and other conditions partially or completely obstructing eustachian tube in adults can also predispose to OME.

Clinical Presentation
Patient will generally complaint of:
- Aural fullness
- Hearing loss in affected ear
- Crackling tinnitus

The patient on examination of ear by otoscope shows retracted, dull pars tensa with abnormal light reflex and fluid level can be seen medial to the tympanic membrane. On pure tone audiometry, conductive hearing loss can be seen on same side.

Diagnosis
OME can be clinically diagnosed with otoscopic examination showing retracted tympanic membrane and if present associated URTI helps confirm the diagnosis. Pure tone audiometry shows conductive hearing loss and impedance can show type 'B' or type 'C' tympanogram.

Treatment
Medical management of OME includes topical nasal decongestants, and oral anti-histaminic. But there is less evidence of an alteration in course of the disease which resolves without treatment in most cases.

Toynbee and Valsalva maneuver are also helpful to relieve eustachian tube obstruction and can help in symptomatic relief of OME. Hearing aids can be prescribed to long term OME patients who have significant conductive hearing loss.

Surgical treatment for OME includes myringotomy which provides a relieving component to pressure change seen in middle ear. Balloon tuboplasty is another method used to resolve eustachian tube obstruction in such patients.

CHRONIC OTITIS MEDIA

Definition
Infection of middle ear mucosa for over 3 months is defined as chronic otitis media (COM). It is classified as:
- Squamous active
- Squamous inactive
- Mucosal active
- Mucosal inactive
- Healed COM

Epidemiology
Lin et al. conducted a study to identify the prevalence of COM in adults (age >15 years) from 1998 to 2007 in 3,223 adult patients and noticed decrease in incidence in adults from 407 to 145 cases per year from 1998 to 2007. The mean age of patients increased from 44.7 to 49.3 years (Yung Song Lin et al).

Etiology and Pathology
Chronic otitis media is caused by recurrent episodes of acute otitis media or OME over time that causes histopathological changes in the middle ear and mastoid mucosa.

In mucosal type of disease, there is chronic inflammation of mucosa with hyperemia and fibrosis is also seen with discharge seen in active cases.

Whereas in squamosal type, active osteitis is causing erosion of mastoid antrum and ossicles causing foul smelling scanty discharge, occasionally blood tinged. There could be presence of keratinized debris of epithelial tissue which form cholesteatoma. Cholesteatoma can be seen commonly occurring in attic. Other sites of occurrence include pars tensa or EAC.

Clinical Presentation

Presentation of disease is varying depending on the type of COM:

1. **Mucosal COM:** Patient will present with chronic history of discharge in active cases, decreased hearing in affected ear, aural fullness and in few active cases tinnitus.
   On otoscopic examination, mucopurulent discharge is seen filling the EAC and middle ear which needs to suction cleaned. Tympanic membrane when visualized shows perforation of pars tensa with intact pars flaccida and no cholesteatoma.
2. **Squamous COM:** In active conditions, patient complaint of scanty foul-smelling discharge that can be blood tinged sometimes. Patient also presents with gradually progressive hearing loss, aural fullness and no pain.
   On otoscopic examination, EAC polyp is commonly seen with pars flaccida retraction and pearly white cholesteatoma in pars flaccida region. In few cases, pars tensa perforation or retraction is also seen and in active cases, serous foul-smelling discharge is seen in EAC.

On pure tone audiometry, mucosal type as well as squamous will show conductive hearing loss of varying degree according to underlying pathology. In squamous type, due to erosion of ossicles, patients might show increased air-bone gap and amount to moderate to severe hearing loss. COM, especially squamous type can also present with complications as depicted in **Table 3.2**.

TABLE 3.2: Complications of squamous type COM.	
Extracranial	Intracranial
Mastoiditis	Brain abscess
Labyrinthitis	Meningitis
Petrositis	Lateral sinus thrombophlebitis
Facial nerve paralysis	Intracranial sepsis
Sensorineural hearing loss	Otic hydrocephalus

Treatment

For active COM, Medical management is required. It includes:
- Regular aural toileting
- Topical antibiotics drops
- Systemic antibiotics if necessary
- Prevention from exposure to moisture.

Surgical intervention is required in patients of mucosal type with pars tensa perforation. Most ENT surgeons prefer to take up the case of tympanoplasty (type according to status of the ossicles) in inactive stage of disease but a few operate wet ear as well.

For squamous disease, high resolution CT scan of temporal bone is necessary before the patient is taken up for surgery to determine the extent of disease, erosion of bone, anatomical anomalies and status of ossicles.

Depending on the clinical picture, hearing loss and HRCT, mastoidectomy is done for the patient especially for removal of cholesteatoma. The primary aim of the surgery is always removal of the disease. Hearing preservation is the secondary goal.

In case the disease is limited and cholesteatoma is not visualized, cortical mastoidectomy can be done.

If cholesteatoma is limited to a certain area and can be removed in complete part, then canal wall up mastoidectomy should be preferred for surgeon. This procedure preserves hearing but revision surgery is required after 6-12 months to evaluate any remnant of disease. Follow up is necessary.

In more extensive disease, open techniques of mastoidectomy are preferred including canal wall down procedure. In canal wall down, the posterior EAC wall is removed to make mastoid, middle ear cavity and EAC as one big single cavity. The recurrence rate with the procedure is less compared to intact canal wall but recurrent debris formation is seen. Patient will also complaint of hearing loss. This procedure is also preferred in patients who would be unable to follow up regularly.

MASTOIDITIS

Definition

Mastoiditis refers to infective pathology involving the mastoid air cell system. It is commonly seen as complication of acute otitis media and chronic otitis media.

Epidemiology

It is the most commonly occurring complication of acute otitis media. Though the frequency of mastoiditis is sharply declined following the widespread introduction of antibiotic use for AOM. Now the estimated incidence of 0.04–0.07% of AOM cases.

Etiology and Pathology

As above mentioned, mastoiditis commonly occur as a complication of AOM due to spread of disease from tympanic cavity to mastoid air cells.

The commonly occurring pathogens are same as AOM including *Staphylococcus aureus, Hemophilus influenzae,* and in few cases *Pseudomonas.* Similar to AOM, eustachian tube dysfunction, allergy and URTI are also the predisposing factors.

The infection course causes accumulation of pus in mastoid air cell system which via aditus is released in tympanic cavity and through perforation seen in EAC. This continuous flow of discharge due inability to clean the mastoid antrum during clinical examination is referred to as **Reservoir sign.**

With progression of disease, the mastoid part of temporal bone is also eroded causing the pus to enter the subcutaneous plane. According to the course of spread, this can be classified as:

- **Bezold's abscess:** Coalescent mastoiditis that break through the mastoid tip and extends into the upper part of neck. Lies deep to sternocleidomastoid and follows posterior belly of digastric.

- **Citelli's abscess:** Refer to abscess formation by extension of disease from mastoid towards occiput.
- **Luc's abscess:** Abscess formed when the pus breaks into the external osseus meatus.
- Postauricular abscess
- Zygomatic abscess

Clinical Features

Patient will present with discharging ear, pain, hearing loss, itching and few will present with fever as well.

On examination, congestion is seen over the mastoid tip. The pinna is pushed laterally and anteriorly. Tenderness over mastoid tip can be elicited with local rise of temperature. In case of abscess, depending on location different abscesses can be identified.

The skin over the mastoid tip is smooth and this is known as **Ironed out appearance.** On transillumination, the pus filled can be visualized called the **Lighthouse effect.**

On otoscopic examination, Perforation of pars tensa can be seen with discharge that could be pulsatile. On aural toileting, the discharge reappears within minutes which is referred to as **Reservoir sign.**

Treatment

- **Medical management:**
  - Topical antibiotic is given to treat the pathology.
  - Systemic antibiotics are required as topical may not be able to reach mastoid air cells.
  - Regular aural toileting should be done.
  - Analgesics and antipyretic for symptomatic relief
  - Antihistamines and nasal decongestants
- **Surgical management:**
  - Incision and drainage of abscess seen under local anesthesia
  - Mastoidectomy to clear the air cells of discharge and provide passage for drainage. Depending on the extent of disease, type of procedure is determined.

OTOSCLEROSIS

Definition

Otosclerosis is a condition affecting otic capsule. Disorganized bone remodelling is seen which causes predominant symptoms of a patient.

Epidemiology

Otosclerosis is most commonly seen in Caucasian population. Female population is more prone to more severe disease and are better surgical candidates (Hussain SM).

Etiology and Pathology

Otosclerosis is a multifactorial disorder with genetic, autoimmune and infective factors. Commonly seen in third decade of life.

Otosclerosis is known autosomal dominant disorder. Fifty percent of the cases are also sporadic. Measles virus is also known to predispose to otosclerosis as measles IgG has been identified in perilymph.

Clinical Presentation and Diagnosis

Patients commonly present with:
- **Hearing loss:** Initially, patient may present with unilateral hearing loss. Few patients develop bilateral. Conductive hearing loss is seen with tuning fork tests. On pure tone audiometry, conductive hearing loss seen with notch on 2000 Hz is known as Carhart Notch.
- **Tinnitus:** Patient complaint of ringing sensation in ear.
- Few patients also present with family history of otosclerosis.
- Fistula test is positive in otosclerosis.

Treatment

Treatment of otosclerosis is:
- **Observation:** In patients with minimal hearing loss, observation, and regular monitoring.
- **Hearing aids:** Unilateral or bilateral hearing aid trial can be given for patients with moderate hearing loss.
- **Surgical intervention:** It includes Stapedotomy for fixed stapes and in few cases stapedectomy is required and replacement with prosthesis.

DISORDERS OF INNER EAR

Various disorders of inner ear include:
- Ototoxicity
- Motion sickness
- Tinnitus
- Labyrinthitis
- Meniere's disease
- Acoustic neuroma

OTOTOXICITY

Definition

Ototoxicity is defined as a process by which the therapeutic drugs and solvents can cause damage to cochlear and vestibular system.

Epidemiology

Ototoxicity is caused by wide range of pharmacological agents which can be dose related and duration of treatment given. According to a study (Ganesan P et al), cisplatin ototoxicity is seen to occur between 23% to 50% in adults and 60% in children. Similarly, ototoxicity with aminoglycosides range to 63% and 6-7% with furosemide.

Etiology

Various ototoxic drugs are as follows:
- Macrolides including Erythromycin, azithromycin, clarithromycin
- Aminoglycosides including amikacin, gentamicin, kanamycin, neomycin, netilmicin, ribostamycin, streptomycin, tobramycin.
- Ampicillin, capreomycin, chloramphenicol, vancomycin, viomycin.
- Colistin (polymyxin E), minocycline, polymyxin B, rifampicin.
- Anticancer trugs including cisplatin, carboplatin, bleomycin, nitrogen mustards.

- Antimalaria drugs including quinine, chloroquine.
- Anti-inflammatory including Salicylates, ibuprofen, naproxen.
- Beta blockers including propranolol, loop diuretic (e.g., furosemide)
- Industrial chemicals including toluene, xylene, styrene.

Pathogenesis
Various modes of drugs to transfuse to inner ear causing ototoxicity include:
- Drugs can transfuse via the round window to enter the inner ear which can enter tympanic cavity via eustachian tube like OME with intact TM.
- CSF forms the perilymph of inner ear. Drug whose concentration can be detected in the CSF can get transfuse into perilymph as well.
- Via Blood stream the drug can reach the ear.
- Commonly the outer hairs cells are affected of the basal turn of cochlea (Ganesan P).

Clinical Features
Patient may present with hearing loss at high frequencies (as the drugs can affect the basal turn of cochlea), tinnitus, disequilibrium, oscillopsia, ear fullness.

Diagnosis
It is made clinically with symptomatology, drug history of patients, examination of ear and audiological investigations. Otoscopic examination may show normal picture of the tympanic membrane with associated symptoms. Pure tone audiometry will show sensorineural hearing loss. Otoacoustic emission might be absent due to involvement of outer hair cells.

Treatment
- Prevention from exposure to ototoxic drugs or decreased duration of treatment.
- Regular audiometric follow up if the condition of patient necessitates ototoxic drugs.
- Dose modulation when patient shows otological symptoms, then regular follow up to monitor the effect of drugs.

MOTION SICKNESS

Definition
Motion sickness is defined as a condition in which due to active motion, the individual complaints of dizziness which may or may not be associated with nausea and/or vomiting.

Epidemiology
Predisposing factors of motion sickness include:
- **Age:** Seen more commonly in children and elderly individual, however can occur at any age.
- **Sex:** More commonly seen in females.
- Vestibular disorders including Meniere's disease (MD), vestibular neuritis, BPPV also predispose to motion sickness.

Etiology and Pathogenesis
Balance of the body is maintained by input from vestibular system, proprioception and visual inputs. Disturbance in input of any system will cause dizziness.

Motion sickness is elicited with low frequency lateral and vertical motion or sense of motion (Akov V et al).

Clinical Presentation
Diagnosis is made clinically. Patient will present with dizziness associated with nausea and vomiting. Patient may present with aural fullness also.

Treatment
- Prevention of episode of motion sickness includes preference of front seat, avoid head movement, focus on stable horizon, deep breathing, other diversional therapies like music etc.
- **Pharmacological treatment:** Anticholinergics including scopolamine; antihistaminic including cinnarizine, betahistidine, promethazine are commonly used medication for motion sickness.

TINNITUS

Definition
Tinnitus refers to perception of extra ringing sound by patient. It can be subjective (perceived by the patient only) or objective (can be heard by examiner as well either unaided or with stethoscope). Tinnitus can also be classified into pulsatile and non-pulsatile.

Epidemiology
Studies show prevalence of tinnitus between 8–25.3% of the population of the United States. Studies conducted in other nations have shown prevalence of tinnitus between 4.6% to 30% (Bhatt JM et al).

Etiology and Pathology
Tinnitus is a symptom associated with underlying disorder. Subjective tinnitus is seen associated with ontological conditions including:
- Impacted wax, acute otitis media, chronic otitis media active, MD, otosclerosis, noise induced hearing loss, acoustic neuroma. Meniere's disease is also associated with pulsatile tinnitus.
- Ototoxic drugs can also cause tinnitus. Anxiety and depression are few psychological factors associated with tinnitus as well.
- Objective tinnitus can be seen in AV shunts, vascular bruit, patulous eustachian tube, dental disorders and TM joint clicking.

Clinical Features
Patients present with ringing sensation. They can also present with symptoms like aural fullness, dizziness, pain in ear, ear discharge depending upon the cause of tinnitus.

Treatment

Tinnitus associated pathological condition resolves if the pathology is treated.

If no cause is found, patient should be reassured and psychotherapy is advised.

Masking can also be tried for tinnitus. Masking using white noise or masking machine can also be used.

LABYRINTHITIS

Definition

Labyrinthitis refers to infective pathology of membranous labyrinthine. Labyrinthitis also presents as a complication chronic otitis media.

Epidemiology

Prevalence of labyrinthitis, in South Korea, varies from 3.1–35.4%. Adults are commonly affected and is mostly seen in females.

Etiology and Pathology

Labyrinthitis is an infective condition which can be due to viral infection, bacterial or systemic disease.

Viral pathologies include cytomegalovirus, rubella, measles and mumps. Ramsay hunt syndrome is also associated with labyrinthitis predisposed in URTI.

Bacterial infection can be due to spread of bacterial pathology to labyrinth in cases of chronic otitis media or bacterial meningitis.

Labyrinthitis is commonly divided into serous labyrinthitis and suppurative labyrinthitis.

Serous is commonly caused when bacterial toxins cross the round window to cause inflammation of labyrinth whereas suppurative labyrinthitis is commonly seen with bacterial infection and occur in associated with untreated otitis media.

Clinical Features

Patient presents with aural fullness, pain in the ear, dizziness seen with hearing loss and discharge according to the type of labyrinthitis, nausea and vomiting.

Dizziness occurs in brief episodes and can be associated with hearing loss as well unlike vestibular neuritis.

On otoscopic examination, presence of cholesteatoma, discharge and tympanic membrane retraction can be seen if the condition is sequelae of AOM or COM.

Rinne's and Weber's tests show presence of sensorineural hearing loss. Romberg's and balance test are performed to see the involvement of labyrinth.

Treatment

Acute labyrinthitis can be treated with medical management with intravenous antibiotics, analgesics, and vestibular suppressants.

Surgery is required for treatment of disease like cholesteatoma is present in tympanic cavity and may predispose to the condition. This includes mastoidectomy according to extent of pathology.

MENIERE'S DISEASE

Definition

Meniere's disease is defined as inner ear pathology of vestibular system due to increase pressure in endolymphatic sac.

Epidemiology

Meniere's disease is more common in adults, with symptoms seen between 20 and 60 years of age. Equal preponderance is there in both the ears but more common in females. Current prevalence rate ranges from as low as 3.5 per 100,000 to 513 per 100,000 (Teixeira LS et al).

Etiology and Pathogenesis

The well-established reason of MD is due to increased pressure in endolymphatic sac. This can be due to increased production or decreased absorption of endolymph. Decreased absorption can be seen if there is block in endolymphatic system as in the endolymphatic duct. Increased production can be seen in patients with hypertension and other systemic causes that will increase endolymphatic production.

Meniere's disease can be classified into cochlear and vestibular depending on the system involved. It can also be classified into:

- **Meniere's syndrome:** The underlying pathology causing increased pressure is well established.
- **Meniere's disease:** Idiopathic

Clinical Features

The patient will present generally with classic triad of symptoms including:

- **Hearing loss:** Fluctuant hearing loss is observed by the patient during the episode of MD which commonly is low frequency hearing loss.
- **Tinnitus:** Tinnitus can occur in between episodes as well but typical 'roaring' type of tinnitus is noticed during the episode.
- **Dizziness:** Episodic vertigo which lasts for 20 minutes to 24 hours and can debilitate the patient for the complete duration.
- Aural fullness.
- Atypical MD may show one or more of the above symptoms without the classic occurrence of triad of symptoms.

Diagnosis

Diagnosis is made clinically. On otoscopic examination, EAC and Tympanic membrane appear normal. Nystagmus can be seen in active episode.

On pure tone audiometry, low frequency hearing loss can be identified generally during the episode. Short increment sensitivity index (SISI) is audiological test used to observe if patient can appreciate 1 dB change in the sound at 20 dB above hearing threshold. In, MD the results vary from 80% and above.

Treatment

Medical management of disease include:
- Regular audiometric follow up to check for remnant hearing loss even after the episode.
- Pharmacological drugs like promethazine, betahistine, cinnarizine, flunarizine act as vestibular sedative agents.
- Carbonic anhydrase inhibitors like acetazolamide can also be used to decrease the production of endolymph. And antihypertensive drugs are prescribed if the patient is hypertensive.
- Tinnitus generally will resolve if the underlying pathology is treated.

In severe cases with closely recurrent episodes, surgical management can be opted for, which includes endolymphatic sac decompression.

ACOUSTIC NEUROMA

Definition

Acoustic neuroma or vestibular schwannoma is tumor of Schwann cells near vestibulocochlear nerve and facial nerve in cerebellopontine angle near internal auditory meatus.

Epidemiology and Etiology

Approximately 8% of all intracranial tumors are acoustic neuroma. It can be unilateral or bilateral. Unilateral is more common and such cases are sporadic. Bilateral acoustic neuroma are genetic and can have syndromic occurrence, for example in neurofibromatosis 2 (NF2). It is a genetic disorder caused due to chromosomal defect on chromosome 22q12.2 (location of neurofibromin 2 gene) which encodes merlin protein (Greene J).

Pathogenesis

Acoustic neuroma arise from junction of glial cells and Schwann cells. The tumor on light microscopy shows spindle cells (Antoni A and Antoni B cells) with fibrillary cytoplasm and elongated nuclei. As the tumor grows compression of nearby structures in the internal acoustic canal causes symptoms in the patients.

Clinical Features

Symptoms in acoustic neuroma is due compression of structures nearby including nerves passing near the cerebellopontine angle including cochlear nerve, vestibular nerve, facial nerve and in later stages trigeminal nerve and glossopharyngeal and vagus nerve as well.

Due to compression of cochlear nerve, patient will complaint of hearing loss which is slowly progressive and retrocochlear sensorineural hearing loss (SNHL) type that can be commonly determined by an objective neurophysiological method called brainstem evoked response audiometry (BERA). It is a non-invasive and the most cost-effective method for diagnosing retrocochlear lesion to identify retrocochlear hearing loss. SNHL is a common disorder resulting from damage to the inner ear.

Patient can also complaint of dizziness due to involvement of vestibular division of nerve. Facial nerve is involved in later stages causing obvious deviation of ipsilateral half of the face (LMN palsy).

Involvement of trigeminal nerve will show paresthesia of face according to involvement of trigeminal nerve division, absent cochlear reflex and neuralgic pain can also ensue. Glossopharyngeal and vagus nerve involvement can cause hoarseness of voice and dysphagia. In later stages with large tumors, cerebellar involvement is also seen due to compression. Patient will have gait ataxia and rarely dysarthria. Involvement of brainstem with large tumors will cause pyramidal tract involvement causing weakness of limbs on ipsilateral side. Raised intracranial pressure can also be seen with very large tumors.

Diagnosis

Clinical picture of the patient and examination can provide acoustic neuroma as differential. Pure tone audiometry (PTA) will show sensorineural hearing loss. BERA can confirm retro cochlear cause hearing loss. But diagnosis of acoustic neuroma is confirmed by MRI showing tumor in cerebellopontine angle.

Treatment

Symptomatic treatment to control dizziness and hearing aid for hearing loss can be prescribed for short duration, but definitive treatment for acoustic neuroma is excision of tumor through middle cranial fossa, trans labyrinthine or retro sigmoid approach.

NURSING MANAGEMENT OF THE PATIENTS UNDERGOING EAR SURGERY

Preoperative Nursing Care

Irrespective of the type and extent of surgery, preoperative preparation of the patients is extremely important for their better outcomes in the postoperative period. The preoperative care basically aims to prepare the patient for a safe transition from surgery to the postoperative recovery room. The following points should be considered:

- The patients undergoing elective surgery will be admitted in the wards few days prior to the surgery. So, prepare and assist the patients for all the preoperative investigations. Inform them the rationales for undergoing all the investigations.
- The word operation as such could be a worrying event for majority of the people especially for those who are undergoing surgery for the first time and even for those who have some bad experience of the previous surgery. So, preoperative preparation will help in minimizing the anxiety level of the patients. Talk to the patients and try to recognize signs and symptoms of anxiety, e.g., alteration in vital signs, sweating, behavior change, aggression etc. Ensure that the patient is aware of the nature of his ear problem, about his operation, and what results are expected postoperatively. They should be completely informed about the kind of procedure they are undergoing, regarding the process of recovery, and duration of hospitalization etc.
- The most difficult time in the preoperative period could be the waiting time for the surgery. Someone should always be sitting with the patients till the patient has been shifted in the operating room. Provide some diversional

therapies in the form of preferred music, watching TV, etc., to the patients.
- Ask the patient to wash hair and to take a good shower with soap and lukewarm water on the day of surgery. This will facilitate the feeling of well-being.
- Ensure that the identified area of the surgery around the ear has been shaved properly. Application of some antiseptic at the proposed incision site may be done as per the institute policy.
- Maintain the NPO status of the patients. For food it should be for six hours and for clear liquids it should be for two hours [The Royal College of Nursing (2005)]. Good oral care should be ensured as the patient if NPO.
- The prescribed preoperative medicines should be administrated with a small amount of water only. All the medicines should be thoroughly reviewed. The medicines causing drowsiness should be administered only after complete preparation of the patient for OT maintain patients' privacy, comfort, and dignity at the time of changing into their theatre clothes.
- Assess the hydration level of the patients especially when there is a change in the operation list and the waiting for the patients has been prolonged. Delay in surgery should be documented in patients' records. There should be good communication between the OT staff and ward staff.
- Ensure that the patients/their carers have signed the informed consent form. It will ensure their understand of the procedure and that they are happily and willfully are in agreement to go ahead with the planned procedure.
- Jewellery, dentures, loose teeth, hearing aids should be removed and handed over to the patients' caregivers.
- Vital signs should be recorded and the abnormal readings should be reported in patients' treatment charts. Knowing the baseline findings will help to recognize the fluctuations and potential complications postoperatively.
- Any kind of allergies should also be documented in patients' record sheets.
- Before the patients are shifted for surgery, a final preoperative checklist should be completed (Kindly refer to Chapter 5 of Volume I for further details).

Postoperative Care

Postoperative care begins when the patient is shifted from the operating table to the recovery room. Postoperative nursing interventions for the patients after ear surgery involve checking vital signs such as blood pressure, heart rate, and temperature; assessing and managing pain; assessing the incision site for bleeding; and monitoring the patients for signs of infection. Nurses need to ensure that the patient's pain is controlled, patient is able to breath properly, there is normal urine output, and all other vital signs are within normal range. Once the patient's condition is stabilized, she/he is shifted to the ward.

For the general postoperative care, kindly refer to Chapter 7 of Volume I.

The specific nursing interventions for the patients undergone ear surgery are as follows:
- Instruct the patients to keep the operated ear up while lying. The head may be elevated to minimize swelling.
- Administer analgesics as per requirement of the patients. All the antibiotics should be administered as prescribed.
- Patients may experience vertigo or light headache at the time of ambulating for the first time after surgery. So, the patient should be well supported and protected from falling.
- If required, the patient may blow the nose very gently one side at a time.
- Sneezing and coughing should be done with the mouth open for at least one week after the surgery.
- The large dressing over the ear will be removed and will be replaced with a smaller dressing the second day after surgery. Further change of dressing will be done as per the type of surgery the patient has undergone.
- After the removal of dressing, the prescribed ear drops are instilled in the ear and a clean cotton ball is placed in the ear canal.
- A small amount of serosanguineous drainage is normal. If it is more, the treating doctor should be informed immediately. The color of the drainage will change from red to yellow to clear, and then will stop within few days.
- Avoid heavy lifting for at least 3–4 weeks especially after stapedectomy.
- The patients may gently shampoo the hair after the dressing is removed. Bending the ears should be avoided. Bending or hitting the affected ears should also be avoided while brushing or combing the hair.
- The patients may resume light walking three days after surgery. Aerobic exercise, weight training, heavy lifting, and straining may be gradually resumed three to four weeks after surgery.
- Instruct the patients not to swim or participate in other water sports or activities for at least four weeks post surgery.
- All the discharge instruction should be given to the patients in writing and any doubt should be clarified before sending the patients home.

GERIATRIC CONSIDERATIONS

Generally, in elderly population, the most common complaint is of hearing loss. They can also have Presbycusis (hearing loss for both lower and higher frequencies). Geriatric population, in general, have co-morbidities including hypertension, diabetes mellitus, asthma, chronic kidney disease, etc. Thus, discharge from ear in patient with diabetes mellitus should raise the suspicion of malignant otitis externa. Malignant otitis externa (MOE) refers to a subtype of otitis externa which is more fulminant and can also include bone erosion of nearby EAC walls. Thus, MOE is more commonly associated with complications including intracranial complications. These patients need to be treated with antibiotic course suitable to the pathogen responsible (most common—*Pseudomonas aeruginosa*), regular cleaning and monitoring of blood sugar levels with proper treatment for diabetes mellitus. Other disorders that can be common in elderly population include wax, foreign body, otitis externa, and chronic otitis media. Chronic otitis media in geriatric population has similar sequelae but surgical management of patients may not show more chances of graft failure.

Case Scenario

1. Patient named XYZ, male, age 29 years old presented to ENT OPD with complaints of excruciating pain, aural fullness and decreased hearing from left ear since 2 days and fever since 1 day. Patient gives history of nasal obstruction, rhinorrhea and postnasal drip since 5 days. On examination of left ear under bull's lamp or head light, Pinna appears normal, EAC shows no congestion but tympanic membrane appears bulged out, congested with obvious yellow dependant point in postero-inferior quadrant. On otoscopy, the findings are confirmed. Right ear was also examined and showed mild congestion of tympanic membrane as well. Routine investigations of patient show leukocytosis with increased neutrophil count on DLC. The patient was started on oral antibiotic, oral antihistaminic, analgesics and nasal decongestants. Patient was called for follow up after 5 days. During follow up patient reports improvement in symptoms and on otoscopic examination, both tympanic membranes appear normal.

2. A 35-year-old female presented in ENT OPD with complaint of active foul-smelling ear discharge from right ear since 5 days. Patient gives history of right ear discharge since childhood which is temporarily relieved with medication. Patient also complaint of tinnitus since 5 days and hearing loss in ipsilateral ear which gradually have progressed since 5–6 years. On examination under bull's lamp, scanty serous discharge is seen in EAC with tympanic membrane retraction. On otoscopic examination, tympanic membrane is clearly visualized with retraction of pars tensa, dimpling in pars flaccida and with white debris like collection seen near pars flaccida. Discharge is foul smelling. Left ear on examination shows normal pinna, EAC and tympanic membrane. Rinne's with 512 Hz shows bone conduction (BC) better than air conduction (AC) in right ear and AC>BC in Left ear. Weber's lateralized to the right ear. Pure tone audiometry shows threshold of 35/45 dB HL in right ear (conductive hearing loss) and normal hearing in left ear. On HRCT temporal bone, slight erosion is seen of posterior wall of middle ear and soft tissue density in mastoid and tympanic cavity with intact ossicles. Patient is treated with topical antibiotics for discharge and later taken up for mastoid exploration under GA.

SUMMARY

Diseases of ear can involve external ear, middle ear or internal ear. The common symptoms include discharge, otalgia, aural fullness, hearing loss, dizziness, and tinnitus, etc. The diagnosis of external and middle ear pathologies is commonly done on clinical basis by history and examination of ear with bull's lamp or head light followed by otoscopic examination. Certain symptoms are specific to a particular disease like the patients with otitis externa present with pain not proportionate to disease, MD show triad of symptoms including hearing loss, tinnitus, dizziness. Patients undergoing surgery should be fully informed about the procedure, and postoperative recovery period. Preparation of the patients psychologically and physically will decrease the risk of postoperative complications leading to speedy recovery.

MULTIPLE CHOICE QUESTIONS

1. Patient presents with right aural fullness, hearing loss, ear pain. On otoscopic examination, wax is seen impacted in the EAC. Next step in management includes:
   a. Topical antibiotics
   b. Aural syringing
   c. Wait and watch
   d. None of the above
2. Amongst the following drugs, which one is not ototoxic?
   a. Furosemide
   b. Metformin
   c. Cisplatin
   d. Gentamicin
3. Patient with acute otitis media presents with ear discharge and history of pain and aural fullness which resolved after ear discharge is seen. Identify the stage?
   a. Stage of suppuration
   b. Stage of resolution
   c. Stage of complication
   d. Stage of tubal occlusion
4. Patient presents with fever, tenderness over mastoid tip with ironed out appearance of skin. On examination, discharge is cleaned with aural toileting and discharge is also seen filling the EAC again. Provisional diagnosis is:
   a. Mastoiditis
   b. Otitis externa
   c. Impacted wax
   d. Chronic otitis media
5. Identify the tympanoplasty when graft is placed over the suprastructure of stapes?
   a. Type 1 tympanoplasty
   b. Type 2 tympanoplasty
   c. Type 3 tympanoplasty
   d. Type 4 tympanoplasty
6. Acoustic neuroma does not present with:
   a. Facial nerve paralysis
   b. Gait ataxia
   c. Absent corneal reflex
   d. Anosmia
   e. Increased Intracranial Pressure
7. Patient with history of discharge from 6 years with mucopurulent discharge from left ear, hearing loss. Otoscopic examination shows subtotal perforation of pars tensa. Provisional diagnosis is:
   a. Otitis externa
   b. Chronic otitis media squamous
   c. Meniere's disease
   d. Chronic otitis media mucosal active
8. Complications of chronic otitis media include:
   a. Lateral sinus thrombophlebitis
   b. Labyrinthitis
   c. Mastoiditis
   d. All of the above.
9. Patient presents to ENT OPD with complaint of hearing loss in left ear for 6–7 months. Patient does not have history of discharge, pain or dizziness. On pure tone audiometry, a notch is observed at 2000 Hz and tympanogram shows type As. What is the diagnosis?
   a. Chronic otitis media
   b. Acoustic neuroma
   c. Otosclerosis
   d. Otitis externa
10. A 55-year-old patient presents to you in OPD with complaint of aural fullness from right ear since 2–3 months and hearing loss and tinnitus since 2 months. Patient also reports history of recurrent episodes of upper respiratory tract infection. On otoscopy, right tympanic membrane shows retraction of pars tensa and bubbles behind the tympanic membrane. What is the diagnosis?
    a. Suppurative stage of acute otitis media
    b. Chronic otitis media
    c. Serous otitis media
    d. Otosclerosis

ANSWERS

1. b	2. b	3. a	4. a
5. b	6. d	7. d	8. d
9. c	10. c		

SUGGESTED READING

1. Akov V, Tadi P. Motion Sickness. [Updated 2021 Sep 29]. In: StatPearls [Internet]. Treasure Island (FL): StatPearls Publishing; 2021.
2. Awad AL, ElTaher M. ENT Foreign Bodies: An Experience. Int Arch Otorhinolaryngol. 2018;22(2):146-51. doi: 10.1055/s-0037-1603922.
3. Bhatt JM, Lin HW, Bhattacharyya N. Prevalence, Severity, Exposures, and Treatment Patterns of Tinnitus in the United States. JAMA Otolaryngol Head Neck Surg. 2016;142(10):959-65.
4. Diseases of the external ear. In: Patrick M Spielmann and S Musheer Hussain (Eds). Logan Turner's Diseases of the Nose, Throat and Ear Head and Neck Surgery, 11th edition. Florida, CRC Press Taylor and Francis Group; 2016. pp. 395-401.

5. Ganesan P, Schmiedge J, Manchaiah V, et al. Ototoxicity: A Challenge in Diagnosis and Treatment. J Audiol Otol. 2018 Apr; 22(2): 59–68.
6. Graham MD. Osteomas and exostoses of the external auditory canal: a clinical, histopathological and scanning electron microscopic study. In Watkinson JC, Clarke RW (ed). Scott-Brown's Otorhinolaryngology Head and Neck Surgery, 8th edition. Florida, CRC Press Taylor and Francis Group, 2018.
7. Greene J, Al-Dhahir MA. Acoustic Neuroma. [Updated 2021 Aug 11]. In: StatPearls [Internet]. Treasure Island (FL): StatPearls Publishing; 2021 Jan.
8. Otosclerosis. In Hussain SM (ed). Logan Turner's Diseases of the Nose, Throat and Ear Head and Neck Surgery, 11th edition. Florida, CRC Press Taylor and Francis Group, 2016 Page 433-441.
9. Pritchard MJ (2009a) Identifying and assessing anxiety in pre-operative patients. Nursing Standard; 23: 51, 35-40.
10. Pritchard MJ (2009b) Managing anxiety in the elective surgical patient. British Journal of Nursing; 18: 7, 416-419.
11. Robinson PM. Secretory otitis media in the adult. Clin Otolaryngol Allied Sci 1987; 12: 297–302. In Watkinson JC, Clarke RW (ed). Scott-Brown's Otorhinolaryngology Head and Neck Surgery, 8th edition. Florida, CRC Press Taylor and Francis Group, 2018.
12. Royal College of Nursing (2005) Perioperative Fasting in Adults and Children. An RCN Guideline for the Multidisciplinary Team. London: RCN.
13. Teixeira LS and Guimaraes AM. Meniere's Disease: Epidemiology. Intechopen.com/chapter/56186. October 2017.
14. Yung Song Lin, Li-Ching Lin, Fei-Peng Lee, Kuan Ji Lee. The prevalence of chronic otitis media and its complication rates in teenagers and adult patients. Otolaryngology-Head and Neck Surgery Volume: 140 issue: 2, page(s): 165-170.

CHAPTER 4

Upper Airway Infections

Vivek K Pathak, Pragya Pathak, Pradeepti Nayak

"Listen to your patient, he is telling you the diagnosis."
—Willam Osler

LEARNING OBJECTIVES

After going through the chapter, the learner will be able to:
- Enumerate and define various types of upper respiratory tract infections based on the anatomical region involved.
- Describe the pathophysiology and the associated clinical features of the different respiratory infections.
- Elaborate various aspects of management like diagnostic, medical, surgical and other non-pharmacological modalities.
- Assess the critical illness of the patients for the emergency interventions.
- Discuss the geriatric considerations for upper airway infections.

TERMS

- **Coryza:** Viral rhinitis
- **Epiglottitis:** Epiglottitis or supraglottic laryngitis is the diffuse inflammation of the supraglottis, especially the inlet, i.e., epiglottis, aryepiglottic folds and the arytenoids.
- **Laryngitis:** Inflammation of the laryngeal mucosa.
- **Peritonsillar abscess:** Collection of purulent discharge in the peritonsillar space.
- **Pharyngitis:** Inflammation of the mucosa of the pharynx including nasopharynx, oropharynx and laryngopharynx.
- **Rhinitis:** Inflammation of the mucosa of the nasal cavity.
- **Sinusitis:** Inflammation of the mucosa of the sinuses.
- **Tonsilitis:** Inflammation of the palatine tonsils.

INTRODUCTION

Upper airway or upper respiratory infections (ARI or URI) are one of the commonest pathologies encountered in medical practice. In developing countries, on an average every child has five episodes of ARI/year accounting for 30-50% of the total pediatric outpatient visits and 20-30% of the pediatric admissions. India is thought to contribute to 700 million episodes of ARI every year alone.

In the current chapter common upper airway infections discussed are common cold, sinusitis, ethinitis, rhinitis, pharyngitis, laryngitis, epiglottitis, tonsillitis, and adenoiditis, peritonsillar abscess.

COMMON COLD

CONCEPT AND DEFINITION

The common cold is a self-limiting, viral infectious disease affecting the upper airway. It is used interchangeably with the terms like coryza, nasopharyngitis and sniffles.

EPIDEMIOLOGY

Common cold is the most common infectious disease in human beings. On an average, adults get 4 to 6 colds per year, while children get 6 to 8 episodes per year.

ETIOLOGY

This illness can be caused by more than 250 viruses. These include rhinovirus, coronavirus, human influenza virus, parainfluenza virus, adenovirus, Epstein-Barr virus, respiratory syncytial virus amongst others. However, the most common cause of common cold is the rhinovirus.

PATHOPHYSIOLOGY

The symptomatology of common cold is associated with a polymorphonuclear response to the invading pathogen causing the cardinal signs of inflammation including hypersecretion of mucoid discharge. Ciliated epithelial cells are the primary cell type involved, although non-ciliated cells are also infected. However, on microbiological examination there is a paucity of virus-infected cells. This is thought to be a result of desquamation of infected cells into the nasal secretions.

CLINICAL MANIFESTATIONS

The symptoms usually occur within 12–72 hours of exposure after the incubation period and may last for over a week.

Signs and Symptoms

1. **Local:** The common symptoms the patients experience are cough, sore throat, nasal congestion, runny nose, sneezing, facial pain, and earache (referred pain).
   - *Nasal discharge*—profuse, yellowish or greenish, mucoid or mucopurulent
   - *Nasal mucosa*—glistening with occasional edema
   - Tender, enlarged cervical lymph nodes
2. **Constitutional symptoms:** Low-grade fever, malaise, headache, irritability, restlessness

DIAGNOSIS

Diagnosis is usually clinical following a thorough history and clinical examination.

MANAGEMENT

The disease is usually mild and self-limiting. The mainstay of treatment includes symptomatic relief and prevention of transmission. Rest and hydration with medications such as nasal decongestants and antihistamines usually suffice as a treatment protocol. Warm saline gargles and steam inhalation may aid in early relief from the symptoms.

Dietetics
- Avoid cold/spicy food
- Avoid consumption of alcohol and smoking

COMPLICATIONS

Otitis media, sinusitis, bronchitis, LRTI.

NURSING MANAGEMENT

- Teach handwashing and other preventive measures.
- Ask the patient to cover nose/mouth while sneezing or coughing. Its better to use disposable tissues.
- During flu season try to avoid going to crowded areas.
- Avoid allergens.
- Maintain good oral hygiene.
- Take nutritious diet.
- Monitor signs and symptoms of infection and report back to your physician in case:
  - Shortness of breath, difficulty breathing
  - Lymphedema
  - Nasal discharge is foul smelling
  - Headache is severe
  - Persisting tenderness or pain in sinuses or periorbital area
  - Fever persisting beyond 2 days or temperature is above 100°F
  - White patches or redness is seen on back of throat
  - Avoid smoking and exposure to smoke
- Encourage use of moist air through humidifier to relieve swollen mucus membrane.
- Minimize exposure to pets.
- Take more of liquids preferably hot.
- Use infection prevention measure to avoid spreading infection.

RHINITIS

CONCEPT AND DEFINITION

Rhinitis is defined as non-specific inflammation of the nasal mucosa. It may be acute or chronic.

ACUTE RHINITIS

Epidemiology

Acute rhinitis is a very common ailment amongst all age-groups. It is more commonly seen in children and those with predisposition to allergies.

Etiology

It may be infective (viral or bacterial) or inflammatory (irritant).

Pathophysiology

Viral rhinitis also called 'coryza' has been covered in a previous segment. Bacterial rhinitis may be primary or secondary to viral rhinitis. It may be caused by *pneumococcus*, *streptococcus* or *staphylococcus*. Diphtheria may also present as rhinitis. Irritant rhinitis is caused due to exposure to dust, noxious gases or even mechanical trauma.

Clinical Manifestations

The symptoms usually occur within hours to days of exposure after the incubation period and may last for over a week. Irritant rhinitis presents immediately on exposure.

It usually presents with irritation in the nose, rhinorrhea, stuffiness and sneezing. In cases of bacterial rhinitis, the nasal discharge may be purulent. There may also be a greyish white membrane in the nose that may bleed on attempt to remove.

Management

The disease is usually mild and self-limiting. The mainstay of treatment includes symptomatic relief and prevention of transmission. Rest and hydration with medications such as nasal decongestants, e.g., xylometazoline, oxymetazoline and antihistamines, e.g., cetirizine, levocetirizine, fexofenadine usually suffice as a treatment protocol. In case of bacterial rhinitis antibiotics like penicillin, cephalosporins or macrolides may be administered.

CHRONIC RHINITIS

Various types of chronic rhinitis are:
1. **Chronic simple rhinitis:** It is caused due to recurrent nasal infection, constant exposure to irritants, nasal obstruction, endocrine and metabolic causes.
   - *Clinical features*: Nasal obstruction, nasal discharge, headache, inferior turbinate hypertrophy, postnasal discharge
   - *Management*: Treatment of the cause, alkaline douching, decongestants, antibiotics.

   Symptomatic management may be done by use of decongestants and antihistamines (to reduce the secretions). Antibiotics like penicillins and cephalosporins may be used in case of secondary bacterial infection. Alkaline nasal douching helps to clear secretions, provides moisturization and reduced edema locally.

2. **Hypertrophic rhinitis:** It is characterized by thickening of the soft tissue of the nasal cavity, especially the turbinates. Most common cause of hypertrophied turbinates is a grossly deviated nasal septum. In this case, there is a roomier cavity on the other side causing 'compensatory hypertrophy'.

   The most common symptom is nasal obstruction. Surgical reduction of the turbinate is the treatment of choice.

- **Rhinitis sicca:** It is an occupational disorder and occurs in people working in dry, hot, dusty environs. It causes dryness, friability and crusting in the nasal cavity. Treatment includes avoidance of the cause, moisturization by topical ointments and douching.
- **Rhinitis caseosa:** It usually occurs in males; unilateral; and the patient presents with purulent and cheesy nasal discharge. Underlying granulation may be formed due to chronic inflammation. There may be some bony erosion.
- **Atrophic rhinitis:** It is the chronic inflammation characterized by atrophy and destruction of the nasal mucosa and underlying neurovasculature.

Etiopathogenesis

It may be primary or secondary:
- **Primary:** It is idiopathic disease. It may be hereditary, racial, due to endocrine abnormalities, nutritional deficiencies, infections or autoimmune. It is usually seen in young to middle aged females.
- **Secondary:** It is due to destructive granulomatous diseases like lupus, syphilis, excessive destruction of the nasal structures due to surgery, chronic infections, and radiotherapy.

Clinical Features

The patient presents with nasal obstruction, foul smell emanating from the nose which the patient does not appreciate 'merciful anosmia', thick greenish crusts, roomy nasal cavities and pale nasal mucosa.

Diagnosis and Management

Diagnosis is clinical. Management is a combination of medical and surgical modalities.

Most important is alkaline nasal douching to remove the crusts and maintain moisture, 25% glucose and glycerine solution to inhibit proteolytic activity, antibiotics, eastradiol spray (to increase vascularity), potassium iodide to increase secretions.

Surgical: Traditional Young's or modified Young's procedure may be used to narrow the nasal cavity and promote healing.

Young's procedure: It entails raising flaps over the septum and lateral wall and suturing them together to close the external nares, thus reducing the size of the nasal cavity, minimizing exposure to air and environment, promoting moisturization and therefore healing. The flaps are usually released after 3 months. In modified Young's procedure the flaps are sutured leaves a small opening of about 3 mm. This modification is more comfortable for the patient assuring compliance.

RHINITIS MEDICAMENTOSA

It develops due to overuse and non prescriptional use of topical decongestants. It causes rebound congestion and nasal obstruction.

VASOMOTOR RHINITIS

This problem develops due to rebound parasympathetic stimulation after a period of sympathetic hyperactivity, as in case of excitement, fear, etc. It causes excessive mucoid nasal discharge and nasal obstruction.

ALLERGIC RHINITIS (AR)

It refers to inflammatory changes in the nasal mucosa to inhaled allergens. Allergic rhinitis is clinically defined as a disorder of the nose induced by allergen exposure causing an IgE-mediated inflammation.

Features

Type II hypersensitivity reaction (Th2 mediated) → production of allergen-specific IgE → Binding to mast cells causing degranulation → release of histamines and other inflammatory mediators

Allergic rhinitis is defined clinically as having two or more symptoms of anterior or posterior rhinorrhea, sneezing, nasal blockage and/or itching of the nose during two or more consecutive days for more than one hour on most days. Prevalence 0.8–39.7%. It can be classified into different types:
1. **Based on duration:** Intermittent/persistent
2. **Based on severity:** Mild/moderate/severe

Risk Factors

- Young, adolescent males
- Family history of atopy (allergic rhinitis, asthma, etc); increased risk by 3–6 times
- **Environmental factors:** Hygiene hypothesis. It is postulated that high exposure to potential allergens early, decreases the probability of developing allergic diseases. It has been seen that occurrence of helminthic infections during early years, large family size, frequent infections all have a protective role against development of allergy.

Etiopathogenesis

It is caused due to Th2-mediated hypersensitivity mediated by IgE. The allergens responsible are numerous. They may be seasonal (pollen, grass etc.), perennial (dust mites, dander etc.), occupational (latex, lab animals, chemicals etc.) or ingested like food and drugs.

Mechanism of Allergy (Fig. 4.1)

Antigen or allergen initially presents to antigen-presenting cells (APCs) like dendritic cells and Langerhans cells in lymphoreticular cells which then activate Th2 cells. These Th2 cells produce interleukins IL4, IL5 and IL13 which mediate inflammatory responses like edema, mucous hypersecretion and respiratory epithelium remodeling. IL4 also activates B cells to form plasma cells and secrete allergen-specific IgE. IgE causes mast cell degranulation and basophil activation on subsequent exposure causing release of histamine, leukotrienes and prostaglandins. This is called priming.

An allergic response occurs in 2 stages. Early/acute phase—may occur within 5 minutes, due to release of vasoactive amines. Late phase—due to stimulation of eosinophils.

Clinical Features

Symptoms and sign may be nasal, ocular, otologic, pharyngeal and laryngeal.

- **Nasal:** Sneezing, clear mucoid, watery nasal discharge, nasal congestion, itching in the nose, Darrier's line—transverse crease over nose with crusting due to repeated wiping of the nose; also called the allergic salute.
- **Ocular:** Itching, edema of the eyelids, cobblestone conjunctiva, conjunctival chemosis, dark circles under the eye "Allergic shiner", epiphora.
- **Dennie Morgan line:** Transverse skin crease under the eye due to Muller muscle spasm
- **Otologic:** Sensation of ear fullness, tympanic membrane retraction, serous otitis media
- **Pharyngeal:** Postnasal drip, granular pharyngitis.
- **Laryngeal:** Hoarseness, edema and at time breathing difficulty and bronchospasm

Complications

Sinusitis, serous otitis media, nasal polyposis, bronchial asthma

Investigations

- Total and differential leukocyte count: raised eosinophila
- Serum IgE

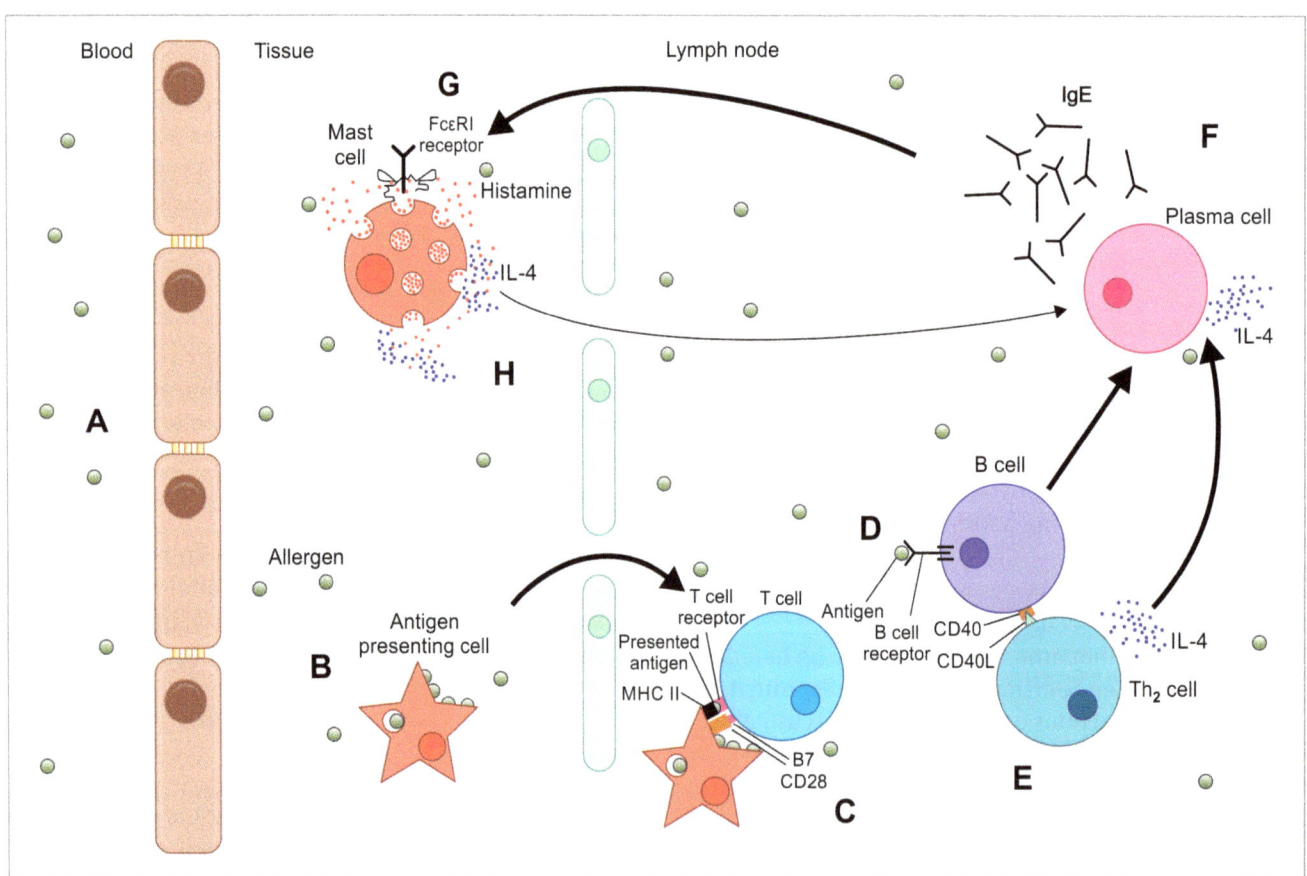

Fig. 4.1: Biochemical mechanism of allergy.

- **Skin prick test:** Positive if on intradermal infiltration of the allergen response within 10-15 minutes (central wheal with surrounding erythema)
- Radioallergosorbent test (RAST)
- Nasal provocation test/nasal allergen challenge
- **Anterior rhinoscopy:**
  - Pale, edematous, bluish mucosa
  - Inferior turbinate hypertrophy/'mulberry' turbinates
  - Clear mucoid discharge

Treatment

It depends on the severity and type of disease. It is staged according to ARIA (allergic rhinitis and its impact on asthma) classification **(Fig. 4.2)**.

As per the modification of ARIA classification of 2010:
- Intra-nasal corticosteroids (INCS) should be considered first line in the management of mild/moderate allergic rhinitis.
- Addition of oral antihistamines (OAH) or intranasal antihistamines (INAH) is a conditional recommendation based on response to initial INCS therapy, patient preference and cost-effectiveness.
- Leukotriene receptor antagonist (LTRA) may be used in conjunction with INCS in place of OAH
- In case of severe AR, a short course of oral corticosteroids (OCS) may be administered for relief.

General Principles in the Management of Allergic Rhinitis (AR)

- **Avoidance of allergen:** Most effective, depends upon patient compliance
- **Antihistamines:** May be first generation or second generation with or without leukotriene receptor antagonists. They ameliorate the acute signs like sneezing, rhinorrhea, nasal block, itching. Most common adverse effect reported is drowsiness, e.g., cetirizine, levocetirizine
- **Anticholinergics:** Used in cases of excessive nasal discharge—ipratropium bromide
- Sympathomimetic drugs—salbutamol, terbutaline
- **Corticosteroids:** Mainstay for treatment of allergic rhinitis.
  - *Topical:* Fluticasone, mometasone, budesonide, etc.
  - *Systemic:* Given as a short course in tapering doses in severe persistent cases.

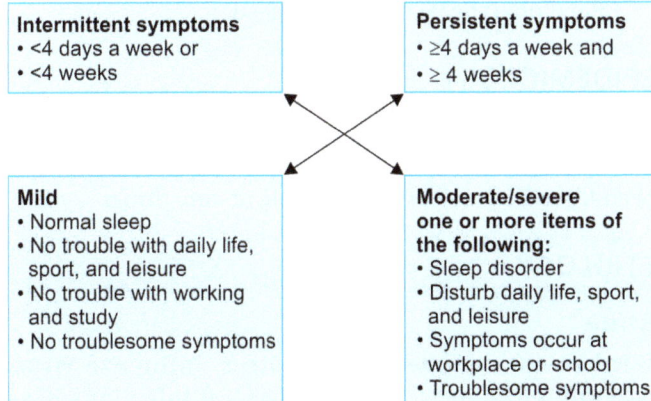

Fig. 4.2: Classification of allergic rhinitis as per the ARIA classification.

- **Mast cell stabilizers:** Prevent mast cell degranulation, e.g., sodium chromoglycate, nedochromil, ketotifen, etc.
- **Leukotriene receptor antagonists:** Montelukast, zafirlukast, etc.
- Anti-IgE—omalizumab
- Immunotherapy

Nursing Interventions

- Demonstrate and inform correct technique of nasal drug administration.
- Try to minimize or avoid exposure to irritants and allergens, e.g., sprays, fumes, etc.
- Demonstrate correct hand hygiene technique to prevent infection transmission in infectious rhinitis.
- In the elderly and high-risk patients, encourage influenza vaccination before flu season after consulting physician.
- Ask the patients to use saline nasal sprays to soften the crusted secretions and sooth nasal mucosa.

Dietetics

- Avoid cold/spicy food
- Avoid consumption of alcohol and smoking

SINUSITIS

CONCEPT AND DEFINITION

Sinusitis refers to the inflammation of the mucosal lining of the paranasal sinuses. These include the maxillary sinus, frontal sinus, ethmoidal sinuses and the sphenoid sinus. In some cases, all the sinuses may be affected causing 'pan-sinusitis'. Since sinusitis rarely occurs without concurrent involvement of the nasal mucosa, the terminology commonly accepted these days is 'rhinosinusitis'. It may be classified as:

- **Acute rhinosinusitis:** It is defined as acute inflammation of the mucosa of the nose and paranasal sinuses.
- **Chronic rhinosinusitis (CRS):** It is defined as inflammation of the nose and the paranasal sinuses lasting at least 8–12 weeks, with at least 2 symptoms, like nasal blockage/obstruction/congestion, nasal discharge (anterior/posterior nasal drip), facial pain/pressure and/or reduction or loss of smell along with either endoscopic signs of disease or relevant CT scan changes. It has been further divided into subtypes:
  - CRS with nasal polyps (CRSwNP)
  - CRS without nasal polyps (CRSsNP)

EPIDEMIOLOGY

Sinusitis is a very common condition with multiple etiologies affecting a large number of patients. Its occurrence has been recorded as early as 1500 BC. According to different reports including CDC, it afflicts almost 10–15% of the population worldwide. Almost 24 million people suffer from this disease every year. In India it is thought to affect 1 in 8 people. Almost 134 million individuals in this country are believed to be suffering from this disease. It is much more common in adults than in children, whose sinuses are not fully developed.

ETIOLOGY

It may be bacterial, viral, fungal, or allergic.
- **Ostial obstruction:** It may be mechanical obstruction of the osteomeatal complex due to anatomic factors or mucosal edema due to inflammation. Conditions that predispose to this include allergy, septal deviation, polyps, HIV infection, foreign body, or any tumors.
- **Non-ostial obstruction:** Cystic fibrosis, lymphoma, leukemia, immunosuppression
- **Direct extension:** Dental infection, facial trauma

PATHOPHYSIOLOGY

The symptomatology of sinusitis is associated with a polymorphonuclear response causing the cardinal signs of inflammation including hypersecretion of mucoid discharge and tenderness over the regions of sinuses. Following a common cold/coryza/rhinitis, a decrease in ciliary function due to the subsequent inflammation allows bacteria to colonize on the mucous membrane surfaces within the sinuses and produce a purulent sinusitis. The organisms usually involved are *H. influenzae, Streptococcus pneumniae, Staphylococcus aureus* and *Streptococcus pyogenes*.

CLINICAL MANIFESTATIONS

Acute: The patients present with nasal discharge, obstruction, pain over the site of sinuses, headache, periorbital pain, fever, symptoms of upper respiratory tract infection, tenderness over the paranasal sinus.
Chronic: The patients complain of nasal discharge, nasal obstruction, facial pain, headache, postnasal discharge, hyposmia, anosmia.
On anterior rhinoscopy: Congested and hypertrophied turbinates, mucosa congested with mucopurulent discharge.

DIAGNOSIS

Clinical history and examination, anterior rhinoscopy, computed tomography of nose and paranasal sinuses.

MANAGEMENT

- **Medical:** Oral antibiotics
  - IV antibiotics
  - Topical nasal steroid sprays
  - Oral antihistamines
- **Surgical:** Functional endoscopic sinus surgery (FESS): This surgical procedure is aimed at clearing the disease from the paranasal sinuses with preservation of the *function* by preserving as much of the normal mucosa as possible.

Basic Steps of FESS:
- Medialization of the middle turbinate and uncinectomy
- Maxillary ostium widening
- Anterior ethmoidectomy
- Sphenoid ostium localization and widening
- Posterior ethmoidectomy

COMPLICATIONS

Mucocele, osteomyelitis, meningitis, extradural abscess, brain abscess, cavernous sinus thrombosis, orbital cellulitis, septic shock.

NURSING MANAGEMENT OF THE PATIENTS

- Propped up position
- Keep the patient comfortable and maintain humidification of air to reduce respiratory effort.
- Advise the patient to take complete course of prescribed antibiotic treatment.
- Increase fluid intake.
- Take steam. Sinus drainage can be removed by increasing environmental humidity.
- Take rest when febrile.
- Follow precautions to avoid coming in contact with people having upper respiratory tract infections.
- Follow healthy practices.
- Informing patients about nasal congestion resulting from side effects of nasal sprays.
- Report if symptoms persist even after taking treatment.

PHARYNGITIS

CONCEPT AND DEFINITION

Pharyngitis refers inflammation of the mucosa of pharynx. It is an extremely common condition with varied etiology. It can be divided into acute and chronic pharyngitis.

Acute Pharyngitis

It refers to acute inflammation of the pharyngeal mucosa. It is most commonly of viral origin.

Chronic Pharyngitis

It is defined as chronic inflammation of the pharynx. It may be divided into two types:
1. **Chronic catarrhal pharyngitis:** It is characterized by posterior pharyngeal wall congestion, mucoid secretions and occasionally thickening of the faucial pillars.
2. **Chronic hypertrophic pharyngitis:** It is characterized by edematous and nodular posterior pharyngeal wall (granular; local lymphoid hyperplasia and thickened lateral pharyngeal bands), congestion.

EPIDEMIOLOGY

Pharyngitis or 'sore throat' is an extremely common illness. It is estimated that at least 15–16% of adults and almost 40% of children have at least one episode of 'sore throat' a year.

ETIOLOGY

Acute

Viral (most common): Rhinovirus, influenza virus, parainfluenza virus, etc. Certain viral infections have

pharyngitis as a part of their clinical presentation as well. These include:
- Herpangina and acute lymphonodular pharyngitis—Coxsackie virus
- Infectious mononucleosis—EBV
- Pharyngoconjunctival fever—adenovirus
- Measles
- Chickenpox—Varicella
- Cytomegalovirus

Bacterial with Group A beta-hemolytic *Streptococcus* deserving special mention due to its progression to rheumatic heart disease and glomerulonephritis in some cases. *C. diphtheriae* and Gonococci may also present initially with pharyngitis. Other rare causes of acute pharyngitis include chlamydia trachomatis, candida, toxoplasma gondii, etc.

Chronic

It is multifactorial, most commonly due to persistent and recurrent infections in the vicinity including rhinosinusitis, tonsillitis and dental infections. Other causes include:
- **Mouth breathing:** It causes increased exposure and dryness of the mucosa predisposing to infection.
- Environmental factors like dust, smoke and industrial effluents.
- Irritants like tobacco in the form of smoking, chewing tobacco or *paan*, alcohol consumption and frequent intake of spicy food.
- Constant hawking and clearing of throat especially in case of professional voice users and patients of GERD.

PATHOPHYSIOLOGY

This is usually infectious, with most cases being of viral origin as in rhinitis. Most of the bacterial cases found are attributable to group A streptococci (GAS). Other causes include allergy, trauma, toxins, and neoplasia.

Acute pharyngitis is characterized by a general polymorphonuclear response to pathogen and the patients present with the signs of inflammation.

Chronic pharyngitis is characterized by mucosal hypertrophy, hypertrophy of the mucinous glands, submucosal lymphoid follicles and the muscular coat of the pharynx. As in cases of mucosa in other regions, the inflammation causes ciliary dysfunction and stasis of secretions, promoting secondary infections as well.

CLINICAL MANIFESTATIONS

Acute
- **Local:** Discomfort in throat in mild cases; dysphagia and severe throat pain in moderate to severe cases
- **Constitutional symptoms:** Low- to high-grade fever depending upon the severity, malaise, headache, irritability, restlessness
- Enlargement of tonsils with exudate and erythema with edema of the soft palate and uvula in severe cases
- Lymphoid follicles and granulations on the posterior pharyngeal wall
- Tender, enlarged cervical lymph nodes

Chronic
- Dry cough
- Foreign body sensation in throat or 'globus'
- Throat discomfort or pain
- Congestion of the posterior pharyngeal wall, granulations and hypertrophy of lymphoid follicles in case of hypertrophic variant, thickening of the faucial pillars.

DIAGNOSIS

Diagnosis is usually clinical following a thorough history and clinical examination. In case of acute pharyngitis, throat swab in cases of bacterial pharyngitis to detect Group A beta-hemolytic *streptococcus* should be done. In cases of diphtheria or *gonorrhea* too, the swab must be taken immediately and sent for microscopy, culture and antibiotic susceptibility.

MANAGEMENT

Acute Pharyngitis
- **General:** Rest, plenty of oral fluids, warm saline gargles, analgesics suffice for viral pharyngitis.
- **Specific:** In case of confirmed streptococcal pharyngitis the treatment of choice remains Penicillin G, 200,000 to 250,000 units orally four times a day for 10 days or benzathine penicillin G, 600,000 units once IM for patient less than 25 kg in weight and 1.2 million units once IM for patients >25 kg. Other antibiotic affective in these cases include cephalosporins and macrolides which may be used in place of penicillin.

Diphtheria is treated by diphtheria antitoxin and administration of penicillin or erythromycin.

Gonococcal pharyngitis is also treated with penicillin or tetracycline.

Chronic Pharyngitis

The causal factor should be identified and addressed.

General measures like warm saline gargles, voice rest may offer some symptomatic relief. Betadine gargles may also be prescribed.

In case of recalcitrant lymphoid granule, chemical cauterization may be attempted under local anesthesia with 4% trichloroacetic acid or 10% silver nitrate.

NURSING INTERVENTIONS

Nurses need to advise the patients on the following points:
- Take measures to prevent spread of infection like proper disposal of used tissues, avoiding contact with people.
- Use of warm saline gargles will relieve pain. Irrigating throat reduces spasm and soreness in throat.
- Observe skin for presence of any rash as pharyngitis may precede some communicable disease like rubella.
- Frequent mouth care will prevent oral inflammation and cracking of lips as well as add to comfort.
- Complete full antibiotic course.
- Observe for any complications.
- Increase fluid intake.

LARYNGITIS

CONCEPT AND DEFINITION

Laryngitis refers to inflammation of the laryngeal mucosa. It may be divided into acute and chronic laryngitis.

Acute Laryngitis

It refers to acute inflammation of the laryngeal mucosa. It may be due to infectious or non-infectious etiology.

Chronic Laryngitis

It is defined as chronic inflammation of the larynx. It may be divided into two types:
1. **Chronic laryngitis without hyperplasia:** Diffuse inflammation of laryngeal mucosa; also called chronic hyperemic laryngitis
   - Laryngeal examination shows general congestion of the larynx; dull, edematous vocal cords and mucoid discharge
   - Symptomatic management usually suffices.
2. **Chronic hyperplastic/hypertrophic laryngitis:** It may be diffuse or localized. Chronic irritation generally causes fibrosis and granuloma formation presenting as a neoplasm. It may present in various forms including Rienke's edema, vocal nodules, vocal polyps, dysphonia plica ventricularis (thickening of false vocal cords; compensatory hypertrophy due to chronic true vocal cord inflammation).
   - Chronic inflammation causes submucosal cellular infiltration and subsequent metaplasia leading to fibrosis and thickening of vocal cords followed by surrounding structures.
   - Affects males more than females, middle-aged
   - Laryngeal examination showed congested, dry laryngeal mucosa; thickened or nodular vocal cords with impaired mobility and cricoarytenoid stiffening in the later stages.
   - Conservative management may ameliorate the condition in the initial stages. Surgical management or stripping may be required in the later stages.
   - *Rienke's edema:* It is the presentation of chronic hypertrophic laryngitis. There is bilateral, symmetrical edema of the vocal cords due to oedema of the subepithelial space (Rienke's space). On laryngoscopic examination, the vocal cords appear symmetrically fusiform with impaired mobility presenting with a low pitched, rough, and hoarse voice.

EPIDEMIOLOGY

Acute laryngitis is more common in children. Women are affected more often than men. It is seen more commonly in the winter season.

ETIOLOGY

Acute

It may be infectious or non-infectious in origin. It is most commonly viral, though there may be secondary bacterial infection. *Streptococcus pneumoniae*, *Haemophilus influenzae* and hemolytic streptococci or *Staphylococcus aureus* are the most commonly isolated bacteria. Conditions like measles, chickenpox and whooping cough also present with laryngitis.

Non-infectious causes include vocal abuse, acid-reflux and laryngeal trauma due to physical or chemical trauma. Procedures such as endotracheal intubation may also result in laryngeal trauma.

Chronic

It is multifactorial, most commonly occur due to incomplete resolution or recurrent attacks of acute laryngitis. Other causes include:
- Persistent and recurrent infections in the vicinity including rhinosinusitis, tonsillitis and dental infection.
- Environmental factors like dust, smoke and occupational exposure to industrial fumes and heavy metals such as in mining and chemical industries.
- Irritants like tobacco in the form of smoking, chewing tobacco or *paan*, alcohol consumption and frequent intake of spicy food.
- Constant coughing as seen in patients with COPD, acid-reflux, etc.
- Vocal abuse

PATHOPHYSIOLOGY

Inflammatory process leads to changes of the laryngeal mucosa causing impairment of the function of the ciliated epithelium. Subsequently, the clearance of mucous produced by the goblet cells is hampered, leading to stasis in and around the vocal cords. It may further cause reactive cough, laryngospasm, dyskeratosis, hyperkeratosis, parakeratosis, acanthosis and cellular atypia.

Acute laryngitis is characterized by a general polymorphonuclear response with the cardinal signs of inflammation.

In chronic laryngitis, initially there may be cellular infiltration in the submucosa. As the disease progresses, the pseudostratified ciliated epithelium of respiratory mucosa undergoes metaplasia to squamous type which further becomes hyperplastic and keratinized. Mucous glands undergo atrophy reducing lubrication and causing dryness of the larynx.

CLINICAL MANIFESTATIONS

Acute

- **Local:** Discomfort in throat, hoarseness, dry cough. Severe cases of laryngitis like membranous laryngitis (diphtheria) may produce dyspnea and dysphagia.
- **Constitutional symptoms:** Low-grade fever, malaise, headache, irritability, restlessness
- **Inflammation and edema:** Epiglottis, aryepiglottic folds, arytenoids, ventricular bands. Vocal cords may become congested and erythematous in severe cases. Mucoid secretions may be found on the laryngeal structures.

Chronic

- Dry, irritating cough

- Hoarseness of voice
- Throat discomfort or pain, hawking (constant clearing of throat due to stickiness)
- Congestion of the posterior pharyngeal wall, granulations and hypertrophy of lymphoid follicles in case of hypertrophic variant, thickening of the faucial pillars.

DIAGNOSIS

Diagnosis is usually clinical following a thorough history and clinical examination. Indirect laryngoscopy or Hopkins endoscopy (rigid – 70/90°) should be performed to confirm the laryngeal signs.

MANAGEMENT

Acute Laryngitis

General: Vocal rest (single most important factor for prognosis, less than complete adherence may lead to delayed recovery. Steam inhalation also helps to alleviate the symptoms. Antitussives may be prescribed to relieve the cough.

Specific: In cases of secondary bacterial infections antibiotics may be given with analgesics to counter the infection and concomitant inflammation. Steroids may be prescribed in cases of severe oedema in cases of chemical or thermal injury.

Chronic Laryngitis

The causal factor, mainly the foci of infection if present should be identified and addressed. Occupational exposure to dust, smoke and fumes should be avoided. Voice rest may be required for a prolonged period of weeks to months. Surgical management many be instituted for hyperplastic cases with stripping of the hyperplastic mucosa.

NURSING INTERVENTIONS

- Provide rest to voice.
- Encourage intake of plenty of fluids to loosen secretions.
- Maintain well-humidified environment.
- Take prescribed expectorants if secretions are present.

EPIGLOTTITIS

CONCEPT AND DEFINITION

Epiglottitis or Supraglottic laryngitis is defined as the diffuse inflammation of the supraglottis, especially the inlet, i.e., epiglottis, aryepiglottic folds and the arytenoids.

EPIDEMIOLOGY

It is commonly seen in children between 2–7 years.

ETIOLOGY

H. influenzae.

PATHOPHYSIOLOGY

Bacterial infection of the epiglottis leads to acute onset of inflammatory edema, beginning on the lingual surface of the epiglottis where the submucosa is loosely attached. Swelling significantly reduces the airway aperture. Edema may rapidly progress to involve the aryepiglottic folds, the arytenoids, and the entire supraglottic larynx. The tightly bound epithelium on the vocal cords halts the spread of edema at this level. Aspiration of oropharyngeal secretions or mucus due to the surrounding edema and 'plugging' can cause respiratory distress and arrest.

CLINICAL MANIFESTATIONS

It may have an abrupt onset and usually progresses rapidly and may prove fatal in the absence of prompt management.
Local: Dysphagia, odynophagia. Patient may present with dyspnea or stridor in case of laryngeal obstruction due to oedema.
- Patient may present with the classical 'tripod sign' where the patient sits leaning forward with open mouth so as to relieve the difficulty in breathing and drooling.

Constitutional symptoms: High-grade fever, irritability
- Swollen, congested and grossly edematous epiglottis
- Indirect laryngoscopy should be avoided so as to avoid precipitation of respiratory distress

DIAGNOSIS

A lateral X ray of neck shows the characteristic 'thumb sign' due to the swollen epiglottis (**Fig. 4.3**).

MANAGEMENT

- Patient requires immediate hospitalization in anticipation of respiratory distress or stridor.
- Immediate securing of the airway, intubation or tracheostomy if required.
- Parenteral antibiotics to counter the infection. Third-generation cephalosporins have been found to be especially effective against *H. influenzae*.
- Intravenous steroids like hydrocortisone reduce the laryngeal oedema to reduce the respiratory distress.
- Adequate hydration, nebulization and humidification.

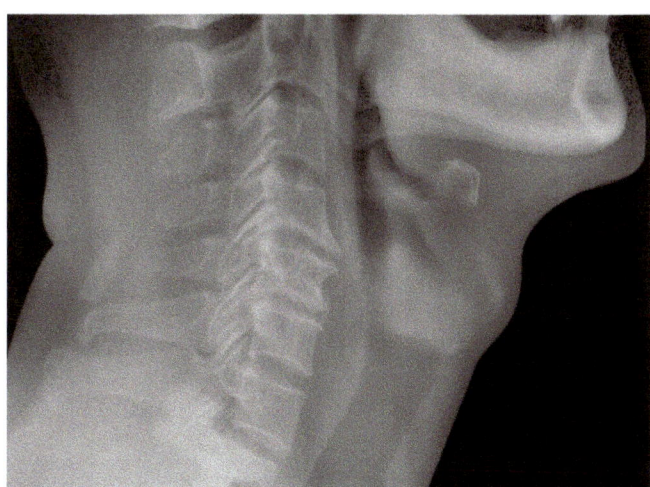

Fig. 4.3: 'Thumb sign' in epiglottitis.

COMPLICATIONS

Respiratory distress, stridor.

NURSING MANAGEMENT OF PATIENTS

- Provide propped up position to patient.
- Assess and monitor respiration of patient.
- Keep the patient comfortable and maintain humidification of air to reduce respiratory effort.

TONSILLITIS

ACUTE TONSILLITIS

It is defined as acute inflammation of the palatine tonsils and its components. It is divided into four subtypes based on the constituent affected:
1. **Acute catarrhal/superficial tonsillitis:** It is a part of generalized pharyngitis.
2. **Acute follicular tonsillitis:** Here the infection spreads into the tonsillar crypts **(Fig. 4.4)**.
3. **Acute parenchymatous tonsillitis:** It is the infection of tonsillar substance making it uniformly enlarged and congested.
4. **Acute membranous tonsillitis:** Caused when the purulent exudate in follicular tonsillitis spreads medially and forms a film over the entire tonsil.

CHRONIC TONSILLITIS

It is defined as chronic inflammation of the tonsil. It is similarly divided into three subtypes:
1. **Chronic follicular tonsillitis:** It is the presence of cheesy material in the tonsillar crypts.
2. **Chronic parenchymatous tonsillitis:** It is the chronically enlarged tonsils due to lymphoid hyperplasia.
3. **Chronic fibrotic tonsillitis:** It is the small, atrophied tonsils due to recurrent attacks.

EPIDEMIOLOGY

Tonsillitis most commonly occurs in school-going children between 5–15 years of age. It may occur in adults but is rarely seen in very young children or the elderly.

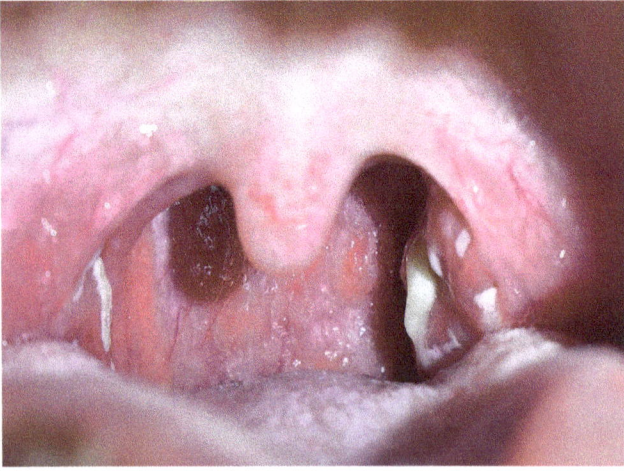

Fig. 4.4: Acute tonsillitis.

ETIOLOGY

Acute Tonsillitis

Most commonly caused by hemolytic streptococci, *Staphylococcus aureus*, pneumococci, or *H. influenzae*.

Chronic Tonsillitis

Usually occurs due to repeated attacks of acute tonsillitis. It may also be due to concurrent chronic infection of the nose, paranasal sinuses or teeth.

PATHOPHYSIOLOGY

It is usually seen secondary to a viral infection. These bacteria may also primarily infect the tonsils. It is generally considered a part of the secondary immune system which responds when exposed to ingested or inspired antigens that pass across the epithelial layer. The immunologic structure is divided into 4 compartments: reticular crypt epithelium, extrafollicular area, mantle zone of the lymphoid follicle and the germinal center of the lymphoid follicle. Membrane cells and antigen presenting cells (APCs) are involved in transport of antigen from the surface to the lymphoid follicle. Antigen is presented to T-helper cells. T-helper cells induce B cells in germinal center to produce antibody. Secretory IgA is the primary antibody produced and is involved in local immunity.

CLINICAL MANIFESTATIONS

Acute Tonsillitis

- **Local:** Throat pain, pain on swallowing, earache due to pain referred from the tonsil, halitosis or bad breath
- **Constitutional symptoms:** High-grade fever, may be associated with chills and rigors, malaise, headache, etc.
- Coated tongue
- **Tonsils:** Congestion of the tonsillar pillars with enlarged, congested tonsils. The purulent exudate in the crypts may present as whitish-yellow spots over the tonsillitis (acute follicular tonsillitis) or as a whitish membrane over the tonsils that is easily removed (membranous tonsillitis).
- Enlarged, tender jugulodigastric nodes

Chronic Tonsillitis

- Recurrent attacks of acute tonsillitis, constant throat irritation, halitosis and difficulty in speech, swallowing and breathing in case of grossly enlarged tonsils.
- Cardinal signs of tonsillitis:
  - Flushing of anterior tonsillar pillar
  - Exudation of yellowish, cheesy material on application of pressure over the anterior tonsillar pillar—'Irwin Moore sign'
  - Enlarged jugulodigastric nodes
- Enlarged tonsils (chronic parenchymatous tonsillitis)

Grades

- **Grade 1:** Tonsils enlarged but not reaching the anterior pillars.
- **Grade 2:** Tonsils enlarged, up to the level of anterior pillars obscuring the posterior pillars.

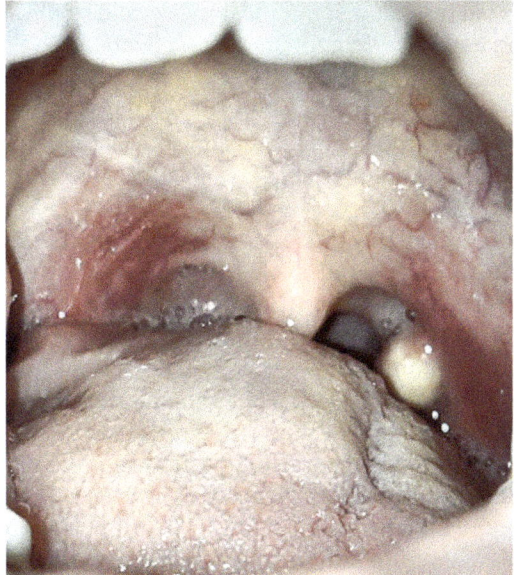

Fig. 4.5: Chronic tonsillitis showing anterior pillar congestion and left tonsillar cyst.

- **Grade 3:** Tonsillar enlargement beyond the level of the anterior pillar
- **Grade 4:** 'Kissing tonsils', gross tonsillar enlargement meeting in the midline.

COMPLICATIONS

Respiratory distress, stridor, Cor pulmonale, obstructive sleep apnea, peritonsillar abscess or 'Quinsy', parapharyngeal abscess, tonsilloliths, tonsillar cysts **(Fig. 4.5)**, rheumatic heart disease and glomerulonephritis (in certain cases of infection by beta hemolytic streptococci).

DIAGNOSIS

- Swab for microscopy and culture sensitivity
- Complete blood count to look for leukocytosis, ESR (usually raised in chronic tonsillitis)
- ECG and ECHO to rule out rheumatic heart disease.
- CT scan to rule out spread of the infection into the peritonsillar space and other complications.

MANAGEMENT

Acute Tonsillitis

- **Antibiotic therapy:** Penicillin is the drug of choice for *streptococcus*. Macrolides may be used if the patient is allergic to penicillin.
- **Anti-inflammatory medications** like NSAIDs to reduce pain and manage fever.
- **Adequate hydration and rest:** Warm saline or betadine gargles may offer symptomatic relief.

Chronic Tonsillitis

It involves concurrent treatment of infections of teeth, nose and sinuses. Tonsillectomy should be performed in case of features of difficulty in swallowing, speech or obstructive sleep apnea.

Tonsillectomy

It refers to surgical extracapsular resection of the tonsils. There are two types of tonsillectomies depending upon the time when it is performed.

1. **Interval tonsillectomy:** It is the most commonly performed procedure. It is done after the attack of acute tonsillitis subsides, about 6 weeks after resolution. It is the preferred procedure as active inflammation poses the risks of heavy bleeding during the procedure.
2. **Hot tonsillectomy:** It is rarely performed these days. It refers to excision of the tonsils during an episode of peritonsillar abscess.

Complications of Tonsillectomy

Bleeding is the most common and most dangerous complications of tonsillectomy. The others are sore throat, otalgia, fever, uvular edema, etc. Atlantoaxial subluxation, mandibular condyle fracture, secondary infection, eustachian tube injury are the less common injuries.

Bleeding in tonsillectomy is divided into 3 types based on when it presents:

1. **Primary hemorrhage:** It presents during the surgery.
2. **Reactionary hemorrhage:** It occurs within 24 hours of the surgery. It is thought to be most commonly due to the presence of a clot that impedes the compression of the bleeding vasculature by superior constrictor muscle. It has also been observed due to slippage of clots or ligatures.
3. **Secondary hemorrhage:** It is usually seen after 24 hours of surgery and may present at any time up to 10 days of the surgery. It usually occurs due to infection.

NURSING MANAGEMENT

- Ask patient and family members to report if any bleeding occurs, which usually occurs within first 24 hours.
- Provide prone position to the patient with head turned towards one side. This position will promote drainage of secretions from mouth.
- Oral airway to be removed from patients' mouth only after returning of swallowing and gag reflex.
- Check and monitor vital signs, and report any rise in pulse and temperature, restlessness and blood in vomits.
- Advise patient to avoid activities causing throat pain like coughing and talking for long.
- Keep articles ready for examination of surgical site near patient bedside. It includes curved hemostat, a light, a mirror.
- Water and ice chips may be given to patient on return of Gag reflex.
- Inform that mild pain in ear may be felt for few days.
- Halitosis may also last for a few days post surgery.
- Advise the patient that mouthwash or warm saline solutions reduce halitosis and remove thick mucus as well.
- Avoid brushing hard to prevent bleeding.
- Avoid rough, spicy and hot food. Patient should be provided liquid to semiliquid diet for few days.
- Inform that the patient may have vomiting, stiff neck, sore throat within first 24 hours. Report any frank bleeding.

ADENOIDITIS

CONCEPT AND DEFINITION

Adenoiditis is defined as the inflammation of the nasopharyngeal tonsils. Nasopharyngeal tonsils or adenoids refers to lymphatic tissue present at the junction of the roof and posterior wall of the nasopharynx.

EPIDEMIOLOGY

It is almost exclusively seen in children as adenoids regress with age.

ETIOPATHOGENESIS

Adenoids tend to enlarge in children in response to infection of the surrounding structures including recurrent bouts of rhinitis, sinusitis or pharyngitis. Allergy may also contribute to adenoid enlargement. Bacterial agents proliferate and infect the adenoids and surrounding tissue resulting in inflammation and increased production of exudates. Symptoms include rhinorrhea, post-nasal drip, nasal obstruction, snoring, fever, and halitosis. Chronic adenoiditis shows many of the same symptoms but on a persistent basis lasting 90 days and is often caused by polymicrobial infections and biofilm formation. Exudates are frequently absent in chronic adenoiditis.

CLINICAL MANIFESTATIONS

- **Local:** Nasal obstruction leading to mouth breathing and snoring, recurrent of chronic rhinitis, change in voice (rhinolalia clausa), epistaxis rarely, ear pain, ear discharge, decreased hearing.
- **General symptoms:** Lack of concentration (aprosexia)
- **Adenoid facies:** High arched palate, crowded teeth, malar hypoplasia (elongated face), pinched nose—due to chronic mouth breathing, blank look.

COMPLICATIONS

Obstructive sleep apnea, cor pulmonale, pulmonary hypertension, cognitive impairment.

DIAGNOSIS

- X-ray nasopharynx, lateral view (soft tissue) shows adenoid enlargement in the nasopharynx.
- Pure tone audiometry and impedance audiometry to rule out hearing loss and fluid in the middle ear.
- Posterior rhinoscopy and diagnostic nasal endoscopy to visualize the grade of adenoid hypertrophy.

MANAGEMENT

Adenoid hypertrophy is one of the few conditions, if diagnosed early, can be resolved completely. Due to the severity of complications, the latest guidelines for adenoid hypertrophy recommend surgical management of the patient by adenoid resection. It may be done by cold steel, laser, co-ablation and debridement under visualization.

Steps of Conventional Adenoidectomy

- Position—supine with extension at neck (with the aid of a bolster at shoulder) and flexion at the atlanto-occipital joint.
- Boyle Davis Mouth gag is applied. The adenoids are palpated and medialized to prevent injury to the eustachian tubes and any anatomically abnormal vasculature.
- St. Clair Thomson's adenoid curette is inserted (pencil/dagger hold), taking care not to injure the uvula and the soft palate and is engaged at the roof of the nasopharynx.
- It is then swept downward along the posterior pharyngeal wall while the neck of the patient is flexed, and the adenoid tissue is scooped out.
- The cage of the curette prevents slippage of the tissue into the airway.
- The adenoids are palpated once more, and the curette may be used again to remove any substantial residual adenoid tissue.
- Hemostasis is achieved.

NURSING CONSIDERATIONS

Follow same as in case of tonsillitis.

PERITONSILLAR ABSCESS

CONCEPT AND DEFINITION

Peritonsillar abscess, also called 'quinsy' occurs as a complication of acute or chronic tonsillitis is defined as collection of purulent material in the peritonsillar space. Peritonsillar space **(Fig. 4.6)** is the space bounded by the tonsillar capsule and the superior constrictor muscle underneath.

EPIDEMIOLOGY

It is paradoxically seen in adults though tonsillitis, as a rule, is commonly observed in children.

ETIOLOGY

The most commonly isolated organisms are *Streptococcus pyogenes* and *Staph. aureus*. Anaerobic organisms have been isolated in some cases. Mixed cultures may also be obtained occasionally.

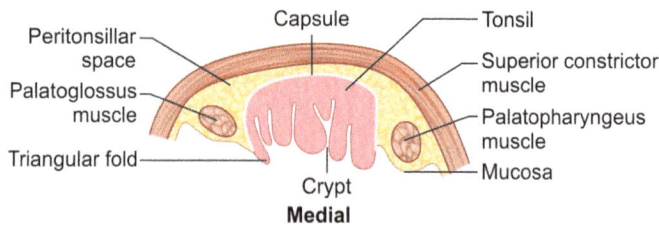

Fig. 4.6: Peritonsillar space.

PATHOPHYSIOLOGY

It occurs mainly after a bout of acute tonsillitis in adults. The involvement of crypta magna allows the infection to spread through the tonsillar tissue into the loose areolar tissue underneath the capsule. This occurs because in adults the tonsils are usually smaller allowing the crypta magna to easily traverse the depth of the tonsil to the peritonsillar space.

Another proposed mechanism is necrosis and pus formation in the capsular area which then obstructs the Weber's glands, resulting in abscess formation. These are minor salivary glands in peritonsillar space which are responsible for clearing debris from the tonsillar area. The occurrence of peritonsillar abscess in patients who have undergone tonsillectomy further supports this theory.

CLINICAL MANIFESTATIONS

It is usually unilateral:
- **Local:** Severe throat pain; pain on swallowing (odynophagia) to the extent that patient may present with drooling); halitosis, thick, muffled voice ('hot potato voice'), referred pain to ipsilateral ear, trismus (due to spasm of the medial pterygoid muscle).
- **Constitutional symptoms:** High-grade fever with chills and rigors, malaise, headache, nausea, constipation
  - The tonsillar pillars, soft palate and uvula are grossly edematous and congested. The tonsils themselves may not be enlarged but are pushed medially. Uvula may be pushed to the opposite side.
  - Tender, enlarged cervical lymph nodes
  - Wry-neck or torticollis—tilting or twisting of neck to the side of the abscess

COMPLICATIONS

Parapharyngeal abscess, laryngitis, respiratory distress, pneumonia, lung abscess, jugular venous thrombosis, hemorrhage, septicemia.

DIAGNOSIS

It is mainly a clinical diagnosis based on the history and examination. Radiological investigation like CT scan may be done to rule out any complications.

MANAGEMENT

- The patient should be hospitalized.
- Immediate securing of the airway.
- Parenteral antibiotics to counter the infection with both aerobic and anaerobic cover.
- Analgesics to counter pain
- Adequate hydration
- In case the abscess has already been formed it needs to be drained surgically by incision and drainage. The point of incision is usually the point of maximum bulge or fluctuation, as in case of any other abscess.
- In case of peritonsillar abscess a stab incision may be given at the junction of the horizontal level of the base of uvula and the anterior pillar.

NURSING MANAGEMENT

- Educate importance of frequent mouthwash, every 1 to 2 hour for 2 to 3 days
- Prescribed topical anesthetic agent can be taken.

OVERALL NURSING CONSIDERATIONS IN URI

Assessment

- Patient must be assessed for fever, cough, hoarseness, fatigue, discomfort, periorbital pain, headache, sore throat.
- Assess patient for history of any allergies or any other illness.
- Inspect nasal mucosa for redness, nasal polyps, swelling or exudates.
- Palpate maxillary and frontal sinuses. Tenderness on palpation indicates inflammation of sinuses.
- Examine throat. Inspect pharynx and tonsils for redness, asymmetry, enlargement, ulceration, drainage.
- Palpate trachea for any deformities or masses. Examine neck lymph nodes for tenderness and enlargement.

Nursing Management

Nursing management of a patient with URI has been discussed separately under each condition.

DIETETIC

- Avoid spicy/cold or any throat irritating foods.
- Stop alcohol and tobacco consumption.
- Consume normal balanced diet.
- Consume adequate amount of water.

GERIATRIC CONSIDERATIONS

The prevalence of URI in the elderly is only marginally more than in other age-groups. However, the rate of complications in these patients is higher. Infection is a major cause of morbidity and mortality in patients over the age of 65 years.

Various biological and societal factors have been posited to play a major role in the same. For instance:
- **'Immunosenescence':** Decreased immunity and increased inflammatory changes that occur with age.
- Reduced response to antibiotics and other therapy for infections
- Atypical symptoms and signs of the disease
- Morphological changes of ageing that increase susceptibility to infections:
  - Impaired mucociliary clearance and age-related ciliary dysmotility
  - Impaired reflexes due to neurodegeneration—cough reflex
  - Gastroesophageal reflux

One subset of the geriatric population thought to be more susceptible to URI include those living in long-term care facilities, like old-age homes. Close quarters and increased transmission lead to higher risk of infection spread in these patients, especially during influenza outbreaks.

Challenges in Management

- Injudicious use of OTC medications.

❖ Difficult to ascertain whether symptoms like hyposmia and dysgeusia are age-related neurodegeneration or a part of the spectrum of the disease process especially in cases of rhinitis, sinusitis, and pharyngitis.

Case Scenario

1. A 10-year-old boy presented with complaints of recurrent bouts of throat pain and difficulty swallowing over the last 3 years. On examination, his tonsils were enlarged with multiple yellow spots over the tonsils. There were multiple bilateral, non-tender swellings over the neck.
    a. What is your diagnosis?
    b. How will you manage this patient?
2. A 3-year-old boy presented to the emergency with tachypnea, tachycardia and respiratory distress. He sat leaning forward, leaning on his hands with an open mouth and drooling. On examination an inspiratory stridor was heard, accessory muscles of respirations were being used. He had a fever of 102°F and refused feeds.
    a. What is your diagnosis?
    b. How will you manage this patient?

SUMMARY

- URI is one of the commonest illnesses encountered in medical practice.
- Coryza is a self-limiting viral illness, generally of viral origin that requires only symptomatic management.
- Inflammation of the nasal mucosa is called rhinitis. It may be classified as acute or chronic rhinitis.
- Atrophic rhinitis is a form of chronic rhinitis where chronic inflammation of the nasal mucosa causes destruction of the neurovasculature and atrophy of the nasal structures.
- Injudicious use of nasal decongestants can cause rebound congestion of the nasal mucosa leading to rhinitis medicamentosa.
- Allergic rhinitis (AR) is a heterogeneous disorder caused due to immune-mediated inflammation of the nasal mucosa. Clinically it is defined as having 2 or more of the following symptoms for 2 or more consecutive days lasting more than an hour on most of the days.
    – Rhinorrhea (anterior/posterior)
    – Sneezing
    – Nasal blockage
    – Itching of the nose
- Management of allergic rhinitis depends upon the severity and frequency of the symptoms as per the ARIA classification.
- Epiglottitis refers to diffuse inflammation of the supraglottic structures and presents with difficulty breathing. It is seen almost exclusively in children and may present with the characteristic 'thumb' sign on lateral radiograph of the neck.
- Tonsillitis refers to inflammation of the palatine tonsils and may be acute or chronic.
- The most common complication of tonsillectomy is hemorrhage.
- Peritonsillar abscess or 'quinsy' usually presents in adults.

MULTIPLE CHOICE QUESTIONS

1. Which of the following is not a cardinal sign of chronic tonsillitis?
    a. Pus in the crypts which can be expressed
    b. Congestion of the anterior tonsil
    c. Congestion of the posterior pillar
    d. Enlargement of cervical lymph nodes
2. Which of the following is not seen in adenoid facies?
    a. Crowding of teeth   b. Elongated face
    c. Protruding tongue   d. Pinched nose
3. Which of the following is not a feature of atrophic rhinitis?
    a. Profuse mucoid discharge
    b. Thick, greenish crusts
    c. Nose block sensation
    d. Foul smell from the nose.
4. Infection by which of the following organisms causing pharyngitis may cause rheumatic heart disease?
    a. *Corynebacterium diphtheriae*
    b. Gonococci
    c. *Chlamydia trachomatis*
    d. Beta-hemolytic streptococci
5. Which endoscope may be utilized for visualization of the larynx?
    a. 0°   b. 30°
    c. 45°   d. 70°
6. Which of the following organisms causes epiglottitis?
    a. *Streptococcus*   b. *Pneumococcus*
    c. *Haemophilus influenzae* d. *Staphylococcus*
7. Tripod sign is a feature of which disease?
    a. Epiglottitis
    b. Acute laryngotracheobronchitis
    c. Acute laryngitis
    d. Peritonsillar abscess
8. Which of the following is not a feature of peritonsillar abscess?
    a. Odynophagia/pain on swallowing
    b. More common in children
    c. Fever   d. Wry neck
9. Which of the following conditions is caused due to overuse of topical nasal decongestants?
    a. Atrophic rhinitis   b. Rhinitis sicca
    c. Rhinitis medicamentosa d. Rhinitis caseosa
10. Which one of the following conditions presents with a 'thumb sign' on lateral neck X-ray?
    a. Acute laryngotracheobronchitis
    b. Epiglottitis
    c. Tonsillitis   d. Adenoiditis

ANSWERS

1. c	2. c	3. a	4. d
5. d	6. c	7. b	8. b
9. c	10. b		

SUGGESTED READING

1. Allan GM, Arroll B. "Prevention and treatment of the common cold: making sense of the evidence". CMAJ : Canadian Medical Association Journal. 2014;186(3):190-9.
2. Common Colds: Protect Yourself and Others". CDC. 6 October 2015. Archived from the original on 5 February 2016. Retrieved 4 February 2016.
3. DeConde AS, Soler ZM. Chronic rhinosinusitis: Epidemiology and burden of disease. Am J Rhinol Allergy. 2016;30(2):134-9. doi: 10.2500/ajra.2016.30.4297. PMID: 26980394.
4. Dhingra PL (Ed). Diseases of Ear, Nose and Throat, 6th Edition. New Delhi; Elsevier; 2014.
5. Geffen L. Common upper respiratory tract problems in the elderly—A guide to clinical diagnosis and prudent prescription. South African Family Practice 2006;48(5),20-3, DOI: 10.1080/20786204.2006.10873390.
6. Linda K Clarke. Management of clients with upper airway disorders. In: Black J. Hawks J Medical surgical nursing. 7th edition. India. Elsevier; 2005. pp. 1796-801.
7. Selvaraj K, Chinnakali P, Majumdar A, Krishnan IS. Acute respiratory infections among under-5 children in India: A situational analysis. J Nat Sci Biol Med. 2014;5(1):15-20. doi:10.4103/0976-9668.127275
8. Watkinson, John C. Scott-Brown's Otorhinolaryngology and Head and Neck Surgery, 8th edition. Boca Raton: Chapman and Hall/CRC; 2018.

CHAPTER 5

Obstruction and Trauma of the Upper Respiratory Airway

Vivek K Pathak, Pragya Pathak, Pradeepti Nayak

"All that wheezes is not asthma."

—Chevalier Jackson

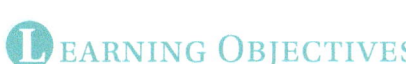 LEARNING OBJECTIVES

After going through the chapter, the learner will be able to:
- Enumerate various causes of upper airway obstruction.
- Describe the pathophysiology and the associated clinical features of airway obstruction at different levels in the airway.
- Describe the pathophysiology and the associated clinical features of airway obstruction due to different causative factors.
- Elaborate various aspects of management including diagnosis, medical and surgical management wherever applicable and other non-pharmacological modalities, if any.
- Identify emergency situations with respect to airway obstruction and institute critical care as per protocol.
- Enumerate the potential complications along with the actions that are necessary to prevent them in patients of upper airway obstruction.
- Describe the nursing care required in various aspects of patient management like diet and nutrition, wound care, pain management and antimicrobial therapy.
- Discuss the geriatric considerations in disorders of upper respiratory airway.

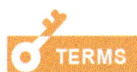 TERMS

- **ANP:** Anterior nasal packing.
- **Epistaxis:** Bleeding from nose.
- **PNP:** Posterior nasal packing.
- **Stridor:** High pitched sound produced by upper airway obstruction.
- **TESPAL:** Transnasal endoscopic sphenopalatine artery ligation.

INTRODUCTION

Upper airway obstruction is defined as narrowing of the airways leading to compromise in respiration and ventilation It may be at level of the upper airway including the nasal cavity, nasopharynx, oropharynx, laryngopharynx and trachea. Airway obstruction produces a distinct sound during respiration called 'stridor'. Stridor is defined as an audible harsh, high-pitched, musical sound on inspiration produced by turbulent airflow through a partially obstructed upper airway.

In the current chapter we will discuss the common causes of laryngeal obstruction including epistaxis, laryngeal obstructions, deviated nasal septum, nasal trauma, nasal polyps, cancer of larynx, and obstructive sleep apnea.

EPISTAXIS

CONCEPT AND DEFINITION

The word epistaxis is etymologically deriving from Greek "epi" meaning upon and "stazi" meaning to drip. It is defined as bleeding from one or both the nasal cavities.

TYPES OF EPISTAXIS

1. **Anterior:** It is more common, less severe, and easy to control. Most commonly involves the Little's area at the antero-inferior part of the nasal septum – Little's area is a confluence of vessels; anterior ethmoidal artery, sphenopalatine artery, greater palatine artery and septal

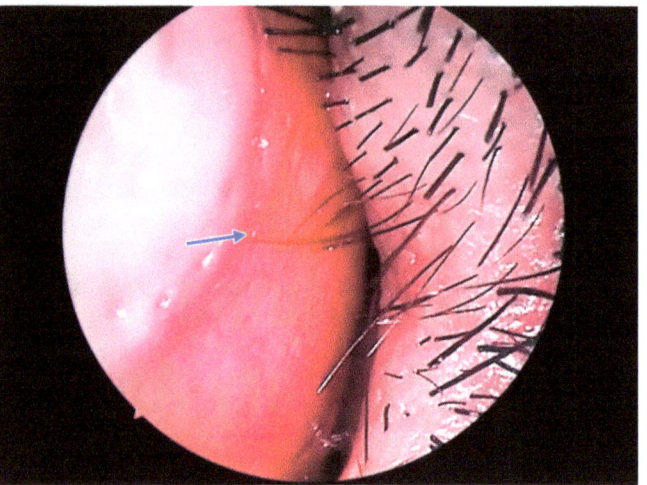

Fig. 5.1: Retrocolumellar vein.

branch of superior labial artery. Sphenopalatine artery is called the 'Artery of epistaxis'.

In children the most common cause of bleeding is injury to the retrocolumellar vein **(Fig. 5.1)**.

2. **Posterior:** It is less common and more severe, difficult to control, may present with per oral bleed or hematemesis. It is generally seen in elderly hypertensives. It is hypothesized that acute hypertensive episodes cause the venous pressure in the 'Woodruff's venous plexuses at the posterior end of the inferior turbinate to rise and causing rupture and bleeding.

EPIDEMIOLOGY

It may occur in any of the age groups due to different etiological factors. It is extremely common. According to reports, everyone suffers from at least one episode of epistaxis in their lifetime.

ETIOLOGY

Local Causes

Trauma, Infections (acute, chronic and granulomatous), foreign body, deviated nasal septum, nasal picking, atmospheric changes-high altitude, benign and malignant neoplasms, juvenile nasopharyngeal angiofibroma.

The most common cause of epistaxis in children includes digital trauma and injury to the retrocolumellar vein. In adults the most common cause are rhinitis and trauma.

Systemic Causes

Hypertension is the most common cause of posterior epistaxis. The other causes include liver diseases, bleeding disorders, vitamin K deficiencies, and renal diseases.

PATHOPHYSIOLOGY

Rupture of vessels inside the nasal cavity due to underlying local or systemic causes like hypertension, trauma, blood thinner medications.

CLINICAL MANIFESTATIONS

Various clinical manifestations include profuse bleeding from unilateral or bilateral nasal cavities, dizziness, features of raised blood pressure, history of trauma, history of bleeding disorders/transfusions.

DIAGNOSTIC EVALUATION

History: Amount of blood loss, duration of blood loss, laterality, medication history, family history of blood dyscrasias and coagulopathy, fever, rashes.
Examination: It involves careful inspection with nasal speculum to determine any raw area in the mucosa of nasal cavity followed by diagnostic nasal endoscopy.
Investigations: Hemoglobin, coagulation profile, renal and liver function tests.

COMPLICATIONS

Various complications include:
❖ Hemorrhagic shock—due to excessive blood loss, more common in cases of posterior epistaxis.
❖ Pressure necrosis—due to the pack, uncommon if adequate care is taken.
❖ Other more uncommon complications include sinusitis, epiphora, and hypoxic ischemic encephalopathy.

MANAGEMENT

❖ **First aid:** Most of the time, bleeding occurs from the little's area and can be easily controlled by pinching the nose with thumb and index finger for about 5–8 min. This compresses the vessels of the little's area.
❖ In Trotter's method **(Fig. 5.2)** patient is made to sit, leaning a little forward over a basin to spit any blood and breathe quietly from the mouth. Cold compresses may be applied to the nose to cause reflex vasoconstriction.
❖ **Cauterization:** Chemical (trichloroacetic acid, 10% silver nitrate), bipolar/unipolar

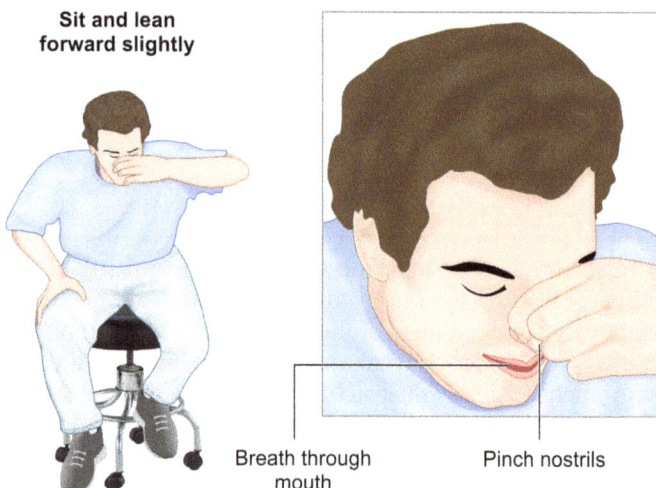

Fig. 5.2: Trotter's method.

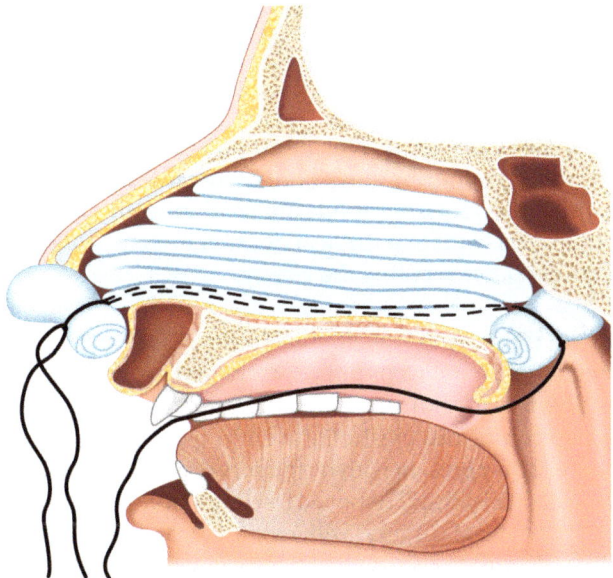

Fig. 5.3: Anterior nasal packing.

- **Anterior nasal packing (Fig. 5.3):** Gauze soaked in ointment, merocele etc.
- **Posterior nasal packing**
- **Transnasal endoscopic sphenopalatine artery ligation (TESPAL):** This procedure is undertaken when the bleeding is not controlled by conventional methods like nasal packing.

Dietetics

Avoid intake of cold food; medications that may precipitate bleeding

NURSING MANAGEMENT OF PATIENTS

- Ask the patient to calm down and relax as bleeding causes lot of anxiety to patient.
- Make patient to sit in popped up position with head bend forward.
- Pinch nose for 10–15 minutes and also inform the patient to pinch nose in case of recurrent bleeding.
- Check and record vital signs of the patients appropriately.
- Ask the patients to avoid forceful blowing nose, do not do nose picking, straining and going to high altitude.
- Move to hospital in case the bleeding do not stop.
- Keep the patient comfortable and maintain humidification of air to reduce respiratory effort.

LARYNGEAL OBSTRUCTION

CONCEPT AND DEFINITION

Laryngeal obstruction refers to any impedance to the airway at the level of the laryngopharynx. It is a critical condition and often life-threatening condition which requires immediate intervention. It may lead to severe hypoxia and subsequent encephalopathy.

ETIOPATHOGENESIS

Various etiological factors causing laryngeal obstruction are shown in **Box 5.1**.

> **BOX 5.1:** Causes of laryngeal obstruction.
>
> - **Traumatic:** Direct or blunt trauma, chemical, thermal, iatrogenic injury
> - **Congenital/developmental/malformations:** Subglottic stenosis, subglottic hemangioma, laryngomalacia, laryngeal cyst, glottic web, vocal cord paralysis (bilateral)
> - **Infections/inflammatory conditions:** Acute laryngotracheobronchitis, acute epiglottitis, laryngeal diphtheria, deep neck space infections, tuberculosis, syphilis
> - **Neoplasms:** Benign (recurrent laryngeal papillomatosis), malignant (carcinoma larynx)
> - **Laryngospasm:** Due to trauma, medications (anesthesia)—may require muscle relaxants and oxygen support
> - **Miscellaneous:** Foreign bodies, granulomas, cyst, pseudotumors, amyloidosis

Traumatic

Any direct blunt or penetrating trauma to the region of the neck causing injury to the larynx and subsequent hematoma, edema or injury to nerves, musculature may cause laryngeal obstruction. Chemical or thermal injury and iatrogenic injury during intubation/endoscopy may also precipitate this condition.

Congenital/Developmental/Malformation

These involve subglottic stenosis, subglottic hemangioma, laryngomalacia, laryngeal cyst, glottic web, vocal cord paralysis (bilateral).

Laryngomalacia

Laryngomalacia is a congenital disorder of the laryngeal cartilages. It is thought to be due to delayed maturation of the cartilages causing supraglottic collapse during inspiration and subsequent airway obstruction. It is the commonest cause of stridor in children and is also the most common congenital anomaly. It is most commonly seen in infants of 6–6 months of age.

There is no race or gender predilection to this pathology.

Pathophysiology

It commonly involves the epiglottis and at times the arytenoid cartilages. The epiglottis becomes 'floppy', curls unto itself giving it the characteristic 'omega' shape associated with laryngomalacia. During inspiration, when the intraluminal pressure decreases, it leads to prolapse of epiglottis producing noisy breathing. This noisy breathing is exaggerated in supine position as the epiglottis falls over the laryngeal inlet due to gravity causing obstruction.

Consequent to the increased respiratory effort, the transthoracic pressure also increases compensatorily. This often leads to an increased incidence of gastroesophageal reflux in these children. The increased intra-thoracic pressure may also lead to pulmonary hypertension due to increased venous return to the pulmonary bed.

Clinical Features

- Noisy inspiratory breathing which may be high or low pitched and is aggravated in the supine position. One of the characteristic features of laryngomalacia is that the noisy breathing usually abated when the child is made prone.

The noise may be exacerbated during episodes of URI, crying, agitation and feeding.
- There may be chocking or gagging during feeds if the child is suffering from concomitant reflux pharyngitis.

Diagnosis

Diagnosis is usually clinical. Flexible laryngoscopy or bronchoscopy may be performed under appropriate anesthesia or sedation to directly observe the larynx (omega epiglottis), collapse of arytenoids during inspiration.

Management

- The pathology is usually self-limiting and remits by the age of 2 years.
- Oxygen saturation of the child should be monitored.
- Anti-reflux therapy may be considered in patients with severe reflux pharyngitis.
- In patients with severe manifestations like cyanotic spells and sleep apnea surgical intervention may be considered. Supraglottoplasty is the procedure of choice in such cases.
- **Supraglottoplasty:** It is a surgical procedure to alter the morphology of the supraglottic structures to widen the airway. It encompasses all surgeries undertaken to modify the airway at the level of the upper larynx to alleviate obstruction.

Vocal Cord Paralysis

Bilateral vocal cord paralysis may be another cause for laryngeal obstruction. It is usually a consequence of bilateral recurrent laryngeal nerve (RLN) injury due to iatrogenic causes. Certain viral infections like varicella may also cause vocal cord paralysis.

RLN supplies all the muscles of the larynx except the cricothyroid muscle. Bilateral RLN injury therefore paralyses all but one muscle of the larynx. Being a tensor, unopposed action of both the cricothyroid muscles causes complete closure of the glottis causing immediate and critical airway obstruction.

In chronic cases however, compensation occurs gradually, and the patient does not usually present with respiratory distress.

Subglottic Stenosis

It refers to narrowing of the subglottic airway at the level of the cricoid cartilage.

Congenital subglottic stenosis is thought to occur due to in utero deformation of the cricoid cartilage.

Clinical Features

Noisy breathing, stridor, weak or hoarse cry. In mild cases, it is usually precipitated by exercise or crying. Severe cases present with stridor.

Management

The first order of management is to secure the airway. The patient may need endotracheal intubation or tracheostomy.

Surgical management includes various procedures depending upon the grade of obstruction. These include endoscopic dilation, cricoid split (posterior or posterior cricoid split), laryngotracheoplasty or cricotracheal resection and anastomosis.

Laryngeal Cyst

It is a rare cause of stridor in newborn babies. It is quite rare and accounts for only about 5% of all benign laryngeal neoplasms. The only modality of management for this condition is complete surgical excision or marsupialization of the cyst after securing the airway.

Glottic Web

Congenital glottic webs are very rare and generally present at the anterior commissure. It results due to failure of absorption of the epithelial web in the laryngotracheal groove. It may present with respiratory distress in neonates. It is usually excised and removed by endoscopic flap technique (microlaryngeal surgery) with or without keel placement.

Subglottic Hemangioma

Hemangiomas are amongst the commonest congenital malformation. Subglottic hemangiomas present in the larynx and subglottic as potentially life-threatening, large neoplastic masses that may completely obstruct the airway. They require surgical excision after securing the airway.

Infections/Inflammatory Conditions

These involve acute laryngotracheobronchitis, acute epiglottitis, laryngeal diphtheria, deep neck space infections, tuberculosis, and syphilis.

Acute Laryngotracheobronchitis

Also called 'croup' is primarily an acute, viral infection of the larynx in children. The word croup is derived from the Anglo-Saxon word *kropan* meaning to "cry in a hoarse voice". It is more commonly seen in males between the ages of 6 months and 3 years.

Etiopathology and Clinical Features

It is caused by the parainfluenza viruses. The infection causes airway edema due to inflammation. The inflammation is usually concentrated in the subglottic region (narrowest part of the airway in children) producing a characteristic harsh, 'seal-like' barky cough. The cough is characteristically more at night. The narrowing of the airway also produces a characteristic inspiratory stridor. Other symptoms include a low-grade fever, rhinorrhea and concomitant pharyngitis. In severe cases the child may present with biphasic stridor, agitation, severe intercostal retractions, cyanosis and even respiratory arrest.

Diagnosis

The diagnosis is usually clinical.
X-ray: The X-ray may show the classical 'steeple' sign due to narrowing of the airway in the subglottic region.

Management

In mild cases, conservative management suffices. Parental guidance, adequate hydration and monitoring the oxygen saturation with symptomatic management of fever with antipyretics usually alleviates the symptoms in less severe cases.

Humidified air helps to reduce the edema in the respiratory tract.

In severe cases careful evaluation and prompt management is imperative. Securing the airway and adequate oxygenation is of primary concern. Corticosteroids and nebulization have been proven to be beneficial in children with respiratory distress.

Laryngeal Diphtheria

It a bacterial disease caused by *Corynebacterium diphtheriae* presenting with constitutional symptoms like fever, chills, malaise, hoarseness, cough, odynophagia, dysphagia and in severe cases, difficult and raid breathing and blood-stained oral and nasal discharge.

It is characterized by formation of thick, greyish membrane due to amassment of the dead necrotic tissue (pseudo-membrane), that bleeds on removal and causes severe respiratory distress.

In case of stridor and airway compromise the patient may need intubation or tracheostomy.

Management is medical with parenteral antibiotics like metronidazole, erythromycin or penicillin. In refractory cases or in patients with allergy to the first line drugs rifampicin or clindamycin may be administered.

It is a potentially life-threatening disease with a mortality of up to 20% in children.

Deep Neck Space Infections

Deep neck space infection (DNI) is defined as the infection of the deep fascia enclosing potential spaces of the neck. Multiple layers of deep cervical fascia encases the contents of the neck to form the potential head and neck spaces, condensation of which forms the fascial planes. These spaces contains adipose tissue and majority of the major neuro-vasculature supplying the head and neck region.

Strong fascial attachments to the hyoid bone anteriorly, provides barrier to downward spread of the infection. So, deep neck spaces are often classified as:
- Those located above the hyoid bone (peritonsillar, mandibular, parapharyngeal, masticator/temporal, buccal and parotid spaces).
- Those located below the hyoid bone (anterior visceral space).
- Those involving the entire neck length (carotid, retropharyngeal, danger, prevertebral spaces).

Deep neck space infections like Ludwig's angina, retropharyngeal and parapharyngeal abscesses can cause acute respiratory distress and may require tracheostomy followed by urgent incision and drainage of the abscess with adequate medical management with parenteral antibiotics.

Neoplasms

Recurrent Laryngeal Papillomatosis (RRP)

It is a rare, benign, recurrent neoplastic disease caused by the human papilloma virus (HPV 6 and HPV 11). HPV causes warty growths to occur in the respiratory larynx causing mechanical obstruction of the airway. It has a bimodal distribution.

- **Juvenile onset (JORRP):** It is more severe and more common and occurs in children under 5 years of age. It is thought to be due to peripartum transmission of the virus. The classical triad of risk factors include mother <20 years of age, vaginal delivery and first-born babies.
- **Adult onset (AORRP):** It is seen in adults in the 3rd and 4th decades. It is thought to be sexually transmitted.

Clinical Features

It presents with upper airway obstruction and the most common presenting symptom is hoarseness of voice. Other symptoms include foreign body sensation in throat, difficulty breathing and noisy breathing (mostly inspiratory stridor).

Diagnosis

Flexible laryngoscopy or bronchoscopy to visualize the growth.

Treatment

Most of the children presenting with RRP eventually require tracheostomy to secure the airway. Unfortunately, there no definitive treatment or cure for this condition as it nearly always recurs. Therapy is aimed at improving voice quality and relieving airway compromise.

Repeated surgical debulking may be required by micro-debridement, cryotherapy or laser. Intralesional cidofovir has been administered with varying success. Long-term interferon therapy is another modality that has been tried with varying results.

CLINICAL FEATURES (LARYNGEAL OBSTRUCTION)

Respiratory distress, stridor, hoarseness, dysphagia, swelling over neck, aspiration, cough.

MANAGEMENT

In these cases, airway management is of prime importance and first line of management. In case of critical patients with rapidly declining SPO_2, cricothyrotomy or tracheostomy must be performed to secure the airway. Medical management may include muscle relaxants, nebulization with bronchodilators and corticosteroids. This is an emergency and prompt intervention must be instituted.

Secondary management consists of the management of the underlying conditions.

Dietetics

Tobacco and alcohol consumption must be strictly avoided.

NURSING MANAGEMENT

Heimlich maneuver/subdiaphragmatic abdominal thrust is performed, which may help to remove foreign body in larynx. So, the nurses should be well aware of these maneuvers.

TRACHEOSTOMY

It is derived from Greek word 'stoma' meaning mouth. It literally means making a hole in the trachea and exteriorizing it.

It provides a definite airway and relieves all forms of laryngeal obstruction. It may be classified in various ways

- Depending upon the indication it may be elective or emergency. It is usually performed under local anesthesia in cases of emergency.
- **Depending upon the level of the tracheostomy:** It may be high tracheostomy, mid-tracheostomy or low tracheostomy. Mid-tracheostomy is performed most commonly through the second and third tracheal rings. High tracheostomy is preferred in cases of laryngeal malignancy.

Steps

- **Position:** Supine with extension of the head and neck
- The incision may be horizontal (better cosmesis, less visualization) or vertical (bad cosmetic results but better visual field). The incision is usually given from just below the lower border of the cricoid cartilage to two finger breadths above the supraclavicular line).
- Division of subcutaneous tissue.
- Vertical incision in deep cervical fascia, followed by retraction of the strap muscles.
- Division of thyroid isthmus (if required)
- Incision on the trachea.
- Insertion of tracheostomy tube.
- Closure of the wound.
  Types of tracheostomy tubes:
  - *Portex:* More expensive, less traumatic, used more commonly
  - *Metallic:* Less expensive, more traumatic
  - The portex tubes may be cuffed or uncuffed. Cuffed tubes are routinely used during tracheostomy to provide secured airway for ventilation and prevent aspiration. Uncuffed tubes are generally used in maintenance of the stoma once the tract is formed after 48–48 hours.

Postoperative Care

Initial post op care includes propped up positioning for the patients, regular humidification, suctioning and oxygen monitoring of the patient

Complications

These may be divided into immediate and late complications.
Immediate complications: Hemorrhage, bronchospasm, apnea and cardiac arrest.
Other complications include dislodgement of the tube, surgical emphysema, pneumothorax, infection, necrosis, tracheoesophageal fistula, tracheal stenosis. The patient may also face difficult decannulation, tracheocutaneous and scarring.

Nursing Responsibilities

- Give Fowlers position to patient, this will assist in breathing.
- Monitor tracheostomy tube for patency and sudden expulsion.
- Monitor patient for any signs of respiratory distress.
- Monitor patient for any complications.
- To handle emergencies, in case of accidental expulsion of tube, all emergency articles must be available at bed side of patient. Tray must contain additional tracheostomy tube, cleaning lotions, scissors, dilator, dressing supplies, double hook retractor. A tray with tracheostomy suctioning articles must be kept ready. In addition, oxygen, respirator, humidifier, Ambu bag and suction machine must be available at patient bedside.
- Provide patient warm, humidified air.
- Practice aseptic measures to prevent respiratory infection. Change tracheostomy dressing daily.
- Advise patient for sufficient fluid intake to keep respiratory tract moist.
- Patient with tracheostomy must be informed about various communication methods to use, e.g., communication board, writing in a diary, using pictures etc.
- Provide teaching to the patients/caregivers regarding care of the tracheostomy tube with permanent tracheostomy before discharge.

DEVIATED NASAL SEPTUM

CONCEPT AND DEFINITION

Deviated nasal septum (DNS) refers to any displacement of the septum from midline.

TYPES OF DNS

1. Anterior dislocation
2. **C shaped deviation:** Due to bowing of the septum to one side
3. **S shaped deviation:** Due to bowing of the septum on both sides at different places, either in antero-posterior or the vertical place. May cause bilateral nasal obstruction
4. **Spur (Fig. 5.4):** Shelf like projection at the bony-cartilaginous junction
5. **Thickening:** Generalized and diffuse thickening of the cartilaginous or bony septum.

EPIDEMIOLOGY

Deviated nasal septum is one of the commonest causes of nasal obstruction. It may be hereditary. Racial predisposition

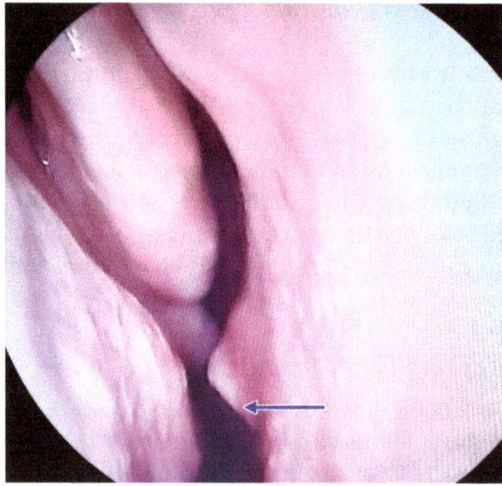

Fig. 5.4: Endoscopic view showing bony spur almost in contact with the inferior turbinate.

has also been reported with Caucasians being more affected by this condition. Almost 70% of the world's populations is thought to have some degree of septal deviation with a majority of them on the left side.

ETIOPATHOGENESIS

Trauma and developmental defects are said to the major causes of a deviated nasal septum.
- ❖ Trauma may be overt as in cases of blows to the face or forgotten if inflicted during childhood. A difficult labor may also cause a deviated nasal septum in the child.
- ❖ An error during the development of the midface may also cause the septum to become deviated.

CLINICAL MANIFESTATIONS

Nasal obstruction including recurrent bouts of rhinitis and mechanical obstruction due to a grossly deviated septum are the most common and major symptom of DNS. The other manifestations include:
- ❖ **Sinusitis:** Due to secondary obstruction of the ostia of the paranasal sinuses.
- ❖ **Headache/facial pain:** Due to concurrent sinusitis, anterior ethmoidal nerve syndrome/Sluder's neuralgia.
- ❖ **Epistaxis:** Due to sharp spur/recurrent rhinosinusitis, external deformity in cases of gross DNS, recurrent otitis media.
- ❖ Other uncommon symptoms include noisy breathing, snoring, sleep apnea, hyposmia and nasal deformity.

DIAGNOSIS

- ❖ **Cold spatula test:** A cold Lac's tongue depressor is placed under the nostrils and the patient is asked to breathe out over it. Decreased fogging of the spatula is observed on the side of the obstruction.
- ❖ **Other tests for nasal patency:** The spatula may be replaced by a cotton wick, the relative movement of which may indicate the site of obstruction.
- ❖ **Cottle's test:** The cheek is pulled away from the nose by placing the flat of the fingers on the cheek of the affected side. If the obstruction gets relived, the prognosis for the patient is good after surgical correction.
- ❖ Paranasal sinus tenderness for concurrent sinusitis.
- ❖ **Anterior rhinoscopy:** Appreciate the type and grade of septal deviation/features of sinusitis
- ❖ Diagnostic nasal endoscopy to confirm findings
- ❖ **X-ray:** Useful only in cases of gross deviation
- ❖ **CT scan (non-contrast) (Fig. 5.5):** To look for the bony deformity

MANAGEMENT

Medical Management

In cases of minor deviation, no intervention is required. If the patient presents with features of sinusitis, it should be treated first before instituting definitive management.

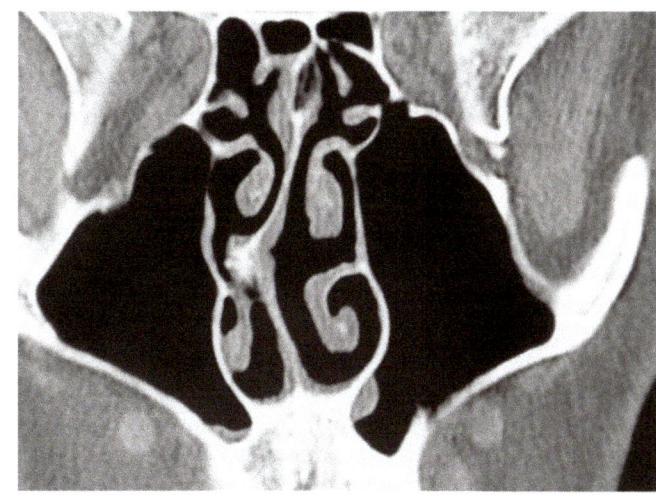

Fig. 5.5: Deviated nasal septum.

Surgical Management

Surgical management should be offered only in case of presence of symptoms. Two types of surgery have been traditionally performed for DNS—submucous resection (SMR) and septoplasty.

The surgery should not be performed in young children as it may hinder or disrupt the development of the nasal framework causing a gross deformity later in life.

Steps of septal correction: (Common to both SMR and Septoplasty):
1. **Killian's incision:** Vertical incision taken a few mm behind the mucocutaneous junction; Freer's incision (hemitransfixion incision)—taken over the caudal dislocation anteriorly
2. Mucoperichondrial and mucoperiosteal flap elevated on one side by anterior and inferior 'tunnelling'

SMR: The flap on the other side is raised by making an incision over the cartilage a few mm behind the first incision or tunnelling behind the columella. The entire septum—cartilaginous and bony is excised and flaps are reposed.

Septoplasty: It is more conservative. Only the deviated parts of the septum are excised, and the flap is raised only on one side.

NURSING MANAGEMENT

- ❖ Provide propped up position
- ❖ Humidification of respired air
- ❖ Monitoring the patient for anterior or posterior nasal bleed
- ❖ If the patient is planned for some surgical procedure, try to reduce his anxiety by informing about the surgical procedure and its need.

NASAL TRAUMA

EPIDEMIOLOGY

Nasal fracture is amongst the commonest features of facial trauma. This is due to the fact the nose is a projecting structure on the face and most prone to exposure during trauma.

ETIOPATHOGENESIS

It is usually traumatic, due to blunt force trauma to face. Depending upon the direction of the impact, the types of fracture may differ, as listed below:
1. **"Jarjaway" fracture:** It occurs due to a blow from the front.
2. **"Chevallet" fracture:** Septal cartilage fracture due blow from below.

CLINICAL MANIFESTATIONS

Local: Nasal bleed/epistaxis, nasal deformity, contusion/abrasions/laceration, localized pain, swelling, nasal obstruction in case of blood clots or gross deformity.
Deformity, edema, tenderness, bony crepitus.

DIAGNOSIS

- **Anterior rhinoscopy:** Active bleeding or blood clots, septal deviation.
- Diagnostic nasal endoscopy to confirm findings
- **X-ray:** Nasal bone (bilateral lateral view) **(Fig. 5.6)** to look for the alignment of the nasal bones look for any dislocation.
- **CT scan:** CT scan offers more details regarding the bones fractured, the type of fracture and helps in formulating a plan of management.

MANAGEMENT

Medical Management

- Control of bleeding
- Analgesics
- **Steroids:** May be used in case of concurrent orbital trauma or severe edema under the cover of antibiotics
- Cold fomentation in case of edema

Surgical Management

Depends on when the patient presents, the clinical features and the type of fracture.
- In case of un-displaced fractures, no surgical management if required

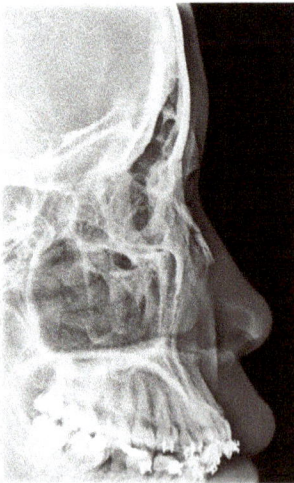

Fig. 5.6: X-ray lateral view showing fracture of the nasal bone.

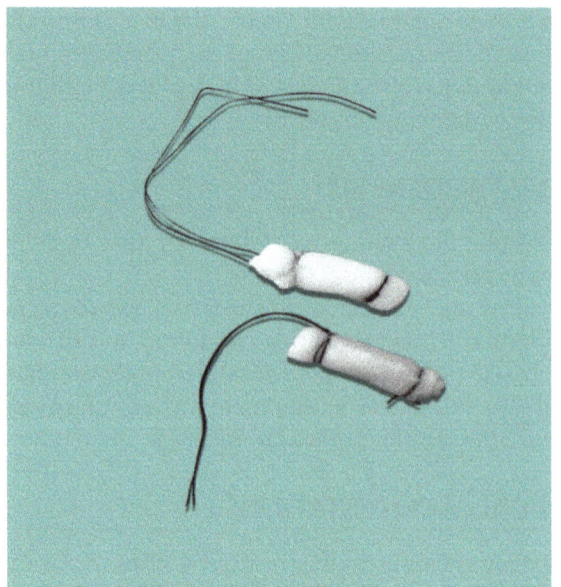

Fig. 5.7: Anterior nasal packs.
(*Courtesy:* Shutterstock).

- In cases of displaced fractures, if the patients present within 6 hours and edema has not set in, they can be taken up for fracture reduction immediately. In case the inflammation has set in, it is allowed to resolve before reduction is attempted.

Technique

- **Under general anesthesia:** Nasal bone out-fracture using Walsham's forceps.
- Asch's forceps are then used to centralize, align and raise the septum wherever required.
- Anterior nasal packing **(Fig. 5.7)** is done and splint applied to hold the position until healing.

NURSING MANAGEMENT

- Patient should be kept in propped up position to help with the pain and edema.
- Monitor for bleeding from nose.

Follow Up

Follow up is required for removal of any sutures and to monitor for any nasal or orbital complications.

NASAL POLYPS

CONCEPT AND DEFINITION

Nasal polyp is defined as prolapse of the nasal mucosa. Nasal polyposis has traditionally been classified as:
- Ethmoidal polyps
- Antrochoanal polyp

EPIDEMIOLOGY

Antrochoanal polyp is usually seen in children at a mean age of 4 years. Ethmoidal polypi are usually seen in adults.

TYPES

Ethmoidal Polyps

Etiopathogenesis

Nasal polyps may occur as a result of chronic inflammatory conditions or disorders of ciliary motility. The common causes are as listed below:
- Chronic rhinosinusitis/allergic fungal sinusitis
- **Asthma/aspirin intolerance:** As a part of Sampter's triad (nasal polypi, asthma and aspirin intolerance)
- Cystic fibrosis
- Motility disorders (Kartagener's syndrome, Young's syndrome)
- **Churg:** Strauss syndrome
  Due to repeated attacks of inflammation, there is oedema of the mucosa which over long term prolapse to form polypi. Ethmoidal polyps generally arise from the lateral nasal wall, mainly the ethmoidal air cells.

Clinical Manifestations

Ethmoidal polyposis is generally bilateral and multiple.
- **Local:** Nasal obstruction leading to mouth breathing, change in voice if extensive—rhinolalia clausa, anosmia/hyposmia, features of allergy, nasal mass
- **General symptoms:** Headache, features of allergy (sneezing, watering from eyes, itching, nasal discharge)

Diagnosis
- **Anterior rhinoscopy:** Smooth, glistening, pale grape like mass, usually sessile. On probing, they are soft, insensitive to touch, do not bleed and the attachment is localized to the lateral wall.
- Diagnostic nasal endoscopy to confirm findings and attachment.
- **X-ray:** PNS may show opacification of the sinuses.
- CT scan may be done to assess the anatomical landmarks, look for the extent of the tumor, any hint of bony erosion or other signs of neoplastic or malignant etiology.

Management
- **Medical management:** During initial stages avoidance of the inciting allergen, antihistamines and nasal steroids may help the edematous mucosa to revert to normal. A short course of oral steroids may be considered in case of acute exacerbation, in the absence of other co-morbidities.
- **Surgical management:** Functional Endoscopic Sinus Surgery remains the only surgical therapy currently recommended for polyposis. It is termed 'functional' as the normal mucosa is to retain the function and preserve the ciliary clearance.
  Other surgical methods previously practiced include polypectomy, intranasal ethmoidectomy, extranasal ethmoidectomy. Caldwell Luc surgery was performed in cases of recurrence.

Antrochoanal Polyp

Etiopathogenesis

Antrochoanal polyp arises from the maxillary sinus. As the word suggests, there are different parts to an antrochoanal polyp. It has an antral (stalk-like), a nasal (flattened) and a choanal (globular) part. It is thought to be infectious in origin and generally seen in young children. Various theories have been proposed to explain the pathophysiology of antrochoanal polyps.

Clinical Manifestations

Ethmoidal polyposis is generally bilateral and multiple:
- **Local:** Unilateral nasal obstruction, change in voice if choanal part obstructs the nasopharynx—rhinolalia clausa, snoring, mouth breathing, nasal mass, mucoid nasal discharge
- **General symptoms:** Headache, features of allergy (sneezing, watering from eyes, itching, nasal discharge)

Diagnosis
- **Anterior rhinoscopy:** Usually not visible unless it is large as AC polyps grow posteriorly. In case of large polyps, we may observe a single, smooth, greyish mass obstructing the nasal cavity, may be reddish pink in case of superimposed infection.
- *Posterior rhinoscopy* to assess the choanal part of the antrochoanal polyp.

Bulge in the soft palate on oral examination in case of large polyps:
- X-ray PNS shows the opacification in the maxillary sinus and corresponding nasal cavity. The choanal part may be identified in the nasopharynx. It can be differentiated from the primary nasopharyngeal masses due to presence of the column of air behind it.
- CT scan may be done to assess the anatomical landmarks, look for the extent of the tumor, any hint of bony erosion or other signs of neoplastic or malignant etiology.

Management

The management of an antrochoanal polyp is surgical removal.

Functional Endoscopic Sinus Surgery

It should be ascertained that the entire mass is removed in its entirely as any remnant may cause recurrence.

Steps
- Medialization of the middle turbinate
- Uncinectomy
- Widening of the maxillary ostium
- Complete excision of the polyp with the stalk.

CARCINOMA LARYNX

CONCEPT AND DEFINITION

Cancer of the larynx is a malignant tumor in and around the larynx (voice box).

TYPES

Supraglottic, glottic, subglottic

EPIDEMIOLOGY

Squamous cell carcinoma is the most common form of cancer of the larynx (95%). Cancer of the larynx occurs more frequently in men than in women, and it is most common in people between the ages of 50–70 years of age.

ETIOLOGY

Carcinogens that have been associated with laryngeal cancer include tobacco (smoke or smokeless) and alcohol and their combined effects, as well as exposure to asbestos, mustard gas, wood dust, cement dust, tar products, leather, and metals. It has been reported that the rates of laryngeal malignancy is 10–15 times higher in smokers than non-smokers.

Other contributing factors include low socioeconomic status, chronic laryngitis, gastroesophageal reflux, nutritional deficiency (riboflavin), and family predisposition/genetic factors.

Some studies have suggested that human papilloma virus (HPV) may also play a role in the etiopathogenesis of laryngeal malignancy.

PATHOPHYSIOLOGY

Persistent carcinogenic exposure causes metaplasia of the epithelial lining of the larynx and mucosa followed by dysplasia. This dysplasia, if unchecked may proliferate leading to rapid seeding of the malignant cells.

Also supraglottis is very richly supplied by lymphatics causing early metastasis into lymph nodes and lungs.

CLINICAL MANIFESTATIONS

Clinical features and presenting complaints differ depending upon the region involved:
- **Glottic tumor:** Voice change, Hoarseness, Hemoptysis, Dyspnea, Respiratory obstruction, Dysphagia, Weight loss, Pain.
- **Supraglottic tumor (Fig. 5.8):** Aspiration on swallowing, Persistent unilateral sore throat, foreign body sensation, Dysphagia, Weight loss, Mass in neck, Hemoptysis
- **Subglottic tumor:** Dyspnea, airway obstruction, dysphagia, weight loss, hemoptysis

COMPLICATIONS

Respiratory distress (hypoxia, airway obstruction), hemorrhage, infection, aspiration.

DIAGNOSIS

History and clinical examination:
- Indirect laryngoscopy
- Direct laryngoscopy and biopsy for histopathological evaluation
- CT scan/MRI—to evaluate the extent, spread and involvement of the malignancy

MANAGEMENT

Treatment of laryngeal cancers depends on the staging of the tumor, which includes location, size, and histology of the tumor and the presence and extent of cervical lymph node involvement. The most widely accepted staging system is the American Joint Committee on Cancer (AJCC) staging **(Tables 5.1 to 5.3).**

Treatment options include Surgery (partial or total laryngectomy) Radiation therapy and Chemotherapy.

With organ and function a priority in recent times, patients with early stage disease (stage I or II' early/intermediate cancer) are usually treated with chemo-radiation therapy with or without surgical intervention like transoral or endoscopic laser resection.

Patients with stage third or fourth or advanced tumors require combined treatment modalities consisting of either surgery or chemoradiation or all three.

Dietetics

Strictly avoid tobacco and alcohol. It has been seen that continued smoking after diagnosis and management is associated with poorer survival outcomes and a higher rate of recurrence.

NURSING MANAGEMENT OF PATIENTS

Nursing Assessment

Assess patient for symptoms as hoarseness, dyspnea, sore throat, dysphagia, burning or pain in throat, swelling in neck. Assess ABG values, pulse oximetry and FiO_2 levels.

Nursing Diagnosis

Preoperative
- Fear and anxiety related to the diagnosis and surgery
- Knowledge deficit related to surgery and postoperative care

Postoperative
- Ineffective airway clearance related to surgical incision in the airway
- Impaired verbal communication related to the removal of larynx

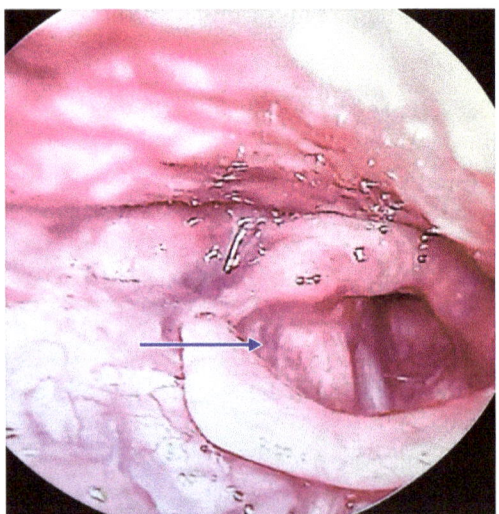

Fig. 5.8: Hopkin's endoscopic picture (70°) showing an ulcer proliferative growth in the larynx.

TABLE 5.1: Tumor staging is based on local extent and prescence/absence of vocal cord fixation, according to AJCC 8th edition. Pathologic T staging is identical to clinical staging.

Glottis

Clinical T stage	Local extent	Vocal cord function
1	Limited to vocal cord: a. Limited to one vocal cord b. Involving both vocal cords	Normal
2	Other laryngeal subsite (supraglottis, subglottis)	+/− Impaired mobility
3	Limited to the larynx. Invasion of paraglottic space or inner cortex to thyroid cartilage	+/− Fixation
4a	Outer cortex of thyroid cartilage and/or tissues beyond larynx (trachea, soft tissues of neck, thyroid, esophagus)	Any
4b	Inoperable disease—prevertebral space invasion, carotid artery encasement, mediastinal invasion	Any

Supraglottis

1	Limited to one supraglottic subsite	Normal
2	More than one supraglottic subsite or glottis or adjacent extraglottic site	No fixation
3	Limited to the larynx. Invasion of preepiglottic space or postcricoid are or inner cortex of thyroid cartilage	+/− Fixation
4a	Outer cortex of thyroid cartilage and/or tissues beyond larynx (trachea, soft tissues of neck, thyroid, esophagus)	Any
4b	Inoperable disease—prevertebral space invasion, carotid artery encasement, mediastinal invasion	Any

Subglottis

1	Limited to subglottis	Normal
2	Extends to vocal cords	+/− Impaired mobility
3	Limited to the larynx. Invasion of inner cortex of thyroid cartilage	+/− Fixation
4a	Outer cortex of thyroid cartilage and/or tissues beyond larynx (trachea, soft tissues of neck, thyroid, esophagus)	Any
4b	Inoperable disease—prevertebral space invasion, carotid artery encasement, mediastinal invasion	Any

TABLE 5.2: Clinical and pathologic nodal staging based on size, number, laterality and presence/absence of extranodal extension (ENE), according to AJCC 8th edition.

Clinical nodal stage	Involvement
X	Not assessed
0	No clinically-positive nodes
1	Single ipsilateral positive node, ≤3 cm
2	Single positive node, >3 but ≤6 cm
2a	Single positive node, >3 but ≤6 cm
2b	Multiple ipsilateral nodes, >3 but ≤6 cm
2c	Contralateral or bilateral nodes, >3 but ≤6 cm
3	Any node >6 cm
3a	>6 cm, ENE (−)
3b	Any lymph node with clinical ENE (+)

Pathologic nodal stage	Involvement
X	Not assessed
0	No regional lymph node metastasis
1	Single ipsilateral positive node, ≤3 cm and ENE (−)
2a	Single ipsilateral positive node, >3 but ≤6 cm and ENE (−) or ≤3 cm and ENE (+)
2b	Multiple ipsilateral nodes, ≤6 cm and ENE (−)
2c	Contralateral or bilateral nodes, ≤6 cm and ENE (−)
3a	>6 cm, ENE (−)
3b	Single ipsilateral node >3 cm and ENE (+), or multiple lymph nodes (any laterality) with ENE (+), or single contralateral lymph node any size and ENE (+)

TABLE 5.3: Stage groupings according to T, N, and M staging, according to AJCC 8th edition. For all subsites, T3–4 disease or any nodal involvement are considered locally advanced.

Grouping	TNM staging
Stage I	T1N0M0
Stage II	T2N0M0
Stage III	T3N0M0 T1–3N1
Stage IVA	T4aN0-1M0 T1–4aN2M0
Stage IVB	T4bN0-3M0 T1–4bN3M0

- Self-care deficit related to pain, fatigue and surgery
- Low self-esteem related to impaired body image secondary to neck surgery
- Knowledge deficit related to care after surgery
- Anxiety and depression related to surgical procedure

Goals

The main goals are to:
- Maintain patent airway
- Reduce the anxiety of patient about surgery
- Maintain hydration and nutrition
- Improve self-care by providing knowledge
- Use effective communication through alternative methods

Nursing Interventions

- **Reduce fear and anxiety** of patient by informing about surgical procedure and its need. Initiate training of patient in communication means planned to be used postoperatively
- **Maintaining patent airway:**
  - Observe and check patients' vitals, difficulty breathing, restlessness
  - Provide Fowler's or semi-Fowler's position after recovery from anesthesia
  - Encourage early ambulation and make patient to turn, take deep breaths and cough and perform suctioning whenever required
  - Provide adequately humidified environment to reduce cough, mucus production and crusting in peri stomal area using nebulizers
  - Teach patient cleaning and changing of laryngectomy tube and removing secretions when stoma has led within 6 weeks postoperatively
- **Using alternative communication methods:**
  - Initiate training of patient in communication means planned to be used postoperatively e.g., picture board, writing slate
  - Provide a call bell within access of patient
  - Do not put infusions in the dominant hand used by patient for drawing, writing
  - Initiate early rehabilitation of patient after laryngectomy
- **Monitoring for complications:**
  - Monitor patient for restlessness, agitation, hypoxia respiratory distress, oxygen saturation
  - Monitor surgical site for bleeding
  - Check the wound for poor healing, infection

Discharge Planning

- Teach patient and family members about clearing secretions and maintaining airway
- Demonstrate cleaning and care of the stoma and peristomal skin
- Explain family members and patient about alternative methods of communication
- Inform about follow ups
- During bathing stoma to be covered
- Maintain humidification using nebulizer
- Demonstrate technique of changing tracheostomy tube safely
- Wear loose clothing and prevent any irritation around stoma with tight clothings
- Inform about signs and symptoms of infection and how to identify them
- Educate about doing frequent mouth care and its need
- Inform measures to handle emergencies as bleeding and dyspnea

In Brief Nursing Care

- Checking vital signs, spO_2, FiO_2
- Giving semi Fowler's to high Fowler's position
- Monitoring oxygen therapy
- Tracheostomy care and suctioning
- Chest physiotherapy and nebulization
- **Nutrition:** Tube feeding—start oral feeding with fluids and semi-soft foods
- Communication—give pen and paper—communication board—constant conversation with the patient
- Rehabilitation, prosthesis and voice therapy wherever applicable.
- Keep the patient comfortable and maintain humidification of air to reduce respiratory effort.

OBSTRUCTIVE SLEEP APNEA

DEFINITION

Obstructive sleep apnea (OSA) is defined as a repetitive obstruction of the upper airway during sleep causing hypoxemia with arterial oxygen desaturation, which leads to a reduced quality of sleep. It is a sleep disorder that involves cessation or significant decrease in airflow despite the presence of breathing effort. It is the most common type of sleep-disordered breathing (SDB) and is characterized by recurrent episodes of upper airway (UA) collapse during sleep.

CRITERIA FOR DIAGNOSIS

Complete obstruction of the airway should occur repeatedly during sleep for more than 10s in the presence of continued movement of the diaphragm, leading to a reduction of greater than 4% in arterial oxygen saturation (SaO_2) from the baseline.

Anatomical and Physiological Reasons for the Development of Sleep Disordered Breathing

Macroglossia and a wide-tongue base, retrognathia, tumors of the upper airway, craniofacial disorders (Pierre Robin syndrome, Down syndrome, Marfan syndrome, Prader-Willi syndrome), neuromuscular disorders, tonsillar hypertrophy, neck girth of 17 inch or more, brachycephalic head form, inferior displacement of the hyoid, adenoid hypertrophy (particularly in children and young adults), high, arched palate (particularly in women), polyps, septal deviation, tumors, trauma, stenosis, retropalatal obstruction-elongated, posteriorly placed palate and uvula, tonsil; retroglossal obstruction.

CLINICAL PRESENTATION

Obesity with BMI >30; neck girth >17 inch; excessive snoring and daytime sleepiness; symptoms of GERD; episodes of breathing cessation during sleep, abrupt awakenings accompanied by gasping or choking, awakening with a dry mouth or sore throat, morning headache, difficulty concentrating during the day, mood changes, such as depression or irritability.

Other systemic examination to rule out hypertension, DM, hypothyroidism:
- The typical appearance of the tongue in a patient with OSA-'crenellations' or indentations on the lateral borders of the tongue (made by the teeth).
- Mallampati score of 4.
- Redundant pharyngeal mucosal folds
- The Epworth Sleepiness Scale (ESS) may be used to assess this condition in patients with day time somnolence. An ESS score of 12 is associated with a greater propensity to fall asleep on the Multiple Sleep Latency Test (MSLT). ESS is useful for evaluating responses to treatment; the ESS score should decrease with effective treatment.

PATHOPHYSIOLOGY

OSA is caused by soft tissue collapse in the pharynx. This occurs due to generation of negative intraluminal pressure during inhalation causing collapse of the surrounding tissue and subsequent airway obstruction.

The pathophysiology of OSA may be technically explained as a consequence of changes in transmural pressure during sleep. Transmural pressure is the difference between intraluminal pressure and the surrounding tissue pressure. If transmural pressure decreases, the cross-sectional area of the pharynx decreases. If this pressure passes a critical point, pharyngeal closing pressure is reached. Excessive pharyngeal critical pressure (Pcrit) causes the tissues to collapse inward causing obstruction.

DIAGNOSTIC INVESTIGATIONS

Polysomnography (gold standard), EEG, DICE (drug induced sleep endoscopy), lipid profile, thyroid profile, craniocorpography.

Indices for sleep-disordered breathing:
- **Apnea-hypopnea index (AHI):** The AHI is defined as the average number of episodes of apnea and hypopnea per hour. It is derived from the total number of apneas and hypopneas divided by the total sleep time. The classification based on AHI is as mentioned below:
  - 5-5 episodes per hour as normal.
  - 5-5 episodes per hour for mild.
  - 5-5 episodes per hour for moderate.
  - More than 30 episodes per hour for severe.
- **Respiratory disturbance index (RDI):** It is defined as the average number of respiratory disturbances [obstructive apneas, hypopneas, and respiratory event-related arousals (RERAs)] per hour.

MANAGEMENT

Medical Management

Weight reduction, CPAP, and treating the underlying cause are the main management strategies.

CPAP is considered the most effective treatment for OSA. It increases the caliber of the airway in the retropalatal and retroglossal regions by increasing the lateral dimensions of the UA and thinning the lateral pharyngeal walls. It helps maintain upper airway patency during sleep, preventing the soft tissues from collapsing.

Complications and adverse effects include sensation of suffocation or claustrophobia, difficulty exhaling, inability to sleep, musculoskeletal chest discomfort, aerophagia, sinus discomfort, pneumothorax and/or pneumomediastinum (extremely rare), pneumocephalus (isolated case report), tympanic membrane rupture (rare). Mask-related problems include skin abrasions, rash, and conjunctivitis. Nasal problems may include rhinorrhea, nasal congestion, epistaxis, and nasal and/or oral dryness.

Despite its suitability CPAP is often not well tolerated by patients and surgical intervention may be required.

Surgical Management

The surgical management depends upon the level of obstruction. The various surgeries performed to alleviate OSA include septorhinoplasty, nasal valvuloplasty, turbinate reduction, maxillomandibular advancement, hypoglossal nerve stimulator, hyoid suspension, uvulopalatopharyngoplasty (UPPP), partial glossectomy and epiglottoplasty.

Nursing Management

- Educate the patients about importance of weight reduction.
- Use CPAP if prescribed.
- In case surgical procedure is planned, inform about surgical procedure to reduce their anxiety and enhance understanding about need of surgery.

GERIATRIC CONSIDERATIONS

Airway obstruction in much more common in elderly as compared to their younger counterparts. Ageing causes:
- Decline in muscle tone
- Reduced immunity
- Chronic illnesses

All these factors predispose to airway obstruction in the geriatric population. Also any symptoms of airway obstruction in a geriatric patient with risk factors like tobacco exposure has a much higher malignant potential as compared to other age groups. The differential diagnoses for airway obstruction varies greatly in different age groups.

Furthermore, management of airway obstruction in the elderly has its own challenges.
- Dental problems like loose teeth and caries can become dislodged and impede suctioning and airway clearance.
- Decreased muscle tone puts them at a risk of iatrogenic trauma during bag mask ventilation and intubation.

- Cognitive dysfunction and impairment of mobility makes positioning a challenge. Also, the former reduces compliance in such patients.
- There could also be difficulty in maintenance of oxygen saturation due to reduced cardio-pulmonary reserve in elderly people.

Case Scenario

1. A 4-year-old boy presented with complaints of right sided nasal obstruction since 6 months. It is associated with purulent nasal discharge. There is no obvious pathology on anterior rhinoscopy. There is no associated history of snoring and mouth breathing. On oral examination there is bulging of the soft palate.
   a. What is your probable diagnosis and why?
   b. What is the etiopathology of the disease.
   c. Discuss the management of the patient including investigations and interventions.
2. A middle aged male presented to the emergency with complaints of hoarseness for 8 months. He now has difficult and noisy breathing over the last 10 days which has become acute over the past 2 days. On presentation, his pulse is 101/min, respiratory rate 26/min, SPO$_2$ is 82% and falling. He has audible and noisy breathing with visible respiratory efforts.
   a. What will you do at the presentation in emergency? Describe briefly.
   b. What is your probable diagnosis?
   c. How will you manage the patient definitively?

SUMMARY

- Airway obstruction refers to narrowing of any part of the airway causing an impediment to the passage of air. It is usually classified as upper or lower airway obstruction.
- One of the main characteristics of upper airway obstruction is production of a high-pitched sound due to turbulence during the flow of air at the region of constriction. This sound is called **'stridor'**. Upper airway obstruction usually produces inspiratory stridor.
- It is a life-threatening condition and requires immediate intervention. Securing the airway is of prime importance and the first line of management.
- In severe obstruction the patient may require intubation or tracheostomy. It is the surgical procedure wherein we make an incision on the trachea and exteriorizing it. It provides a definite airway and relieves all forms of laryngeal obstruction.

MULTIPLE CHOICE QUESTIONS

1. **All are true about ethmoidal polyps, *except*:**
   a. Multiple
   b. Bilateral
   c. Allergic etiology
   d. More commonly seen in the first decade of life
2. **The best way to diagnose laryngomalacia is:**
   a. Symptoms and signs of disease only
   b. Soft tissue lateral view neck
   c. Direct laryngoscopy under general anesthesia
   d. Flexible laryngoscopy
3. **The treatment of antrochoanal polyps is:**
   a. Wait and watch
   b. Systemic steroids
   c. Endoscopic sinus surgery
   d. Antihistamines
4. **Sluder's neuralgia is seen in which of the following conditions:**
   a. Nasal polyps
   b. Spur
   c. Hypertrophic inferior turbinate
   d. Concha bullosa
5. **Arteries in Kiesselbach's plexus are all, *except*:**
   a. Anterior ethmoidal
   b. Greater palatine
   c. Superior labial
   d. Posterior ethmoidal
6. **All are causes of stridor, *except*:**
   a. Laryngomalacia
   b. Croup
   c. Asthma
   d. Carcinoma larynx
7. **Indication for high tracheostomy is:**
   a. Carcinoma larynx
   b. Bilateral vocal cord paly
   c. Prolonged intubation
   d. Subglottic stenosis
8. **Which of the following is the etiological factor for acute laryngotracheobronchitis?**
   a. *Haemophilus influenzae*
   b. Respiratory syncytial virus
   c. Parainfluenzae virus
   d. *Streptococcus pneumoniae*
9. **Gold standard for the management of OSA is:**
   a. Uvulopalatopharyngoplasty
   b. Septoplasty
   c. CPAP
   d. Glossectomy
10. **All are true for supraglottic cancer, *except*:**
    a. Hoarseness is the first symptom
    b. Most aggressive of all laryngeal malignancies
    c. High incidence of nodal metastasis
    d. Commonest site is the epiglottis

ANSWERS

1. d	2. c	3. c	4. b
5. d	6. c	7. a	8. c
9. c	10. a		

SUGGESTED READING

1. Calder I, Pierce A. Core topics in Airway Management. Cambridge: Cambridge University Press; 2016.
2. Cathain EO, Gaffey MM. Upper Airway Obstruction. [Updated 2020 Oct 22]. In: StatPearls [Internet]. Treasure Island (FL): StatPearls Publishing; 2021.
3. Chan DK, Truong MT, Koltai PJ. Supraglottoplasty for occult laryngomalacia to improve obstructive sleep apnea syndrome. Arch Otolaryngol Head Neck Surg. 2012;138(1):50-4.
4. Cooper T, Benoit M, Erickson B, El-Hakim H. Primary Presentations of Laryngomalacia. JAMA Otolaryngol Head Neck Surg. 2014.
5. Daly R. Diagnosing and managing patients with inducible laryngeal obstruction. Nursing Times. 2020;116(12):38-40.
6. Dhingra PL (Ed). Diseases of Ear, Nose and Throat, 6th Edition. New Delhi: Elsevier.
7. Edge S, Byrd DR, Compton CC, Fritz AG, Greene FL, Trotti A. American Joint Committee on Cancer—Head and Neck cancer staging 2007, 7th edition. Philadelphia: Springer; 2010.
8. Kashima HK, Shah F, Lyles A, Glackin R, Muhammad N, Turner L. A comparison of risk factors in juvenile-onset and adult-onset recurrent respiratory papillomatosis. Laryngoscope. 1992;102(1):9-13.
9. Linda K. Clarke. Management of clients with upper airway obstructions. In: Black J. Hawks J. Medical surgical nursing. 7th edition. India. Elsevier; 2005. pp. 1802-3
10. Say SDS. (2018, November 8). Airway Obstruction in The Elderly: What You Need to Know. SSCOR. Retrieved January 13, 2022, from https://blog.sscor.com/airway-obstruction-in-the-elderly-what-you-need-to-know.
11. Watkinson, John C. Scott-Brown's Otorhinolaryngology and Head and Neck Surgery, 8th edition. Boca Raton: Chapman and Hall/CRC; 2018.

CHAPTER 6

Speech Defects and Speech Therapy

Sanjay Munjal, Anuradha Sharma

"Speech is power: Speech is to persuade, to convert, to compel."

—Ralph Waldo Emerson

LEARNING OBJECTIVES

After going through the chapter, the learner will be able to:
- Discuss various disorders of speech impairment.
- Enumerate the classification and causes of articulation disorders.
- Appreciate various assessment and treatment methods for congenital and adult voice disorders.
- Explain the prevention, assessment, and intervention methods for the normal non-fluency and stuttering disorders.
- Discuss the geriatric considerations in speech disorders.

TERMS

- **Articulation:** Production of speech sounds using the mouth, lips, and tongue.
- **Communication:** Exchange of information between individuals by speaking, writing, or using some other medium.
- **Fluency:** Ability to speak with good flow, accuracy, and proper expression.
- **Language:** The comprehension and/or use of a spoken (listening and speaking), written (reading and writing), and/or other communication symbol system.
- **Speech:** The communication or expression of thoughts in spoken words
- **Voice:** The sound produced by humans and other vertebrates using the lungs and the vocal folds in the larynx, or voice box.

INTRODUCTION

Speech disorder in children and adults is a widespread disabling problem. These disorders can impact the communication skills of the people which further may influence their personal and professional life. The most common speech disorders both in children and adults are articulation disorders, voice disorders, and fluency disorders. Children with speech sound disorders can have problems in the phonological representation of the sounds which may affect their speech clarity. The speech intelligibility varies depending on the characteristic features and other associated problems. Individuals with facial structural anomalies, cleft lip and palate, malocclusions, and neuromuscular disorders may have severe difficulties in speech.

Another speech disorder commonly seen is voice disorder which can be classified as acquired and congenital. The primary treatment of individuals with congenital laryngeal abnormalities is medical and surgical. These infants must be closely monitored for the possible development of abnormal voice. Congenital abnormal larynx may develop as mass lesions or structural abnormalities. Acquired voice disorders such as vocal nodules, polyps, etc., can be treated with various techniques of speech therapy directly. These types of voice disorders are more prevalent in adults as compared to children.

Fluency disorders are characterized by core behaviors and secondaries present in an individual's speech. Primary (core) behaviors may include prolongations, repetitions, pauses, and blocks. Secondaries are learned behaviors that individuals develop over time. Secondary behaviors may be present in the form of poor eye contact, avoidance, eye blinking, shaking of hands or legs. All these behaviors can have a major impact on individuals' personality. "Stuttering" is usually confused with "normal disfluency", which typically emerges when children are acquiring language. Some therapy techniques are indirect, where the speech pathologist works with the caregivers and modifications are made in the home environment. Direct therapy is also given where the therapist works on the client depending on the nature of the speech problems.

Individuals face extreme difficulties while giving interviews for jobs as speech disorders can hamper communication abilities, success rate, academic achievements, career, and confidence. So it is very important to know about such types of disorders and the possible management options available for the particular disorder.

SPEECH DEFECT

"It can be defined as a condition that interferes with the mental formation of words or their physical production". In India prevalence of speech disorders is more as compared to developed countries. Konadath et al. (2017) reported the prevalence of speech defects to be 6.07% in India's rural area, where the population strength was 15,441.

Speech defects can be classified as:
- Speech sound disorders (articulation disorders)
- Voice disorders
- Fluency disorders

ARTICULATION DISORDERS

"Articulation is an acquisitional process that also involves the gradual development of the ability to move the articulators in a precise and swift manner".

Articulation disorder can be described as a speech sound disorder that incorporates problems in the production of speech sounds (Elbert and Gierut, 1986). It can also be defined as "disturbances in the speech-motor processes, which results in the production of sounds that are remarkably distinct from usual productions".

Speech sound errors (also called SODA errors) can be divided into 4 categories **(Fig. 6.1)**:

1. **Omissions:** Production of some sounds is not there; whole syllables or classes of sounds might be missing; e.g., di' for dish or 'at for bat.
2. **Additions:** One or more sound or sounds are added to the target word; e.g., tomomato for tomato.
3. **Distortions:** Sounds are changed or altered.
4. **Substitutions:** When one or more sounds are replaced for other; e.g., lat instead of rat

Incidence and Prevalence
The prevalence ranges from 2–25% of children between 5–7 years of age [Law, Boyle, Harris, Harkness, and Nye (2000)].

Etiology
Etiology can be classified as organic, non-organic, or mixed. Organic causes have a known structural, physiologic, neuromuscular, sensory, or cognitive deficit in the vocal tract or related structures. The non-organic cause has no apparent structural abnormalities, and mixed causes include both organic and non-organic factors.

Structural, Physiologic and Neurological Causes

Various structural, physiological and neurological causes of articulation disorders are:
- **Teeth:** Malocclusions of teeth may contribute to misarticulations.
- **Tongue:** Structural deviations like ankyloglossia (also called tongue-tie in which small, thick or tight band of tissue tethers the bottom of the tongue's tip to the floor of the mouth), aglossia (congenital defect in which tongue is completely absent or partially developed), macroglossia (unusually large tongue), microglossia (abnormally small tongue), etc., may compromise speech intelligibility and articulation.
- A cleft palate can also result in misarticulation.
- Dysarthria and apraxia are two other major neuromuscular problems that lead to articulation disorders.

Sensory Perceptual Factors

Various sensory perceptual factors responsible for articulation disorders are hearing impairment, auditory perception, oral/sensation perception, and visual acuity."

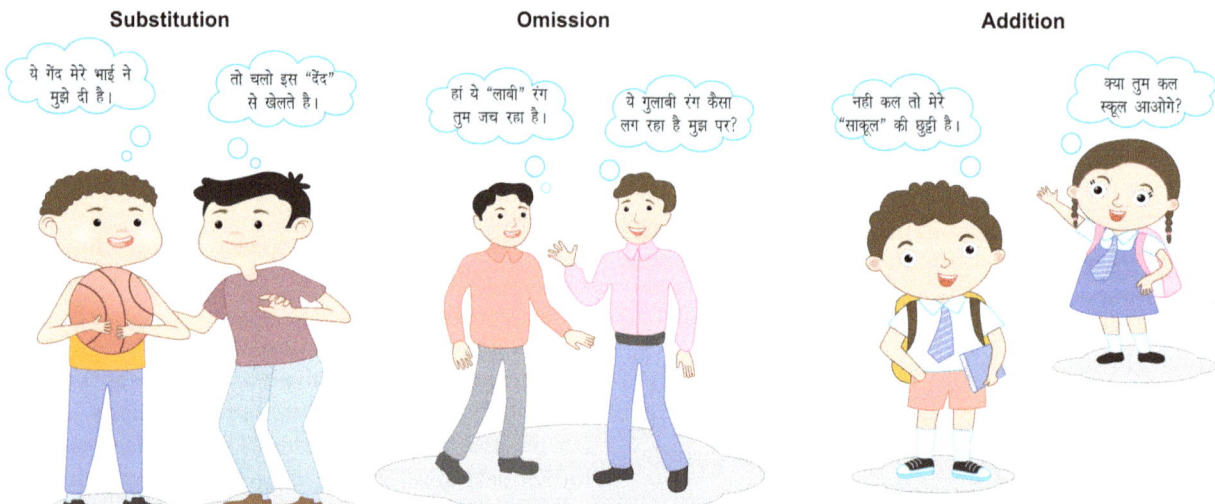

Fig. 6.1: Speech sound disorders.

Cognition

Cognition can also interfere in the production of accurate speech sounds when the intelligence quotient is lower than the normal range.

Genetic Components/Surroundings/Psychosocial Issues

These issues like limited speech models, inappropriate speech stimulation and reinforcement, lack of motivation, episodes of trauma, and other emotional responses can affect the speech in an individual.

Interpersonal Factors

Age, sibling status, socioeconomic status, and gender play a significant role in the development of children's speech."

Other Factors

Other factors such as cleft lip and palate, apraxia of speech, dysarthria, mental retardation, cerebral palsy, Down's syndrome, stuttering, voice disorders can be associated with inaccurate speech productions.

Assessment of Articulation Disorders

Whenever speech sound disorder is suspected, screening is carried out for a child's comprehensive speech and language assessment. The screening aims to identify individuals who require further speech-language evaluations and referral for other professional services.

Screening generally involves:
- Assessment of oral mechanism to screen the strength and range of motion of oral structures
- Examination of orofacial structures for the identification of facial asymmetry and other abnormalities (e.g., cleft lip and palate, malocclusion, etc.)
- Informal assessment of speech and language reception and expression.

Single-word testing provides information about the production of almost all the consonants in the language. However, the production of the consonants may or may not be the same in connected speech. Therefore, it is important to carry connected speech testing. It provides information about the articulation of sounds in connected speech using various tasks (e.g., narrating a story, picture portrayal, typical discussion about a subject of interest) and with various individuals (e.g., friends, teachers, guardians, etc).

Speech Therapy for Speech Sound Disorder

"Articulation treatment procedure focuses on teaching one sound at a time and then moving to words, phrases and sentences, reading and then conversation the function of sounds. It is based on the principle of phonetic placement of sound ". Prognosis is usually good if treated at an earlier age. Articulation disorders are often treated by teaching the child how to produce the sound physically. Then they are asked to practice its production until it becomes natural. The target word is selected according to the stimulability of the child. Initially, auditory and visual feedback is given to the child so that he/she can differentiate between correct and incorrect sounds. They have to practice the target word first in isolation, vowel combination, and then at word level in all the positions (initial, medial and final). When the child can speak the target sound at the word level, he/she is asked to practice at sentence-level and then at story level so they can speak correctly and clearly in connected speech. Finally, the focus is on the generalization of the sound so that the child can communicate clearly in any context and all the situations while having a conversation with others.

VOICE DISORDERS

When the quality, pitch, loudness, or flexibility of a person's voice differs significantly from the voice of others of similar age, cultural group, and sex, voice disorder can be suspected. According to the American Speech and Hearing Association (ASHA) "voice disorder is present when an individual expresses concern about having an abnormal voice that does not meet daily needs even if others do not perceive it as different or deviant". Voice disorders can be present by birth or they can also be acquired.

Congenital Voice Disorders

Voice disorders present at birth resulting from the laryngeal anomaly are referred to as congenital voice disorders. Primary management with congenital laryngeal anomalies is medical and surgical, but these children should be carefully monitored for the possible development of voice disorders. Symptoms include respiratory difficulties due to airway obstruction, hoarseness, or a weak or aphonic cry and dysphagia. Congenital anomalies can be either mass-size lesions or structural anomalies. It can be classified into supraglottic anomalies, glottic anomalies, and subglottic anomalies."

Supraglottic Anomalies

Saccular cysts: These cysts are usually small in size and are filled with fluids, appear in the larynx (ventricle). Congenital cysts have the same origin as laryngoceles.

Glottic Anomalies

Vocal cord paralysis: It can be due to birth trauma when the recurrent laryngeal nerve is stretched during various delivery procedures (commonly forceps and breech delivery) or it can be associated with central nervous system anomalies.

Vocal cord immobility: Vocal cords' restricted movement is the most common congenital disorder. It can lead to feeding issues, breathiness while crying, and choking.

Laryngeal webs: It is a type of occluded larynx due to the formation of a mesh of connective tissue in the subglottis, glottis, and supraglottis regions. Congenital webs of the larynx have adverse effects on both respiration and phonation.

Subglottic Anomalies

Subglottic hemangiomas: Large, purplish-red, sessile tumors below the glottis are called as subglottic hemangioma. These types of anomalies are not seen commonly and these lesions are generally treatable. It can cause obstruction in the airway passage in children. Sometimes they might spread sub-mucosally into other regions of the larynx.

Laryngeal cleft: It is a vertical split between the laryngeal (cricoid cartilage) and the esophageal region, forms due to incomplete fusion of the cricoid lamina. The cleft might be restricted to the laryngeal area or form a laryngo-tracheoesophageal cleft.

Acquired Voice Disorders

Vocal Nodule (Fig. 6.2), "Nodes, Singer's Nodes, Screamer's Nodes"

"Nodules are benign growths that develop on the epithelium of the vocal folds as a result of vocal hyperfunction and inflammation". The vocal cords close with high muscular tension, when these abnormal collision forces are generated, it results in the damage of tissues.

Etiology of Acquired Voice Disorders

Trauma to the vocal folds is the most common cause of nodules. Gastroesophageal reflux disease and laryngo-pharyngeal reflux have also been implicated in around 2/3rd of speakers with nodules. Some conditions like chronic cough, dehydration in vocal folds, an endocrine disorder, allergies, infection in the larynx, throat clearing, and upper respiratory tract infections can also be the causes of the development of vocal nodules.

Appearance and Site

The vocal nodes commonly occur on both folds. These nodules are present with a wide base, bright white in color. They generally emerge at a medial position between the anterior 1/3rd and posterior 2/3rds of the vocal fold or the point of the maximum amplitude of vocal cords vibration.

Clinical Characteristics

Characteristics of vocal nodules range from mild to serious symptoms and incorporate hoarseness, breathiness, brought down pitch, strain, vocal exhaustion. Often, individuals report that their voice quality is best early in the first part of the day and worsens as time passes. Some patients have complaints of sore throat or pain in the neck region that might radiate towards the ear or to the chest area. Some clients experience foreign body sensations in the "throat". Problems in the production of higher pitches are a common difficulty, specifically faced by singers.

Perceptual Sign

A hoarse and breathy voice is the most remarkable sign of nodules. The severity of the hoarse and breathy component depends on the size of the nodule.

Laryngoscopy Findings

Stroboscopic examination shows a reduction in mucosal waves, all through the vocal cord, and completely absent in the region of nodes. The stroboscopic examination helps in revealing the voice parameters such as reduced fundamental frequency and increase in aperiodicity. A typical "hourglass" pattern of the incomplete glottis is seen, and a glottal chink might be present. The area around the nodes may be swollen, inflamed and red.

Management

Voice therapy is the preferred course of treatment for nodules. Surgical intervention should be avoided if possible to minimize the risk of damage to the layers of lamina propria. Initially, trial therapy can be given for 42 days to reduce the swelling and edema. The voice rest should be given until re-epithelialization of the vocal folds occurs, usually approximately three days.

Vocal Fold Polyps (Fig. 6.3)

Polyps are generally caused by single vocal fold trauma in which excessive vocalizations lead to hemorrhaging of superficial layer lamina propria at the maximum glottal contact point. This hemorrhaging condition finally results in polyp formation. Initially, the polyp is small and sessile but becomes pedunculated as the disorder advances. Low pitch rough voice with restricted pitch range are the key signs of the disorder. The patient usually reports a lump in his/her throat. Inhaled allergens and smoking are also among the contributing factors for vocal fold polyps.

Clinical Characteristics

The characteristics are similar to that of vocal nodes, although polyp usually happens unilaterally. There is breathiness and

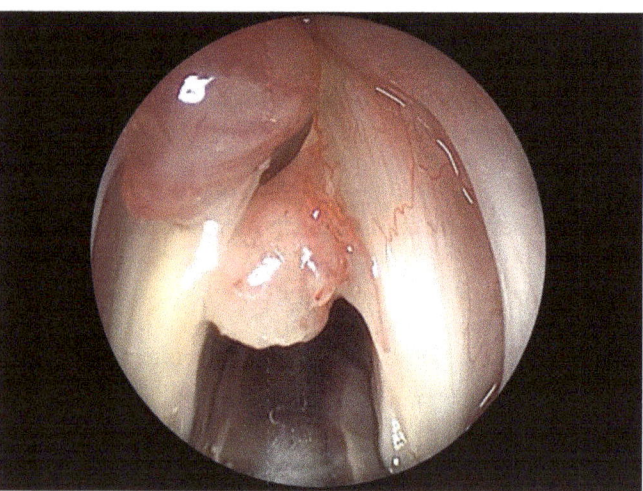

Fig. 6.2: Vocal fold nodule.

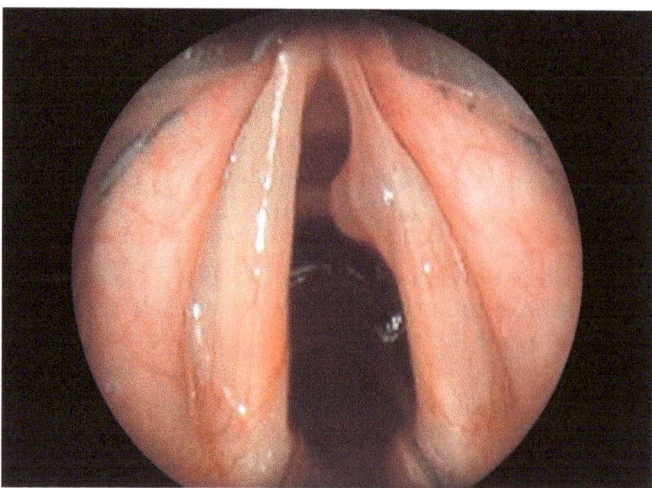

Fig. 6.3: Unilateral polyp (see the right vocal fold).

roughness in voice due to restricted vocal fold movement. The abnormality in voice characteristics depends on the size of the polyp.

Perceptual Signs

Along with vocal tract discomfort features, individuals with polyp have a feeling of 'something in the throat' ("Globus sensation"). Individuals have a problem in clearing sputum from the larynx. A hoarse and breathy voice is also a common sign.

Laryngoscopic Findings

Polyps are usually large with a wide base and a stalk-like structure is also attached to the vocal cords. The size of polyp can range from a small "blood blister" to a large "pedunculated mass". The polyp can be visualized easily if it is present on the outer edge of the vocal cords. Some large polyps are still not fully visualized as they hang into the subglottis and are superiorly into the glottis while production of voice.

Management

Management depends upon the size and shape of the polyp. For small and translucent polyp voice therapy is the first treatment of choice. While large and fibrotic polyp are mostly treated by surgery. Microflap and epithelial cordotomy are the widely used surgical techniques. Voice therapy is then applied to stabilize voice characteristics, improving lifestyle and diminishing the possibility of reoccurrence.

Vocal Cord Cyst (Fig. 6.4)

Cyst arises in the larynx whenever the duct of the mucous gland gets blocked. The blockage leads to the accumulation of keratin and sebum in the sac of the duct. Excessive use of voice, laryngopharyngeal reflux, allergy, and infection of the respiratory tract are among the underlying causes of this disorder. It mainly arises at the interior surface just below the free edge.

Perceptual Signs and Symptoms

Hoarse voice and reduced pitch are the common signs. The individuals might report a "tired" voice.

Laryngoscopy Findings

It may be difficult to identify the cyst. Bouchayer et al., reported that on examination 10% of their population had clear cyst. However, 55% of the patients had signs indicating the presence of a cyst. Sometimes on endoscopic examination light reflection is seen from the area where the cyst is present. On laryngoscopy increased mass and dilated capillaries are seen.

Management

Surgical management is the best treatment of choice for vocal fold cyst. Voice therapy is generally followed after the surgical procedure to stabilize voice characteristics.

Reinke's Edema (Fig. 6.5)

Reinke's edema or polypoid degeneration is a condition in which voice trauma leads to disruption in the collagen architecture and eventually result in the development of thick gelatinous fluid within Reinke's space. Due to the increased mass of vocal folds, voice is mostly low pitch and hoarse. In advance stages, vocal cords start occluding the airway, and the patient reports shortness of breath as the main symptom. On laryngoscopy, diffuse swelling of the vocal fold is seen.

Appearance and Site

It incorporates a superficial layer, "Reinke's space", which is usually bulged and, primarily on VF's superior layer.

Signs and Symptoms

Reduced pitch and hoarse voice are common symptoms. The client might report shortness of breath if the size of the lesion is large as it can block the airway passage. Some of the patients complain of a reduction in the pitch range and increased effort to phonate.

Laryngoscopic Findings

On examination large fluid-filled boggy structures can be observed. They are usually present literally on the entire length of vocal cords. Reinke's edema appears similar to a wide-based polyp covering VF's entire length in some aspects.

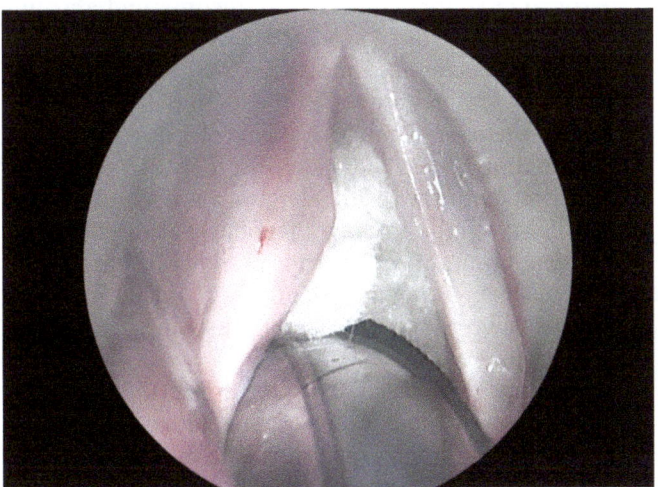

Fig. 6.4: Vocal cyst.

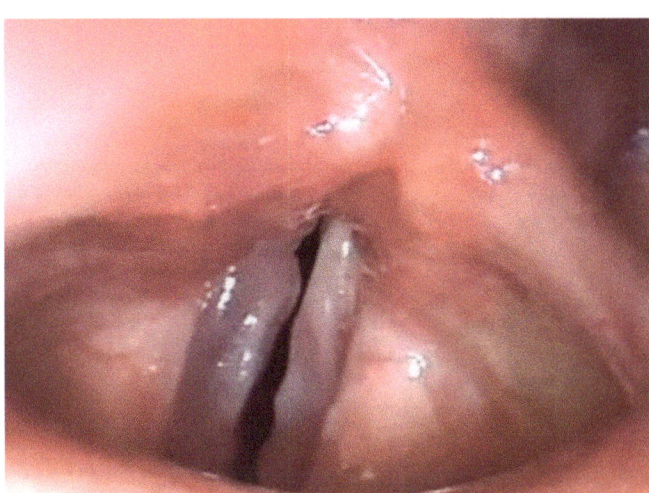

Fig. 6.5: Reinke's edema covering entire length of vocal folds.

Perceptual Characteristics

It results in a very low pitch and is associated with the severity of the lesion. The range of pitch is also affected due to an increase in the mass of vocal folds. Edema reduces the potential to increase VF tension leading to a reduction in loudness.

Management

Voice programs which include vocal reeducation and eliminating causative factors such as irritants are most responsive to this condition. Surgical management involves the removal of redundant vocal fold mucosa. Smoking and laryngopharyngeal reflux can cause delayed and abnormal recovery. Indirect and voice therapy approaches may help restore the patient's vocal quality as far as possible.

Sulcus Vocalis (Fig. 6.6)

It is a voice disorder in which furrow or depression develops at the medial edge of the vocal fold. This furrow can be localized or diffused covering the entire length of the cord. It can be congenital or acquired. Depression or furrow may be confined to a single superficial layer or can even extend to the ligament. Furrow generally gives a spindle-like configuration.

Causes

During embryonic development, incomplete development of layers of vocal folds may result in the congenital sulcus. Patients with congenital sulci typically have a lifelong history of disordered voice. Acquired sulcus may be related to age, degeneration, vocal fold weakness, repeated chronic inflammation, infection, and laryngeal surgery.

Perceptual Signs and Symptoms

It results in a stiff and compromised mucosal wave. Voice is low-pitched and strained. Due to glottal incompetence, patients put extra effort to achieve optimum loudness which can lead to increased laryngeal muscle tension.

Laryngoscopy Findings

A sulcus might be seen as a furrow or line along with the upper medial edge of the vocal cords. The furrow may be present on the full length of the vocal cord. The groove may be deep or shallow. The sulcus is located in the superficial layer of the lamina propria, which reduces the mass of the cover but may increase its stiffness.

Management

Treatment involves a combination of voice therapy and surgical management. Alone therapy may not be that effective in eliminating the voice difficulties caused due to sulcus/scar. Hence, surgical treatment might be required which include implantations of substances like human collagen, hyaluronic acid, bovine, autologous fat, fibroblasts, and bioinjection. To increase the flexibility of vocal cords open surgical procedures are also recommended.

Voice Therapy

Voice therapy is based on three main principles:
1. **Remove obstacles:** It involves removing the underlying causes that are obstructing normal laryngeal functions. It ranges from teaching proper voice usage to manually manipulating the position of the larynx.
2. **Provide feedback:** Optimum feedback is essential for effective voice therapy. Feedback can be auditory, visual, or tactile.
3. **Individualized therapy:** Voice therapy should be planned according to the age, occupation, motivation, voice needs, and general health of the patients.

Various voice therapies are discussed as follows:
- **Hygienic voice therapy:** It is generally the initial step in most voice rehabilitation programs. It includes eliminating vocal abusive behaviors such as screaming, whispering, vocal noises, throat clearing, shouting, coughing, and inadequate hydration. Vocal abusive and unhygienic voice behaviors are identified in this program. Modification of such behaviors can reduce the vocal symptoms without manipulating the other subsystems of voice. The nodules resolve by reducing the vocal abusive behavior, and the voice may improve.
- **Relaxation:** It primarily focuses on decreasing the excessive muscular tension by providing a relaxed way to phonate. Chewing and yawn sigh are the main techniques that are helpful in relaxation.
- **Voice rest:** It is an indirect voice therapy technique that is based on the assumption that avoiding phonation promotes self-healing. Depending upon the severity and associated factors clinician can recommend absolute voice rest or modified voice rest. Confidential voice rest can also be given in some patients which involves the usage of a low breathy voice for communication.
- **Throat clearing:** Gradually throat clearing becomes a habit in individuals with voice disorders due to sputum secretion associated with allergies, flu, and cold or as a secondary symptom of laryngopharyngeal reflux. This behavior occurs primarily in the presence of mass lesions and vocal cord edema. "Silent cough" technique along with relaxation has been suggested to eliminate this kind of behavior.
- **Hydration:** The vocal hygiene program not only considers elimination and modification of traumatic vocal behaviors, but it must also attend to the health of the tissue lining of the true vocal folds and larynx. Internal hydration is an

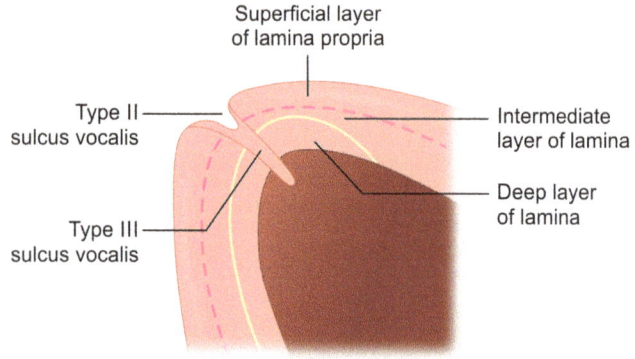

Fig. 6.6: Sulcus vocalis.

essential component of good vocal hygiene. Literature has shown that laryngeal dehydration leads to increased stress on the vocal system during phonation. Over a period of time, this stress/strain can cause vocal fatigueness, or the development of some pathology in the larynx, or both. The hydration program is helpful for all individuals with voice disorders. Usually, 1–1.5 liter water is recommended per day. The appropriate amount of water varies depending on the type of lesion and lifestyle of the person. Vocal cords should remain moist for their smooth movement. Alcohol and caffeine consumption should be avoided as these can cause dehydration.

- **Symptomatic voice therapy:** Symptomatic voice therapy was introduced by Boone et al. Its primary goal is to focus on the modification of the abnormal perceptual voice components of the subject's voice. Elimination of abuse, Chant talk, Counseling, Auditory feedback, Masking, Yawn-sigh, Relaxation, Open mouth approach, and Laryngeal massage are a few of the techniques used by many speech and language pathologists to eliminate the individuals' difficulties. Management program involves evaluation of the present voice abnormalities and using facilitation methods/approach to bring stability in the phonation. "Symptomatic voice therapy" can be most effective when voice issues are because of inappropriate use of vocal elements.

- **Physiologic voice therapy:** Physiologic voice therapy programs are devised to alter or modify the voice-producing mechanisms' underlying physiology directly. Physiologic voice therapy is a holistic approach for treating voice problems that involve techniques to improve the balance between the supraglottic resonatory structures, laryngeal, and respiratory system. Primarily abnormal physiologic activities are modified by using this method and exercises. Accent method of voice therapy, vocal function exercises (VFE), the manual laryngeal musculoskeletal tension reduction technique (MLMTRT), and resonant voice therapy (RVT), are the different therapy techniques used in the management of voice issues. **Accent method of voice therapy** can improve both speech and voice production. It is also used to treat other disorders like stuttering. It primarily focuses on pulmonary output, reduction of glottis waste, decreases muscle tension and also helps to stabilize the vibrations of the vocal cords. **Vocal function exercises (VFE)** help in recalibration of laryngeal mechanism. These also maintain balance amongst phonatory system. The exercises which can be used in therapy for the treatment of voice disorders include Warm up: sustaining vowel "ee" for as long as possible; Stretching: Pitch glides starting from highest note to lowest note and Contraction: Pitch glides starting from lowest note to highest. **Manual laryngeal musculoskeletal tension reduction technique** primarily focuses on the relaxation of excessive muscle tensions. Excessive muscle tension can affect the function of larynx; therefore it is important to relax these muscles for normal phonation. **Resonant voice therapy** helps in the production of better phonation by enhancing the sensations of vibrations which are felt on the teeth, lips and nose.

Its focus is on easy phonation without excessive force. It also includes voiced and voiceless humming that is shaped into words and sentences.

FLUENCY DISORDERS

"Normal fluency is characterized by the ease and ongoing flow of speech muscular movement and the resultant speech sounds. Speech produced fluently consists of suitable dimensions of (1) rate, (2) continuity, and (3) tension effort". Therefore, different stages of the speech system should function properly and in close coordination.

The various causes of fluency disorders can range from a delay in developmental milestones, emotional personality, short temperament, tension, and frustration. Some other indirect causes can be non-realistic parental demands, positive family history, and minor brain damage/head trauma. The main characteristics of fluency disorders are frequent sound repetitions, prolongations, blocks, irregular rate and rhythm of speech, insertion of a vowel between words **(Fig. 6.7)**. The patients might also show avoidance or refusal to talk to strangers or in a gathering. Sometimes they develop fear in speaking certain sounds. When the subject is trying to come out of stuttering moments with effort, abnormal facial grimacing (eye blinking, raising eyebrows, etc.) can also be observed.

Normal Non-fluency (NNF)

Kindergarten children usually have problems with a speech concerning motor planning and execution; this generally results in disfluencies related to speech development (also called "normal non-fluency" or "other disfluencies"). These types of disfluencies are usually a part of normal speech and language development and are temporarily seen at a very young age when children are at the learning stage.

The term disfluency refers to speech disorganization regardless of whether they occur to be normal or abnormal speech events **(Table 6.1)**.

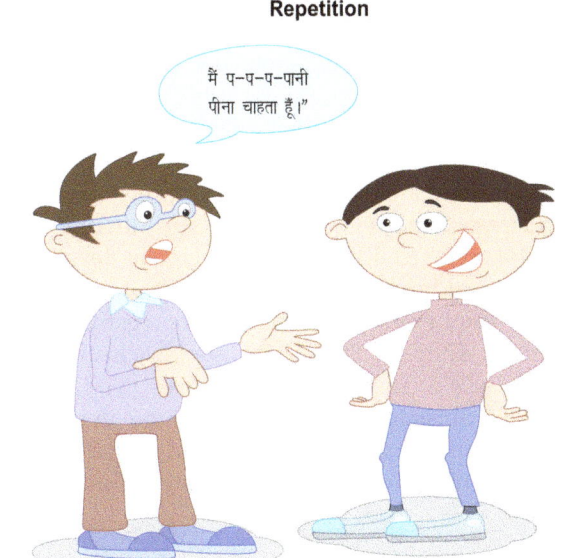

Fig. 6.7: Repetitions, one of the most common characteristics seen in fluency disorder.

TABLE 6.1: Types of disfluencies seen in NNF.

Types of normal disfluency	Example
Part-word Repetition	Ca…cake
Single syllable word repetition	I…I don't want
Multisyllabic word repetition	Reena…Reena is going to market
Phrase repetition	Bhanu is coming…..…Bhanu is coming to play
Interjections	Rakesh is going to the…uh…circus
Revision-incomplete phrase	My ball…. Where is Diana?
Prolongation	She is gooooo….good
Tense pause	I don't want to go (lips together, no sound) out

Normal disfluencies transpire all through adolescence and adulthood. It starts sooner than 1.6 years of age and tops between ages two to three years. It gradually reduces after that yet additionally changes in form. A few sorts of disfluencies, for example, reiterations decline after 3 years, yet different disfluencies, like revisions, might increase. The frequency of disfluencies, recurrence of redundancies, and interpositions are the highlights that separate typical NNF from stuttering. Yairi found that kids somewhere in the range of 2 and 3.5 years showed an increment in amendment and expression reiteration, along with a decrease to some degree in part-word repetitions and interjections.

Revisions, interjections, and repetitions are mostly seen in normal developing children and might increase further as a significant characteristic of their disfluencies with age.

Secondaries are not present in normal disfluent children. Literature has revealed that a typically developing child also shows "tense pauses" occasionally, but this type of tension does not seem to be a response to their disfluencies. If in case children show pauses or interjections frequently, then they should undergo evaluation of stuttering.

Prevention and Counseling

Some young children who begin to stutter recover without treatment. Sometimes early intervention is needed to prevent the development of chronic problems. Once stuttering has become firmly established, it becomes more difficult for the child to deal with it. It has a significant effect on the individual's personal and social life. Since children with normal non-fluency are unaware of their disfluencies, it is better to treat them before it develops into stuttering. Parents should be counseled regarding the typical development of speech and language in children. Clinicians usually tell parents not to make the child aware regarding his/her disfluencies. They should not give repetitive instructions to the child, for e.g., speak properly, why are you talking like this?...etc. Counseling plays an essential role in preventing stuttering as proper guidance is required for the parents by a speech therapist to learn how to deal with normal non-fluency.

Developmental Stuttering

It is generally a developmental disorder that begins at an early age and continues into adult age in at least 20% of the affected individuals. The typical onset of non-fluent speech is 3 years. Although there is variability, primary stuttering behaviors usually consist of word or syllable repetitions, while secondary behaviors such as tension, avoidance, or escape behaviors are absent. With young stutterers, disfluency may be episodic, and periods of stuttering are followed by periods of relatively decreased disfluency.

Neurogenic Stuttering

"The person with neurogenic stuttering has difficulty with rhythm and cannot produce speech fluently and smoothly. Usually, the person(s) knows precisely what they want to say, but they cannot speak it because of involuntary disruptions, prolongation, or halting of a sound. When this type of speech disfluencies occurs in the presence of acquired neurological problems, it is diagnosed as Stuttering Associated with Acquired Neurological Disorders (SAAND)". — WHO.

Assessment of Stuttering

Assessment of stuttering primarily focuses on identifying the type and severity of overt (repetitions, prolongations, blocks) and covert behaviors (when a person who stutters hides his or her dysfluencies from others by substituting or omitting the word). It generally involves taking a relevant history and recording an adequate speech sample of the individual's speech. Scales like Stuttering Severity Instrument (SSI), Stuttering Prediction Instrument (SPI), and Dysfluency Type Index (DTI) are then used to index frequency and type of stuttering. Situational variability should also be kept in mind while assessing the patient with stuttering.

Decisions regarding the treatment of stuttering:
Based on the observations and diagnosis, a clinical decision is made regarding what type of treatment is required. The treatment could be direct or indirect, or together. The prognostic indicators vary widely from client to client. This information should be intimated to the concerned person, guardian or parents. Parent counseling and or comprehensive treatment program can be carried for individuals based on different evaluation procedures.

Management of Stuttering

Van Riper's approach is called MIDVAS; "motivation, identification, desensitization, variation, approximation, and stabilization" can be used to modify stuttering.

- **Motivation:** It is the initial and very important stage. The speech and language pathologist plays a very important role as a guide during the first phase. It is crucial for both speech therapist and client to build a rapport with each other so that client can comfortably express his or her feelings regarding the speech problems. The therapist should motivate the client to stay positive and the client should participate actively for better results and fluent speech.
- **Identification:** This stage focuses on awareness training and encouraging the patient to identify stuttering behaviors. The aim is to eliminate denial and to modify the primary and secondary behaviors.
- **Desensitization:** This stage involves addressing associated negative suspicions and emotions of stuttering. Techniques like relaxation and adaptation are usually included in speech therapy sessions.

- **Variation:** It is followed by desensitization. This stage involves modification of anticipated stuttering behaviors in various settings. This phase is followed after desensitization.
- **Approximation:** At this stage additional techniques are incorporated in therapy to achieve maximum fluency. Most commonly cancellation, preparatory sets, and pullout techniques are used.
- **Stabilization:** Once optimum fluency is attained, therapy sessions can be terminated. At this final stage, the patient gains a positive self-image and starts self-monitoring of stuttering.

Regulated Breathing

Regulation of respiration is designed to help people who cannot speak fluently, to create awareness in them regarding their stuttering moments. In this method, the clinician trains the client to regulate the airflow during conversation or while speaking so that he/she can prevent the occurrence of stuttering. This method incorporates awareness, relaxation, motivation, and generalization training. Literature has revealed that regulation of breathing is a useful method for decreasing the disfluencies in both children and adults. Reports regarding regulated breathing have indicated a decrease in stuttering without a reduction in speech rate.

Cognitive Behavioral Therapy (CBT) for Stuttering

Cognitive behavior therapy (CBT) is the leading treatment for social anxiety disorder, and it also helps in stuttering modification therapy. CBT is based upon the relationship between thoughts, feelings, and behaviors. The therapy focuses on the factors that are causing distress and leading to stuttering. Therapy teaches the elimination of avoidance behaviors, confrontation of fears, and changing negative or unhelpful thinking patterns.

Menzies, Onslow, Packman, and O'Brian have described the symptoms to discover the client's cognitive symptoms and her/his strengths to help speech-language pathologists in management programs. Also, most individuals with stuttering symptoms suffer from feelings of shame and guilt. Therefore, CBT can be incorporated with fluency techniques within the treatment.

GERIATRIC CONSIDERATIONS IN SPEECH DISORDERS

Speech problems are commonly seen in the geriatric population. However, data about the prevalence of voice disorders are not well documented in elderly people. Hoarse voice, vocal exhaustion, strained voice, breathy voice, reduced loudness and pitch are some of the common vocal symptoms in geriatric population. These symptoms may be associated with anatomical and physiological changes in larynx due to ageing process. Most common conditions associated with voice problems in geriatric group are vocal fold paralysis, functional dysphonia (voice problems in the absence of structural or neurologic pathology), laryngopharyngeal reflux, and vocal polyps. With ageing the rate of speech might reduce. Among the fluency disorders, neurogenic stuttering can be seen in elderly population followed by brain injury. However, articulation errors are seen in association with other neurological disorders only. Speech sound disorders without any associated disorder are not seen in elderly population.

Rehabilitation interventions including vocal hygiene program, vocal function exercises, and resonant voice training could be effective in the elderly patients.

Case Scenario

1. A 4-year-old girl was very good in academics. However, her speech intelligibility was not that good. Her parents reported to ENT department with a complaint of lack of speech clarity. She was then referred to audiologist and speech pathologist for further evaluation. Detailed audiological assessment was done to rule out any type of hearing difficulties. The child was not having any other associated problems. So speech therapy sessions were planned for the child for a complete assessment of types of errors at different levels (words, sentences, story, and conversation). Substitutions and omissions were observed in the child's speech after administering standardized tests. Parents were counseled regarding the nature of the speech problem of the child and regular speech therapy was recommended. The child followed regular speech sessions and practiced as advised. The prognosis was very good and speech therapy was effective in the case.
2. A 35-year-old female came with a chief complaint of change in voice and foreign body sensation in the throat. She was a teacher by profession and it became very difficult for her to deliver the lectures because of her voice problem. ENT examination revealed that the client was having bilateral vocal nodules and she was referred to a speech pathologist for further management. The patient was counseled regarding the vocal hygiene program and complete voice rest was recommended initially. Relaxation exercises were also demonstrated. After speech therapy sessions she was again referred back to ENT for stroboscopy. On examination, it was found that the patient had improved significantly. She continued with teaching with some modifications as recommended by the speech pathologist.
3. A 2.5-year-old male child named Yash had disfluent speech. His parents reported that the child is not able to speak properly. They also reported that sometimes the child speaks fluently and sometimes it becomes difficult for him to speak. A complete audiological assessment was done to rule out the hearing loss. The audiological reports were normal. A detailed case history was taken and an assessment was done for the identification of the type of fluency disorder. He was found to have normal non-fluencies. No secondary behaviors were observed during the session. Only part word repetitions were seen at the conversation level. Parents were counseled regarding normal speech and language development. The speech pathologist recommended not to make the child aware of his disfluencies and parents were asked to report after three weeks. In the follow-up session parents reported that the child has improved.

SUMMARY

Speech disorders can have an adverse effect on the quality of life of individuals. Early identification and management are a must for such disorders. Speech and language pathologist plays a very important role in the treatment and management of different types of speech disorders. The various types of speech disorders can be eliminated with the help of speech therapy. Certain cases with associated structural deficits, other medical professionals' attention is also required for better treatment and outcomes. Speech pathologists depend on various characteristic features for making the differential diagnosis. They also consider the risk factors and warning symptoms that point to which patient would get benefit from the treatment. Depending on the type and severity of the disorders speech therapy techniques vary considering the client's difficulties and major concerns.

MULTIPLE CHOICE QUESTIONS

1. Replacement of one or more sounds with another sound is termed as:
   a. Addition
   b. Substitution
   c. Distortion
   d. Omission
2. Ankyloglossia can be defined as:
   a. Unusual small tongue
   b. Unusually large tongue
   c. Tongue-tie
   d. Partially developed tongue
3. Malocclusion of teeth mainly results in:
   a. Voice disorder
   b. Articulation disorder
   c. Normal non-fluency
   d. Stuttering
4. Which of the following is not a congenital voice disorder?
   a. Laryngeal cleft
   b. Subglottic hemangiomas
   c. Laryngeal web
   d. Vocal nodules
5. When the mucus gets trapped, it can result in …………?
   a. Vocal polyp
   b. Vocal nodules
   c. Vocal cyst
   d. Laryngeal web
6. Vocal fold paralysis is a:
   a. Supraglottis anomaly
   b. Glottis anomaly
   c. Subglottic anomaly
   d. Both a and b
7. Expand SSI:
   a. Stuttering severity instrument
   b. Stuttering severity index
   c. Stuttering severity identification
   d. Stuttering severity indicator
8. The client demonstrates newly learned behavior outside the clinical setup. What is it called?
   a. Extension
   b. Motivation
   c. Generalization
   d. Stabilization
9. MIDVAS approach is used to treat which of the following disorder/s?
   a. Misarticulation
   b. Acquired voice disorders
   c. Stuttering
   d. Congenital voice disorders
10. Part word repetitions are commonly seen in:
    a. Developmental stuttering
    b. Neurogenic stuttering
    c. Acquired stuttering
    d. Normal non-fluency

ANSWERS

1. a
2. c
3. b
4. d
5. c
6. b
7. a
8. c
9. c
10. d

SUGGESTED READING

1. American Speech-Language-Hearing Association. (1993). Asha (Vol. 35). The Association.
2. Andrews G, Tanner S. Stuttering treatment: An attempt to replicate the regulated-breathing method. Journal of Speech and Hearing Disorders. 1982;47(2):138-40.
3. Arnold GE. Vocal nodules and polyps: Laryngeal tissue reaction to habitual hyperkinetic dysphonia. Journal of Speech and Hearing Disorders. 1962;27(3):205-17.
4. Barlow JA, Gierut JA. Minimal pair approaches to phonological remediation. In Seminars in speech and language 2002;23(01):57-68. Copyright© 2002 by Thieme Medical Publishers, Inc., 333 Seventh Avenue, New York, NY 10001, USA. Tel.:+ 1 (212) 584–4662.
5. Benninger MS, Alessi D, Archer S, Bastian R, Ford C, Koufman J, et al. Vocal fold scarring: current concepts and management. Otolaryngology—head and neck surgery. 1996;115(5):474-82.
6. Boone DR, McFarlane SC, Von Berg SL, Zraick RI. The voice and voice therapy. 10th, edition Pearson.
7. Bouchayer M, Cornut G, Loire R, Roch JB, Witzig E, Bastian RW. Epidermoid cysts, sulci, and mucosal bridges of the true vocal cord: a report of 157 cases. The Laryngoscope. 1985;95(9):1087-94.
8. Elbert M, Gierut JA. Handbook of clinical phonology: Approaches to assessment and treatment. London: Taylor and Francis; 1986.
9. Hamdan AL, Sataloff RT, Hawkshaw MJ. Non-Laryngeal Cancer and Voice. Plural Publishing; 2020.
10. Jaryszak EM, Collins WO. Microdebrider resection of bilateral subglottic cysts in a pre-term infant: a novel approach. International journal of pediatric otorhinolaryngology. 2009;73(1):139-42.
11. Kandoğan T, Özüer Z. Acoustic difference in voice of the patients with and without organic lesion in functional voice disorders. InKBB-Forum. 2007;6(2):26-9.
12. Konadath S, Chatni S, Lakshmi MS, Saini JK. Prevalence of communication disorders in a group of islands in India. Clinical epidemiology and global health. 2017;5(2):79-86.
13. Ladouceur R, Côté C, Leblond G, Bouchard L. Evaluation of regulated-breathing method and awareness training in the treatment of stuttering. Journal of Speech and Hearing Disorders. 1982;47(4):422-6.
14. Law J, Boyle J, Harris F, Harkness A, Nye C. Prevalence and natural history of primary speech and language delay: findings from a systematic review of the literature. International Journal of Language and Communication Disorders. 2000;35:165-88.
15. Martins RH, Santana MF, Tavares EL. Vocal cysts: clinical, endoscopic, and surgical aspects. Journal of Voice. 2011;25(1):107-10.
16. Menzies RG, Onslow M, Packman A, O'Brian S. Cognitive behavior therapy for adults who stutter: A tutorial for speech-language pathologists. Journal of Fluency Disorders. 2009;34(3):187-200.
17. Murry T, Abitbol J, Hersan R. Quantitative assessment of voice quality following laser surgery for Reinke's edema. Journal of Voice. 1999;13(2):257-64.
18. Ransom ER, Antunes MB, Smith LP, Jacobs IN. Microdebrider resection of acquired subglottic cysts: case series and review of the literature. International Journal of Pediatric Otorhinolaryngology. 2009;73(12):1833-6.
19. Remacle M, Degols JC, Delos M. Exudative lesions of Reinke's space. An anatomopathological correlation. Acta Oto-rhino-laryngologicaBelgica. 1996;50(4):253-64.
20. Salmen T, Ermakova T, Schindler A, KO SR, Göktas Ö, Gross M, et al. Efficacy of microsurgery in Reinke's oedema evaluated by traditional voice assessment integrated with the Vocal Extent Measure (VEM). Acta OtorhinolaryngologicaItalica. 2018;38(3):194.
21. Starkweather CW. Fluency and stuttering. Prentice-Hall, Inc; 1987.
22. Van Riper C. Speech correction. Prentice-Hall; 1972.
23. Van Riper C. The treatment of stuttering. Prentice Hall; 1973.
24. Woods DW, Twohig MP. Habit reversal treatment manual for oral-digital habits. In Tic disorders, trichotillomania, and other repetitive behavior disorders Springer, Boston, MA; 2001. pp. 241-67.
25. World Health Organization. Manual of the international statistical classification of diseases, injuries, and causes of death: based on the recommendations of the ninth revision conference, 1975, and adopted by the Twenty-ninth World Health Assembly. World Health Organization; 1977.
26. Yairi E. Disfluencies of normally speaking two-year-old children. Journal of Speech, Language, and Hearing Research. 1981;24(4):490-5.

CHAPTER 7

Deafness and its Management

Sanjay Munjal, Md Noorain Alam

"Blindness cuts us off from things, but deafness cuts us off from people."
—Hellen Keller

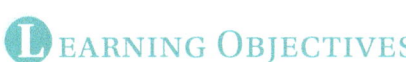 LEARNING OBJECTIVES

After going through the chapter, the learner will be able to:
- Get acquainted with the meaning of hearing impairment.
- Discuss the epidemiology of hearing impairment.
- Enumerate the classification and causes of hearing impairment.
- Appreciate various assessment methods of the hearing impairment.
- Discuss various interventions for the impaired hearing.

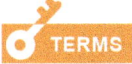 TERMS

- **Acoustic:** Related to sound.
- **Acoustic reflex:** A protective mechanism that involves automatic contraction of the stapedial muscle of the middle in response to loud sounds.
- **American sign language:** A manual communication system used mainly by persons who are congenitally deaf.
- **Audiogram:** A graphic presentation of the hearing test showing hearing levels in dB at various frequencies.
- **Audiometry:** Measurement of hearing using pure tones and speech stimuli.
- **Auditory brainstem response (ABR):** An objective test that detects and measures the electrical activities up to the level of the brainstem in response to the acoustical stimulation of the ear.
- **Bone conduction:** Transmission of sound waves directly to the cochlea by the skull bones.
- **Cerumen:** Ear wax
- **Cochlear implant:** A surgically implanted device that bypasses the external and middle ear directly and stimulates the auditory nerve in persons with severe to profound hearing loss.
- **Conductive hearing loss:** Hearing impairment due to outer and or middle ear problems.
- **Decibel:** A unit of sound intensity or loudness.
- **Hertz (Hz):** A unit of frequency of the sound which also signifies the number of cycles per second.
- **Intensity:** The power or pressure magnitude of sound.
- **Otosclerosis:** A condition in which the footplate of stapes becomes affixed to the oval window causing hearing loss as the vibrations are not effectively transmitted to the inner ear.
- **Presbycusis:** The hearing loss associated with ageing.
- **Speechreading:** Identifying the spoken words visually by observing the speaker's facial expressions, gestures, lip movements.
- **Stapedectomy:** A treatment of otosclerosis in which stapes is surgically removed and replaced with a prosthesis.

INTRODUCTION

Out of five senses, hearing is vital, helping to connect to others and experience our surroundings. It also helps to detect a danger that was crucial for our survival even during the stone age. Hearing plays a central role in communication. For verbal communication to take place, the listener needs to understand the message spoken by the speaker. Similarly, the speaker also hears his/her verbal output, which provides him/her feedback about the correct spoken message.

Hence, the speaker's, as well as the listener's hearing, should remain intact for effective communication to take place. In case of impaired hearing, communication gets affected, and the ability to communicate ideas, emotions, and thoughts to others gets affected. Hearing is one of the basic needs of human beings. Inability to hear the sounds may require extra concentration by the listener which is tiring. It may also cause frustration and confusion in both the listener and speaker leading to avoidance of social gatherings by the persons with impaired hearing. The interpersonal relationship may also get affected due to hearing loss.

DEAFNESS OR HARD OF HEARING

Hearing loss or hearing impairment is the partial or total inability to hear sound in one or both ears. Deafness has been defined by the WHO as a complete loss of the ability to hear from one or both ears. Generally, it refers to the severe to a profound degree of hearing loss, which suggests very minimal or no hearing. Persons with deafness typically do not have a residual hearing to communicate, even with hearing aids. Hearing devices like cochlear implants may help them to hear and learn to speak. Such people may benefit from visual cues like sign language or lip-reading. Based upon the time of onset of hearing loss, people with deafness are divided into two groups, the congenitally deaf and the adventitiously deaf. Congenital means the deafness was present at the time of birth, while adventitiously deaf means the hearing was lost through illness or accident. Similarly, prelingual deafness means deafness was congenital or before the child learns to speak, and post-lingual deafness means deafness occurred after the child has already developed spoken language skills.

Hard of hearing has been defined as complete or partial loss of hearing from one or both ears. The degree of hearing loss may range from mild to severe. People with hard of hearing have enough residual hearing and may use it for communication purposes with hearing aids or other amplification devices like FM systems.

IMPACT OF HEARING LOSS

Hearing impairment negatively affects the physical, cognitive, behavioral, and social functions and the overall quality of life. Lack of proper diagnosis and hearing loss management severely impacts quality of life, autonomy, mental well-being, social integration, and participation. During childhood, hearing loss can lead to delayed speech and language skills, learning problems in school, social isolation, and social stigmatization. Persons with hearing loss have difficulty in obtaining, performing, and keeping an occupation. Hearing loss can be associated with various psychological and cognitive conditions like depression, isolation, and dementia in the elderly population of more than 65 years of age. Older persons who have hearing loss have higher rates of hospitalization, death, and fall, and dementia, and depression compared to the same age population with normal hearing.

EPIDEMIOLOGY OF HEARING LOSS

Hearing loss is one of the most frequent sensory deficits and globally has the fourth highest cause of disability. According to the World Health Organization, the prevalence of disabling hearing loss (hearing loss greater than 40 dB in the better hearing ear in adults (15 years or more) and a hearing loss greater than 30dB in the better hearing ear in children (0–14 years) in the year 2020 has been estimated to be 466 million which is about 6.1% of world's population. Out of this, the number of adults and older adults suffering from hearing loss is estimated to be 432 million (91%). The number of children with disabling hearing loss is approximately 34 million (9%). The total number of hearing-impaired persons will be over 900 million people by 2050. The annual global cost of untreated hearing loss poses an annual global cost of US$ 750 billion (WHO, 2020). According to statistics, 1–2 babies per 1,000 newborns have a profound hearing impairment. As per WHO (2018) data, the prevalence of disabling hearing impairment in India is around 63 million (6.3%). The estimated prevalence of adult-onset deafness in India is about 8%, and childhood-onset deafness is around 2%.

Age has the strongest association with hearing loss among adults in 20–69 years of age. 16.8% of 18 years and older reportedly have difficulty hearing without a hearing aid. Percentage of hearing loss increases with age. It has been estimated that 5.5% of adults in the age range of 18–39 years and 19% of adults in the age range of 40–69 years have hearing loss. Disabling hearing loss affects approximately one-third of persons over 65 years. Men are almost two times likely to have hearing loss than women among adults aged 20–69. Worldwide, the prevalence of hearing loss in the old age-group is greatest in South Asia, Asia-Pacific, and sub-Saharan Africa.

CLASSIFICATION OF HEARING LOSS

Classification of hearing loss is essential for the selection of tests used to assess the hearing further. It also helps for the selection of any medical and or audiological intervention. Hearing loss may be classified based on the **type, degree, and configuration** of the hearing impairment.

Hearing impairment occurs due to the abnormal structure and or function in the auditory system. It is mainly quantified in terms of hearing threshold levels, i.e., the lowest level in decibel or dB across different frequencies at which a signal is just detected by the person at least 50% of the time. The gold standard for measuring thresholds is Pure Tone Audiometry (PTA), suitable for adults and children older than four years of age. The thresholds are plotted on a chart known as an audiogram.

The X-axis of the audiogram represents frequency octaves from 250 Hz to 8000 Hz, and Y-axis represents the intensity in dB (HL) starting from 0–120 dBHL. The pure tone signals are presented through air-conduction (AC) mode, i.e., the signal passes from the outer ear to the middle ear and then the inner ear. AC test is followed by bone conduction (BC) mode, i.e., signal directly stimulates the inner ear. Hearing thresholds obtained through AC and BC tests are used to quantify the degree, types, and configuration of hearing loss.

Types of Hearing Loss

There are mainly three types of hearing loss, i.e., conductive hearing loss, sensorineural hearing loss, and mixed hearing loss.

A. Conductive Hearing Loss

Conductive hearing loss occurs when the lesion impairs the conduction of sound from the environment to the external and the middle ear. On an audiogram (**Fig. 7.1**), it is indicated when the air conduction thresholds are elevated, i.e., above 25 dBHL, but the bone conduction thresholds are within normal limits below 25 dBHL. Conductive hearing loss is often about 60 dB. Any lesion in the external or middle ear that blocks the flow of sound to the inner ear causes conductive hearing loss.

B. Sensorineural Hearing Loss

Sensorineural hearing loss occurs when the lesion is either in the inner ear or cochlea or auditory nerve and auditory pathway. On an Audiogram (**Fig. 7.2**), it is indicated when both the air conduction thresholds and bone conduction thresholds are elevated, i.e., above 25 dBHL, and both the thresholds are the same or having a difference less than 10 dB.

C. Mixed Hearing Loss

Mixed hearing loss occurs due to the combined presence of conductive and sensorineural hearing loss. On an Audiogram (**Fig. 7.3**), it is indicated when both the air conduction thresholds and bone conduction thresholds are elevated, i.e., above 25 dBHL and having an AC and BC difference of 10 dB or more.

D. Central

Any interference with sound transmission from the brainstem to the auditory cortex is termed as central hearing loss. Central hearing loss may lead to problems in auditory comprehension, auditory discrimination, auditory learning, and difficulty in language development.

Degree of Hearing Loss

Hearing loss may also be classified based on hearing loss severity, which corresponds to the hearing threshold on different frequencies. Generally, the degree of hearing loss is decided by taking an average of three frequencies, i.e., 500 Hz, 1000 Hz, and 2000 Hz, also known as speech frequencies. Hearing loss in the range of 26-40 dB is considered mild, 41-55 dB moderate, 56-70 dB moderately severe, 71-90 dB severe, and greater than 90 dB profound.

Degrees of hearing loss, the associated handicap, and educational needs of children with hearing impairment are shown in **Table 7.1**.

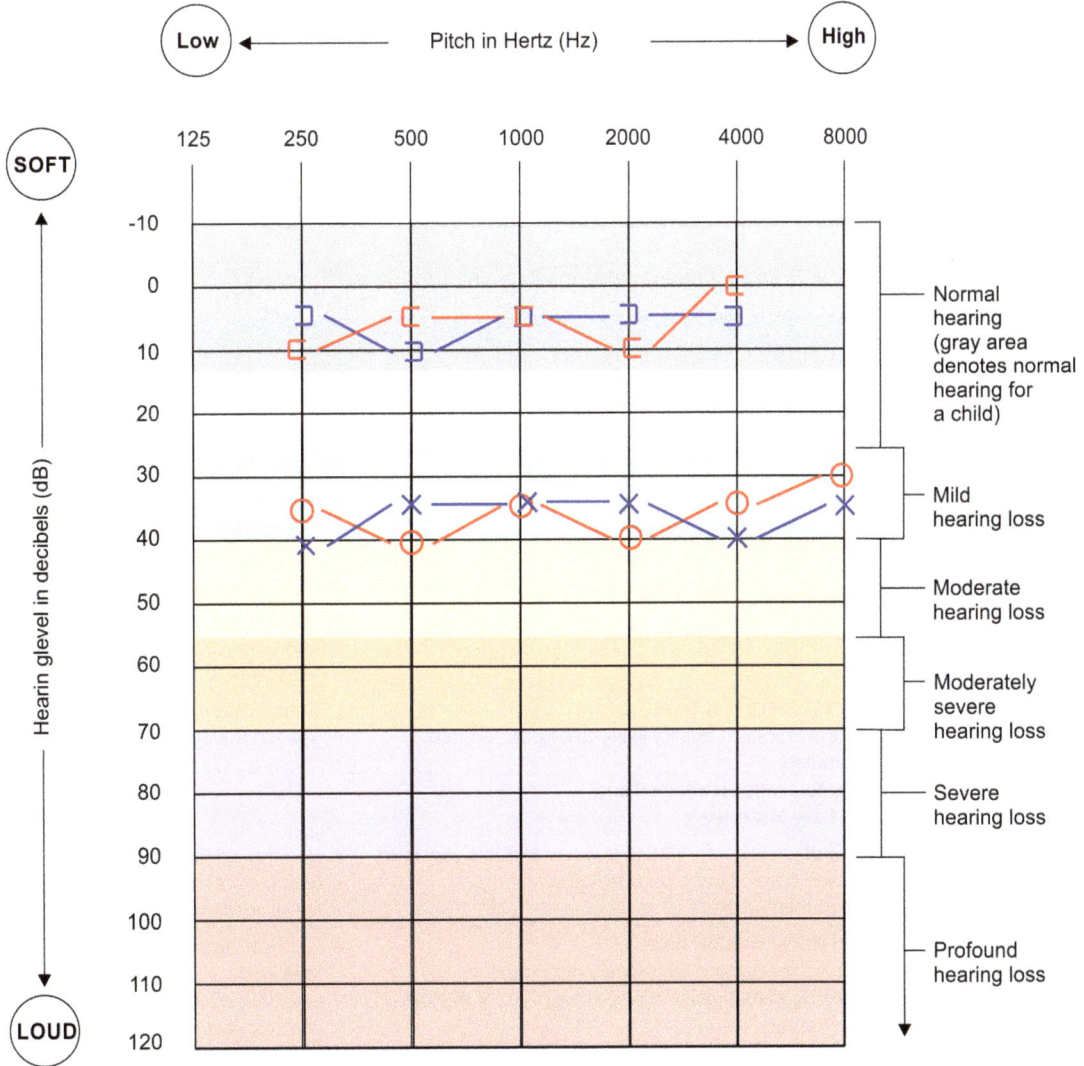

Fig. 7.1: An audiogram showing bilateral conductive hearing loss.

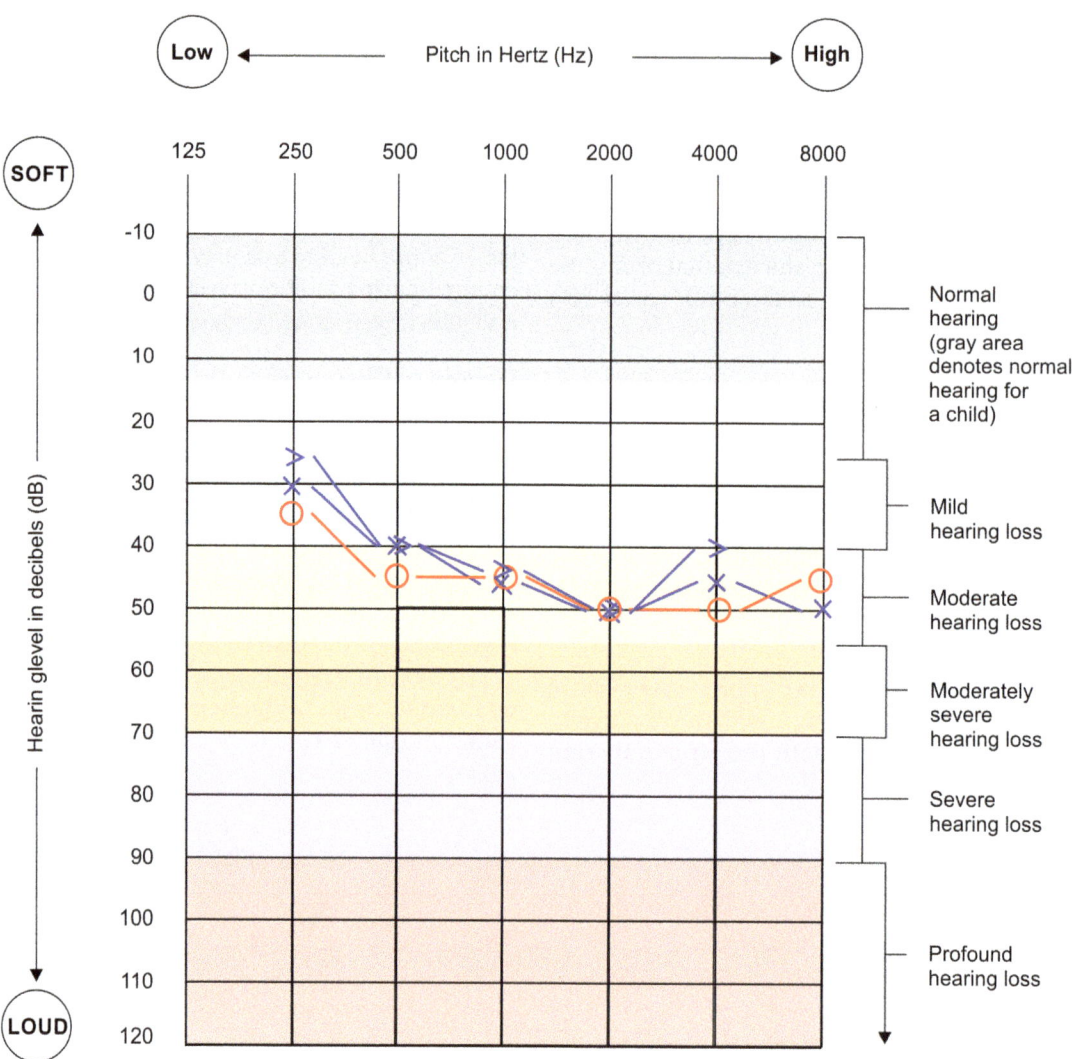

Fig. 7.2: An audiogram showing bilateral sensorineural hearing loss.

TABLE 7.1: Degree of hearing loss, associated handicap and educational needs of children with hearing impaired.		
Degree of hearing loss (Average thresholds of 500 Hz, 1000 Hz, and 2000 Hz)	*Associated handicap and behaviors without amplification*	*Educational needs*
0–15 dB HL (Normal hearing)	Can detect all aspects of the speech signal	No special needs
16–25 dB (Slight)	• May miss up to 10% of speech in noise • May respond inappropriately • Peer social interaction affected	• Medical management of ears • The teacher needs to be made aware of the impact on instruction
26–40 dB (Mild)	• May miss up to 50% of speech • Self-esteem affected	• Hearing aid or personal FM unit and preferential seating • May need special language, vocabulary, and reading help
41–55 dB (Moderate)	• 50% of speech may be missed • Voice and speech quality likely to be poor, limited vocabulary • Communication is affected and • May have low esteem	• Amplification • Speech therapy and special education
56–70 dB (Moderately severe)	• 100% of speech information is lost unless it is very loud • Delayed speech and poor intelligibility • Social isolation likely	• Hearing aid essential • Resource teacher or special class likely needed for all academic areas
71–90 (Severe)	• Loud voices possibly heard • Delayed speech and language if prelingual • Declining speech abilities and atonal voice if the loss is post lingual	• Full-time amplification essential • Special class with caregiver's choice of method emphasized (auditory/verbal, signing, or total communication)
91+ (Profound)	• Sound vibration felt rather heard • Visual cues primary for communication	• Special school for the deaf • Some mainstreaming, • Possible candidacy for cochlear implants

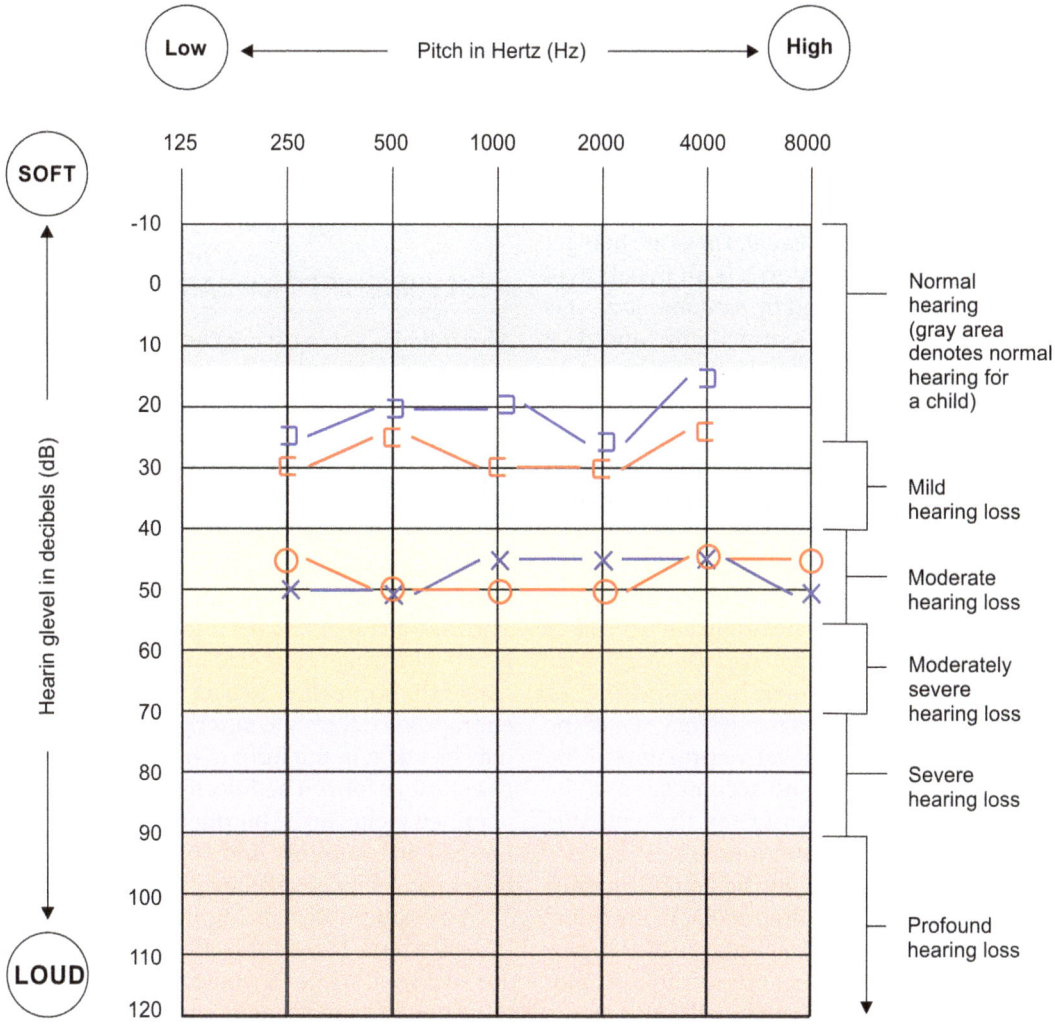

Fig. 7.3: An audiogram showing bilateral mixed hearing loss.

Configuration of Hearing Loss

Hearing losses may also be classified according to the audiogram's shape or pattern across the tested frequency range. The configuration of hearing losses suggests which sounds are heard best by the person with impaired hearing. A hearing loss classification has been proposed by Carhart (1945) and Lloyed and Kaplan (1978) **(Box 7.1)**.

> **BOX 7.1:** Hearing loss as per audiogram's shape.
>
> - **Flat type:** A flat type of hearing loss suggests that hearing loss across frequency spectrum is relatively the same, i.e., hearing loss varies <5 dB/octave.
> - **Gradual sloping or sharply sloping:** The hearing loss rise or fall/octave in the range of <5–12 dB or <15–20 dB are called **gradual sloping or sharply sloping**, respectively.
> - **Precipitously sloping:** A hearing loss of more than 25 dB rise or fall/octave is called **precipitously sloping**.
> - **Rising type:** More than 5 dB decrease in threshold per octave is called **rising type**.
> - **Peaked/saucer type:** If the loss is 20 dB or more at the extreme frequencies but not on the mid frequencies, it is called the **peaked/saucer type**.
> - **Trough type:** A 20 dB or more significant loss in the mid frequencies (1–2 kHz), but not at the extreme frequencies (500 or, 4kHz), is known as **trough type**.
> - **Notched type:** In the case of the 20 dB or more loss at one frequency with adjacent normal or near-normal thresholds, it is called a **notched type**.

CAUSES OF HEARING LOSS

There are prenatal, perinatal, and postnatal causes of hearing loss. The Joint Committee on Infant Hearing, 2019, has listed few risk factors associated with hearing loss. Prenatal risk factors include a family history of hearing impairment, birth asphyxia, presence of a syndrome, NICU admission of more than five days, administration of aminoglycosides, TORCH infection (Toxoplasmosis, Others including Syphilis, Rubella, Cytomegalovirus, Herpes), congenital abnormalities including craniofacial malformations, and hydrocephaly, microcephaly, etc. The peri- and postnatal risk factors for hearing loss include infection like bacterial meningitis and encephalitis, head trauma, and developmental delays like delayed speech and language development.

Now we will study the causes of hearing loss based on the types of hearing loss.

Conductive Hearing Loss

Congenital causes of conductive hearing **loss** related to the outer ear are outer ear anomalies, microtia, and atresia, often present together. Microtia means smaller than normal size pinna. Anotia implies the absence of pinna. Narrowing of the ear canal is known as aural stenosis. Similarly, there may be abnormal development of middle ear structures like the tympanic membrane and ossicles.

Acquired causes related to the outer ear are impacted cerumen (accumulation of wax in the ear canal) that causes conductive hearing loss of up to 45 dB and produces itching, tinnitus, and vertigo. Cerumen can be removed using irrigation of the ear with water, a blunt curette, and suction. Foreign bodies may block the canal and cause hearing loss. Growth and tumors such as exostoses are the frequently occurring tumors of the external ear canal. These are benign, skin-covered bony growth. Otitis externa is an infection of the outer ear canal, primarily caused by *pseudomonas*. It is also known as swimmer's ear as it is commonly caused by swimming in inadequately maintained swimming pools. It causes an excessive amount of pain, swelling, discharge, itching, and conductive hearing loss. It is generally treated with antibiotic drops or creams. Furuncle is a *Staphylococcus* infection of a hair follicle of the ear canal which is treated with oral antibiotics.

Middle ear infections or otitis media are the inflammation of the middle ear and are among the most prominent causes of conductive hearing loss. It occurs in almost 75% of children below five years of age. *Streptococcus pneumoniae* and *Haemophilus influenzae* are mainly responsible for otitis media. It is primarily related to the dysfunction of the eustachian tube, which causes a negative pressure in the middle ear. The fluid is produced and accumulated in the middle ear cavity and builds up pressure on the tympanic membrane leading to tympanic membrane perforation. Before three months, the stage is called acute otitis media, after which it is known as chronic otitis media. In the initial stage, the discharge from the ear is clear watery called serous otitis media and in the late stage, it becomes yellow in color known as a purulent discharge that smells bad. Otitis media is treated with antibiotics and surgery.

Another acquired cause of conductive hearing loss is otosclerosis, a condition when the ossicular chain's bone becomes spongy. It usually affects the oval window and stapedial footplate. The patients typically have progressive hearing loss with tinnitus. There is often an increased bone conduction threshold at 2000 Hz, known as Carhart's notch (Carhart,1950). It can be treated either by surgery (stapedectomy) or in older patients with hearing aids.

The ossicular chain's dislocation can occur due to physical trauma after an accident or may be in chronic otitis media leading to necrosis of ossicular bones. Cholesteatoma is a cystic mass of epithelial cells that occlude the middle ear and produce enzymes that may destroy nearby bones. Tymapnosclerosis occurs as a result of repeated middle ear infections. It is presented as white chalky calcium plaques on the pars tensa part of the tympanic membrane. The conductive hearing loss sometimes is reversible, like after removal of wax or with the use of medication or surgery.

Sensorineural Hearing Loss

Congenital causes of sensorineural hearing loss include genetic hearing loss (syndromic and nonsyndromic), congenital infections (e.g., Rubella, CMV). Acquired causes include infections (measles, mumps, toxoplasmosis, meningitis, syphilis), ototoxicity (aminoglycosides, loop diuretics, cytotoxic drugs, antimalarials), noise-induced hearing loss, and presbyacusis (age-related hearing loss).

Mixed Hearing Loss

Mixed hearing loss occurs as a result of sensorineural hearing loss combined with otitis media or some congenital causes leading to abnormal development of the middle ear and inner ear. A brain tumor may cause central hearing loss, vascular changes in the brain, acquired/congenital brain damage, or central lesions.

ASSESSMENT FOR HEARING

A qualified audiologist carries out hearing assessments. The audiologists are allied health professionals with bachelor or master's degrees from the institute recognized by the Rehabilitation Council of India, a statutory body under the Ministry of Social Justice and Empowerment, Government of India.

Once a patient is referred to the audiologist for the hearing assessment, they review the case history and perform the otoscopic examination of the patient's ears. The case history includes information that provides insight into the hearing status and related factors. It contributes to diagnostic impression, to plan audiological management and appropriate referrals to other professionals. The case history may be taken in the form of interviews and recorded in the case history form. The information which is required to be obtained includes the pertinent medical and family history, the patient's auditory and communicative status, and any history which may be related to his auditory functioning.

Assessment of hearing includes both subjective and objective tests. In the subjective tests, the patient's responses are required, while in objective tests, patients don't have to respond to the acoustic signal presented to them. A test battery is needed where the findings of one test are verified or ruled out by another test result.

Following are the main audiological tests for the assessment of hearing disorders:

Behavioral Tests

❖ **Behavioral observation audiometry (BOA):** It is used for very young children (below one year) or older children who are difficult to test, like children having behavioral issues. As shown in **Figure 7.4**, calibrated noisemakers

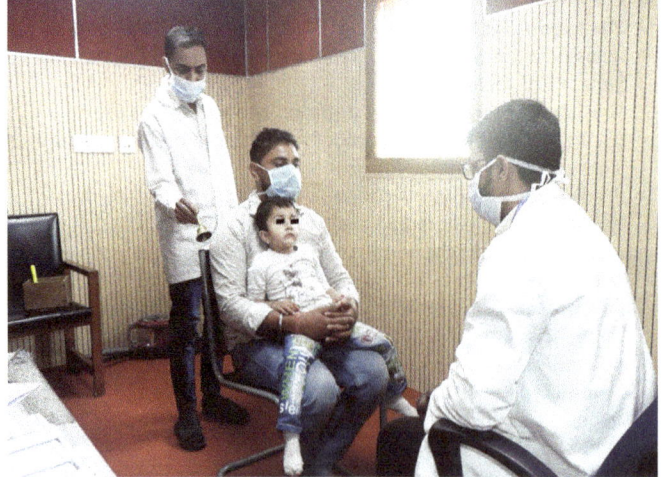

Fig. 7.4: Behavioral observation audiometry (BOA) test of a child using noisemakers.

ranging from low, mid, and high frequencies (e.g., a bell for high frequency and drum for low frequency) are presented at variable distances. Test signals like speech or speech noise can be delivered through an audiometer with sound field capability. The hearing level of the child is estimated by observing the behavior change as a response to the noise presented. Eye widening, head turn, startle, eye blink, change in breathing pattern, etc., are the observed few behavior changes.

- **Visual reinforcement audiometry:** In this test, the child in the age range of 5 months to 2 years old is tested by presenting a signal by the audiometer using insert earphones, bone conduction vibrator, or sound field speaker(s). Flashing light or puppet is used as a reward once the child looks in the direction of an incoming signal.
- **Conditioned play audiometry:** This test is administered to assess hearing in children in the range of 2–5 years. The child is taught to respond to sound by doing some activity e.g., by placing a peg in a pegboard, tossing a block in a box, stacking blocks, or other game-type activities in response to an auditory stimulus (speech or frequency-specific). The signals (either speech or tonal) are presented by the audiometer using insert earphones, bone conduction vibrator, or sound field speaker(s).
- **Pure tone audiometry (PTA):** It is considered the gold standard test of hearing. The subject has to indicate each time he or she hears the tone. Usually, children above five years of age and adults may perform pure tone audiometry. The hearing threshold, i.e., the minimum level of sound heard at least 50% of the times, is measured for the frequency octaves ranging from 250 Hz to 8 kHz for air conduction and from 250 to 4 kHz for bone conduction. The pure tones are presented by an audiometer to both ears separately using headphones (TDH39 or TDH49), insert receivers (ER-3A) for air conduction, and Radio ear B71 transducer for bone conduction testing, and the subject is asked to give a signal in the form of hand raising or pressing a button whenever he/she hears the tone **(Fig. 7.5)**. The hearing thresholds are plotted on a graph known as an audiogram. The audiogram has frequency octaves (in Hz) on X-axis and intensity on Y-axis (in dBHL). The audiogram provides information about the degree, type, and configuration of hearing loss.
- **Speech audiometry:** Speech audiometry employs the speech stimuli, either words or phrases, to assess the auditory system. It is also used as a cross-check to the hearing thresholds obtained in the pure tone audiometry test.

Following tests are mainly used:
- *Speech detection threshold (SDT):* The minimum level at which the speech signal is detected at least 50% of the time. Phrases or connected speech are used for this purpose.
- *Speech reception threshold (SRT):* It is the minimum level at which the spondee words (Bisyllabic words with equal stress on each syllable like "Airplane") are repeated by the listener at least 50% of the times.
- *Word recognition score (WRS) or speech discrimination score (SDS):* It is the percentage of correctly repeated monosyllabic words that are phonetically balanced having consonant vowel consonant (CVC) structure and the initial and final consonants in each word appear by their frequency of use in these positions. Phonetically balanced (PB) words are presented at the suprathreshold level or level which is most comfortable for the listeners. This test is useful in getting information about the patients' communication abilities and helps differentiate between cochlear and retrocochlear disorders.

Objective Tests

- **Impedance audiometry:** This test provides information about the middle ear's status, and is performed using the impedance audiometer **(Fig. 7.6)**. The test consists of tympanometry and reflexomtery.
  - *Tympanometry:* This test assesses the tympanic membrane's mobility characteristics with the change in the middle ear pressure. The result is plotted on a graph known as tympanogram with pressure plotted in decapascals (daPa) or mmH_2O on X-axis and acoustic admittance in mmhos (or equivalent volume in mL) plotted on Y-axis. The pressure of 226 Hz probe tone (1 kHz in cases of infants of <6 months) is first raised to +200 daPa and decreased till -400 daPa. Tympanograms have been classified **(Fig. 7.7)** according to middle ear pressure and static compliance measures in the test (Jeger, 1970).

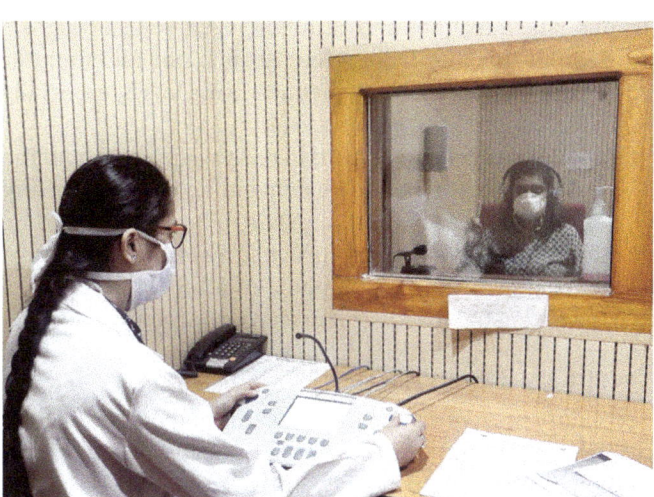

Fig. 7.5: Pure tone audiometry (PTA) test.

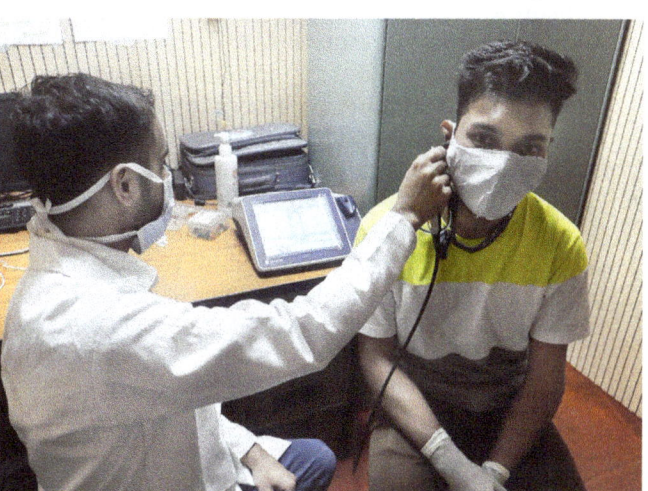

Fig. 7.6: Impedance audiometry test of an adult.

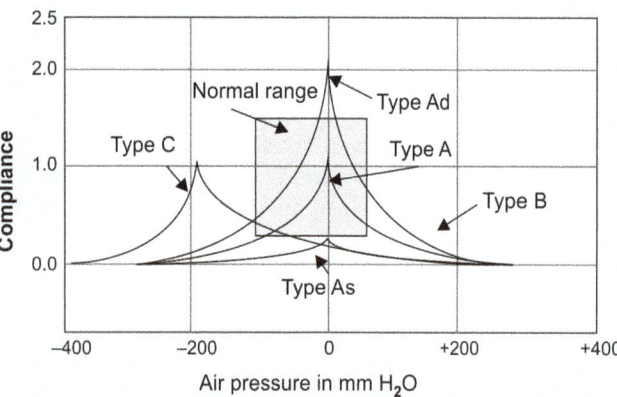

Fig. 7.7: Types of tympanograms adapted from Jerger (1970).

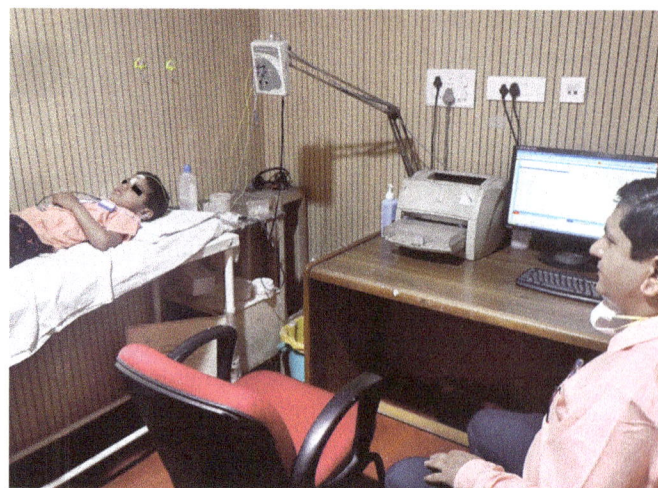

Fig. 7.8: Auditory brainstem response (ABR) test of a child.

The middle ear pressure is the level of pressure where the tympanogram shows maximum acoustic admittance—the normal value of the middle ear pressure ranges between ± 100 deca pascal (daPa). Static compliance is the value that suggests the amount of acoustic energy being transferred from the middle ear to the inner ear. The normal value of static compliance ranges from 0.28 to 1.75-milliliter (mL).

Type A: Normal values of static compliance and middle ear pressure. Present in normal middle ears and some cases of otosclerosis.

Type A_s: 'S' stands for 'shallow'. In this type, there is a reduced value of static compliance (<0.28 mL) with normal middle ear pressure. Type A_s is present in otosclerosis and tympanic sclerosis cases.

Type A_D: 'D' stands for 'Deep.' Increased value of static compliance (>1.75 daPa) with normal middle ear pressure. Type A_D is present in hypermobile tympanic membrane or ossicular disarticulation.

Type C: A type tympanogram with negative middle ear pressure (<-100 daPa). This type is present in cases of eustachian tube dysfunction.

Type B: In this type no peak is present or it is a flat type. It is present in cases of impacted cerumen, middle ear effusion, or tympanic membrane perforation.

> *Reflexometry test* assesses the stapedial reflex at the suprathreshold level. Elevated and absent reflexes indicate pathologies at different levels in the auditory pathway.

- **Auditory brainstem response (ABR):** This is an objective test to assess the auditory nerve's neural synchrony. It suggests the auditory pathway's integrity up to the brainstem level and is widely used to screen hearing and estimate hearing loss in children **(Fig. 7.8)**.
- **Otoacoustic emissions (OAEs):** This test is sensitive to outer hair cell functioning. OAE measures the outer hair cell functioning. It is widely used for the screening of hearing in children. Mainly two types of OAEs are used to assess hearing transient evoked OAEs (TEOAEs) and distortion product OAEs (DPOAEs).

PREVENTION OF HEARING LOSS

Prevention can be defined as "action to reduce or eliminate or reduce the onset, causes, complications, or recurrence of the disease."According to WHO, 40% of hearing loss in children is preventable. The first three years of life are considered crucial for the development of the child, especially the speech-language development. If the hearing impairment is identified and managed later than three years, it will cause irreversible damage. Hence, this time window is known as the critical period for development. Congenital hearing loss needs to be detected by one month of age, adequately diagnosed by three months, and receive the intervention by six months. This protocol is known as 1-3-6 guidelines.

World Health Organization has classified prevention of hearing loss in three stages: Primary, secondary and tertiary prevention.

Primary Prevention

This involves the prevention of the manifestation of the disability. It requires action to reduce the occurrence of the disorder. Primary prevention for hearing loss include:

- **Immunization programs:** Immunization in children against the infections which lead to hearing loss like rubella, meningitis, mumps, and measles.
- **Improved prenatal, perinatal and postnatal care:** It involves steps to prevent low birth weight, prematurity, birth asphyxia, cytomegalovirus, and neonatal jaundice. Actions include improved nutrition, safe birth awareness, awareness of hygienic practices, and treatment of neonatal infections and jaundice.
- **Regulations and legislation:** Regulations and monitor the use of ototoxic medicines and noise levels, especially in recreational and sports areas.
- **Raising awareness:** Actions to raise awareness about the healthy ear care practice like avoiding insertion of any substance like an earbud, any sharp object or oil, avoiding noise, using a helmet to prevent head trauma, use of hearing protectors, avoidance of ototoxic medicines, preventing the marriage between close relatives, etc.

Secondary Prevention

Secondary prevention means screening and diagnosing the disorder. Screening means the identification of a portion of the population which have a high probability of having the disorder. Screening services are crucial for the early identification and management of the disorders. Most of the hearing screening team comprises of the audiologist and ENT specialist.

Hearing screening programs can vary depending on the target population. In newborns, the hearing screening program can be universal, i.e., all the newborns are screened or can be targeted like screening of infants admitted in the neonatal intensive care unit. It is very important as we can identify and manage the infants at the early stage to reduce the impact of the hearing loss including the delayed speech and language development. Similarly, a hearing screening program in the school-going population is helpful as hearing loss in schoolchildren may lead to speech disorders. Also, hearing screening programs are targeted at the elderly population and people working in industrial setups as they are at high risk of hearing loss.

Tertiary Prevention

Tertiary prevention is aimed at reducing the impact of the already present disorder. Individuals diagnosed with hearing loss are provided medical or surgical treatment or audiological management. Surgical treatment includes cochlear implants, middle ear implants, bone-anchored hearing aids, etc. The audiological intervention involves providing or prescribing hearing aids and or assistive listening devices like FM system, TV listening system, and telephone amplifier based on the individual needs.

HEARING AIDS AND IMPLANTABLE DEVICES

HEARING AIDS

These are sound amplification devices that help people with hearing impairment. The hearing aids components include **a microphone** a transducer that picks up the sound and converts the acoustic signal into an electrical signal. The electrical signal is sent to the **amplifier,** which amplifies it, i.e., increases its intensity and sends it to the **receiver,** which converts the amplified electrical signal back into an acoustic signal. The acoustic signal is then sent to the ear using an **earmold**. An earmold is an object which is inserted into the ear. A **battery** provides the power to the hearing aid to carry out its function.

The difference between the input signal levels and the amplified output signal level of a hearing aid is called a hearing aid gain. Any hearing aid can produce a wide range of gains, but the **volume control** provides some degree of control to the hearing aid wearer. The greatest sound magnitude produced by a hearing aid is called Maximum Power Output **(MPO).** Beyond the maximum power output, the amplified signals are clipped off, also called peak clipping. Many hearing aids use **compression** or **automatic gain compression** (AGC) circuit that slows down the amplification rate so that the clipping level is never reached. Compression also helps in preventing the loud sound from becoming uncomfortable for persons with loudness recruitment problems.

Directionality in Hearing Aids

The hearing aids' microphone may be omnidirectional, equally sensitive to sound coming from all directions or directional, sensitive to sounds coming from a specific direction, and less sensitive to sound coming from the other directions.

Types of Hearing Aids

With the advanced technologies the size of hearing aids have become smaller and signal processing technique has shifted from analog to digital.

Body Hearing Aids

Body of hearing aids contains all their components except the receiver and earmold in a case that is placed in a chest pocket or clipped to a shirt **(Fig. 7.9)**. The wire connects the case to the receiver and earmold.

Advantages of Body Hearing Aids

- ❖ These are the most powerful hearing aids hence preferred in patients with severe to profound hearing loss. However, nowadays behind the ear types of hearing aids are also capable of providing equivalent gain.
- ❖ The battery and controls size is larger in body hearing aids; these are preferred in cases with reduced manual dexterity in elderly patients and younger children.
- ❖ As the microphones and receiver are placed further apart, there is less chance that the amplified signal to be picked up by the microphone and reamplified to produce the acoustic feedback, a whistling-like sound. So chances of acoustic feedback are less in body hearing aids.

Disadvantages of Body Hearing Aids

- ❖ Body hearing aids are not preferred because of their large size, which causes cosmetic undesirability.
- ❖ As the aid's location is on the body rather than on the ear, it picks up the noise as clothing brushes across the case.
- ❖ Also, the body affects the intensity and spectrum of sound reaching the microphone. It is called body baffle and body shadow.

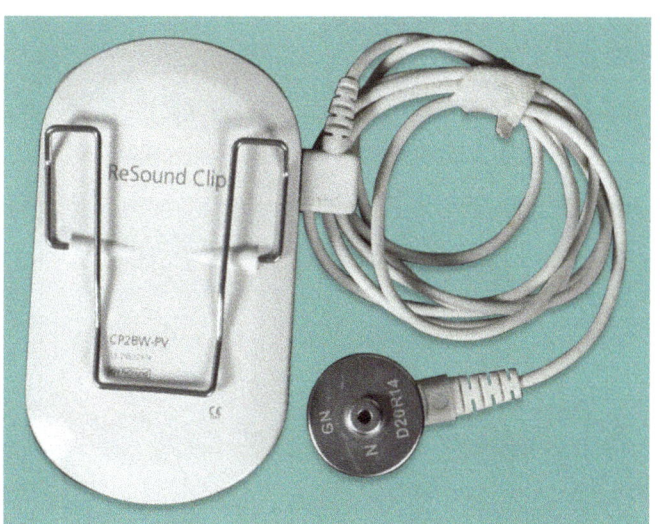

Fig. 7.9: Body hearing aid.

Ear Level Hearing Aids

The ear-level hearing aids have all the components placed in a small package to be worn in or near the ear. Behind the ear, in the ear, in the canal, and receiver in the ear are the different types of ear-level hearing aids.

Behind the Ear (BTE)

This hearing aid **(Fig. 7.10)** has all the components placed in a crescent-shaped plastic case worn behind the pinna. The sound from the receiver is transmitted through a plastic tube to the earmold in the patient's ear. These are preferred in young children as with the increase in age, the canal size grows, and the earmolds need to be replaced frequently, and this can be easily achieved using BTEs. Nowadays, **Mini BTE** hearing aids are available, useful in relatively less occlusion fitting in the ear.

In the Ear (ITE)

In ITEs, the hearing aid components are placed in a shell that is fitted in the outer part of the ear. It fills the whole concha of the pinna and extends into the ear canal.

In the Canal Aids (ITC) and Completely in the Canal (CIC) Aids

ITC and CIC hearing aids are very small and the hearing aid is fitted 1–2 mm inside of the ear canal entrance **(Fig. 7.11)**. Advantages of CIC hearing aids include taking advantage of pinna and concha effect in localization of sounds, deeper insertion allows for more gain and output, own speech is heard more natural. Also, they have a cosmetic advantage.

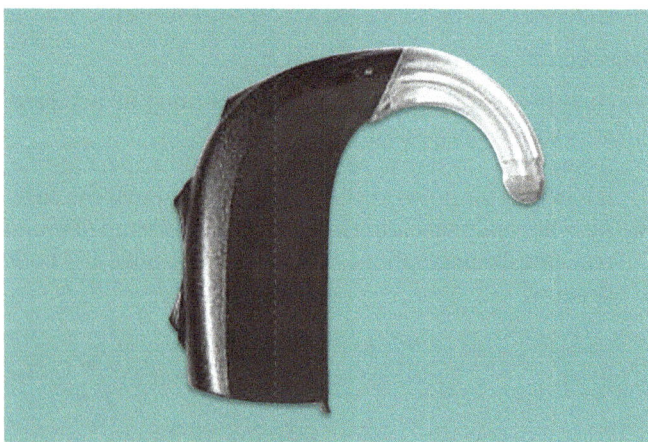

Fig. 7.10: Behind the ear (BTE) hearing aid.

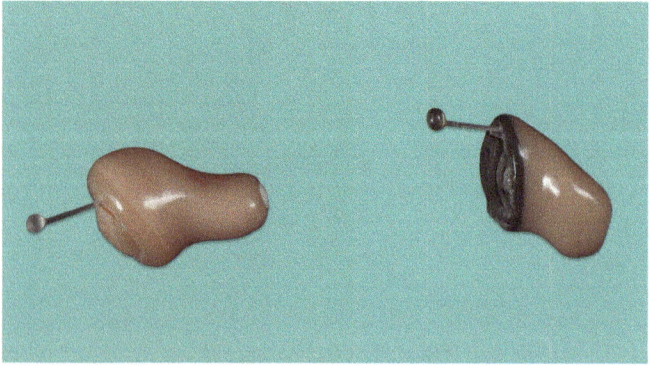

Fig. 7.11: ITC and CIC types of hearing aids.

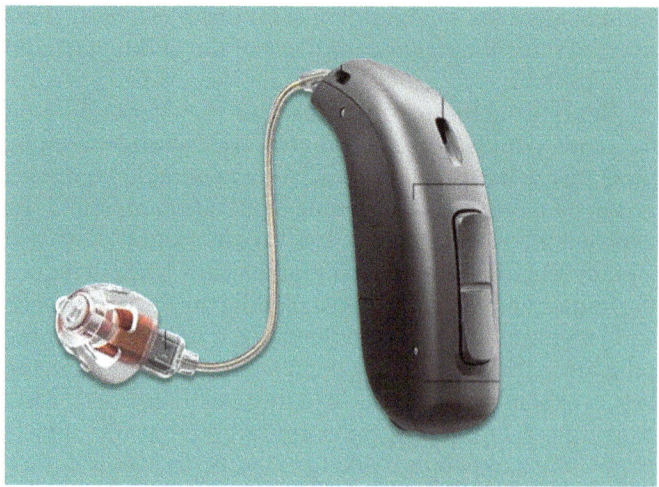

Fig. 7.12: Receiver in the ear hearing aid (RIC).

Receiver in the Canal (RIC)

RIC hearing aids are similar to BTEs in shape, but the receiver is placed apart in the ear canal **(Fig. 7.12)**. RICs' advantages include the relatively open fitting with the special domes, which are placed over the receiver. Hence less occlusion effect and own speech is perceived more natural. Also, as the microphone and receiver are apart, fewer chances for the acoustic feedback to take place. It is more suitable for a person with sloping hearing loss.

Technologies in the Hearing Aid

Based on signal processing technologies, there are three types of hearing aids:

Conventional Analog Hearing Aids

In the analog hearing aids microphone converts the acoustic signal into an electrical signal which is amplified by the amplifier and is converted back to an acoustic signal. The aid amplifies both speech and noise and may be uncomfortable in a noisy situation. Some adjustments are possible. This technology is cheaper than other types of technologies.

Programmable Analog Hearing Aids

These hearing aids have a microchip that allows an audiologist to program the aid for different listening environments, e.g., the hearing aid may have the first program setting for a quiet listening situation and a second program for the noisy listening situation. The chip is digitally programmed, which controls the functions of the amplifier but the signal remains analog during the amplification process.

Digital Hearing Aids

These hearing aids use digital sound processing (DSP). In DSP, the signal entering the microphone is first converted into a digital signal (binary digits 0 and 1) by an analog to digital converter (ADC). The signal is thereafter analyzed, and algorithms are used to reduce the noise from the signal and then amplified by the amplifier. After the signal processing, the signal is transformed back into an analog signal using the digital to analog converter (DAC).

HEARING AID SELECTION AND FITTING

There are six steps involved in hearing aid selection and fitting (ASHA, 1998):

1. **Assessment stage:** It involves determining the degree and type of hearing loss and candidacy for hearing aid, which includes the audiometric test result, self-assessment, and communication, mental, motivation, sociological, and physical status of the patient.
2. **Treatment planning stage:** Audiologist, patient, and family review findings to identify the needs, set rehabilitation goals, plan intervention and understand the treatment benefits and limitations, and cost.
3. **Selection stage:** Hearing aids are selected based on their amplification characteristics, known as electroacoustic characteristics (e.g., frequency-gain response, etc.) and other monoaural or binaural; style and size characteristics.
4. **Verification stage:** Hearing electroacoustic measurement and real ear measurement are carried out. Real ear measurements include programming the hearing aid with prescriptive targets (frequency-based gain according to specific formula) and measuring the hearing aid gain in the patient's ear. It is also determined if the hearing aids are comfortable providing the proper audibility, etc.
5. **Orientation stage:** Post-hearing aid fitting, the patient is counseled about the use and care, realistic expectations. Also, further rehabilitation intervention if needed is planned.
6. **Validation stage:** Intervention outcome is assessed using self-assessment tools and assessment of speech perception.

IMPLANTABLE HEARING DEVICES

When conventional hearing aids are not beneficial for the person with hearing impairment, implantable devices are needed for such patients due to medical or audiological reasons. Implanted devices are indicated in the patients whose hearing loss is beyond the gain range of a hearing aid, who have a malformation of the ear, or have chronic otitis media that cannot be treated otherwise by ear surgery.

Cochlear Implants

A cochlear implant is a surgically implanted device that bypasses the external and middle ear and stimulates the cochlea's auditory neurons. The device provides the hearing sensation to children as well as adults with severe to profound hearing loss.

An implant has the following parts:
- **External parts (Fig. 7.13):** This part sits behind the ear—
  - **A microphone,** which picks up sound from the surroundings and transduces it into an electrical signal.
  - A **speech processor** analyzes the sound and converts it into a code representing various aspects of the sound.
  - A **transmitter** that sends the encoded signal to the implanted device via electromagnetic or radio-frequency signal.
- **Internal parts (Fig. 7.14):** This part is surgically placed under the skin:

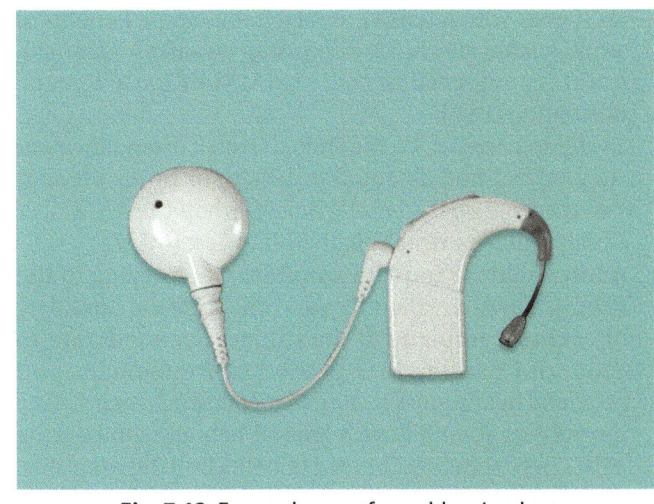

Fig. 7.13: External parts of a cochlear implant.

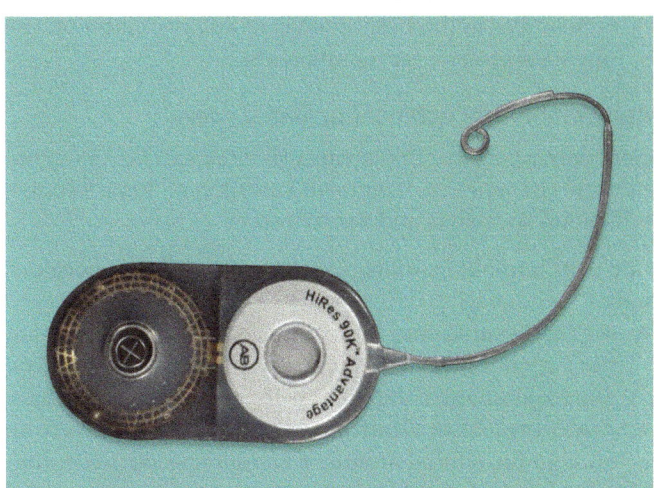

Fig. 7.14: Internal parts of a cochlear implant.

- A **receiver** that picks up the signal from the external transmitter
- An **electrical stimulator** converts the signal into electric impulses. It has an **electrode array** which is a group of electrodes that sends these electrical impulses to different auditory nerve regions.

There are three Food and Drug Association (FDA)-approved cochlear implant companies. These are the:
1. Cochlear Corporation (Australia), e.g., Nucleus 22 and 24 systems which have 22 electrodes
2. Advanced Bionics (America), e.g., Neptune systems have 16 electrodes
3. Med-El (Austria), e.g., Sonata systems that have 24 electrodes which are arranged in 12 pairs.

Candidacy Criteria for Cochlear Implants

- **Pediatric cochlear implant candidacy:** Food and Drug Administration America (FDA) has prescribed the candidacy criteria for cochlear implantation in children. According to these guidelines, the hearing loss degree should be bilateral profound sensorineural hearing loss in children (9–24 months) and severe to profound hearing loss in children (2–17 years). There should be limited benefits with hearing aids. The limited benefits may be considered if there is a lack of progress in auditory skills even with intensive aural rehabilitation. Benefits of amplification may be assessed using tests like Meaningful Auditory Integration Scale (MAIS) or Early Speech Perception (ESP).

In children aged 2–17, the limited benefit of amplification may be defined as equal or less than thirty percent correct score on the Lexical Neighborhood Test (LNT) or Multisyllabic Lexical Neighborhood Test (MLNT).

❖ **Adult cochlear implant candidacy:** According to the FDA, adults (more than 18 years of age) are the candidate of cochlear implants if the subject has moderate to profound hearing loss in the low frequencies and profound hearing loss in the mid to high frequencies. Also, the subject should have a limited benefit with hearing aids. There should be limited benefits from hearing aids. The limited benefits may be considered if the subject scores 50% correct or less in the ear to be implanted and 60% or less in the best-aided listening condition on the open-set sentence recognition test.

Assessment for Cochlear Implant Surgery

Generally, a cochlear implant team includes an ENT surgeon, Audiologist, Speech-Language Pathologist, Psychologist, Education specialist, and Social worker.

Cochlear implant candidacy involves the following evaluation:

❖ **Medical evaluation:** It is comprised of an assessment of the patient's overall medical condition, the case history, and assessment of the cause of the patient's hearing loss.
❖ **Audiological evaluation:** It consists of a pure-tone audiogram, administration of various speech perception tests such as word and sentence recognition, and assessment of benefits of hearing aids and hearing aid trial for three to six months.
❖ **Psychological evaluation:** In children, the psychosocial evaluation includes developmental and educational assessments and family assessments.

Many factors determine the overall benefits in children. These include the child's age at onset of deafness, age of implantation, cochlear implant usage duration, and therapy duration. Generally, children need to undergo speech therapy and auditory training for two years or more to achieve speech and language skills. Auditory verbal therapy (AVT) training is a special form of teaching cochlear implanted children to learn to listen and talk.

Bone Anchored Hearing Aids

Bone anchored hearing devices (BAHA) **(Fig. 7.15)** are an ideal solution for assisting patients with chronic otitis media, absent external acoustic canal (atresia), small (microtia), or absent (anotia) pinna, as well as single-sided deafness. Anders Tjelsstrom first introduced BAHA in 1977 (Mudry and Tjellstrom, 2011). The device works on the osseointegration principle. The surgery involves a titanium screw, which is also known as an abutment, is inserted into the bone behind the ear. The abutment osseointegrates with the skull bone, and thus, the abutment becomes part of the skull bone. A sound processor is then attached to the abutment. The sound is picked by the sound processor's microphone and

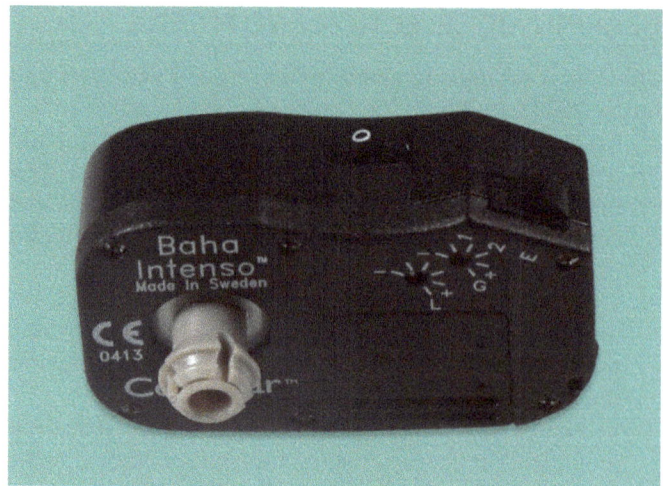

Fig. 7.15: Bone-anchored hearing aid (BAHA).

is transmitted to the abutment, which vibrates and transmits the signal to the inner ear using bone conduction. Currently, three companies are manufacturing the Bone-anchored Hearing System—the Baha (Cochlear), the Ponto (Oticon), and the Alpha 1 (Sophono). The FDA candidacy criteria for BAHA is for use in patients (1) having conductive or mixed hearing loss and can still benefit from sound amplification, (2) with bilaterally symmetric conductive or mixed hearing loss, (3) with sensorineural deafness in one ear, and normal hearing in the other, and (4) who cannot or will not wear a contralateral routing of signals (CROS) hearing aid. The minimum age criteria are five years and older.

Middle Ear Implant

The middle ear implant is used in adults with moderate to severe sensorineural, conductive, or mixed hearing loss. MED-EL company (Austria) manufactures the Vibrant Soundbridge middle ear implant. The implant consists of a surgically implanted vibrating ossicular prosthesis (VORP) which has a floating mass transducer (FMT) attached to the ossicular chain. The receiver of VORP is placed underneath the skin behind the ear. The audio processor sends the signal to the receiver of VORP transcutaneously via electromagnetic signals that are converted to oscillations by the FMT. These oscillations then transmit to the inner ear for the perception of sound. Middle ear implant reduces the feedback (whistling sound) as well as occlusion effect (block sensation and increase in the intensity of low-frequency sound) commonly encountered with conventional hearing aids.

EDUCATIONAL APPROACHES FOR THE DEAF

There are mainly two types of communication modes for deaf children. The oral approach advocates reliance on hearing and spoken language, while the manual approach relies primarily on sign language for communication. Based on these two approaches, other methods have been developed. These include:

❖ **Acoupedic method:** This mainly relies on hearing ability and eliminating the visual cues. They stress on the use of residual hearing through amplification and auditory training.

- **Oral/aural methods:** This approach relies on developing spoken language, i.e., speech, speech reading, and writing with or without natural gestures.
- **Speech reading:** It is the ability to understand speech through observing lip movements and facial expressions.
- **Total communication:** It combines both the manual and oral methods. Speech, speech reading, and amplification are used simultaneously with a sign language system.
- **American sign language (ASL) or Indian sign language (ISL):** It is a true manual, ideographic sign language with its own vocabulary, grammar, and word order.

Case Scenario

1. **Pediatric:** Payal was an intelligent and affectionate girl as a child. However, her language development was slow and her speech lacked precision. Her parents visited a pediatrician at the age of two years with a concern of delayed speech and language development. With some clap sound, the pediatrician assessed her hearing and observed that Payal was responding. The pediatrician counseled the parents to increase speech stimulation and that Payal had normal hearing. As time passed Payal started talking with the help of watching the speaker's lip movement. However, she struggled in following the conversation. When she joined the school, the teacher noticed that Payal had difficulty following the instructions. She advised the parents to consult an Audiologist. With proper audiological tests, Payal was diagnosed with severe high-frequency sensorineural hearing loss. She was fitted with bilateral behind the ear hearing aids. As her hearing loss was identified late Payal had to struggle to communicate and had delayed speech and language development. She needed speech therapy to improve her communication skills with hearing aids.
2. **Adult:** Mr Mehta is 45-year-old male who suddenly lost hearing in both ears. The audiologist performed the audiological tests and he was diagnosed with bilateral profound sensorineural hearing loss. Hearing aids were not providing any benefits to him. He had to leave the job as hearing loss made it difficult for him to continue. The ENT doctor advised him to get cochlear implant surgery done. He underwent cochlear implant surgery and now hears all types of sounds as he was hearing before the occurrence of the hearing loss. He has rejoined the job and enjoying conversation with his colleague and clients.

SUMMARY

Hearing loss is the most prevalent sensory disorder. It affects speech-language skills, reading writing abilities, psychosocial and emotional development as well as the employability of a child. In a recent WHO report globally, 1 in 4 persons will be having hearing loss by 2050. There are many pre, peri, and postnatal causes of hearing loss that may occur at any age. But many of these causes are preventable and if identifies and managed early its impact may be decreased. The treatment options include medical and assistance using hearing aids and implantable devices like cochlear implants, BAHA, middle ear implants, etc.

MULTIPLE CHOICE QUESTIONS

1. Hearing is very important because:
    a. It is essential for verbal communication
    b. It helps to connect to the surrounding
    c. It alerts about the dangers
    d. All of the above
2. What is the relation between the terms "deafness" and "hard of hearing"?
    a. Both are the same and can be used interchangeably.
    b. Deafness means profound hearing loss, hard of hearing means mild to severe hearing loss
    c. Hearing aids do not help the deaf person but can be used for heard of hearing persons.
    d. Both b and c
3. According to the World Health Organization by 2050, how many persons will be affected by disabling hearing loss?
    a. One in ten
    b. One in five
    c. One in four
    d. One in three
4. An audiogram represents on X and Y-axis:
    a. Frequency and intensity respectively
    b. Intensity and frequency respectively
    c. The minimum and maximum range of hearing
    d. None of the above
5. What is the finding of sensorineural hearing loss on the audiogram?
    a. Both AC and BC are affected and there is no gap between AC and BC
    b. Both AC and BC are affected there is a gap between AC and BC
    c. Only AC is affected but BC remains normal
    d. Only BC is affected but AC remains normal
6. Hearing loss ranging from 71–90 dBHL is classified as:
    a. Profound hearing loss
    b. Moderate hearing loss
    c. Moderately severe hearing loss
    d. Severe hearing loss
7. Ageing and noise exposure are major causes of which type of hearing loss?
    a. Conductive hearing loss
    b. Mixed hearing loss
    c. Sensorineural hearing loss
    d. Central hearing loss
8. Osseointegration is the basic principle of which implantable device?
    a. Cochlear implant
    b. Middle ear implant
    c. Bone-anchored hearing aid
    d. All of the above
9. Which part of the cochlear implant transmits the electrical signal to auditory neurons?
    a. Speech processor
    b. Transmitting coil
    c. Receiver coil
    d. Electrode
10. Which tests are used in hearing screening in infants:
    a. Pure tone audiometry
    b. Reflexomtery
    c. Otoacoustic emission and auditory brainstem response
    d. None of the above.

ANSWERS

1. d	2. d	3. c	4. a
5. a	6. d	7. c	8. c
9. d	10. c		

SUGGESTED READING

1. American Speech-Language-Hearing Association. Guidelines for Hearing Aid Fitting for Adults [Guidelines]www.asha.org/policy]; 1998.
2. Carhart R. Clinical application of bone conduction audiometry. Archives of Otolaryngology. 1950;51:798-808.
3. Carhart R. An improved method for classifying audiograms. Laryngoscope. 1945;55:640662.
4. Clark J G. Uses and abuses of hearing loss classification. Asha. 1981;23:493-500.
5. Connolly JL, Carron JD, Roark SD. Universal newborn hearing screening: Are we achieving the Joint Committee on Infant Hearing (JCIH) objectives. Laryngoscope. 2005;115:232-6.

6. Contrera KJ, Betz J, Genther DJ, Lin FR. Association of hearing impairment and mortality in the National Health and Nutrition Examination Survey. JAMA Otolaryngol Head Neck Surg. 2015;141:944-6.
7. Davis A, McMahon CM, Pichora-Fuller KM, Russ S, Lin F, Olusanya BO et al. Aging and Hearing Health: The Life-Course Approach. The Gerontologist. 2016;56(Suppl 2):S256-67.
8. Fisher D, Li CM, Chiu MS, et al. Impairments in hearing and vision impact on mortality in older people: the AGES- Reykjavik Study. Age Ageing. 2014;43:69-76.
9. Flexer C. Class room management of children and minimal hearing loss. Hear J. 1995;48:54-8
10. Gallacher J, Ilubaera V, Ben-Shlomo Y, et al. Auditory threshold, phonologic demand, and incident dementia. Neurology. 2012;79:1583-90.
11. Garbaruk ES, Koroleva IV. Newborns Audiological Screening in Russia: Problems and Prospects: Textbook. St. Petersburg: Research Institute LOR; 2013. p. 6.
12. Garg S, Chadha S, Malhotra S, Agarwal AK. Deafness: Burden, prevention, and control in India. Natl Med J India. 2009;22:79-81.
13. GBD 2015 Disease and Injury Incidence and Prevalence Collaborators. Global, regional, and national incidence, prevalence, and years lived with disability for 310 diseases and injuries, 1990–2015: a systematic analysis for the Global Burden of Disease Study 2015. Lancet. 2016;388:1545-602.
14. Genther DJ, Frick KD, Chen D, Betz J, Lin FR. Association of hearing loss with hospitalization and burden of disease in older adults. JAMA. 2013;309:2322-4.
15. Hoffman HJ, Dobie RA, Losonczy KG, Themann CL, Flamme GA. Declining Prevalence of Hearing Loss in US Adults Aged 20 to 69 Years. JAMA Otolaryngology-Head and Neck Surgery. December 2016 online.
16. Jerger JF. Clinical experience with impedance audiometry. Archives of Otolaryngology. 1970;92:311-24.
17. Joint Committee on Infant Hearing 1994 position statement. Pediatrics. 1994;95:152.
18. Klein JO. Otitis media. Clinical Infectious Diseases. 1994;19:823-33.
19. Li CM, Zhang X, Hoffman HJ, Cotch MF, Themann CL, Wilson MR. Hearing impairment associated with depression in US adults, National Health and Nutrition Examination Survey 2005–2010. JAMA Otolaryngol Head Neck Surg. 2014;140:293-302.
20. Lin FR, Ferrucci L. Hearing loss and falls among older adults in the United States. Arch Intern Med. 2012;172:369-71.
21. Lin FR, Metter EJ, O'Brien RJ, Resnick SM, Zonderman AB, Ferrucci L. Hearing loss and incident dementia. Arch. Neurol 2011;68:214-20.
22. Lin FR, Yaffe K, Xia J, et al. Hearing loss and cognitive decline in older adults. JAMA Intern Med. 2013;173:293-9.
23. Livingston G, Sommerlad A, Orgeta V, Costafreda SG, Huntley J, Ames D. Dementia Prevention, Intervention, and Care. Lancet. 2017;390(10113):2673-734.
24. Lloyd L, Kaplan H. Audiometric interpretation: a manual of basic audiometry: Press; 1978.
25. Mener DJ, Betz J, Genther DJ, Chen D, Lin FR. Hearing loss and depression in older adults. J Am Geriatr Soc. 2013;61:1627-9.
26. Mudry A, Tjellström A. Historical background of bone conduction hearing devices and bone conduction hearing aids. Adv Otorhinolaryngol. 2011;71:1-9.
27. National Public Health Partnership. Preventing chronic disease: a strategic framework. Background paper. Melbourne, Australia: National Public Health Partnership; 2001.
28. Northern J Downs M. Hearing in children, 4th edition Baltimore, Md. Williams and Wilkins; 1991.
29. The Joint Committee on Infant Hearing. Year 2019 Position Statement: Principles and Guidelines for Early Hearing Detection and Intervention Programs. The Journal of Early Hearing Detection and Intervention. 2019;4(2):1-44.
30. Viljanen A, Kaprio J, Pyykko I, et al. Hearing as a predictor of falls and postural balance in older female twins. J Gerontol A Biol Sci Med Sci. 2009;64:312-7.
31. WHO. World Report on hearing. https://apps.who.int/iris/bitstream/handle/10665/339913/9789240020481-eng.pdf?sequence=1. Accessed date 26 Mar 2021.
32. World Health Organization. Deafness and hearing loss [Online]. Available https://www.who.int/news-room/fact-sheets/detail/deafness-and-hearing-loss(2020) Accessed: 06-Sep-2020
33. World Health Organization. Deafness and hearing loss [Online]. Available https://www.who.int/pbd/deafness/activities/strategies/en/(2021). Accessed on 09-Feb-2021.
34. World Health Organization. Facts about deafness (online). Available https://www.who.int/pbd/deafness/facts/en/. Accessed on 09-Feb-2021.
35. Zelaya CE, Lucas JW, Hoffman HJ. Self-reported hearing trouble in adults aged 18 and over: the United States, 2014. US Department of Health and Human Services, Centers for Disease Control and Prevention, National Center for Health Statistics; 2015.

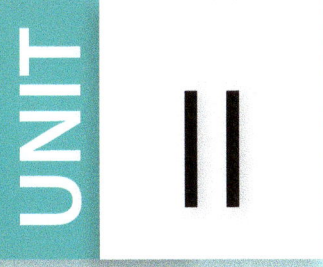

UNIT II

Disorders of Eye

OUTLINE

8. **Review of Anatomy and Physiology: Eye**
   Tulika Gupta, Tanvi Soni, Daisy Sahni

9. **Assessment and Diagnostic Evaluation of Eye**
   Anshul Chauhan, Gagandeep Kaur, Priyanka Verma, Lakshya Kumar, Mona Duggal

10. **Ophthalmic Surgical Instruments**
    Manpreet Singh, Manpreet Kaur, Aditi Mehta

11. **Ocular Pharmacology and Lasers**
    Himanshi Singh, Parul Chawla Gupta, Jagat Ram

12. **Refractive Errors**
    Himanshi Singh, Parul Chawla Gupta, Jagat Ram

13. **Cataract**
    Ranjan Kumar Behera, Parul Chawla Gupta, Jagat Ram

14. **Disorders of Eyelid and Lacrimal System**
    Manu Saini, Tanvi Soni

15. **Orbital Disorders**
    Manu Saini, Tanvi Soni

16. **Disorders of Cornea**
    Surbhi Khurana, Parul Chawla Gupta, Ranjan Kumar Behera, Jagat Ram

17. **Glaucoma**
    Faisal Thattaruthody, Neha Chauhan, Madhuri Akella

18. **Disorders of Conjunctiva**
    Surbhi Khurana, Parul Chawla Gupta, Ranjan Kumar Behera, Jagat Ram

19. **Disorders of Retina and Vitreous**
    Atul Arora, Reema Bansal, Vishali Gupta

20. **Disorders of Sclera and Uvea**
    Atul Arora, Reema Bansal, Vishali Gupta

21. **Neuro-ophthalmology**
    Shweta Chaurasia, Kajree Gupta

22. **Strabismus**
    Shweta Chaurasia, Shagun Korla, Kiran Kumari

23. **Ocular Injuries**
    Surbhi Khurana, Parul Chawla Gupta, Ranjan Kumar Behera, Jagat Ram

24. **Eye Banking, Ocular Prosthesis and Rehabilitation**
    Ranjan Kumar Behera, Parul Chawla Gupta, Jagat Ram

25. **Community Ophthalmology**
    Mona Duggal, Anshul Chauhan

CHAPTER 8

Review of Anatomy and Physiology: Eye

Tulika Gupta, Tanvi Soni, Daisy Sahni

"The eyes are the window to the soul."

—**William Shakespeare**

LEARNING OBJECTIVES

After going through the chapter, the learner will be able to:
- Identify the parts of eye including the lacrimal apparatus.
- Define the parts of eye including the lacrimal apparatus.
- Understand their structure and functions.
- Comprehend the visual pathway.

TERMS

- **Cornea:** Anterior-most transparent layer in front of eye and allows light to enter in eye.
- **Fovea centralis:** Pit-like structure in retina where only photoreceptors are cones and forms the sharpest image of object.
- **Limbus:** Junction of cornea and sclera.
- **Retina:** Innermost layer of eyeball responsible for vision processing.

INTRODUCTION

Eyes are the organ of sight and are present in the bony orbits, located one on each side. Orbits are pyramidal in shape and made of seven different bones. It has a wide base opening anteriorly and extends into the posterior medial direction and apex transmits the optic nerve to the cranial cavity. The orbit contains eyeball, extraocular muscles for movement of eyeball, vessels, nerves, lacrimal gland, fascia and fat.

EYEBALL AND ITS APPENDAGES

Eye is a sense organ designed to capture and focus an image on retina and transmit to brain via optic nerve. **Eyeball** is an inch-wide sphere having anterior and posterior poles; equator is an imaginary circumferential line in the middle of the two poles **(Fig. 8.1)**.

Each eyeball is protected by a pair of eyelids and is suspended by extraocular muscles and fascial sheaths in a bony cavity known as orbit. There are 6 extraocular muscles: 4 recti and 2 obliques. The anterior portion which is transparent is formed by cornea and posterior opaque portion is formed by sclera. Their junction is called limbus

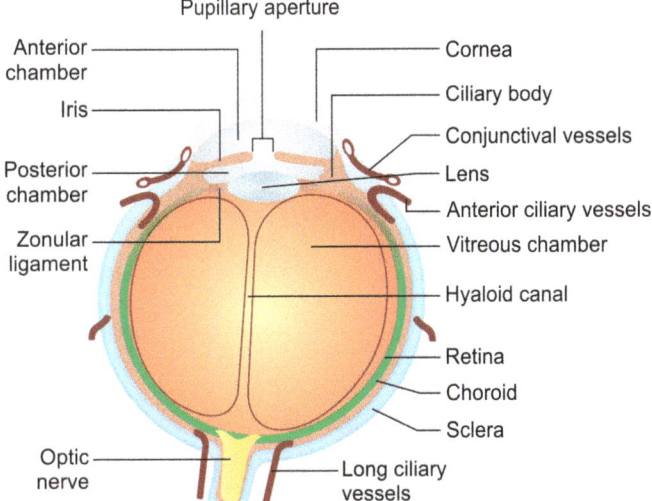

Fig. 8.1: Structure of eye.

which is marked by external scleral sulcus. The anterior portion of sclera is covered by conjunctiva which is reflected on the inner aspect of eyelids. The cornea and conjunctiva are always kept moist by tear film which is produced in lacrimal

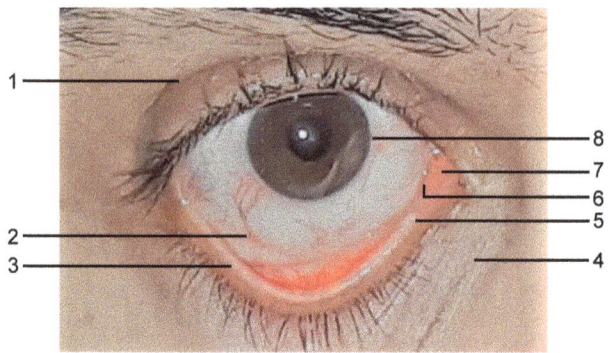

Fig. 8.2: Surface anatomy of eyelid margin and conjunctiva: 1. Eyelid, 2. Inferior fornix (exposed by pulling lower eyelid), 3. Eyelid margin showing opening of meibomian glands, 4. External landmark for lacrimal sac, 5. Lower punctum, 6. Plica seminularis, 7. Caruncle, 8. Limbus.

gland and drained by lacrimal passages. The healthy tear film contains three layers: Mucinous, aqueous, and lipid layers. Eyebrows, eyelids, conjunctiva and lacrimal apparatus are collectively called as ocular appendages **(Fig. 8.2)**.

Extraocular Muscles (Fig. 8.3, Table 8.1)

There are six small ribbon-like muscles which move the eyeballs in tandem; out of which four are straight muscles (recti) named according to their location medial rectus, lateral rectus, superior rectus and inferior rectus and two oblique muscles, superior and inferior oblique. All the muscles take origin at the posterior aspect near the apex of the orbit, except the inferior oblique which arises from the floor of the orbit anteriorly. All the muscles insert in the sclera; the recti insert anterior to the equator of the eyeball while both the oblique muscles insert posterior to it. All the muscles are supplied by the oculomotor nerve (III cranial nerve) except superior oblique which is supplied by the trochlear nerve (IV cranial nerve) and lateral rectus, which is supplied by the abducent nerve (VI cranial nerve). Adduction of the eyeball is caused by medial rectus, assisted by the superior and inferior recti, abduction is caused by lateral rectus and assisted by the superior and inferior oblique muscles; elevation of the eyeball by the superior rectus and inferior oblique and depression is by the inferior rectus and superior oblique muscles. Normally both the eyes move together and

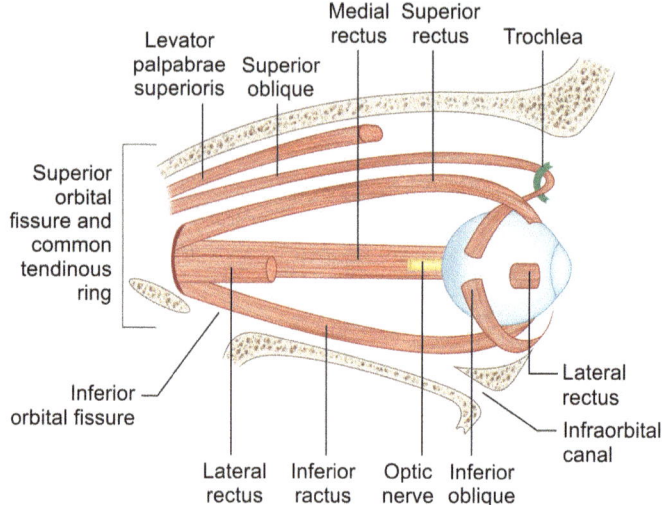

Fig. 8.3: Sagittal section showing origin and insertion of extraocular muscles.

to the same extent this is known as the conjugate movement.

Lacrimal Glands

Lacrimal glands are situated laterally in the roof of each orbit and secrete a lacrimal fluid which has lubricating and protective function. Lacrimal gland is supplied by the lacrimal nerve. Their secretions are released by small ducts into the upper conjunctiva, spreads over the conjunctiva with every blink as a tear film and lubricates the conjunctival covering of the eyeball and eyelids. The lacrimal fluid then drains via the lacrimal canaliculi into the nasolacrimal sac present near the medial puncta of the eye and then to the nose via the nasolacrimal duct.

Eyelids

Eyelids or palpebrae shield the eyeball from injury and bright light. The interior surface of the conjunctival sac is filled and with tear film is present between the eyelids and eyeball to and keep them moist. The palpebral fissure is space between the two eyelids. Each eyelid is formed by thin skin with glands of Zeis (sebaceous) and Molls (sweat), subcutaneous tissue, orbicularis oculi muscle fibers, tarsal plate with meibomian glands, and conjunctiva. The free edge of the eyelid has two

TABLE 8.1: Extraocular muscles.

Muscle	Origin	Insertion (sclera)	Blood supply
Superior rectus	Superior part of annulus of Zinn and optic nerve sheath	7.7 mm from limbus	Lateral muscular branch of ophthalmic artery
Inferior rectus (shortest recti)	Inferior part of annulus of Zinn	6.5 mm from limbus	Infraorbital artery and medial muscular branch of ophthalmic artery
Medial rectus	Medial part of annulus of Zinn and optic nerve sheath	5.5 mm from limbus	Medial muscular branch of ophthalmic artery
Lateral rectus	Lateral part of annulus of Zinn	6.9 mm from limbus	Lacrimal artery and lateral muscular branch of ophthalmic artery
Superior oblique	Bone above and medial to optic foramen	Upper and outer part behind equator	Lateral muscular branch of ophthalmic artery
Inferior oblique	Orbital plate of maxilla	Lower and outer part behind equator	Infraorbital artery and medial muscular branch of ophthalmic artery
Levator palpebrae superioris	Lesser wing of sphenoid	Lid crease and anterior surface of tarsus	Lateral muscular branch of ophthalmic artery

or more layers of hair, the eyelashes. The palpebral fissure is closed by approximation of eyelids by contraction of orbicularis oculi skeletal muscle supplied by the facial nerve (VII cranial nerve). Elevation of the upper eyelid is done by a muscle named levator palpebrae superioris muscle, innervated by the oculomotor nerve (EN III).

Conjunctiva

Conjunctiva is a transparent mucus membrane which lines the inner side of each eyelid from the free edge to its attached edge, then it reflects back to cover the front of sclera and cornea. Lines of reflection are known as superior fornix and inferior fornix. Palpebral conjunctiva is adherent to the tarsal plate of the eyelids and is very rich in blood vessels. While the bulbar conjunctiva is loose over the sclera to facilitate eyeball movements.

Conjunctival Sac

Conjunctival sac lines the ocular surface and has three parts: bulbar part, forniceal part and palpebral part. It is formed by non-keratinized epithelium. The palpebral portion lines the lids extending to fornices and reflects on eyeball as bulbar conjunctiva. It merges with corneal epithelium. Beneath the bulbar conjunctiva is thin fascia of connective tissue known as *Tenon's capsule*. It fuses with episcleral tissue at limbus and extends posteriorly as muscle sheath ending in distal part of optic nerve. Episcleral tissue is a loose vascular connective tissue layer between anterior sclera and bulbar conjunctiva.

Volume of conjunctival sac: Approx. 30 µL and average eye drop volume is 40–70 µL. Hence most of the drug is washed out after instillation.

Coats of Eyeball

Eyeball is made of three concentric layers from outside to inside namely: Corneoscleral envelope, uvea and retina.

Corneoscleral Coat

It is the outermost fibrous coat which is tough and inelastic. Anterior sixth is formed by cornea and posterior five-sixths is sclera.

Cornea

Cornea is ellipsoid in shape with vertical diameter of 10.6 mm and horizontal diameter of 11.75 mm. Refractive index of cornea is 1.376. It consists of 6 layers **(Table 8.2)**. Cornea is transparent and avascular structure. Its primary function is to allow the entry of the light rays inside the eyeball and it also refracts the entering light rays. It is highly intersected by branches of the ophthalmic division of trigeminal nerve (sensory).

Sclera

Sclera is present in the posterior five-sixths part of the outer coat of the eyeball. It is a thick, tough, white and opaque layer consisting of interwoven collagen fibers of variable diameter. It provides shape and protection to eyeball and receives insertion of extraocular muscles. Its outer surface is covered by thick facial layer the Tenon's capsule. Optic nerve can be seen emerging from the posterior aspect of sclera

TABLE 8.2: Layers of cornea and key features.

Corneal layer	Key features
Epithelium	• Non-keratinized stratified squamous epithelium • Defect in this layer is stained using fluorescein dye
Bowman's membrane	• Condensed portion of anterior stroma • Does not regenerate after trauma • Not a true membrane
Stroma	• Collagen fibers encased in mucopolysaccharides and ground substance • Accounts for 90% of corneal thickness
Dua's layer	• Pre-Descemet acellular layer. • Type 1 bubble in deep anterior lamellar keratoplasty (DALK) is formed between Dua's layer and stroma
Descemet's membrane	• Basement membrane of endothelium • Can regenerate after injury
Endothelium	• Hexagonal cells lining the Descemet's membrane • Cells can be visualized using specular microscopy

inferomedial to the posterior pole is known as cribriform plate. The emerging fibers of the optic nerve make this area sieve, like and weakest point of sclera. Posteriorly sclera is continuous with the dural sheath of the optic nerve. The anterior rim of sclera is continuous with cornea at corneoscleral junction known as **limbus.** So, limbus is a junction of the opaque sclera and the transparent cornea. It contains a trabecular network and the canal of Schlemm which drains the aqueous humor. The aqueous humor flow from posterior chamber to anterior chamber and then onto the canal of Schlemm, from here to aqueous veins and ultimately to the episcleral veins. An obstruction in the flow of aqueous humor will increase intraocular pressure leading to the glaucoma.

On the inner aspect, sclera is lined by highly vascular uveal tissue. **Uvea** comprises **iris, ciliary body and choroid**. Of these, iris forms a diaphragm-like structure with central aperture known as pupil. **Crystalline** lens is biconvex structure located just behind the iris and centered on pupil. Underneath the uveal tissue lies the nervous layer known as **retina**.

Endophthalmitis: It is defined as inflammation of inner layers of eyeball (retina and choroid) with exudation in vitreous cavity.
Panophthalmitis: It is defined as acute suppurative inflammation involving sclera with or without extension of inflammation into orbit.

Iris

Iris is the circular, pigmented contractile diaphragm which has an opening named pupil at the center. It lies between anterior and posterior chamber and peripherally iris is attached to ciliary body where it is thinnest. It is the anterior most and visible part of uveal tract. It has stromal layer anteriorly and double epithelial layer posteriorly. The iris is comprised of rich vascular stroma, smooth muscles and pigment; latter determines the color of the iris. The iris contains two smooth muscles, sphincter pupillae which is in the shape of concentric rings and contracts the pupil. The dilator pupillae muscle is radially arranged around the entire circumference of the iris. It dilates the pupil on contraction. The sphincter pupillae is supplied by the parasympathetic nerves and dilator pupillae by the sympathetic nerves.

Any pathology in the sympathetic pathway will result in Horner syndrome. The iris controls the amount of light entering the eye by altering the size of the pupil. Paralysis of III cranial nerve results in fixed dilated pupil.

Ciliary Body

The ciliary body is a complete ring present behind the limbus, triangular in cross section and extending from anterior rim of choroid to the posterior margin of the iris. Its outer scleral surface contains smooth ciliaris muscle which is circularly arranged around the entire circumference of the ciliary body and is innervated by parasympathetic nerves through the oculomotor nerve. The inner surface has smooth posterior part pars plana and rough part pars plicata. Pars plicata is formed by ciliary processes. Ciliary body suspends the lens with the help of suspensory ligament of lens, which is mainly attached to the grooves between the ciliary processes. Accommodation is the process by which the lens becomes rounder to focus a nearby object or flatter to focus a distant object. Contraction of the ciliaris muscle relaxes the suspensory ligament of lens which makes the lens more convex for near vision. The ciliary processes contain rich capillary network which secretes aqueous humor.

Choroid

Choroid is the large posterior part, which is separated from the sclera by suprachoroidal lamina. It is firmly attached to the retina by Bruch's membrane and is posteriorly continuous with the arachnoid membrane of the optic nerve. This is mainly a vascular membrane and is rich in melanin pigment. Rich vascularity of the choroid is responsible for red eye which occur, with flash photography.

Retina

Retina is the inner most layer and consists of outer pigment epithelium and the inner neural, in between the two there is intraretinal space which is obliterated in the adult. But it remains a weak area prone to retinal detachment. It is the inner photosensitive layer and is concerned with processing of visual information. It corresponds to the extent of choroid. It consists of multiple layers which can be broadly classified as external layer of visual cells (photoreceptors), middle layer of bipolar cells and inner layer of ganglion cells. Axon of ganglion cells constitutes the optic nerve and runs into central nervous system exiting the globe at optic disc. The retina is divided, anterior 1/3 of which is light insensitive and 2/3rds into posterior optic part of retina, which ends at a crenated edge known as ora serrata behind the ciliary body, and beyond this non-nervous pigmented epithelium of retina covers the ciliary body and iris. The optic part of retina is light sensitive and is composed of ten layers made up of neurons and supporting glial cells; the first layer is adjacent to the choroid—retinal pigment epithelium, outer limiting membrane, the layer of rods and cones, outer nuclear layer, outer plexiform layer, inner nuclear layer, inner plexiform layer, ganglion cell layer, nerve fiber layer, and inner limiting membrane. Rods and cones are photoreceptors, rods are sensitive to dim light (scotopic vision) and cones are more sensitive to colors and photopic vision. The rods and cones contain a

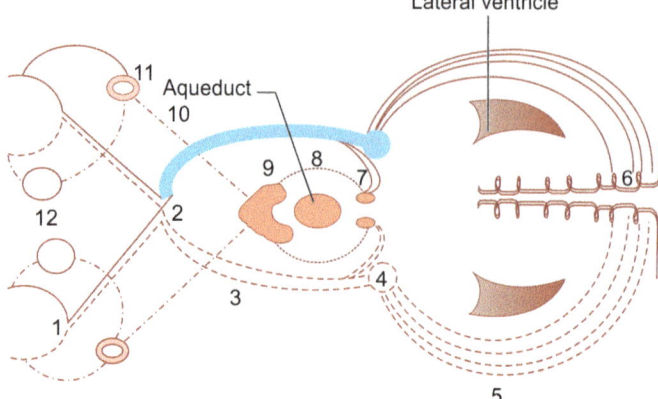

Fig. 8.4: Optic nerve pathway and light reflex pathway. Optic nerve pathway from fixation area to occipital cortex and light reflex pathway from fixation area to ciliary ganglion. 1. Fovea, 2. Optic chiasma, 3. Optic tract, 4. Lateral geniculate body, 5. Optic radiation, 6. Occipital cortex, 7. Pretectal nucleus, 8. Internuncial fibers, 9. Edinger–Westphal nucleus, 10. Oculomotor nerve, 11. Ciliary ganglion, 12. Accessory ganglion.

TABLE 8.3: Parts of the optic nerve.	
Part of optic nerve	Features
Intraocular (optic disc/ optic nerve head)	Portion of optic nerve lying within the sclera 1 mm long
Intra-orbital	Part from globe to optic foramen 25–30 mm long
Intracanalicular	Traverses optic canal in lesser wing of sphenoid 6 mm long
Intracranial	From optic canal to optic chiasma 5–16 mm (10 mm average)

photopigment, which has 11-cis retinaldehyde and opsin. The light isomerizes the retinaldehyde to all-trans configuration and generates the receptor potential. This information is transferred to the bipolar cells present in inner nuclear layer and then to the ganglion cells. The axons of the ganglion cells collect at the optic disc to form the optic nerve which carries the information through optic chiasma and optic tract, to the visual area in the cerebral cortex **(Fig. 8.4)**. It gives rise to the optic nerve. Optic nerve is 50 mm long from globe to chiasma and is divided into four portions **(Table 8.3)**.

Optic Disc

Optic disc is a circular depressed area of about 1.5 mm in the retina where axons of ganglion cells converge to form optic nerve; to exit the eyeball these fibers penetrate the sclera forming the lamina cribrosa. The optic disc lacks rods and cones and is therefore a blind spot. The central retinal artery and vein pass through the optic nerve. Macula lutea is a pale-yellow area (due to xanthophyll pigment accumulation in ganglion cells) near the posterior pole, it has small, depressed area known as *fovea centralis* located 3 mm lateral (temporal side) to the optic disc along the visual axis. Fovea has the maximum concentration of cones (no rods or capillaries) that are arranged to an angle so that light directly impinges on the cornea without passing through the other layers of the retina and is linked to a single ganglion. This is the spot of keenest vision in the eye.

Interior of Eyeball

Interior of the eyeball is divided into anterior and posterior segments by the lens. The anterior segment is further divided by iris into anterior chamber situated between the cornea and iris and posterior chamber present between the iris and the lens; both the chambers are filled by the aqueous humor and are continuous through the pupil. The aqueous humor is secreted in the posterior chamber by the ciliary processes and absorbed by the venous sinuses or canals of Schlemm present at the iridocorneal angle. The posterior segment of eyeball present behind the lens and surrounded by the retina, is filled with jelly like vitreous humor which holds the retina in place and supports the lens.

Lens

Lens is a transparent biconvex disc-shaped structure made up of a capsule, anterior epithelium and fibers. It is highly compressible and can increase its convexity to adapt for the near vision. Lens is suspended by the suspensory ligaments from the ciliary body. It contains mainly water (98%), hyaluronic acid and collagen. Its function is to focus the light rays entering into the eye by bending them; lens is the only structure in the eye which can vary its dioptric power. Blood supply of eye is derived from ophthalmic artery which is a branch of internal carotid artery. Retina receives blood supply from central retinal artery (branch of ophthalmic artery).

Site of intravitreal injection: 3 mm from limbus (aphakia), 3.5 mm (pseudophakia), 4 mm (phakic eye)

Compartments and Fluids in Eyeball

Anterior chamber is a fluid-filled space bounded anteriorly by cornea and posteriorly by iris. It is about 2.5 mm deep (range 2.6 to 4.4 mm). It is filled with approximately 250 μl of aqueous humor. Peripheral recess of anterior chamber is known as angle. Angle is bounded anteriorly by corneosclera and posteriorly by root of iris and ciliary body. It gives access to drainage structures and is visualized in gonioscopy. In this region on the inner aspect of sclera is canal of Schlemm which is the site for drainage of aqueous humor. Just below the canal of Schlemm, there is triangular shaped sponge work of connective tissue known as trabecular meshwork. The trabecular meshwork extends from peripheral termination of Descemet's membrane to narrow strip of scleral tissue just anterior to ciliary body known as scleral spur.

Posterior chamber is space between posterior surface of iris with part of ciliary body and lens and zonules containing 6 μL of aqueous humor. Posterior four fifth of eyeball cavity (space between lens and vitreous) is filled by vitreous humor which is transparent jelly like and is about 4 mL in volume. Aqueous humor is a clear transparent fluid which maintains intraocular pressure and plays important role in metabolism by proving substrates and removing metabolites from cornea and lens. Normal intraocular pressure is 10-20 mm Hg. It is measured using *tonometry*. Rise in intraocular pressure either due to increased resistance to aqueous outflow through trabecular meshwork or change in dynamics balance between production and outflow leads to *glaucoma*.

Vitreous humor is optically clear, provides a support system for globe stabilization and forms a pathway for nourishment of retina.

VISUAL PATHWAY

The optic nerve is the second cranial nerve and is made up of axons of the ganglion cells of retina. It exits the retina at the optic disc and the eyeball by piercing sclera at the cribriform plate. Outside the eyeball the nerve is covered by the meninges of the brain and it passes posteriorly and medially to exit the orbit through its apex traverses the optic canal to enter the cranial cavity. In the cranial cavity, optic nerves of both sides join to form a flattened optic chiasma. Within the chiasma there is crossing over of nasal (medial) fibers of both retina to the opposite side while the fibers from the temporal (lateral) half of each retina continue to remain on the same side. Fibers then form optic tracts; each optic tract contains ipsilateral temporal and contralateral nasal fibers or visual information from the opposite half of the visual field. Each optic tract relays its information to the lateral geniculate body of the thalamus where they relay further send the information by a fiber bundle called, optic radiation to the visual or striate area in the occipital lobe of the cerebral cortex.

PHYSIOLOGY OF VISION

It involves initiation of vision at photoreceptors, transmission of sensation via optic nerve pathway (**Fig. 8.4**) and visual perception in cortex. Light reflex is contraction of pupil when light enters the eye (direct light reflex) and simultaneous contraction of pupil of other eye (consensual reflex).

Visual field is the elliptical area seen by both the eyes with peripheral small crescents of monocular vision on both sides. Light travels in a straight light, in order to see any object, the light reflected by the object has to be focused on the retina. The eye is constructed to achieve this objective, there are many refractive structures in the eyeball which bend the light so that it can focus on retina. The transparent cornea allows the entry of the light rays into the eyes at the same time its regular structure bends the rays (refracts) and directs them towards the pupil. Pupil protects the eye from the bright light by contacting and thus controlling the amount of light entering inside. Both aqueous and vitreous humor have refractive power but lens is unique in this regard as it can adapt its refractive power (15 diopters). The light rays coming from the near objects are not parallel and require more bending (or refraction) in order to focus on retina. Thus, lens increases its refractive power by increasing its convexity. This is achieved by contraction of ciliaris muscles which leads to relaxation of suspensory ligament of lens and lens becomes more convex and adapted for near vision. On the other hand, parallel light rays from distant objects are bent less by opposite action. Thus, all the refractive medias of the eyeball function to focus the light on fovea centralis. Scattered light is absorbed by the choroid so as to avoid blurring of the image formed.

SUMMARY

Thorough knowledge of ocular anatomy and physiology has clinical implications. Understanding of surgical anatomy is imperative for better collaboration between surgeons and assistants. Familiarity with ocular physiology aids in understanding the medical management of ocular disorders.

MULTIPLE CHOICE QUESTIONS

1. What is innermost layer of eyeball responsible for vision processing?
   a. Choroid
   b. Retina
   c. Sclera
   d. Cornea
2. What is the corneoscleral junction called?
   a. Optic nerve
   b. Ciliary body
   c. Sclera
   d. Limbus
3. What is blind spot?
   a. Fovea
   b. Optic nerve head
   c. Pupil
   d. Lens
4. What are the structures forming boundaries of posterior chamber?
   a. Iris, lens and zonules
   b. Lens, choroid and retina
   c. Cornea and iris
   d. Sclera and choroid
5. Blood supply of eye is derived from which artery?
   a. Middle cerebral artery
   b. Anterior communicating artery
   c. Maxillary artery
   d. Ophthalmic artery
6. Which of the following cranial nerves do not supply the extra-ocular muscles?
   a. III cranial nerve
   b. IV cranial nerve
   c. V cranial nerve
   d. VI cranial nerve
7. Identify the false statement regarding the optic nerve:
   a. It is the II cranial nerve
   b. It is formed by axons of the ganglion cells
   c. At the chiasma temporal fibers cross
   d. Optic tract is from lateral geniculate body to the cortex
8. The uveal tissue consists of:
   a. Retina, choroid and sclera
   b. Retina, iris and sclera
   c. Choroid, ciliary body and sclera
   d. Choroid, ciliary body and iris

ANSWERS

| 1. b | 2. d | 3. b | 4. a |
| 5. d | 6. c | 7. c | 8. d |

SUGGESTED READING

1. Agrahari V, Mandal A, Agrahari V, et al. A comprehensive insight on ocular pharmacokinetics. Drug Deliv Transl Res. 2016;6(6):735-54.
2. Bron AJ. Vortex patterns of the corneal epithelium. Trans Ophthalmol Soc U K. 1973;93(0):455-72.
3. Dua HS, Faraj LA, Said DG, Gray T, Lowe J. Human corneal anatomy redefined: a novel pre-Descemet's layer (Dua's layer). Ophthalmology. 2013;120(9):1778-85.
4. Durand ML. Endophthalmitis. Clin Microbiol Infect. 2013;19(3):227-234. doi:10.1111/1469–0691.12118.
5. Williams PL, Warwick R, Dyson M, Bannister LH. Gray's anatomy, 37th edition. Edinburgh: Churchill Livingstone; 1989.
6. Izzotti A, Saccà SC, Longobardi M, Cartiglia C. Sensitivity of ocular anterior chamber tissues to oxidative damage and its relevance to the Pathogenesis of Glaucoma. Invest Ophthalmol Vis Sci. 2009;50(11):5251-8.
7. Snell RS, Lemp MA. Clinical Anatomy of the Eye. Hong Kong: Blackwell Scientific; 1989.
8. Takahashi Y, Watanabe A, Matsuda H, Nakamura Y, Nakano T, Asamoto K, et al. Anatomy of secretory glands in the eyelid and conjunctiva: a photographic review. Ophthalmic Plast Reconstr Surg. 2013;29(3):215-9.
9. T Thoft RA, Friend J. The X, Y, Z hypothesis of corneal epithelial maintenance. Invest Ophthalmol Vis Sci. 1983;24(10):1442-3.
10. Wolff E. Anatomy of the Eye and Orbit, 7th edition. London: HK Lewis; 1976.
11. Yanoff M, Duker JS, Augsburger JJ. Ophthalmology. Edinburgh: Mosby Elsevier; 2009.

CHAPTER 9

Assessment and Diagnostic Evaluation of Eye

Anshul Chauhan, Gagandeep Kaur, Priyanka Verma, Lakshya Kumar, Mona Duggal

"Your eyes could be the windows to your health."
—**American Academy of Ophthalmology (AAO)**

Learning Objectives

After going through the chapter, the learner will be able to:
➤ Describe comprehensive eye examination.
➤ Discuss the importance of history taking procedures.
➤ Describe the procedures involved in eye evaluation.
➤ Distinguish between various eye assessment and diagnostic evaluation procedures.

TERMS

- **Anterior segment evaluation:** It includes cornea, iris lens, conjunctiva and eye lids. Assessment of these structures using slit-lamp biomicroscopy is an integral part of ophthalmic examination.
- **Comprehensive eye examination:** It consists of a series of tests that assess the posterior and anterior segment of eye health performed either by optometrist or an ophthalmologist.
- **Fundus fluorescein angiography (FFA):** It is a valuable tool in the diagnosis and management of a large number of fundus disorders. The examiner studies the changes produced by various fundus disorders in the flow of fluorescein dye along the vasculature of the retina and choroid.
- **Intraocular pressure (IOP):** It is the pressure exerted by intraocular fluids on the coats of the eyeball. The normal IOP varies between 10 and 21 mm of Hg (mean16 ± 2.5 mm of Hg). The normal level of IOP is essentially maintained by a dynamic equilibrium between the formation and outflow of the aqueous humor.
- **Optical coherence tomography (OCT):** It is a non-invasive, high-resolution diagnostic imaging platform that uses light waves to generate in vivo, cross-sectional images of ocular tissues.
- **Posterior segment evaluation:** This is essential to diagnose the diseases of the vitreous, optic nerve head, retina and choroid.
- **Visual acuity (VA):** It is a measure of the eye's ability to distinguish shapes and details of objects at a given distance.

INTRODUCTION

An eye examination is a series of tests performed to assess vision and ability to focus on and discern objects. It also includes other tests and examinations pertaining to the eyes. Diagnostic tests are approaches used in clinical practice to identify with high accuracy the disease of a particular patient and thus to provide early and proper treatment. A comprehensive eye examination (CEE) by an ophthalmologist or optometrist is important part of caring for our eyes, vision and overall general wellbeing. Early diagnosis and treatment of the eye disorders can prevent vision loss. There are number of common eye diseases that can be detected by simple means such as torch light examination. Patients' signs and symptoms in addition to professional judgment determine the tests to be conducted. Other methods like use of visual acuity chart for vision assessment are low cost and easy to use. In order to carry out an eye examination we need a professional who is skilfully trained to carry out patient-centered eye examination.

Nurses have to juggle different tasks each day in order to meet the expectations and needs of their patients and colleagues—especially when working in a busy hospital.

Nurses have the potential to significantly contribute in ophthalmology and the visual sciences. They are also a critical element in healthcare system because they can deliver up-to-date knowledge between health-caregivers, such as general physicians. Nurses are greatly able to assist in providing referrals to patients who need subspecialty services and subsequently this will contribute to saving healthcare expenditures since patients would receive proper management. They could perform their duties in an effective manner, they are likely to require special training. Nurses could support the process of categorizing eye pathologies as emergency or ordinary medical situations and perform triage by identifying benign and malignant conditions.

ASSESSMENT

A routine CEE should be patient centric so that adequate focus is given to their requirement, belief and their preferences. It will help to drive towards patient-cantered care to screen and detect common eye diseases, whereby reducing morbidity and associated cost with the disease. A CEE should not always be done with a patient presenting with ocular symptoms but also those reporting for routine eye examination. A patient-centered care should focus on.

- **Care recipient:** Note the patient features (physical and behavioral) when they enter the room. Look for any signs of discomfort that indicates eye pain and assist the people with disabilities (visual and other).
- **Maintaining pleasant communication to develop trust:** Effective communication is the mainstream that establishes the trust with the patients. Express empathy without being emotionally overwhelmed, stay respectful. Always listen to the patient and be considerate with people with impairments (hearing, visual or learning).
- **History taking:** Request the person to elicit the reason for their visit as this will help the examiner to look for the required information and patient concerns. The required data can then be filled on the prescribed formats (online or offline). The patient should be asked about the patients' presumptions about their expected treatment and their outcome.
- **Eye examination and vision assessment:** Start eye examination and explain to the patient what further tests are necessary, time required and cost involved. Analyze the patient for referral to higher facilities and ensure adequate information is given to them before they take up referral.
- **Treatment plan discussion with family:** Family members should be made aware of the tests performed, diagnosis, treatment and prognosis. Repeat if patients or unable to understand anything and allow enough time to ask questions. Ask the person if there is anything they do not understand and allow enough time to the patients to make decisions as they are likely to cooperate once they fully understand the clinical conditions.

Before starting a procedure:
- Wash hands thoroughly before and after procedure.
- Use of gloves during the procedures is advised.
- Clean/wipe the equipment before and after use.
- Lighting should be appropriate in the room.
- Explain the procedure clearly.

History Taking

History recording is a structured process of determining patient's problem in a systematic order to collect relevant information. This information helps us to form the hypothesis for the underlying diagnosis. Further investigations are suggested to either confirm or disagree upon the hypothesis based on history recording **(Table 9.1)**.

TABLE 9.1: Good history recording components.

Components	What to record	Importance
Personal and demographic data	Name	Identification, follow-up
	Age and gender	Ruling out disease associated specifically with age and gender
	Address and contact number	Follow-up and identification of areas with endemicity
	Education	Assessment of health literacy and understanding level of patient
	Occupation	Assessment of daily visual needs
Reason for visit or presenting complaint	Redness, soreness, pain	This enlists the main reason for visit to the eye care facility
	Decreased distance vision in unilateral or bilateral	
	Diplopia (double vision), swelling of eyelid	
History of presenting complaint	Onset, progression, duration of complaint, severity, unilateral or bilateral, associated symptoms, past medical suggestions and medications	Probing more will help in elaborating presenting complaint in detail
Past eye history	Past similar complaints	For differential diagnosis, deciding treatment plan
	History of trauma	
	Past eye surgery	

Contd...

Contd...

Components	What to record	Importance
General medical history	Diabetes, hypertension, cardiovascular diseases, arthritis, HIV	Ocular diagnosis can be achieved appropriately based on medical history and other specialties For example, neuro-ophthalmology Treatment plan can be modified based on the general medical history
Family eye history	History of glaucoma, retinoblastoma, diabetes, hypertension	Important to know if their genetic predisposition of inherited disease
Medication history	Past and present medication for medical and eye conditions	• Some medications may be important etiology for ocular conditions • Drug use compliance and reasons for non-compliance
Allergy history	Any drug allergies in the past	Alternate medication as per allergy history
Social history	Smoking	Dry eye, cataract age-related macular degeneration (AMD), Graves, uveitis
	Alcohol	Dry eye, fetal alcohol syndrome, ocular trauma, diplopia, Wernicke's encephalopathy

EYE EXAMINATION

EXTERNAL OCULAR EXAMINATION

Visual Acuity

Visual acuity (VA) is a measure of the eye's ability to distinguish shapes and details of objects at a given distance. VA measurement is a part of eye examination which needs precise measurement unless leading to incorrect decisions and management. That is why it is important to assess VA consistently in order to detect changes in vision.

Requirements to record VA:
- ❖ **Equipment:**
  - ➢ Snellen E chart, C chart **(Figs. 9.1 and 9.2)**
  - ➢ Occluder, card or tissue
  - ➢ Pinhole occlude **(Fig. 9.3)**
- ❖ **How to record VA:**
  - ➢ Proper light condition to illuminate the chart (if wall chart is used)
  - ➢ Explain the importance of procedure to the patient.

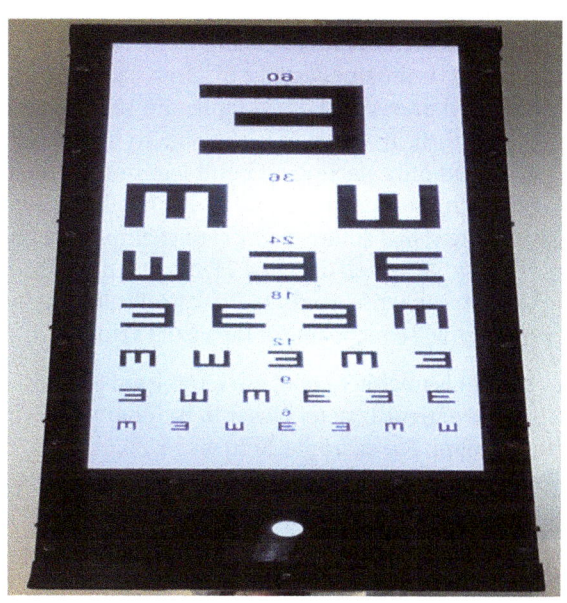

Fig. 9.2: Tumbling E-chart.

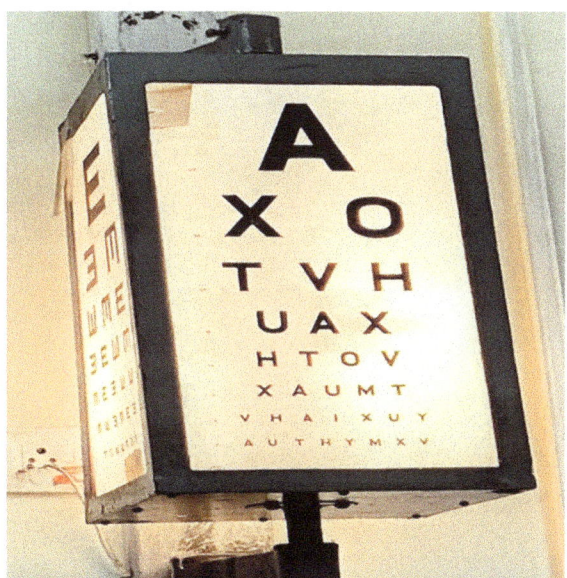

Fig. 9.1: Snellen visual acuity chart (drum chart).

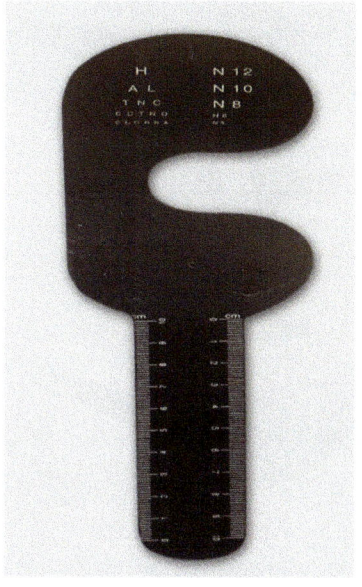

Fig. 9.3: Pinhole-occluder.

- Explain to the patient to tell clearly if they are unable to see properly.
- *Patient positioning:* Six meters distance from Snellen or E chart in sitting or standing position
- Start with right eye (RE) without spectacles (one eye at a time).
- While doing this, patient should cover left eye (LE) with plain occluder, or if not available tissue can be used (avoid touching by hand).
- Tell the patient to read from left to right and use tumbling E chart or C chart for those who cannot read letters.
- *Using E or C chart:* Ask the patient to point direction of the letter E (upward, downward, left or right). In case of C chart ask for the direction in which it is opening. Three out of four orientation should therefore be correctly identified by the patient.
- *Recording VA:* It is expressed as fraction, e.g., 6/18. The numerator (top number) displays the distance of the patient from the chart (6 meter). Denominator (bottom number) is the smallest line of letter-size that a person can read precisely. For example, the 18 line (6/18) or 6 line (6/6). If a person is not able to read a full line and read only starting and end letter of the line, you can record this visual acuity by adding the alphabet P with the visual acuity record. For example, if a person is only able to read only first 2 letter at 4th line from the top you can write it as 6/18 P +2. It will allow to record more precise recording of the visual acuity.

When patient is unable to read top letter from 6 meter:
- Move the patient 1 meter closer to the chart until able to see top letter. For example, 5/60 and 4/60.
- Visual acuity can also be calculated through counting finger (CF) by holding fingers at a distance of 5 meters or 4 meters. For example, VA = CF 5 m, VA = CF 4 m
- If unable to count fingers at 1 meter then wave hand and check whether patient is able to see hand movements (HM); VA = HM
- If unable to see HM, then record perception of light (PL) by shining torch light in the eye and ask them to see. For example, VA = PL and VA = NPL (non-perception of light)

Autorefractometry

An autorefractor **(Fig. 9.4)** is used to provide measurement of refractive error to provide glasses and lenses for correction. This can provide information which will tell whether patient will have spherical or cylindrical correction. It is easy to use and can be a good alternative in busy clinical practice. Its ease of use makes it advantageous to use for screening large number of people, for research purposes. But it can show some variations or unreliable results, high refractive error, cataract, and people with small pupil, so requires subjective verification.

Intraocular Pressure (IOP)

Tonometry is used to detect raised pressure in the eyes which predicts the patients at risk or with glaucoma. Tonometer can be categorized into two category, which are contact tonometer and non-contact tonometer. Goldmann and Perkins applanation tonometry (contact tonometer) ocular response analyzer (non-contact tonometer), Schiotz tonometer, pneumotonometer, tonopen (indentation tonometry **(Figs. 9.5 and 9.6),** rebound tonometer, pascal dynamic contour tonometer.

Refraction

Refraction is defined as the act of determining the focal condition (myopia, hypermetropia, and astigmatism) of the eye and its corrections by optical devices, usually spectacles or contact lenses. It also tells us about the refractive error (RE) which means the lens power used to correct it. SI Unit of power of a lens is Diopter.

Refraction is an eye exam that measures the type (myopia, hypermetropia, and astigmatism) and the amount of refractive error (RE). It also determines the required lens power needed to compensate for it **(Figs. 9.7 and 9.8)**.

Myopia (nearsightedness): It is a type of refractive error in which near objects are clear but far objects are blurred.

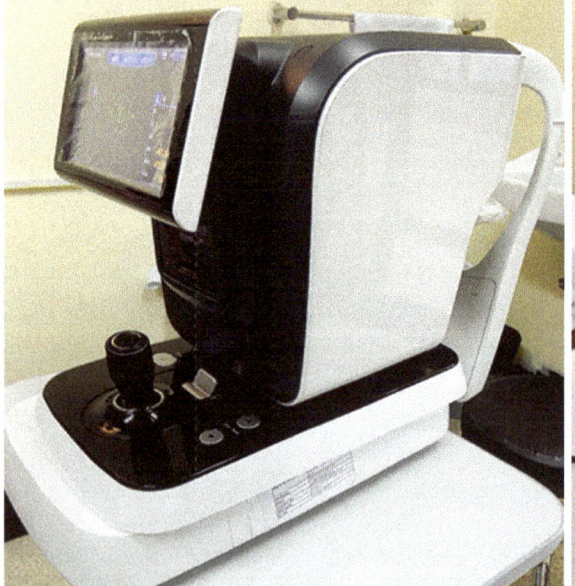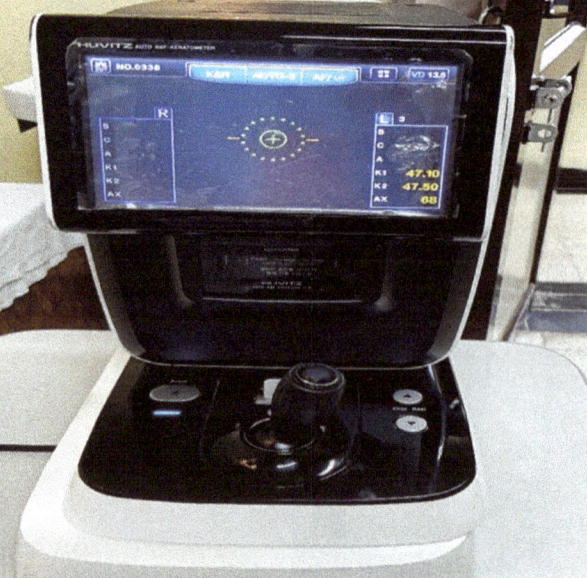

Fig. 9.4: Auto-refractometers.

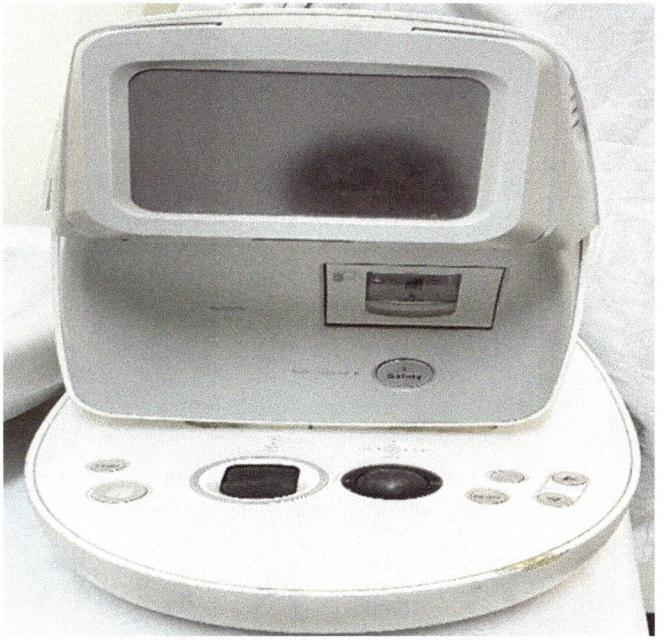

Fig. 9.5: Non-contact tonometer.

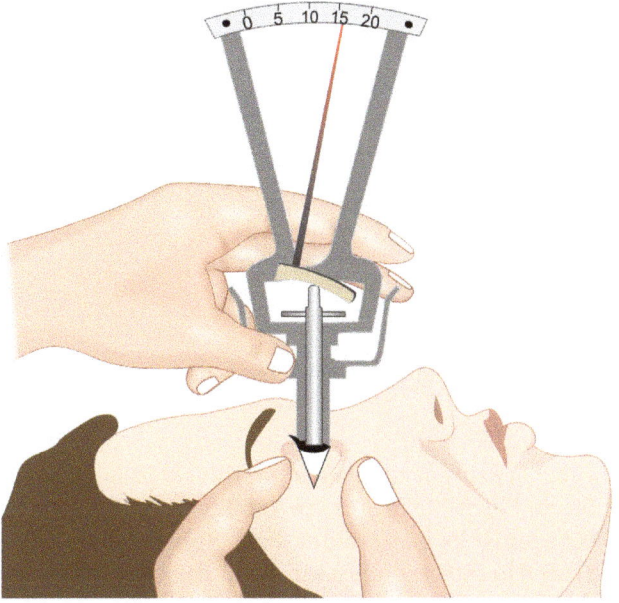

Fig. 9.6: Schiotz tonometer.

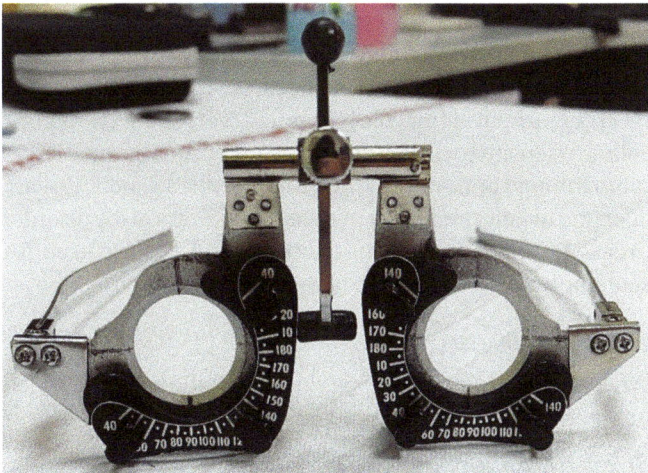

Fig. 9.7: Trial frame.

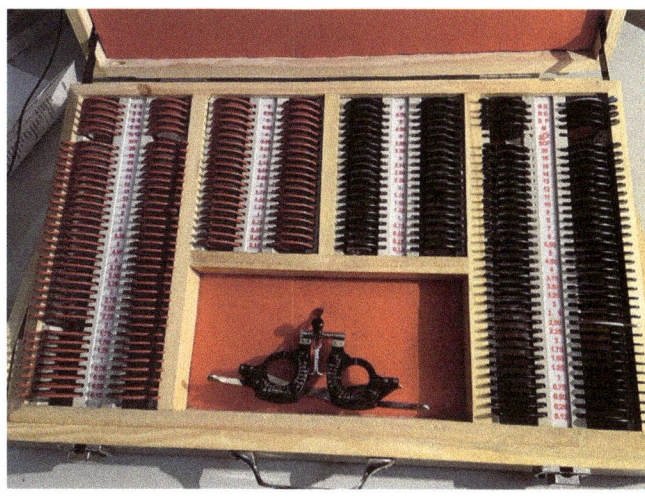

Fig. 9.8: Trial set

Hypermetropia (farsightedness): It is a type of refractive error in which far objects appear clear but close objects are blurred.

Astigmatism is an irregular curvature of eye's cornea or lens that causes improper refraction.

Torchlight Eye Examination

It is the simplest method to perform external eye examination. It helps us to inspect eye, eyelids, conjunctiva, sclera, cornea, iris and pupil. Eye movements, eye symmetry, redness, discharge, size, and shape of pupil can be observed upon **(Table 9.2)**.

Direct Ophthalmoscope

The direct ophthalmoscope **(Fig. 9.9)** is a small handheld instrument device used to examine the back of patient's eye. The ophthalmoscope is most suitable to use and serves handy. It can be used for detection of foreign body, pupil irregularity and light reflexes.

Some incorporations like cobalt blue filter allows corneal abrasions ulcers visible after fluorescein insertion.

TABLE 9.2: Key parts to examine during torch light examination.	
Eye parts to be examined	*What is to be examined*
Eyelids	• Normal movement and position • Any swelling or lumps • Opening and closing of eyelids is normal • Protrusion of eyes • Redness or discharge
Conjunctiva (white part of the eye)	• Redness • Growth or raised areas
Cornea (clear part of the eye)	• Foreign body • White or grey areas on the cornea
Pupil	• Color: Black is normal, grey or white indicates cataract • Shape: Circular • Size of pupil: Normally size of pupil reduces when torch is shone at it, look for opposite scenario

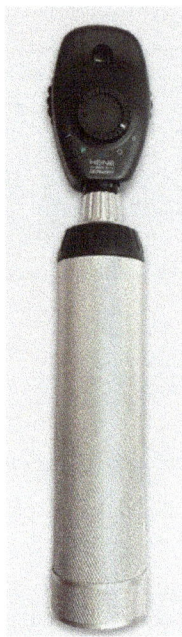

Fig. 9.9: Direct ophthalmoscope.

Indirect Ophthalmoscope

Indirect ophthalmoscope **(Fig. 9.10)** is an instrument worn on head or attached to spectacles and is used to examine the back of the eye. This optical instrument works on the principle of light transmission from headset to fundus through a condensing lens. The light is reflected back from lens that creates a laterally inverted image observed through stereoscopic viewing system.

Visual Field Test

Visual field test, perimetry tells us about how wide of an area of an eye can see when focused on a central point. It is also called as confrontation test, individual eye is tested for all four quadrants (superior and lower, nasal and temporal). While performing this test, the patient is asked to focus on examiner finger (target) from periphery to center and patient is asked to tell when they see the finger.
Tools: Central 30-2 full threshold Humphrey visual field analyzer **(Fig. 9.11)**, frequency doubling perimeter, Amsler Grid, Goldmann kinetic perimeter.

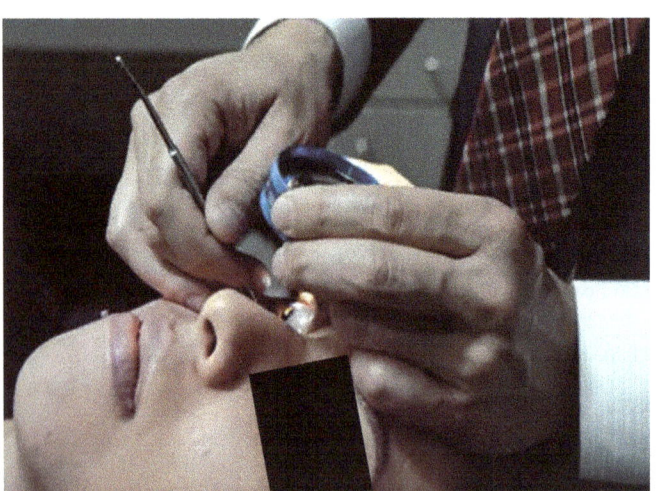

Fig. 9.10: Indirect ophthalmoscopy.

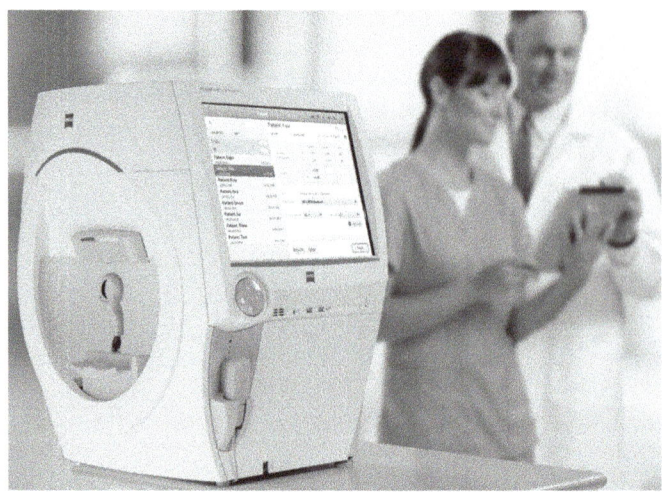

Fig. 9.11: Humphrey visual field analyzer.

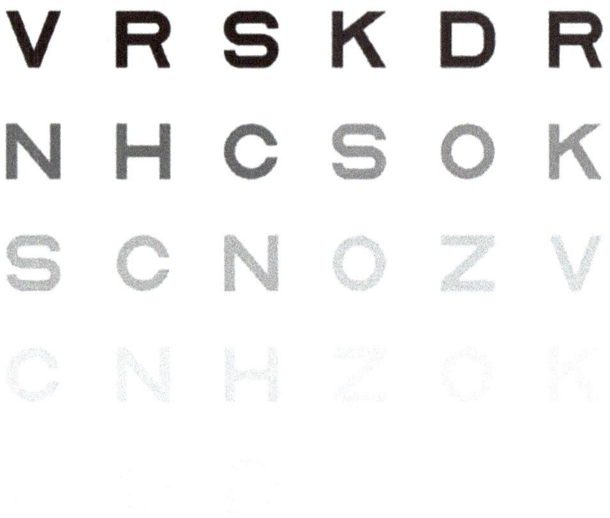

Fig. 9.12: Pelli-Robson chart.

Contrast Sensitivity

Contrast sensitivity measures the threshold between the visible and invisible means eye's ability to clearly detect an object against its background. Pelli–Robson chart is **(Fig. 9.12)** used to detect contrast sensitivity. Diabetic retinopathy (DR), glaucoma and cataracts present with reduced contrast sensitivity.

Color Vision

It is defined as the inability to distinguish between different shades of color. The color vision occurs in our eyes due to cone receptor present at (macula) central part of retina. These cone cells are sensitive to different colors and send information to brain through optic nerve. Color blindness is a genetic disease affecting mostly men. Most people are unaware of the disorder unless tested. Color vision charts **(Fig. 9.13)** are used for screening and detecting the type of blindness.

Binocular Vision

When a normal person looks at something, the image is formed on the fovea of both eyes independently, but the person only sees a single image. Binocular single vision is the name for this condition. In other words, bilateral single vision is when both eyes work together to make a single image in your mind.

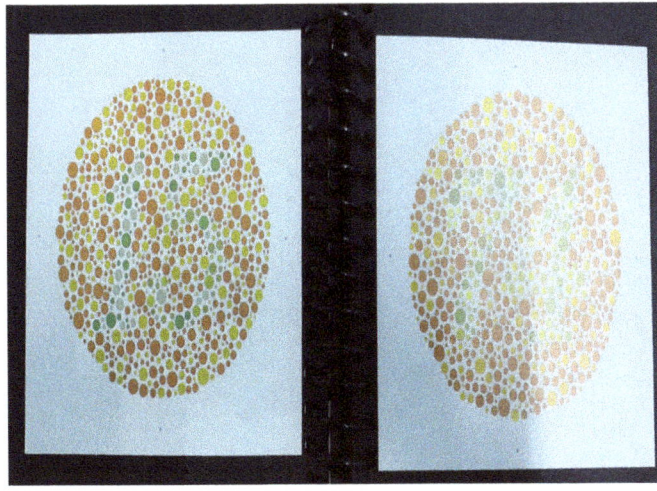

Fig. 9.13: Ishihara chart.

Red filter test, worth four dot test, Baglioni's striated glasses test, Hirschberg test is used to test binocular vision.

Strabismus

Strabismus (squint) is a condition in which the eyes are not lined up properly. If the affected eye's strabismus is not handled early, it can cause permanent loss of vision. This is called amblyopia, which is another name for "lazy eye." There is a chance that the child's vision will always be worse in the eye that is turned inward.

The eye a person wants to look at is called the "fixing eye," and the eye that is looking somewhere else is called the "deviated eye."

ANTERIOR AND POSTERIOR SEGMENT EVALUATION

Slit-lamp Biomicroscopy for Anterior Segment

Slit-lamp **(Fig. 9.14)** is useful in examining anterior and posterior segment of the eye. Anterior segments involve conjunctiva, cornea, anterior chamber, pupil and posterior segment involves iris, lens, retina.

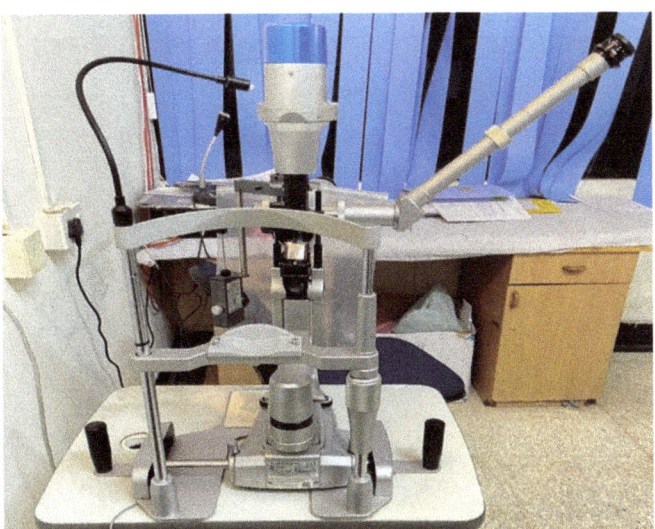

Fig. 9.14: Slit-lamp.

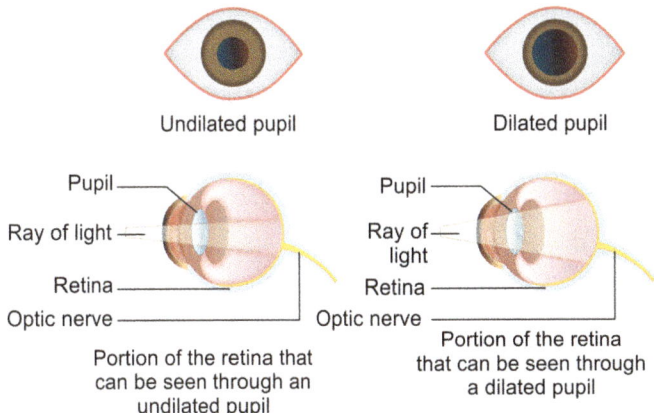

Fig. 9.15: Effects of dilation.

What is Eye Dilation?

It is defined as a temporary change in the pupil size under the effect of anticholinergic agents which block the effect of acetylcholine a neurotransmitter released by parasympathetic nerve cells. Under the effect of dilating agent, pupil size is increased.

It makes clinical examination of posterior segment of the eye easier **(Fig. 9.15)**. For example, tropicamide, atropine.

Indications

- ❖ **Age:** Examining eyes with small pupil in patients with old age, cloudy media and meiosis prevents clear view of the back of the eye.
- ❖ **Trauma:** To rule out intraocular injury after a trauma, dilated fundus examination is required. External appearance may not present best accurate picture of an eye internally so requires dilation.
- ❖ **Predisposing systemic diseases:** Conditions requiring monitoring of fundus to see visible changes over time also require dilated fundus examination. For example, diabetes, hypertension.

Contraindications

Careful history of angle-closure glaucoma, intraocular lens implants should be interrogated before dilation as may aggravate the conditions.

B-scan (Ultrasonography)

B-scan (USG) **(Fig. 9.16)** is a simple, ocular assessment more specifically back of the eye. It is noninvasive procedure used in detection of choroidal detachment, trauma, tumors, etc. B-scan can generate sound waves up to frequency of 10 MHz. During the procedure patient is instructed to look straight so that the probe is perpendicular to the area being examined.

Optical Coherence Tomography (OCT)

Optical coherence tomography (OCT) **(Fig. 9.17)** is a non-invasive test through which ophthalmologist can see retina's individual layers. It helps in estimation of layers thickness under cross-sectional images. OCT works with light waves passing through eyes and is helpful in evaluating the changes caused by glaucoma on fibers of optic nerve. It fails to see changes where light cannot enter eyes like in cataract and vitreous hemorrhage.

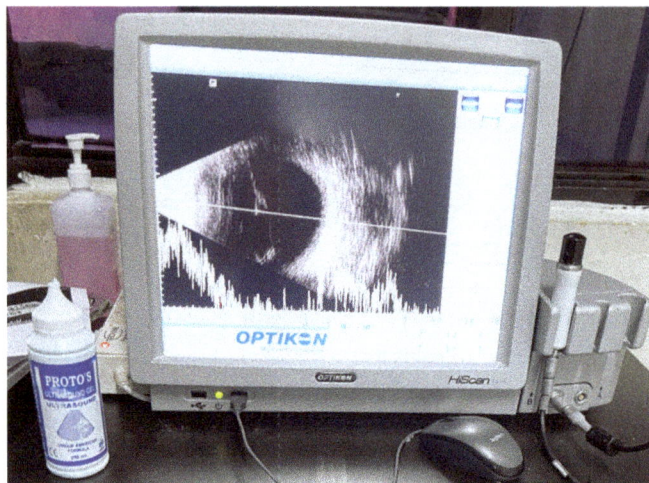

Fig. 9.16: B-scan.

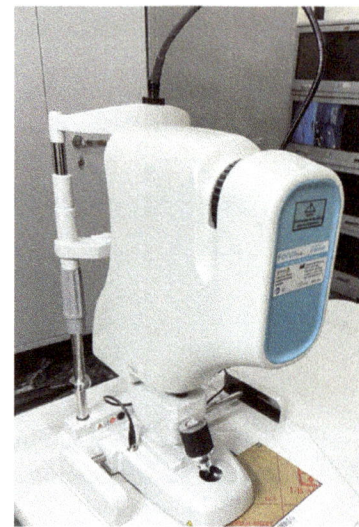

Fig. 9.18: Fundus camera.

Indications

It is indicated in many disorders of the ocular fundus: diabetic retinopathy, vascular occlusions, Eales' disease, central serous retinopathy, cystoid macular edema.

Technique

The technique of FFA comprises rapidly injecting 5 mL of 10% solution of sterile sodium fluorescein dye in the antecubital vein and taking serial photographs (with fundus camera) of the fundus of the patient who is seated with pupils fully dilated. The fundus camera has a mechanism to use blue light (420–490 nm wavelength) for exciting the fluorescein present in blood vessels and to use a yellow-green filter for receiving the fluorescent light (510–530 nm wavelength) back for photography. The first photograph is taken after 5 seconds, then every second for the next 20 seconds, and every 3–5 seconds for the next one minute. The last pictures are taken after 10 minutes (**Fig. 9.19**). FFA is a safe procedure with some minor side effects including discoloration of skin and urine, mild nausea, and rarely vomiting. Anaphylaxis or cardiorespiratory problems are extremely rare. However, a syringe filled with dexamethasone and antihistaminic drug along with other measures should be kept ready to deal with any complications.

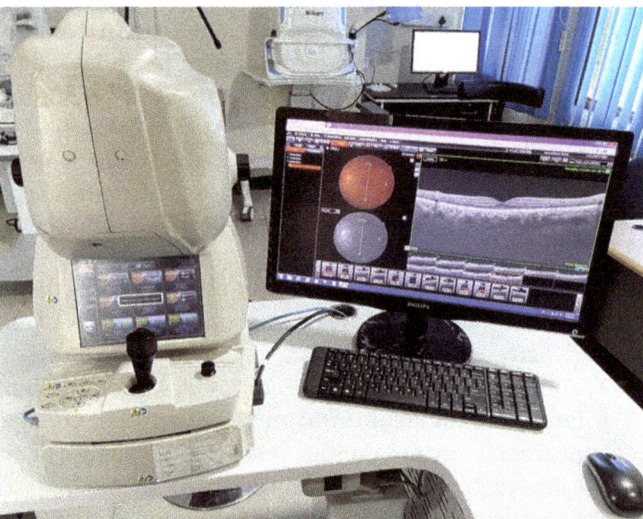

Fig. 9.17: Optical coherence tomography.

Fundus Photography

A fundus camera is a specialized low power microscope with an attached camera. It allows ophthalmologist to retrospectively review the images later in time. This digital imaging system allows good resolution and reproducible images that are available immediately for review. This is widely used technology where multiple images can be stored and also great advancements are being done towards good resolution and accuracy. There are two types of fundus photography including standard and wide view. Standard view can provide up to a view of 30–50°, whereas wide field can provide up to 200° retinal view. Types of fundus photography include standard view and wide field. The camera shown in **Figure 9.18** has a field of view of 45°.

Fundus Fluorescein Angiography (FFA)

Fundus fluorescein angiography (FFA) is used for the diagnosis and management of a large number of fundus disorders. Basically, FFA gives information by allowing the examiner to study the changes, produced by various fundus disorders, in the flow of fluorescein dye along the vasculature of the retina and choroid.

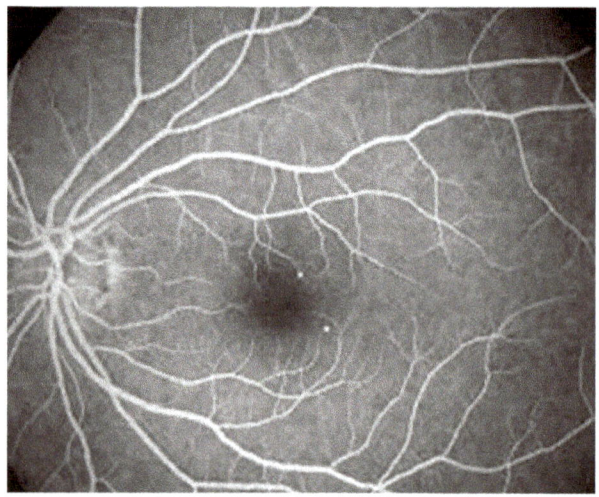

Fig. 9.19: Fluorescein angiogram.

NURSING CONSIDERATIONS

Nurses have the potential to significantly contribute in ophthalmology and the visual sciences. Ophthalmic nurses could play a significant role in the process of teaching people, providing proper diagnoses, administration and even management of many cases of medical conditions.

Case Scenario

Sant Ram is a 66-year-old male driver from Ludhiana city Punjab who had been diagnosed with type 2 diabetes mellitus (T2DM) five years ago without diabetic retinopathy at the baseline. He presently visited to district hospital with low vision problem. A detailed history was recorded including duration of diabetes, glycemic control, current medications, and medical and ocular history. Initial examination included VA assessment, IOP measurement, and examination of the peripheral retina. All these examinations were performed by the duty nurse posted at eye clinic. Then slit-lamp biomicroscopy was done by the ophthalmologist posted at the clinic and he further suggested for OCT and if required FFA. OCT appointment was indicated to provide high-resolution imaging of the vitreous and retina. This imaging modality is used to quantify retinal thickness, to diagnose and monitor macular edema, and to monitor response to treatment. Fluorescein angiography (FA) is also indicated for detecting macular edema or ischemia in patients with unexplained vision loss.

The patient was diagnosed with proliferative diabetic retinopathy (PDR) in right with macular edema changes and mild non-proliferative diabetic retinopathy (NPDR) in the left eye based on the test result findings.

SUMMARY

A careful CEE helps screen and diagnose common eye diseases, therefore reducing morbidity and associated costs with eye diseases. It can be done if a patient reports with ocular symptoms to seek medical advice or during a simple routine eye checkup. Number of eye diseases can simply be detected by torchlight examination or visual acuity testing which are not very costly and easy to do.

MULTIPLE CHOICE QUESTIONS

1. Ishihara chart is used in the diagnosis of:
   a. Diplopia
   b. Color vision deficiency
   c. Corneal thickness
   d. None of the above
2. At what distance visual acuity is usually recorded?
   a. 1 meter
   b. 3 meter
   c. 1.5 meter
   d. 6 meter
3. OCT is helpful in the diagnosis of:
   a. Changes in optic nerve due to glaucoma
   b. See retinal layers
   c. Thickness of layers
   d. All of the above.
4. Raised IOP is seen typically in:
   a. Astigmatism
   b. Glaucoma
   c. Cataract
   d. Diabetic retinopathy
5. Perimetry is another name for:
   a. Retinoscopy
   b. Gonioscopy
   c. Visual field test
   d. None of the above
6. Retinoscopy is best defined as:
   a. Visualization of retina alone
   b. Visualization of the retina and all other posterior segment contents
   c. Objective measurement of refractive error of patient
   d. Subjective measurement of refractive error of patient
7. SI unit of power of a lens is:
   a. Diopter
   b. Snellen
   c. Meter
   d. Centimeter
8. Under the effect of anticholinergic agents, pupil will:
   a. Constrict
   b. Dilate
   c. Remain same
   d. None
9. Slit-lamp is used in examining:
   a. Anterior segment
   b. Posterior segment
   c. Both a and b
   d. None of the above
10. B-scan can generate sound waves up to frequency of:
    a. 15 MHz
    b. 40 MHz
    c. 20 MHz
    d. 10 MHz

ANSWERS

1. b	2. d	3. d	4. b
5. c	6. c	7. a	8. b
9. c	10. d		

SUGGESTED READING

1. Aironi VD, Gandage SG. Pictorial essay: B-scan ultrasonography in ocular abnormalities. The Indian Journal of Radiology and Imaging. 2009;19(2):109.
2. Baumal CR, Duker JS. Current management of diabetic retinopathy. Elsevier Health Sciences; 2017.
3. Benjamin WJ. Borish's Clinical Refraction-E-Book. Elsevier Health Sciences; 2006. pp. 790-989.
4. Bowling B. Kanski clinical ophthalmology: A systematic approach, 8th edition. Elsevier; 2016. p. 2.
5. Bowling B. Kanski clinical ophthalmology: A systematic approach, 8th edition. Elsevier; 2016. p. 25.
6. Boyd K. Smoking and Eye Disease. [online] American Academy of Ophthalmology (2021). Available at: <https://www.aao.org/eye-health/tips-prevention/smokers> [Accessed 20 December 2021].
7. Color vision deficiency [Internet]. American Academy of Ophthalmology. 2020 [cited 2021Dec20]. Available from: https://www.aoa.org/healthy-eyes/eye-and-vision-conditions/color-vision-deficiency?sso=y.
8. du Toit R, Wolvaardt E. Putting patients first: how to carry out a patient-centred eye examination. Community eye health. 2019;32(107):43.
9. du Toit R. How to do a person-centered eye health consultation. Community eye health. 2015;28(90):36.
10. Eye examination [Internet]. Wikipedia. 2007 [cited 2021Dec20]. Available from: http://en.wikipedia.org/wiki/Eye_examination
11. Farsightedness: What is hyperopia? [Internet]. American Academy of Ophthalmology. 2020 [cited 2021Dec20]. Available from: https://www.aao.org/eye-health/diseases/hyperopia-farsightedness
12. Foster A, Morjaria P. Examining the eye. Community eye health. 2019;32(107):41.
13. Hadavand MB, Heidary F, Heidary R, Gharebaghi R. Role of ophthalmic nurses in prevention of ophthalmic diseases. Medical Hypothesis, Discovery and Innovation in Ophthalmology. 2013;2(4):92.
14. Helveston EM, Moodley A. How to check eye alignment and movement. Comm Eye Health. 2019;32(107):55.
15. Kanski JJ, Bowling B. Clinical ophthalmology: a systematic approach. Elsevier Health Sciences; 2011.
16. Khurana AK. Comprehensive Ophthalmology, 4th edition India: New Age International Publisher; 2007. p. 480.
17. Khurana AK. Comprehensive Ophthalmology, 4th edition India: New age international publisher; 2007. pp. 487-88.
18. Levine LE. Mydriatic effectiveness of dilute combinations of phenylephrine and tropicamide. American Journal of Optometry and Physiological Optics. 1982;59(7):580-94.
19. Marsden J, Stevens S, Ebri A. How to measure distance visual acuity. Community Eye Health. 2014;27(85):16.

20. Moradi M. Importance of ophthalmic nursing in primary healthcare systems. Medical Hypothesis, Discovery and Innovation in Ophthalmology. 2016;5(1):1.
21. Muhammad N. How to examine the front of the eye. Community Eye Health. 2019;32(107):48.
22. Pelli DG, Bex P. Measuring contrast sensitivity. Vision research. 2013;90:10-4.
23. Peragallo J, Biousse V, Newman NJ. Ocular manifestations of drug and alcohol abuse. Current opinion in ophthalmology. 2013;24(6):566.
24. Sorana D Bolboaca. "Medical Diagnostic Tests: A Review of Test Anatomy, Phases, and Statistical Treatment of Data", Computational and Mathematical Methods in Medicine, Vol. 2019, Article ID 1891569, 22 pages, 2019. http:doi.org/10.1155/2019/1891569.
25. Takusewanya M. How to take a complete eye history. Community eye health. 2019;32(107):44.
26. Trevino RC. Pupillary dilation in clinical practice. Can J Optom. 1988;50:167-75.
27. Turbert D. Near sightedness: What Is Myopia? [online] American Academy of Ophthalmology (2021). Available at: <https://www.aao.org/eye-health/diseases/myopia- nearsightedness> [Accessed 20 December 2021].
28. Visual field test [Internet]. American Academy of Ophthalmology. 2020 [cited 2021Dec20]. Available from: https://www.aao.org/eye-health/tips-prevention/visual-field-testing.
29. Wang MY, Asanad S, Asanad K, Karanjia R, Sadun AA. Value of medical history in ophthalmology: a study of diagnostic accuracy. Journal of current ophthalmology. 2018;30(4):359-64.
30. What is astigmatism? [Internet]. American Academy of Ophthalmology. 2020 [cited 2021Dec20]. Available from: https://www.aao.org/eye-health/diseases/what-is-astigmatism.
31. Wolvaardt E, Hennelly M. Eye Health. Community eye health journal. 2020;33(110):41.
32. Yadav S, Tandon R. Comprehensive eye examination: what does it mean. Community Eye Health. 2019;32(107):S1.

CHAPTER 10

Ophthalmic Surgical Instruments

Manpreet Singh, Manpreet Kaur, Aditi Mehta

"You are only as strong as the tools in your toolbox."

—Michael Bastian

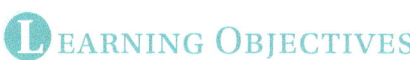

After going through the chapter, the learner will be able to:
- Define ophthalmic surgical instruments.
- Describe the actions of various ophthalmic surgical instruments.
- Recognize the importance of instrument naming.
- Enumerate the classification of surgical instruments.
- Discuss the materials of surgical instruments.
- Understand the sterilization process of instruments.

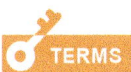

- **Autoclaving:** An effective method of sterilizing the surgical instruments and other items.
- **Disinfection:** A process of eliminating the majority of pathogens from the surface of equipment or tools.
- **Sterilization:** A process in which all pathogens including the spores and other forms of life are deactivated.

INTRODUCTION

The surgical instruments are a vital component of the operation theater armamentarium. Generally, the instruments are smaller in size in ophthalmological procedures, and sometimes the tips/business ends of instruments are not visible to the naked eye. Hence, it becomes challenging for the assistant nursing officer for accurate identification of 'on trolley' instruments. Therefore, remembering the name of the ophthalmic surgical instrument goes a long way in an efficient operation theater management.

IMPORTANCE OF INSTRUMENT NAMING

Knowing the name of a surgical instrument builds a proficient intraoperative understanding between the assistant nursing officer and surgeon. Additionally, the name acknowledges its inventor and minimizes the errors inside the operation theater. The instrument nomenclature may follow any of the following—the appearance of instrument (cat's paw, mosquito forceps, ribbon retractors, etc.), name of inventor/doctor, its function (scissors, retractors, clamps, etc.), or based on the name of surgery (ptosis clamp, chalazion clamp and curette, etc.).

DEFINITION OF A SURGICAL INSTRUMENT

It is a specially designed tool or device used to perform or facilitate specific actions during surgery. A good surgical instrument helps to achieve the best surgical outcomes with efficiency and minimum possible complications.

ACTIONS PERFORMED BY SURGICAL INSTRUMENTS

The specific actions performed by the surgical instruments are enumerated in **Table 10.1**.

Generally, the instruments used in majority of the operation theaters are made up of stainless steel, titanium, tungsten carbide, diamond and optic fibers. Of these, the most common material used is stainless steel due to its easier maintenance, low-cost and availability. As the instruments undergo wear and tear over a period of time, replacing the old instruments with new ones remains a better idea than

TABLE 10.1: Types of actions performed by surgical instruments.

	Actions	Type of instruments
1.	Holding or grasping of tissue	Forceps, holders, clamps
2.	Cutting, incising, punching or breaking	Scissors, knives, blades, awls, chisels, rongeur, punches
3.	Retraction or separation	Retractors, speculums, hooks
4.	Aspiration, irrigation, draining or injection	Needles, suction tips, catheters, syringes, cannulas, drains
5.	Probing and dilatation	Probes, stylet, dilators
6.	Cautery or hemostasis	Fire-heated or electricity-based instrument
7.	Apposition	Tissue glues, sutures, stickers, staplers

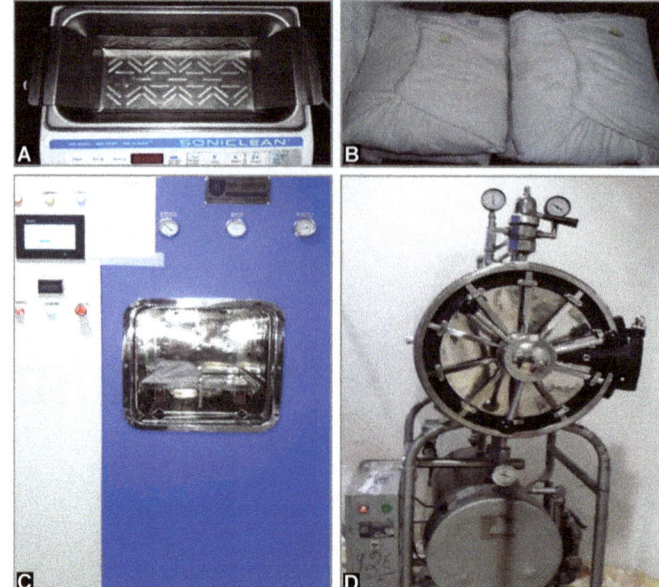

Figs 10.1A to D: (A) The ultrasonic cleaner for the removal of microdebris from the tip of fine instruments. Caution: Titanium instruments should not be put in ultrasonic cleaners; (B) Linen packed set of surgical instruments/gowns/drape sheets; (C) Digital modern autoclave with indicators; (D) Horizontal traditional steam autoclave.

getting them repaired or serviced. However, the expensive instruments can be considered for service or repair for its efficient use.

CLASSIFICATION OF INSTRUMENTS

The Spaulding's Classification

The Spaulding's classification of instruments based on cleaning process and the cleaning product is highlighted in **Table 10.2**.

The cycle of Instrument Sterilization

This cycle of sterilization for the operation theater instruments consists of the following steps in a specific order:

- **Cleaning:** Cleaning of the surgical instruments is to be done for removing blood, threads, dirt, pus and mechanical debris. The ideal fluid for cleaning is distilled water as it will not leave any residue after drying. The mechanical cleaning is done using brush and running tap water. The ultrasonic cleaner (used for fine instruments) is advisable for smaller instruments **(Fig. 10.1A)**. The use of magnifiers is also advocated to prevent damage to the fine tips of instruments.
- **Drying:** A hot air blower is used for faster drying of the instruments. Normal air drying is also performed at few centers. At this stage, the instruments are checked for any corrosion, malalignment, cracks, pits, etc.
- **Packing:** The instruments are packed in linen **(Fig. 10.1B)** or plastic packs and made ready for the sterilization process. In this process, the chemical or biological indicators of sterilization are inserted or applied over the packs for the assessment of sterilization adequacy.
- **Sterilization:** The types of sterilization include—autoclaving **(Figs. 10.1C and D)**, plasma sterilization, chemical sterilization and UV sterilization. The most common one is autoclaving. The details of sterilization are compiled in **Table 10.3**.
- **Storage:** The sterilized items can be stored for a particular period called as shelf-life. Generally, the longest shelf-life is for plasma sterilized items, i.e., 6 months, while the items after autoclaving have a shelf-life of 72 hours (in 20–24°C and <60% humidity).
- **Monitoring of effective sterilization:** This is done via the chemical or biological indication strips applied over the sterilized items. The sterilized packets or items should be kept at minimum of 3 feet high above the ground.

For further details about each step, a chapter has been contributed by us in our textbook of "Ophthalmic instruments and surgical tools" (Singh M et al.; and Thakur S et al.).

The most common type of sterilization used for surgical instruments is autoclaving. The steps of autoclaving include thorough cleaning of instruments and arranging those in a

TABLE 10.2: Spaulding's classification of instruments.

Classification		Instruments	Cleaning process	Cleaning product
Critical	Entering inside bloodstream, sterile body cavities, or sterile tissue	Implants, blades, needles, cannulas, phacoemulsification handpieces, ophthalmic intraocular probes, vitrectomy cutters, instruments for intraocular use.	Sterilization	Sterilizing agent or process
Semicritical	Comes in contact with mucous membranes, non-sterile regions or non-intact skin	Nasal endoscopes, tips of tonometer's, the probe of contact/immersion biometry and pachymeter, fluorescein strips, Schirmer's strips, Castroviejo calipers, gonio lens, speculum	High-level disinfection	Chemical disinfectant
Noncritical	Comes in contact with intact skin	Blood pressure cuffs, rulers, ultrasonography probes, exophthalmometers, prisms,	Low- level disinfection	Soap and water

TABLE 10.3: Various methods/techniques for sterilization of surgical instruments and tools.

Technique	Merits	Demerits	Time and temperature	Ideal for
Autoclave (pressurized steam)	• Inexpensive • Highly effective • Rapid • Nontoxic	• Rubber, plastic—can melt • Unsuitable for powder, oils, ointment, etc. • Closed glass chambers	20–60 minutes 121–180°C	• Operating metallic surgical instruments • Gowns, drapes, dressings
Hot air oven (dry heat)	• Noncorrosive • Inexpensive • Nontoxic	• Less effective • Longer duration	60–80 minutes 340°F	• Metallic instruments • Powder, oils, etc. • Open glass vials
Ethylene oxide (ETO)	• Plastic handle blades • Wires • Heat-labile tubes • Ready-to-use pack • Longer storage	• Toxic • Caution for handlers (Carcinogenic, explosive) • Expensive • Long aeration time • Long cycle time	6–12 hours	• Phaco tubings vitrectomy cutters • Acrylic orbital implants • Plastic eye shields • Cryoprobes • Optical-fiber light pipe • Silicone stents • Conformers
Plasma (hydrogen peroxide)	• Short cycle time • Longer storage • Ready to use • Wires • Plastic, heat-labile material	• Special packing needed • Expensive equipment	75–80 minutes	Same as of ETO
Chemical disinfectants	• Quick and ready method • Inexpensive	• Toxic to mucosa and conjunctiva • Not for any intraocular instrument • Proper lumen rinsing before use • Needs thorough wash for all items	3–4 hours	• Plastic, glass, airways, etc. • Nasal packing forceps • Nasal endoscope tips

perforated steel tray. The stacking of instruments should be avoided, and the unlocking of joints should be ensured for the better penetration of steam. Adjust the time, pressure, and temperature of the autoclave machine and start the cycle. After completion of the cycle, the autoclave lid should be opened with caution only after the gauge reaches the zero mark. Sufficient drying time (15–20 minutes) should be given. The instruments and packs should be considered adequately sterilized if dry.

COMMONLY USED INSTRUMENTS FOR THE ROUTINE OPHTHALMIC SURGERIES

The commonly used instruments for the routine ophthalmic surgeries have been compiled in the following **(Table 10.4)**.

TABLE 10.4: Commonly used instruments for the routine ophthalmic surgeries.

Surgery	Instruments
Routine ophthalmic OPD	Beer's or Barraquer's cilia forceps, Lim's forceps **(Fig. 10.2C)**, Vanna's scissors, punctum dilator, Irrigation cannula, McPherson's forceps, universal speculum, Foerster's sponge-holding forceps **(Fig. 10.2D)**, dressing forceps **(Fig. 10.2E)**
Eyelid and oculoplastic surgeries	Adson forceps, Jeweller forceps, Chalazion clamp **(Figs. 10.2G and H)**, artery/hemostatic forceps, Berke's ptosis clamp, Putterman's forceps, Knapp's retractor, Mule's evisceration scoop, Well's enucleation spoon, Kerrison's bone punch
Squint surgeries	Moorfield's forceps, superior rectus-holding forceps, Jameson's or Green's muscle hook **(Fig. 10.2F)**, globe fixation forceps

Contd...

Contd...

Surgery	Instruments
Conjunctiva	Moorfield's forceps, Bishop-Harmon tissue forceps, Piers-Hoskins forceps, Colibri forceps, plain forceps, conjunctival scissors **(Fig. 10.2B)**
Cornea and refractive surgery	Colibri forceps, corneal flap forceps in LASIK, globe fixation forceps, Carlson DSEK graft
Suturing	Kelman-Mcpherson's forceps, Harms tying forceps, Castroviejo's needle holder, Bishop-Harmon, plain forceps
Glaucoma	Kelly Descemet membrane punch, Harms trabeculotome, muscle hook, tying forceps
Iris	Iris forceps, Lim's forceps, De Wecker's scissors
Lens	Utrata capsulorhexis, irrigation and aspiration cannulas, Lim's forceps, IOL implantation forceps (Neuhann/Shepard/Tenner)
Retina	Landers vitrectomy lens forceps, end-grasping microforceps, Liebermann's eyelid speculum **(Fig. 10.2A)**, ILM peeling forceps

NURSING CONSIDERATIONS

The operation theater nursing officer must know the above-mentioned information about the surgical instruments and ophthalmic operation theater functions. The surgical instruments constitute the most important part of surgery and are directly responsible for the type of outcomes. Hence, proper care and maintenance of surgical instruments is vital for the efficient working of OT. As a matter of fact, if a doubt arises regarding the sterility of any equipment (like microscope handle covers, etc.), surgical instrument, or

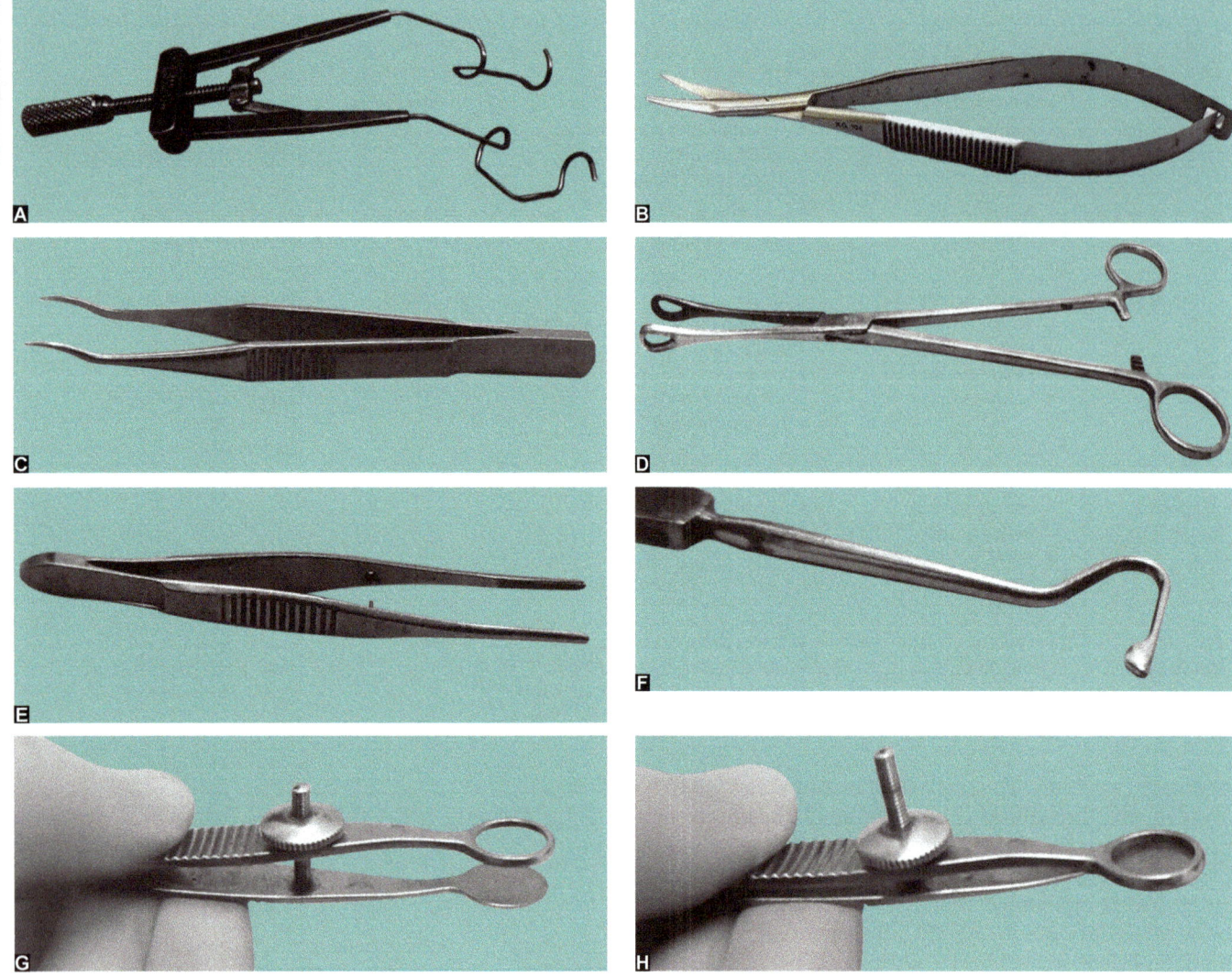

Figs. 10.2A to H: (A) Universal (can be used for either of eyes) eyelid speculum (Liebermann's); (B) Castroviejo's conjunctival scissors; (C) Lim's forceps; (D) Foerster's sponge-holding forceps; (E) A non-toothed Bonaccolto's forceps; (F) Jameson's muscle hook; (G) Open Lambert's chalazion clamp; (H) Closed chalazion clamp.

surgeon's gown or gloves, we should believe it to be unsterile and repeat all the steps of sterilization.

Case Scenario

Surgery: External dacryocystorhinostomy for the blocked nasolacrimal duct.
- **Points to consider:** To keep the local anesthesia and adrenaline-soaked sponges/gauze pieces handy considering intraoperative bleeding.
- **Instrument related:** Bone Rongeur or punches should be sharp and well-maintained as the bone removal would be easier and precise. The nursing officer should be ready to remove the pieces of the bone from the Kerrison's bone punch and provide it readily to the surgeon.
- **Postoperative instrument cleaning:** As the external dacryocysto-rhinostomy procedure witness more bleeding than other ophthalmic surgical procedure, all the instruments should be thoroughly cleaned under running tap water and the visible dirt and blood should be removed. The fine instruments should be cleaned in an ultrasonic cleaner.
- Checking the cutting-edges of the bone punches under magnification is a desired step. Instrument lubrication at the joints makes the movement smooth and easy.

SUMMARY

In summary, a nursing officer should be well-versed with all the nuances of the surgical instruments for the efficient working of the operation theater. Nicely maintained surgical instruments provide the best quality surgical results and keep the harmony of the operation theater.

MULTIPLE CHOICE QUESTIONS

1. The nomenclature of surgical instruments is NOT based on:
   a. Name of the scientist
   b. Shape of the instrument
   c. Action of the instrument
   d. Material of the instrument
2. The Spaulding's classification is based on:
   a. Chemical used in sterilization
   b. Temperature of the steam
   c. Atmospheric pressure
   d. Level of disinfection needed

3. The correct cycle of sterilization is:
   a. Packing → autoclaving → cleaning
   b. Autoclaving → cleaning → packing
   c. Cleaning → packing → autoclaving
   d. Cleaning → autoclaving → packing
4. The principle autoclave parameters are:
   a. 121–180°C for 20–60 minutes
   b. 121–180°C for 60–90 minutes
   c. 91–101°C for 20–60 minutes
   d. 91–101°C for 60–90 minutes
5. The name 'Universal' for an instrument signifies:
   a. Developed by universal company
   b. Developed for all surgical procedures
   c. Developed for use in either eye surgery
   d. Developed by the WHO

ANSWERS			
1. d	2. d	3. c	4. a
5. c			

SUGGESTED READING

1. Singh M, Kaur M, Gautam N, Yangzes S. Basics of Surgical Instruments. Springer Nature Singapore Pte Ltd. In: Ichhpujani P, Singh M (Eds). Ophthalmic Instruments and Surgical Tools, Current Practices in Ophthalmology; 2019. pp. 23-30.
2. Singh M, Malhotra J. Instrument Sterilization and Care. Springer Nature Singapore Pte Ltd. In: Ichhpujani P, Singh M (Eds). Ophthalmic Instruments and Surgical Tools, Current Practices in Ophthalmology; 2019. pp. 1-10.
3. Thakur S, Seth NG, Balyan M, Ichhpujani P. Anterior segment surgery instruments. Springer Nature Singapore Pte Ltd. In: Ichhpujani P, Singh M (Eds). Ophthalmic Instruments and Surgical Tools, Current Practices in Ophthalmology; 2019. pp. 31-50.

CHAPTER 11
Ocular Pharmacology and Lasers

Himanshi Singh, Parul Chawla Gupta, Jagat Ram

"I shut my eyes and all the world drops dead; I lift my eyes and all is born again."
—Sylvia Plath

LEARNING OBJECTIVES

After going through the chapter, the learner will be able to:
- Describe various drugs and routes of administration of drugs in eye.
- Describe the associated actions of drugs and their clinical applications.
- Elaborate various lasers and their mechanism of action in treating various disorders of eye.
- Discuss geriatric considerations with regard to ocular pharmacology.

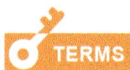

- **LASER:** Light Amplification by Stimulated Emission of Radiation.
- **Obscuration:** The action of hiding or concealing something.
- **Pharmacodynamics:** Study of the biological effects of drugs and their mechanisms of action.
- **Pharmacokinetics:** Study of drug absorption, distribution, metabolism, and excretion of drugs.
- **Photoablation:** Process of breakage of the chemical bonds by laser that hold tissue together essentially vaporizing the tissue.
- **Photocoagulation:** Denaturation of tissue proteins by heat generated by laser.
- **Photodisruption:** Disruption of tissues due to the rapid ionization of molecules caused by exposure to laser light.

INTRODUCTION

Ocular pharmacology is the study of interaction and reaction of drugs with ocular tissues. It is broadly divided into two categories:
1. **Pharmacokinetics:** It is the study of distribution, absorption, metabolism, and removal of drugs. Data is gathered for optimal dosage and minimize side effects for better therapeutic outcomes
2. **Pharmacodynamics:** It is the study of mechanism of action and biological effects of drugs. Absorption of the drug is its movement from site of administration to the target tissue for the desired effect. Factors affecting the absorption of drug are:
    - *Drug concentration and solubility:* Higher concentration will have better penetration.
    - *Viscosity:* higher viscosity will increase the contact time and hence retention time of drug in the eye.
    - *Lipid solubility:* Highly lipid soluble drugs will have better penetration.

MODES OF ADMINISTRATION (FIG. 11.1)

Ocular drugs can be administered by four methods:
1. **Topical instillation:** It is the most common route of administration of drugs. The drugs can be given topically in the form of the eyedrops, gels, or ointments.
2. **Periocular injections:** These include administration of drug around the eye tissues. It includes subconjunctival, sub-Tenon, retrobulbar and peribulbar injections.
3. **Intraocular injections:** When the drug is injected directly inside the eye for achieving maximum concentration of drug at the target tissue.

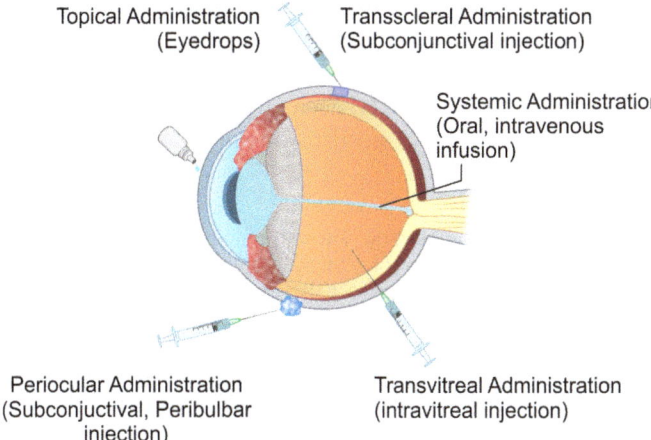

Fig. 11.1: Modes of administration of ocular drugs.

4. **Systemic administration:** The penetration of systemically administered drugs in the eye mainly depends on the eye's blood–aqueous barrier. It includes oral intake, intramuscular and intravenous injections of various drugs.

COMMON DRUGS USED IN OPHTHALMOLOGY

Common drugs used in ophthalmology are categorized into following categories:

- **Anti-infective agents:**
  - *Antibacterials (antibiotics):* Amoxicillin, gentamicin, ciprofloxacin
  - *Antifungals:* Natamycin, voriconazole, amphotericin-b
  - *Antivirals:* Acyclovir, gancyclovir, foscarnet
- **Mydriatics and cycloplegics agents:** Tropicamide, phenylephrine, cyclopentolate
- **Anti-glaucoma drugs:** Timolol, brimonidine, dorzolamide
- **Anti-inflammatory and immunosuppressive agents:**
  - *Corticosteroid:* Betamethasone, dexamethasone, loteprednol, prednisolone
  - *Nonsteroidal anti-inflammatory drugs:* Indomethacin, ketorolac, nepafenac
  - *Immunosuppressive and antimitotic drugs:* Cyclosporine, tacrolimus, methotrexate
- **Anti-allergic and vasoconstrictor drugs:** Olopatadine, cromolyn sodium, naphazoline
- **Lubricating agent and artificial tears:** Carboxymethylcellulose, hydroxyethylcellulose

LASERS IN OPHTHALMOLOGY

LASER stands for 'Light Amplification by Stimulated Emission of Radiation'. A laser system consists of a transparent crystal rod or a gas or liquid-filled cavity constructed with a fully reflective mirror at one end and a partially reflective mirror at the other. Surrounding the rod or cavity is an optical or electrical source of energy that will raise the energy level of the atoms within the cavity or rod to a high and unstable level. From this, the atoms spontaneously decay back to a lower energy level, releasing the excess energy in the form of light which is amplified to an appropriate wavelength. Properties of laser light are:

- **Coherence:** Each wave is in phase with the other near it.
- **Collimation:** All the rays are exactly parallel.
- **Monochromatic:** It consists of a narrow beam of a single wavelength and thus, is always colored and can never be white.
- **Polarized in one plane:** Easy to pass through media

The difference between LASER and light rays is depicted in **Table 11.1**.

Types of Lasers

1. **Solid state:** Nd:Yag, ruby
2. **Gas lasers:** Argon, krypton, neon, helium
3. **Excimer:** Argon fluoride

Laser Tissue Interactions

Laser interaction with various tissues of the eye may be classified into following categories **(Fig. 11.2)**.

Clinical Application of Laser in Ophthalmology

- **Diabetic retinopathy:** Laser causes photocoagulation of proteins resulting in adhesion of chorioretinal layers

TABLE 11.1: Different characteristics of LASER and light rays.

Laser	Light
Monochromatic	Polychromatic
Stimulated emission	Spontaneous emission
Highly energized	Poorly energized
Parallelism	High divergence
Coherence	Noncoherent
Sharp focus	Poor focus

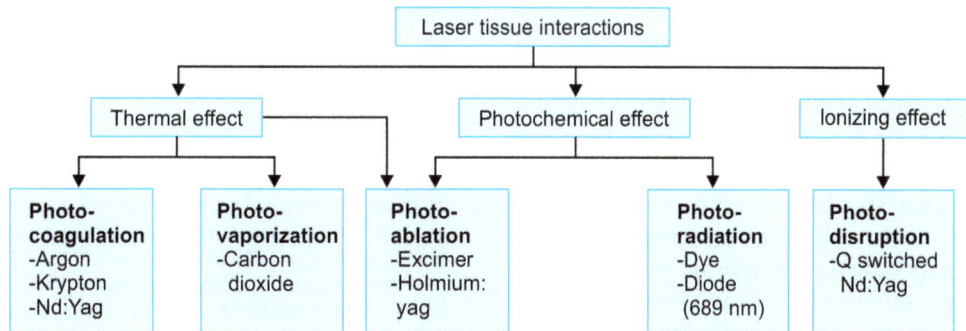

Fig. 11.2: Various laser tissue interactions and the type of laser involved.

decreasing the release of hypoxic factors that causes damage to retina.
- **Laser iridotomy in glaucoma:** Laser is used to create a hole in the iris, thereby allowing aqueous humor to traverse directly from the posterior to the anterior chamber and, consequently, relieve a pupillary block in case of glaucoma.
- **Posterior capsulotomy:** When there is obscuration of visual axis due to development of white opaque layer behind the artificial intraocular lens, laser is used to create an opening in the white layer to clear the visual axis.
- **Retinal breaks:** Seals the break by causing chorioretinal adhesions.
- **Laser-assisted cataract surgery or refractive surgery:** Laser helps in breaking the hard cataractous nucleus into smaller pieces by photodisruption. In case of refractive surgery, laser energy is used to create the corneal flap and flattening of the corneal surface by photoablation.

Complications of Laser
- **Accidental corneal or retinal burns:** Excessive laser spots or laser energy can inadvertently cause burn to retina or corneal surface.
- **Intraocular hemorrhage:** Laser can accidently hit new retinal vessels causing bleeding.
- **Localized opacification of lens:** Laser energy can cause damage to lens fibers causing cataractous changes.
- **Decrease in visual acuity and color vision:** Laser can cause mild temporary edema and can cause decrease in sharpness of vision and color vision clarity.

GERIATRIC CONSIDERATIONS

The dose for older adults should be titrated monitoring the side effects of the drugs. A low level of compliance has generally been seen in older adults. Apart from advancing age, the other associated factors may be functional and cognitive impairment, lack of family and social support, multiple morbidities, polypharmacy, etc.

Specific interventions should be planned in order to improve the adherence and compliance amongst them.

NURSING CONSIDERATIONS

All the 'Rights' of medication administration through eye remain the same as has been practiced for the other routes of medication administration. The eyes of the patients should be assessed for new or unusual redness or drainage. The patients should also be asked for unusual irritation, burning, stinging, etc., which should not be there after few minutes of administration of the eye drops. When instilling eye drops especially to the elderly patients, the nurse should ensure that the correct drop or ointment is instilled in the correct eye. They should perform hand hygiene and wear gloves preferably. In order to prevent contamination, they should avoid touching the dropper tip to the patient's eyelashes. Contact lenses should be removed before administering the eye drops and a wait period of at least 10 minutes before reinserting the contact lenses should be followed. Excess drop should be wiped off to avoid excoriation of the surrounding skin and a gap of at least 5 minutes should be given before instilling the second type of drops. They must also be aware of the patient's allergies, as well as any history of any drug interactions in the past.

Case Scenario
A 10-year-old boy complaining of itching, redness, watering from eyes was diagnosed with allergic conjunctivitis by the physician, what is the best mode of delivery of drug in such patient?
Answer: Topical drug administration.

SUMMARY

A good understanding of basic pharmacokinetic and pharmacodynamic principles of drugs helps practitioners to understand effects of these drugs in the patients, and their significant side effects. Nurses should have good knowledge of pharmacology for any drug they give to their patients in practice. Lasers have become very important tool for preventing and treating various eye diseases and hence have become an indispensable tool in ophthalmology.

MULTIPLE CHOICE QUESTIONS

1. What is systemic ocular medication?
   a. Injections to the eye
   b. Eye drops
   c. Medication that has ocular side effects
   d. A pill taken orally to treat certain eye conditions
2. Pharmacokinetics—true is:
   a. Study of absorption of drug
   b. Study of effect of drug
   c. Study of biological action of drug
   d. Study of dosage of drug
3. Which of the following is NOT the topical route of drug administration?
   a. Eyedrops
   b. Ointments
   c. Subconjunctival injection
   d. Gels
4. Which of the following is NOT the characteristic of laser?
   a. Coherence
   b. Collimation
   c. High divergence
   d. Monochromatic
5. Which of the following is NOT the thermal effect in laser tissue interactions?
   a. Photocoagulation   b. Photoablation
   c. Photovaporization   d. Photodisruption

ANSWERS
1. d   2. a   3. c   4. c
5. d

SUGGESTED READING
1. Amanda L, Needham Y. Pharmacological issues in ophthalmology. International Journal of Ophthalmic practice; 2012;3:43-7.
2. Park Y, Ellis D, Mueller B, Stankowska D, Yorio T. Principles of Ocular Pharmacology. Handb Exp Pharmacol. 2017;242:3-30.
3. Krauss JM, Puliafito CA. Lasers in ophthalmology. Lasers Surg Med. 1995;17(2):102-59.

CHAPTER 12

Refractive Errors

Himanshi Singh, Parul Chawla Gupta, Jagat Ram

"Knowledge is the eye of desire and can become the pilot of the soul."

—Will Durant

LEARNING OBJECTIVES

After going through the chapter, the learner will be able to:
- Define refraction.
- Enumerate various types of refractive errors in eye.
- Describe the pathophysiology and the associated clinical manifestations.
- Elaborate various aspects of management of refractive errors.
- Discuss geriatric considerations with regard to refractive errors.

TERMS

- **Ametropia:** Presence of refractive error.
- **Astigmatism:** Refractive power of the eye being different in different meridians.
- **Emmetropia:** Absence of a refractive error.
- **Hypermetropia:** Long-sightedness.
- **Myopia:** Short-sightedness.

INTRODUCTION

Refraction of light is the process of change in the path of light ray, when it goes from one medium to another. More the difference in optical density between the two media, more will be the deviation of light.

Emmetropia is a condition where parallel rays of light coming from far are focussed on retina with accommodation at rest. Ametropia is the condition where eye does not bend light properly resulting in a defocused image.

EPIDEMIOLOGY

Blindness due to refractive error is reported to be almost 0.2% in India, blindness being defined as visual acuity <3/60 in the good eye. (*Source:* National survey of blindness 1986–89 and 2001–02).

TYPES OF REFRACTIVE ERRORS (FIGS. 12.1A TO D)

1. **Myopia:** Nearsightedness also known as short sightedness where light focuses in front of the retina instead of on retina which causes far objects to be blurred.
2. **Hypermetropia:** Farsightedness also known as long-sightedness where light focuses behind the retina instead of retina resulting in an inability to seen near objects clear.
3. **Astigmatism:** Refractive power of the eye being different in different meridians causing inability of the light from a point of a distant object to form a single point of an image.

PATHOPHYSIOLOGY

- **Abnormal corneal curvature:** Steep cornea in myopia and flat cornea in hypermetropia. A 1 mm change in the

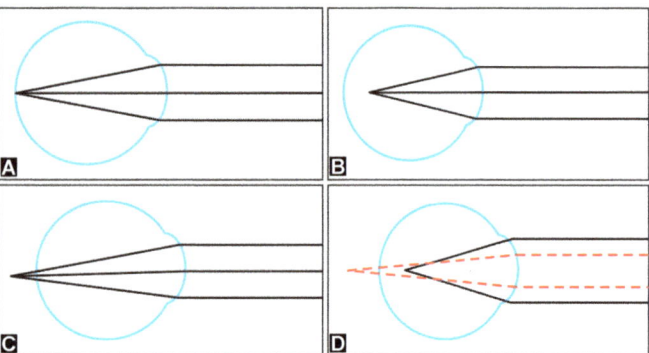

Figs. 12.1A to D: Line diagram depicting refraction in: (A) An emmetropic eye; (B) A myopic eye; (C) A hypermetropic eye; (D) An astigmatism eye.

radius of curvature of the cornea produces a 6 D refractive change.
- **Abnormal size of eyeball:** Presence of longer than normal axial length in myopia and shorter than normal axial length in hypermetropia. A 1 mm elongation produces approximately 3 D of myopia and 1 mm shortening 3 D of hypermetropia.
- **Abnormal index of refraction:** Abnormal refractive indices of the media. Higher refractive index can cause myopia, while a lower refractive index can cause hypermetropia.

CLINICAL MANIFESTATIONS

- Doubling of vision
- Blurriness
- Halos around bright light
- Squinting—to achieve the greater clarity of stenopaeic vision.
- Headache
- Eye strain fatigue pain in or around the eyes
- Eye irritation

A myope's complaint is difficulty to see far objects clearly whereas hypermetropes complaint is difficulty to do near work very well.

DIAGNOSTIC MODALITIES

- **History taking:** As in details what all complaints the patients have regarding vision.
- **Corneal topography:** This computerized test maps the curve of the cornea, showing problem with eye surface like swelling or scarring.
- **Slit-lamp examination:** A microscope to focus light on affected eye to look for any surface abnormalities.
- **Retinoscopy:** A technique for objective measurement of refractive error of a patient's eye.

MANAGEMENT

Medical Management

- **Identify and treat the underlying cause**
- **Prescription of spectacle correction:** Concave lenses are used for myopic correction and convex lenses are used for hypermetropic correction to focus the image on the retina.

Attention must be paid to the use of suitable correcting spectacles. Myopia must never be overcorrected with spectacles.
- **Contact lenses:** They have the advantage of providing a wider field and larger image size compared to glasses in patients with high myopia.

Surgical Management

Refractive Surgery

It is the surgical improvement of refractive state of the eye to eliminate the dependency on glasses or contact lenses.
- **Keratomileusis:** Reshaping corneal surface surgically to change its optical power. Various procedures are:
  - *Radial keratotomy:* Radial keratotomy (RK) refers to making deep (90% of corneal thickness) radial incisions in the peripheral part of cornea leaving the central 4 mm optical zone. These incisions after healing flatten the central cornea thereby reducing its refractive power. This procedure gives good correction in low to moderate myopia (2 to 6 D).
  - *Laser in-situ keratomileusis (LASIK):* In this technique first a flap of 130–160 micron thickness of anterior corneal tissue is raised with the help of an automated microkeratome. Nowadays, femtosecond laser is being used for more accurate and smooth flaps. After creating a corneal flap midstromal tissue is ablated directly with an excimer laser beam, ultimately flattening the cornea. Hyperopic LASIK is effective in correcting hypermetropia up to +4D.
- **Intraocular lens implantation or intraocular lens replacement surgery:** Phakic refractive lens (PRL) or implantable contact lens (ICL) is considered now for correction of myopia of >8D. In this technique, a special type of intraocular lens (IOL) is implanted in the anterior chamber or posterior chamber anterior to the natural crystalline lens.

GERIATRIC CONSIDERATIONS

Refractive error is one of the most common causes of loss of vision in older adults. The uncorrected refractive error may significantly impact their ability to perform basic activities of daily living which can adversely affect their quality of life.
Presbyopia: It is also known as age-related long-sightedness or far-sightedness, is a normal component of ageing. It can happen even if already caused by loss of flexibility of the crystalline lens in the eye.

NURSING MANAGEMENT

The general pre- and postoperative management of all the eye surgeries remain the same. The specific preoperative care of the patients includes:
- **Preparation of the patient:**
  - Ask the patients to stop wearing the contact lenses before surgery. The timeframe may vary for around 2–3 weeks for the soft contact lenses and around 4 weeks for the hard lenses.
  - The patient should not be suffering from any other eye disease.

- It is important that the patients undergoing refractive surgery understand the benefits, potential complications and limitations associated with the procedure. So, preoperative counseling regarding all these aspects along with postoperative follow-up and compliance with medications is very important.

❖ **Postoperative care:**
- To check for compliance of glasses or contact lenses
- Restore maximum functional ability of the eye in activities of daily living.
- Psychosocial support for enhancing self-image.

Case Scenario

A 50-years-old male complaining of difficulty in reading newspaper since one year, however, he is able to see clearly distant objects, what kind of refractive error is it?

Answer: Hypermetropia or farsightedness

SUMMARY

Eyes not able to focus parallel rays of light on the retina are termed as ametropic and the condition is known as ametropia. Commonly seen refractive errors in population are myopia, hypermetropia and astigmatism. Timely optical correction is required to restore the maximum visual potential of the eye.

MULTIPLE CHOICE QUESTIONS

1. **Myopia is:**
   a. Corrected with convex glasses
   b. Light falls in back of retina
   c. Corrected with concave glasses
   d. Farsighted
2. **Hypermetropia is:**
   a. Corrected with convex glasses
   b. Light falls in front of retina
   c. Corrected with concave glasses
   d. Shortsighted
3. **Which of the following is the best term that implies perfect vision?**
   a. Ammetropia
   b. Emmetropia
   c. Myopia
   d. Astigmatism
4. **What is the name for a condition where the unequal curvature of the cornea is unable to focus light on the retina, resulting in light rays focusing at different meridians?**
   a. Ammetropia
   b. Emmetropia
   c. Myopia
   d. Astigmatism
5. **According to the National Survey of Blindness, blindness is defined as visual acuity in the good eye less than:**
   a. 1/60
   b. 2/60
   c. 3/60
   d. 6/60

ANSWERS

1. c
2. a
3. b
4. d
5. c

SUGGESTED READING

1. American Academy of Ophthalmology. Refractive errors and refractive surgery; 2013.
2. Hinkle JL, Cheever KH. Textbook of Medical Surgical Nursing, 13th edition. Wolters Kluwer; 1862.
3. Millodot M. Dictionary of Optometry and Visual Science; 7th edition Oxford, UK: Butterworth-Heinemann; Elsevier; 2009. p. 116.
4. Optics and refraction (David Miller section editor). In: Yanoff M, Duker IS (Eds.). Ophthalmology. London: Mosby; 1999.
5. Sheeladevi S, Seelam B, Nukella PB, Modi A, Ali R, Keay L. Prevalence of refractive errors in children in India: a systematic review. Clin Exp Optom. 2018;101(4):495-503.

CHAPTER 13

Cataract

Ranjan Kumar Behera, Parul Chawla Gupta, Jagat Ram

"Good eye service is the right of everybody, not just the wealthy who can afford it."
—**Unknown**

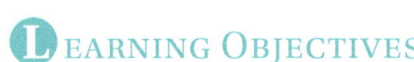 Learning Objectives

After going through the chapter, the learner will be able to:
- Understand the concept of cataract.
- Enumerate the types of cataracts.
- Enlist the risk factors of cataracts.
- Explain the pathophysiology of cataract.
- Assess the diagnostic findings of cataract.
- Describe the management of cataract.

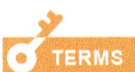 **TERMS**

- **Congenital cataract:** Disturbance in lens development that occurs before birth.
- **Cortical cataract:** Lens opacity occurring due to increased water content of lens cortex.
- **Lamellar cataract:** Type of developmental cataract in which opacity occupies a discrete zone in the lens.
- **Phacoemulsification:** Ophthalmic surgery involving ultrasonic energy to emulsify the cataractous lens.
- **Polar cataract:** Cataract which involves the central part of either the anterior/posterior capsule.
- **Subcapsular cataract:** Cataract involving the central part of the anterior/posterior cortex just below the capsule.

INTRODUCTION

Any opacity in the lens is defined as a cataract or capsule. It can occur due to formation of opacity in the fibers of the lens or due to degeneration of the normal transparent lens fibers. The opacity usually occurs naturally due to age related degenerative process but can also occur because of trauma, congenital causes, or metabolic disorders etc. It usually becomes significant when it starts interfering with vision.

CONCEPT AND DEFINITION

A cataract is the clouding of the naturally clear lens of the eyes that gradually degrades the vision quality. In other words, it is an ocular condition involving the opacity of the lens (**Fig. 13.1**).

Most of the cataracts develop gradually with an undisturbed change in vision. People are often unaware that they have cataracts because the change in their vision is always so gradual. As the cataract grows larger, lens becomes more clouded and the cataract will eventually disrupt vision, i.e., the cloudier the lens, the worse vision gets. Cataracts generally affect both eyes, but not evenly. The cataract in one eye may be more advanced than the other causing a visual difference between the two eyes. It is the most common cause of reversible blindness in the world, and it is the third leading cause of preventable blindness.

EPIDEMIOLOGY

Cataracts are common in the ethnic groups particularly Caucasians and African Americans and they have a typical onset between 5th to 6th decade of life. It is gradual and progressive over time. The incidence is equal in male and female.

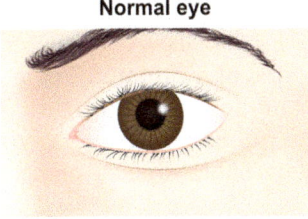
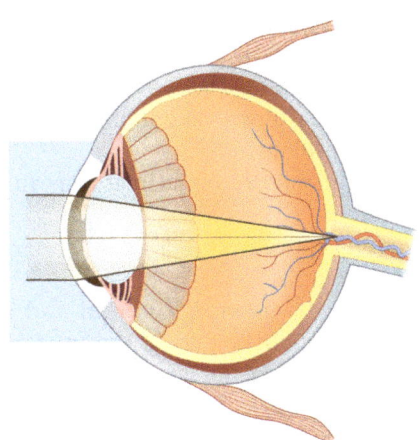

Fig. 13.1: Cataract.

RISK FACTORS FOR CATARACT FORMATION

Associated ocular conditions
- Myopia
- Infection (e.g., uveitis)
- Retinitis pigmentosa
- Retinal detachment
- Retinal surgery

Nutritional factors
- Obesity
- Poor nutrition
- ↓ Antioxidants

Ageing
- Loss of lens transparency
- Accumulation of yellow brown pigment
- Aggregation of lens protein
- ↓ Oxygen uptake
- ↑ Sodium and calcium
- ↓ Vitamin C, protein and glutathione

Physical factors
- Dehydration
- Perforation of lens
- UV radiation and X-ray

Systemic diseases
- Down syndrome
- Diabetes
- Renal disorders
- Musculoskeletal disorders

Miscellaneous
- Long-term use of corticosteroids
- Poisoning
- Deposition of calcium, iron, copper, mercury, gold and silver
- Cigarette smoking

PATHOPHYSIOLOGY (FLOWCHART 13.1)

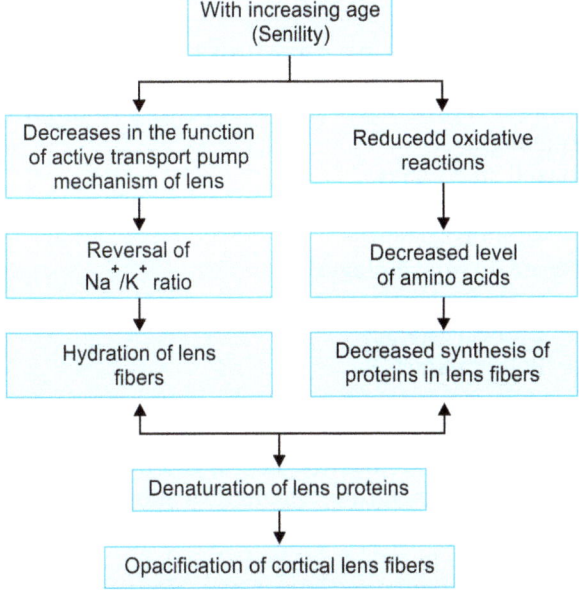

Flowchart 13.1: Pathophysiology of cataract.

CLINICAL MANIFESTATIONS

❖ Painless, blurry vision is characteristic feature of cataract **(Fig. 13.2)**.
❖ In cataract, the scattering of light is common, the person may experience reduced contrast sensitivity, sensitivity to glare, and reduced visual acuity.
❖ Color shift
❖ Myopic shift

Fig. 13.2: Blurred vision in cataract.

- Astigmatism
- Brunescens
- Monocular diplopia
- Reduced light transmission.

DIAGNOSTIC EVALUATION

- Slit lamp examination to provide magnification and visualize opacity of lens.
- Tonometry to determine IOP and rule out other conditions.
- Direct and indirect ophthalmoscopy to rule out retinal disease.
- Perimetry to determine the scope of visual field.

CLASSIFICATION OF CATARACT

Cataracts can be classified according to etiology or morphology.
- **Based on etiology:**
  - Congenital and developmental cataracts
  - Acquired cataracts
- **Based on morphology:**
  - Subcapsular cataract
  - Cortical cataract
  - Polar cataract

Congenital and Developmental Cataracts

If any disturbance occurs during the normal natural growth of the lens, it can result in formation of congenital or developmental cataracts. When this disturbance occurs before birth, it is called congenital cataract and when it occurs between infancy and adolescence, it is known as developmental cataract. The embryonic or fetal nucleus gets involved in congenital cataracts whereas infantile or adult nucleus, capsule or deeper parts of cortex gets involved in developmental cataracts.

Etiology

- **Idiopathic:** One third of cases are sporadic.
- **Heredity:** One third of the cases are hereditary. They may be associated with systemic disorders like Down's syndrome.
- Maternal and fetal factors also play an important role in this type of cataracts.

Almost 40% of all bilateral cataracts and 60% of all unilateral cataracts are idiopathic. As a rule, unilateral cataracts are not associated with systemic abnormalities and are not heritable whereas bilateral cataracts are often inherited.

Types of Congenital Cataract

Lamellar or zonular type of cataract is the most common type of congenital cataract (**Fig. 13.3**). The lens opacity basically occupies a discrete zone of the lens. This can occur due to genetic or environmental causes:
- **Genetic form:** Autosomal dominant variety
- **Environmental form:**
  - TORCH infection-rubella infection can cause lamellar cataract.
  - Vitamin D deficiency
  - Hypocalcemia.

The cataract is usually bilateral and causes vision impairment. It usually occurs in the zone of fetal nucleus surrounding the embryonic nucleus and 2 rings of opacity are visible. This type of cataract may be associated with small linear opacities called riders (like spokes of a wheel) seen towards the lens equator.

Other Types of Congenital/Developmental Cataracts

- **Polar cataract:**
  - *Anterior polar cataract:* Involves central zone of anterior capsule and adjoining cortex.
  - *Posterior polar cataract:* Involves posterior capsule. It may be associated with persistent fetal vasculature (**Fig. 13.4**).
- **Sutural cataract:** Punctate opacities seen around anterior and posterior Y sutures of the lens and do not affect vision.
- **Blue dot cataract:** Rounded bluish punctate opacities in the peripheral part of adolescent nucleus cortex and do not affect vision (**Fig. 13.5**).
- **Total congenital cataract:** Consists of pearly white cataract and is progressive, associated with TORCH infections.

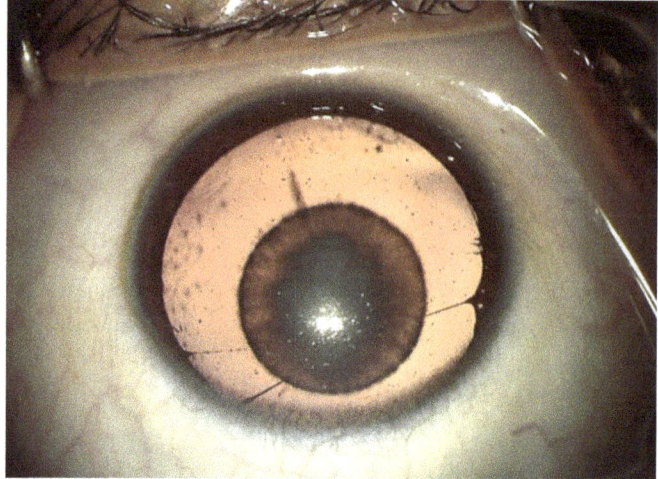

Fig. 13.3: Lamellar cataract.
(*Courtesy:* Prof Jagat Ram—AEC, PGIMER).

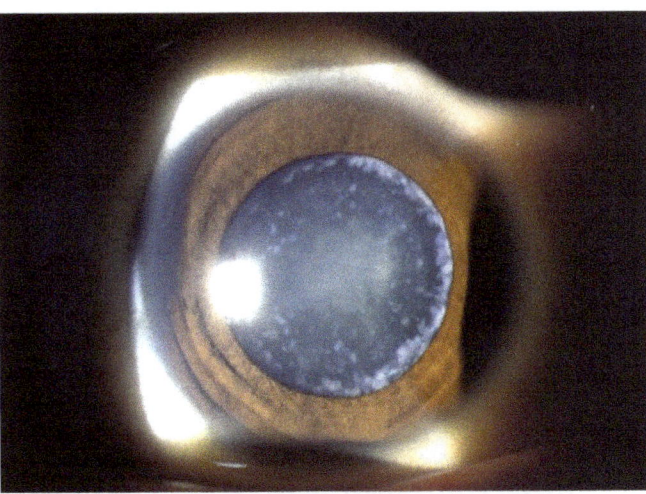

Fig. 13.4: Blue dot cataract.
(*Courtesy:* Prof Jagat Ram—AEC, PGIMER).

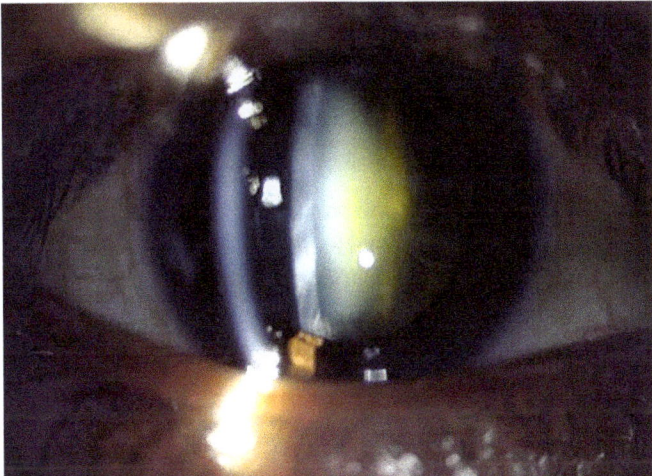

Fig. 13.5: Nuclear sclerosis.
(*Courtesy:* Prof Jagat Ram—AEC, PGIMER).

- **Persistent fetal vasculature (PFV):** Unilateral condition occurring due to failure of regression of hyaloid vascular system that provides nutrition to the lens during its development. Lens in these cases opacifies over a period with 2/3rd eyes with PFV being microphthalmic. A fibrovascular stalk may be seen extending behind the lens till the optic disc in such cases.

- **Subcapsular cataract:** Appear as granular opacities in the posterior pole of cortex adjacent to posterior capsule. It can be age related or chronic steroid use **(Fig. 13.6)**.
- **Cortical cataract:** Opacities located in the cortical layer of the lens. It appears as wedge like opacities arising from the periphery and sparing the central visual axis.

Diagnostic Evaluation

- **Ocular examination:** Assess density of cataract, assess visual function (retinoscopy, fixation reflex) and associated ocular anomalies.
- **Laboratory tests:** TORCH titers, urine examination (galactosemia, Lowes syndrome), serum calcium levels.

Management

Timing of Surgery

- Unilateral dense cataracts should be removed as early as possible followed by optical correction to prevent lazy eye.
- Bilateral cataracts should be removed within 6 weeks of birth, other eye to be operated within days after the first eye is operated.
- Visually insignificant cataracts can be observed.

The pediatric cataracts are usually soft and can be removed by irrigation and aspiration, posterior capsulorhexis and anterior vitreous needs to be removed to prevent posterior capsular opacification post operatively. Foldable acrylic lenses are preferred for implantation and decision of IOL implantation depends on the axial length of the eye. Post operatively, these children should be prescribed glasses/contact lenses depending on their refractive error to prevent amblyopia.

Acquired Cataract

In this the already formed normal lens fibres undergo degeneration due to age related changes causing opacification resulting in senile cataract. It is of two types—cortical and nuclear cataract.

Etiology

Usually occurs after the age of 50 years with a slightly higher prevalence in females. Longer duration of exposure to UV radiations has been implicated in early onset and maturation

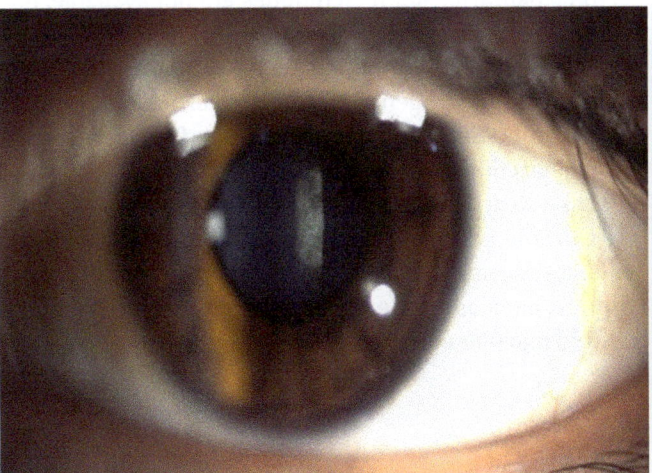
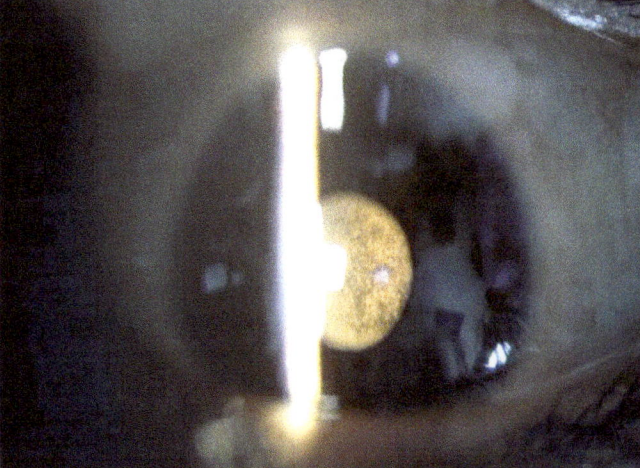

Fig. 13.6: Posterior subcapsular cataract.
(*Courtesy:* Prof Jagat Ram—AEC, PGIMER).

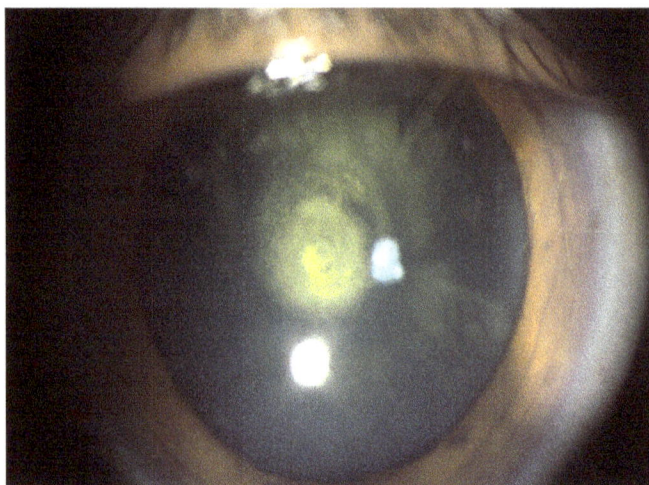

Fig. 13.7: Posterior polar cataract. (*Courtesy:* Prof Jagat Ram—AEC, PGIMER).

of cataract. Smoking and dietary deficiency of certain amino acids and vitamins have been associated with cataract.

The decreased levels of total proteins, amino acids and potassium in the crystalline lens have been implicated in the causation of cortical cataract whereas age related nuclear sclerosis associated with dehydration and compaction has been associated with nuclear cataract **(Fig. 13.7)**.

Stages of Cataract Formation (Pathophysiology)

- **Lamellar separation:** Separation of cortical fibres by fluid.
- **Incipient cataract:** Early detectable opacities with clear areas.
- **Immature senile cataract:** Greyish white appearance of lens but cortex is clear.
- **Mature senile cataract:** Complete lens opacification with involvement of cortex. Lens appears pearly white.
- **Hypermature senile cataract:**
  - *Morgagnian hypermature cataract:* Liquefaction of entire cortex, nucleus settles at bottom.
  - *Sclerotic hypermature cataract:* Disintegration of cortex and shrinking of lens with wrinkling of anterior capsule.

Clinically patient presents with diminution of vision, glare, black spots in front of eyes, etc.

Diagnostic Evaluation

Clinical examination includes:
- Detailed history along with medical conditions if any
- Visual acuity testing to assess vision
- Intraocular pressure
- Slit lamp examination to assess grade of cataract and other ocular structures

Preoperatively investigations such as blood pressure, blood sugar levels, ECG to rule out any abnormality as these can have serious implications during surgery.

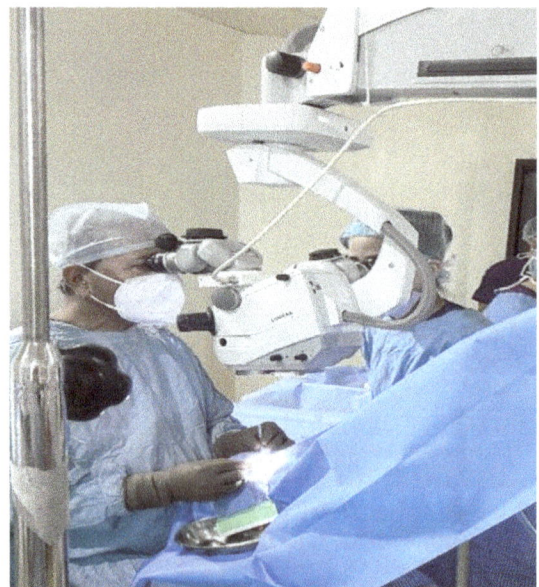

Fig. 13.8: Phacoemulsification procedure being performed by an expert.

Management

Preoperative Planning

Intraocular lens (IOL) type and power planning is essential using keratometry and axial length so that patient is visually satisfied post-surgery. Preoperatively patient is counselled to put antibiotics and pupil dilator medications to prevent infection and have good view of the cataract intraoperatively.

Surgical Procedure

Various types of cataract surgery can be planned depending upon the hardness of cataract, surgeon comfort and availability of machines and equipment.

- **Extracapsular cataract surgery:** Cataractous nucleus removed via limbal incision using wire Vectis and lens spatula but requires sutures, risk of astigmatism post surgery.
- **Small incision cataract surgery:** Cataract nucleus removed via partial thickness scleral incision (6–7 mm), no need for suture, less risk of astigmatism. It is the most widely practiced technique in centres where phacoemulsification techniques are not available, ideal for hard cataracts. It is done under local anesthesia.
- **Phacoemulsification:** Cataractous lens emulsified using acoustic energy generated due to piezoelectric crystal in the probe. Self-sealing incisions make faster recovery and patient comfort. Can be done under topical anesthesia but has a steep learning curve **(Fig. 13.8)**.

Complications of cataract surgery include—corneal edema, descemet membrane detachment, posterior capsular rupture, nucleus drop, endophthalmitis, retinal detachment, cystoid macular edema, etc.

NURSING MANAGEMENT

Preoperative Nursing Responsibilities

- Written and informed consent
- Assessment of the blood studies including—complete blood count, liver function test, kidney function test, blood sugar and vital signs.
- Administration of dilating eye drops every 10 minutes for four doses at least 1 hour before surgery.
- Prophylactic administration of antibiotics, corticosteroids, and anti-inflammatory drugs to prevent postoperative infection and inflammation.
- Earlier it was practiced withholding anticoagulants 5-7 days prior surgery to reduce the risk of retrobulbar hemorrhage. However, a recent study showed that the risk of adverse events for patients who continued anticoagulant therapy before cataract surgery was very low (0.1–0.8%).
- Educate the patient about surgery to reduce anxiety.
- Check the preoperative checklist and transfer the patient to the operating room.

Postoperative Management

- Assess the vital signs of the patient.
- Reassure the patient.
- Before discharge, provide the verbal and written instructions about the eye protection, medication administration and recognizing the signs of complications.
- Ask patient to always wear glasses or metal eye shield following surgery as instructed by physician.
- Tell the patient to always wash hands before touching or cleaning the postoperative eye.
- Ask patient to clean postoperative eye with clean tissue, wipe the closed eye with single stroke from inner canthus to outer canthus.
- Tell patient to avoid lying on the affected eye side at night after surgery
- Instruct patient to take mild analgesic agent like acetaminophen as prescribed.

GERIATRIC CONSIDERATIONS

Preoperatively, any history of medication should be taken which may have intraoperative implications, e.g., tamsulosin. They need to take their antihypertensive and antidiabetic drugs prior to surgery. If they are unable to do so, a responsible family member should do the same.

Case Scenario

A 55-year-old female, known case of severe rheumatoid arthritis on oral steroids, presented with diminution of vision for 3 months, no other h/o systemic illness. On examination, BCVA was 6/24 both eyes and slit lamp examination revealed both eye posterior subcapsular cataract. She underwent RE phacoemulsification with posterior chamber IOL implantation.

SUMMARY

Any opacification in the lens apparatus can impair vision. This is more important in children as they are not able to communicate about diminution of vision, so early intervention and postoperative refractive rehabilitation is important. In adults, proper preoperative planning is necessary to avoid any untoward complications and provide refractive satisfaction post surgery. As the life expectancy improves this is likely to burden the healthcare system. The major barrier in the path of its treatment is the cost and lack of knowledge.

MULTIPLE CHOICE QUESTIONS

1. Which is the most common type of congenital cataract?
   a. Lamellar cataract
   b. Blue dot cataract
   c. Sutural cataract
   d. Total white cataract
2. Liquefaction of the entire cortex with nucleus settling at bottom is:
   a. Immature senile cataract
   b. Mature senile cataract
   c. Sclerotic cataract
   d. Morgagnian cataract
3. What is the cut off limit of visual acuity below which cataract surgery is indicated?
   a. 6/9
   b. 6/12
   c. 6/24
   d. 6/60
4. Which preoperative medication need to be put prior to a normal cataract surgery?
   a. Antibiotic and steroid
   b. Antibiotic and antiglaucoma
   c. Antibiotic and dilators
   d. Steroid and antiglaucoma
5. Which surgical procedure for cataract can be done under topical anesthesia, has fastest visual recovery with self sealing incisions but long learning curve?
   a. Intracapsular cataract extraction
   b. Extracapsular cataract extraction
   c. Phacoemulsification
   d. Small incision cataract surgery

ANSWERS

1. a   2. d   3. b   4. c
5. c

SUGGESTED READING

1. Gupta P, Zheng Y, Ting TW, Lamoureux EL, Cheng CY, Wong TY. Prevalence of cataract surgery and visual outcomes in Indian immigrants in Singapore: the Singapore Indian eye study. PloS one. 2013;8:e75584.
2. Khurana AK, Khurana A, Khurana BP. Diseases of the Lens. Comprehensive Ophthalmology, 5th edition. New Delhi: New Age International (P) Limited; 2012. pp. 177-216.
3. Ram J, Brar GS. Pediatric Cataract Surgery, 1st edition. New Delhi: Jaypee Brothers Medical Publishers (P) Ltd; 2007.

CHAPTER 14

Disorders of Eyelid and Lacrimal System

Manu Saini, Tanvi Soni

"The intricate dance of the eyelid and lacrimal system underscores the harmony of our ocular world, where even the slightest malfunction can cast a shadow upon the window to our vision."

—Unknown

LEARNING OBJECTIVES

After going through the chapter, the learner will be able to:
- Identify specific pathologies that affect the structure and function of these tissues.
- Develop approach towards diagnosis and management of common eyelid and lacrimal system pathologies.
- Discuss the nursing considerations in disorders of eyelid and lacrimal system.

TERMS

- **Dacryocystitis:** Inflammation of lacrimal sac which can be acute, subacute and chronic.
- **Ectropion:** Outward turning of eyelid margin.
- **Entropion:** Inward turning of eyelid margin and tarsal plate.
- **Eyelid malignancies:** Malignancy arising from layers of eyelid or adnexal structures.
- **Ptosis:** Drooping of upper eyelid margin when eye is looking in primary gaze.

INTRODUCTION

The eyelid acts as a shutter to the eyeball and protects the eye from injury, dryness, and excessive light. The blinking action of the eyelids evenly distributes the tear film across the eye.

DISORDERS OF EYELIDS

The functions of the eyelids are adequate lubrication of exposed portion of globe and protection of globe. Some of the common eyelid disorders are discussed here **(Box 14.1)**.

MALPOSITION OF EYELID AND LASHES

Ectropion

Ectropion is an abnormal eversion of the lid margin away from the globe. Without normal lid globe apposition, corneal exposure, tearing, keratinization of the palpebral conjunctiva, and visual loss may result. The most common cause for the ectropion is laxity of lid tissues due to ageing, scarring of the lid skin, and orbicularis muscle laxity as in facial nerve palsy **(Fig. 14.1)**. Ectropion can be rectified by surgical correction depending upon the etiology.

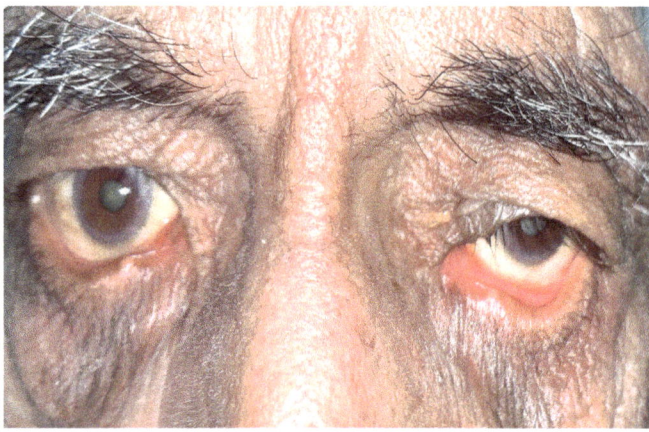

Fig. 14.1: Clinical photograph showing bilateral severe ectropion with laterally displaced lacrimal punctum.

> **BOX 14.1:** Disorders of eyelid and lacrimal system.
>
> A. **Disorders of eyelids**
> - *Malposition of eyelid and eyelashes:*
>   - Ectropion
>   - Entropion
>   - Trichiasis
>   - Ptosis/blepharoptosis
>   - Lid retraction
> - *Inflammatory diseases of eyelid:*
>   - Blepharitis
>   - Preseptal cellulitis
>   - Xanthelasma
> - *Benign lesion of eyelid:*
>   - Cyst of moll (apocrine hydrocystoma)/sebaceous cyst
>   - Squamous papilloma
>   - Melanocytic nevus
> - *Malignant lesion of eyelid:*
>   - Basal cell carcinoma
>   - Sebaceous cell carcinoma
>   - Squamous cell carcinoma
>
> B. **Disorders of the lacrimal drainage system**
> - Congenital nasolacrimal duct obstruction

Nursing Consideration

Patients may develop periocular dermatitis. Prepare the patient for surgery and intraoperatively be aware of risk of entropion.

Entropion

Entropion is inward turning of eyelid margin against the globe **(Fig. 14.2)**. The lower eyelid is more frequently affected. When the lid turns in, the eyelashes and/or lid skin rub against the cornea, creating irritating red-eye with associated photosensitivity. If untreated it may lead to corneal ulceration and infection. The condition may be due to congenital, spasticity of preseptal orbicularis oculi, laxity of lower lid retractors, or shortening of the conjunctiva. Like, ectropion it is addressed by surgical correction of the causative factor.

Trichiasis

It is misdirected eyelashes, rubbing against the ocular surface in the absence of entropion. The condition is often associated with chronic blepharitis or injury to the eyelid or conjunctiva. Trichiasis should be differentiated from distichiasis, which is the congenital condition of partial or complete accessory rows of eyelashes, exit from the posterior lid margin at or near the Meibomian gland orifices.

Trichiasis can present as foreign body sensation, watering, and pain. If the condition persists, may lead to scarring of the cornea. Treatment of trichiasis consists of removal of eyelashes by epilation, electrolysis (electrical energy to destroy the hair follicle), or cryosurgery (extreme cold to destroy the hair follicle).

Nursing Considerations in Entropion and Trichiasis

Complaint of foreign body sensation in a patient with entropion suspect eyelash rubbing the cornea. Ensure adequate lubrication with gels and high viscosity lubricating drops. Address trichiasis by epilation. Make the patient understand the risk of corneal exposure and keratitis if left untreated. Prepare the patient for surgical procedure as advised by surgeon. Intraoperatively risk of overcorrection and ectropion is there. At discharge instruct the patient to return to the clinic on developing foreign body sensation.

Ptosis/Blepharoptosis

Ptosis is defined as drooping of the upper eyelid **(Fig. 14.3)**. It can be congenital, neurogenic as in third nerve palsy, Horner's syndrome, involutional (senile), mechanical (mass over lid), or myogenic (myasthenia gravis). The majority of patients with blepharoptosis have either congenital blepharoptosis caused by dystrophy in the levator muscle or involutional blepharoptosis related to ageing changes in the levator aponeurosis or muscle. Congenital ptosis may also be associated with blepharophimosis syndrome, Marcus-Gunn jaw-winking syndrome, and other systemic causes of muscle weakness. Levator function and severity of ptosis determine the selection of surgical technique.

True ptosis needs to be differentiated from pseudoptosis where lid droop is not because of levator malfunction like seen in microphthalmos, contralateral lid retraction, enophthalmos, hypotropia, and ptosis gets corrected when the causative factors are removed.

Nursing Considerations

Patient should be prepared for advised surgery. Postoperative risk of exposure keratitis should be explained in case of over correction. Patient should be advised on the technique of

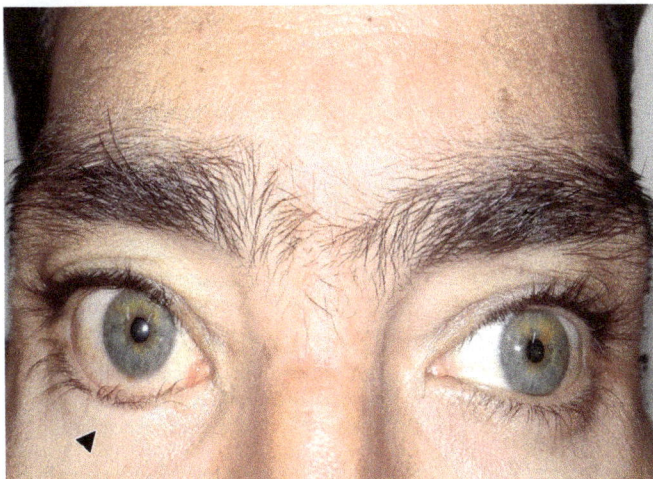

Fig. 14.2: Clinical photograph of right eye lower eyelid entropion shown with arrowhead.

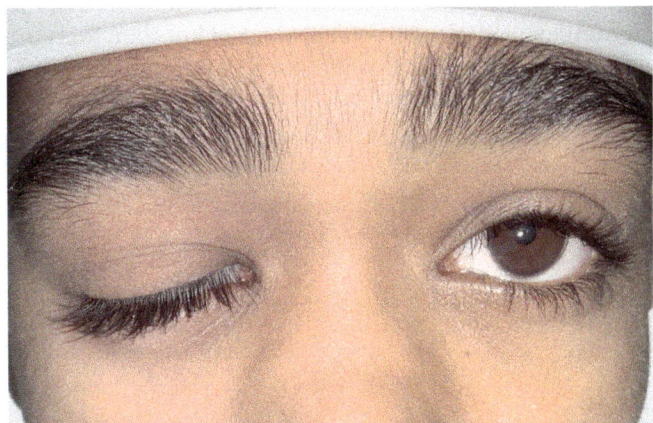

Fig. 14.3: Clinical photograph of right eye congenital severe ptosis in a 10-year-old child.

application of frost suture over forehead using small pieces of adhesive tape over forehead. In pediatric cases, ptosis correction should be followed by refraction and amblyopia therapy if needed.

Lid Retraction

Eyelid retraction is usually secondary to thyroid disorders, trauma, proptosis, seventh nerve palsy, or neurological abnormalities affecting the third nerve. Exposure of cornea, bulbar conjunctiva in lower eyelid retraction can cause dryness, exposure keratitis, and corneal ulcer. Although conservative treatment, such as the use of artificial tears, can be sufficient in mild to moderate cases, surgery is required for severe symptoms.

INFLAMMATORY DISEASE OF EYELID

Blepharitis

Blepharitis, defined as inflammation of the eyelids is associated with irritation, hyperemia, foreign-body sensation, and crusting of the eyelids. Blepharitis can present with a range of signs and symptoms and seen in various dermatological conditions, including seborrheic dermatitis, rosacea, and eczema. Anterior blepharitis (near the eyelashes) is generally of staphylococcal or seborrheic origin, and posterior blepharitis (inner margin, touches the eye) results from the Meibomian gland dysfunction. A topical broad-spectrum antibiotic to the eyelid margins can be useful in staphylococcal blepharitis. Meibomian gland dysfunction can be treated with warm compresses followed by eyelid massage and expression of the liquefied secretions and systemic tetracyclines unless contraindicated.

Nursing Considerations

Cleaning the eyelids in blepharitis should be done using baby shampoo diluted with water and it should be applied using cotton buds. Explain the patient chronic nature of the disease and long duration (weeks) for response to treatment.

Preseptal Cellulitis

Preseptal cellulitis describes an infection of the eyelid and superficial periorbital soft tissues without the involvement of the globe and orbit typically present with eyelid edema and erythema, features characteristic of cellulitis (**Fig. 14.4**). Contiguous spread of infection from the soft tissues of the face and ocular adnexa and extension of infection from the paranasal sinus is the important causative factors for preseptal cellulitis. The primary management of preseptal cellulitis

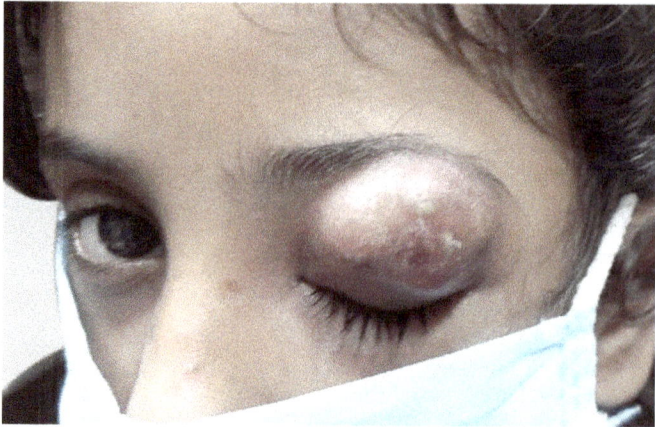

Fig. 14.4: Clinical photograph of an 8-year-old child present with left upper lid, preseptal cellulitis, abscess formation following episode of stye.

focuses on appropriate antibiotic therapy, which should be modified based on clinical response and microbiology report. Surgical intervention required in associated foreign body or eyelid abscess.

Most common frequently occurring mass on the eyelid are depicted in **Table 14.1**.

Xanthelasma

Xanthelasmas are yellowish papules and plaques caused by a localized accumulation of lipid deposits commonly seen on the eyelids (**Fig. 14.6**). Treatment options include superficial excision, CO_2 laser ablation, or topical 100% trichloroacetic acid.

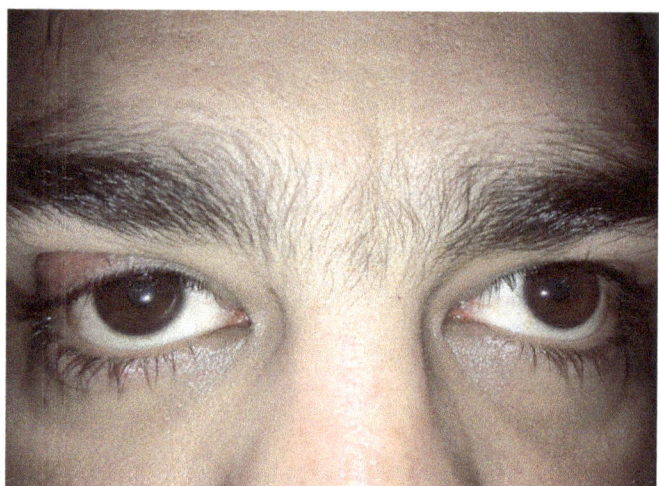

Fig. 14.5: Clinical photograph of right eye showing upper and lower eyelid chalazion in adult male.

TABLE 14.1: Most frequent occurring mass on eye lid.

Type of lesion	Origin	Clinical features	Management
Chalazion (**Fig. 14.5**)	Chronic non-infectious granulomatous inflammation of the Meibomian gland	Chronic, painless nodular mass over lid; located away from the lid margin	Warm compresses and topical antibiotics, incision and curettage in persistent cases
External hordeolum (Stye)	Acute infection of hair follicle of eyelashes and adjacent glands of Zeis or Moll	Painful, acute localized swelling at lid margin; usually pyogenic.	Hot compression, topical antibiotics; incision and drainage if required. Oral antibiotics if preseptal cellulitis accompanied
Internal hordeolum (Stye)	Acute infection of Meibomian gland	Painful, acute localized swelling at lid margin; usually pyogenic	Oral antibiotics with topical antibiotics; incision and drainage if needed

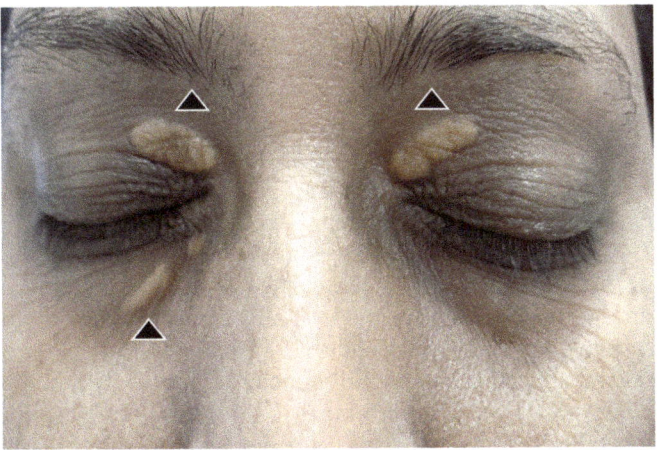

Fig. 14.6: Clinical photograph of bilateral xanthelasma (arrow head) in a 50-year-old female with lipid dysfunction.

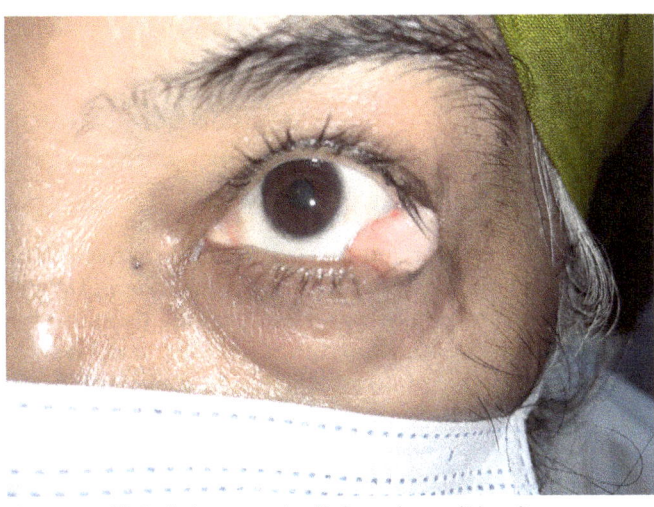

Fig. 14.7: Clinical photograph of left eye lower-lid malignant tumor.

BENIGN LESIONS OF EYELID

Cyst of Moll (Apocrine Hydrocystoma)/Sebaceous Cyst

Cyst of Moll (apocrine hydrocystoma) is nontender, translucent, small retention cyst of lid margin apocrine gland. Whereas non-translucent cystic lesion at lid margin represents obstructed sebaceous glands associated with the lash follicle. Treatment is surgical excision.

Squamous Papilloma

Squamous papilloma is sessile or pedunculated, solitary or multiple, most common benign lesion of old age. Pedunculated papilloma has a rough, convoluted, cerebriform surface. Treatment involves surgical excision or CO_2 laser ablation.

Melanocytic Nevus

The tumors are usually brownish pigmented, thick, range from flat to elevated nodular pigmented growth in the lid margin, may extend to the tarsal conjunctiva. Kissing nevus and hairy nevus are the two characteristic verities described. Evidence of change in size, growth requires surgical intervention.

MALIGNANT LESION OF EYELID

Frequent occurring malignant tumors of the eyelid are described in **Table 14.2**. Treatment required biopsy for confirmation followed by wide local excision of the lesion.

LACRIMAL SYSTEM

Watering is the most common ophthalmic complaint and it can be due to hypersecretion or due to obstruction in the lacrimal outflow pathway. True epiphora refers to watering due to obstruction in the lacrimal outflow pathway, while hyerlacrimation refers to excessive watering due to reflex irritation of ocular surface. It is also important to differentiate between anatomical and functional lacrimal pathway obstruction. Anatomical obstruction refers to any structural pathology in the lacrimal outflow pathway. Conditions like punctal and canalicular stenosis and block, nasolacrimal duct obstruction (NLDO), are the causes of anatomical obstruction. In functional dysfunction, the lacrimal outflow pathway is normal anatomically, with a patent syringing. However, there is a failure of the lacrimal pump mechanisms like in punctal ectropion, eyelid laxity, facial nerve palsy.

DISORDERS OF THE LACRIMAL DRAINAGE SYSTEM

Disorders of the lacrimal drainage includes: Atresia of lacrimal puncta, congenital mucocele of lacrimal sac and most common occurring congenital nasolacrimal duct obstruction.

Dacryoadenitis

It is the inflammation of lacrimal gland. It can be infectious or noninfectious. Infectious cases are acute and respond to appropriate antibiotic therapy. Noninfectious cases are

TABLE 14.2: Malignant lesion of eyelid.				
Malignant tumor of eyelid	Common site	Clinical features	Mode of spread	Pathognomonic histological features
Basal cell carcinoma	Medial canthus/lower lid	Nodular, central ulceration with pearly white rolled out margins with telangiectasia	Local	Palisading peripheral cells
Sebaceous cell carcinoma	Upper lid	Nodule, yellowish appearance, multifocal, more chances of recurrence	Local, intraepithelial, lymph nodes	Foamy cytoplasm
Squamous cell carcinoma	Lower lid (pre-existing actinic keratosis) **(Fig. 14.7)**	Ulcerate with thickened margins, keratosis	Local, lymph nodes	Keratin pearls

chronic and evaluation is done for any systemic cause like sarcoidosis, tuberculosis, syphilis and lymphoma.

Dacryocystitis

It can be acute or chronic inflammation of lacrimal sac due to obstruction in lacrimal drainage system. Acute dacryocystitis patient needs relief of pain and infection. Nursing care is directed towards compliance with the prescribed antibiotics, analgesia and maintenance of ocular hygiene. In chronic dacryocystitis patients present with complain of persistent watering and patient is advised to undergo dacryocystorhinostomy (DCR). Patient is prepared for surgical procedure which can be done endoscopically or externally by giving skin incision in region of lacrimal sac. The surgical procedure is done for opening a new tear drainage path in nasal cavity. Postoperatively patient needs to be observed for active bleed from nasal cavity. Antibiotic application is done over the suture site. If there is stent placement patient should be instructed not to pull out the stent and avoid forceful blowing of nose.

Congenital Nasolacrimal Duct Obstruction

Epiphora due to congenital nasolacrimal duct obstruction (CNLDO) will present since shortly after birth. CNLDO is usually caused by imperforate valve of Hasner (lower end of nasolacrimal duct) and the symptom of watering is mostly constant in these patients. Pressure over the lacrimal sac can cause mucopurulent material to regurgitate through the punctum confirming a diagnosis of chronic dacryocystitis or lacrimal mucocele.

Fluorescence dye disappearance test is a physiological test for checking the function of the lacrimal outflow pathway and is extremely useful in children and good screening test, with complaint of watering who are not suitable for other diagnostic procedures like irrigation and probing. Few drops of fluorescein dye instilled in the conjunctival sac. The dye disappears within 5 seconds if lacrimal outflow is patent (**Fig. 14.8**). A positive test indicates dysfunction in the lacrimal outflow pathway. However, this test cannot differentiate a functional from anatomical obstruction and cannot pinpoint the site of anatomical block. Patients with a positive test need further evaluation with other test—irrigation and probing. On the other hand, adult patients can undergo diagnostic irrigation and probing to establish the diagnosis.

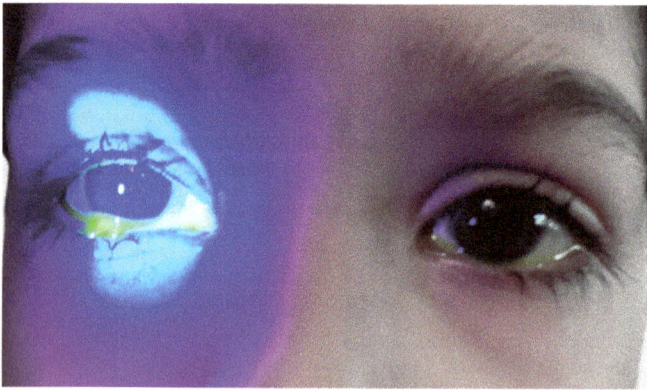

Fig. 14.8: Clinical photograph of bilateral congenital NLDO showing positive fluorescence dye disappearance test.

Management

The most common outcome of CNLDO is the spontaneous resolution without the surgical intervention. Topical antibiotics are needed when there is purulent discharge and conjunctivitis or associated acute dacryocystitis. Pediatricians should instruct the parents on proper massage of the nasolacrimal sac region. First described by Crigler in 1923, this technique has been shown to increase the rate of nonsurgical resolution of the obstruction. When resolution does not occur probing and irrigation of nasolacrimal duct system is the treatment of choice. If nasolacrimal system does not remain patent, many ophthalmologists repeat the probing once or twice before attempting the more complicated procedures, silicon tube intubation or dacrocystorhinostomy.

> **Case Scenario**
>
> A 42-year-old male presented to the eye care services with a one-day history of trauma to the right lower lid. On examination, the patient had a full thickness lower lid laceration with canalicular involvement. The rest of the examination was unremarkable (**Fig. 14.9**).
>
>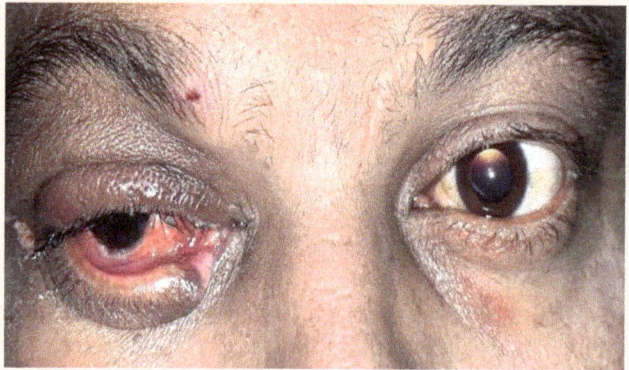
>
> **Fig. 14.9:** Clinical photograph of a 42-year-old male following a dog bite to the lower lid.
>
> The diagnosis is post-traumatic full thickness laceration of the right eye's lower lid with canalicular tear.
>
> **Management:** The patient was given a tetanus toxoid injection, thorough cleaning of the wound followed by primary repair of the lid defect and canalicular repair.

SUMMARY

Eyelid pathologies directly affect the ocular surface and should be treated with utmost care. There is a risk of development of corneal ulcer and dry eye if left untreated. Lacrimal drainage system obstruction should be diagnosed at an early stage and treated according to age of patient.

MULTIPLE CHOICE QUESTIONS

1. What would be the diagnosis if a mother comer with history of watering and discharge since birth in 6-month-old baby?
    a. Ectropion
    b. Congenital nasolacrimal duct obstruction
    c. Conjunctivitis
    d. Ptosis
2. Structures forming upper eyelid are:
    a. Tarsal plate
    b. Levator palpebrae superioris
    c. Muller's muscle
    d. All of the above
3. Misdirection of eyelashes is known as:
    a. Distichiasis
    b. Trichiasis
    c. Meibomitis
    d. Tylosis

4. What is the surgical treatment for chronic dacryocystitis?
   a. Pars plana vitrectomy
   b. Enucleation
   c. Evisceration
   d. Dacryocystorhinostomy
5. Drooping of upper eyelid is known as:
   a. Exophthalmos
   b. Proptosis
   c. Ptosis
   d. Tylosis

ANSWERS

1. b 2. d 3. a 4. d
5. c

SUGGESTED READING

1. Cates CA, Tyers AG. Outcomes of anterior levator resection in congenital blepharoptosis. Eye (Lond). 2001;15:770-3.
2. Hurwitz JJ. The Lippincott-Raven Publishers. Lacrimal System; 1996.
3. Kashkouli MB, Mirzajani H, Jamshidian-Tehrani M. Reliability of fluorescein dye disappearance test in assessment of adults with nasolacrimal duct obstruction. Ophthal Plast Reconstr Surg. 2013;29(3):167-9.
4. Kim KH, Baek JS, Lee S, Lee JH, Choi HS, Kim SJ, et al. Causes and Surgical Outcomes of Lower Eyelid Retraction. Korean J Ophthalmol. 2017;31(4):290-8.
5. Laftah Z, Al-Niaimi F. Xanthelasma: An update on treatment modalities. J Cutan Aesthet Surg. 2018;11:1-6.
6. Lavrich JB, Nelson LB. Disorders of the lacrimal system apparatus. Pediatr Clin North Am. 1993;40(4):767-76.
7. Lee S, Yen MT. Management of preseptal and orbital cellulitis. Saudi Journal of Ophthalmology. 2011;25:21-9.
8. Lemp MA, Nichols KK. Blepharitis in the United States 2009: a survey-based perspective on prevalence and treatment. Ocular Surface. 2009;7(Suppl 2):1-14.
9. O Collin JR, Allen L, Castronuovo S. Congenital eyelid retraction. BJO. 1990;74:542-4.
10. O'Donnell BA, O Collin JR. Distichiasis: management with cryotherapy to the posterior lamella. BJO. 1993;77:289-92.
11. Turnbull AMJ, Mayfield MP. Blepharitis. BMJ. 2012;344:e3328.
12. Weber RK. Atlas of lacrimal surgery. New York: Springer; 2007.
13. Wong CY, Fan DS, Gohty, Lam DS. Long-term results of Palmaris longus frontalis sling in children with congenital ptosis. Eye. 2005;18(5):546-8.
14. Wong VA, Beckingsale PS, Oley CA, Sullivan TJ. Management of myogenic ptosis. Ophthalmology. 2002;109:1023-31.

CHAPTER 15

Orbital Disorders

Manu Saini, Tanvi Soni

"Orbital diseases, with their intricate interplay of anatomy and pathology, remind us of the delicate balance that exists within the depths of the eye socket, where the complexities of vision and health converge."

—Unknown

LEARNING OBJECTIVES

After going through the chapter, the learner will be able to:
- Describe common ocular pathologies involving orbit.
- Differentiate between orbital and preseptal cellulitis.
- Enumerate and identify common orbital tumors.
- Choose appropriate imaging studies and understand the principles of medical and surgical management in orbital pathology.
- Discuss the nursing considerations in various orbital disorders.

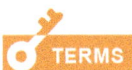

TERMS

- **Enucleation:** Surgical removal of entire globe.
- **Evisceration:** Surgical removal of entire contents of eyeball apart from scleral tissue.
- **Exenteration:** Removal of whole orbit (globe, eyelid and content of orbit).
- **Orbital cellulitis:** Periorbital infection involving structures posterior to the orbital septum.
- **Preseptal cellulitis:** Periorbital infection involving structures anterior to orbital septum.
- **Proptosis:** Protrusion of eyeball.

INTRODUCTION

The orbital inflammatory disease (OID) represents inflammatory conditions of the orbit which can be infectious or noninfectious. The differential diagnosis includes infection, systemic inflammatory conditions and neoplasms, other concomitant medical conditions **(Table 15.1)**. Acute OID presents with proptosis, extraocular motility disturbance, pain, erythema, and chemosis.

The orbital diseases are identified by accurate clinical history followed by good clinical examination. Imaging modalities help in precisely locating the lesion, and establishing the differential diagnosis that guides in management.

INFECTIOUS ORBITAL INFLAMMATION

It is further classified as preseptal (limited anterior to orbital septum) and orbital cellulitis (extending beyond orbital septum) **(Table 15.2)**.

ORBITAL TUMORS

Orbital tumors are rare but can affect children as well as adults **(Fig. 15.3)**. Benign tumors like dermoid cyst and vascular malformations can be observed if there is no immediate threat to vision and are cosmetically acceptable. Orbit has dense network of both central and peripheral nervous systems. Tumors can arise from second, third, fourth, fifth and sixth cranial nerves as well as from sympathetic and parasympathetic nervous system. Orbital metastasis in systemic malignancies is important for prognosis as their presence is associated with poor survival **(Table 15.3)**. A brief understanding of location of orbital tumors can help in making a differential diagnosis **(Fig. 15.3)**.

IMAGING IN ORBITAL PATHOLOGY

X-ray and computerized tomography (CT) scan are done for better bony structure imaging. CT helps in delineation of the

TABLE 15.1: Orbital inflammatory disease differential diagnosis.

Structure affected	Clinical features	Imaging findings	Possible diagnosis
Lacrimal gland	**Dacryoadenitis** Painful, firm, erythematous mass in the lateral upper lid, and possible ptosis	Diffuse lacrimal gland enlargement	Epithelial neoplasm, lymphoma
Extraocular muscles (EOM)	**Myositis** Dysthyroid orbitopathy presents with lid retraction, lateral flare, lid lag and other lid signs **(Fig. 15.1)**. Inferior rectus being most frequently affected EOM	Bilateral EOM inflammation, enlargement, involving surrounding fat and tendon sparing	Dysthyroid orbitopathy
Extraocular muscles	**Myositis**	Unilateral EOM inflammation, enlargement, surrounding fat and tendon involvement	Pseudotumor/non-specific idiopathic orbital inflammatory disease
Orbital/ periorbital fat	**Cellulitis** Orbital cellulitis accompanied by fever, leukocytosis, and a clinical history of head and neck infection **(Fig. 15.2)**. Carotid cavernous fistula (CCF) have enlarged superior ophthalmic vein (SOV), abnormal fullness of cavernous sinus, or, in larger fistulas, flow voids MRI. Cavernous sinus thrombosis (CST) presents with enlarged SOV	Enhancing periorbital tissues with possible intraconal extension	Orbital cellulitis, carotid cavernous fistula (CCF), cavernous sinus thrombosis (CST)
Orbital apex	Orbital apicitis, Tolosa-Hunt syndrome Paralysis of cranial nerves III, IV, V1, and VI	Ill-defined, enhancing lesion at orbital apex, variably involving middle cranial fossa and cavernous sinus	Meningioma, other dural infiltrative process
Periscleral	Perisclerites Present as uveitis or sclerites/episcleritis	Scleral thickening with periscleral edema and fluid in Tenon's capsule	Endophthalmitis

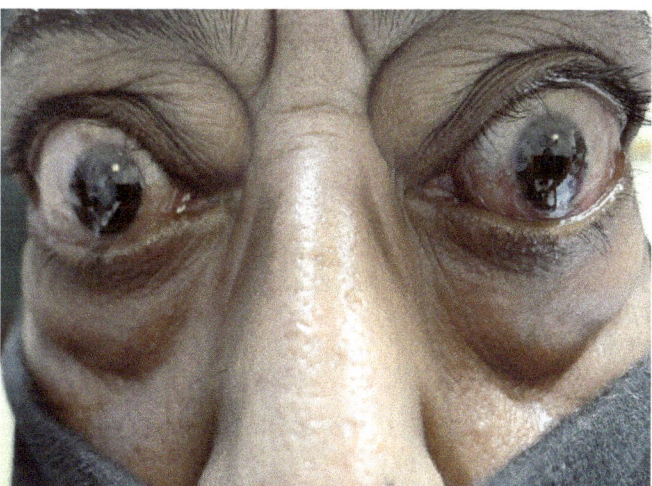

Fig. 15.1: Clinical photograph of bilateral symmetrical thyroid-associated orbitopathy in a chronic smoker.

TABLE 15.2: Infectious orbital inflammatory disease.

	Preseptal cellulitis	Orbital cellulitis
Location of inflammation	Anterior to orbital septum	Extending beyond orbital septum
Symptoms	Painful eyelid swelling	Painful eyelid swelling with decreased vision
Signs: • Visual acuity • Pupillary reaction • Conjunctiva • Extraocular motility	• Normal • Normal • Normal • Normal	• Decreased • Relative afferent pupillary defect (RAPD) • Chemosis • Decreased
Prognosis	Good (If untreated it can progress to orbital cellulitis)	• Poor (untreated) • Risk of blindness, cavernous sinus thrombosis, mortality
Management	Responds to oral antibiotics	Intravenous antibiotics

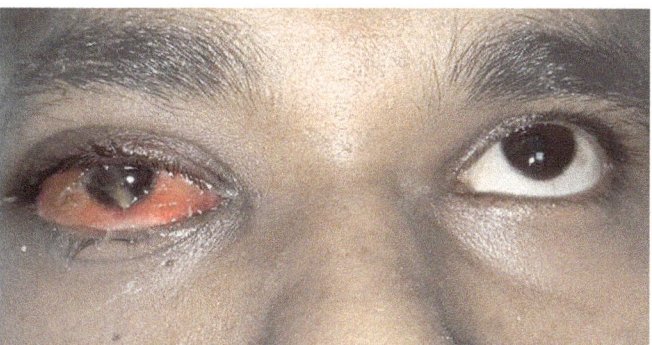

Fig. 15.2: Clinical photograph of right eye post-traumatic orbital cellulitis showing proptosis, chemosis, limitation of extraocular movements, corneal penetrating injury with exudates in anterior chamber.

shape, location and extent of orbital lesions in the orbit. It is the technique of choice in orbital trauma and bony tumors **(Fig. 15.4)**. Magnetic resonance imaging (MRI) is non-invasive technique which is better for soft tissue delineation and imaging of orbitocranial junction. However, in some cases both may be required for astute management.

PROPTOSIS

Proptosis is the protrusion of the eyeball away from the orbit. Generally, a 2 mm or greater asymmetry between the protrusion of a patient's eyes is considered abnormal. The 6 P's (**Pain, Progression, Proptosis, Pulsation, Palpation and Periocular changes**) of the orbital history and physical

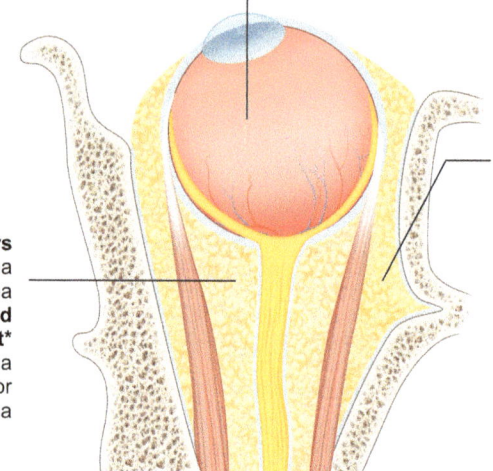

Fig. 15.3: Differential diagnosis of orbital tumors on the basis of location.

*Metastasis to orbit—can present as intraconal or extraconal.
**Leukemia, lymphoma—extraconal more often than intraconal.

TABLE 15.3: Types of orbital tumors.	
Category (based on origin of tumor)	Type of tumor
Congenital	Dermoid cyst
Vascular malformations	• Infantile capillary hemangiomas • Cavernous hemangiomas • Lymphatic malformations • Arteriovenous fistula
Neural tumors	• Optic nerve glioma • Neurofibroma • Meningioma • Schwannoma
Mesenchymal tumors	Rhabdomyosarcoma
Lymphoproliferative disorders	• Lymphoma • Langerhans cell histiocytosis • Xanthogranuloma
Lacrimal gland tumors	• Pleomorphic adenoma • Adenoid cystic carcinoma • Malignant mixed tumor
Metastatic tumors	• Neuroblastoma • Leukemia • Breast carcinoma • Prostate carcinoma • Bronchogenic carcinoma

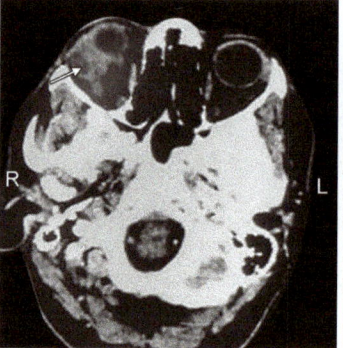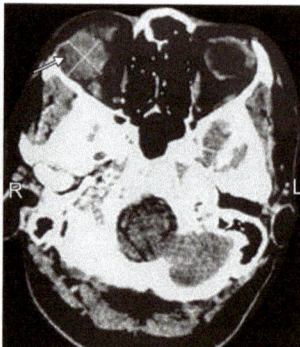

Fig. 15.4: Computed tomography showing right superior-temporal heterogenous orbital mass with fossa formation of lateral orbital wall suggesting possibility of lacrimal gland tumor.

- ❖ **Enucleation:** Surgical removal of globe sparing the extraocular muscles.
- ❖ **Exenteration:** Surgical removal of orbital contents and all the involved surrounding structures including eyelid and bone.

NURSING CONSIDERATIONS

- ❖ In orbital cellulitis patient demands in-patient care.
- ❖ Monitor vitals (heart rate, saturation and temperature) of patient and alert the clinician if patient complains of rapid deterioration of vision, sudden pain and headache.
- ❖ Arrangement of imaging (CT) and strict compliance of intravenous antibiotic schedule should be followed.
- ❖ Laboratory investigations should include complete blood counts, renal function test and liver function test (depending on type of antibiotics used).
- ❖ All the surgical procedures to be carried out are psychologically affecting the patient.
- ❖ It is important for the nursing personnel to educate the patient preoperatively regarding the outcome of surgical procedure.

examination are helpful to create a quick and easy framework for the diagnosis.

SURGICAL PROCEDURES IN ORBITAL PATHOLOGY

In a painful blind eye due to underlying malignancy, uncontrolled glaucoma, infection or trauma, surgeon can opt for removal of eye. Following surgical procedures can be done:

- ❖ **Evisceration:** It is the removal of intraocular contents and sparing sclera.

- They need to highlight the need for placement of ocular prosthesis later.
- Postoperatively patient may need antiemetics and adequate analgesia.
- Pressure bandage and cleaning of ocular socket followed by instillation of antibiotic should be thoroughly explained to the patient.
- If a conformer is placed, patient should be taught the technique of cleaning and placement of conformer in socket.
- **Technique of insertion of ocular prosthesis:** After taking consent from patient and explaining the procedure, nursing personnel should wash hands. Pull the upper eyelid upwards and insert the prosthesis in upper fornix. Lower eyelid should be everted and lower edge of prosthesis is inserted in lower fornix.
- **Technique of removal of ocular prosthesis:** After washing hands, evert the lower eyelid and prosthesis comes out.
- Prepare the patients for discharge with all the instructions given in writing.

Case Scenario

A 35-year-old male presents with acute onset left eyelid swelling, pain, redness, and proptosis following a wooden prick to the pre-existing lid lesion. He had a low-grade fever at the presentation. His best corrected visual acuity was 20/40. On examination, the patient had upper eyelid tense swelling (**Fig. 15.5A**, oval-shaped marking) with a lesion on the medial side. The anterior segment and fundus examination were within normal limits. A CT scan of the head and orbit (**Figs. 15.5B and C**) revealed a heterogenous, irregular superiortemporal preseptal cystic lesion with anterior orbit involvement.

Diagnosis: Left eye post-traumatic upper lid abscess with orbital cellulitis.

Management: Topical and intravenous antibiotics (combination of linezolid, ceftriaxone, and metronidazole) were started and upper lid abscess drainage was performed under aseptic conditions. The patient responded well and was symptom-free after ten days of the treatment.

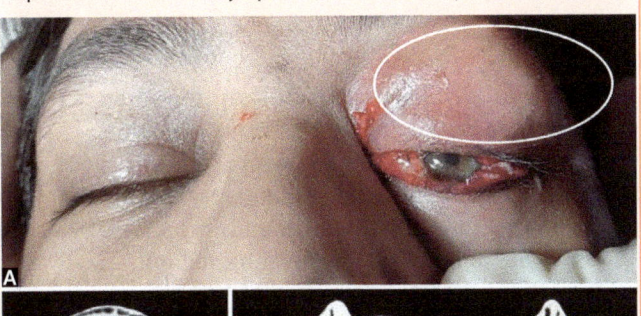
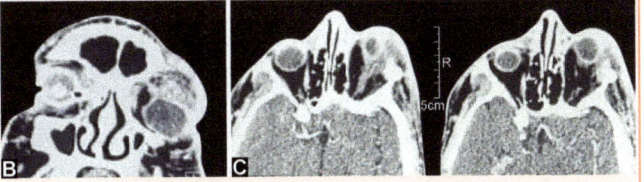

Figs. 15.5A to C: Clinical photograph.

SUMMARY

Orbit is a complex bony structure which contains eyeball, extraocular muscles, nerves and connective tissue. Also, it is surrounded by paranasal sinuses and cranium. The implications of orbital pathology are grave and need immediate attention, e.g., cases like orbital cellulitis which can be life-threatening.

MULTIPLE CHOICE QUESTIONS

1. Most common cause of bilateral proptosis in adults:
    a. Thyroid ophthalmopathy
    b. Leukemia
    c. Cavernous hemangioma
    d. Retinoblastoma
2. What is the difference between orbital and preseptal cellulitis?
    a. Involvement of structures posterior to orbital septum (orbital) and anterior to orbital septum (preseptal)
    b. Involvement of orbital tissue (orbital) and involvement of eyelid (preseptal)
    c. Both are same
    d. None of the above
3. What is evisceration?
    a. Removal of eyelid
    b. Removal of lacrimal sac
    c. Removal of whole eyeball including sclera
    d. Removal of eyeball excluding sclera
4. Most common muscle involved in thyroid ophthalmopathy:
    a. Superior rectus   b. Medial rectus
    c. Inferior rectus   d. Lateral rectus
5. Which orbital wall is most likely to be involved in blow-out fracture?
    a. Roof   b. Floor
    c. Medial wall   d. Lateral wall

ANSWERS

1. a   2. a   3. d   4. c
5. b

SUGGESTED READING

1. Kapur R, Sepahdari AR, Mafee MF, Putterman AM, Aakalu V, Wendel LJ, et al. MR imaging of orbital inflammatory syndrome, orbital cellulitis, and orbital lymphoid lesions: the role of diffusion-weighted imaging. AJNR Am J Neuroradiol. 2009;30:64-70.
2. Pakdaman MN, et al. Orbital inflammatory disease: Pictorial review. World J Radiol. 2014;6(4):106-15.
3. Rootman J. Diseases of the orbit: A multidisciplinary approach. 2nd edition. Philadelphia: Lippincott Williams & Wilkins; 2003.
4. Topilow NJ, Tran AQ, Koo EB, Alabiad CR. Etiologies of proptosis: A review. Intern Med Rev (Wash DC). 2020;6(3):10.18103/imr.v6i3.852. doi:10.18103/imr.v6i3.852

CHAPTER 16

Disorders of Cornea

Surbhi Khurana, Parul Chawla Gupta, Ranjan Kumar Behera, Jagat Ram

"Although cornea is just about the size of a postage stamp and lacks the neurobiological sophistication of the retina and the dynamic movement of the lens yet without its clarity the eye would not be able to perform its necessary functions."

—Unknown

LEARNING OBJECTIVES

After going through the chapter, the learner will be able to:
- Enumerate various corneal disorders.
- Understand diagnostic tests of various corneal disorders.
- Discuss the management of various corneal disorders.
- Discuss the nursing interventions of various corneal disorders.

TERMS

- **Corneal ulcer:** Corneal epithelial defect with infiltrates.
- **Epithelial defect:** Any break in the integrity of the cornea.
- **Infective conjunctivitis:** Conjunctivitis caused due to bacterial or viral causes.
- **Keratoplasty:** Corneal transplantation.

INTRODUCTION

The cornea is a transparent, convex structure, which is surrounded by sclera; the anatomical junction of both is called the limbus. The corneal thickness is more in the periphery as compared to the center. Anatomically, it consists of five layers; the epithelium, Bowman's membrane, stroma, Descemet membrane and the endothelium. Recently, the sixth layer, called Dua's layer, has been hypothesized and is known to be between the stroma and Descemet membrane. Histologically, it consists of three layers; the epithelium, substantia propria, and the endothelium.

The cornea is the most important refractive surface of the eye, with a refractive index of 1.38 and tear film as the anterior refractive surface. Various factors maintain the transparency of the cornea, like avascular nature, dehydrated stage, and uniform arrangement of the collagen fibrils.

- ❖ **Blood supply:** The normal cornea is avascular, with no lymphatics. Nutrition is derived from the aqueous, the limbal capillaries and the oxygen in the tear film.
- ❖ **Nerve supply:** The nerve supply of the cornea is from the ophthalmic division of the trigeminal nerve, mainly by its branch-long ciliary nerve. Due to the dense nerve supply, the cornea is an extremely sensitive structure.
- ❖ **Oxygen supply:** The metabolism of the cornea is mainly aerobic. Oxygen is used by keratocytes, endothelium and the epithelium. The tear film mainly supplies oxygen, and glucose is mainly supplied by the aqueous.
- ❖ **Functions:** The main functions of the cornea are focusing the light by refraction, maintenance of transparency, protection of the eye and maintenance of the structural integrity of the globe. Tear film and sodium-potassium ATPase pumps help in these functions. In case of any injury or inflammation, the normally avascular cornea can become vascularized, and transparency or integrity of the cornea can be lost.

DISEASES OF THE CORNEA AND THEIR RELEVANT TERMINOLOGY

- ❖ **Keratitis:** Any inflammation in the cornea is called keratitis. It can be superficial if it is anterior to the bowman's layer and deep if it involves stroma.

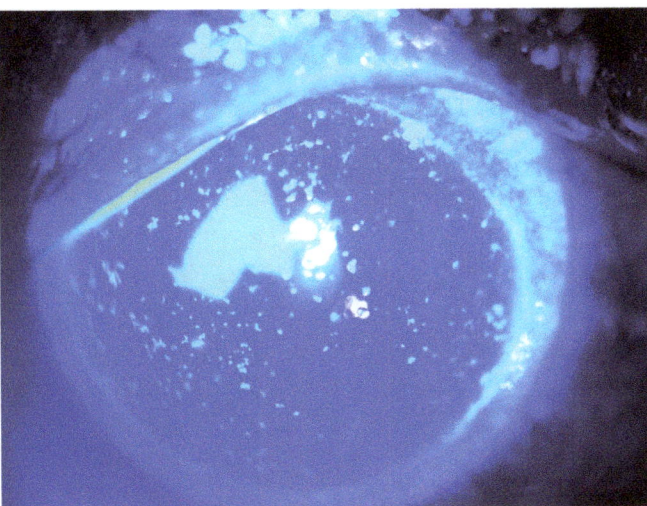

Fig. 16.1: Image showing epithelial defect stained with fluorescein and seen under cobalt blue filter.

- **Epithelial defect:** Any loss in integrity of the corneal epithelium is called an epithelial defect, and it can be stained by fluorescein stain 1% and viewed with a cobalt blue filter light **(Fig. 16.1)**.
- **Corneal ulcer:** If the epithelial defect is associated with corneal infiltrates, it is called a corneal ulcer.
- **Corneal opacity:** All the above problems can cause corneal scarring or opacity after their healing, which is seen as a white opacity in the cornea.
  Corneal opacity can be nebular, macular or leucomatous, depending upon its severity.
  - If iris details are clearly visible, it is called nebular opacity.
  - If iris details are obscured, but iris and pupillary margins are visible, it is called macular opacity.
  - In cases with complete obscuration of the anterior chamber details, it is called leucomatous opacity or leucoma.
  - If the iris is stuck to the opacity, it is called adherent leucoma.
- **Corneal edema:** It is caused by the accumulation of fluid in between the collagen fibrils, causing haziness of the cornea. It first appears in the epithelium, then involves stroma, and causes pain and foreign body sensation.
- **Filamentary keratopathy:**
  - It is formed by corneal filaments, which are attached to the cornea at one end and are free at the other end.
  - It produces symptoms of foreign body sensation, irritation and pain.
  - *Causes:* It is seen in dry eye disease, viral diseases and long-standing degenerative conditions. It is commonly seen in dry eye disease associated with systemic diseases like Rheumatoid arthritis, Sjogren syndrome, etc.
  - *Treatment:* Lubricants, N-acetylcysteine.

CLINICAL FEATURES IN CORNEAL DISEASES

- **Symptoms:** The common symptoms of corneal diseases are decreased vision, pain, lacrimation, photophobia, foreign body sensation, irritation and 'whiteness' of the cornea.
- **Signs:** The common signs to be looked for in corneal diseases are circumcorneal or diffuse congestion, corneal oedema, infiltrates, epithelial defect, vascularization or change in shape or curvature of the cornea.

INFECTIOUS KERATITIS

Infectious keratitis, also known as **'Corneal Ulcer'**, can be caused by various organisms like bacteria, fungi or parasites.

Clinical Features

- Patients usually complain of pain, foreign body sensation and decreased vision.
- The common clinical signs are congestion, epithelial defect, infiltrates, necrotic slough, hypopyon, corneal abscess and corneal thinning.
- A hypopyon consists of a collection of polymorphonuclear leucocytes in the inferior part of the anterior chamber, with a mesh of fibrin.
- A careful slit lamp examination is essential in all patients with corneal ulcers to assess the extent of involvement. A slit lamp diagram can help to evaluate the improvement or worsening in subsequent visits.

Diagnosis

The diagnosis is based on clinical examination and microbiological reports. All the corneal ulcers should be subjected to scrapings using a sterile disposable blade or needle, subjected to microscopy with Gram, Giemsa and KOH stain, and plated on culture plates like blood agar, chocolate agar, non-nutrient agar with *Escherichia* coli, and Sabouraud dextrose agar.

Bacterial Keratitis

Causes

- Bacterial keratitis can be commonly caused by *Staphylococcus, Streptococcus, Pseudomonas* and *Neisseria gonorrhoeae.*
- The principal mode of entry is through the corneal epithelium, from a break or direct invasion.
- Certain predisposing factors can include chronic dacryocystitis, dry ocular surface, ocular trauma, use of contact lenses, prolonged use of topical steroids, lid abnormalities and poor ocular hygiene.

Fungal Keratitis

- It is the most common keratitis in tropical countries, rural areas, and immunocompromised individuals.
- *Aspergillus, Fusarium* and *Candida* commonly cause it.
- Fungal ulcers are typically seen after trauma with the vegetative matter.

Clinical Features

- The symptoms in these ulcers are much less than the signs.
- Fungal ulcers are dry-looking ulcers with feathery margins, and have fixed, convex hypopyon **(Fig. 16.2)**.

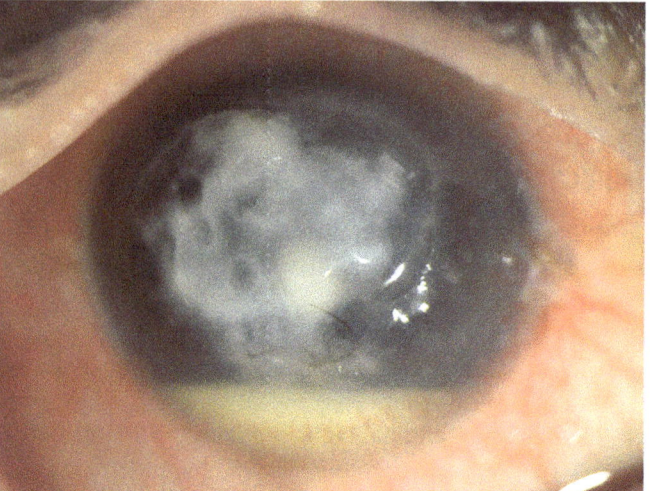

Fig. 16.2: Image showing a fungal ulcer with hypopyon.

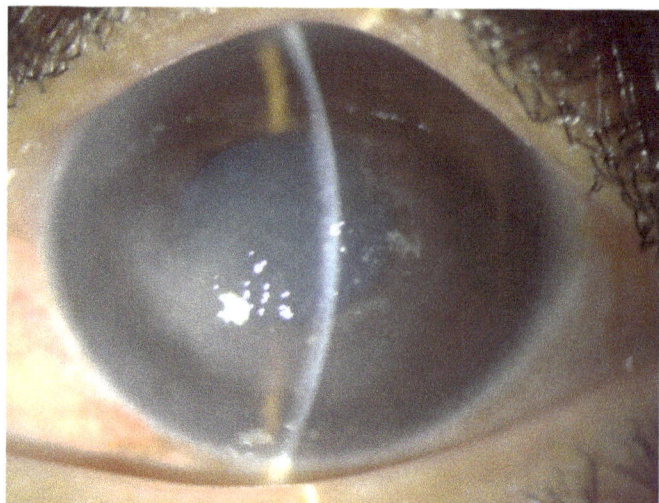

Fig. 16.3: Image showing corneal edema with keratic precipitates, suggestive of disciform keratitis.

Viral Keratitis

It can be caused by herpes simplex or adenovirus.

Herpetic Keratitis

It is caused by herpes simplex virus, with the mode of infection as oral or genital transmission.

Epithelial Keratitis

The most characteristic pattern seen **in dendritic ulcers**, seen as a branching ulcer.

Stromal Keratitis

It is associated with decreased vision and seen as stromal edema with Descemet folds.

It can also be seen as **disciform keratitis**, where corneal oedema is associated with underlying keratic precipitates **(Fig. 16.3)**.

Endotheliitis

Sometimes the inflammation is limited to the corneal endothelium with associated keratic precipitates and corneal edema, called as endotheliitis. It can be associated with iritis in a few cases.

Complications of Corneal Ulcer

- ❖ **Desmetocele:** Sometimes, the ulcer can rapidly invade all the layers superficial to the Descemet membrane, which causes herniation of the Descemet due to intraocular pressure, causing desmetocele.
- ❖ **Corneal perforation:** Perforation can occur through the thinned out area or desmetocele, and cause sudden leakage of aqueous from the perforation and shallow/flat anterior chamber.
- ❖ **Others:** Secondary glaucoma, cataract, choroidal detachment and staphyloma are various other complications of corneal ulcers.

Treatment of Infectious Keratitis

Control of infection, symptomatic relief, and prevention of complications form the mainstay of treatment.

Bacterial Keratitis

- ❖ **Antimicrobials:** Fortified eye drops for both gram-positive and gram-negative bacteria are given, like a cephalosporine in combination with an aminoglycoside. Fluoroquinolone eye drops can also be given.
- ❖ Atropine 1% is given to decrease the pain associated with ciliary spasms.
- ❖ Antiglaucoma therapy is required as well.
- ❖ Steroids can be given in severe infections to decrease the inflammation under extreme supervision.

Fungal Keratitis

- ❖ Topical natamycin, voriconazole and amphotericin B are given in fungal ulcers.
- ❖ Oral antifungal agents can be given in severe ulcers or if there is suspicion of endophthalmitis.

Surgical Management

- ❖ Urgent keratoplasty is required in cases with uncontrolled infection or large corneal perforation.
- ❖ In eyes with a corneal scar and no visual potential, corneal tattooing can be done.
- ❖ In eyes with small corneal perforation, tissue adhesives like N-butyl 2-ethyl cyanoacrylate can be used to seal the perforation.

Viral Keratitis

- ❖ The treatment of herpes simplex is comprised of topical and systemic antivirals, topical steroids and supportive therapy, including lubricants and cycloplegics.
- ❖ Commonly used topical antivirals are acyclovir 3%, idoxuridine 5% and trifluridine 1%, and systemic are acyclovir and valacyclovir.
- ❖ Topical steroids are contraindicated in epithelial keratitis.
- ❖ Oral antivirals may be required to continue for the long term to prevent recurrence.

HERPES ZOSTER OPHTHALMICUS

It is caused by varicella zoster virus. After infection with chickenpox in childhood, this virus stays dormant in Gasserian ganglion. It is reactivated whenever there is decreased immunity and affects the area supplied by the ophthalmic division of the trigeminal nerve.

Clinical Features

- It is nearly always unilateral and does not cross the midline.
- The onset is accompanied by fever, neuralgic pain and vesicular eruptions over the affected area.
- It can cause punctate lesions, iridocyclitis, neurotrophic keratitis, oculomotor nerve paralysis and retinal necrosis.

Treatment

- Oral antivirals are required for 10 days.
- Topical lubrication might be required for the associated dry eye.
- Neurotrophic ulcers might require tarsorrhaphy.

ACANTHAMOEBA KERATITIS

Clinical Features

- It is a devastating infection, usually seen in contact lens users.
- It causes severe ocular pain, ring infiltrates, and perineural infiltration (Fig. 16.4).

Treatment

Comprises of polyhexamethyl biguanide 0.02% and propamidine 0.1%.

IMMUNOLOGICALLY MEDIATED DISEASES

Phlyctenular Keratitis

- Phlyctenular keratoconjunctivitis is nodular affection occurring as an allergic response to endogenous allergens.
- Type IV cell mediated delayed hypersensitivity reaction to tuberculin and *Staphylococcus* proteins.
- Exudation and infiltration of leukocytes occurs in deeper layers of conjunctiva followed by eventual nodular ulceration of cornea.
- Treatment involves topical steroids, antibiotic drops, ruling out TB and other parasitic infections along with general health and dietary measures.

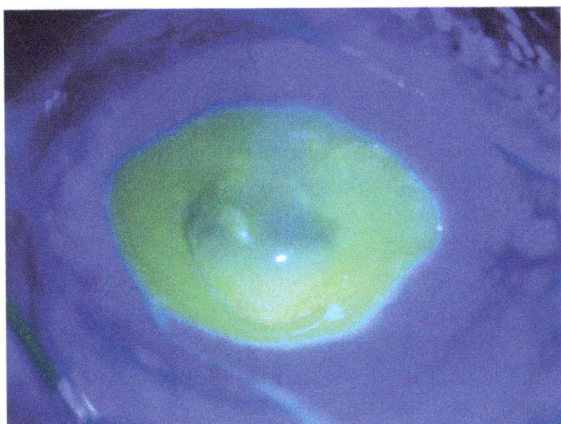

Fig. 16.4: Image showing ring ulcer, in patient with acanthomeba keratitis.

Marginal Keratitis

- There are multiple lesions commonly seen at the cornea, near the point of contact with lid margins.
- These lesions are known to be caused due to immunological reaction to *Staphylococcus* and are situated with a clear interval from the limbus.
- The treatment comprises of treatment of blepharitis, lid scrubs, topical antibiotics and steroids.

Mooren Ulcer

- It is a rare, degenerative superficial ulcer starting at the margin, progressing circumferentially and then involving the entire cornea.
- The etiology is unknown, with autoimmune lysis and collagenolysis.
- The ulcer undermines the epithelium at the advancing margin, forming an overhanging edge.
- It is a diagnosis of exclusion after ruling out all other causes of peripheral ulcerative keratitis.
- Treatment comprises of steroids, resection of the conjunctiva and management of the corneal perforation.

CORNEAL DYSTROPHIES

Corneal dystrophies are bilateral, non-inflammatory and hereditary diseases of the cornea without any vascularization. They can affect any layer of the cornea.

Epithelial and Subepithelial Dystrophies

- They can be asymptomatic or have recurrent corneal erosions, pain, lacrimation and photophobia.
- Epithelial basement membrane dystrophy and Cogan microcystic epithelial dystrophy are the common types of these dystrophies.

Bowman Layer Dystrophies

These are autosomal dominant dystrophies, causing recurrent corneal erosions, with Reiss Buckler dystrophy and Theil-Behnke dystrophy as the common types.

Stromal Dystrophies

- The three types of stromal dystrophies are granular, lattice and macular dystrophy.
- In granular dystrophy, abnormal deposition of hyaline material forms the opacities.
- Lattice dystrophy has the deposition of amyloid material. Both of these dystrophies are dominantly inherited.
- Macular dystrophy, a recessively inherited dystrophy, has the deposition of glycosaminoglycans (Fig. 16.5).

Endothelial Corneal Dystrophy

The most common endothelial dystrophy is Fuch's endothelial dystrophy. It is seen in older people, commonly females, due to abnormal hyaline excrescences on the Descemet's membrane. The changes can be seen as black areas on specular microscopy. It can cause epithelial and stroma edema, and require treatment with hypertonic saline. Keratoplasty may be needed in advanced stages.

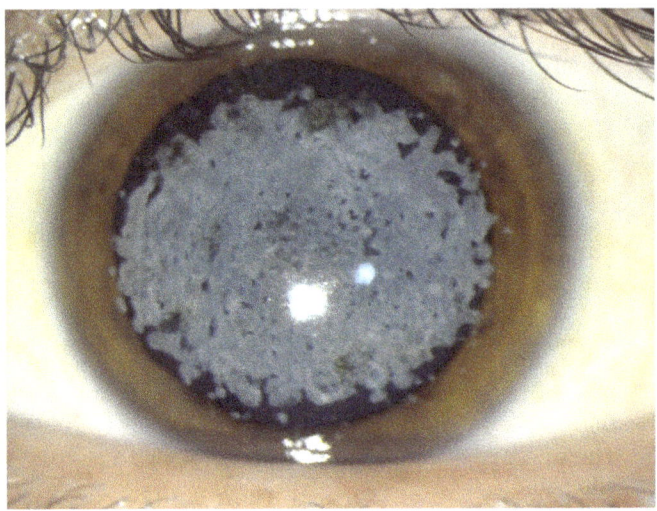

Fig. 16.5: Image showing macular corneal dystrophy.

OTHER DEGENERATIVE DISEASES

Arcus

- **Arcus Senilis** is the lipid deposition in the corneal periphery in a concentric ring-like manner in elderly people.
- Arcus juvenilis is a similar pathology occurring in young people below the age of 40 years.

Band-shaped Keratopathy

It is caused by the deposition of calcium salts in the central interpalpebral area of the cornea, in patients with chronic uveitis, oil-filled eyes or in hypercalcemia. It can be treated by scraping it off and by dissolution with sodium edetate.

ECTATIC CONDITIONS

Keratoconus

It is the most common corneal ectatic disorder, with its onset in pubertal age. It is a bilateral disorder causing thinning of the cornea, progressive forward bulge and conical protrusion.

Clinical Features

- The apical protrusion can be seen as a conical bulge in the lower lids when the patient looks down, called as Munson sign.
- A brownish ring, called as Fleischer ring, can be seen at the base of the cone, along with thin vertical lines on the cornea, called Vogt's striae.
- Irregular astigmatism is seen in retinoscopy, and the diagnosis is made by inferior steepening, corneal thinning and inferior-superior asymmetry seen on corneal topography.
- The thin cornea may sometimes spontaneously rupture, causing acute hydrops characterized by sudden onset of decreased vision due to corneal edema.
- Keratoconus can also develop in patients with vernal or allergic keratoconjunctivitis due to excessive rubbing of the cornea.

Treatment

- Rigid contact lenses and glasses are used for visual rehabilitation in these cases.
- **Corneal cross-linking:** In patients with progression of the disease, cross-linking of the cornea using riboflavin and UV-A light is indicated to strengthen the cornea. It helps in the formation of bonds between the collagen fibrils, hence the process of strengthening.
- **Corneal transplantation:** In advanced cases not amenable to cross-linking or in patients with corneal scarring due to hydrops, corneal transplantation is required. Both full-thickness penetrating keratoplasty or anterior lamellar keratoplasty can be done. In penetrating keratoplasty, all the layers of the host cornea are transplanted to the recipient. Anterior lamellar keratoplasty is a recent technique where the endothelium and Descemet membrane of the host is left intact, and only the anterior layers of the donor are transplanted, hence improving the chances of survival of the graft.

Keratoglobus

It is a congenital condition, causing hemispherical protrusion of the cornea and generalized thinning.

Pellucid Marginal Degeneration

It is an ectatic disorder causing bilateral thinning of the inferior cornea, usually from 4 to 8 o'clock. The overlying epithelium is intact.

Terrien Marginal Degeneration

It is a bilateral ectatic disorder which causes thinning of the cornea, initially superiorly. The advancing edge may have lipid deposition with vascularization.

MISCELLANEOUS CONDITIONS

Exposure Keratopathy

- It occurs in patients with the inability to close their eyes completely, causing drying of the corneal epithelium, making the cornea prone to infections.
- **Causes:** It can occur in patients with proptosis, in coma, or in paralysis of the orbicularis muscle, causing an inability to blink.
- **Treatment:** The treatment consists of frequent lubrication, and closure of the lid using a tape or tarsorrhaphy.

Neurotrophic Keratitis

- In patients with trigeminal nerve paralysis, the cornea is anaesthetized, hence causing desquamation of the corneal epithelium and formation of a non-healing epithelial defect and corneal ulcer later.
- The absence of pain is mostly noticed.
- Treatment comprises of intensive lubrication, ointments and tarsorrhaphy.

Pseudophakic Bullous Keratopathy

- It is seen after complicated cataract surgery due to damage of the corneal endothelium, causing corneal decompensation and edema.
- It is also commonly seen in patients with Fuch's endothelial dystrophy.
- A good quality viscoelastic is required to protect the endothelium during cataract surgery.

- Treatment aims at decreasing the edema using hypertonic saline eye drops and ointment, bandage contact lens to decrease the irritation and keratoplasty in advanced cases.

SURGERIES

Keratoplasty

'Corneal transplantation' is coined as keratoplasty. It can be full thickness or lamellar keratoplasty.

- **Penetrating keratoplasty:** All the layers of the cornea are transplanted in penetrating keratoplasty **(Fig. 16.6)**.
- Lamellar keratoplasty can be anterior or posterior. DALK (deep anterior lamellar keratoplasty) is the most common anterior keratoplasty where the Bowman's layer and stroma are transplanted. In posterior lamellar keratoplasty, the Descemet membrane can be transplanted, with deep stroma and endothelium or with endothelium alone.
- **Steps:** After preparing the donor cornea, the host bed is prepared by trephination of the cornea. It is followed by transplantation the donor cornea to the recipient bed using non-absorbable sutures.

REFRACTIVE PROCEDURES

Laser-assisted in Situ Keratomileusis (LASIK)

It is the most commonly done refractive procedure. An excimer laser is used in this procedure to ablate the cornea after the formation of a superficial corneal flap, hence affecting the corneal curvature and causing correction of the refractive error.

Small Incision Lenticule Extraction (SMILE)

It is a newer technique in which a lenticule of the cornea is taken out. This alters the shape of the cornea, hence correcting the refractive error.

Both procedures can correct myopia, hyperopia and astigmatism.

NURSING INTERVENTIONS

The nursing staff can be trained to identify the basic corneal disorders and can advise the patients for early consultation and treatment. In case of infectious corneal disorders, the nurses can help in proper compliance and instillation techniques of antibiotic drops to the admitted patients.

GERIATRIC CONSIDERATIONS

Elderly should take care to avoid any kind of trivial trauma to the eye which can cause serious corneal disorders and can impact the quality of life. Timely referral is necessary in case of any kind of corneal injury to prevent long term complications. Protective eye glasses can be used by the elderly to prevent any kind of corneal trauma.

SUMMARY

Cornea is an essential part of the eye which helps in image formation of an object and helps us in seeing things clearly. Since cornea is avascular, late presentations of corneal disorders can result in scarring and can impact life quality. Early detection and early treatment of corneal disorders is the key for leading a good quality of life.

MULTIPLE CHOICE QUESTIONS

1. All of the following are characteristics of corneal dystrophies, *except*:
   a. Unilateral
   b. Absence of vascularization
   c. Hereditary
   d. Bilateral
2. Which of the following is common in contact lens use?
   a. Fungal keratitis
   b. Herpetic keratitis
   c. Mooren's ulcer
   d. Acanthamoeba keratitis
3. Which of the following is not a stromal dystrophy?
   a. Macular dystrophy
   b. Fuch's dystrophy
   c. Granular dystrophy
   d. Lattice dystrophy
4. Which of the following is not seen in fungal keratitis?
   a. Dendrite
   b. Hypopyon
   c. Infiltrates
   d. Congestion
5. Which of the following is characteristic of fungal keratitis?
   a. Hypopyon
   b. Absent corneal sensations
   c. Feathery margins of the infiltrate
   d. Photophobia

ANSWERS

1. a   2. d   3. b   4. a
5. c

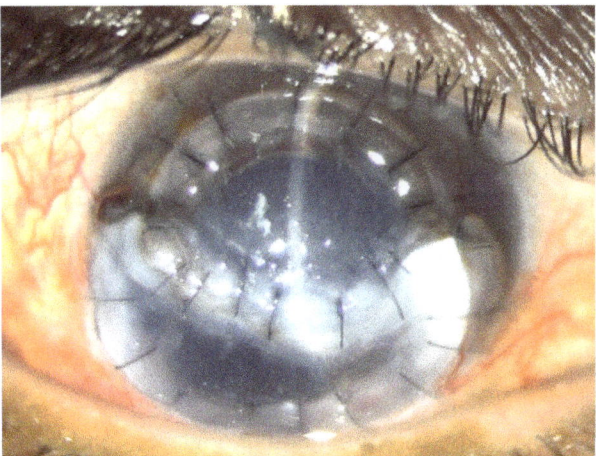

Fig. 16.6: Image showing keratoplasty.

SUGGESTED READING

1. Abreu EB, Novaes GA, Fernandes BF, et al. Corneal stromal dystrophies: a clinical pathologic study. Arq Bras Oftalmol. 2012;75:390-3.
2. Brad Bowling. Kanski's Clinical Ophthalmology a Systemic Approach, 8th edition, Elsevier, Edinburgh; 2016.
3. Dua HS, Faraj LA, Said DG, et al. Human corneal anatomy redefined: a novel pre-Descemet's layer (dua's layer). Ophthalmology. 2013;120:1778-85.
4. Kaye S. Herpes simplex keratitis: bilateral effects. Invest Ophthalmol Vis Sci. 2015;56:4907.
5. M. Green, A. Apel, F. Stapleton. Risk factors and causative organisms in microbial keratitis. Cornea. 2008;27:22-7.
6. Puy P, Stoica BT, Alejandre N, et al. Temporal pellucid marginal degeneration displaying high "with-the-rule" astigmatism. Can J Ophthalmol. 2013;48:e142-e4.
7. Rabinowitz YS: Keratoconus [review]. Surv Ophthalmol. 1998;42:297-319.
8. Solomon A: Corneal complications of vernal keratoconjunctivitis. Curr Opin Allergy Clin Immunol. 2015;15:489-494.
9. Wallang BS, Das S. Keratoglobus. Eye (Lond). 2013;27:1004-12.
10. Zhu AY, Eberhart CG, Jun AS. Fuchs endothelial corneal dystrophy: a neurodegenerative disorder? JAMA Ophthalmol. 2014;132:377-8.

CHAPTER 17

Glaucoma

Faisal Thattaruthody, Neha Chauhan, Madhuri Akella

"Glaucoma is the thief of sight. Each day it steals from you precious memories-not of what was, but of what's to come."
—**Jeremiah Lim**

LEARNING OBJECTIVES

After going through the chapter, the learner will be able to:
- Define glaucoma.
- Discuss the epidemiology of glaucoma.
- Enumerate the classification of glaucoma.
- Explain the management of glaucoma.

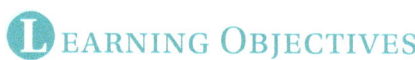

- **Antiglaucoma medications:** Medications used to lower the intraocular pressure.
- **Childhood glaucoma:** Glaucoma occurs in babies and children.
- **Closed angle glaucoma:** Type of glaucoma where drainage angle is formed by the cornea and peripheral iris is narrowed or blocked.
- **Glaucoma:** A group of eye conditions that irreversibly damage the optic nerve.
- **Gonioscopy:** Technique of evaluation of anterior chamber angle.
- **Intraocular pressure:** The pressure exerted by various fluids inside the eye.
- **Open angle glaucoma:** Most common form of glaucoma where the drainage angle remains opened.
- **Optic disc:** Round area on back surface inside the eye formed by the axons of retinal ganglion cells.
- **Perimetry:** Systematic measurements of visual field function.
- **Primary glaucoma:** An isolated and idiopathic form of glaucoma.
- **Secondary glaucoma:** Any form of glaucoma in which there is an identifiable cause for increased pressure.
- **Tonometry:** Method used to determine the intraocular pressure.
- **Trabeculectomy:** Type of glaucoma surgery in which an alternate pathway is created between anterior chamber and sub-Tenon's space to bypass the diseased natural pathway.
- **Visual field:** Portion of space or surroundings seen when eye is fixed straight at a point.

DEFINITION AND EPIDEMIOLOGY

Glaucoma is the leading cause of irreversible blindness globally, and the term is comprised of a group of optic neuropathies with characteristic morphological changes in the retinal nerve fiber layer and optic nerve head which are associated with visual field loss. The estimated prevalence of primary open angle glaucoma (POAG) and primary angle closure glaucoma (PACG) is 60.5 million worldwide by 2010. The main goal of treatment is to reduce intraocular pressure (IOP), as it is the most common modifiable factor associated with disease progression in eyes with glaucoma. Other risk factors include age more than 40-years, family history of glaucoma, myopia, thin cornea, ocular trauma, long-term use of steroids, and systemic illness like diabetes mellitus, hypertension, migraine, or any peripheral vascular occlusive diseases.

APPLIED ANATOMY

The major ocular structures concerned with glaucoma are the ciliary body, anterior chamber angle, aqueous outflow system, retinal ganglion cells and optic nerve head.

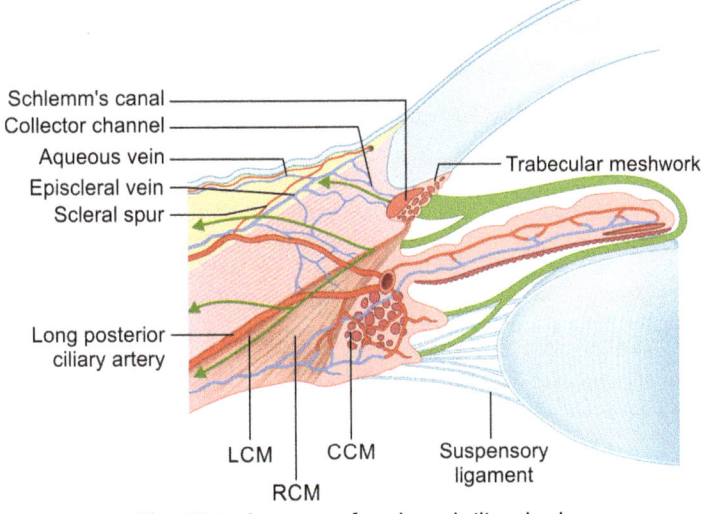

Fig. 17.1: Anatomy of angle and ciliary body.

[LCM: longitudinal ciliary muscle; CCM: circular (fibers) ciliary muscle; RCM: radial ciliary muscle]

Ciliary Body

It is the anterior continuation of the choroid and is triangular on the cut section **(Fig. 17.1)**. The ciliary body has two parts. The anterior part is called pars plicata, which contains 70-80 fingers-like projection called ciliary processes **(Fig. 17.1)**. These processes are the site of aqueous production. Pars plana, which is the posterior smooth part of ciliary body.

Anterior Chamber Angle

Anterior chamber angle (ACA) is formed anterior to posterior by Schwalbe's line (termination of Descemet's membrane of the cornea), trabecular meshwork (TM), scleral spur (SS), ciliary body band (CBB), and root of iris **(Fig. 17.1)**. Clinically, the anatomy of the angle is assessed by gonioscopy and the widths are graded to various levels. The angle width varies in different individuals and plays a major role in the pathomechanism of glaucoma in adults.

Aqueous Outflow System

It includes the TM, Schlemm's canal (SC), collector channels or aqueous vein, and episcleral and conjunctival veins **(Fig. 17.2)**. The TM is a sieve-like structure that bridges the Schwalbe's line (SL) and SS. It may be divided into three portions: (a) Uveal meshwork; (b) Corneal meshwork; and (c) Juxtacanalicular tissue. The SC is a 360° endothelial lined tube present circumferentially in the scleral sulcus.

APPLIED PHYSIOLOGY

Aqueous humor is a dynamic intraocular fluid produced by the ciliary processes (by the inner nonpigmented epithelial cells) at an average rate of 1.5–4 µL/min. It is a clear watery fluid filling both the anterior and posterior chamber of the eyeball. It is not only important for maintaining intraocular pressure but also plays a vital role in the metabolism of the cornea and lens. Normal aqueous consists of water 99%, proteins (0.04%), and traces of Na^+, K^+, Cl^-, amino acids, lactic acid, and bicarbonate, etc.

Aqueous Humor Drainage

The aqueous humor flows from the posterior chamber to the anterior chamber (AC) via the pupil then it leaves the eye by two pathways **(Flowchart 17.1)**.

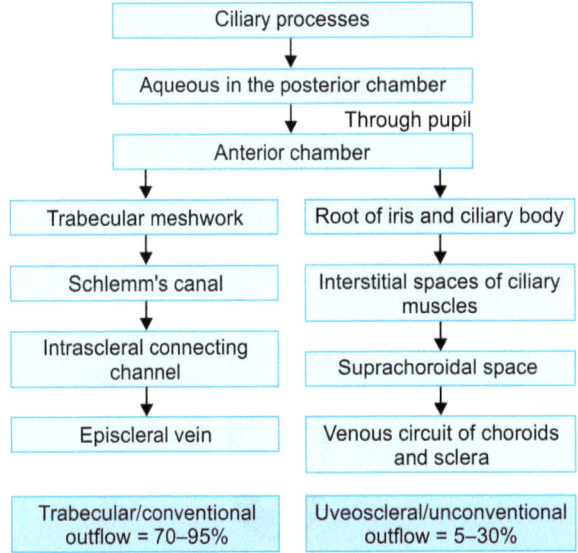

Flowchart 17.1: Aqueous outflow pathways.

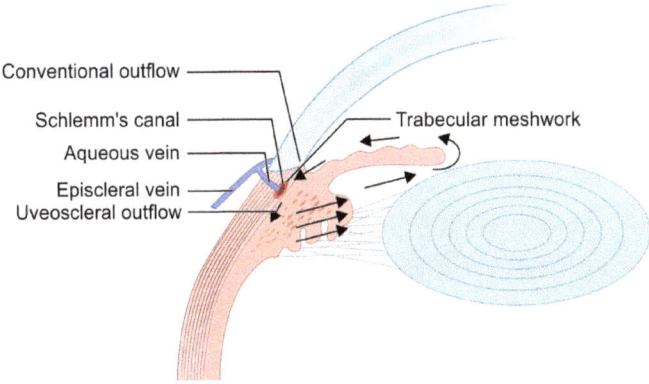

Fig. 17.2: Shows anatomy aqueous outflow.

RISK FACTORS OF GLAUCOMA

- Thin cornea
- Older age
- Family history of glaucoma
- African American race
- Cardiovascular disease
- Diabetes mellitus
- Migraine syndromes
- Eye trauma
- Nearsightedness (myopia)
- Prolonged use of topical or systemic corticosteroids

PATHOPHYSIOLOGY

See **Flowchart 17.2**.

DIAGNOSTIC EVALUATION

Intraocular Pressure and Tonometry

Intraocular pressure refers to the pressure exerted by various intraocular fluids on the coats of the eye. The "normal" IOP may be defined as "that pressure that does not lead to glaucomatous damage of the optic nerve head". The normal IOP varies between 10 and 21 mm Hg (average is 15.5 ± 2.57). The mean IOP measured under general anesthesia in children by Perkin's tonometer is <8 mm Hg before 3 months and <12 mm Hg between age 6 to 9 months, then a gradual increase in IOP is 1mm Hg/year up to 12 years. Target pressure or IOP is a range of IOP on treatment that would stabilize glaucoma or prevent further glaucomatous damage. Various factors affecting IOP can be genetics, environment (physical, smoking, drug, and dietary exposure), sex (in older age groups females have greater increase in mean IOP with age), age, diurnal (higher IOP in the morning), postural, and systemic parameters like hypertension and diabetes mellitus.

The term tonometry refers to the measurement of IOP and the instrument used is called a tonometer. The principle is based on the deformation of the globe (indentation and applanation/flattening). The most widely used monometers are the Schiotz indentation tonometer **(Fig. 17.3B)**, non-contact tonometer (NCT) **(Fig. 17.3C)**, and Goldmann applanation tonometer **(Fig. 17.3A)**. Other monometers

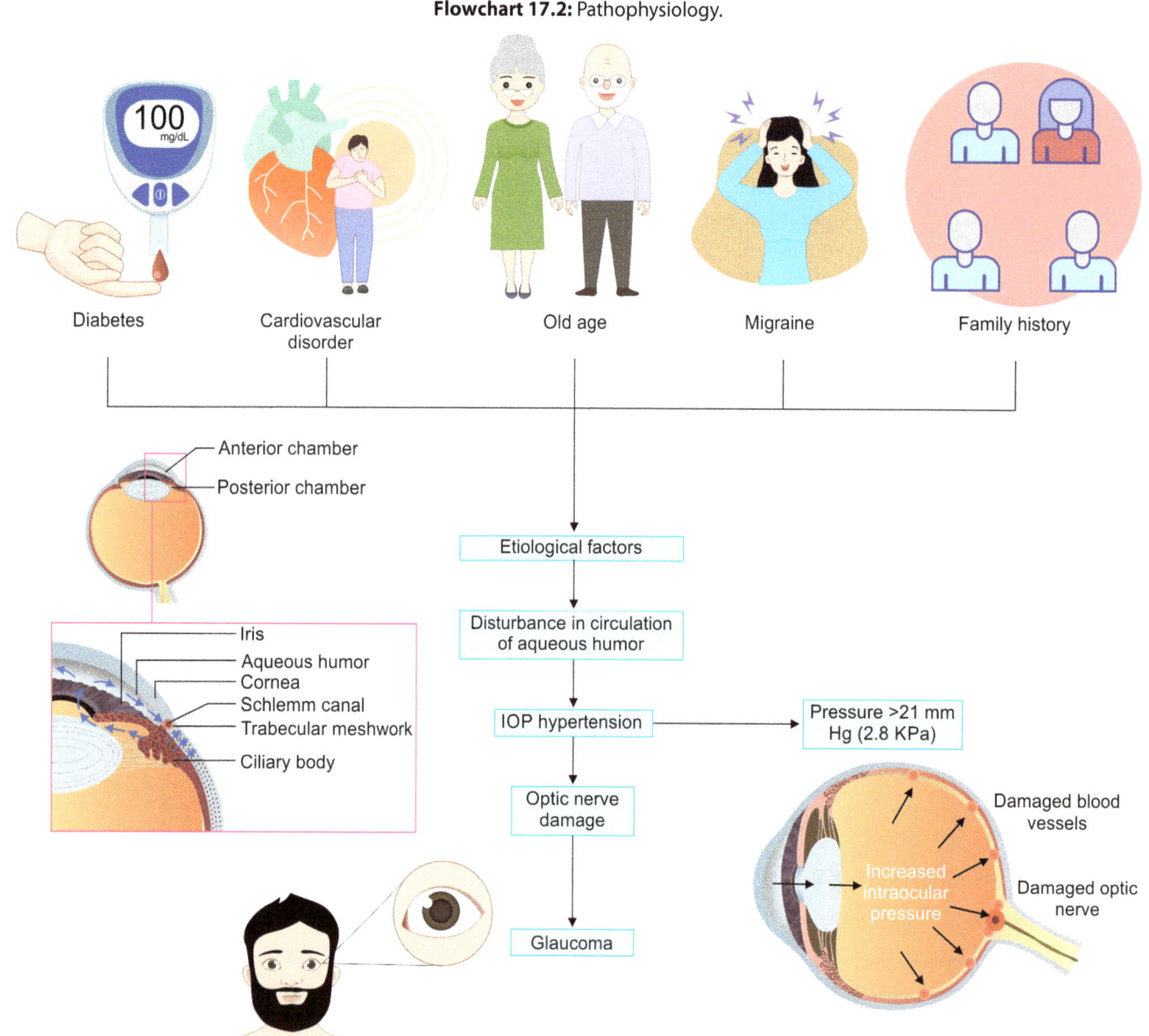

Flowchart 17.2: Pathophysiology.

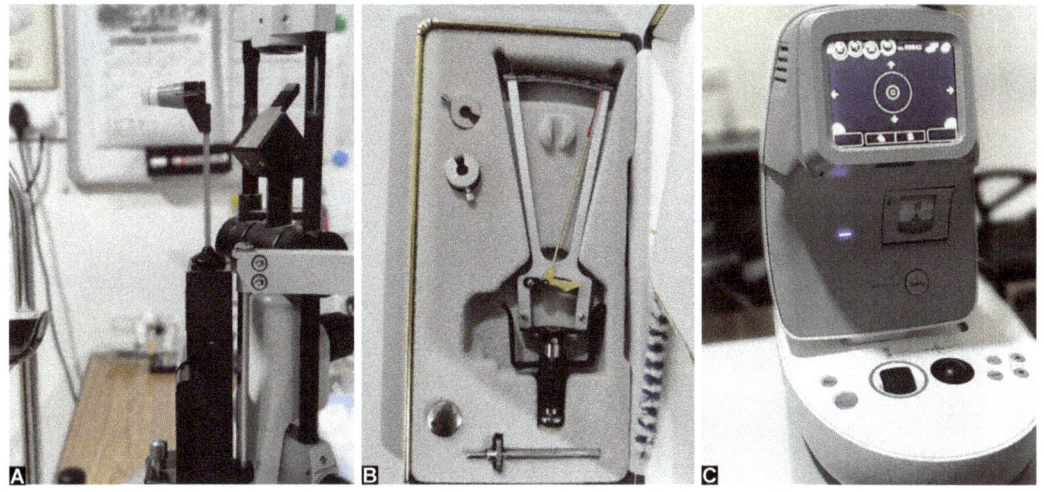

Figs. 17.3A to C: Commonly used tonometers: (A) GAT attached to a slit lamp; (B) Shiotz indentation tonometer; (C) Noncontact tonometer.

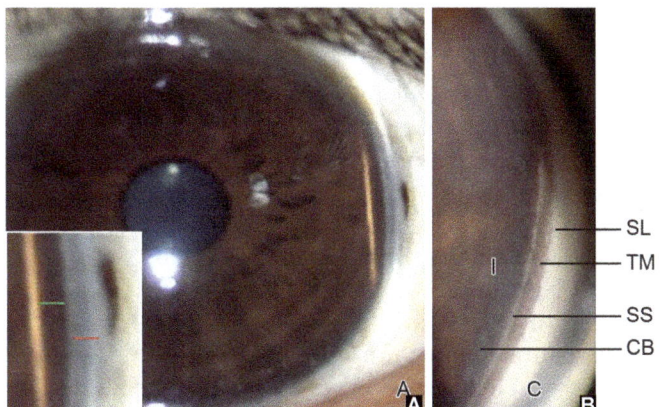

Figs. 17.4A and B: (A) Shows anterior chamber depth evaluation by van Herick method. Insight shows a magnified view; Red line shows the peripheral corneal thickness and the green line shows anterior chamber depth; (B) Shows the anatomy of anterior chamber angle by indirect gonioscopy: I = iris, CBB = ciliary body band (in this eye CBB is widened due to blunt trauma), SS = scleral spur, TM = trabecular meshwork, SL = Schwalbe's line, and C = cornea.

are Perkins's tonometer, Tono-Pen, Pascal dynamic contour tonometer, Rebound tonometer, etc. Goldmann Applanation Tonometry (GAT) is the gold standard technique in glaucoma practice.

Assessments of Anterior Chamber Depth and Anterior Chamber Angle

Assessment of peripheral anterior chamber (AC) depth by slit-lamp examination and anatomy of the AC by gonioscopy is an essential part of the evaluation of all glaucoma. The peripheral AC depth is measured commonly by the van-Herick technique by comparing the peripheral AC depth to the adjacent cornea **(Figs. 17.4A and B)**. When the peripheral anterior chamber depth is <1/4th of corneal depth the angle is potentially occludable.

Gonioscopy is the clinical biomicroscopic technique of evaluating the ACA of the eye with the use of a special contact lens known as the gonioscope. Gonioscopy can be broadly divided into two viz, direct and indirect gonioscopy. It is helpful diagnostically, prognostically, and therapeutically in glaucoma. Direct techniques utilize gonio lenses (e.g., Koppe, Barken, Thorpe, and Swan-Jacob) through a hand-held microscope or operating microscope. The indirect method uses gonioprism with a slit lamp to obtain an inverted view of angle in sitting position. There is a various grading system of anterior chamber angle of which Shaffer system is now commonly used. In the Shaffer system, the widest open-angle is grade-4 and the closed-angle is grade-0.

Clinical Appearance and Glaucomatous Changes in Optic Nerve Head

The clinical appearance of the optic nerve head (the distal portion of the optic nerve, which is directly susceptible to IOP elevation) is generally vertically oval, with a pale central depression termed as optic disc cup **(Figs. 17.5A and B)**. The tissue between disc margin and cup is called the neuroretinal rim (NRR) and it contains axons of the retinal ganglion cells. The NRR is typically thickest at the inferior quadrant, followed by the superior and then nasal quadrant, and the temporal quadrant being the thinnest. Evaluation of optic disc and peripapillary nerve fibers are at most important in glaucoma because they provide the most important early evidence of glaucomatous optic neuropathy. Commonly occurred morphological changes in glaucoma include focal thinning of NRR, concentric thinning, deepening of the cup, disc hemorrhage, and increased tortuosity of peripapillary retinal vessels. Other changes include thinning of retinal nerve fibers and broadening of peripapillary atrophy.

Perimetry and its Importance

Perimetry is the term used to describe the measurement of the visual field. It is vital in glaucoma management including diagnosis and monitoring progression and the instrument is called the perimeter. The commonly used perimeters are the Humphrey field analyzer and Octopus. **Figure 17.6** shows a printout of Humphrey standard 24–2 singe field. Common visual field changes in glaucoma are nasal step, arcuate scotoma, ring scotoma, central or paracentral scotoma, etc.

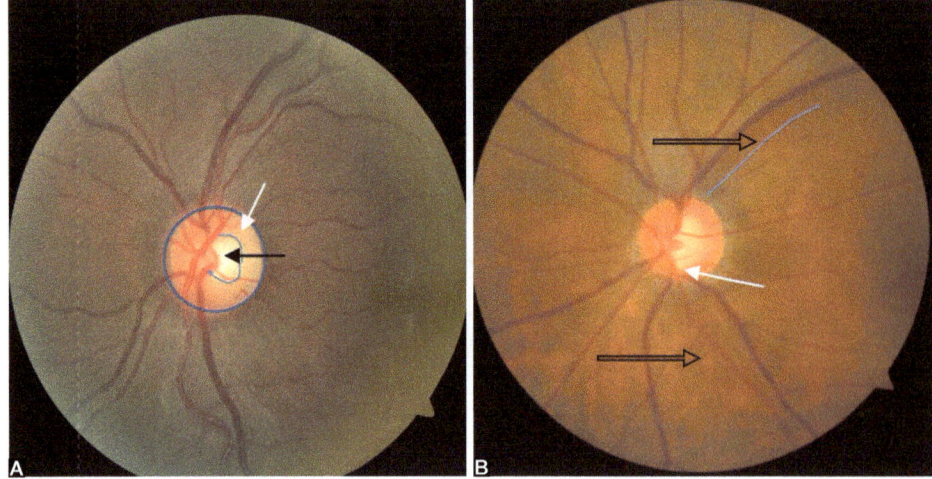

Figs. 17.5A and B: (A) A normal-looking optic disc showing NRR (white arrow) and optic disc cup (black arrow) of a left eye; (B) showing glaucomatous changes like increased cup disc ratio, focal thinning (white arrow), and thinning of retinal nerve fiber bundle (black arrow).

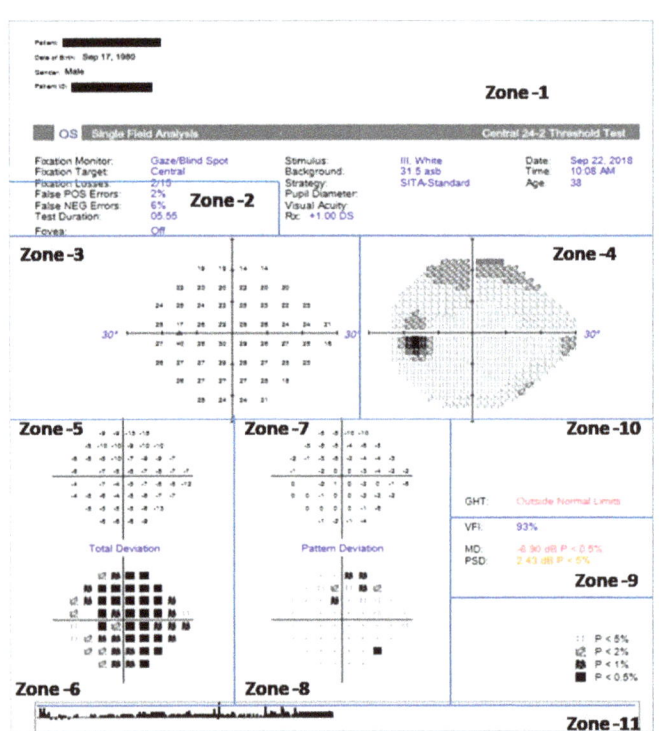

Fig. 17.6: For better understanding Humphrey single field print out is divided into 11 zones: Zone-1—patient data/test data, Zone-2—reliability indices, Zone-3—raw data, Zone-4— gray scale, Zone-5—total deviation numerical plot, Zone-6—total deviation probability plot, Zone-7—pattern deviation numerical plot, Zone-8—pattern deviation probability plot, Zone-9—global Indices, Zone-10—glaucoma hemifield test, Zone-11—gaze tracker.

CLASSIFICATIONS AND VARIOUS TERMINOLOGY OF GLAUCOMA

For better understanding the glaucoma can be categorized into childhood glaucoma and glaucoma in adult. For classification of childhood glaucoma CGRN (Childhood Glaucoma Research Network) classifications is used. The details are depicted in **Flowchart 17.3**.

Clinical Features of Glaucoma

Various presenting signs and symptoms of glaucoma depend upon the types of glaucoma and its severity.

1. **Primary congenital glaucoma:** Symptoms include lacrimation, photophobia, blepharospasm, and eye rubbing. Signs include corneal enlargement **(Fig. 17.7)**, corneal haziness, Descemet's tear (Haab's striae), and bluish sclera. IOP may or may not be very high.
2. **Primary open-angle glaucoma:** POAG is usually insidious and asymptomatic in the initial stage of illness. At the advanced stage, patients can present with significant loss of visual acuity or narrowing of the visual field. Some patients may experience mild headaches, blurring of vision, or early-onset presbyopia. On ocular evaluation usually normal anterior chamber (relative afferent pupillary defect may be present in advanced disease), elevated IOP, and characteristic optic disc changes with corresponding visual field changes.
3. **Primary angle-closure glaucoma:** Acute angle-closure glaucoma (acute congestive glaucoma) is characterized by severe ocular pain, redness, watering, and decreased vision. Often patients have vomiting or nausea. Signs include conjunctival congestion, corneal edema, shallow AC, closed angles. IOP is markedly elevated.
4. **Chronic angle closure glaucoma:** In chronic angle-closure glaucoma patients have had a history of intermittent episodes of blurring, colored halos, redness. The IOP may be elevated and the eyes may have mild congestion. The optic disc shows glaucomatous changes with corresponding changes in the visual field

TREATMENT OF GLAUCOMA

Glaucoma is the leading cause of irreversible blindness, and hence early diagnosis and treatment is most important. Currently, IOP is the only modifiable risk factor for glaucoma, hence treatment strategies are targeted to reduce the IOP. The objective of treatment is to control IOP, halt or reduce the

Flowchart 17.3: Classification of glaucoma.

```
                    Glaucoma
                   /        \
    Childhood glaucoma (CGRN)   Glaucoma in adult
```

- **Primary childhood glaucoma**
  - **IA**: Primary congenital glaucoma-'buphthalmos' (isolated angle anomalies)
    - Neonatal onset (<1 month)
    - Infantile onset (>1month to 24 months)
    - Late onset (>2 years)
  - **IB**: Juvenile open angle glaucoma (no buphthalmos, no associated ocular anomaly/syndrome)
- **Secondary childhood glaucoma**
  - **IIA**: Associated with ocular anomalies, e.g., aniridia, Axenfeld-Rieger anomaly, Peters anomaly, micophthamia, congenital aphakia, etc.
  - **IIB**: Associated with systemic anomalies/syndrome, e.g., Lowe's syndrome, Marfan's syndrome, neurofibromatosis.
  - **IIC**: Associated with acquired ocular conditions, e.g., uveitic glaucoma, post-traumatic glaucoma steroid-induced glaucoma following ocular surgery other than congenital cataract surgery.
  - **IID**: Glaucoma following congenital cataract surgery

- **Primary glaucoma:** Glaucoma not associated with any ocular or systemic anomaly.
  - **Open angle spectrum (open angle by gonioscopy and age of onset >40 years)**
    - Glaucoma suspect (IOP >21 mm Hg or glaucomatous optic disc changes or visual suspicious of early glaucomatous changes).
    - Normal-tension glaucoma: Glaucomatous optic disc changes with corresponding visual field changes in the absence of elevated IOP.
    - Ocular hypertension: IOP >21 mm Hg on multiple occasion on applanation tonometry with normal optic disc and visual field.
    - Primary open angle glaucoma: IOP >21 mm Hg on multiple occasion on applanation tonometry along with glaucomatous optic disc changes and corresponding visual field changes.
  - **Angle closure spectrum**
    - Primary angle closure suspect (PACS): Occludable angle (posterior trabecular meshwork is not seen at least 270°) on gonioscopy.
    - Primary angle closure (PAC): Raised IOP with occludable angle or evidence of angle closure like pigmentation, peripheral anterior synechiae, iris atrophy or glaucoma fleckens. No optic disc or field changes
    - Primary angle closure glaucoma (PACG): PAC along with glaucomatous optic disc and corresponding field changes.
- **Secondary glaucoma:** Glaucoma secondary to other ocular or systemic illness which can be secondary closed/open angle, e.g., pseudoexfoliation glaucoma, pigmentary glaucoma, lens-induced glaucoma, steroid-induced glaucoma, angle recession glaucoma, uveitic glaucoma, aphakic glaucoma, glaucoma following posterior segment surgery, neovascular glaucoma, postkeratoplasty glaucoma and glaucoma secondary to intraocular tumor.
- **Juvenile open angle glaucoma:** Age <40 years with open angle and without any ocular anomalies.

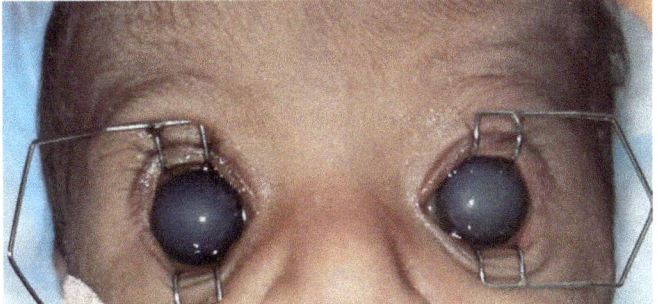

Fig. 17.7: An infant with enlarged (buphthalmos) and hazy cornea.

optic nerve damage/visual loss and ensuring good quality of life at an affordable cost. The treatment can be medical, laser, or surgical, but medical therapy is the first option and thus should be considered in most glaucoma.

Medical Treatment

The goal of medical management is to achieve the desired target level of IOP using the minimum number of medications. Medical treatment should be started as monotherapy, and ≥20% IOP reduction from baseline is targeted. Four to six weeks after commencing the monotherapy, its efficacy, safety and tolerability must be reassessed. Classification and other details of commonly used medications are listed in **Table 17.1**.

Laser Procedures in Glaucoma

Peripheral iridotomy, selective laser trabeculoplasty, and cyclodestructive procedures are commonly used laser procedures in glaucoma. Peripheral iridotomy by Nd-YAG laser is the first-line of treatment in primary angle-closure glaucoma and is the most widely used laser procedure in

TABLE 17.1: Commonly used medications in glaucoma.

Class/medication	Mechanism of action	Daily dose	Adverse effect
Prostaglandin analogues • Latanoprost • Bimatoprost • Travaprost	Increases uveoscleral outflow	• 0.005% eyedrop at bed time • 0.03/0.01% eyedrop at bed time • 0.004% eyedrop at bed time	Conjunctival hyperemia, local irritation, iris pigmentation, hypertrichosis, cystoids macular edema
Beta blockers • Timolol • Betaxolol	Reduces aqueous production	• 0.25/0.5% drop BD • 0.25/0.5% drop BD	Ocular allergy, stinging sensation, bradycardia and hypotension
Alpha agonist: Brimonidine	Reduces aqueous production Increases uveoscleral outflow	0.2/0.15/0.1% drops TID	Irritation, allergy, drowsiness and dry mouths
Cholinergic agonistics: Pilocarpine	Increases trabecular outflow	0.5–2% drops TID	Miosis, browache and follicular conjunctivitis
Topical carbonic anhydrase inhibitors: • Dorzolamide • Brinzolamide	Increases trabecular outflow	2% drops TID 1% drops TDS	Stinging, burning Blurred vision, dryness
Rho-kinase inhibitors: • Ripasudil • Netarsudil	Increases trabecular outflow	0.4% drops BD 0.02% OD	Blepharitis, hyperemia
Systemic therapy: Carbonic anhydrase inhibitors, (e.g., acetazolamide) **Hyperosmotic agent:** • Glycerol • Mannitol	Reduces aqueous production Dehydrates the vitreous	250 mg tablet QID 1.5 g/kg in 50% of solution 1–1.5 g/kg 20% solutions	Paresthesia, fatiguability, gastritis and renal stones. Hypokalemia Hyperglycemia, diarrhea Hypertension, renal failure and cardiac failure, electrolyte imbalance

glaucoma. Selective laser therapy by a frequency-doubled by Nd-YAG (Neodymium-doped Yttrium Aluminum Garnet) laser is used in open-angle glaucoma, and some cases of PACG following peripheral iridotomy and it enhances the trabecular outflow. The cyclodestructive procedure through various routes by diode or argon laser is commonly used in end-stage glaucoma.

Surgical Management

Indication for glaucoma surgery includes inability to maintain the target IOP, intolerant to medications, progression of glaucoma even with maximum medication, poor affordability for medication, and primary congenital glaucoma.

Angle procedures like goniotomy or trabeculotomy are routinely done in primary congenital glaucoma. Trabeculectomy with antimetabolite (5 fluorouracil/mitomycin C) augmented is the gold standard procedure in various glaucomas in adults. Other commonly done procedure includes glaucoma drainage device implantation. The implant can be valved (e.g., Ahmed glaucoma valve) or nonvalved device (Baerveldts implants) and a common indication is failed trabeculectomy. Trabeculectomy or drainage implants makes an alternate pathway that is between the AC and sub-Tenon space. All these surgical procedures can have intraoperative, early postoperative or delayed postoperative complications. Prompt detection and timely management of complications is most important as a few of them are potentially blinding.

GERIATRIC CONSIDERATIONS

Glaucoma can occur at any age but it is more common in the aged population, and it is one of the leading causes of blindness for people more than 60 years of age. Glaucoma can be considered as a disease of ageing population, as age advances the risk also increases. As the age increases the optic nerve is less able to withstand insults such as an increase in IOP. Apart from that in the aged population, the blood flow to the optic nerve is also compromised due to atherosclerotic changes in significant vessels, which cause the optic disc more vulnerable to glaucomatous damage. The first-line treatment for POAG is eye drops. Most glaucomatous patients need multiple medications at multiple times in a day. The side effects of these medications are more in the elderly population. Other comorbidities like dementia and parkinsonism cause poor compliance and adherence to these medications. Socioeconomic problems like loneliness, poor accessibility to medication, lack of employment, other psychological issues, and various other systemic medications may also affect treatment compliance and adherence. So overall the management of glaucoma in geriatric population is more complicated than the younger people.

NURSING MANAGEMENT

Preoperative and Postoperative Management

It is the nursing responsibility to take meticulous history and make proper diagnosis before proceeding surgery. Surgery is always proceeded by extensive discussion and counseling with patients and his/her relatives regarding indication, nature of the surgery, postoperative management and follow-ups, possible complications. The attending nurse have definite role in counseling pertaining to above points, and can explain to patients and relatives that the procedure is not visual gain or visual recovery and is aimed to further decrease the glaucomatous progression. Preoperatively the attending nurse should check the patient's vital signs and make the patient comfortable in the operation room. Often patients with high IOP need preoperative intravenous infusion of 20% mannitol (1.5 g/kg) over 30-60 minutes 1-1.5 hour prior to procedure. Preinfusion and postinfusion recording of BP is mandatory. In the postoperative recovery room the attending nurse can follow the instructions given by the anesthetists (in case of general anesthesia) pertaining to vital sign monitoring and patients positioning, etc. After recommended time in recovery room patient can be discharged with proper advises after consulting with treating physician. The attending nurse should stress the postoperative instruction like requirement to systemic analgesic drugs as when required, discontinuation of all preoperative antiglaucoma medications in the operated eye, and care of operated eye from trauma and timing of next visit to hospitals. All patients should be explained about good postoperative ocular hygiene (gentle wipe of eyelashes with sterile wet cotton), use of protective glasses and timely instillation of postoperative medication.

Nursing Considerations

- Maintaining normal intraocular pressure
- Inform the patient about the extent of vision loss and damage of optic nerve.
- Keep a record of eye pressure measurements and visual field test results to monitor the progress.
- Assess for potential side effects of eye medications if any.
- Educate the patient about glaucoma, eyedrop compliance and importance of follow up
- Manage the anxiety of the patient.
- Ensure patient safety.

Follow-up of Glaucoma Patients

By definition glaucoma is a chronic disease and most of the patient will require a lifelong follow-up. All follow-up visits should include comprehensive glaucoma evaluation, assess the efficacy and safety of medication or surgical procedure, and treatment should be titrated individually. The follow-up frequency usually depends upon severity of glaucoma, response to treatment or patient profile and should be individualized.

Case Scenario

1. A 75-year-old male farmer by occupation referred to you with a diagnosis of glaucoma since 6 months. On history patients complained of painless progressive loss of vision.
   - Describe detailed history pertained to glaucoma which you would like to take.
   - Describe comprehensive ocular evaluation related to his case.
   - Describe the difference in symptoms and signs in open angle and acute angle closure glaucoma.
   - What is your plan of management if anterior chamber angles were opened?
   - Describe the indication for surgery in this patient.
   - Narrate the importance of counseling before glaucoma surgery.
2. A mother brought her 1 week old baby with compliance of hazy and large cornea.
   - Describe the symptoms and signs of congenital glaucoma.
   - If you are working in the neonatal ICU, how will you alert the parents about the possibilities of congenital glaucoma?
   - Describe how will you examine the patient?
   - Narrate the classification of childhood glaucoma.

SUMMARY

- The term glaucoma is comprised of a group of optic neuropathies with characteristic morphological changes in the RNFL and optic nerve head which are associated with visual field loss. The main goal of treatment is to reduce intraocular pressure. The major ocular structures concerned with glaucoma are the ciliary body, anterior chamber angle, aqueous outflow system, retinal ganglion cells and optic nerve head. IOP is maintained by a delicate balance between aqueous production and its outflow. Aqueous fluid is produced by ciliary processes of ciliary body and it drained by trabecular (conventional) or uveoscleral (unconventional) pathways. GAT is the gold standard for measuring IOP. Gonioscopy should a part of evaluation. Assess the structural and functional damage for diagnosing and classifying the glaucoma. For convenience and easy understanding glaucoma can be categorized into glaucoma in children and glaucoma in adults. The first line management of glaucoma is medical except some particular entities.
- Indication for glaucoma surgery includes inability to maintain the target IOP, intolerant to medications, progression of glaucoma even with maximum medication, poor affordability for medication, and primary congenital glaucoma.

MULTIPLE CHOICE QUESTIONS

1. **Aqueous humor is secreted by:**
   a. Cornea
   b. Iris
   c. Lens
   d. Ciliary processes of the ciliary body
2. **Normal IOP in adults varies from:**
   a. 0–10 mm Hg
   b. 10–21 mm Hg
   c. 21–30 mm Hg
   d. 30–41 mm Hg
3. **Gold standard technique for IOP measuring is:**
   a. Noncontact tonometer
   b. Goldmann applanation tonometer
   c. Shiotz tonometer
   d. Perikin's tonometer
4. **Name one cholinergic agonistic glaucoma medication:**
   a. Pilocarpine
   b. Timolol
   c. Latanoprost
   d. Dorzolamide
5. **Most widely practiced laser procedure in glaucoma:**
   a. Diode laser cyclophotocoagulation
   b. Iridoplasty
   c. Trabeculoplasty
   d. Iridotomy

ANSWERS

1. d   2. b   3. b   4. a
5. d

SUGGESTED READING

1. Allingam RR, Damji KD, Freedman S, Moroi SE, Rhee DJ. Shields textbooks glaucoma, 6th edition. Lippincott Williams & Wilkins; 2011.
2. Khurana AK, Khurana B. Glaucoma. Comprehensive Ophthalmology, 5th edition. New age International Publications (P) limited publishers; 2012.

3. Bresson-Dumont H. La mesure de la pression intra-oculaire chez l'enfant [Intraocular pressure measurement in children]. J Fr Ophtalmol. 2009;32(3):176-81.
4. Classification developed by members of CGRN and vetted by consensus committee of WGA in July 2013.
5. Kingman S. Glaucoma is second leading cause of blindness globally. Bull World Health Organ. 2004;82:887-8.
6. Quigley HA, Broman AT. The number of people with glaucoma worldwide in 2010 and 2020. Br J Ophthalmol. 2006;90:262-7.
7. Stamper RL, Lieberman MF, Darke MV. Beckers- Schaffer's diagnosis and therapy of the glaucomas; 8th edition. Elsevier; 2009.
8. Sihota R, Angmo D, Ramaswamy D, Dada T. Simplifying "target" intraocular pressure for different stages of primary open-angle glaucoma and primary angle-closure glaucoma. Indian Journal of Ophthalmology. 2018;66(4):495-505.
9. Dada T, Sharma R, Sobti A. Gonioscopy: A text and Atlas. First edition; Jaypee Brothers Medical Publishers; 2013.
10. Tielsch JM, Sommer A, Katz J, et al. Racial variations in the prevalence of primary open-angle glaucoma. The Baltimore Eye Survey. JAMA. 1991;266:369-74.
11. Weinreb RN, Aung T, Medeiros FA. The pathophysiology and treatment of glaucoma: a review. JAMA. 2014;311(18):1901-11.
12. Wong TY, Loon SC, Saw SM. The epidemiology of age related eye diseases in Asia. Br J Ophthalmol. 2006;90:506-11.

CHAPTER 18

Disorders of Conjunctiva

Surbhi Khurana, Parul Chawla Gupta, Ranjan Kumar Behera, Jagat Ram

"Where words are restrained, the eyes often talk a great deal."
—Samuel Richardson

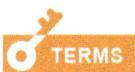 EARNING OBJECTIVES

After going through the chapter, the learner will be able to:
- Understand various disorders of conjunctiva.
- Diagnose 'red eye'.
- Manage common causes of ocular redness.
- Define infective and degenerative conditions of conjunctiva.

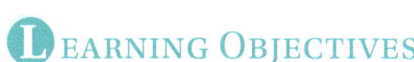

- **Allergic conjunctivitis:** Conjunctivitis due to allergy or atopy, can be seasonal or perennial.
- **Conjunctivitis:** Inflammation of the conjunctiva.
- **Infective conjunctivitis:** Conjunctivitis caused due to bacterial or viral causes.
- **Punctate keratitis:** Damage of corneal epithelium in pinpoint pattern.
- **Tear film:** Thin fluid layer covering outer mucosal surface of eye.

INTRODUCTION

The conjunctiva is a mucous membrane, which lines the surface of eyelids and the eye. It is divided into two parts; bulbar conjunctiva and palpebral conjunctiva. The conjunctiva is covered with a tear film, consisting of outermost lipid layer, middle aqueous layer and innermost mucin layer.

- **Functions:** The conjunctiva has various functions like; tear film production, washing away debris, maintenance of a smooth ocular surface for proper refraction of light rays for clear image formation at the retina. Presence of rich blood supply, lymphoid tissue in the mucosa and secretion of IgA antibodies has a defensive action against infective agents.
- **Nerve supply:** Branches of ophthalmic division and maxillary division of trigeminal nerve.
- **Blood supply:** Marginal arcade of the eyelid, peripheral arcade of the eyelid, posterior conjunctival artery and the anterior conjunctival artery.
- **Lymphatic drainage:** Submandibular and preauricular lymph nodes.

CLINICAL FEATURES IN CONJUNCTIVAL DISORDERS

- At the time of presence of any conjunctival disorder, the common symptoms are foreign body sensation, redness, stickiness, watering and sometimes photophobia.
- Conjunctival disorders usually do not cause any problems in vision.
- Sometimes, there can be a growth on the conjunctiva, localized or extending to the cornea.
- It is important to look for signs like hyperemia, discharge, and tear film while assessing the conjunctiva.
- Conjunctival inflammatory reactions could be in the form of papillae, follicles or granulomas. Follicles are localized aggregations of lymphocytes in the sub-epithelial adenoid layer. Papillae are caused by hyperplasia of the normal vasculature system **(Fig. 18.1)**.
- **Subconjunctival hemorrhage:** Sometimes, there can be subconjunctival hemorrhage. It can be due to trivial trauma or can be in the elderly due to fragile vessels, or in those with hypertension, or after ocular trauma or surgery.

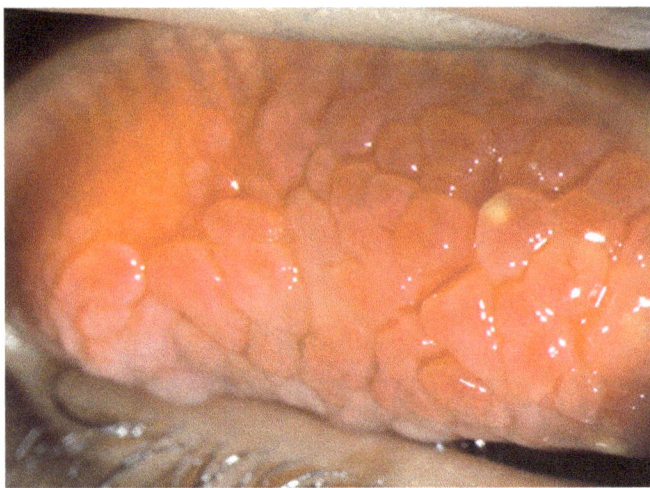

Fig. 18.1: Image showing papillae.

It is important to rule out bleeding disorders in case of recurrent hemorrhage.
- **Chemosis:** Sometimes, the conjunctiva can be edematous, called chemosis, as in cases with acute inflammation or abnormal blood circulation.

CONJUNCTIVAL DISORDERS

CONJUNCTIVITIS

The most common conjunctival disorder is conjunctivitis, which is inflammation of the conjunctiva. It can be of allergic or infectious origin. Acute conjunctivitis, with <4 weeks duration, is usually infective; for example, bacterial, viral or chlamydial.

Bacterial Conjunctivitis
- Bacterial conjunctivitis is characterized by mucopurulent discharge and diffuse congestion.
- It is highly infectious and transmissible through discharge.

Causes

The most common cause of bacterial conjunctivitis is staphylococcus aureus. Other causative organisms are *Neisseria gonorrhoeae, Corynebacterium diphtheriae, E. coli,* etc.

Gonorrheal Conjunctivitis
- It is usually transmitted by genital infection and has purulent discharge.
- It always involves the cornea, with the ability of the organism to invade intact corneal epithelium.
- It may be associated with corneal ulcers and perforation.
- Coinciding urethritis is the rule.
- Gram-negative diplococci are seen in culture.
- Enlarged preauricular lymph nodes can be seen.

Treatment

Intensive topical antibiotic therapy is required, along with treatment of urethritis. Cycloplegics are given in case of corneal involvement. Intramuscular ceftriaxone can also be used. Consultation for the venereal disease should be taken, and treatment of sexual partners is required.

Diphtheria
- It causes membranous conjunctivitis, with involvement of the upper respiratory tract.
- A membrane is formed on the conjunctiva and respiratory tract.
- Mucopurulent discharge is seen with serosanguinous involvement.

Treatment
- Prompt administration of anti-diphtheria serum is required, along with antimicrobial treatment. Penicillin is the drug of choice in such cases.
- Removal of membranes can cause symblepharon.

Angular Conjunctivitis
- **Most common cause:** Moraxella.
- Diplobacilli are seen in culture.

Clinical Features

Dirty white discharge at the angles of the eye, along with irritation and discharge.

Treatment

Tetracycline ointment 2-3 times a day for 10-14 days.

Viral Conjunctivitis

Viral infections usually have serous discharge and cause a follicular reaction. It can be due to adenovirus or herpes virus.

Epidemic Keratoconjunctivitis

It is usually caused by adenovirus, most commonly serotypes 8 and 19.

Clinical Features
- The patient usually has foreign body sensations, watering and stickiness.
- It is characterized by follicles, serous discharge, pseudo-membranes and preauricular lymphadenopathy.
- There can be corneal complications like punctate keratitis and subepithelial opacities causing photophobia.
- The disorder is highly infectious and occurs in epidemics.
- Cleaning slit lamps, ophthalmic devices and tonometers is paramount in preventing widespread disease.

Diagnosis

Detection of adenoviral antigen in the conjunctival swab.

Management
- Hand hygiene and surface disinfection play a major role in preventing transmission.
- The treatment focuses on supportive care, like cold compresses, topical decongestants and lubricants.
- Topical steroids may be required in cases with subepithelial infiltrates.
- Adenovirus can also cause pharyngoconjunctival fever.

Hemorrhagic Conjunctivitis

It is caused due to picornavirus and enterovirus 70.

Herpetic Keratoconjunctivitis
- It is usually caused by the herpes virus, due to primary infection by the virus.
- It causes follicular reaction with dendritic keratitis.
- The condition is acute, with a decrease in corneal sensation.
- Treatment comprises of topical acyclovir 3% or vidarabine 3%, antibiotics and lubricants.

Chronic Conjunctivitis
Conjunctivitis of more than 4 weeks duration is called chronic conjunctivitis.

Trachoma
Causes
It is caused by Chlamydia trachomatis type A, B and C.
- It is endemic in various parts of the world like the Mediterranean, Middle east, South West and Central Asia.
- Predisposing factors: children, females
- It is seen in unhygienic conditions
- It spreads by transfer of conjunctival secretions through infected towels, hands or clothes.

Clinical Features
- It mainly causes non-specific symptoms like watering, irritation, and photophobia in acute stages.
- It affects the lids, conjunctiva and cornea in chronic stages.
- It causes lid abnormalities, like entropion, ectropion, and trichiasis.
- The follicular reaction is seen in the upper tarsal conjunctiva, conjunctival scarring, pannus formation and Herbert pits.
- Hebert pits are sequelae of limbal follicles.
- Cicatrization of follicles is seen in the later stages.

Course
Reinfections are common.

Treatment
- Treatment for trachoma is recommended as **SAFE strategy**; Surgery for cicatricial ectropion and trichiasis, Antibiotics, Facial cleanliness to prevent infection, and Environmental hygiene.
- The antibiotic treatment includes topical azithromycin 1% ointment and oral azithromycin.

Ophthalmia Neonatorum
- It is also called neonatal conjunctivitis.
- It is an infectious disease occurring in newborns, with discharge in one or both eyes in the first week of life due to transmission of infection from the mother to the child from the birth passage.
- It can be caused by *Neisseria gonorrhoeae* or *Chlamydia trachomatis*.
- Corneal involvement may be seen in the gonococcal disease, whereas chlamydial disease is less severe.
- If left untreated, it may also cause pneumonia or otitis.

Diagnosis
Conjunctival swabs are stained with Gram and Giemsa stain. Gram-negative intracellular diplococci are seen in *Neisseria*, whereas polymorphonuclear leucocytes and lymphocytes may be seen in Chlamydial disease.

Treatment
It is according to the results of Gram and Giemsa stain. Chlamydia is treated with a suspension of erythromycin or azithromycin.
- *Neisseria* is treated with injectable ceftriaxone or topical erythromycin.
- Sometimes, it may be chemical conjunctivitis due to the toxic reaction of the neonate or silver nitrate used. No treatment is required in these cases.

Allergic Conjunctivitis
- It can be seasonal conjunctivitis, perennial conjunctivitis, vernal keratoconjunctivitis, atopic keratoconjunctivitis or contact dermatoconjunctivitis.
- It is caused due to type I hypersensitivity reaction to pollen and other allergens, causing an increase in IgE levels.
- Itching is the main feature, with white ropy discharge.
- Patients have symptoms throughout the year of perennial conjunctivitis.

Treatment
It requires the removal of allergen. Mast cell stabilizers (olopatadine, cromolyn sodium), and topical decongestants (naphazoline) may provide symptomatic relief. Topical steroids might be required in case of severe allergies.

Vernal Keratoconjunctivitis (VKC/Spring Catarrh)
- It is a recurrent, bilateral, allergic conjunctivitis; commonly seen in young children, especially males.
- It is seen in the hot or spring season.

Clinical Features
- Severe burning, itching, and photophobia.
- It can be of three types—palpebral, limbal or mixed. Palpebral VKC has mostly features involving the lid, limbal VKC affects limbus predominantly, and mixed VKC has features of both.
- Limbal VKC causes gelatinous thickening of the cornea.
- It causes a papillary reaction, punctate keratitis, and corneal epithelial ulceration in the form of shield ulcer and keratoconus **(Fig. 18.2)**.
- The papillary reaction is the predominant clinical sign.
- It is a self-limiting disease which wanes off after 18 years of age.
- It can cause gelatinous thickening of the limbus, called Horner Trantas spots, due to the collection of eosinophils.

Treatment
- Treatment of this disease is purely symptomatic, with cold compresses, mast cell stabilizers, topical steroids and lubricants.
- Topical decongestants might be required.
- Medications are prescribed in a titrating manner, with minimum medications in the beginning and

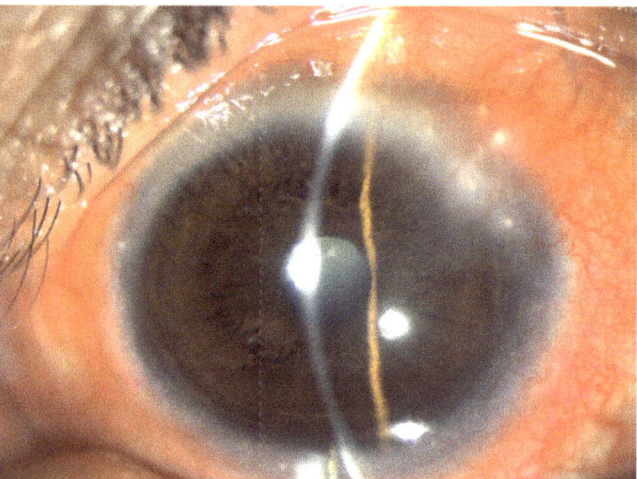

Fig. 18.2: Image showing a patient with vernal keratoconjunctivitis.

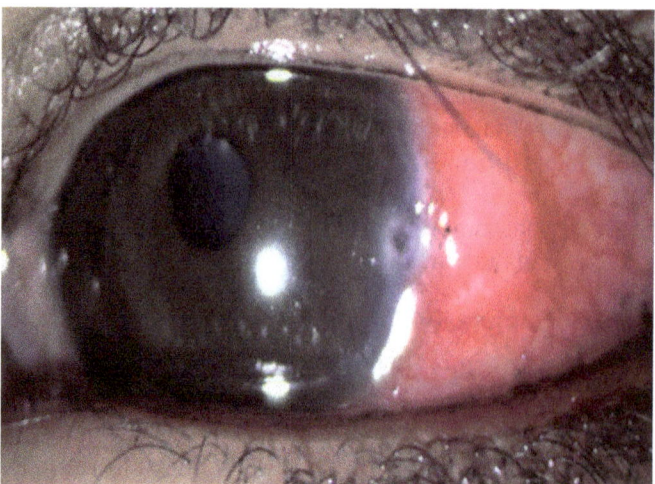

Fig. 18.3: Anterior segment photo showing phlyctenular conjunctivitis.

increased if the symptoms increase. Patients are kept on a maintenance dose.
- Sometimes, supratarsal steroid can be required in the presence of a giant papillary reaction or shield ulcer.
- In cases with shield ulcers, debridement of the ulcer is required, with amniotic membrane transplantation/bandage contact lens in a few instances.
- Chronic rubbing of the eye should be avoided.
- Oral antiallergics and/or steroids might be required in severe cases.

Complications

Keratoconus, corneal scarring, tarsal conjunctival scarring.
- Keratoconus is one of the most common complication seen in children with VKC.
- The use of chronic steroids should be avoided as they can cause cataracts and glaucoma.

Atopic Keratoconjunctivitis

It is seen in young adults in association with eczema, asthma, or allergic rhinitis. It is similar to VKC but has a more chronic, severe and complicated course.

Phlyctenular Keratoconjunctivitis

- One or two raised nodules are seen near the limbus (**Fig. 18.3**).
- Phlycten is usually surrounded by congestion.
- The disease is prevalent in regions where tuberculosis is endemic.
- The epithelium over the phlycten becomes necrotic in later stages and can form ulcers which heals rapidly.
- It can involve the cornea, if left untreated.
- It has been hypothesized that it is due to an allergic response to endogenous bacterial agents like *Mycobacterium tuberculosis*.
- Systemic evaluation for tuberculosis is required in these cases.

Treatment

Topical steroids, lubricants in only conjunctival disease. If it involves cornea, antibiotics and cycloplegics are required as well.

Stevens-Johnson Syndrome

It is a disorder caused by type II hypersensitivity reaction caused by an immunological reaction to drugs or infectious agents, like antiepileptics, NSAIDs, antibiotics, antimalarials, mycoplasma, or chlamydia.

Clinical Features

- It is a fatal disease, causing fever, malaise, erythematous and bullous reactions in the skin and mucous membranes of the body, including ocular surface.
- It can cause a complete epithelial defect, with infiltrates and symblepharon.

Treatment

- It is considered an emergency.
- It needs immediate identification of the offending drug, followed by maintenance of the airway.
- Topical lubricants, antimicrobials and release of adhesions are required for active ocular disease.

Surgical

Amniotic membrane transplantation in early stages might help to prevent devastating sequelae.

In later stages, lid margin deformities need to be corrected. Punctal Occlusion for dry eye, or mucous membrane grafting may also be required.

Complications

Severe dry eye, symblepharon, lid margin keratinization, entropion, persistent epithelial defects, corneal ulcers, corneal perforations, corneal vascularization.

Chemical Conjunctivitis

- It happens due to a toxic reaction to topical drugs like gentamicin, neomycin, idoxuridine, brimonidine and other drugs containing preservatives like benzalkonium chloride.
- It is believed to be due to type IV hypersensitivity reaction.
- It is essential to stop the offending drug when this happens.

DEGENERATIVE CHANGES IN THE CONJUNCTIVA

Pinguecula

- It is a triangular patch in the conjunctiva near the limbus.
- It is usually seen in elderly people, after exposure to strong sunlight or dust.
- It does not require any treatment.

Pterygium

- It is a triangular growth of the conjunctiva, which crosses the limbus and covers some parts of the cornea **(Fig. 18.4)**.
- The condition is common in dry, sunny areas.
- Pinguecula is a precursor of pterygium.
- It can be atrophic or fleshy, depending upon the type of mass.

Clinical Features

- It occurs in the interpalpebral area, with exposure to sunlight and dust as the risk factors.
- It is often bilateral and, more commonly, on the nasal side.
- It destroys the superficial layers of the cornea, like the epithelium and Bowman's layer.
- It causes decreased vision due to astigmatism and obstruction of the visual axis.
- Flattening is seen over the horizontal axis.
- It is usually thick and fleshy in the early stages and becomes atrophic in later stages.

Treatment

- Treatment comprises of its removal if it causes decreased vision, involves the pupillary area or due to cosmetic reasons.
- Recurrence is common after its removal. Amniotic membrane transplantation, conjunctival graft or mitomycin C has been known to decrease the recurrence.

Tumors of the Conjunctiva

- There can be different tumorous conditions of the conjunctiva like ocular surface squamous neoplasia, limbal dermoid, lymphoma, Kaposi sarcoma, or nevus **(Fig. 18.5)**.

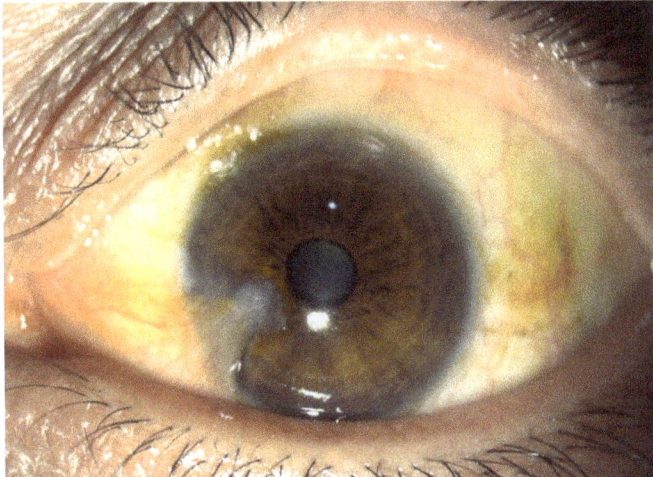

Fig. 18.4: Image showing pterygium extending on to cornea.

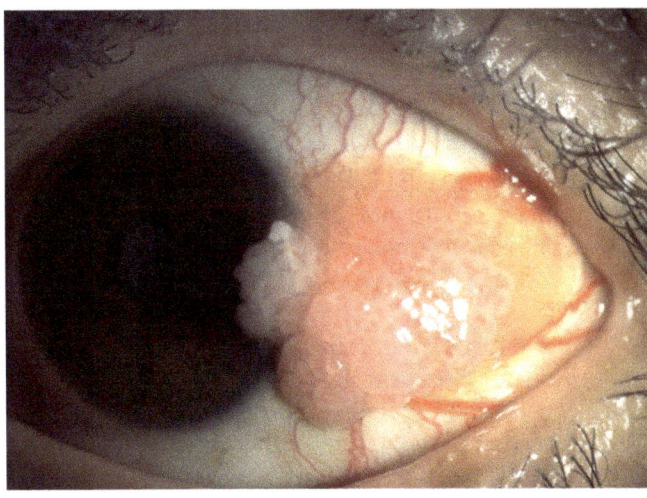

Fig. 18.5: Image showing a tumor on the conjunctiva.

- Dermoid and dermolipomas are congenital tumors seen on the conjunctiva. Dermoids are congenital tumors seen at the limbus. They have keratinized epithelium and hair on their surface.
- Various other tumors which can be seen are papillomata, pyogenic granuloma, or basal cell carcinoma.
- Lid tumors can also invade the conjunctiva.
- Nevus and malignant melanoma are pigmented tumors.

Xerosis (Xerophthalmia)

- It is a dry, lustreless condition of the conjunctiva which can be caused by a deficiency of mucin.
- It is most commonly caused by vitamin A deficiency and can be accompanied by night blindness.
- The epithelium stops the production of mucin, and the conjunctiva becomes epidermoid, like that of skin.
- Local treatment consists of the instillation of lubricant drops and ointments, with the systemic treatment comprising of vitamin A supplementation.
- Proper care of the nutrition has to be taken.

Keratoconjunctivitis Sicca (Sjogren Syndrome)

It is caused due to deficiency of the aqueous component of the tear film.

Causes

It is commonly seen in women after menopause and can be associated with rheumatoid arthritis.

Clinical Features

It causes chronic irritation, foreign body sensation and photophobia.

Treatment

Control of the systemic disease and intensive lubrication.

Dry Eye Disease

It produces chronic discomfort due to repeated breakdown of the tear film, as it is unstable.

Causes

- **Deficiency of tears:** Sjogren syndrome
- **Deficiency of mucus:** Goblet cell deficiency in avitaminosis, *Steven Johnson* syndrome, old trachoma.

- Corneal surface irregularities
- Decreased wetting due to lid paralysis

Signs
- Punctate keratitis
- Tear film break-up time <10 seconds
- Schirmer's test <10 mm
- Increase in tear osmolarity

Treatment
- Intensive lubrication, using preservative-free lubricant eye drops and ointment. Frequency varies from 4–12 times a day depending upon the severity of the disease.
- Preservation of the natural tears can be done through punctal occlusion
- Evaluation for any systemic disease, and treatment, if present.

Symblepharon

It is adhesion between bulbar and palpebral conjunctiva after both the surfaces are raw due to any chemical and thermal burn or cicatrizing diseases like Stevens-Johnson syndrome.

Conjunctivochalasis

It is seen in older adults due to lax conjunctiva, causing folds of conjunctiva over the lid margin. It can be asymptomatic or cause foreign body sensation, warranting treatment by lubricants or removal.

Argyrosis

It is discoloration of the conjunctiva by prolonged treatment with silver salts used for the treatment of chronic conjunctivitis or trachoma.

NURSING CONSIDERATIONS

Nursing staff can train patients how to maintain ocular hygiene, timely administration of eyedrops and its proper technique. In cases of neonatal conjunctivitis, nurses can be the first responders in identifying the disease so that the child can receive timely treatment which can prevent child blindness and infant mortality.

GERIATRIC CONSIDERATIONS

Elderly suffering from dry eye should undergo regular checkups to assess ocular health and adjustment of ocular medications to maintain corneal hydration. They should also undergo systemic examination to rule out any connective tissue disorders like arthritis which can worsen dry eye if not treated.

Case Scenario
1. A newborn developed eye discharge from both eyes approximately 2 days after birth. The eye discharge was copius, yellowish in color and matting the eyelashes which prevented eye opening. Conjunctival swabs revealed Gram negative diplococci on Gram staining.
2. It is a case of neonatal conjunctivitis due to *Neisseria* due to infected maternal birth passage. Child needs to be started on IV ceftriaxone to prevent systemic illness and corneal perforation along with topical erythromycin.

SUMMARY

Conjunctiva is one of the most dynamic parts of the eye. Its extensive blood supply, lymphatics and secretion of antibodies helps in clearing offending agents at a faster rate as compared to cornea. However, its exposure to environmental irritants make it vulnerable to repeated infections and local damage causing degenerative disorders.

MULTIPLE CHOICE QUESTIONS

1. Which one of the following is chronic conjunctivitis:
    a. Adenoviral conjunctivitis
    b. Bacterial conjunctivitis
    c. Neonatal conjunctivitis
    d. Trachoma
2. Which one of the following is not the treatment of vernal keratoconjunctivitis:
    a. Mast cell stabilizers
    b. Steroids
    c. Antibiotics
    d. Lubricants
3. Which of the following is a degenerative disease?
    a. Conjunctivitis
    b. Pterygium
    c. Stevens-Johnson syndrome
    d. Argyrosis
4. All of the following are differential diagnosis of red eye, *except*:
    a. Conjunctivitis
    b. Ophthalmia neonatorum
    c. Pingecula
    d. Stevens-Johnson syndrome
5. All of the following are tumors of the conjunctiva, *except*:
    a. Melanoma
    b. Lymphoma
    c. Dermoid
    d. Pingecula

ANSWERS

1. d   2. c   3. b   4. c
5. d

SUGGESTED READING

1. Cronau H, Kankanala RR, Mauger T. Diagnosis and management of red eye in primary care. Am Fam Phys. 2010;81:137-44.
2. Dart JK. The 2016 Bowman Lecture Conjunctival curses: Scarring conjunctivitis 30 years on Eye (Lond). 2017;31:301-32
3. Gokhale NS. Systematic approach to managing vernal keratoconjunctivitis in clinical practice: Severity grading system and a treatment algorithm. Indian J Ophthalmol. 2016;64:145-8.
4. Kohanim S, Palioura S, Saeed HN, et al. Acute and chronic ophthalmic involvement in Stevens-Johnson syndrome/toxic epidermal necrolysis—a comprehensive review and guide to therapy. II. Ophthalmic disease. Ocul Surf. 2016;14:168-88.
5. Owen CG, Shah A, Henshaw K, Smeeth L, Sheikh A. Topical treatments for seasonal allergic conjunctivitis: systematic review and meta-analysis of efficacy and effectiveness. Br J Gen Pract. 2004;54:451-6.
6. Ryder EC, Benson S. Conjunctivitis. In: StatPearls. Treasure Island (FL): StatPearls Publishing LLC; 2020.
7. Shields CL, Shields JA. Tumors of the conjunctiva and cornea. Surv Ophthalmol. 2004;49:3-24.
8. Singh SK. Pterygium: epidemiology prevention and treatment. Community Eye Health. 2017;30(99):S5-S6.
9. Varu DM, Rhee MK, Akpek EK, Amescua G, Farid M, Garcia-Ferrer FJ, et al. conjunctivitis preferred practice pattern®. Ophthalmology. 2019;126:P94–P169.
10. Wotherspoon AC, Hardman-Lea S, Isaacson PG. Mucosa-associated lymphoid tissue (MALT) in the human conjunctiva. J Pathol. 1994;174(1):33-7.

CHAPTER

19

Disorders of Retina and Vitreous

Atul Arora, Reema Bansal, Vishali Gupta

"Within the complex fabric of visual perception, vitreoretinal diseases weave challenges that test both science and compassion, reminding us that every thread of knowledge and care is essential in illuminating the path towards sight and clarity."
—Atul Arora

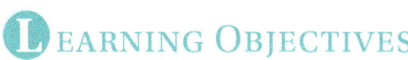

After going through the chapter, the learner will be able to:
- Learn basics of individual retinal pathologies.
- Understand pathophysiology, clinical features, diagnosis and management aspects of each individual disease.
- Discuss the nursing management of disorders of retina and vitreous.

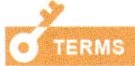

- **Choroidal neovascular membrane (CNVM):** Pathological growth of new blood vessels that arise from choriocapillaris layer of choroid and grow in sub-retinal pigment epithelium and sub-retinal space.
- **Cystoid macular edema (CME):** Retinal thickening of the macula due to collection of fluid in outer plexiform layer.
- **Elschnig spots:** Black spots surrounded by bright yellow or red halos seen on the retina during fundoscopy.
- **Fundus autofluorescence (FAF):** A noninvasive retinal imaging modality based on detection of fluorophore (lipofuschin) in retinal pigment epithelium.
- **Fundus fluorescein angiography (FFA):** An invasive retinal imaging modality to examine the retinal circulation.
- **Intraocular pressure (IOP):** Fluid pressure inside the eye.
- **Neovascular age-related macular degeneration (NAMD):** An advanced form of age-related macular degeneration resulting in severe vision loss.
- **Optical coherence tomography (OCT):** Noninvasive imaging technique that uses light waves to take cross-section images of retina.
- **Optical coherence tomography angiography (OCTA):** Noninvasive imaging technique to visualize retinal and choroidal vasculature.
- **Pars plana vitrectomy (PPV):** Vitreoretinal surgery technique to access the posterior segment of eye.
- **Siegerts streaks:** Line of pigment spots seen along choroidal arteries in the fundus in advanced hypertensive retinopathy.
- **Ultrasonography (USG):** A diagnostic technique that utilizes high frequency sound waves to image internal structures of eye.
- **Venous beading:** Irregular constriction and dilatation of venules in the retina.

INTRODUCTION

This chapter provides brief overview about common vitreoretinal pathologies. Retina, the innermost layer of the eyeball, consists of a thin, transparent membrane—neurosensory retina and a pigmented layer: retinal pigment epithelium (RPE). Vitreous humor consists of transparent gel that fills the vitreous cavity. Vitreoretinal pathologies can be grouped into vascular disorder, macular disorders, retinal dystrophies and degenerations and retinal detachment.

Vascular Disorders
- Diabetic retinopathy
- Hypertensive retinopathy

- Retinal vein occlusions
- Retinal artery occlusions
- Retinopathy of prematurity

Macular Disorders
- Age-related macular degeneration (ARMD)
- Epiretinal membranes, vitreomacular traction, macular hole
- CSCR and pachychoroid spectrum of diseases

Retinal Detachment

Retinal Dystrophies and Degenerations
- **Diffuse photoreceptor dystrophy:**
  - Retinitis pigmentosa
  - Cone dystrophies
  - Cone-rod dystrophies
- **Macular dystrophies:**
  - Adult-onset vitelliform lesions
  - Best disease or best vitelliform dystrophy
  - Stargardt disease
  - Pattern dystrophies

VASCULAR DISORDERS OF RETINA

Vascular diseases of retina include diabetic retinopathy, hypertensive retinopathy, vein occlusions, central or branch retinal artery occlusions and retinopathy of prematurity.

DIABETIC RETINOPATHY

Diabetes mellitus is a major cause of avoidable blindness. Diabetic retinopathy (DR) is one of the complications of uncontrolled diabetes. Chronic hyperglycemia leads to progressive dysfunction of retinal vasculature and structural damage to neural retina. Various risk factors of DR include: duration of diabetes, poor metabolic control, hypertension, smoking, obesity and dyslipidemia. In addition, pregnancy may accelerate the changes of diabetic retinopathy.

Pathophysiology of DR

Patients with Type I diabetes mellitus show changes of diabetic retinopathy 5–10 years after being diagnosed with diabetes. Patients with Type II diabetes mellitus on the other hand may have retinopathy changes at the time of diagnosis of the disease. Screening for diabetic retinopathy is therefore recommended at the time of diagnosis of Type II diabetes mellitus. Chronic hyperglycemia causes biochemical and physiologic changes resulting in endothelial damage. Pathological changes noticed are capillary basement membrane thickening and loss of pericytes. These pathological changes lead to retinal edema and exudation due to decompensation of endothelial barrier. Progressive microvascular damage results in capillary occlusion, retinal nonperfusion and ischemia. Vascular endothelial growth factor (VEGF) released from retinal pigment epithelium (RPE) cells and vascular endothelium induces retinal neovascularization and progression to proliferative diabetic retinopathy.

Clinical Features

Microaneurysms are the earliest clinical lesions to be picked up on fundus examination. Deep (dot and blot) and superficial (flame-shaped) retinal hemorrhages; hard exudates (waxy looking bright yellow lipid deposits); retinal thickening due to retinal edema, beading, looping and dilatation of veins; intraretinal microvascular abnormalities (IRMAs) are the other clinical findings seen in diabetic retinopathy. In advanced stages, signs of neovascularization: neovascularization of disc (NVD) and neovascularization elsewhere (NVE); and fibrovascular proliferation (FVP) appear. Contraction of FVP lead to TRD and severe visual loss.

Classification of DR

Diabetic retinopathy has been classified based on presence/absence of neovascularization. Early stages of DR are characterized by presence of dot-blot retinal hemorrhages; hard exudates beading, looping and dilatation of veins and IRMAs but lack neovascularization: nonproliferative diabetic retinopathy (NPDR). Later, as the disease progresses, neovascularization appears and the disease is referred as proliferative diabetic retinopathy (PDR).

Nonproliferative Diabetic Retinopathy
- **Mild NPDR:** Presence of microaneurysm only.
- **Moderate NPDR:** Presence of retinal hemorrhages; microaneurysms, cotton-wool spots, venous beading, or IRMA criteria not met for more severe retinopathy.
- **Severe NPDR:** Presence of one the following, in the absence of PDR:
  - More than 20 intraretinal hemorrhages in each of four quadrants
  - Definite venous beading in two or more quadrants
  - Prominent IRMA in one or more quadrants
- **Very severe NPDR:** Presence of two or more of the following, in the absence of PDR:
  - More than 20 intraretinal hemorrhages in each of four quadrants
  - Definite venous beading in two or more quadrants
  - Prominent IRMA in one or more quadrants

Proliferative Diabetic Retinopathy

Presence of neovascularization is the hallmark of PDR.
- **High-risk PDR:** Presence of one or more of the following (Fig. 19.1):
  - Neovascularization at or within one disc diameter of the optic disc [NVD] (1/4–1/3 disc area in size) with or without vitreous hemorrhage or preretinal bleed.
  - NVD <1/4–1/3 disc area with vitreous and/or preretinal hemorrhage.
  - Neovascularization elsewhere (NVE) with vitreous and/or preretinal hemorrhage.
- **Clinically significant diabetic macular edema (CSME) (Fig. 19.2):** DME is referred as CSME if one of the following three criteria is fulfilled upon fundus examination with slit-lamp using 90 D lens:
  1. Thickening of the retina at or within 500 microns of the center of the fovea

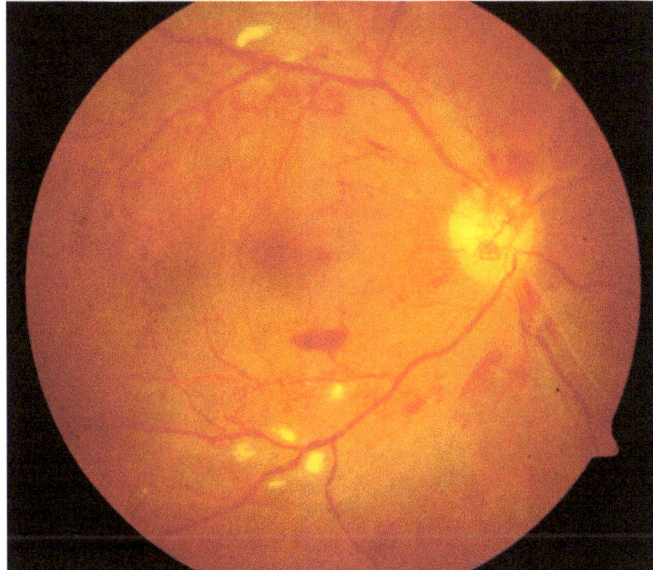

Fig. 19.1: Fundus photograph of right eye of a diabetic patient showing neovascularization at disc (NVD) of size >1/3 disc area (high-risk PDR).

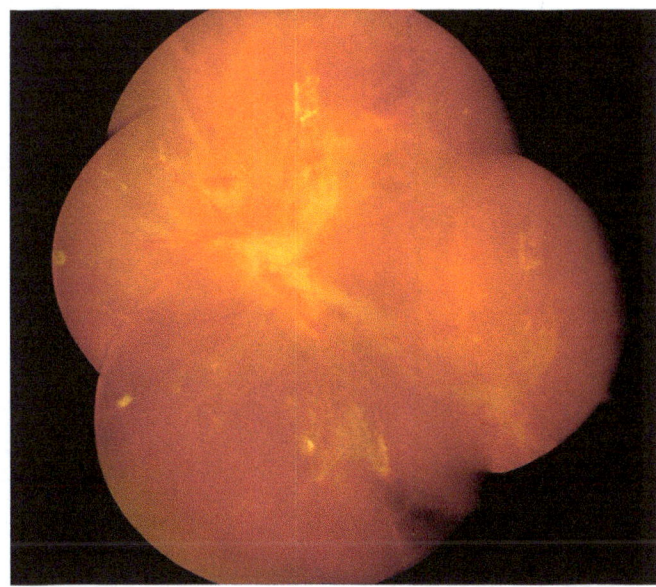

Fig. 19.3: Fundus photograph showing fibrovascular proliferation at disc with tractional retinal detachment (advanced diabetic retinopathy).

Fundus fluorescein angiography (FFA) aids in picking up subtle neovascularization and also to guide laser therapy for DME.

Management

Management of DR involves correcting the deranged metabolic profile. Good glycemic control along with control of hypertension, correction of dyslipidemia goes a long way in preventing progression of DR.

Intravitreal anti-VEGF or steroid injections are useful in treating CSME while macular photocoagulation is done in cases of DME away from foveal center.

Panretinal photocoagulation (PRP) is done in cases of PDR. Surgical intervention is required in cases of vitreous hemorrhage and tractional retinal detachment.

HYPERTENSIVE RETINOPATHY

Systemic hypertension is known to cause end organ damage in heart, kidneys, and brain. Eye is also affected in both chronic as well as acute rise in blood pressure. Hypertension results in damage to retina, choroid, and optic nerve. Retinal changes include narrowing of arterioles, retinal hemorrhages (flame-shaped or dot-blot), and cotton-wool spots. Acute rise in blood pressure (malignant hypertension) results in loss of autoregulation of choroidal vasculature resulting in hypertensive choroidopathy characterized by Elschnig spots, Siegert's streaks and exudative retinal detachment. Malignant hypertension also causes disc edema and optic neuropathy. **Figure 19.4** shows bilateral hypertensive retinopathy in a patient with essential hypertension.

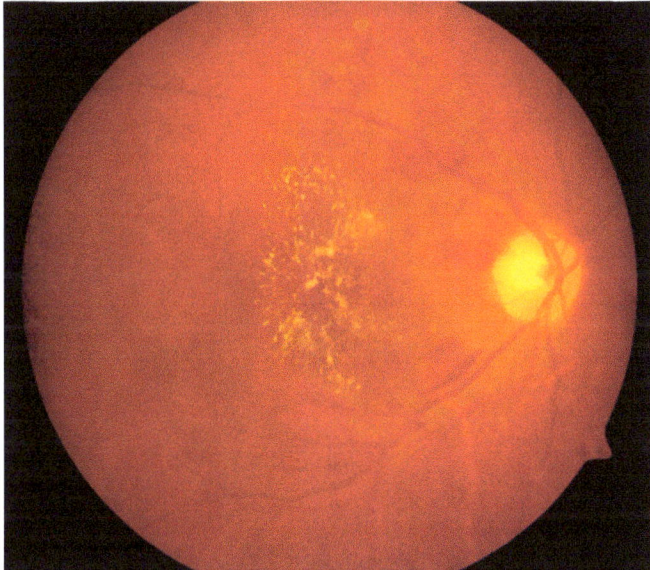

Fig. 19.2: Fundus photograph of right eye of a patient with Type II diabetes mellitus showing moderate nonproliferative diabetic retinopathy with retinal thickening and hard exudates suggestive of clinically significant macular edema (CSME).

2. Hard exudates at or within 500 microns of the center of fovea associated with adjacent retinal thickening.
3. Development of a zone of retinal thickening one disc diameter or larger in size, at least a part of which is within one disc diameter of the foveal center.

Diabetic Macular Edema (Fig. 19.3)

It is the retinal thickening/edema as a result of abnormal retinal vascular permeability in diabetic retinopathy. DME is associated with presence of hard exudates which are precipitates of plasma lipoproteins.

Diagnosis

Diagnosis of diabetic retinopathy is clinical. Optical coherence tomography (OCT) is helpful quantifying DME and monitoring response to treatment.

Diagnosis

The diagnosis is clinical based on fundus examination and clinical signs described above.

Management

Treatment involves controlling blood pressure with anti-hypertensive drugs and dietary modifications like salt restriction, etc.

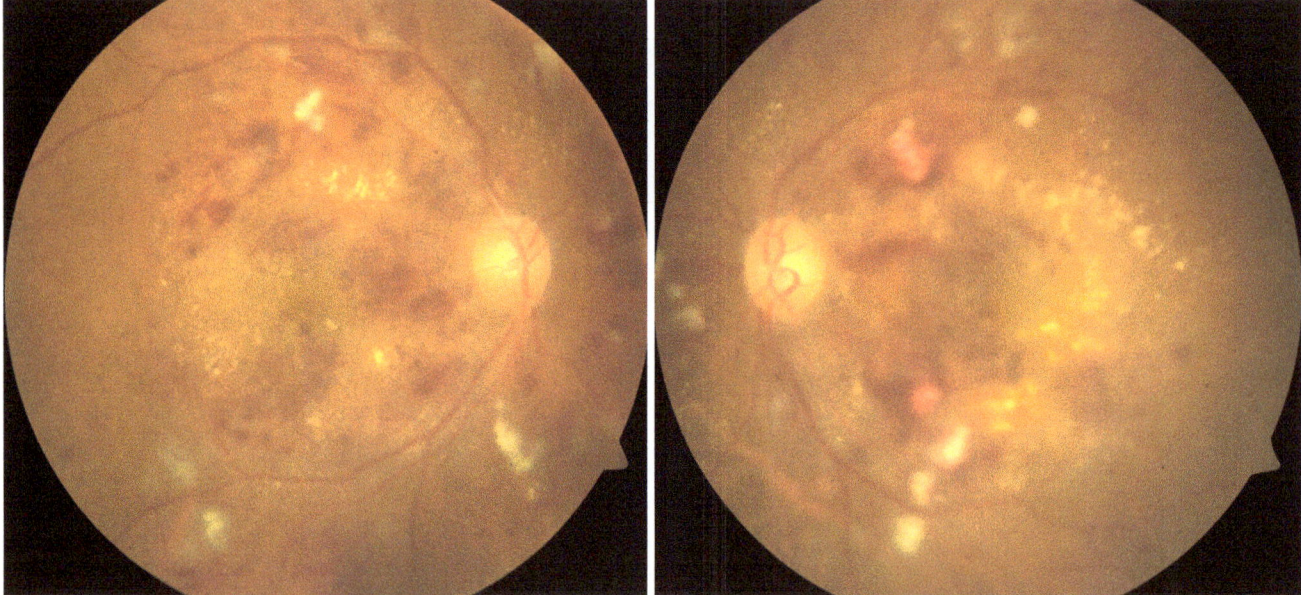

Fig. 19.4: Bilateral hypertensive retinopathy in a patient with essential hypertension.

Uncontrolled hypertension acts as risk factor for branch retinal artery occlusion (BRAO), branch retinal vein occlusion (BRVO), central retinal vein occlusion (CRVO), and retinal arterial macroaneurysms.

RETINAL VEIN OCCLUSION

Definition

Occlusion is a blockage in an artery or vein. The flow of blood from the retina is often blocked because of a blot clot. This condition is called retinal vein occlusion (RVO).

Risk Factors

Risk factors of RVO include advancing age, hypertension, smoking, dyslipidemia and glaucoma.

Pathophysiology

Thickened/sclerotic arterial wall causes compression of retinal veins sharing the same adventitia (e.g., just behind the lamina cribrosa in CRVO and at arteriovenous crossings in BRVO) resulting in vascular occlusion. Additionally, hyperviscosity of blood in polycythemia, homocysteinemia and hyperlipidemia or raised intraocular pressure may impede blood flow.

Classification of RVO

RVO can be broadly classified as CRVO and BRVO.

Central Retinal Vein Occlusion

It is the occlusion of central retinal vein just behind the lamina cribrosa. The more proximal the occlusion, more severe is the presentation and more is the risk of ischemia.

Non-ischemic CRVO (NI-CRVO)

Three-fourths of CRVO is of non-ischemic (NI) variety. Congestion and tortuosity of retinal veins, flame-shaped hemorrhages, mild macular edema and/or mild papilledema and absence of RAPD are the presenting features of NI-CRVO. **Figure 19.5** shows fundus photograph of left eye of a patient

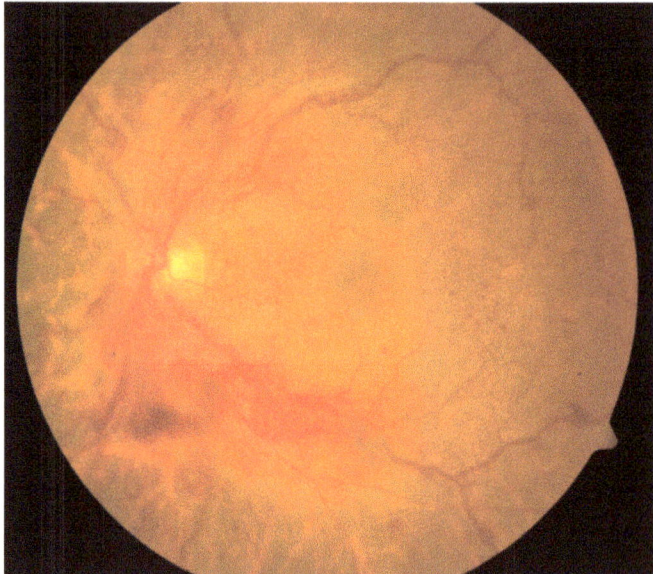

Fig. 19.5: Fundus photograph of left eye showing dilated and tortuous veins along with flame-shaped hemorrhages indicating CRVO.

with CRVO. Dilated and tortuous veins along with flame-shaped hemorrhages can be appreciated.

Ischemic CRVO (I-CRVO)

The clinical features of ischemic CRVO are more severe than NI-CRVO. Visual acuity is less than 6/60, an afferent pupillary defect is present and there is marked venous dilation, extensive hemorrhages, and cotton-wool spots.

Causes of decreased vision in CRVO include macular edema, macular ischemia and neovascular glaucoma. Neovascular glaucoma also known as 90-day glaucoma is seen in I-CRVO and occurs due to severe ischemia resulting in neovascularization of iris and secondary angle closure.

Management includes control of systemic risk factors like hypertension, dyslipidemia, and homocysteinemia. Intravitreal anti-VEGF injections are useful in treating cystoid macular edema while neovascular complications like INV

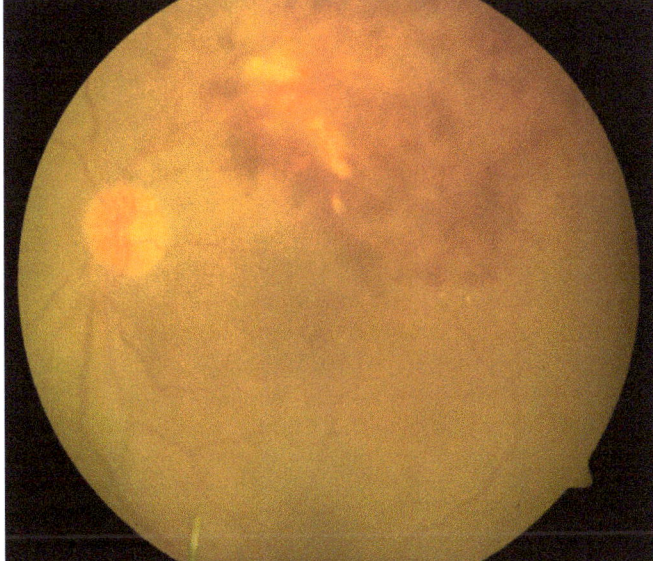

Fig. 19.6: Fundus photograph of left eye showing dilated and tortuous veins, flame-shaped hemorrhages and cotton wool spots restricted to superotemporal quadrant-superotemporal BRVO.

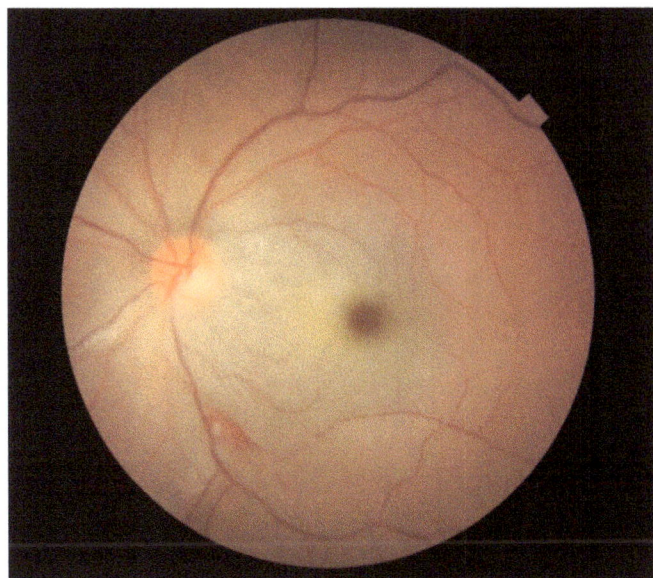

Fig. 19.7: Fundus photograph of left eye showing pale retina with cherry-red spot in a patient with CRAO.

and NVG are managed by scatter laser potocoagulation and anti-glaucoma medications.

Branch Retinal Vein Occlusion (BRVO)

It is the occlusion of branch of central retinal vein at arteriovenous (AV) crossing due to compression by thickened arterial wall. The superotemporal quadrant has maximum number of (AV) crossings and hence is most commonly involved. Venous dilation and tortuosity; retinal hemorrhages and cotton-wool spots are restricted to the drainage area of the occluded vein **(Fig. 19.6)**. Macular edema, macular ischemia, and retinal hemorrhage over the macular area result in acute decrease in visual acuity while complications like vitreous hemorrhage and tractional retinal detachment due to retinal neovascularization are responsible for decreased vision in longer term.

Management

Like CRVO, treatment involves control of systemic risk factors like hypertension, dyslipidemia and intravitreal anti-VEGF injections and/or macular photocoagulation for CME. Scatter laser photocoagulation is reserved for neovascular complications.

RETINAL ARTERY OCCLUSION

Occlusion of central retinal artery or its branch is seen in patients suffering from hypertension, cardiovascular/cerebrovascular diseases.

Pathophysiology

Atherosclerosis and thrombosis of central retinal vein; thromboembolism from the carotid artery or as a result of coronary artery disease are responsible for causing retinal arterial occlusions. Less commonly, inflammatory causes like giant cell arteritis, polyarteritis nodosa, systemic lupus erythematosus and Wegner's granulomatosis may result in arterial occlusion are other causes of CRAO.

Classification
Central Retinal Artery Occlusion (CRAO)

It is the obstruction of central retinal artery at the level of lamina cribrosa. The patient presents with sudden painless loss of vision. Fundus examination shows pale/white retina with markedly attenuated arterioles. Segmented blood column could be seen in retinal veins (*cattle trucking*). Vascular choroid is visible through the thin retina at the center of macula resulting in cherry-red spot **(Fig. 19.7)**. Later in course there occurs retinal atrophy along with consecutive optic atrophy. The affected eye has poor visual prognosis.

Management of CRAO

The management is directed at identifying and eliminating the inciting cause so as to prevent systemic complications like stroke, myocardial infarction, etc. A meticulous cardiac and carotid evaluation is warranted. Supportive measures like IOP-lowering drugs, ocular massage, anterior chamber paracentesis, etc., to dislodge the embolus and enable reperfusion may be beneficial in limited number of cases.

Branch Retinal Artery Occlusion (BRAO)

In BRAO, the occlusion occurs distal to lamina cribrosa in one of the branches of central retinal artery **(Fig. 19.8)**. The patient complains of visual field defect in the area of retinal arterial branch. The management is similar to that of CRAO.

RETINOPATHY OF PREMATURITY

Retinopathy of prematurity (ROP) is a proliferative disease seen in developing retina of premature neonates. Due to advancements in neonatal care, a greater number of preterm and low birth weight babies are being saved. This has resulted in increase in number of babies with ROP to epidemic levels. Because of its association with the use of supplemental oxygen and better neonatal care, ROP is considered as man-made disease.

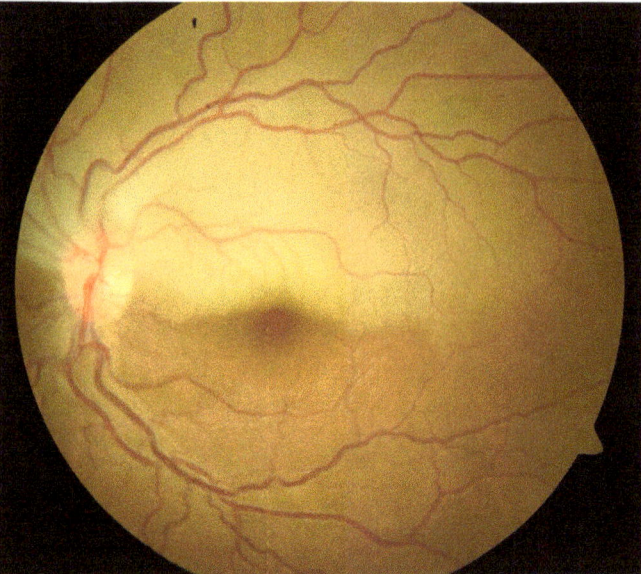

Fig. 19.8: Occlusion of superotemporal branch of central retinal artery resulting in white/edematous retina. Note the area of retina in inferotemporal quadrant with intact arterial supply.

Pathophysiology

In-utero development of retinal blood vessels is a hypoxia-driven process. When a child is born preterm, angiogenesis stops as there occurs decline in hypoxic drive especially when supplemental oxygen is administered. Consecutively, the peripheral avascular retina suffers hypoxic injury and starts producing angiogenic factors like VEGF, and IGF1. This results in growth of abnormal blood vessels out of retina into the vitreous cavity. Later when VEGF levels decline, there occurs angio-fibrotic switch leading to fibrosis and contraction of neovascular fronds resulting in tractional retinal detachment.

ROP Screening

Screening of all the neonates at risk of developing ROP is essential to pick up the disease early and initiate timely treatment. The first screening examination for ROP is advocated to be done by 'day 30' of life, irrespective of the gestational age. Early screening at 2–3 weeks of age is recommended for infants <28 week or <1,200 g.

ROP is classified into different stages depending upon clinical signs/presentation. Also, depending upon location of demarcation line/ridge/FVP from optic disc/fovea, the disease is classified into different zones **(Tables 19.1 and 19.2)**.

NURSING CONSIDERATIONS

- ❖ Screening for ROP is done in neonatal care units, neonatal ICU or in OPD.
- ❖ The baby should not be fed for at least an hour before screening.
- ❖ Commercially available topical dilator drops are diluted to halve their concentration. 0.4% tropicamide and 2.5% phenylephrine are used.
- ❖ Equipment required for screening includes: Indirect ophthalmoscope, 20 or 28 D lens, infant eye speculum, wire vectis/infant scleral depressor. Infant eye speculum and wire vectis/infant scleral depressor should be autoclaved beforehand and 20 or 28 D lens should be washed with soap and water.

TABLE 19.1: Revised international classification of retinopathy of prematurity.

Zone	Zone I	Area within a circle with radius equal to twice the distance from the optic disc to the fovea
	Zone II	Area extending from the border of Zone I to the nasal ora serrata
	Zone III	Remaining crescent of temporal retina beyond Zone II
Stage	Stage 1	Flat grayish-white demarcation line at the junction of the vascular and avascular retina
	Stage 2	Elevated ridge at the junction of the vascular and avascular retina
	Stage 3	Ridge with extraretinal fibrovascular proliferation.
	Stage 4	4A—Subtotal retinal detachment not involving the fovea 4B—Subtotal retinal detachment involving the fovea
	Stage 5	Total retinal detachment
Aggressive posterior ROP (APROP)		Characterized by flat intraretinal neovascularization and vascular loops in posterior Zone I or posterior Zone II associated with rapidly evolving plus disease
Plus disease*		2 quadrants (6 or more clock hours) of dilation and tortuosity of the posterior retinal blood vessels Presence of rigid pupil, vitreous haze or neovascularization of the iris **Preplus:** Vascular abnormalities that are insufficient for the diagnosis of plus disease but demonstrate more arteriolar tortuosity and more venous dilation than normal *Plus disease was defined by Early Treatment for Retinopathy of Prematurity Cooperative Group (ETROP) study

TABLE 19.2: ETROP recommendations for laser treatment.

Laser treatment is recommended for	Zone I, Stage 1, 2 or 3 ROP with plus Zone I, Stage 3 ROP without plus. Zone II, Stage 2 or 3 ROP with plus. Aggressive posterior ROP (APROP) in any zone

- Strict hand hygiene should be maintained: hands should be washed with soap and water before and after handling each baby.
- Babies admitted in NICU/NNU need monitoring by a neonatologist during the screening procedure.
- Council the parents regarding regular follow up of the baby.

MACULAR DISORDERS

Macular disorders comprise of age-related macular degeneration (ARMD), vitreomacular surface—vitreomacular traction, macular hole and epiretinal membrane, and central serous chorioretinopathy (CSCR).

AGE RELATED MACULAR DEGENERATION (ARMD)

Age-related macular degeneration (ARMD) is a chronic, progressive degenerative disorder of macula resulting in loss of central vision. ARMD is the leading cause of blindness in the developed world in people over 50 years of age.

Pathophysiology

Good nutrition, smoking and exposure to sun light are important risk factors of developing AMD. Ageing results in reduced density and increased turn-over of photoreceptors. However, RPE is overwhelmed and unable to process the metabolic by products from degenerating photoreceptors resulting in accumulation of lipofuscin deposits between the plasma membrane of the RPE and the Bruch membrane as well as on either side of the basement membrane of the RPE. Clinically these deposits appear as drusens. Drusen are subretinal pigment epithelial deposits that are characteristic of but not uniquely associated with AMD. ARMD is associated with two types of drusen that have different clinical appearances and different prognoses. Progressive involutional changes result in atrophy of RPE. RPE atrophy and damage to underlying Bruch's membrane leads to growth of neovessels from choriocapillaris into sub-RPE and sub-retinal space resulting in wet AMD (CNVM).

Clinical Features

Dry AMD: Druse is the prototypical lesion of AMD. Drusen appear as round, yellow, subretinal lesions in post-equatorial retina. RPE abnormalities like hyperpigmentation and atrophy are other findings of dry AMD. In advanced stages, focal areas of RPE atrophy coalesce to form geographic atrophy resulting in loss of central vision (**Fig. 19.9**).

Wet AMD: Presence of CNVM is the hallmark of the neovascular AMD. Patients present with acute onset of decrease in vision and/or metamorphopsia. Fundus examination is done for subretinal or intraretinal hemorrhage, fluid and/or presence of hard exudates (**Fig. 19.10**). Disciform scar is seen in advanced cases.

Diagnosis

Diagnosis of AMD is clinical. Optical coherence tomography (OCT) is useful in diagnosing as well as monitoring response to therapy in wet AMD.

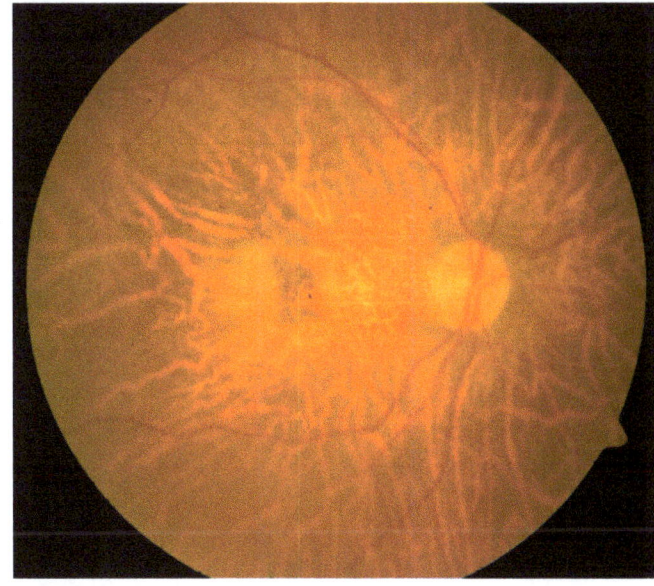

Fig. 19.9: Fundus photograph of right eye of a patient with advanced ARMD. The macular area shows RPE atrophy with visible underlying choroidal vessels (geographic atrophy).

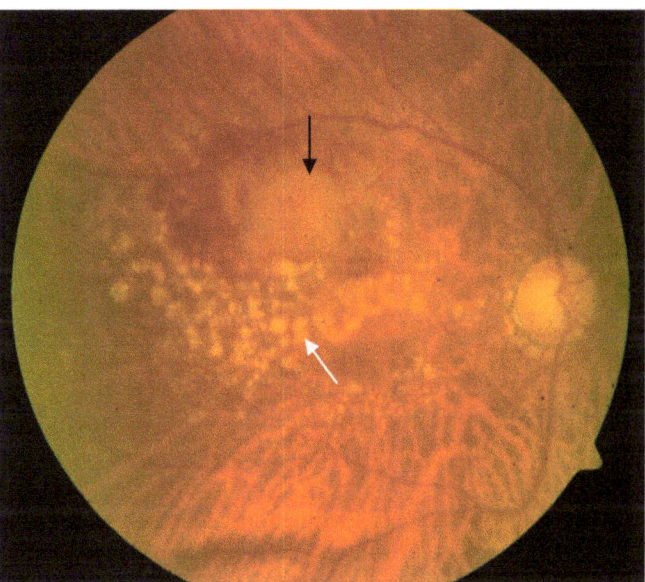

Fig. 19.10: Fundus photograph of a patient with wet ARMD. The macular area shows greenish yellow neovascular membrane with overlying hemorrhage (black arrow). Numerous large sized drusens can be seen all around (white arrow).

Management

The classification and treatment recommendations for ARMD are depicted in **Table 19.3**. Management includes lifestyle modifications like smoking cessation, reduced intake of lipids and including colored fruits and vegetables in diet. Micronutrients supplementation with AREDS II formulation comprising vitamins C (500 mg) and E (400 IU), lutein (10 mg), zeaxanthin (2 mg), zinc oxide (80 mg) and cupric oxide (2 mg) is recommended in patients with intermediate and advanced AMD. Intravitreal anti-VEGF injections are required for treatment of wet AMD.

TABLE 19.3: Age-related eye disease study; classification and treatment recommendations for ARMD.

Classification	Clinical characteristics	Treatment
Early	Presence of numerous small drusens (<63 μ) with few intermediate sized drusens (63–125 μ)	Observation, 6 monthly follow up, smoking cessation
Intermediate	Presence of numerous intermediate sized drusens (63–125 μ) with few large drusens (>125 μ) and/or Geographic atrophy not involving macular center	AREDS II formulation
Advanced	Geographic atrophy not involving macular center Presence of CNVM (wet AMD)	AREDS II formulation Intravitreal anti-VEGF for wet AMD

EPIRETINAL MEMBRANE, VITREOMACULAR TRACTION AND MACULAR HOLE

Epiretinal Membrane

Epiretinal membrane (ERM) is an avascular, fibrocellular membrane formed as a result of proliferation of glia or hyalocytes. ERMs may be idiopathic (more common) or occur secondary to inflammation or ocular procedures like laser photo coagulation, cryopexy, retinal surgery, etc.

Clinical Features

Metamorphopsia and/or decreased vision are the presenting complains of a patient. More commonly ERM is detected incidentally on fundus examination in otherwise asymptomatic patient. The membrane may be thin, transparent appearing as a mild sheen on the retinal surface (cellophane retinopathy) or may become highly thickened and opaque, obscuring underlying retinal details and causing distortion and wrinkling of retinal surface.

Diagnosis

The diagnosis is clinical. OCT is helpful in doubtful cases and also gives information about integrity of retinal layers and the amount of retinal surface distortion caused by ERM.

Management

Mild, asymptomatic cases with good visual acuity are best kept under observation. Pars plana vitrectomy with ERM peeling is useful in symptomatic patients.

Vitreomacular Traction

Incomplete anomalous posterior vitreous detachment results in focal or broad vitreomacular adhesions with/without traction and distortion of foveal contour. The VMT disorders include:
❖ Vitreomacular adhesion (VMA)
❖ Vitreomacular traction (VMT) syndrome
❖ Macular hole

Vitreomacular adhesion (VMA): Posterior hyaloid is adherent to fovea without causing any traction or distortion of foveal contour. VMA itself is asymptomatic but acts as precursor of VMT and macular hole.
Vitreomacular traction (VMT) syndrome: Abnormally adherent posterior hyaloid resulting in distortion of foveal contour, cystic edema, and tractional foveal detachment.
Decreased visual acuity and metamorphopsia are the presenting complaints. Surgical intervention is required in symptomatic patients with decreased visual acuity.

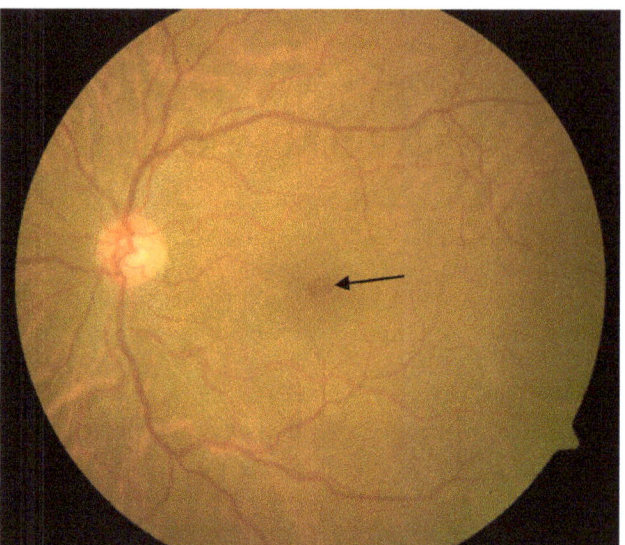

Fig. 19.11: Fundus photograph of left eye of a patient depicting full thickness macular hole (black arrow).

Macular Hole

A full thickness defect in neural retina formed at the center of macula **(Fig. 19.11)**.

Pathophysiology

Idiopathic macular hole: Idiopathic macular holes form as a result of tractional forces exerted by anomalous perifoveal vitreous detachment.
Secondary macular hole: Secondary causes of macular hole include trauma, high myopia, electric shock or laser pointer injury. Alport syndrome, X-linked juvenile retinoschisis, Stargardt disease, best macular dystrophy are other less common causes of secondary macular hole.

Clinical Features

Patients present with decline in central vision and metamorphopsia. Diagnosis is clinical. OCT is useful for confirming the diagnosis.

Management

Surgical intervention is the mainstay of treatment. Small macular hole with visual acuity better than 6/12 can be kept under observation.

CSCR AND PACHYCHOROID SPECTRUM OF DISEASES

The term "pachychoroid" is used to describe a group of macular diseases presenting with a thick choroid.

Pachychoroid is characterized by dilatation of veins in Haller's layer of choroid along with attenuation of choriocapillaris.

Pachychoroid spectrum of diseases include:
- **Pachychoroid pigment epitheliopathy (PPE):** Alterations of the retinal pigment epithelium without neurosensory detachment. PPE is considered as a form fruste of CSC.
- **Central serous chorioretinopathy (CSCR):** Serous detachment of neural retina in the macular region due to chorioretinal pathology.
- **Pachychoroid neovasculopathy (PNV):** Type 1 choroidal neovascularizations above focal areas of pachychoroid.
- **Polypoidal choroidal vasculopathy (PCV):** Exudative maculopathy characterized by presence of polyp (appear clinically as sub-retinal orange-red nodules).

Pathophysiology

The individual entities in the pachychoroid spectrum of diseases represent a continuum of single pathological process. Hyperpermeability and stasis in large choroidal vessels result in their engorgement and dilatation. Subsequently, RPE is overwhelmed in maintaining homeostasis resulting in pachychoroid pigment epitheliopathy (PPE). Next, areas overlying choroidal hyperpermeability demonstrate CSC-defining neurosensory detachments. Impaired RPE-Bruch's complex heralds' formation of choroidal neovascularization above focal areas of pachychoroid (PNV). Excess endoluminal stress due to high flow rates in choroidal circulation can lead to aneurysms resulting in PCV.

RETINAL DETACHMENTS

Retinal detachment refers to the separation of neurosensory retina from the pigment epithelium.

CLASSIFICATION

Rhegmatogenous Retinal Detachment

Rhegmatogenous retinal detachments (RRD) is the most common type of retinal detachment. "Rhegma" is a Greek term meaning "break". Thus in RRD fluid/liquefied vitreous enters subretinal space through a break in neurosensory retina.

Risk factors of RRD include pathological myopia, acute posterior vitreous detachment, trauma and peripheral retinal lesions like lattice degeneration, meridional folds and enclosed or a bays.

The patient presents with acute onset decrease in vision associated with photopsia and floaters. The intraocular pressure is usually lower in the affected eye as compared to the fellow eye. Fundus examination reveals clumps of pigmented cells in vitreous cavity referred as "tobacco dust" or "Shafer sign". The detached retina has convex contour, corrugated appearance and undulates with ocular movements **(Fig. 19.12)**. The retina appears smooth, thin and atrophic with fixed folds resulting from proliferative vitreoretinopathy (PVR) in long-standing RRD.

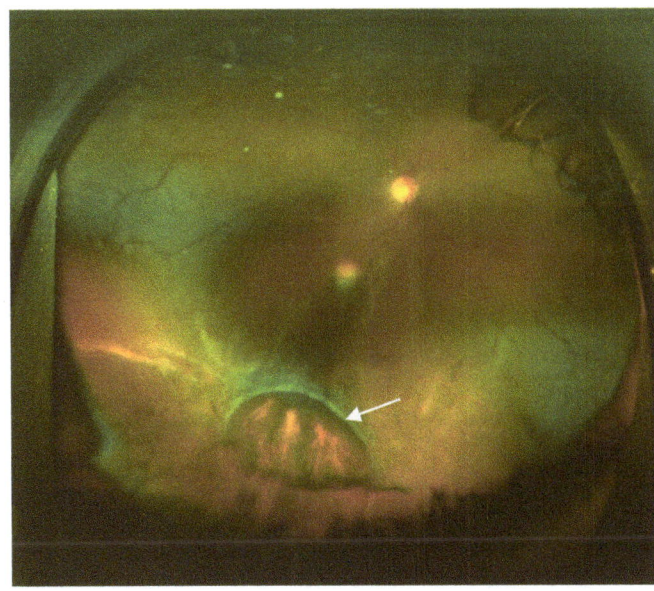

Fig. 19.12: Wide field fundus photograph showing right rhegmatogenous retinal detachment with large retinal break (white arrow).

Management

Management of RRD is surgical. Surgical options include:
- Scleral buckling,
- Pars plana vitrectomy with/without encirclage or
- Pneumatic retinopexy

Basic principles RD surgery include:
- **Finding and sealing of retinal breaks:** All the retinal breaks, are localized and sealed by creating chorioretinal irritation around the break. Cryo or photocoagulation is used to induce aseptic inflammation between retina and choroid.
- **SRF drainage:** SRF drainage is done either externally via sclerotomy or internally by creating a retinotomy. It allows apposition between neurosensory retina and RPE.
- **Removing traction around the break so as to maintain the chorioretinal adhesion:** This can be accomplished by either by an expant (silicone sponge or solid silicone band) or by directly removing the vitreous traction by pars plana vitrectomy followed by internal tamponade.

Tractional Retinal Detachment

Tractional detachments (TRDs) result from contraction of proliferative membranes and is seen in pathologies like proliferative diabetic retinopathy, fibrovascular proliferation secondary to BRVO, retinal vasculitis, and familial exudative vitreoretinopathy (FEVR).

TRD characteristically has smooth concave surface with smooth contour and is immobile. If TRD develops retinal break, it loses its concave surface and assumes a convex shape resulting in combined RD.

Management is surgical. Pars plana vitrectomy is done to release the traction internally. Combination of vitrectomy and a scleral buckling release the traction and seal the break is required in cases of combined RD.

Exudative Retinal Detachment

Exudative detachment results from disruption of outer blood retinal barrier. Fluid accumulates into subretinal space creating a large exudative retinal detachment.

Etiological causes include systemic conditions like malignant hypertension, toxemia of pregnancy, blood dyscrasias or ocular pathologies like inflammation (VKH, sympathetic ophthalmia, posterior scleritis), vascular diseases (central serous retinopathy) and neoplasms (choroidal melanoma, retinoblastoma). Exudative detachments have smooth retinal surface, are convex and demonstrate shifting fluid. Management of exudative retinal detachment requires treatment of the primary cause.

NURSING MANAGEMENT

- **Patient teaching:**
  - Eye surgery is most often done as an outpatient procedure s patient education is vital.
  - Signs and symptoms of complications, especially increased IOP and infection
- Promote the comfort of the patient.
- Patient may need to lie in a special position with pneumatic retinoplexy

Preoperative Care

If the patient is undergoing surgery prepare the patient for surgery.
- Written and informed consent
- Instruct the patient to keep the detached area of the retina in dependent position.
- Cover eye of the patients with some sterile patch.
- Facilitate cleaning the patient's face with antibacterial solution.
- Instruct the patient not to touch the eyes to avoid contamination.
- Administer preoperative medications as ordered.
- To avoid postoperative complications, caution the patient to avoid jerky movements of the head. Also encourage the patient not to cough or sneeze or to perform other straining activities that will increase intraocular pressure.
- Obtain informed consent from the patients/caregivers.
- Make sure regarding the availability of all the things required during surgery.

Postoperative Care

- Administer the prescribed medication for pain, nausea, and vomiting, etc.
- Provide quiet environment to the patient. Encourage diversional activities, such as listening to music, etc.
- Encourage ambulation and independence as per the patient's tolerance.
- Teach proper technique administration of eye medications. If possible, this may be taught in the preoperative period if the patient's condition permits.
- Advise patient to avoid straining or bending the head below the waist for few weeks postoperatively. Also advise the patient to avoid driving till the clearance from ophthalmologist.

Prepare the Patient for Discharge from the Hospital

- Ensure the correct technique of administration of eye drops. Ask the patient or his/her caregivers to demonstrate the correct technique for instilling eye drops.
- Demonstrate and ask them for the return demonstration on eye care. Instruct the patient to follow all the infection control practices at home. Ask him/her to wash their hands before and after removing the dressing.
- Teach the patient to use warm or cold compresses for comfort several times a day.
- The patient may be asked to wear either an eye shield or glasses during the day, during naps, and at night.
- Ask the patient to avoid vigorous activities and heavy lifting exercises till the time getting clearance from the ophthalmologist.
- Teach the patient to recognize the symptoms of retinal detachment such as floating spots, flashing lights, and progressive shadows and to consult their treating doctors immediately.
- Inform the patient regarding the date, time and place of follow up. Also advise them the importance of regular follow up.
- Provide all the instructions in writing only. Also ask the patients/caregivers to repeat the instructions given to them to ensure that they have understood each and every thing.

RETINAL DYSTROPHIES AND DEGENERATIONS

RETINAL DYSTROPHY

Retinal dystrophies and degenerations can be grouped into diffuse photoreceptor dystrophy and macular dystrophies.

Diffuse Photoreceptor Dystrophy

Retinitis Pigmentosa

Retinitis pigmentosa (RP) is a hereditary disease characterized by diffuse involvement of photoreceptors. Primarily rods are involved. Cones may be involved in advanced stages. Patients present with complains of delayed dark adaptation and difficulty in seeing in dark (nyctalopia). In advanced cases, there occurs constriction of peripheral fields resulting in tubular vision. Fundus examination reveals arteriolar narrowing, waxy pallor of optic disc, and bone spicule-like pigmentary changes (**Fig. 19.13**). Diagnosis is clinical based on fundus findings.

Electroretinogram (ERG) shows extinguished waveforms indicating photoreceptor loss. In absence of definitive therapy, management of RP is largely supportive comprising of low vision aids and treatment of CME with oral or topical carbonic anhydrase inhibitors. Recently, gene therapy targeting RPE-65 has been approved by FDA for treatment of RP.

Cone Dystrophies

Cone dystrophies include a heterogeneous group of diseases. Rod photoreceptor may be secondarily involved in some cases resulting cone-rod dystrophies. Usual age at onset is late

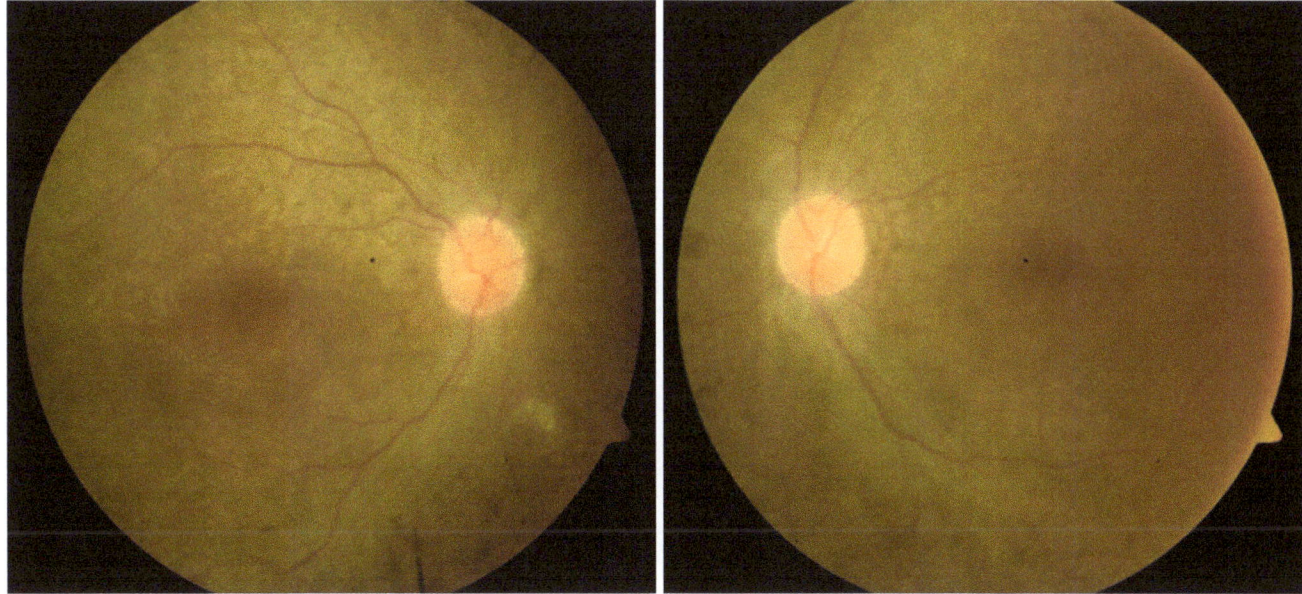

Fig. 19.13: Fundus photographs of right and left eye of a patient with retinitis pigmentosa showing waxy pallor of optic disc, arteriolar narrowing, and diffuse pigmentary changes.

teens or early adulthood. Patients present with progressive loss of visual acuity and color discrimination. Fundus examination shows symmetric bulls-eye maculopathy.

ERG shows extinguished photopic ERG response with near-normal rod response. Additionally, the cone flicker response is delayed.

Macular Dystrophies

Stargardt Disease

Stargardt disease is the most common juvenile macular dystrophy. Mutations in ABCA4, PRPH2, STGD4 and ELOVL4 genes have been implicated in pathogenesis of Stargardt disease. Majority of cases are autosomal recessive while autosomal dominant and X-linked inheritance has also been reported. Patients present with loss of the central visual acuity. Fundus findings include discrete, yellowish, round or irregular lesions at the level of the RPE termed as "flecks" **(Fig. 19.14)**. Another hallmark finding is "dark or silent choroid" on fluorescein angiography due to blocking of choroidal fluorescence by lipofuscin pigment.

Best Vitelliform Dystrophy

Best vitelliform dystrophy or Best disease is characterized by deposition of yellowish/vitelliform deposits in the macular region. Best disease is caused by an autosomal dominant BEST1 (or VMD2), gene. BEST 1 encodes for bestrophin protein, a transmembrane chloride channel located in basolateral plasma membrane of RPE. An abnormal electro-oculogram (EOG) with normal ERG is characteristic of Best disease.

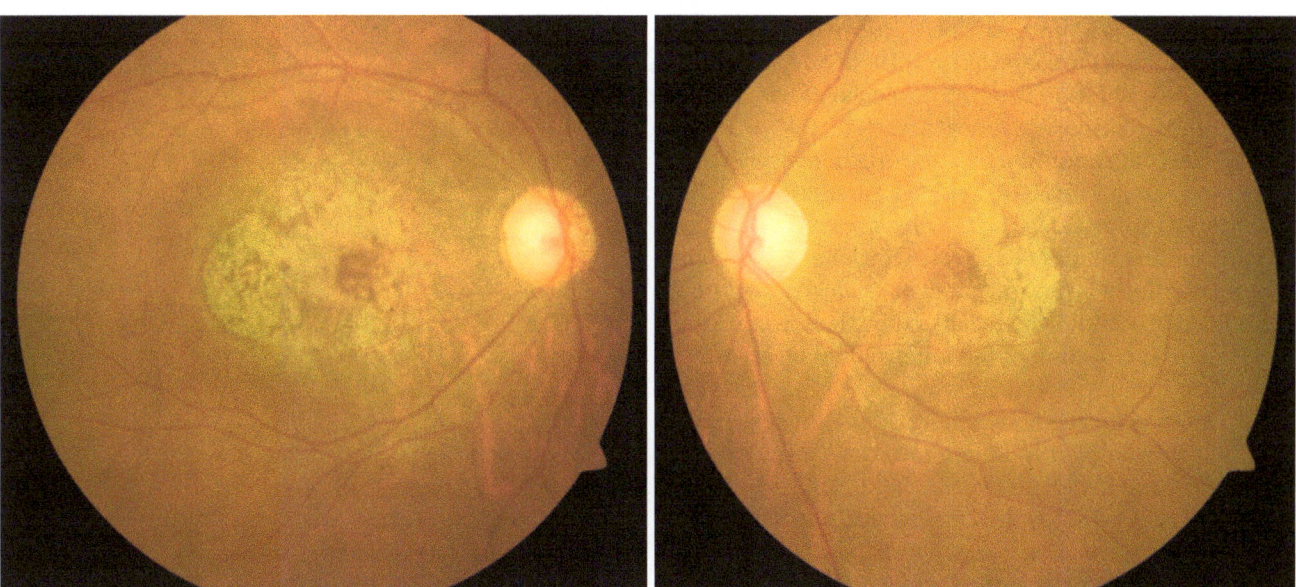

Fig. 19.14: Fundus photographs of right and left eye of a patient with Stargardt disease. Note the bronze-beaten appearance of macula with relatively normal looking retinal periphery.

Pattern Dystrophies

Pattern dystrophies are comprised of group of disorders characterized by:
- Various patterns of yellow or orange pigment deposition in the macular area.
- Autosomal dominant inheritance (most commonly involving mutations in PRPH2).
- Asymptomatic presentation with lesions detected incidentally during routine ophthalmoscopy or complains of mild blurring of visual acuity and/or metamorphopsia.

Pattern dystrophies may be classified into four major patterns according to the distribution of pigment deposits:
1. **Adult-onset foveomacular vitelliform dystrophy:** Adult-onset vitelliform dystrophy is the most common pattern dystrophy. The disease presents in fourth to sixth decade of life. Blurred vision and metamorphopsia may be presenting complaints or the lesions may be picked up incidentally upon fundus examination which shows bilateral round, yellow subfoveal lesions.
2. **Butterfly-type pattern dystrophy:** Butterfly-type pattern dystrophy is characterized by bilateral butterfly-shaped pigmentation in the macular region.
3. **Reticular-type pattern dystrophy:** Reticular pigment of pigmentary changes in macula gives "fish-net" appearance.
4. **Fundus pulverulentus:** Pattern dystrophy characterized by granular appearance of macula.

RETINAL DEGENERATION

Retinal degeneration refers to progressive deterioration of retina due to progressive loss of retinal cells.

Types of Retinal Degeneration

1. **Lattice degeneration:** It is the most common type of peripheral retinal degeneration with incidence of 6–10% in general population and 15–20% in myopic patients. Spindle-shaped area of retinal thinning with atrophic vessels arranged in a lattice pattern with/without pigmentation is the characteristic of lattice degeneration. Lattice degeneration is usually associated with retinal holes and predispose to retinal detachment.
2. **Snail tract degeneration:** A variant of lattice degeneration characterized by frostlike snow-flake areas.
3. **Acquired retinoschisis:** Retinoschisis refers to splitting of neurosensory retina at the level of the inner nuclear and outer plexiform layers. Acquired or *senile retinoschisis is* a bilateral condition characterized by shallow, thin and transparent elevation of the inner retinal layers which produce absolute field defects.
4. **Diffuse chorioretinal degeneration:** Diffuse areas of retinal thinning with depigmentation of underlying choroid. Seen in myopic eyes.
5. **Peripheral cystoid retinal degeneration:** A common degeneration seen in geriatric population.
6. **White-without pressure areas:** Greyish translucent appearance of retina seen without scleral indentation.

GERIATRIC CONSIDERATIONS

Understanding geriatric considerations for vitreoretinal diseases is crucial for nursing students who will be caring for elderly patients. Diabetic retinopathy, vein occlusions, arterial occlusions, age-related macular degeneration (AMD), and retinal degeneration are prevalent among the elderly. Diabetic retinopathy poses the risk of vision loss due to microvascular damage caused by diabetes. Vein and arterial occlusions can lead to retinal ischemia, necessitating prompt intervention to prevent irreversible damage. AMD, a leading cause of blindness, is characterized by central vision loss, affecting daily activities. Retinal degeneration, encompassing various conditions, can result in progressive visual deterioration. Nursing care for geriatric patients with vitreoretinal diseases involves close monitoring, medication administration, lifestyle education, and facilitating access to specialized care, ultimately aiming to preserve and enhance their visual function and overall quality of life.

Case Scenario

1. A 55-year-old male referred to you with a diagnosis of diabetic retinopathy. He was diagnosed with diabetes mellitus 10 years back and he gives history of poorly controlled blood sugars. Recently he noticed gradual onset painless, progressive decrease in vision in both the eyes.
   - Describe how you will approach this patient.
   - What is metabolic syndrome? Describe how will you rule out dyslipidemia, hypertension and investigate nephropathy?
   - What clinical findings you will observe and how will you classify diagnosis of DR?
   - What laboratory investigations you would order?
   - What will be your plan of management if diagnosis is PDR with HRC and patient also has CSME?
   - How would you follow-up the patient?
2. A mother brought her 4-week-old baby who was born at 32 weeks gestational age and 1,400 grams birth weight.
   - Describe the clinical findings of retinopathy of prematurity.
   - If you are a working nursing in the neonatal ICU how will you alert the parents about the possibilities of ROP?
   - Describe how will help in ROP screening?
   - Narrate the classification of ROP.

SUMMARY

Pathological conditions involving retina include vascular disorders, disorders of macula, retinal detachment, retinal dystrophies and degenerations. Each subtype has varied clinical symptoms and signs. Meticulous clinical examination and ancillary investigations like OCT, FFA and FAF are useful for diagnosis and follow up of patients with retinal pathologies.

MULTIPLE CHOICE QUESTIONS

1. All of the following are clinical features of central retinal vein occlusion, *except*:
   a. Neovascularization elsewhere (NVE)
   b. Neovascularization of iris (NVI)
   c. Flame-shaped hemorrhages
   d. Cotton wool spots
2. Risk factors of retinopathy of prematurity (ROP) include:
   a. Prematurity
   b. Low birth weight

c. Oxygen supplementation
d. All of the above

3. **Pachychoroid spectrum of disease include all, *except*:**
   a. CSCR
   b. PCV
   c. PNV
   d. ARMD

4. **Management options for CSME include:**
   a. Anti-VEGF agents
   b. Macular photocoagulation
   c. Intravitreal steroid injection
   d. All of the above

5. **Clinical signs of CNVM include all, *except*:**
   a. Retinal hemorrhage
   b. Intraretinal fluid
   c. Hard exudates
   d. Microaneurysm

ANSWERS

1. a
2. d
3. d
4. d
5. d

SUGGESTED READING

1. Age-Related Eye Disease Study 2 Research Group. Lutein + zeaxanthin and omega-3 fatty acids for age-related macular degeneration: the Age-Related Eye Disease Study 2 (AREDS2) randomized clinical trial. JAMA. 2013;309(19):2005-15.
2. Antonetti DA, Klein R, Gardner TW. Diabetic retinopathy. N Engl J Med. 2012;366(13):1227-39.
3. Brown DM, Campochiaro PA, Bhisitkul RB, et al. Sustained benefits from ranibizumab for macular edema following branch retinal vein occlusion: 12-month outcomes of a phase III study. Ophthalmology. 2011;118(8):1594-602.
4. Brown DM, Kaiser PK, Michels M, et al; ANCHOR Study Group. Ranibizumab versus verteporfin for neovascular age-related macular degeneration. N Engl J Med. 006;355(14):1432-44.
5. Campochiaro PA, Brown DM, Awh CC, et al. Sustained benefits from ranibizumab for macular edema following central retinal vein occlusion: twelve-month outcomes of a phase III study. Ophthalmology. 2011;118(10):2041-9.
6. Central Vein Occlusion Study Group. A randomized clinical trial of early panretinal photocoagulation for ischemic central vein occlusion. The Central Vein Occlusion Study Group N report. Ophthalmology. 1995;102(10):1434-44.
7. Cheung CMG, Lee WK, Koizumi H, et al. Pachychoroid disease. Eye (Lond). 2019;33:14e33.
8. Cideciyan AV, Hauswirth WW, Aleman TS, et al. Human RPE65 gene therapy for Leber congenital amaurosis: persistence of early visual improvements and safety at 1 year. Hum Gene Ther. 2009;20(9):999-1004.
9. Davis MD, Fisher MR, Gangnon RE, et al. Risk factors for high-risk proliferative diabetic retinopathy and severe visual loss: Early Treatment Diabetic Retinopathy Study report 18. Invest Ophthalmol Vis Sci. 1998;39(2):233-52.
10. Davis MD, Gangnon RE, Lee LY, Hubbard LD, Klein BE, Klein R, et al; Age-Related Eye Disease Study Group. The Age-Related Eye Disease Study severity scale for age-related macular degeneration: AREDS Report No. 17. Arch Ophthalmol. 2005;123(11):1484-98.
11. Duker JS, Kaiser PK, Binder S, de Smet MD, Gaudric A, Reichel E, et al. The International Vitreomacular Traction Study Group classification of vitreomacular adhesion, traction, and macular hole. Ophthalmology. 2013;120(12):2611-9.
12. Early Treatment Diabetic Retinopathy Study Research Group Photocoagulation for diabetic macular edema. Early Treatment Diabetic Retinopathy Study report number 1. Arch Ophthalmol. 1985;103:1796-806.
13. Early Treatment for Retinopathy of Prematurity Cooperative Group. Revised indications for the treatment of retinopathy of prematurity: results of the early treatment for retinopathy of prematurity randomized trial. Arch Ophthalmol. 2003;121:1684-94.
14. Fuller JJ, Mason JO III. Retinal vein occlusions: update on diagnostic and therapeutic advances. Focal Points: Clinical Modules for Ophthalmologists. San Francisco: American Academy of Ophthalmology; 2007, module 5.
15. Heier JS, Brown DM, Chong V, et al. Intravitreal aflibercept (VEGF trap-eye) in wet age-related macular degeneration. Ophthalmology. 2012;119(12):2537-48.
16. International Committee for the Classification of Retinopathy of Prematurity. The International classification of retinopathy of prematurity revisited. Arch Ophthalmol. 2005;123:991-9.
17. National Neonatology Forum, India. Evidence-based Clinical Practice Guidelines. Available at: http://www.nnfi.org/images/pdf/nnf_cpg_consolidated_filejanuary 102011.pdf. Accessed on 19 May 2017.
18. Nguyen QD, Brown DM, Marcus DM, Boyer DS, Patel S, Feiner L, et al; RISE and RIDE Research Group. Ranibizumab for diabetic macular edema: results from 2 phase III randomized trials: RISE and RIDE. Ophthalmology. 2012;119(4):789-801.
19. Pascolini D, Mariotti SP. Global estimates of visual impairment: 2010. Br J Ophthalmol. 2012;96(5):614-8.
20. The Diabetic Retinopathy Study Research Group indications for photocoagulation treatment of diabetic retinopathy: Diabetic retinopathy study report no. 14, International Ophthalmology Clinics: Winter. 1987;27(Issue 4):239-53.
21. Wilkinson CP, Ferris FL 3rd, Klein RE, et al. Proposed international clinical diabetic retinopathy and diabetic macular edema disease severity scales. Ophthalmology. 2003;110:1677-82.
22. Wong TY, Mitchell P. Hypertensive retinopathy. N Engl J Med. 2004; 351:2310-7.

CHAPTER 20

Disorders of Sclera and Uvea

Atul Arora, Reema Bansal, Vishali Gupta

"Uveitis: A realm where the eye's silent battles unfold, revealing the profound interplay between inflammation and perception, teaching us that even in darkness, understanding can ignite the light of healing."

—**Atul Arora**

Learning Objectives

After going through the chapter, the learner will be able to:
- Discuss the inflammatory pathologies of scleritis and uveitis.
- Understand stepwise systematic approach for the diagnosis of disorders of sclera and uvea.
- Discuss the management of disorders of sclera and uvea.

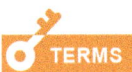

TERMS

- **Band-shaped keratopathy (BSK):** Whitish discoloration of cornea due to deposition of calcium hydroxyapatite crystals in basement membrane, Bowman's layer and anterior stromal lamellae of the corneal epithelium.
- **Choroidal neovascular membrane (CNVM):** Pathological growth of new blood vessels that arise from choriocapillaris layer of choroid and grow in sub-retinal pigment epithelium and sub-retinal space.
- **Cystoid macular edema (CME):** Retinal thickening of the macula due to collection of fluid in outer plexiform layer.
- **Evisceration:** It is a surgical technique by which all intraocular contents are removed while preserving the remaining scleral shell, extraocular muscle attachments, and surrounding orbital adnexa.
- **Fundus autofluorescence (FAF):** A non-invasive retinal imaging modality based on detection of fluorophore (lipofuschin) in retinal pigment epithelium.
- **Fundus fluorescein angiography (FFA):** An invasive retinal imaging modality to examine the retinal circulation.
- **Indocyanine green (ICG) angiography (ICGA):** An invasive imaging modality to examine the circulation of choroid.
- **Intra ocular pressure (IOP):** Fluid pressure inside the eye.
- **Keratic precipitates (KPs):** Inflammatory cellular deposit on corneal endothelium.
- **Optical coherence tomography (OCT):** Non-invasive imaging technique that uses light waves to take cross-section images of retina.
- **Optical coherence tomography angiography (OCTA):** Non-invasive imaging technique to visualize retinal and choroidal vasculature.
- **Pars plana vitrectomy (PPV):** Vitreoretinal surgery technique to access the posterior segment of eye.
- **Synechiae:** These are the adhesions that are formed between adjacent structures within the eye usually as a result of inflammation.
- **Ultrasonography (USG):** A diagnostic technique that utilizes high frequency sound waves to image internal structures of eye.

INTRODUCTION

Sclera forms the outermost tunic of the posterior five-sixth part of eyeball. Sclera is avascular tissue formed by criss-crossing collagen fibers. Throughout its course, it is enveloped by a vascularized layer of connective tissue—tenons capsule. This chapter provides brief overview about pathological conditions involving sclera and uveal tissue.

OVERVIEW OF DISORDERS OF SCLERA AND UVEA

I. **Inflammations of the sclera**
   1. *Episcleritis:*
      - Diffuse episcleritis
      - Nodular episcleritis
   2. *Scleritis:*
      - Anterior scleritis
        - Non-necrotizing scleritis
        - Necrotizing scleritis
      - Posterior scleritis
II. **Inflammation of uvea: Uveitis**
   1. *Anatomical classification:*
      - Anterior uveitis
      - Intermediate uveitis
      - Posterior uveitis
      - Panuveitis
   2. *Endophthalmitis*
   3. *Panophthalmitis*

INFLAMMATION OF THE SCLERA

Episcleritis

It is the inflammation of the episclera (outermost layer of sclera) and overlying tenon's capsule. Sclera tissue as such is spared in episcleritis and is not involved in episcleritis.

Etiology

Episcleritis may be associated with systemic conditions like gout, rosacea and psoriasis. Episcleritis may also result from hypersensitivity reaction to endogenous tubercular or streptococcal toxins.

Clinical Picture

The patient presents with redness, mild pain or ocular discomfort.

Clinical Types

1. **Diffuse episcleritis:** Characterized by diffuse involvement of episclera. Usually, the inflammation involves one to two quadrants.
2. **Nodular episcleritis:** A red to pink colored flat nodule surrounded by localized congestion.

Treatment

Treatment involves a short course of topical steroids for 2–4 weeks. Systemic nonsteroidal anti-inflammatory drugs (NSAIDs) such as indomethacin or flurbiprofen may be required in severe cases.

Scleritis

It is the inflammation of sclera proper. Scleritis is almost always associated with underlying systemic condition and is a serious and visually debilitating condition.

Clinical Features

Moderate to severe pain which makes the patient wake up at night is the presenting and the most characteristic symptom. Localized or diffuse redness, photophobia, watering and decreased vision are other symptoms observed in scleritis.

Classification

Scleritis is classified as anterior scleritis and posterior scleritis.

Anterior Scleritis

There is involvement of sclera anterior to the ora serrata. Anterior scleritis is further classified into:

Non-necrotizing anterior scleritis

It may be diffuse or nodular:
- ❖ **Diffuse scleritis:** Diffuse inflammation involving one or more quadrants of anterior sclera. The inflamed region appears blood red or gives salmon pink appearance **(Figs. 20.1A and B)**. It is the most common type of scleritis.
- ❖ **Nodular scleritis:** It presents with elevated hard whitish nodule with surrounding area of severe congestion and redness **(Fig. 20.1C)**.

Necrotizing anterior scleritis

Characterized by severe localized inflammation along with areas scleral necrosis and thinning. Underlying uveal tissue becomes visible giving brownish hue.

Posterior Scleritis

It involves inflammation of sclera posterior to the ora serrata. Clinical features include exudative retinal detachment, choroidal folds and limitation of ocular movements.

DISORDERS OF UVEAL TISSUE

Uveal tissue represents the middle vascular coat of the eyeball. It comprises of three parts, namely, iris, ciliary body and choroid.

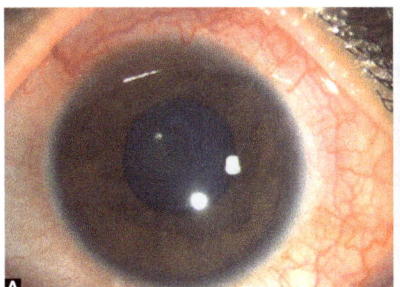 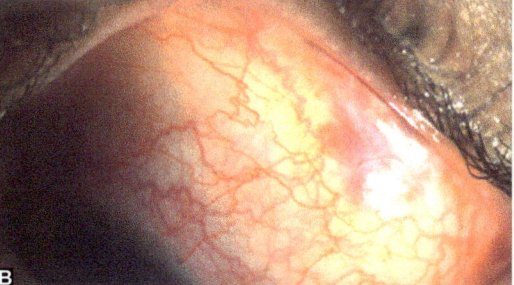 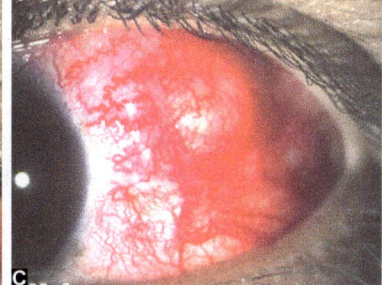

Figs. 20.1A to C: (A and B) A patient with granulomatous polyangiitis presenting with diffuse anterior scleritis; (B) Shows with elevated hard nodule with surrounding area of severe congestion and redness in a patient with nodular scleritis.

Uveitis

Uveitis refers to inflammation of the uvea. The adjacent tissues such as retina, vitreous, sclera and cornea are usually involved in uveitis.

There have been efforts to classify uveitis based on anatomy (the portion of the uvea involved), clinical course (acute, chronic, or recurrent), etiology (infectious or non-infectious), and histology (granulomatous or non-granulomatous). The Standardization of Uveitis Nomenclature (SUN) Working Group in 2005 developed anatomical classification system, descriptors, standardized grading systems, and terminology for uveitis which is now widely followed worldwide.

Clinical Features of Uveitis

The site of inflammation determines the signs and symptoms produced by uveitis. Additionally, the rapidity of onset (sudden or insidious) and the persistence of inflammation affects the clinical presentation.

Anatomical Classification of Uveitis

As per the anatomical classification, uveitis is classified into four categories:
1. **Anterior uveitis:** Inflammation of the uveal tissue involving iris and/or ciliary body.
2. **Intermediate uveitis:** Inflammation of the pars plana and peripheral part choroid. It is also known as 'pars planitis'.
3. **Posterior uveitis:** Inflammation of the choroid (choroiditis) posterior to the pars plana. When associated with inflammation of retina the term *'chorioretinitis'* is used.
4. **Panuveitis:** Inflammation involving the whole of the uvea.

Anterior Uveitis

Symptoms: Pain, photophobia, redness are the presenting features of acute anterior uveitis. Pain and photophobia result from acute inflammation of the iris and associated ciliary spasm. Congestion of circumcorneal vessels results in redness. Chronic anterior uveitis on the other hand has asymptomatic course and the patients present with decreased vision due to complications—band-shaped keratopathy and/or cataract.

Signs: Clinical signs include anterior chamber (AC) cells, flare, endothelial dusting, keratic precipitates (KPs) **(Figs. 20.2A and B)**, iris nodules and/or posterior synechiae.

Intermediate Uveitis

Symptoms: Patients present with floaters and blurred vision. Vitreous cells/membranes cast a shadow when light traverses vitreous cavity resulting in symptoms of floaters. Vitreous opacities along with cystoid macular edema (CME) result in blurred vision.

Signs: Clinical signs include vitreous haze, cells, snowballs, peripheral retinal vascular sheathing/neovascularization.

Posterior Uveitis

Symptoms: Presenting features of posterior uveitis are decrease in visual acuity associated with floaters, metamorphopsia, and/or scotoma.

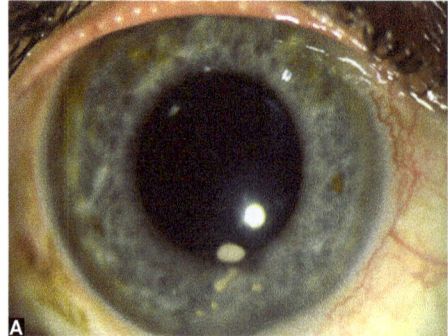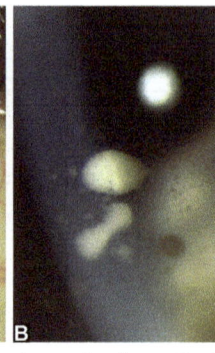

Figs. 20.2A and B: (A) Anterior segment photograph of a patient with granulomatous anterior uveitis; (B) Large keratic precipitates on endothelial surface can be seen in blown up image.

Signs: Fundus examination may reveal vitreous cells, membranes, retinitis and/or choroiditis lesions, CME, retinal vascular sheathing, neovascularization.

Complications and Sequelae of Uveitis

1. **Complicated cataract:** It is a common complication of chronic anterior uveitis.
2. **Secondary glaucoma:** Secondary glaucoma can result from different mechanisms:
   - Clogging of trabecular meshwork with exudates and inflammatory cells
   - Inflammation of trabecular meshwork (trabeculitis).
   - Pupillary block due to posterior synechiae
   - Steroid induced glaucoma
3. **Band-shaped keratopathy:** Whitish band shaped opacification of exposed part of cornea due to deposition of calcium hydroxyapatite crystals. It occurs as a complication of chronic anterior uveitis.
4. **Cyclitic membrane:** In chronic intermediate uveitis, long-standing exudates in the pars plana region organize, undergo fibrosis resulting in formation of fibrotic membrane over ciliary body.
5. **Retinal complications:** These include cystoids macular edema, macular atrophy, choroidal neovascular membrane (CNVM) and tractional retinal detachment.
6. **Phthisis bulbi:** Chronic uveitis leads to ciliary body shut down resulting in soft, shrunken and eventually atrophic globe (phthisis bulbi).

Investigations and Systematic Approach to Diagnosis

A thorough clinical examination allows a clinician to make an accurate anatomical (anterior/intermediate/posterior uveitis) and pathological (granulomatous/non-granulomatous) diagnosis. This narrows down the list of differential diagnoses and subsequently definitive diagnosis can be made with the help of limited number of laboratory investigations **(Flowcharts 20.1 and 20.2)**.

Diagnostic Investigations

Fluorescein Angiography (FA)

Fluorescein dye (10–20% sodium fluorescein) is injected intravenously that reaches the retinal vessels. Upon stimulation with blue light at a wavelength of 465–490 nm, a yellow-green light (520–530 nm) is emitted which is picked up by fundus camera.

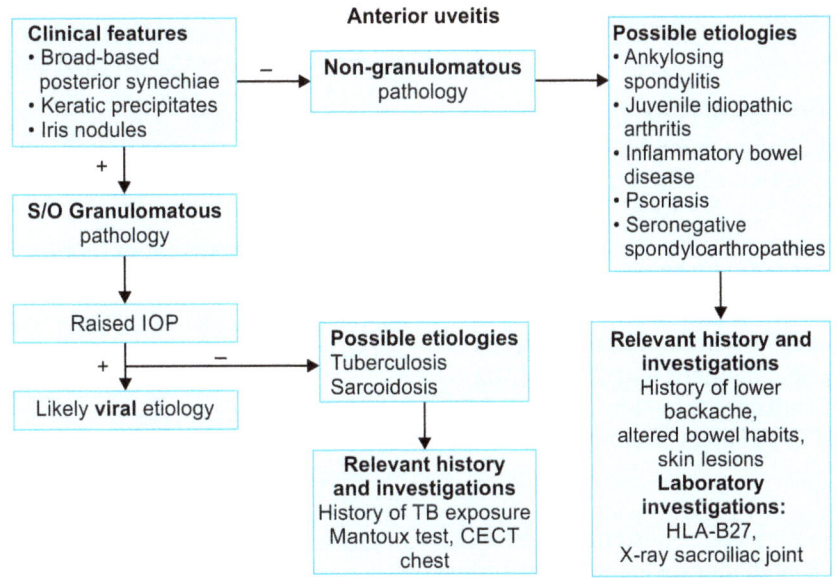

Flowchart 20.1: Systematic approach to a patient presenting with acute anterior uveitis.

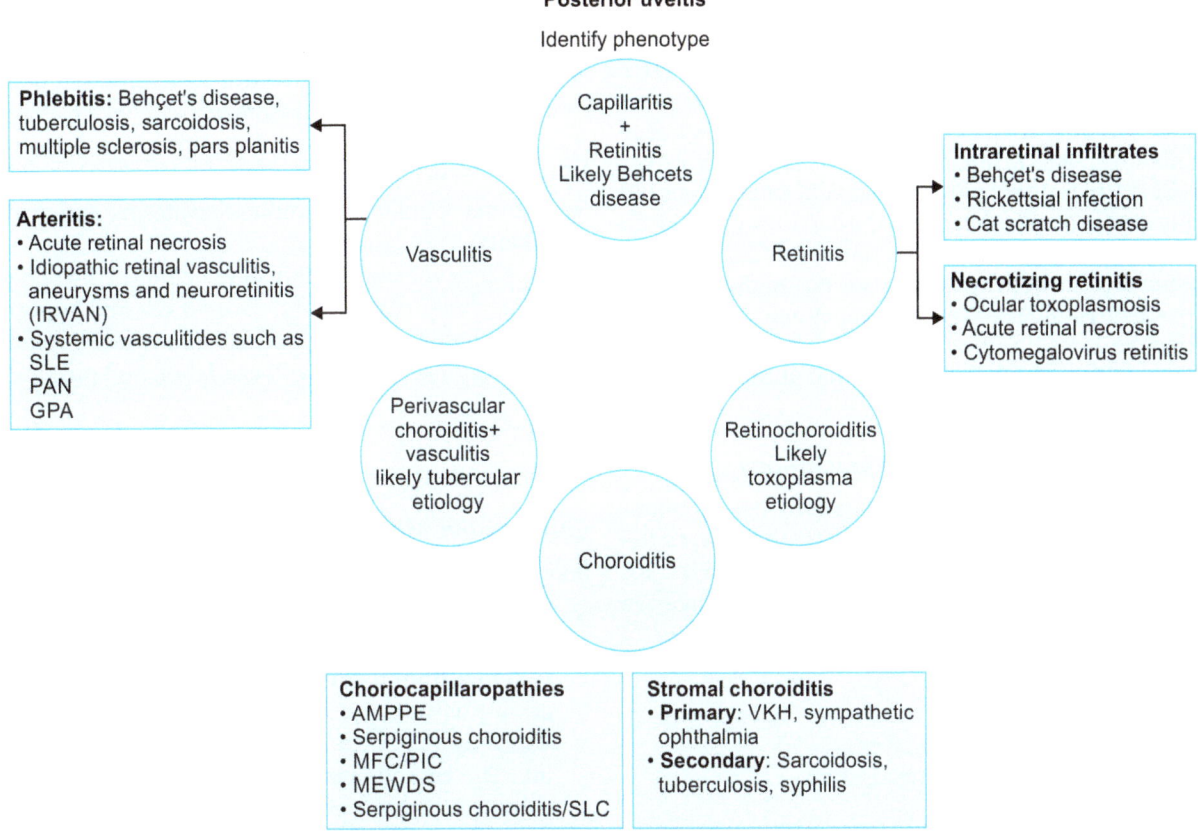

Flowchart 20.2: Systematic approach to establishing etiological diagnosis in a patient of posterior uveitis by identifying clinical phenotype.

FA is useful for making diagnosis and also to monitor response to treatment in retinal vasculitis; guiding scatter laser photocoagulation in occlusive vasculitis with retinal neovascularization. Sympathetic ophthalmia, Vogt Kayanagi Harada (VKH) syndrome; white dot syndromes and several retinochoroidopathies have characteristic appearance on FA.

FFA Procedure

Patient preparation, adverse effects and nursing considerations: FFA procedure is explained to the patient. The pupils are dilated using phenylephrine 5% with tropicamide 0.8%. A 23-gauge butterfly cannula is inserted into an antecubital vein and is held securely by adhesive tape. Sodium fluorescein dye (5 mL of 10–20 % fluorescein) is injected rapidly while cannula remains in place during the procedure for any emergency condition. Adverse reactions range from mild symptoms like nausea, vomiting, sneezing, and pruritis to life-threatening complications—laryngeal edema, bronchospasm, anaphylaxis, and circulatory shock. It is necessary to have access to emergency medications and equipment like laryngoscope, AMBU-bag for resuscitation. Nursing personnel should make sure regarding the availability and working condition of all the equipments. All the health care professionals should be trained in cardiopulmonary resuscitation (CPR).

Indocyanine Green (ICG) Angiography

ICGA uses highly protein bound dye that does not escape from the choriocapillaris and is useful for studying choroidal pathologies.

Fundus Autofluorescence (FAF) Imaging

FAF is a non invasive imaging modality based on fluorescent properties of lipofuscin. It plays an important role in assessment of retinal pigment epithelium (RPE)—photoreceptor complex in inflammatory chorioretinopathies involving outer retina, RPE, and inner choroid.

Ultrasonography (USG)

It provides useful information about posterior segment in presence of media opacities hindering the view of fundus. Vitreous opacities, choroidal thickening, retinal detachment can be easily picked up by USG.

Optical Coherence Tomography (OCT)

OCT allows cross sectional imaging of retina and choroid using low-coherence interferometry. Modern day OCT provides high resolution images of retina enabling detailed evaluation of retinal architecture. OCT is useful to diagnose and monitor response to treatment in uveitic cystoid macular edema (CME); pick up subclinical choroidal granulomas and allows pin-point localization of lesions in retino-choroiditis. Serial choroidal thickness measurements on OCT is useful in monitoring disease activity and recurrence in diseases like Vogt-Koyanagi-Harada (VKH) and sympathetic ophthalmia. VKH disease is defined as a bilateral granulomatous panuveitis with or without extraocular manifestations affecting young adults.

Optical Coherence Tomography Angiography

Optical coherence tomography angiography (OCT) angiography is a novel, non-invasive technique that allows the visualization of retinal vasculature without the need for dye injection. OCTA has the potential to replace invasive investigations like FA and ICGA in near future.

Treatment

Medical Therapy

The goal of medical therapy of uveitis is to:
❖ Control inflammation
❖ Reduce the risk of vision threatening complications like cataracts, glaucoma, CME, and hypotony.

Steroids and Immunomodulatory Agents

Zero tolerance to inflammation is the dictum. Corticosteroids are the best drugs to control acute inflammation. Route and dose are tailored individually depending upon the anatomical distribution (anterior/intermediate/posterior uveitis); systemic involvement and the immune status of the patient. Second-line immunomodulatory drugs are considered in patients with persistent inflammation or multiple recurrences.

Role of Cycloplegic Drugs

Topical cycloplegic drugs are useful for preventing the formation of posterior synechiae or aid in breaking already formed syneciae. They also reduce the symptoms of pain and photophobia by relieving ciliary spasm. 1% atropine sulfate, 2% homatropine or 1% cyclopentolate eyedrops are commonly used topical cycloplegic drugs.

Surgical Management of Uveitis

Surgical intervention is required for complications like complicated cataract, chronic hypotony, vitreous hemorrhage or tractional retinal detachment.

ENDOPHTHALMITIS

Endophthalmitis is the inflammation of the inner coats of eye i.e., uveal tissue and retina associated with accumulation of exudates in the vitreous cavity and/or anterior chamber.

Etiology

❖ **Exogenous endophthalmitis:** Etiological causes include exogenous infection following perforating injuries, infected corneal ulcers or postoperative infections following intraocular surgeries.
❖ **Endogenous endophthalmitis:** Infective organism reaches the eye via bloodstream.

Clinical Features

Symptoms: Ocular pain, redness, watering and significant visual loss.
Signs: Clinical examination shows *conjunctival* chemosis, circumcorneal congestion, Corneal edema, hypopyon in anterior chamber. Fundus examination shows yellow glow and vitreous cavity filled with exudation and pus.

Treatment

An early and aggressive therapy is warranted.

Conservative Management

Role of Antibiotic Therapy

❖ **Intravitreal antibiotics and diagnostic vitreous tap** is done under topical anesthesia from the area of pars plana (4–5 mm from the limbus). Usually antibiotics covering gram positive and gram-negative bacteria are used: Vancomycin 1 mg in 0.1 mL and ceftazidime 2.25 mg in 0.1 mL. The vitreous sample is sent for bacterial and fungal culture and smear examination.
❖ **Topical antibiotics** are started with frequency of (every 30 minute to 1 hourly). Fluoroquinolones (Moxifloxacin) has good ocular penetration and is frequently used.
❖ **Systemic antibiotics** have limited role in the management of endophthalmitis, but is preferred by most retina specialists. Ciprofloxacin intravenous infusion 200 mg BD or orally 500 mg BD for 5–7 days is commonly used.

Role of Steroid Therapy

Steroids limit the tissue damage caused by inflammation. Steroids are started 24–48 hours after instituting antibiotic therapy.

Supportive Therapy

Cycloplegic drugs: Topical cycloplegic drugs reduce the symptoms of pain and photophobia by relieving ciliary spasm. 1% atropine sulcate or 2% homatropine are commonly used topical cycloplegic drugs.

Role of Vitrectomy

Pars plana vitrectomy is performed if the patient shows no improvement with medical therapy for 48–72 hours or in cases of severe disease with visual acuity reduced to light perception. Vitrectomy helps in removal and debulking of vitreous exudates, toxins and inflammatory mediators and aids in better penetration of antibiotics.

Nursing Considerations

Obtaining a good vitreous sample is important. A 10-cc syringe connected to the vitrectomy cutter and manual aspiration is used to collect sample. 4–6 mL of vitreous sample is obtained and transported immediately for microbiological testing: gram stain, KOH mount, bacterial and fungal culture.

PANOPHTHALMITIS

It involves purulent inflammation involving all ocular coats including the Tenon's capsule. Panophthalmitis results from progression of inflammation/infection in cases of endophthalmitis. Mode of infection and causative organisms are similar to that of endophthalmitis.

Clinical Features

Severe ocular pain with complete loss of vision and restriction of ocular movements are the hallmarks of panophthalmitis. In late stages globe perforation may occur at limbus with purulent discharge.

Treatment

There is little scope for conservative management and of globe salvage. Trial of broad spectrum antibiotics along with anti-inflammatory and analgesics can be used for control of inflammation and prevent further spread of infection. *Evisceration* should be performed in case of no response to medical therapy to avoid the risk of dissemination of infection.

GERIATRIC CONSIDERATIONS

Understanding geriatric considerations of uveitis is paramount for healthcare practitioners who care for elderly patients. Uveitis, characterized by inflammation of the eye's uveal tract, can pose unique challenges in the ageing population. As the immune system undergoes changes with age, elderly individuals might experience atypical uveitis symptoms or exhibit systemic conditions that complicate uveitis management. Additionally, the use of systemic medications to manage uveitis requires vigilant monitoring due to potential interactions with medications for other chronic conditions. Careful assessment, tailored treatment plans, regular follow-ups, and patient education are pivotal in addressing uveitis in geriatric individuals, ensuring the preservation of their visual function and overall well-being.

Case Scenario

1. A 35-year-old male referred to you with a diagnosis of acute anterior uveitis. On history patient complained of redness, photophobia and pain in his right eye for a week.
   - Describe detailed history pertained to onset and duration of symptoms.
   - Describe comprehensive ocular evaluation related to his case. Look for circumcorneal congestion, signs of anterior segment inflammation—cells, flare, keratic precipitates, posterior synechiae, pigment on anterior lens surface.
   - Look for any sign of inflammation in posterior segment
   - What is your plan of management if it is first episode of acute anterior uveitis?
   - Describe specific history you will take to rule out different possible etiologies.
   - Describe investigations you would order if any and treatment you will prescribe.
2. A 55-year-old woman presents with redness and throbbing pain in her left eye. The pain is so severe that she wakes up in middle of night. She has recently been diagnosed with granulomatous polyangitis (GPA).
   - Describe the symptoms and signs of scleritis
   - If you are a working nurse in the Uveitis Clinic how will you perform Phenylephrine test to differentiate scleritis from episcleritis?
   - Describe how will you investigate and treat the patient?

SUMMARY

Pathological conditions involving sclera and uvea predominantly include inflammatory conditions. A meticulous clinical examination and stepwise systematic approach is needed to diagnose and manage these inflammatory pathologies.

MULTIPLE CHOICE QUESTIONS

1. **Presentation of ocular tuberculosis include:**
   a. Choroiditis b. Vasculitis
   c. Anterior uveitis d. All of the above
2. **Features of viral anterior uveitis include all, *except*:**
   a. Raised intraocular pressure
   b. Keratic precipitates
   c. Iris atrophy d. Iris heterochromia
3. **All of the following are associated with non-granulomatous anterior uveitis, *except*:**
   a. Sarcoidosis b. Ankylosing spondylitis
   c. Psoriasis d. Inflammatory bowel disease
4. **Which of the following is not a sign of anterior uveitis?**
   a. Cells in anterior chamber b. Flare
   c. Vitritis d. Keratic precipitates
5. **Signs of intermediate uveitis include:**
   a. Snow-balls b. Cystoid macular edema
   c. Vitritis d. All of the above

ANSWERS

1. d   2. d   3. a   4. c
5. d

SUGGESTED READING

1. Jabs DA, Nussenblatt RB, Rosenbaum JT; Standardization of Uveitis Nomenclature (SUN) Working Group. Standardization of uveitis nomenclature for reporting clinical data. Results of the First International Workshop. Am J Ophthalmol. 2005;140(3):509-16.
2. Results of the Endophthalmitis Vitrectomy Study. A randomized trial of immediate vitrectomy and of intravenous antibiotics for the treatment of postoperative bacterial endophthalmitis. Endophthalmitis Vitrectomy Study Group. Arch Ophthalmol. 1995;113(12):1479-96.

CHAPTER 21

Neuro-ophthalmology

Shweta Chaurasia, Kajree Gupta

"The face is a picture of the mind with the eyes as its interpreter."
— Marcus Tullius Cicero

Learning Objectives

After going through the chapter, the learner will be able to:
- Understand the anatomy and function of neurovisual pathway and their defects.
- Discuss basic tests of optic nerve function.
- Know the etiopathogenesis and symptoms of common pathologies of optic nerve.

Terms

- **Optic disc:** Anterior most part of optic nerve or point of exit for ganglion cell axons leaving the eye seen as circular area at the posterior most part of retina.
- **Optic nerve:** Nerve carrying sensory impulses from retina to visual centers in brain.
- **Pupillary reaction:** Reflex response of pupils to light.
- **Visual cortex:** Primary cortical region from brain which receives, integrates, and processes visual information from retina.

INTRODUCTION

The eyes are embryologically an extension of the brain. Neuro-ophthalmology is the study of the eye and its connections with the neurological apparatus. Numerous pathologies of the brain and neurological pathways affect visual function and produce secondary changes within the eye. Similarly, pathology of optic nerves may be initial manifestation of systemic disease and have wide ranging life-threatening consequences requiring urgent attention. For the better understanding of the concept let us discuss first the applied anatomy, physiology and related diagnostic assessments.

APPLIED ANATOMY AND PHYSIOLOGY

Afferent Visual Pathways

Optic Pathway

It consists of four neurons in order **(Fig. 21.1)**:
1. Rods and cones
2. Bipolar cells
3. Ganglion cells
4. Geniculo-calcarine neurons

Retina

Light enters the eye and passes through the optical elements of the eye to reach the retina. Within the photoreceptor layer, the rods and cones initiate the retinal signal and is then processed to the bipolar cells to the ganglion cells. The action potential passes forward to the axons of ganglion cells which converge to form optic nerve and exit the eye.

The ratio of photoreceptor cells to ganglion cells is high in retinal periphery (>1000:1) and lowest at the fovea (1:1) (each ganglion cell is stimulated by a single cone) contributing to higher resolution.

The ganglion cells in the retina have a retinotopic arrangement. Fibers from nasal retina travel directly to reach the disc. Temporal fibers arch in arcuate fashion and reach the disc either at the superior or the inferior pole. Those from the macula enter the disc on its temporal side as the papillomacular bundle. Involvement of the papillomacular

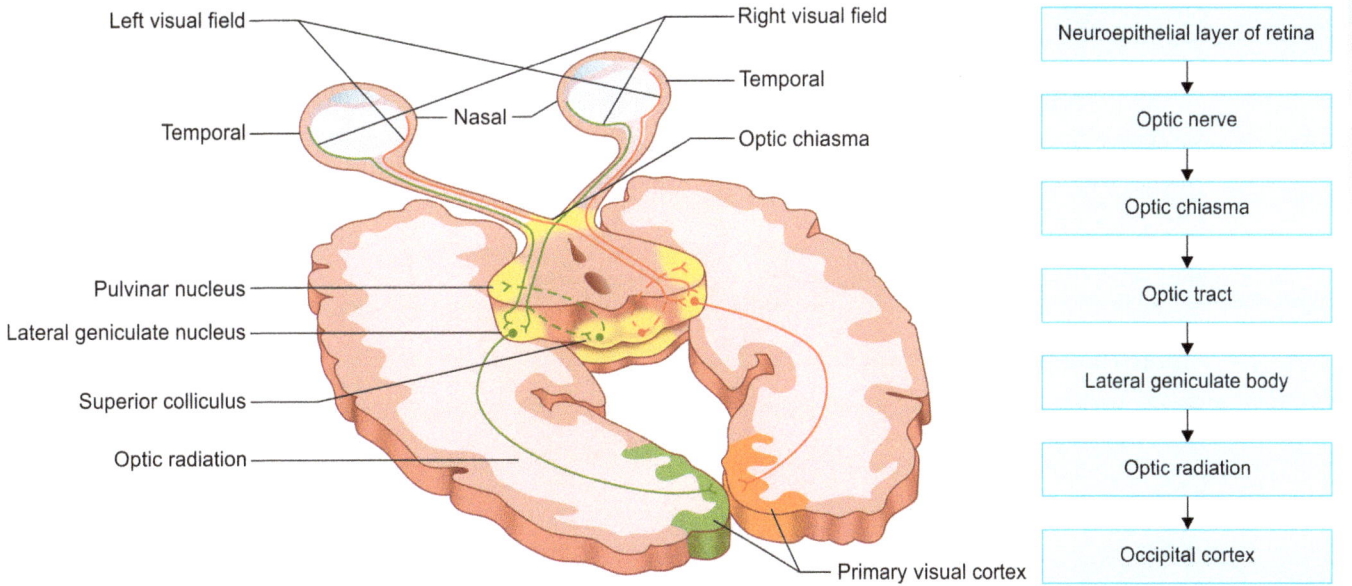

Fig. 21.1: Optic pathway.

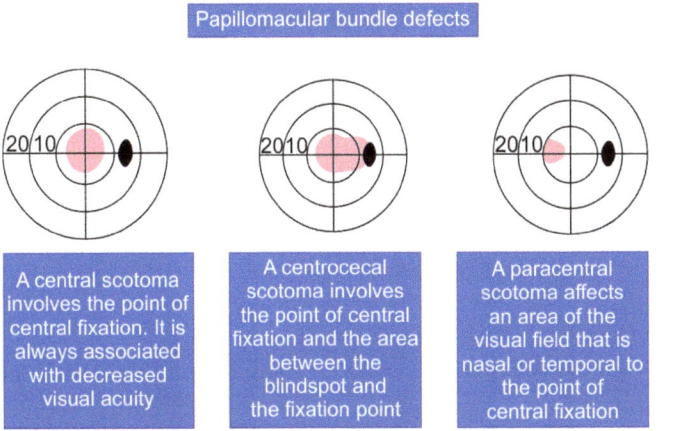

Fig. 21.2: Visual field defects due to papillomacular bundle loss.

bundle can result in central, centrocecal or paracentral scotoma **(Fig. 21.2)**.

The blind spot is a physiological scotoma located 17° from the fovea occurs because the optic disc is devoid of photoreceptors. It measures approximately 5° × 7°.

Optic Nerve

Begins at the optic nerve head consists of 1.2 million retinal ganglion cell axons.

Parts

- Intraocular—1 mm seen as optic disc.
- Intraorbital—30 mm from globe to optic foramen at orbital apex, acquires dural sheath and myelin.
- Intracanalicular—6 mm passes through optic canal and is fixed to it.
- Intracranial—5–16 mm exits the optic canal and reaches the optic chiasm. Injury to optic nerve causes unilateral visual field loss.

Optic Chiasm

Approximately 53% of fibers from the nasal retina decussate to other side to join fibers from temporal retina of contralateral side.

It lies superior to the sella turcica which is a bony structure that houses the pituitary gland **(Fig. 21.3)**. The diaphragm sellae forms the roof of the sella turcica. Because it lies very close to the pituitary gland, the chiasm is affected early in the course of diseases of the pituitary such as adenomas, apoplexy, others tumors such as meningioma and craniopharyngiomas.

Clinical Significance

The optic chiasm consists of fibers from nasal retina which cross over to the other side. Since the nasal retinal fibers receive stimuli from temporal visual field, any insult to optic chiasm results in vision loss in bilateral temporal fields which is referred to as heteronymous bitemporal hemianopia.

Based on its relationship with the sella turcica, anatomical variations of the optic chiasm are described:
- Normo-fixed (majority; 85%) chiasm is situated directly above the diaphragm sellae.
- Pre-fixed (7.5%) when it is anteriorly displaced and is located above tuberculum sellae.
- Post-fixed (8%) when it is posteriorly displaced and located above the dorsum sellae.

Key Points

- Pituitary tumors growing from below compress the inferonasal fibers first, hence begin with superotemporal quadrantanopia before involving both temporal fields.
- Craniopharyngioma growing from below compress the superonasal fibers first hence begin with inferotemporal quadrantanopia before involving both temporal fields.

Optic Tract

- Extends from optic chiasm to lateral geniculate body (LGB)
- LGB is relay center in the thalamus for the visual pathway LGB is located in posterior thalamus and divided into 6 layers: 2 magnocellular (receive input from smaller P-type ganglion cells which are sensitive to spatial resolution and color perception) and 4 parvocellular (receive input from M-type ganglion cells which detect motion) **(Fig. 21.4)**.

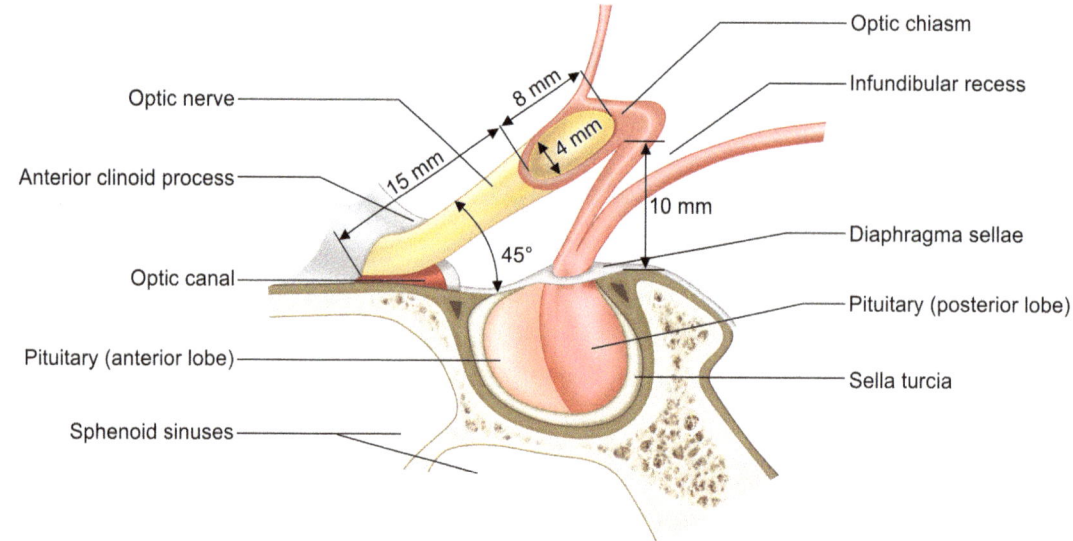

Fig. 21.3: Optic chiasma anatomy.

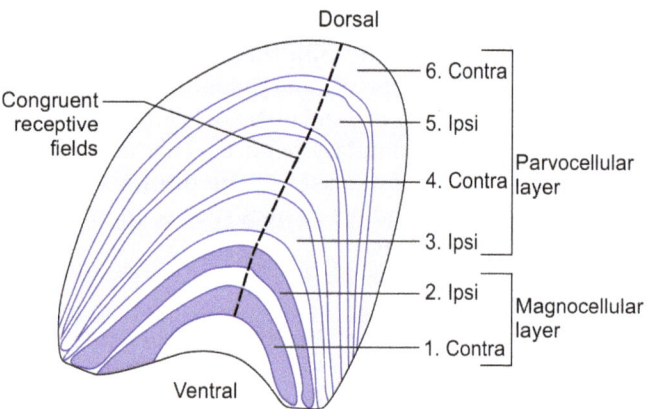

Fig. 21.4: The lateral geniculate nucleus.

- Layers 2, 3 and 5 receive information from the eye on same side.
- Layers 1, 4 and 6 receive information from eye on the contralateral side.

Clinical Significance

Lesions produce homonymous hemianopia (visual field defect that involves either both right or both left halves and respects the vertical midline).

Optic Radiations

Fibers from the LGN travel posteriorly to the visual cortex through the retrolenticular portion of internal capsule and are called as optic radiations.

Clinical Significance

Injury to these fibers produces homonymous hemianopia. It is typically more congruous than anteriorly located lesions.
- Temporal radiations—carry inferior fibers causing pie in the sky field defect.
- Parietal radiations—carry superior fibers causing pie in the floor field defect.

Primary Visual Cortex

The axons that leave the LGN or fibers from optic radiations terminate into V1 visual cortex. The axons from magnocellular and the parvocellular layers go to layer 4 in V1. Other than primary visual cortex axons from LGN also travel to higher cortical areas V2 and V3 (**Fig. 21.5**).

Clinical Significance

- More weightage is given to central vison since 80% of cortex receives input from the macula.
- Posterior circulation stroke involving visual cortex causes a field defect where the macula is spared.
- Head injury causes macular involving homonymous congruous field defects.

Lesions of the Visual Pathway

A number of defects in field of vision (**Fig. 21.6**) may occur due to injury anywhere along the visual pathway. Various clinical presentations can be present depending on the location of defect in afferent visual pathway (**Table 21.1**).

Lesions of the Optic Nerve Anterior to Chiasm

Mono-ocular Blindness

Complete or partial loss of vision in one eye.

Cause

Optic atrophy, optic neuritis, traumatic optic neuropathy.

Clinical features

- Ipsilateral anopia (loss of vision)
- Loss of direct pupillary reaction (same side)
- Loss of consensual pupillary reaction (other side)
- Near or accommodation reflex is present

Junctional Scotomas

Right eye blindness + contralateral left upper quadrantanopia: Seen in sphenoid meningioma (**Fig. 21.7**).

Junctional scotoma formed in lesion of proximal (posterior) part of optic nerve near chiasma due to involvement of Willebrand of knee where inferonasal fibers goes to contralateral optic nerve before crossing to contralateral optic tract.

Lesions Affecting the Chiasma

Bitemporal heteronymous hemianopia:

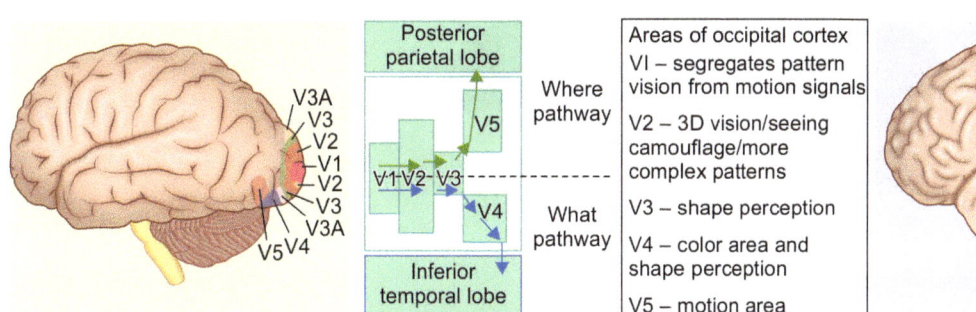

Fig. 21.5: The primary visual cortex.

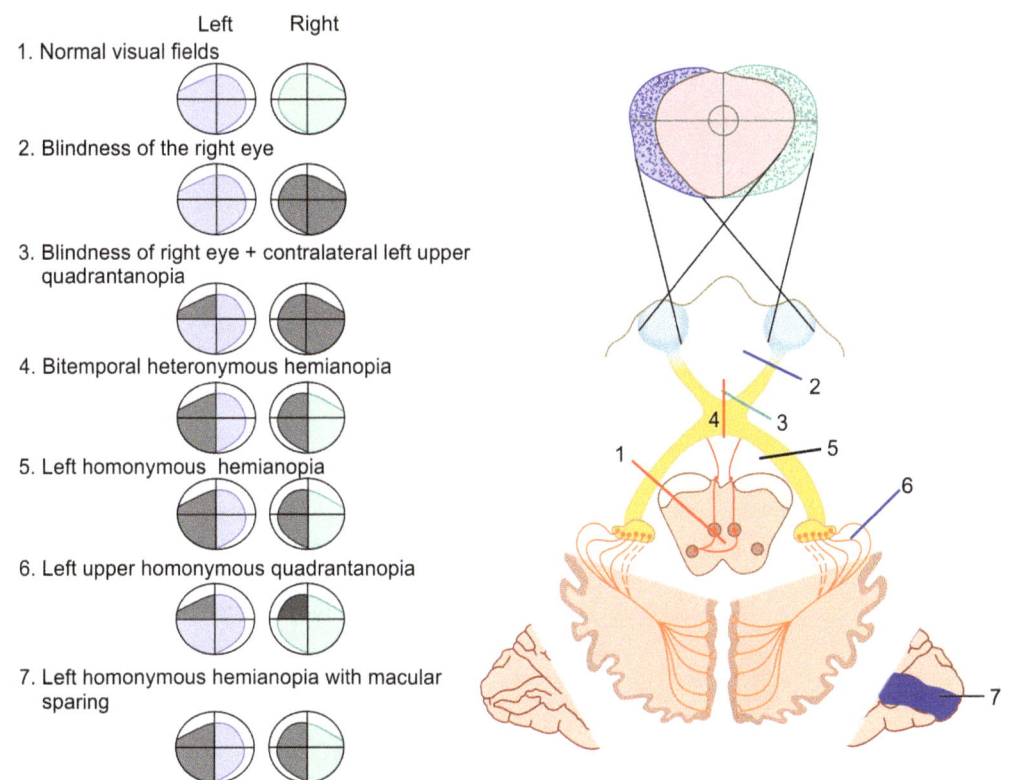

Fig. 21.6: Types of visual field defects and site of lesion.

TABLE 21.1: Differences in clinical features between various locations of afferent visual pathway.

	Optic nerve	Chiasm	Retro-chiasm
Deficit	Monocular	Binocular	Binocular
Acuity	Diminished	Variable	Normal
Pupil (light)	Sluggish	Variable	Normal
Field pattern	Central scotoma	Bitemporal hemianopia	Homonymous hemianopia
Optic disc	Variable pallor	Variable pallor	Normal

Causes

Pituitary adenomas, pituitary apoplexy, meningioma, craniopharyngioma, optic nerve glioma.

Clinical Features

Lesions of optic chiasma (**Fig. 21.8**):
- ❖ **Central chiasmal lesion:**
  - ➢ Bitemporal hemianopia
  - ➢ Bitemporal hemianopic paralysis of pupillary reflex
  - ➢ Partial descending optic atrophy
- ❖ **Lateral chiasma lesion:**
  - ➢ Binasal hemianopia
  - ➢ Binasal hemianopic paralysis of pupillary reflex
  - ➢ Also leads to partial descending optic atrophy
- ❖ **Right homonymous hemianopia (Fig. 21.9):** Lesions of the left optic tract such as tumors, aneurysms, stroke
  Clinical features:
  - ➢ Contralateral incongruous homonymous hemianopia
  - ➢ Contralateral hemianopic pupil (Wernicke's reaction)
  - ➢ Afferent pupillary conduction defect present
  - ➢ Partial descending optic atrophy
- ❖ **Left upper homonymous quadrantanopia:** Lesions of right lateral geniculate body such as stroke, tumors, trauma (extremely rare)
  - ➢ Clinical features of injury to LGB
  - ➢ Incongruous homonymous hemianopia (**Fig. 21.10**)
  - ➢ Pupillary reflexes not affected
  - ➢ Optic atrophy
- ❖ **Lesion of optic radiations (Fig. 21.11):** Any part may be involved.

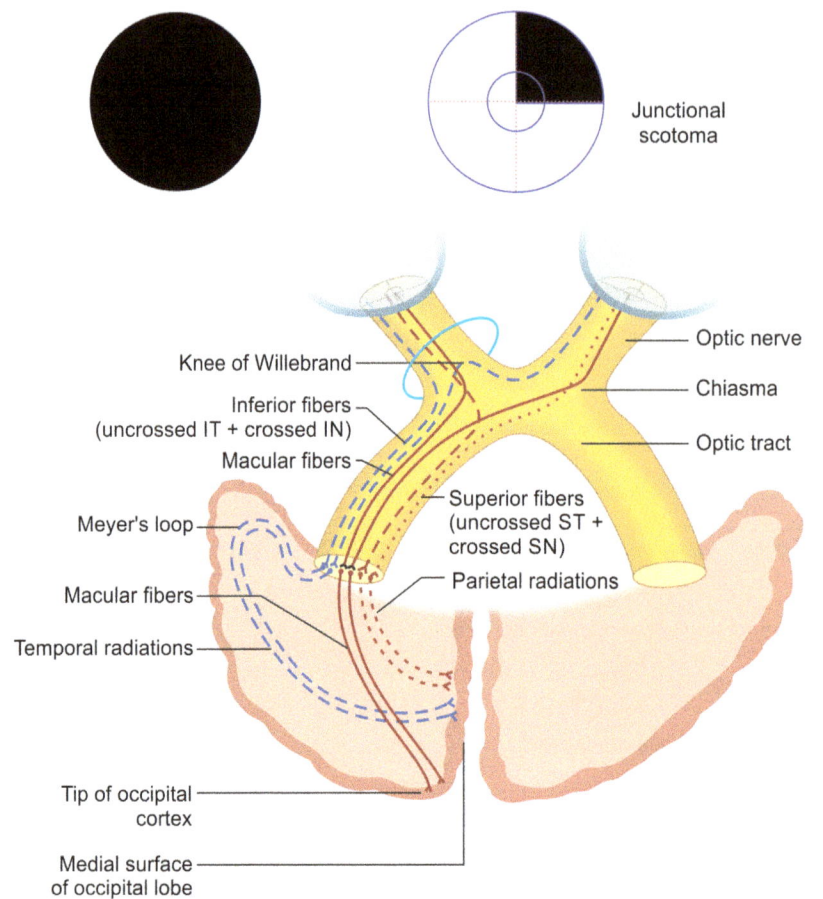

Fig. 21.7: Junctional scotoma due to involvement of Willebrand knee of optic chiasma.

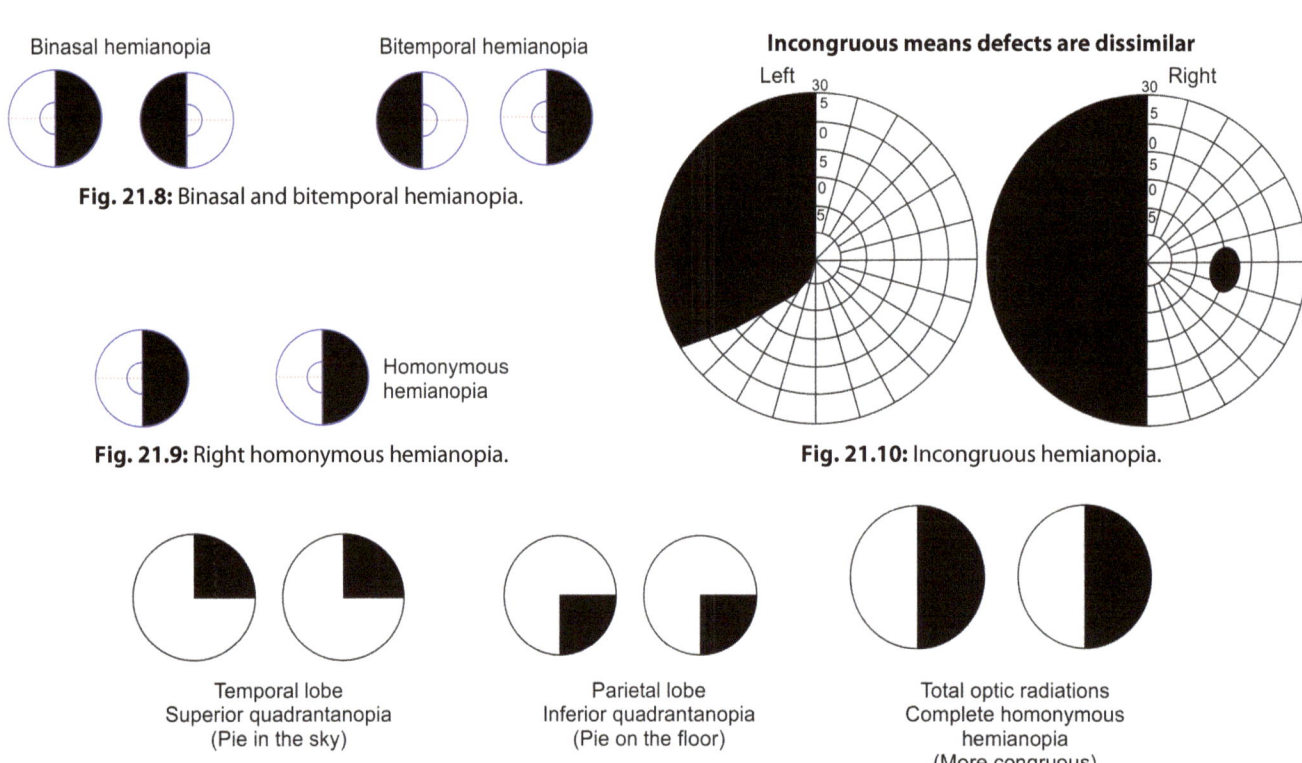

Fig. 21.8: Binasal and bitemporal hemianopia.

Fig. 21.9: Right homonymous hemianopia.

Fig. 21.10: Incongruous hemianopia.

Fig. 21.11: Visual field defects due to involvement of optic radiation.

- **Field defects in lesions of visual cortex (Fig. 21.12):** Lesions of occipital cortex such as posterior stroke, head trauma

Common Causes of Lesions of Visual Cortex

- Vascular lesions in territory of PCA
- Trauma—gunshot injury of fall on the back of head
- Cerebral tumors—primary or metastatic

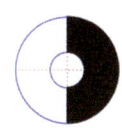 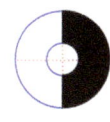 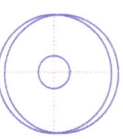 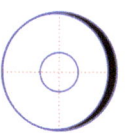

Tip of occipital cortex	Tip of occipital cortex	Anterior most part of visual cortex
Central homonymous hemianopia	Homonymous hemianopia with macular sparing	Contralateral temporal crescentic field defect

Fig. 21.12: Visual field defect due to involvement of visual cortex.

Efferent Visual System

Visual acuity drops off 50% at 2-degree eccentricity. Images are clearest when held within 0.5 degree from fovea.

Basic Circuit

- **Cortical/frontal eye field:** Planning
- **Basal ganglia, thalamus, superior colliculus:** Modulation supranuclear
- **Cerebellum:** Optimization

} Supranuclear

Brainstem nuclei: PULSE and STEP signal generators—nuclear

- Cranial nerve infranuclear
- EOM

} Supranuclear

Types of Eye Movements

- Visual fixation
- Saccades
- Smooth pursuit
- Vestibular
- Optokinetic
- Vergence

Fixation System

The fixation system is utilized in looking at a stationary object. Fixation system originates in the occipital lobe. It maintains fixation of stationary objects without retinal adaptation.

Saccadic System

Saccades are rapid, brief conjugate eye movements that are characterized by their high velocity (400–800°/s) and ballistic nature. These shift the line of gaze from one part of visual field to another while trying to acquire a new object of interest. Frontal eye fields (FEFs) control the voluntary saccades whereas involuntary saccades are initiated by superior colliculus. Both receive additional information inputs from the cortical and subcortical structures of brain which in-turn stimulate horizontal and vertical brainstem gaze centers.

Pursuit System

The smooth pursuit system are slow eye movements (30–40°/s) that come into play while tracking a moving object (of interest) with eyes fixated on it and corrects for any retinal slip. The smooth pursuit system is driven by the visual motion sensed by the striate cortex through pathways that connect the cortical centers in the temporal and the frontal lobe with pursuit-related areas in the brainstem and the cerebellum. Recent evidence also implicates role of superior colliculus in inducing smooth pursuit.

Upward pursuit pathways decussate in the posterior commissure before projecting to the final common pathway. A lesion in the posterior commissure thus causes upward gaze palsy. Fibers for the downward gaze pass ventral to the cerebral aqueduct and are thus spared in posterior commissural lesions.

Vestibular System

The vestibular system stabilizes the eyes on object of interest during brief head motions. This is achieved by compensatory eye movements of similar velocity to the head motion but in an opposite direction. This eye movement termed as vestibulo-ocular reflex (VOR) is produced by the semicircular canals, vestibular nuclei, and flocculonodular lobe of the cerebellum. These vestibulo-ocular movements do not let the image slide away from its position on the retina as the head moves by moving the eyes in a reverse direction.

Optokinetic System

Optokinetic system takes over from vestibular system when the head movements are of large amplitude and too rapid in nature. The pathways are similar to that of the smooth pursuit system.

Vergence System

It is required during the depth tracking of an object. This system has its origins in the parietal, occipital, and frontal regions.

Pathways for Coordinating Conjugate Eye Movements

The motor system of the eye aims for stable, clear binocular vision through.

- Gaze shift
- Gaze stabilization

The pathways for saccades and pursuits reach the brainstem from supranuclear pathways which enable conjugated movements of the eyes.

Gaze Control

- **Vertical: Midbrain**
  - The primary vertical gaze center lies in the rostral interstitial MLF (riMLF)
- **Horizontal: Pons**
  - The primary horizontal gaze center lies in parapontine reticular formation (PPRF) in the brainstem.

Gaze Disorders

Internuclear Ophthalmoplegia

It is a disorder of ocular movement in which the interneuron called medial longitudinal fasciculus (MLF) is damaged. The MLF connects the nucleus of cranial nerve 3 of same side with parapontine reticular formation (PPRF) and cranial nerve 6 of the contralateral side. Information from higher cortical centers travels via the PPRF to ipsilateral 6th nerve and lateral rectus muscle and to contralateral medial rectus via MLF. Horizontal eye movement is produced when the ipsilateral lateral rectus and contralateral medial rectus are activated.

Etiology

Demyelination due to multiple sclerosis is common in young females. Stroke is more common in elderly. Other causes include trauma, tumors, inflammatory causes such as sarcoidosis, Behcet's disease, infectious causes such as cryptococcus, Lyme disease.

Clinical Features

- **Symptoms:** Patients complain of acute onset diplopia in a particular gaze. Visible squint may be present.
- **Signs:** An adduction deficit may be complete or partial on ipsilateral side with an abducting saccade on contralateral side on attempting to gaze towards the side opposite the lesion **(Fig. 21.13)**.

Management

Neuroimaging such as CT scan or MRI to find out the etiology such as stroke, multiple sclerosis is done. Management of stroke with antiplatelets and control of hypertension, diabetes, with consultation of neurologist. If multiple sclerosis is the cause, then immunosuppressive treatment is required. Management of inflammatory or infectious causes with high dose intravenous steroids may be helpful.

Vertical Gaze Palsy

- **Supranuclear gaze palsy/Steele-Richardson-Olszewski syndrome characterized by:**
  - Progressive supranuclear palsy typically vertical but in particular downward limitation of eye movement.
  - There is an associated paralysis of convergence.

  It is late onset tauopathy. It is called supranuclear because tau proteins assimilate in basal ganglia and brainstem which lie above nuclei controlling movement of eyes therefore called supranuclear.
- **Parinaud (dorsal midbrain) syndrome:** The dorsal midbrain is usually affected. Tumors in the area of the pineal gland such as germinoma and pineocytoma are

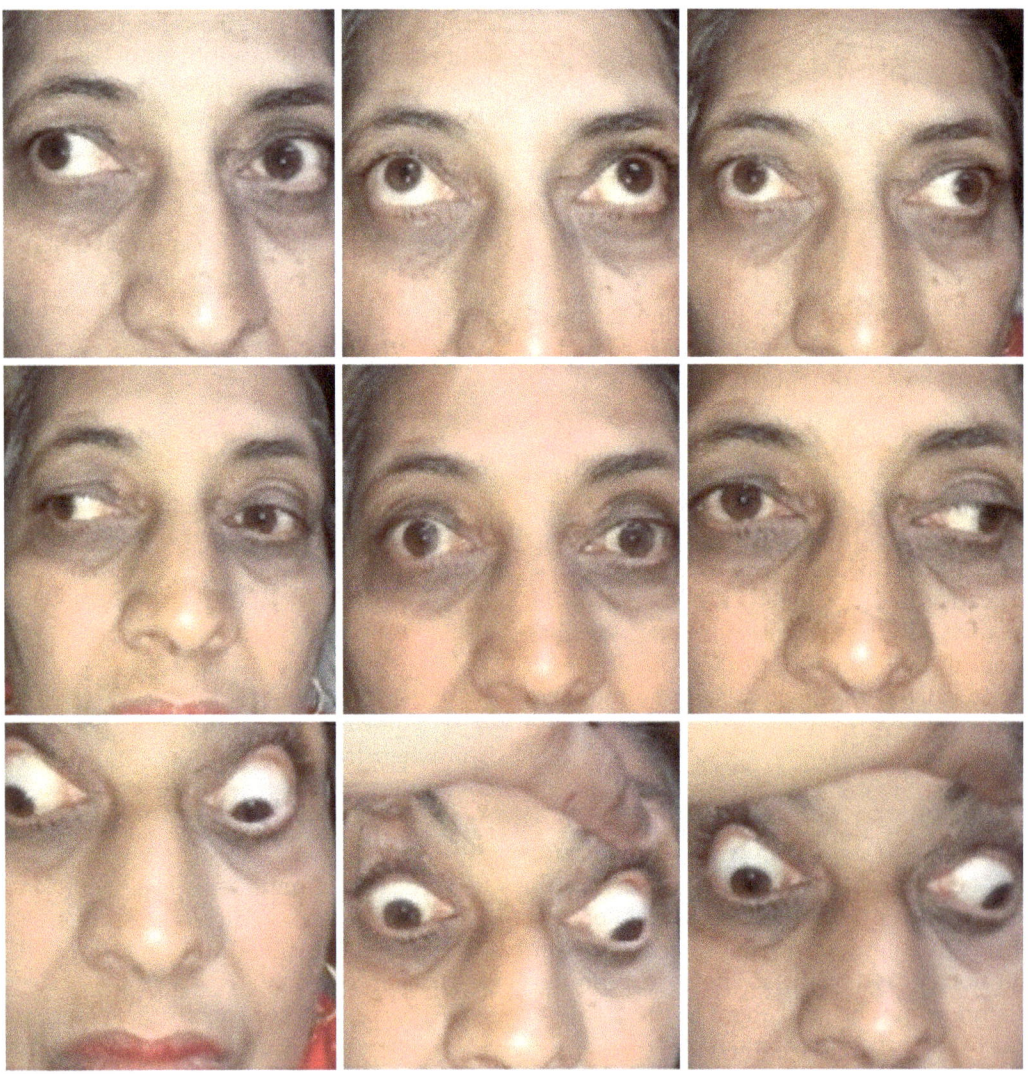

Fig. 21.13: Right internuclear ophthalmoplegia showing right eye adduction deficit and an abduction saccade in left on attempted levoversion.

the most common causes but may also be due to ischemic stroke or hemorrhage.

Clinical Features
- Up-gaze palsy with eyes in downgaze called as sun setting sign.
- Convergence-retraction nystagmus characterized by irregular, oscillatory movements.
- Light reflex is poor, but pupil constricts with convergence (light near dissociation)
- Bilateral lid retraction (Collier)
- Convergence insufficiency
- Ataxia
- Papilledema

Treatment consists of addressing the underlying condition.

CRANIAL NERVES (NEUROANATOMY AND APPLIED)

Third Cranial Nerve

It is primarily a motor nerve and also contains parasympathetic supply. It innervates the following muscles.
- Levator palpebrae superioris
- Superior rectus
- Inferior rectus
- Medial rectus
- Inferior oblique

Anatomy (Fig. 21.14)

- **Nuclear complex**: Situated in the midbrain at the level of superior colliculus. It consists of paired and unpaired nuclei.
- **Fasciculus**: Fibers from the nucleus travel ventrally through the cerebral peduncle to emerge from midbrain. These enter the interpeduncular space.
- **Basilar**: The rootlets emerge from the midbrain and join to form the nerve. It passes in between the posterior cerebral and superior cerebellar arteries.

Lesions here commonly cause isolated 3rd nerve palsy. Common causes include aneurysm of posterior communicating artery and head trauma (extradural or subdural hematoma).
- **Intra-cavernous**: It then enters the cavernous sinus and travels in the lateral wall of the sinus. It lies in superior relation to the 4th nerve. It divides into superior and inferior branches in the anterior part of sinus and passes through superior orbital fissure into the orbit.

Here 3rd nerve palsy commonly occurs with involvement of 4th, 5th, 6th nerve.
- **Intra-orbital**: Superior division supplies the superior rectus and levator muscles. Inferior division supplies the medial rectus, inferior oblique and inferior rectus muscles.

Pupillomotor Fibers

These parasympathetic fibers supplying the iris sphincter are present peripherally in the superomedial part of the 3rd nerve **(Fig. 21.15)**.
- **Surgical lesions**: Aneurysms, trauma characteristically involve the pupil.
- **Medical lesions**: Microangiopathy in hypertension and diabetes spare the pupil.

Signs of 3rd Nerve Palsy (Figs. 21.16 and 21.17)

- Ptosis
- **Down and out eye**: Abduction and depression in primary position
- Limited adduction, elevation, depression with normal abduction
- Dilated pupil and defective accommodation **(Fig. 21.18)**
- Limitation of movements on adduction, elevation and depression. Abduction is normal.

Fourth Nerve

It supplies the superior oblique muscle.

It emerges from dorsal aspect of brain (susceptible to head trauma) **(Fig. 21.19)**:
- **Nucleus**: Situated in midbrain at the level of inferior colliculi inferior to 3rd nerve nucleus. It lies ventral to aqueduct of Sylvius.
- **Fasciculus**: Axons travel posteriorly around the aqueduct and decussate in the anterior medullary velum.

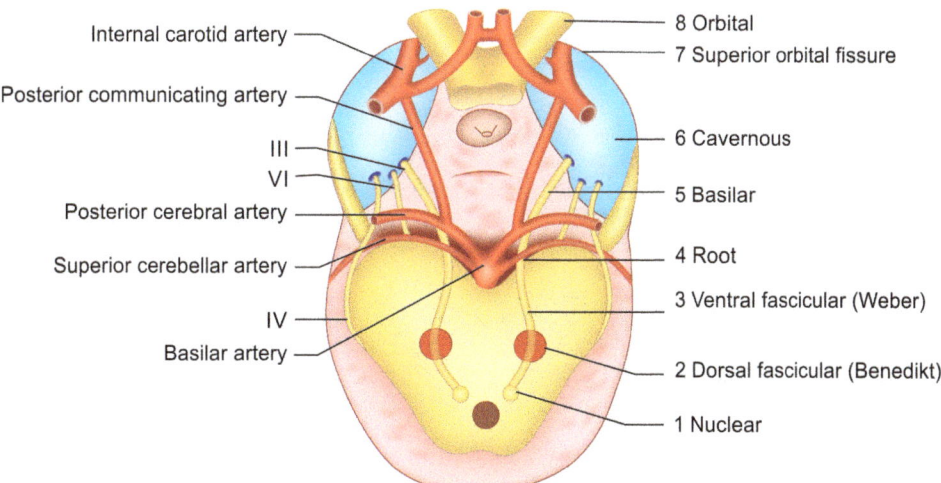

Fig. 21.14: 3rd nerve anatomy.

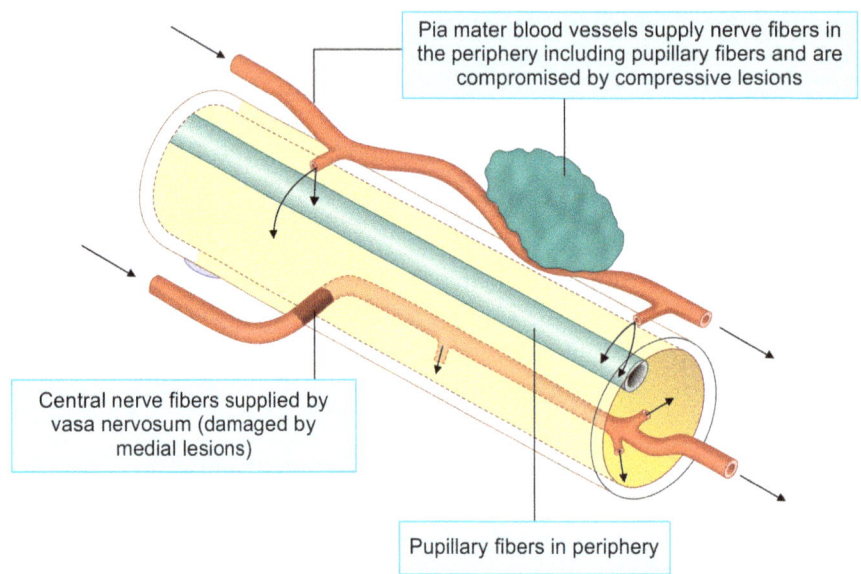

Fig. 21.15: Pupillary fibers located in periphery of 3rd nerve.

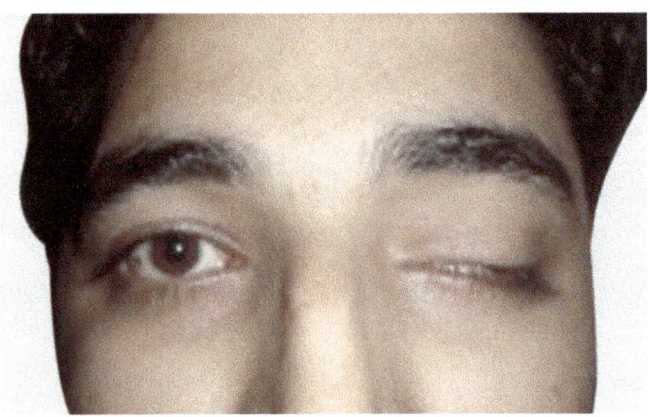

Fig. 21.16: Severe left eye ptosis in a patient with left 3rd nerve palsy.

- **Trunk:** Exits the brainstem from dorsal side and curves laterally around the brainstem, then passes between the posterior cerebral artery and superior cerebellar artery. It then enters the cavernous sinus by piercing the dura.
- **Intra-cavernous part:** Runs in the lateral wall of the sinus below the 3rd nerve and above the 5th nerve. It then passes through the superior orbital fissure into the orbit.
- **Intra-orbital part:** Supplies superior oblique 4th nerve palsy (**Fig. 21.20**).

Causes

Idiopathic, trauma microvascular lesions, tumors, aneurysms.

Signs of 4th Nerve Palsy

- Head tilt in direction away from affected muscle
- Ipsilateral hypertropia and excyclotorsion
- Positive Parks-Bielchowsky 3 step test

Sixth Nerve

It gives motor supply to the lateral rectus muscle.

Anatomy (Fig. 21.21)

- **Nucleus:** Lies at the level of the mid-pons. The fibers leave the brainstem ventrally at the pontomedullary junction.
- **Basilar part:** Enters the prepontine cistern close to the base of the skull. It pierces the dura passes over the tip of the petrous bone through the Dorello canal (below the petroclinoid ligament) to enter the cavernous sinus.

Raised intracranial pressure causes downward displacement of brainstem which stretches the 6th

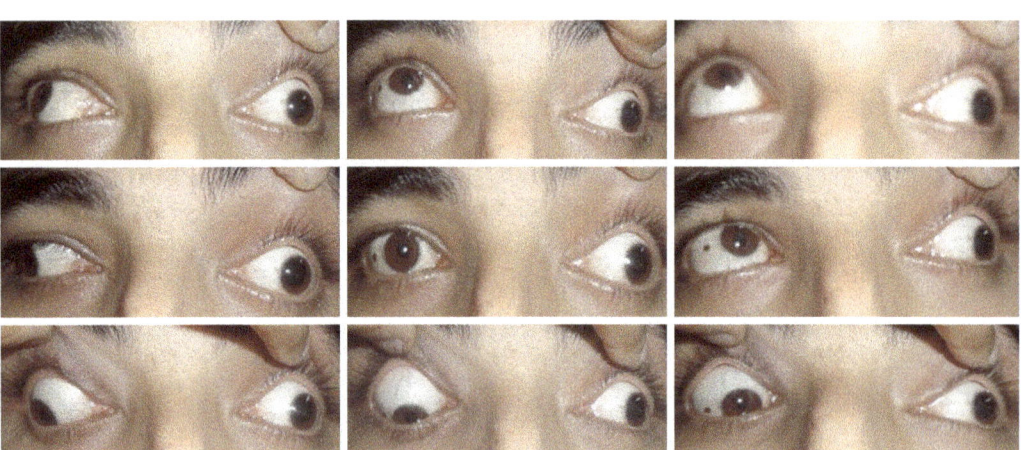

Fig. 21.17: Left eye 3rd nerve palsy: Primary position shows down and out left eye.

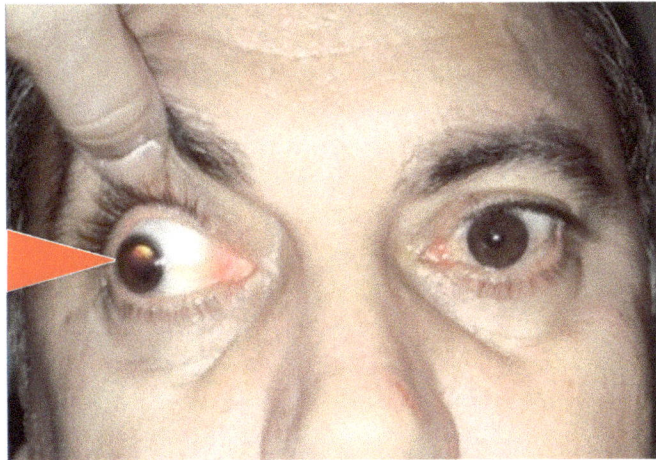

Fig. 21.18: Pupil involving right 3rd nerve palsy with ptosis and 'down and out' eye in primary position.

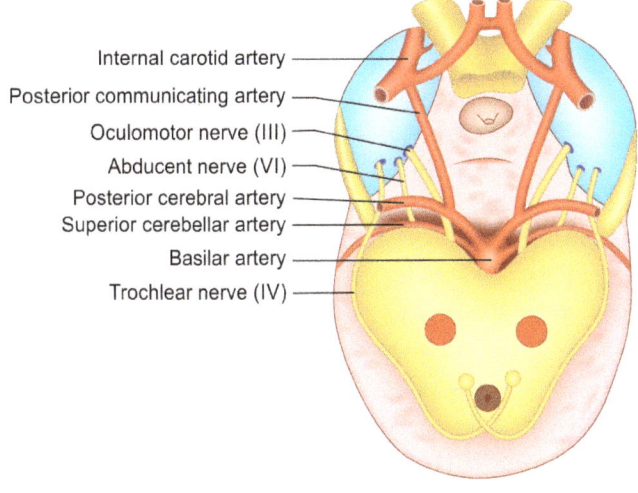

Fig. 21.19: 4th nerve anatomy.

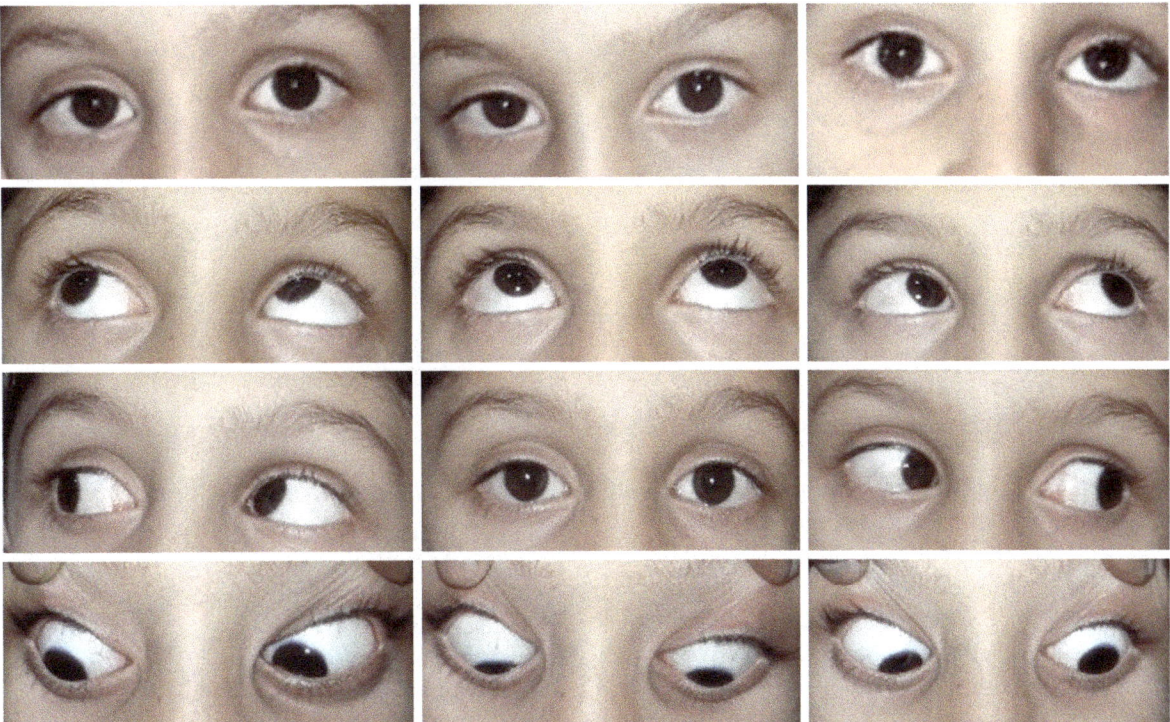

Fig. 21.20: Left superior oblique paralysis. The upper left photograph demonstrates face turn to right and head tilt to right. On tilting head to left, there is worsening of left hypertropia which improves on tilt to right. In the 9 cardinal gazes, eyes appear aligned in primary position, but left superior oblique underaction is seen on dextrodepression and inferior oblique overaction seen on dextroelevation and dextroversion.

nerve at the petrous tip, which causes 6th nerve paresis and is a false localizing sign.
- **Intra-cavernous part:** Runs through the middle of the sinus and is closely situated to the internal carotid artery.
- **Intra-orbital part:** It enters through the superior orbital fissure to innervate lateral rectus muscle.

Signs of 6th Nerve Palsy (Fig. 21.22)
- Limitation of abduction
- Normal elevation, depression and adduction

Investigations in Cranial Nerve Palsies
Measurement of blood pressure, blood sugar levels, lipid profile to assess vascular risk factors.

Indications for Neuroimaging in the form of CT Scan or MRI
- Children with nerve palsies
- Patients less than <50 years
- Patients >50 years of age without vasculopathic risk factors
- Multiple cranial nerve palsies
- CT angiography if suspicion of aneurysm is present.

Treatment of Cranial Nerve Palsies
Nerve palsies are initially observed in microvascular causes. Most resolve within weeks or months. If diplopia is present, it can be treated temporarily by fogging or prisms. Surgical improvement of ocular motility and squint is indicated if spontaneous improvement does not occur after 6–12 months. In case of specific causes such as aneurysms,

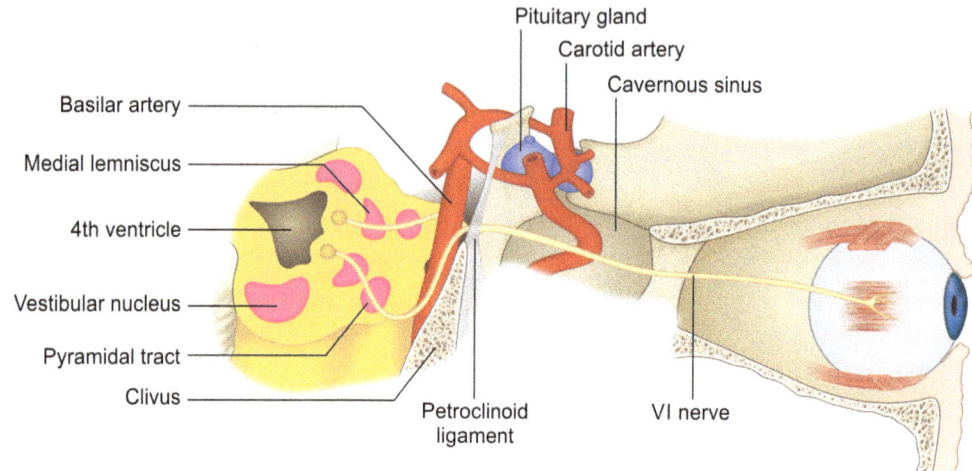

Fig. 21.21: 6th nerve anatomy.

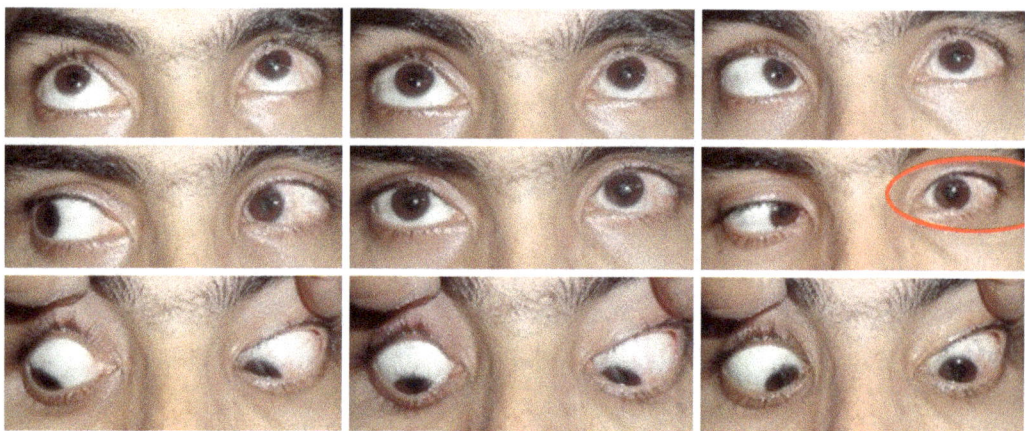

Fig. 21.22: Left 6th nerve palsy showing limitation of abduction. Normal elevation, depression and adduction.

the specific cause is treated first. Squint surgery should always be performed before ptosis surgery.

Multiple Cranial Nerve Palsies

The orbital apex is the posterior most part of orbit where 4 orbital walls converge at the craniofacial junction. It contains 3 main orifices within the sphenoid bone **(Fig. 21.23)**.

- **Superior orbital fissure:** It is the aperture between the lesser and greater wings of the sphenoid. It is comma-shaped, appearing bulbous inferiorly and thin superolaterally. It communicates between orbit and middle cranial cavity.
- **Inferior orbital fissure:** Lies between lateral wall and floor of orbit.
- **Optic foramen:** It lies within lesser wing of sphenoid. The optic nerve, ophthalmic artery and sympathetic arteries pass through it.

Annulus of Zinn

- It is a fibrous ring formed by the common origin of the 4 rectus muscles.
- It encircles the optic foramen and the central portion of the superior orbital fissure.
- The portion of the orbital apex enclosed by the annulus is called the oculomotor foramen. It encircles central part of superior orbital fissure, dividing it into superior, middle, inferior parts.

Structures Passing Through Superior Orbital Fissure

- Superior part **(Fig. 21.24)**:
  - Trochlear nerve
  - Frontal nerve
  - Lacrimal nerve
  - Superior ophthalmic vein
  - Recurrent branch of lacrimal artery
- **Middle part:**
  - Oculomotor nerve (superior and inferior branches)
  - Nasociliary nerve
  - Abducent nerve
  - Fibers from internal carotid sympathetic plexus
- **Inferior part:** Inferior ophthalmic vein

Optic Canal

Posterior continuation of optic foramen through which orbit connects with middle cranial fossa. The lateral wall is shortest, medial wall is longest.

Structures passing through it:
- Optic nerve and its meningeal covering
- Ophthalmic artery
- Sympathetic arteries

Cavernous Sinus (Fig. 21.25)

- Cavernous sinus is a paired structure.
- It is the space between the superior orbital fissure anteriorly, the petrous apex posteriorly.

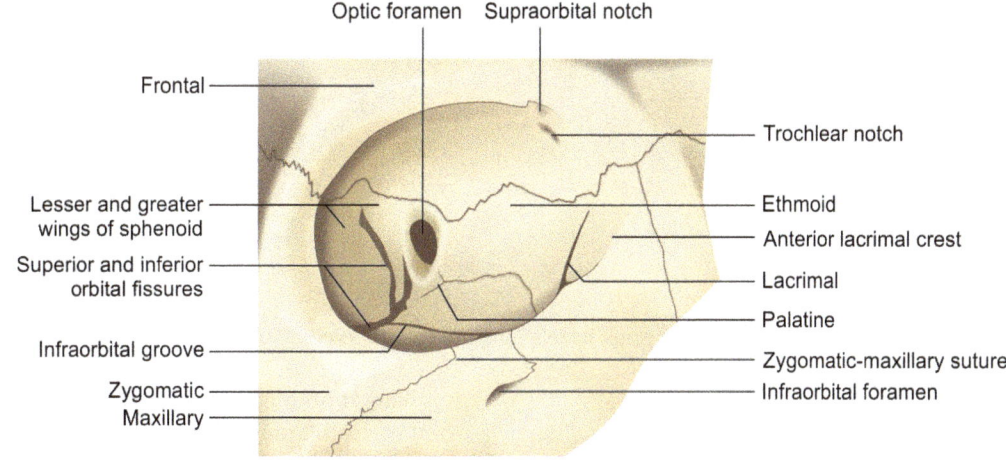

Fig. 21.23: Orbital anatomy.

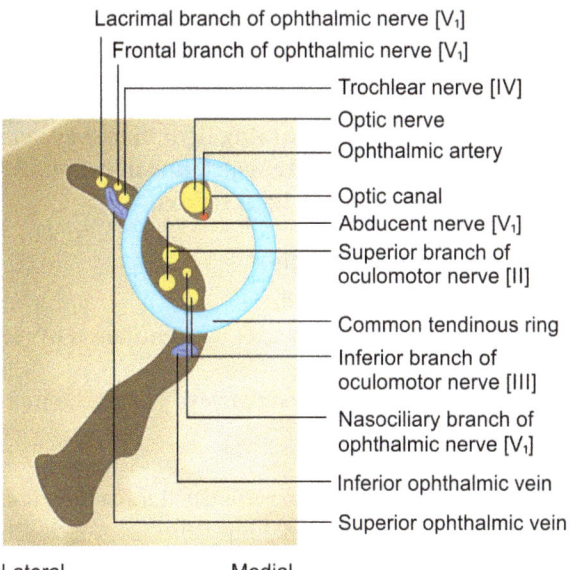

Fig. 21.24: Structure passing through superior orbital fissure.

- The middle cranial fossa inferolaterally where the meningeal and periosteal layers of the dura meet and fuse.
- It measures 8-10 mm in anteroposterior length, and 5-7 mm in height.
- **Contents:** The internal carotid artery, abducent nerve and plexus of sympathetic nerves around ICA pass through the cavernous sinus.
- The 3rd, 4th and 5th (V1 and V2 branches) nerves pass through lateral wall of the sinus.

Superior Orbital Fissure Syndrome

- Involves structures passing through the central annulus of Zinn, as well as those above the annulus
- Multiple cranial nerve palsies involving the oculomotor, trochlear, and abducens nerves, ophthalmic division of the trigeminal nerve

Key point: Does not involve optic nerve

Orbital Apex Syndrome

- Lesions at the apex involving both the superior orbital fissure and the optic canal
- It involves dysfunctions of cranial nerves as seen in the superior orbital fissure syndrome

Key point: Optic nerve involvement present

Cavernous Sinus Syndrome

- More posterior involvement
- Features of the orbital apex syndrome
- Horner's syndrome (oculo-sympathetic fiber involvement)
- Trigeminal nerve (maxillary division)
- Commonly bilateral

Etiology of Orbital Syndromes

- **Inflammatory:** Thyroid orbitopathy, sarcoidosis, Wegener's granulomatosis, giant cell arteritis, orbital inflammatory pseudotumor, Tolosa Hunt syndrome
- **Infectious causes:** Fungal, bacterial (*Streptococcus, Staphylococcus, Actinomyces*, gram-negative bacilli, anaerobes), spirochetes (*Treponema*), viruses (herpes zoster)
- **Vascular causes:** Carotid cavernous aneurysm, carotid cavernous fistulas, cavernous
- **Neoplastic causes:** Neural tumors (neurofibroma, meningioma, schwannoma), head and neck tumors, metastasis (lung, breast, melanoma, renal cell), hematologic (Burkitt lymphoma, NHL, leukemia)
- Trauma

Pituitary Apoplexy

Pituitary apoplexy is a potentially life-threatening disorder due to acute ischemic infarction or hemorrhage of the pituitary gland. It usually occurs in a pre-existing pituitary adenoma when there is rapid growth of neoplastic cells which outgrow blood supply and results in hemorrhagic infarction.

Clinical Features

Headache usually severe and sudden onset retro-orbital in location. Impaired visual acuity or visual field, diplopia, ptosis, facial numbness. Consciousness may be impaired with altered mental status, nausea and vomiting, endocrine abnormalities.

Investigations

X-ray of skull may enlargement of the pituitary fossa and erosion of the sellar floor and dorsum sellae. On CT scan a recent hemorrhage can appear as a single or multiple hyperdense lesions with no or little contrast enhancement.

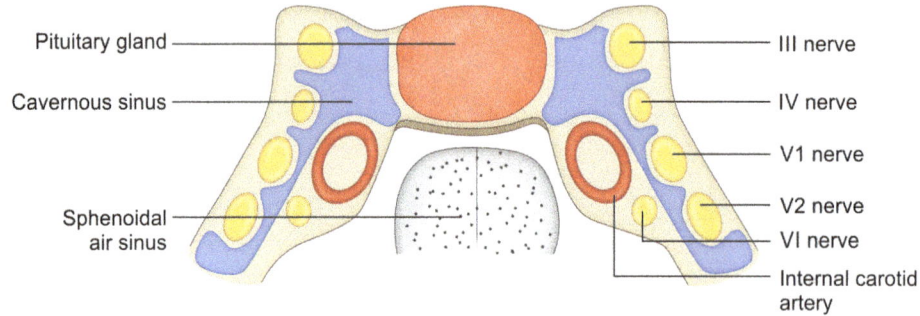

Fig. 21.25: Cavernous sinus, its relations and structures passing through it.

Management

It is an emergency and requires adequate measures for fluid and electrolyte imbalance, corticosteroid replacement therapy and supportive measures.

PUPILLARY REFLEXES

Light Reflex

The light reflex begins from the photoreceptors both rods and cones in the retina. From the optic nerve, the fibers reach the optic chiasma where the nasal fibers decussate and enter the optic tract. From the optic tract the fibred separate from the visual fibers and reach the pretectal nucleus. After relaying in the pretectal nucleus, the fibers decussate and travel to the Edinger-Westphal nucleus on either side. From these nuclei, the fibers enter 3rd nerve, relay and ciliary ganglion and go on to supply the iris sphincter muscle which causes pupillary constriction.

Pupillary Light Reflex Pathway (Parasympathetic Innervation Pathway) (Figs. 21.26 and 21.27)

The role of parasympathetic system comes into play when excessive light enters the eye and the pupil constricts to decrease the amount of light entering the eye.

- **Afferent pathway—optic nerve:** From the ganglion cells, the impulses reach the optic nerve and through it travel to bilateral pretectal nucleus in midbrain. The impulses then travel to the Edinger-Westphal nucleus.
- **Efferent pathway—oculomotor nerve:** From the Edinger-Westphal nucleus impulses travel through the oculomotor nerve to the **ciliary ganglion** (postganglionic sympathetic). From here impulses reach the pupillary sphincter muscle to cause constriction.

Key point: **The pretectal nucleus supplies both Edinger-Westphal nucleus; hence, shining light in one eye causes ipsilateral and contralateral constriction of the pupil. This is known as the consensual light reflex.**

Near/Accommodation Reflex

It is a combination of three effects:
1. Convergence of the optic axis by stimulation of medial rectus
2. Accommodation increased convexity of lens to increase its refractive power
3. Miosis

Its initial part is common with the light reflex. It starts from retinal ganglion cells which send impulses via the optic nerve, optic chiasma and optic tract where most of the fibers of optic tract synapse into LGB nucleus of thalamus. Second order neurons from LGB carry impulses to optic radiations, visual cortex and prefrontal cortex from which fibers pass through internal capsule to reach midbrain

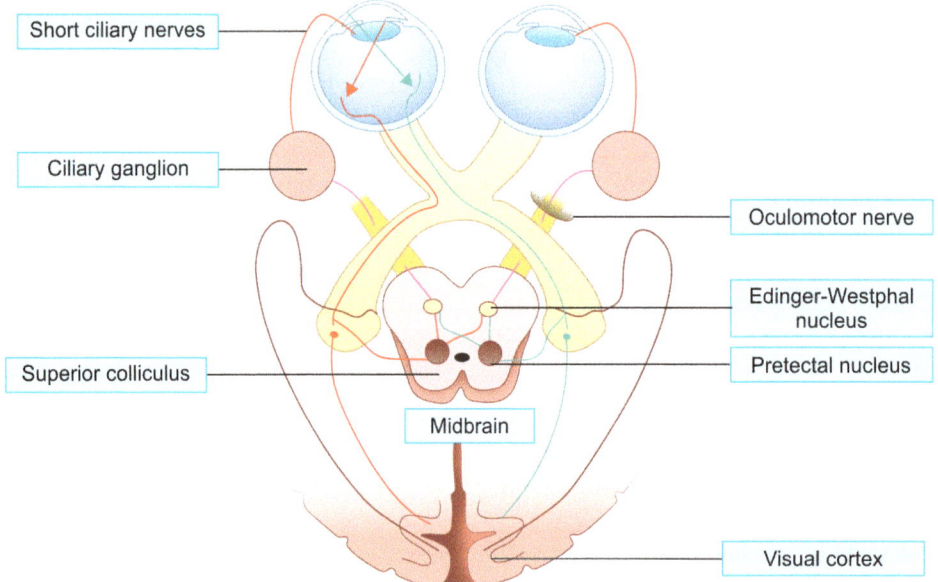

Fig. 21.26: Light reflex pathway.

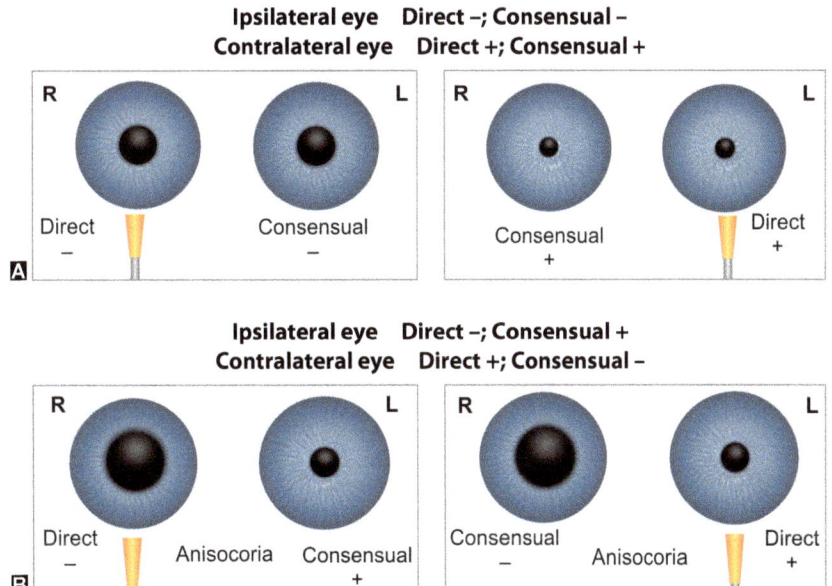

Figs. 21.27A and B: Direct and indirect light reflexes to detect either afferent pupillary defect (A) or efferent pupillary defect (B).

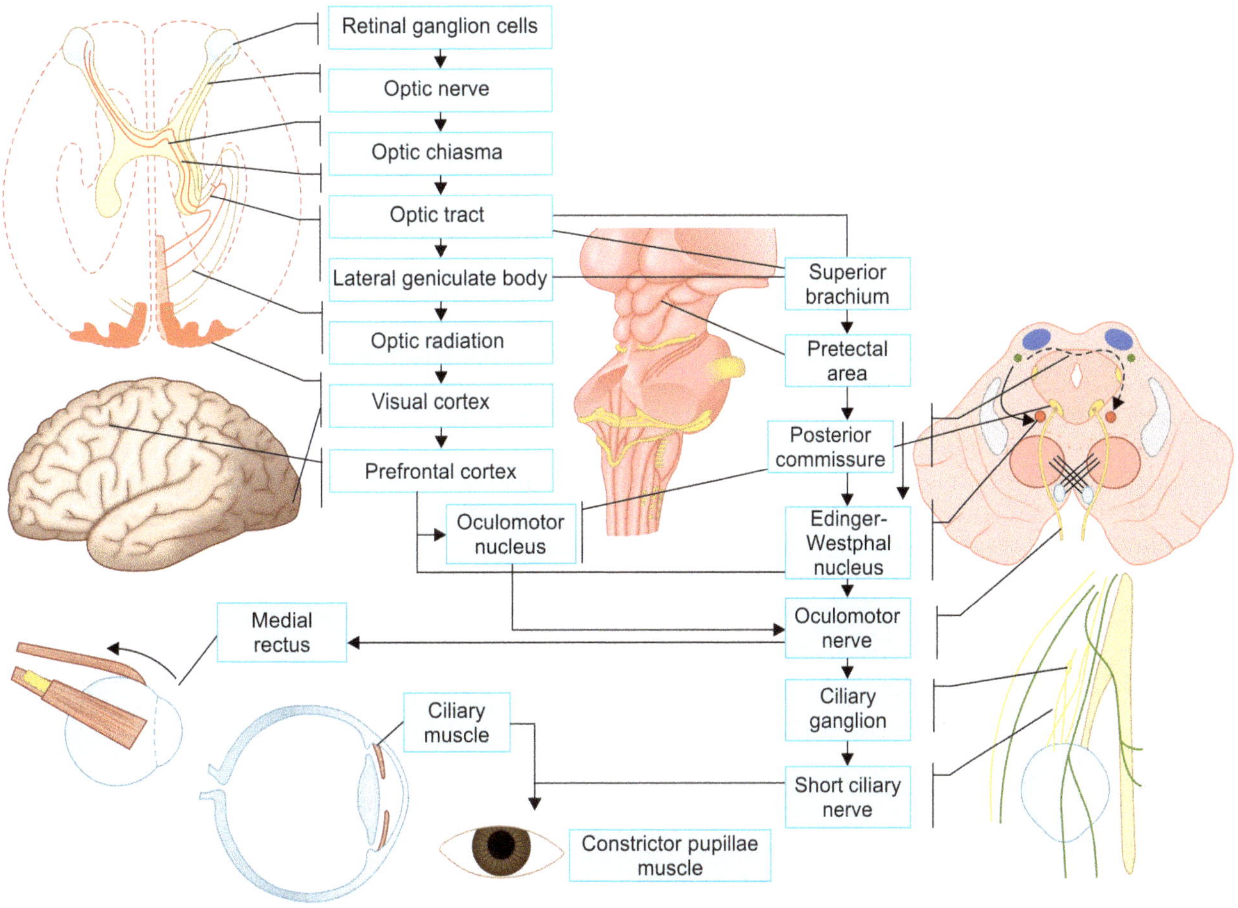

Fig. 21.28: Near reflex pathway shown in blue color and pupillary light reflex shown in green color.

where it synapses with EWN and oculomotor nucleus. Fibers from oculomotor nucleus supply medial rectus cause convergence of both eyes. Preganglionic parasympathetic efferent fibers from EDW nucleus accompany oculomotor nerve and synapse in ciliary ganglion. Post-ganglionic fibers arising from ciliary ganglion pass with short ciliary nerve to supply constrictor pupillae similar to pupillary light reflex but here in accommodation near reflex post ganglionic fibers also supply ciliary muscles in addition to constrictor pupillae **(Fig. 21.28)**.

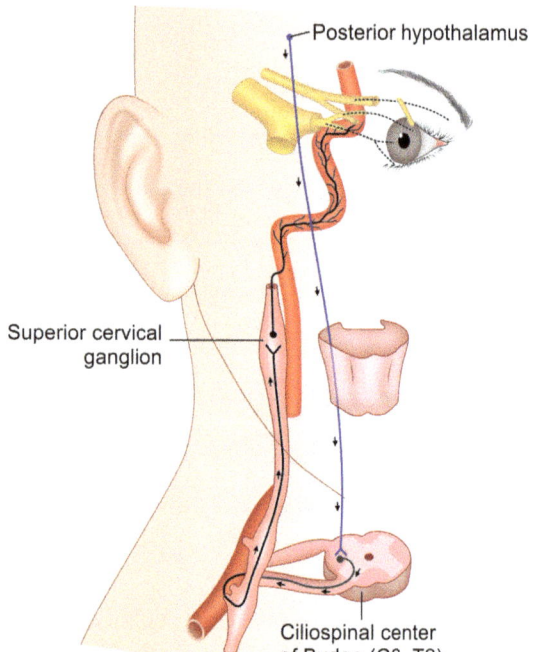

Fig. 21.29: The sympathetic visual system.

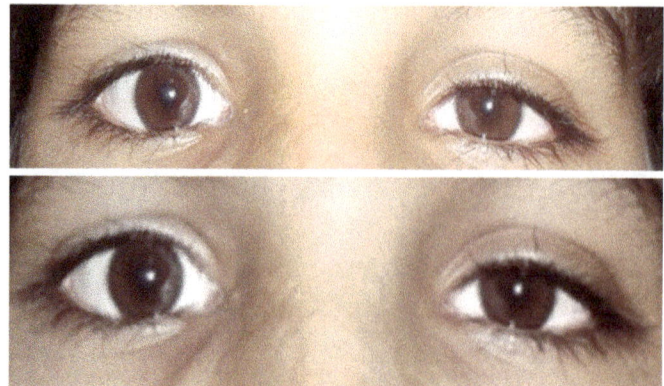

Fig. 21.30: Left eye shows mild ptosis with slight reverse ptosis (elevation of inferior lid) with anisocoria (miotic pupil in left eye).

Clinical Features

It occurs usually unilaterally. Features include **(Fig. 21.30)**:
- **Mild ptosis:** Due to weakness of Muller's muscle
- **Miosis:** Due to unopposed action of sphincter pupillae
- **Anhidrosis:** Reduced ipsilateral sweating
- **Pseudo-enophthalmos:** Appearance of eyeball being displaced inside the orbit due to unilateral ptosis
- Anisocoria is accentuated in dim light because the Horner's pupil dilates slowly in comparison to normal pupil.
- Heterochromia in congenital cases wherein the Horner's pupil iris is lighter
- Inferior ptosis (elevation of inferior eyelid)

Diagnostic Evaluation

Imaging in the form of CT or MR angiography allows examination of the aortic arch to circle of Willis and exclude neck, apical lung, skull base and thyroid lesions. An acute Horner's pupil should be considered an emergency.

Treatment

Treatment of the cause is first line management. Surgery can be considered for ptosis as per the patient's requirement.

Argyll-Robertson Pupil

- Bilateral asymmetric involvement
- Small irregular pupils
- Preserved vision
- Negative light and positive near reflex (light near dissociation)
- Unlike tonic pupil. Do not maintain increased tone to near targets, with normal and brisk re-dilation
- Damage to dorsal aspect of Edinger-Westphal nucleus of midbrain
- Due to neurosyphilis, DM, neurosarcoidosis, chronic alcoholism, multiple sclerosis, herpes zoster

Adie's Tonic Pupil

- Damage to parasympathetic ciliary ganglion
- Unilateral large dilated pupil
- Poor light response
- In near response, slow tonic contraction of pupil, with slow radiation and segmental paralysis of iris sphincter

The Sympathetic Visual System

The main response with respect to eyes is pupillary dilation and elevation of eyelids.

Sympathetic supply to eye consists of three neurons **(Fig. 21.29)**:
1. First order neuron—starts in posterior hypothalamus. From here travel through brainstem to C8 and T2 spinal cord and terminate in the intermediolateral horn called ciliospinal center of Budge.
2. Second order neuron reach from the spinal cord to the superior cervical ganglion of the neck in close proximity to the lung apex.
3. Third order neuron ascends from the superior cervical ganglion along the internal carotid artery and joins the ophthalmic division of the trigeminal nerve. Sympathetic fibers reach the ciliary body and dilator pupillae muscle through the nasociliary nerves and long ciliary nerves.

PUPILLARY ABNORMALITIES

Horner's Syndrome/Oculosympathetic Palsy

Causes

Most common—isolated Horner's is postganglionic, microvascular etiology
- **First order neuron:** Lesions due to stroke, tumors, cervical cord lesion, demyelination, diabetic autonomic neuropathy.
- **Second order neuron (preganglionic):** Lesions caused by lung tumor (Pancoast tumor at lung apex), carotid/aortic aneurysm or dissection, thyroid tumor, enlarged lymph nodes, trauma, post-surgery.
- **Third order neuron (postganglionic):** Lesions caused due to internal carotid artery dissection, nasopharyngeal tumor, cavernous sinus mass, otitis media.

- May be associated with loss of deep tendon reflexes (Adie's syndrome)
- **Causes:** Idiopathic, trauma, viral infection, ocular surgery, tumors

Efferent Pathway Defects

- Absent ipsilateral direct and consensual light reflex and near reflex
- Contralateral consensual reflex preserved.
- Ipsilateral fixed and dilated pupil

Causes

- Brainstem lesion (tumors, strokes)
- Fascicular 3rd nerve lesion
- Ciliary ganglion lesion
- Neuropathic (DM)

Light-Near Dissociation

Light reflex is impaired but near response remains intact.

Causes

- Bilateral complete afferent pathway defect
- Lesion in midbrain at level of pretectal area
- Damage to short ciliary ganglion or short ciliary nerve with regeneration of accommodation fibers into sphincter pupillae
- Aberrant regeneration in DM, alcoholism, amyloidosis

DIAGNOSTIC EVALUATION FOR NEURO-OPHTHALMOLOGY

History Taking

Chief Complaints

- **Vision loss/blurring:**
  - Unilateral vs bilateral
  - Speed of onset of vision loss—sudden in ischemic events, subacute over days to weeks in optic neuritis, gradual over months to years in compressive lesions
  - History of trauma (compressive optic neuropathy)
- **Binocular double vision/diplopia:**
  - Intermittency in myasthenia gravis; constant in paralytic squint
  - Horizontal/vertical/torsional—can be due to in 3rd, 4th, 6th nerve paralysis.
  - Absent in slow progressing disorders like CPEO.
- **Visual field defects:**
  - Homonymous hemianopia in pituitary adenomas and other sellar lesions
  - Altitudinal field defects in ischemic optic neuropathy
  - Enlarged blind spot in papilledema.
- Drooping of upper eyelid—3rd nerve paralysis, Horner's syndrome, myasthenia gravis
- Poor color discrimination suggestive of optic nerve pathology such as ethambutol toxicity, optic neuritis

Associated Conditions

- Headache—raised intracranial tension.
- Pain on ocular movement in optic neuritis
- Weakness in any other part of body—stroke, multiple sclerosis
- Nystagmus—in midbrain lesions and vestibular causes

Systemic History

Diabetes, hypertension, cardiac disease, multiple sclerosis, tuberculosis.

Diet History

Vegetarians more likely to have vitamin B_{12} deficiency in nutritional optic neuropathy, history of alcohol intake in toxic optic neuropathy. History of drug intake—antitubercular drug therapy (ethambutol).

Clinical Examination

Visual Acuity Testing

BCVA may be reduced for both distance—Snellen chart (**Fig. 21.31**) and near—Jaegar's chart (**Fig. 21.32**), e.g., optic neuritis, optic atrophy, ischemic optic neuropathy or may be normal in some instances, e.g., papilledema.

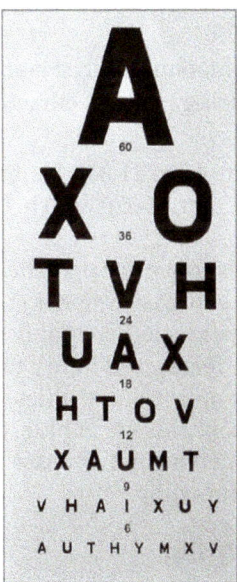

Fig. 21.31: Distance—Snellen's chart.

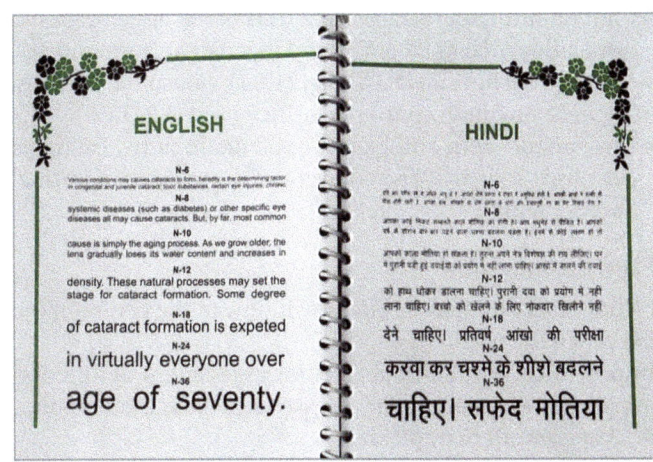

Fig. 21.32: Near—Jaeger's chart.

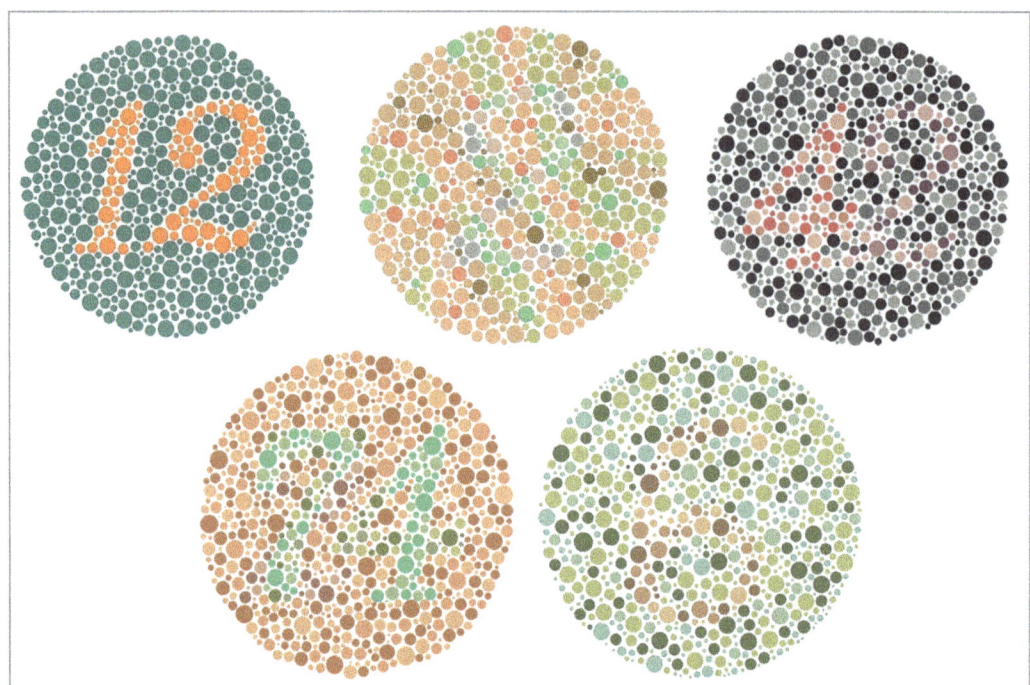

Fig. 21.33: Ishihara plate.

Color Vision Testing

Poor color discrimination/contrast sensitivity—suggestive of optic nerve pathology such as ethambutol toxicity, optic neuritis.

Tests: Ishihara plates **(Fig. 21.33)**, Lantern test, Farnsworth Munsell 100 hue test, Farnsworth D-15 test, Nagel's anomaloscope.

Color vision is disproportionately affected compared with BCVA in optic nerve disease whereas color vision decrease proportionately as per visual acuity and in macular diseases. One of the earliest features of injury to optic nerve is red desaturation. Most optic neuropathies manifest defects in red-green perception. Defects in blue-yellow function are usually seen in glaucoma and diseases of macula but may be seen in optic neuropathy.

Contrast Sensitivity Test

- It is another test to evaluate optic nerve function. It can be used to assess visual function when visual acuity is normal. However, it is not specific for disorders of optic nerve and may be abnormal in the presence of media opacities such as cataracts and macular abnormalities.
- **Tests:** Pelli Robson chart **(Fig. 21.34)**, sinusoidal gratings, Spaeth Richman contrast sensitivity test (SPARCS).
- In patients with amblyopia, optic neuropathy, cataracts contrast sensitivity is reduced in the presence of normal visual acuity.

Pupil Examination

Light enters our eyes through a window in the center of the iris called the pupil.

Importance: It is an important for assessment of function in patients with neurologic diseases and decreased vision.

- **Assessment of pupil size:**
  - Normal resting pupil size depends on age of patient, surrounding light, wakefullness of patient.

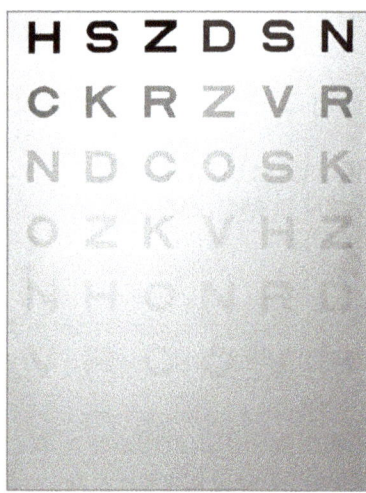

Fig. 21.34: Pelli Robson chart.

  Diameter should be measured in dark, light and during near response
  - In ambient light, the size of the normal pupil is approximately 3–4 mm. Normally, the pupil constricts in bright light and dilates in dark room due to light reflex.
  - *Constricted pupil:* Horner's syndrome, brainstem stroke, drugs—clonidine, phenothiazines, opiates, narcotics, muscarinics, insecticides
  - *Dilated pupil:* Adies tonic pupil
  - *Fixed dilated:* 3rd nerve paralysis, sphincter tear
  - *Anisocoria:* Unequal pupillary size **(difference of more than 0.4 mm)**; may occur from damage to iris dilator or sphincter muscle or abnormality in their innervation.
- **Reaction to light (pupillary reflexes) (Figs. 21.27A and B):**
  - *Direct pupillary light reflex:* Pupillary constriction when light is shown directly on that eye.

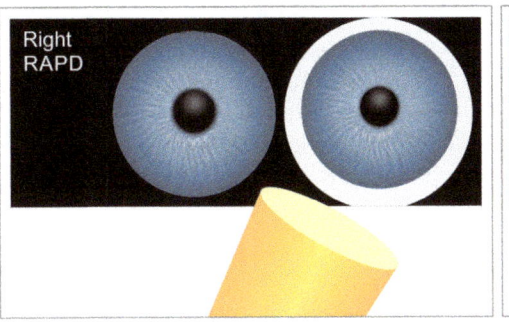 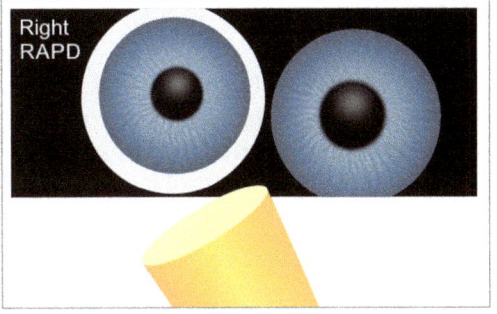

Fig. 21.35: Swinging flashlight test for assessment of RAPD.

- *Consensual pupillary light reflex:* Pupil constricts when light is shown in another eye. Both these reflexes are normal when they are similar in between the two eyes.
- **Relative afferent pupillary defect:** When the eye with abnormal optic nerve function is shown light into, the direct and consensual reflex in response is slower and smaller than the response when light is shown in eye with normal nerve conduction. Relative afferent pupillary defect (RAPD) demonstrated by Swinging Flashlight test. RAPD is a defect in the pupillary reaction of one eye compared to that of the other eye due to defect in the afferent pupillary pathway.
- **Swinging flashlight test:** It is performed when (RAPD) is suspected **(Fig. 21.35)**. It is performed by comparing the light reflex in both eyes after swinging light back and forth from one pupil to the other. When light is shown on a pupil, normally there is a direct and consensual reflex. RAPD is present when there is paradoxical dilation in the affected pupil on exposing to light after the healthy eye has been exposed.
  - *Grades of RAPD*
    - Grade 1: Weak initial constriction followed by greater re-dilatation
    - Grade 2: Initial stall followed by greater re-dilatation
    - Grade 3: Immediate pupillary dilatation
    - Grade 4: Immediate pupillary dilatation following prolonged illumination of the good eye
    - Grade 5: Immediate pupillary dilatation with no secondary constriction

  RAPD may occur due to damage anywhere along the visual pathway from retina to optic tract.
  - *Near response:* Pupils constrict to near response (accommodative target) due to near reflex
  - *Light-near dissociation* occurs when the greatest constriction of pupil to bright light is lesser than that which occurs during the near response.
  - *Causes:*
    - Damage to the afferent visual pathway (retina or optic nerve)
    - Damage to pretectal nucleus: Dorsal midbrain syndrome, Argyll-Robertson pupil)
    - Aberrant regeneration: Adie's pupil, aberrant third nerve regeneration
- **Confrontation test:**
  - It is a rapid way to grossly measure field of vision.

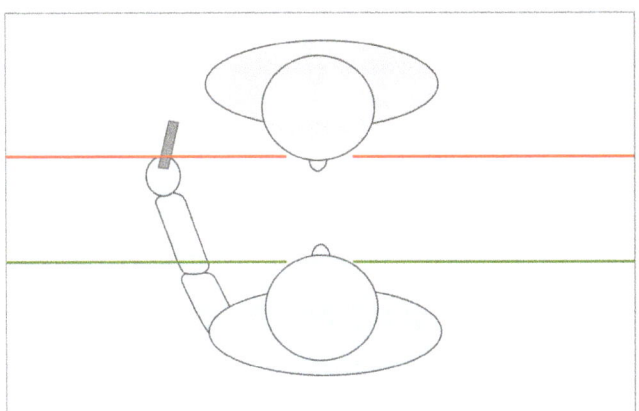

Fig. 21.36: Confrontation test.

- In this test, the patient is examined at the same eye level as the examiner. The patient is asked to close right eye to test left field of vision. The examiner closes his left eye. An outstretched finger is then gradually brought from periphery to center in all 4 fields, i.e., superior, nasal, inferior, and temporal **(Fig. 21.36)**. The examiner compares the patient's field to his own.
- Make sure the patient has one eye occluded and is looking at your nose. Make sure you are putting the target in the patient's visual field not yours.

Slit Lamp Evaluation of Anterior Segment and Posterior Segment

It is a must to carry out detailed evaluation as they often give diagnostic clues.
- **Anterior segment evaluation for:**
  - Cells for signs of uveitis
  - Assessment of pupil
  - Heterochromia (abnormally lighter in acquired Horners' syndrome)
  - Angle recession, transillumination defects, sphincter tear for signs of trauma
- **Posterior segment is evaluated on the slit lamp with a 90 diopter lens. We look for:**
  - Vitreous cells
  - Optic disc edema
  - Peripapillary hemorrhages
  - Disc pallor
  - Macular star
  - Features of hypertensive/diabetic retinopathy.

Direct and Indirect Ophthalmoscopy for Fundus Evaluation

The detailed fundus examination is done to look at the optic disc, macula, retinal periphery, retinal vessels. Ophthalmoscopy is clinical examination of the fundus by means of an ophthalmoscope. It is discussed in chapter on retina.

Oculomotor Evaluation

- Hirschberg test/corneal light reflex test
- Cover uncover test
- **Ocular movements:** These tests have been described in chapter on squint evaluation.
- **Testing of other eye movements:**
  - *Visual fixation and gaze holding:* The patient can be asked to look straight ahead on an object.
  - *Saccades:*
    - Rapid, eye movement that shifts the center of gaze from one part to another
    - Clinical pearl: Evaluate latency, accuracy, conjugacy and velocity
    - Importance: Saccades slow in nerve paralysis
  - *Smooth pursuit:*
    - Helps in maintaining fixation of small moving objects.
    - It can be abnormal in cerebellar or basal ganglia disorders (e.g., parkinsonism, progressive supranuclear palsy
    - A smoothly moving object (like pendulum) in front is used to test these
  - *Optokinetic nystagmus:*
    - It stabilizes the eyes relative to the external world by compensating for head movement
    - Vestibulo-ocular movements can be appreciated by moving the head from side to side while fixating on an object; the eyes automatically maintaining the image of the object on the same location on retina
    - It can also be tested by using an OKN drum which is a rotating cylinder with vertical black and white stripes in front of patient. The eyes follow a stripe until it rotates out of view followed by a quick refixation saccade in the direction opposite to the moving drum, followed once again by smooth pursuit of a stripe. This is called optokinetic nystagmus
    - It is a normal reflex. It should not be confused with pathological nystagmus.
  - *VOR suppression:* Maintain fixation during sustained head rotations or translations
  - *Vergence (convergence):* Achieve fixation of images at varying distance from eye by making disconjugate movements

Nystagmus

- It is the involuntary to and fro oscillatory movement of eyes. It is characterized by the:
  - Plane of movement: Horizontal, vertical, torsional
  - Amplitude of excursion: Coarse, fine
  - Frequency: High, low, moderate
- It is classified as:
  - Jerk: Slow and fast movement
  - Pendular: Both movements are slow
  - Mixed: It is a combination of both with a jerky type of nystagmus in lateral gaze and pendular type in primary position

Importance

It may be physiological in response to optikokinetic drum or inside a moving bus/train. Pathological nystagmus may be congenital, sensory nystagmus, associated with squint, brainstem lesions, midbrain lesions, drugs such as lithium and phenytoin.

Physiological Nystagmus

- **End-point nystagmus:** Occurs as a fine jerky nystagmus when eyes are moved too far laterally or in gaze extremes.
- **Optokinetic nystagmus:** occurs normally when viewing outside while sitting inside a moving vehicle or in response to moving objects like an OKN drum. It is used for testing VA in the very young and for detecting functional blindness.

Vestibular Nystagmus

Abnormalities in the input from vestibular nuclei to gaze centers in brain produce a jerk nystagmus. The vestibular nuclei initiate the slow phase and the brainstem initiates the fast phase. It can be evoked by caloric stimulation.

- When cold water is poured into the left ear the patient develops nystagmus towards right (fast phase to opposite side)
- When warm water is poured into the left ear, left jerk nystagmus occurs (fast phase to same side) [COWS pneumonic cold-opposite, warm-same].

Peripheral vestibular nystagmus due to pathological causes include diseases like labyrinthitis, Ménière's disease, infection of middle or inner ear.

Infantile (Congenital) Nystagmus

It occurs withing first year of life either due to a motor problem or low vision with the nystagmus itself causing poor vision. It may be associated with systemic disorders of the nervous system. Nystagmus is usually minimal at the null point and may develop a compensatory head posture.

Sensory Deficit Nystagmus

Early onset vision impairment may be due to congenital cataract, albinism, corneal opacity, macular hypoplasia, Leber's congenital amaurosis, achromatopsia which produces nystagmus in proportion to severity of vision loss.

Congenital Motor Nystagmus

It is an idiopathic low amplitude pendular nystagmus in primary position that may turn into a jerky form on lateral gaze. Family history is usually present. It presents 2–3 months after birth.

Characteristics are given by pneumonic

- C—Convergence and eye closure dampens
- O—Oscillopsia absent
- N—Null zone present

- G—Gaze position does not change direction of nystagmus
- E—Equal amplitude and frequency in each eye
- N—Near acuity is good
- I—Inversion of optikokinetic response
- T—Turning of head to achieve null point
- A—Abolishes in sleep
- L—Latent (occlusion) nystagmus occurs

Spasmus Nutans

It is a benign idiopathic disorder presents with high frequency small amplitude horizontal nystagmus between 3 and 18 months. It consists of a triad of:
- Nystagmus
- Head bobbing
- Torticollis

Neuroimaging usually MRI is warranted to reveal pathology in anterior visual pathway.

Acquired Nystagmus

- **Latent nystagmus:** It is latent in that it increases on covering one eye. The fast phase is towards the fixing eye. A manifest nystagmus may occasionally have a latent component in addition so that when one eye is covered the amplitude of nystagmus increases (manifest-latent nystagmus). It is seen in patients of infantile esotropia and dissociated vertical deviation.
- **Periodic alternating nystagmus:** It is called alternating because it periodically reverses direction. The amplitude and frequency of nystagmus first increase and then decrease in the active phase. An interlude then follows of around 4–20 sec. During this period the eyes are steady a similar cycle then occurs in the opposite direction, the whole cycle lasting 1 to 3 min. It may be seen in diseases of cerebellum, ataxia telangiectasia or drugs (phenytoin).
- **Convergence-retraction nystagmus:** It is a jerk nystagmus. Extraocular muscle usually medial recti co-contraction causes this. An OKN drum downwards may also produce it. It is seen in dorsal midbrain syndrome.
- **Downbeat nystagmus:** As the name suggests, the fast phase is in the downward direction producing vertical nystagmus. It may be caused by lesions at the foramen magnum such as syringobulbia, demyelination, drugs such as phenytoin and lithium, Arnold-Chiari malformation, Wernicke's encephalopathy and hydrocephalus.
- **Upbeat nystagmus:** The fast phase beats upwards producing vertical nystagmus. Seen in Wernicke's encephalopathy, certain medications, posterior fossa lesions.
- **See-saw nystagmus:** One eye elevates and intorts while the other depresses and extorts. This is repeated with other eye producing pendular nystagmus. It occurs due to tumors around sella turcica, syringobulbia, brainstem stroke.

CRANIAL NERVE EXAMINATION

Apart from oculomotor, trochlear abducens, all other cranial nerves should be examined to look for involvement and to localize the lesion, i.e., olfactory, optic, trigeminal, facial, vestibulocochlear, glossopharyngeal, vagus, spinal accessory, hypoglossal.

Systemic sensory and motor evaluation should be done in all cases with nerve palsies/other sensory deficits.

ANCILLARY TESTS/INVESTIGATIONS

- **Perimetry:** It is used to diagnose and monitor various causes of visual field defects and localization of the lesion. Neuro-ophthalmic field defects usually follow the vertical meridian.
- **Fluorescein angiography:** Optic nerve pathologies—optic neuritis, ischemic optic neuropathy
  - *Optical coherence tomography:* Spectral Domain OCT technology is used to assess the thickness of retinal nerve fiber layer (RNFL) around the optic disc and macular ganglion cell loss **(Fig. 21.37)**.
    - Increased thickness of RNFL is seen in optic neuritis, papilledema, acute ischemia, and idiopathic intracranial hypertension.
    - Thinning of RNFL occurs due to loss of ganglion cells is seen in optic atrophy, toxic and nutritional neuropathies.

    Macular ganglion cell layer thickness is also measure using OCT. Loss of ganglion cells in the macula is an indicator of optic nerve damage.
  - *Visual evoked potential:* It measures the electrical signal produced in the brain when eyes are stimulated. An intact visual pathway produces a normal VEP response.

    The stimulus is either a flash of light (flash VEP) or an alternation black-and-white checkerboard pattern (pattern VEP). Multiple tests are performed, and the average potential is calculated.

    Latency and amplitude are assessed.
    - lash VEP—has multiple positive and negative waves-
    - Pattern reversal VEPs—mainly 2 negative waves (N75, N135) and 1 positive wave (P100). These waves appear at 75 ms, 135 ms and 100 ms after the stimulus, respectively **(Fig. 21.38)**.

Clinical Use

- Assess visual function in infants.
- Determine visual prognosis before planning surgery.
- Evaluation of optic neuropathy.
- Malingering.

OPTIC NEURITIS

It is an acute inflammation of the optic nerve that leads to varying degrees of permanent visual impairment.

CLASSIFICATIONS

1. **Retrobulbar neuritis:** Most common. The optic disc appears normal.

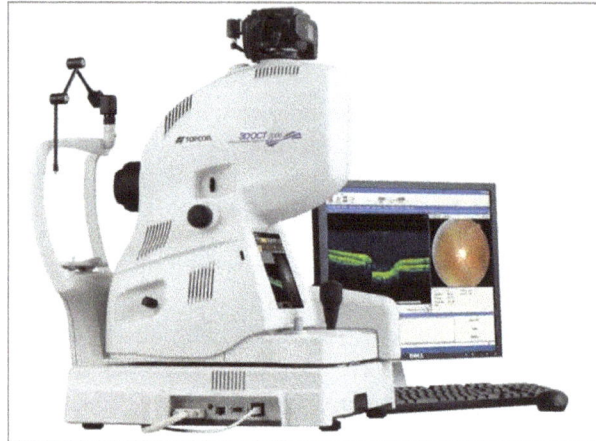

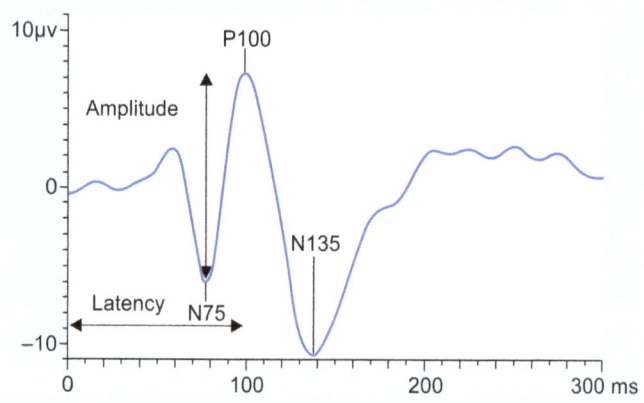

Fig. 21.38: Pattern visual evoked potential.

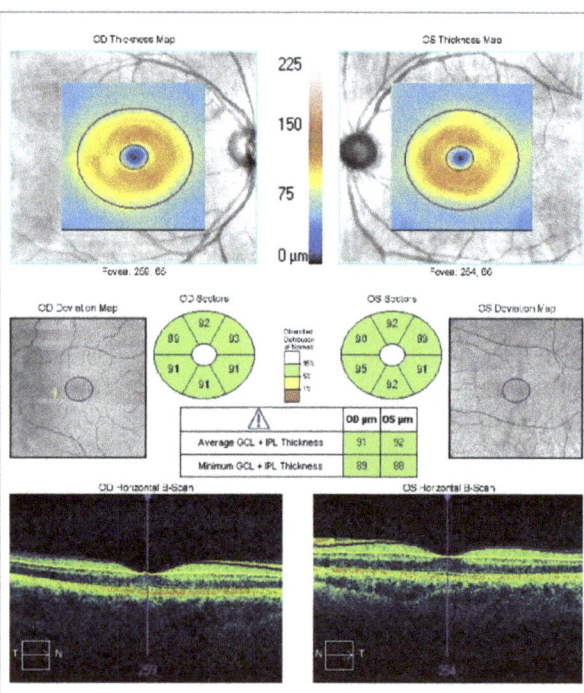

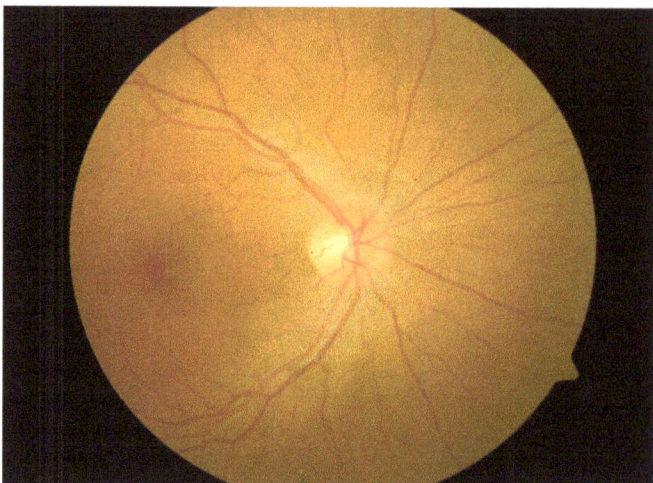

Fig. 21.39: Shows papillitis. Blurring of nasal disc margin indication optic disc edema along with hyperemia.

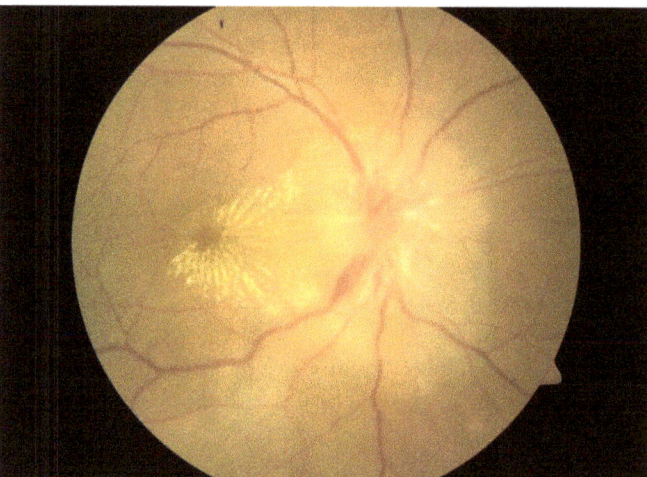

Fig. 21.40: Shows neuroretinitis. There is optic disc edema with disc hemorrhages and incomplete macular star formation.

2. **Papillitis (Fig. 21.39):** There is edema of the optic disc along with hyperemia. Vitreous cells and hemorrhages may be present.
3. **Neuroretinitis (Fig. 21.40):** It is the least common type. Essentially, it is considered as demyelinating disease. It is characterized by papillitis and a macular star figure with inflammation of the retinal nerve fiber layer.

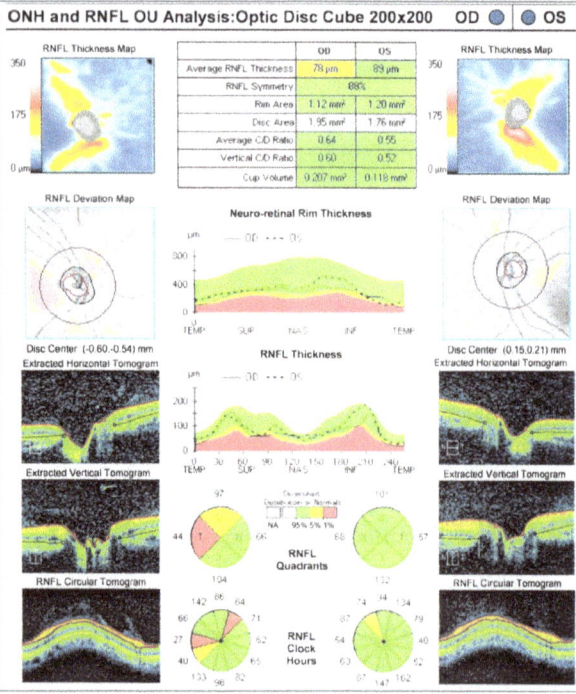

Fig. 21.37: Optical coherence tomography and ganglion cell analysis (GCC) and retinal nerve fiber layer (RNFL) scans.

CAUSES

CNS demyelination	Infectious or para-infectious	
Multiple sclerosis (most common cause)	**Viral:** Adenovirus, measles, rubella, varicella-zoster	After immunization
Neuromyelitis optica spectrum disorder Myelin oligodendrocyte glycoprotein (MOG) syndrome	**Bacterial:** Tuberculosis, Strep. Infection, cat scratch disease, syphilis Lyme disease, herpes zoster, cryptococcal meningitis	Noninfectious Inflammatory diseases—sarcoidosis, polyarteritis nodosa, systemic lupus erythematosus

TYPES

Typical optic neuritis	Atypical optic neuritis
Isolated/idiopathic	Neuromyelitis optica spectrum disorder (NMOSD) (*AQP4, MOG, both negative)
MS associated (typical MS lesion in brain)	• Autoimmune • Chronic relapsing inflammatory optic neuropathy (CRION) • Reactive (postinfection or vaccination)

MS-related Optic Neuritis

Symptoms

- Women more commonly affected usually in 3rd/4th decade.
- Mono-ocular diminution of vision, subacute onset with loss over hours to 7–10 days.
- Associated with pain on ocular movements (painful visual loss).
- Peak visual loss within 2 weeks, improves thereafter.
- Patients may experience colored flashes or sparkles (phosphenes).

Signs

- Decreased visual acuity (6/18 to 6/60), may be worse (no PL).
- Relative afferent pupillary defect
- Impaired color vision and contrast sensitivity out of proportion to severity of vision loss.
- Optic disc may appear normal or there may be disc edema with or without macular star formation.
- Other eye may show temporal disc pallor suggestive of previous optic neuritis.
- Visual field defects in central 30°, altitudinal, centrocecal scotomas are common.

Key Points

- ON present in 50% of patients with MS
- Presenting feature in 20% of MS
- Recurrent ON involving same/fellow eye

Investigations

MRI is mandatory in all patients of optic neuritis.
- MRI brain (T2-weighted with FLAIR with Gadolinium contrast) with 2 mm optic nerve cuts on STIR imaging shows optic nerve enhancement. There may be characteristic periventricular white matter lesions in the brain (Dawson's fingers) which are white matter plaques indicative of multiple sclerosis.
- Lumbar puncture may show oligoclonal bands on protein electrophoresis of cerebrospinal fluid.
- Visual evoked potential are abnormal and show delay in conduction with reduced amplitude.
- In infectious cases a complete blood count, serology for syphilis, *Bartonella henselae, Borrelia, Herpes* and *Cryptococcus* will be required to investigate for cause.

Management

- Patients with multiple sclerosis experience a relapsing-remitting cause. Intravenous methylprednisolone 1 g daily for 3 days may help to speed up recovery in severe vision loss and delay the onset of multiple sclerosis in the short-term. However, it does not affect final visual outcome. It is followed by oral steroids 1 mg/kg/day for 11 days. Oral steroids should not be started before intravenous therapy.
- In case of infectious causes the etiological agent must be treated with antimicrobials.

Infective Optic Neuritis

- Optic nerve could be due to direct infection or inflammation, ischemia or edema.
- Infection may affect selectively optic disc or adjacent retina (neuroretinitis), vitreous, sinus or meninges.
- Causes could be *Tuberculosis,* cat scratch disease, syphilis, *Cytomegalovirus.*
- Nonspecific presentations.

Tuberculosis

- Involvement of optic nerve results because of the involvement of contiguous retina (retinal vasculitis) or choroid (choroidal granuloma or patches of choroiditis).
- Fluorescence angiography detects active lesions in such cases.

Cat Scratch Disease

- Causes neuroretinitis in which optic disc edema is accompanied by macular edema with retinal exudates in the shape of a star centered around the fovea.
- **Causative organism:** *Bartonella henselae* and *B. quintana*
- Generally, it infects children and young adults
- Unilateral acute visual loss
- Antecedent illness
- Branch artery occlusion
- Multiple white retinal lesions
- History of exposure to cats not necessary
- Self-limited with good prognosis
- Treatment is not necessary

Syphilis

- Great mimicker
- Optic nerve involvement can be anterior or retrobulbar or neuroretinitis in secondary or tertiary phases of disease.
- **Laboratory test:** Venereal Disease Research Laboratory (VDRL) followed by *Treponema pallidum Hemagglutination* (TPHA)
- Treatment in line with neurosyphilis (injectable penicillin)

Virus

- Optic neuropathy in herpes simplex virus type 1 or type 2 may occur in association with acute retinal necrosis or less commonly with herpes encephalitis.
- Optic nerve involvement may be concomitant or follow retinal infection.

Toxoplasmosis

- About 5% of patients with toxoplasmosis may have optic nerve involvement.
- Present with isolated papillitis or as juxtapapillary or chorioretinitis.
- Atypical in immunocompromised with rapid progression.

Cryptococcal Disease

- May cause papilledema due to meningitis.
- **Causative agent:** Cryptococcal neoformans
- Especially in HIV patients
- Treatment antifungals
- Poor prognosis

ISCHEMIC OPTIC NEUROPATHY

Ischemia of the optic nerve may occur in different locations and may be due to a numerous causes:

- Anterior ischemic optic neuropathy (AION) involves 1 mm segment of the optic nerve head also known as the optic disc. There is variable disc edema. It has two types: Nonarteritic and arteritic AION.
- Posterior ischemic optic neuropathy (PION) includes conditions that cause ischemia in the any part of the optic nerve posterior to the optic disc. It is not associated with disc edema.

NONARTERITIC ISCHEMIC OPTIC NEUROPATHY

It is caused by occlusion of the short posterior ciliary arteries resulting in infarction of the optic nerve head. Most of the cases of AION are nonarteritic. Males and females are equally affected and patients are usually above 50 years of age. Most cases are idiopathic but associated with certain risk factors.

Risk Factors

Small disc with crowding of the optic nerve head with small or absent physiological cup (disc at risk with cup to disc ratio < 0.3), hypertension, diabetes mellitus, hyperlipidemia, collagen vascular disease, hyperhomocysteinemia, sleep apnea syndrome, nocturnal hypotension, drugs such as sildenafil.

Clinical Features

Symptoms

Sudden onset painless unilateral loss of vision over hours or days frequently noticed on waking up in the morning.

Signs

- Moderate to severe visual impairment
- Dyschromatopsia/impaired color vision proportional to visual acuity loss. Pupillary abnormality in the form of relative afferent pupillary defect.
- Altitudinal and quadratic visual field defects, inferior being most common **(Fig. 21.41)**.
- Optic disc edema which may be diffuse or sectoral. It is commonly associated with disc hyperemia. Peripapillary splinter hemorrhages are seen in three-quarters of patients.

Diagnostic Investigations

- Diagnosis of NAION is a clinical one.
- Assessment of blood pressure, lipid profile, blood sugars. Additional laboratory tests for hypercoagulable states for patients under 50 years of age may be considered. Atypical features may require neuroimaging to rule out optic neuritis.

Management

There is no definitive treatment. Any underlying systemic condition such as hypertension, diabetes, dyslipidemia should be treated. Aspirin is frequently prescribed but has not been shown to improve vision or reduce the risk of involvement of the fellow eye.

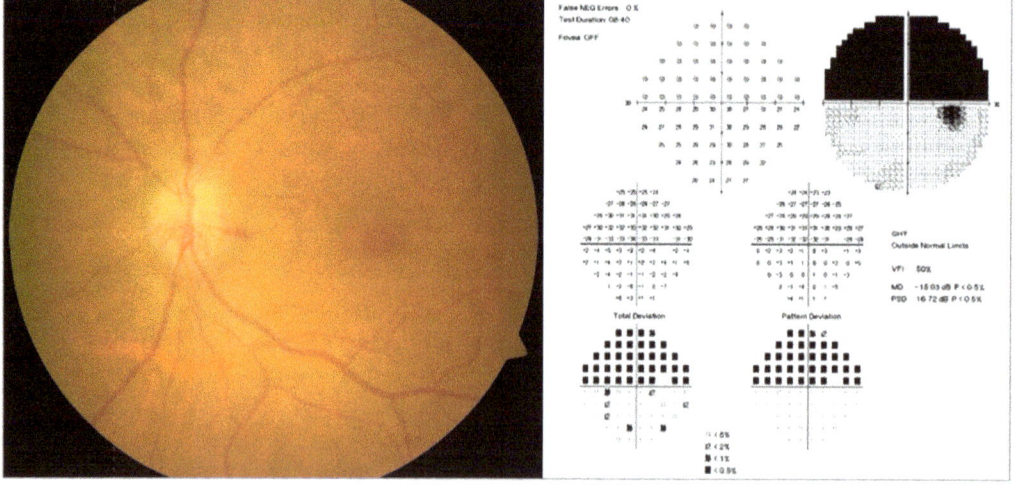

Fig. 21.41: AION showing inferior disc edema sectoral with hyperemia and splinter hemorrhages around disc. Corresponding superior altitudinal field defect.

ARTERITIC ISCHEMIC OPTIC NEUROPATHY

It is less common seen in elderly patients above 50 years of age (more commonly above 70). Women are affected more than men. Giant cell arteritis is the main cause which a granulomatous necrotizing arteritis affecting large and medium-sized arteries particularly the superficial temporal, ophthalmic, posterior ciliary and vertebral arteries.

Clinical Features

Symptoms

- Sudden painless unilateral vision loss which may be preceded by transient vision loss (amaurosis fugax)
- Headache
- Scalp tenderness noticed while combing hair
- Jaw claudication (cramp-like pain on chewing.
- Nonspecific symptoms such as weight loss, fever, night sweats, malaise

Signs

- Severe vision loss with visual acuity < 6/60
- A relative afferent pupillary defect
- Altitudinal visual field defect
- Chalky white pallor of the optic disc with edema is the hallmark and helps in differentiating from nonarteritic AION which is commonly associated with hyperemia. The disc edema is commonly diffuse but segmental involvement with peripapillary disc hemorrhages may occur.
- Superficial temporal arteritis is characterized by thickened, nodular, tender arteries.
- Nonpulsatile superficial temporal artery is strongly suggestive of giant cell arteritis (GCA), but pulsation is usually present initially.
- Scalp gangrene may occur in severe cases.

Diagnostic Investigations

- Erythrocyte sedimentation rate is usually high >60 mm/hour.
- C-reactive protein is raised.
- Complete blood count may show anemia and elevated platelets.
- Temporal artery biopsy should be done if GCA is suspected from ipsilateral side of the involved eye. A negative biopsy does not rule out GCA and should not prevent treatment. At least 2.5 cm of artery should be examined as skip lesions could be present in which inflamed segments of arterial wall are interspersed with normal areas.
- Color Doppler

Treatment

Intravenous methylprednisolone 1 g/day for 3 days followed by 1 mg/kg/day with gradual tapering after 3 days should be started as soon as possible to prevent blindness of other eye. It should never be delayed for biopsy.

NUTRITIONAL/TOXIC OPTIC NEUROPATHY

It is a bilateral symmetric optic neuropathy characterized by gradual and progressive vision loss due to nutritional deficiency or exposure to toxins. Risk factors include inflammatory bowel disease, vegetarian diets, bariatric surgery, malnutrition, alcoholism, parenteral nutrition without adequate vitamin supplementation.

ETIOLOGY

Due to deficiency certain water-soluble neurotrophic vitamins required to maintain the health of the nervous system:

- Vitamin B_1 (thiamine)
- Vitamin B_2 (riboflavin)
- Vitamin B_6 (pyridoxine)
- Vitamin B_{12} (cobalamin)
- Vitamin B_9 (folate)
- Copper

These vitamins are involved in the process of oxidative phosphorylation in the mitochondria and production of energy in the form of adenosine triphosphate (ATP). Decreased ATP with oxidative stress leading to mitochondrial dysfunction is caused by their deficiency which in turn causes accumulation of free radicals.

Toxic substances most commonly causing include:

- **Alcohol:** Methanol
- **Antitubercular:** Ethambutol, isoniazid, streptomycin
- **Anticancer:** Tamoxifen, vincristine, methotrexate
- **Antibiotics:** Sulfonamides, chloramphenicol, linezolid
- **Antimalarials:** Quinine, hydroxychloroquine, chloroquine
- **Antiarrhythmic:** Amiodarone, digitalis
- **Heavy metals:** Lead, mercury, thallium

These cause mitochondrial injury and formation of free radicals.

SYMPTOMS

- Insidious onset
- Bilateral painless
- Blurring of vision
- Peripheral neurological symptoms such as sensory loss and paresthesia's, gait disturbances

SIGNS

- Variable decreased visual acuity
- Color vision deficit disproportionate to the reduction in visual acuity
- Pupillary reaction is normal with no relative afferent pupillary defect (RAPD)
- Bilateral symmetric centrocecal scotomas may occur.
- Optic disc in early stages may be normal or swollen. Temporal disc pallor which is often subtle and thinning

of the papillomacular bundle retinal nerve fiber layer (RNFL).
- In late stages diffuse optic disc pallor and thinning of RNFL in all quadrants is found.

DIAGNOSTIC INVESTIGATIONS

- Complete blood count—to look for anemia
- Serum vitamin B_{12}, B_9, B_1, B_2
- Serum protein levels
- Serum homocysteine (raised in vitamin B_{12} and folate deficiency) and serum methylmalonic acid (raised in vitamin B_{12} deficiency but normal in folate deficiency)
- Screening for blood levels of formic acid and cyanide if suspected.
- Heavy metal screening if suspected.
- Urinalysis to look for specific toxins.

MANAGEMENT

- Treatment of the cause forms the mainstay of treatment
- In both B_{12} and folate deficiency, it is essential to treat the B_{12} deficiency first to avoid precipitation subacute combined degeneration of the spinal cord. Alcohol and tobacco should be stopped.
- In case of methanol poisoning, sodium bicarbonate should be given to correct metabolic acidosis and ethanol forms the mainstay of treatment as antidote. In severe acidosis hemodialysis is done. Intravenous pulse steroids have been used to salvage vision.
- Inciting drugs such as ethambutol, amiodarone should be discontinued.
- In case of heavy metal exposure, the source should be removed and treated with chelating agents.

LEBER'S HEREDITARY OPTIC NEUROPATHY

It is the most common inherited mitochondrial disorder. Young males are typically affected. It usually begins as a unilateral disease but eventually becomes bilateral. It is caused by a maternally inherited mitochondrial DNA point mutation most commonly in the MT-ND4 gene at 11778 nucleotide position.

CLINICAL FEATURES

Symptoms

Slowly progressive painless blurring of vision. It is usually unilateral although some patients may present with bilateral vision loss when they present when the second eye has already involved.

Signs

- Reduced visual acuity
- Abnormal red-green differentiation
- Reduced contrast sensitivity
- A relative afferent pupillary defect may be present.
- Disc hyperemia with obscuration of disc margin in typical cases.
- Swelling of the peripapillary nerve fiber layer pseudo disc edema.
- Dilated capillaries on the disc surface which may extend onto the adjacent retina (telangiectatic microangiopathy).
- Optic atrophy in late stages **(Fig. 21.42)**

Investigations

Genetic testing to look for common causative mutations may be done. Fluorescein angiography to rule out true edema of optic disc (which shows leakage in comparison to pseudo-disc edema which does not).

Management

There is no established treatment. Supplements such as vitamin B_{12} and C, coenzyme Q10, and lutein are recommended. Patients should be asked to avoid alcohol and tobacco. Idebenone may be effective in some. Low vision aids can be provided early. Genetic counselling to affected family members and maternal relatives should be done.

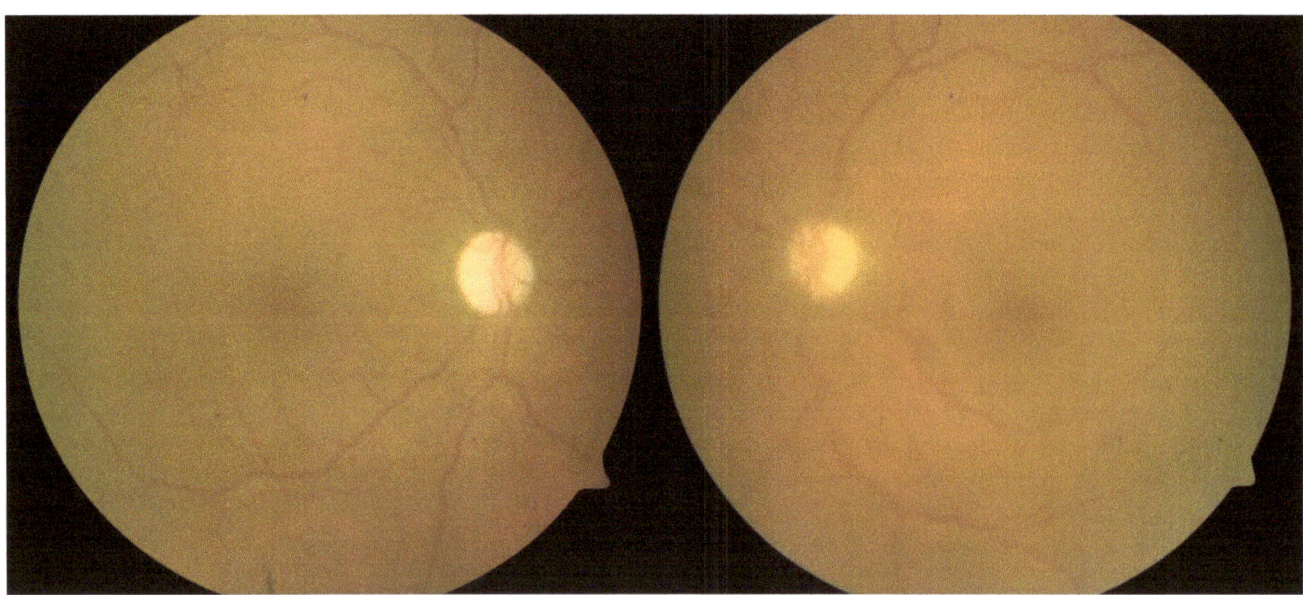

Fig. 21.42: LHON with bilateral optic atrophy and loss of RNFL in papillomacular bundle.

PAPILLEDEMA

It is defined as optic disc swelling due to raised intracranial pressure (ICP). Obstruction to outflow of cerebrospinal fluid due to tumors, cysts, stenosis of aqueduct of Sylvius, craniosynostosis, infections (meningitis) may cause this or may be idiopathic.

CLINICAL FEATURES

- Visual symptoms are usually absent or mild in early stages.
- Transient obscuration of vision for few seconds.
- Horizontal diplopia may occur due to 6th nerve paresis. This is a false localizing sign.
- Headaches waking up the patient from sleep tend to occur early in the morning. These may be generalized or localized.
- Nausea and projectile vomiting (vomiting not preceded by nausea) may occur.
- Altered consciousness which gradually worsens.

CLASSIFICATIONS

Frisen scale is used for grading of papilledema (**Fig. 21.43**).

Stage 0: Normal optic disc	Blurring of nasal, superior and inferior poles radial nerve fiber layer (NFL) without NFL tortuosity
Stage 1: Very early papilledema	Obscuration of the nasal border of the disc. No elevation of the disc borders
Stage 2: Early papilledema	Obscuration of all borders. Elevation of nasal border. Complete peripapillary halo
Stage 3: Moderate papilledema	Obscuration of all borders. Obscuration of one or more segments of major blood vessels leaving the disc
Stage 4: Marked Papilledema	Elevation of the entire nerve head. Obscuration of all borders. Peripapillary halo. Total obscuration on the disc of segment of a major blood vessel
Stage 5: Severe papilledema	Dome-shaped protrusions representing anterior expansion of the optic nerve head. Total obscuration of a segment of a major blood vessel may or may not be present. Obliteration of the optic cup

MANAGEMENT

Depends on underlying cause. If meningitis with infectious cause is present, treatment of specific etiology whether viral, bacterial or tubercular with antimicrobials is required. Surgical removal of space-occupying lesion may be required. Treatment of idiopathic intracranial hypertension (IIH) is discussed below.

IDIOPATHIC INTRACRANIAL HYPERTENSION/ PSEUDOTUMOR CEREBRI

It is characterized by elevated intracranial tension which by definition has no identifiable cause. 90% are women and are obese. It occurs usually in the 3rd decade of life. It is associated with the use of exogenous substances such as vitamin A, retinoic acid, tetracycline, minocycline, doxycycline, lithium and corticosteroids. Sleep apnea has been associated.

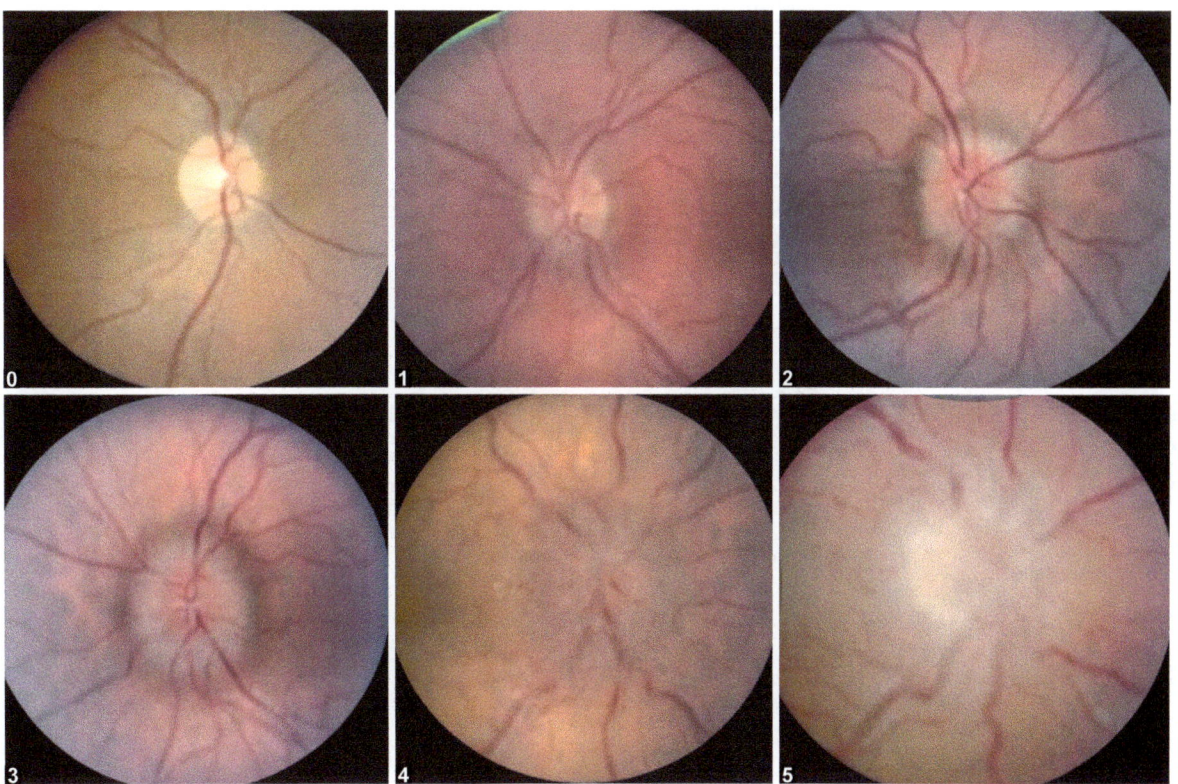

Fig. 21.43: Various stages of disc edema.

(*Source:* Frisén L. Swelling of the optic nerve head: a staging scheme. J Neurol Neurosurg Psychiatry. 1982;45:13).

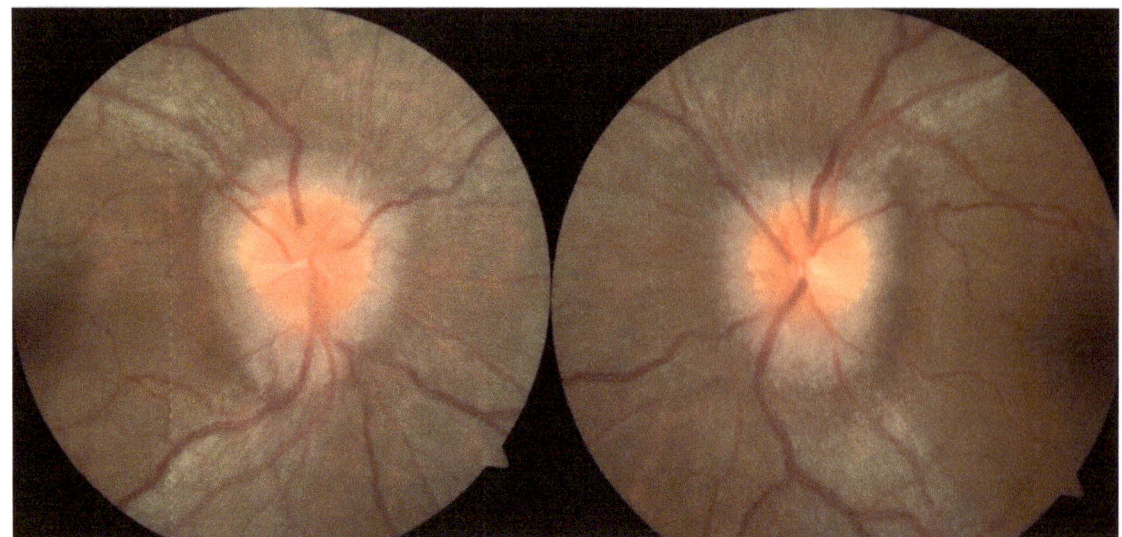

Fig. 21.44: Papilledema in a patient with IIH.

CLINICAL FEATURES

- Headache is common.
- Neck and back pain, transient visual obscurations, diplopia, pulsatile tinnitus, nausea may occur.

Signs

All patients usually have papilledema **(Fig. 21.44)**. 6th cranial nerve paresis may be associated. Visual acuity is usually normal and visual field testing may reveal enlarged blind spot.

Diagnostic Investigations

Neuroimaging is essential to rule out other causes of raised intracranial tension. So, MRI and magnetic resonance venography must be done to rule out these disorders. Characteristic MRI findings include flattening of globes, enlarged optic nerve sheaths, partially empty sella **(Fig. 21.45)**.

Treatment

Weight loss is advised. Medical management to lower raised intracranial tension includes acetazolamide (first-line treatment), furosemide or topiramate.

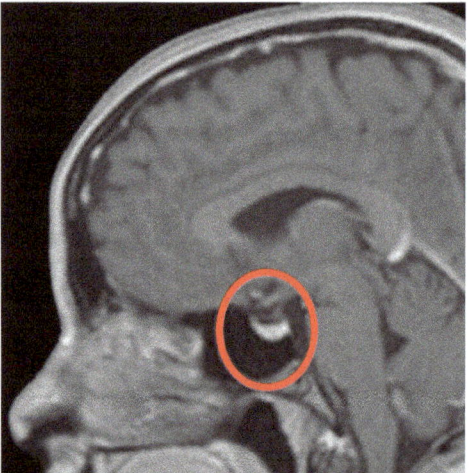

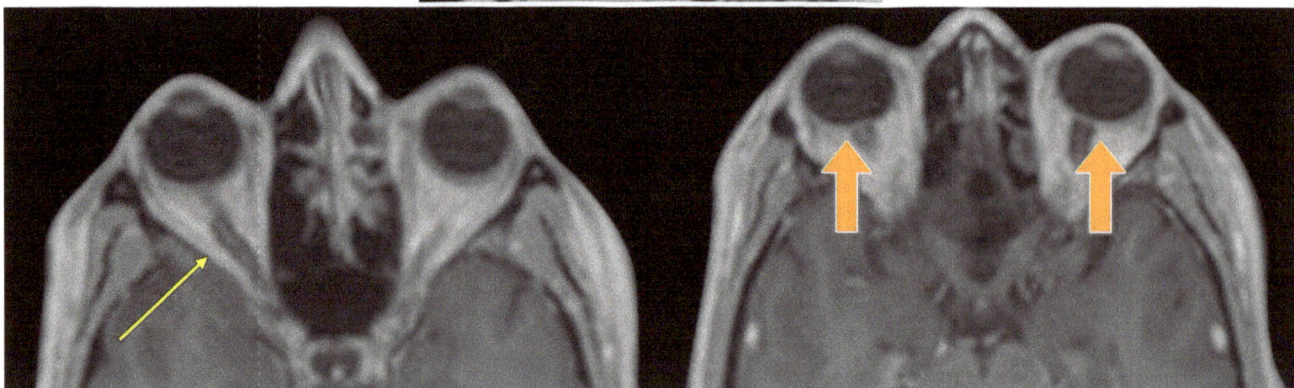

Fig. 21.45: MRI shows partially empty sella in sagittal section (red circle). Lower left image shows tortuous optic nerve sheath (yellow arrow). Lower right image shows posterior flattening of globes (orange arrows).

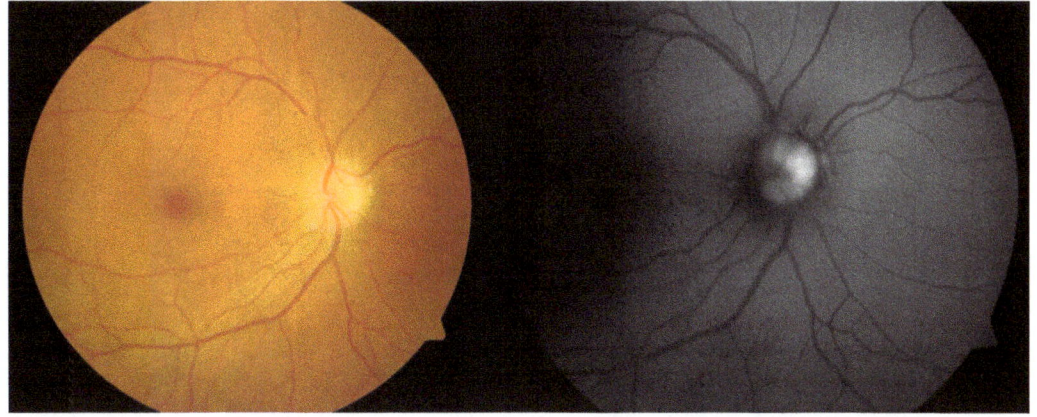

Fig. 21.46: Optic disc drusen showing pseudo disc edema and a 'lumpy bumpy' appearance of optic nerve head. Autofluorescence image on right clearly shows the drusen as hyperautofluorescent.

PSEUDO-DISC EDEMA

It is the anomalous elevation of one or both optic discs without edema of the retinal nerve fiber layer. It is important to distinguish from true disc edema which could be the first sign of a disease which may cause vision loss, neurological impairment or death. It may be due to a number of causes.

1. Optic nerve head drusen **(Fig. 21.46)**
2. Congenital anomalies such as myelinated nerve fibers, hypoplastic disc, tilted disc, Bergmeister papillae (incompletely regressed posterior end of hyaloid artery). Morning glory disc anomaly, small optic disc.
3. Optic disc infiltration by neoplasia or inflammatory cells.
4. Systemic causes such as Down's syndrome, Leber's Hereditary optic neuropathy, Kenny syndrome, Alagille syndrome.

In true disc edema, swelling of the peripapillary nerve fiber layer obscures underlying retinal blood vessels. In pseudo disc edema there is no such obscuration. This is the most important distinguishing feature. Spontaneous venous pulsations when present indicate that there is no raised intracranial tension and indicate that it is pseudo disc edema. Optic disc drusen give a lumpy bumpy appearance with visible retinal vessels.

OCULAR MYOPATHIES

MYASTHENIA GRAVIS

It is an autoimmune disease that affects voluntary muscles of the body due to antibodies against acetylcholine receptor (ACh) at postsynaptic neuromuscular junction (NMJ) causing impaired impulse transmission. Ocular myasthenia affects only the ocular muscles. Muscle weakness increases with sustained muscle activation, and improves after rest.

Clinical Features

Symptoms

Patient complains of worsening muscle weakness in the evening, worsening with use and improving with rest. The most frequently muscles affected are levator palpebrae superioris causing ptosis, extraocular muscles, orbicularis oculi, muscles of facial expression, mastication, and speech.

The edrophonium (Tensilon test) is used for diagnosis. Positive test consists of elevation of ptotic eyelid 2–5 minutes after administration of edrophonium.

Management

Medical Therapy

- Acetylcholine inhibitors such pyridostigmine and neostigmine reduce breakdown of acetylcholine by acetylcholinesterase enzyme at the NMJ. Oral steroids are used as adjunctive therapy.
- Immunomodulators are given in refractory cases.

Surgery

Removal of thymus gland is recommended in symptomatic cases.

CHRONIC PROGRESSIVE EXTERNAL OPHTHALMOPLEGIA

Chronic progressive external ophthalmoplegia (CPEO) is a hereditary myopathy affecting the extraocular muscles. It is a chronic, bilateral, typically symmetric, progressive, external (sparing pupils) ophthalmoplegia. It occurs most commonly due to deletions in mitochondrial DNA. Ptosis usually the first sign is bilateral and symmetric. External ophthalmoplegia is symmetric and begins in young adulthood and gradually progressive **(Fig. 21.47)**. Diplopia may occur. Systemic associations include cardiac conduction abnormality, pigmentary retinopathy with a salt and pepper fundus. Serum lactate, creatinine kinase, and cerebrospinal fluid (CSF) lactate may be elevated. Electromyography shows myotonic and myopathic potentials. Muscle biopsy shows 'ragged red fibers' on Gomori's trichrome stain. Electrocardiography demonstrates cardiac conduction defects, pacemaker implantation may be required. Genetic testing may be done. Diplopia is treated with prism lenses. Squint surgery may be done once disease becomes stable but it may recur even after surgery. Ptosis surgery is done after squint surgery.

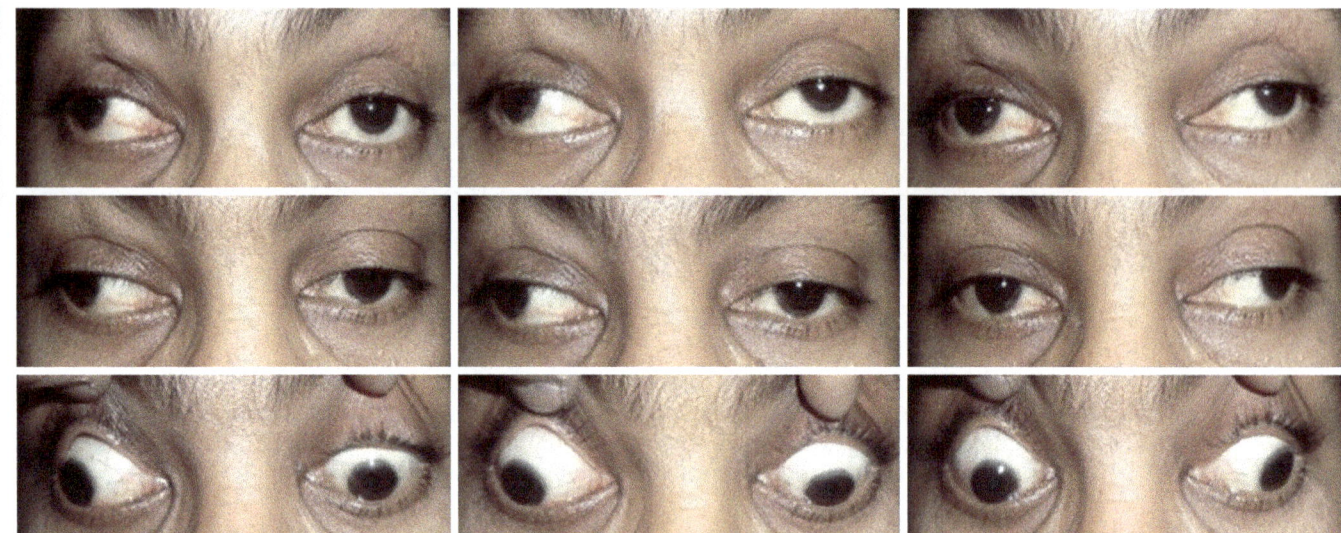

Fig. 21.47: CPEO showing bilateral ptosis with right exotropia in primary position. There is bilateral limitation of movement in all positions of gaze.

GERIATRIC CONSIDERATIONS

1. **Stroke:** Elderly patients often suffer multiple ailments such as hypertension, diabetes, hypercholesterolemia resulting in atherosclerosis and ultimately occlusion of arteries with one of the manifestations being stroke. Such patients have wide-ranging symptoms but may only present with diplopia due to 3rd/4th/6th nerve paresis. Neuroimaging is not indicated in these cases and the manifestation are due to microvascular occlusion and require management of underling comorbidities. However pupil involving 3rd nerve palsies require neuroimaging to rule out compressive lesions.
2. **Progressive supranuclear palsy:** A disease of elderly, tauopathy present with vertical ophthalmoplegia more in downgaze. Symptomatic treatment and physical therapy are mainstay. Mirror prism glasses and botox injections may help but prognosis is poor.
3. **Giant cell arteritis:** Usually seen in patients older than 50 years, it presents with acute onset unilateral vision loss with scalp tenderness, headache, jaw claudication. It is an ophthalmic emergency.
4. **Nonarteritic ischemic optic neuropathy:** Most common optic neuropathy in patients older than 50 years associated with systemic comorbidities such as hypertension and diabetes. It presents with sudden onset painless unilateral vision loss. Control of systemic risk factors plays an important role to prevent vision loss in contralateral pathway.

NURSING MANAGEMENT

Assessment

- **Gather patient history:** Obtain a comprehensive medical history, including any neurological or ophthalmological conditions, previous treatments, surgeries, and medications.
- **Perform a neurological assessment:** Evaluate cranial nerve function, reflexes, motor and sensory function, coordination, and gait.
- **Conduct an ophthalmological assessment:** Assess visual acuity, visual fields, pupillary responses, extraocular movements, and any other relevant eye-related assessments.
- **Explore symptoms:** Thoroughly assess the patient's chief complaints, such as diplopia, vision changes, eye pain, nystagmus, and any other neurological or ophthalmological symptoms.
- **Evaluate the patient's cognitive and emotional status:** Assess how the condition impacts the patient's mental and emotional well-being.

Nursing Diagnosis

- Risk for falls related to visual disturbances and impaired coordination.
- Impaired sensory perception (visual) related to the neuro-ophthalmological condition.
- Deficient knowledge about the condition and its management.
- Anxiety related to changes in vision or diagnosis uncertainty.

Nursing Interventions

- Administer prescribed medications and monitor for any adverse effects.
- Provide information about the neuro-ophthalmological condition, its management, medications, lifestyle modifications, and safety precautions.
- Assist with visual field assessments and document the results.
- Offer emotional support, address concerns, and provide counseling to patients and their families.
- Implement fall prevention strategies and ensure a safe environment for the patient.

SUMMARY

1. Any neuro-ophthalmological case must be approached in a step manner with detailed history, careful neuro-ophthalmological examination, required investigation to reach out to the diagnosis and appropriate management.
2. Knowledge of topographic neuro-anatomy and its clinical implication is MUST in any neuro-ophthalmological case.

MULTIPLE CHOICE QUESTIONS

1. From which retina layers does the visual pathway begin:
   a. Retinal nerve fiber layer
   b. Ganglion cell layer
   c. Photoreceptor layer
   d. Retinal pigment epithelium
2. Pupil involving third nerve palsy may be seen in which of the following conditions:
   a. Diabetes
   b. Hypertension
   c. CNS tumors
   d. Myasthenia gravis
3. MRI is superior to CT in all of the following, *except*:
   a. Acute infarct
   b. Acute hemorrhage
   c. Demyelinating disease
   d. Parenchymal abnormalities
4. Which of the following is not helpful is distinguishing disc edema from disc drusen?
   a. Ultrasound
   b. Fundus autofluorescence
   c. Disc elevation
   d. Fluorescein angiography
5. Which is the most common optic neuropathy in patients above 50 years of age?
   a. Traumatic
   b. Demyelinating
   c. Compressive
   d. NAION
6. Which of the following is not a risk factor for pseudotumor cerebri?
   a. Oral contraceptives
   b. Obesity
   c. Weight loss
   d. Tetracyclines
7. Which is not a feature of dorsal midbrain syndrome (Parinaud's syndrome)?
   a. Convergence retraction nystagmus
   b. Lid retraction
   c. Upgaze palsy
   d. Light-near dissociation
8. A lesion in left temporal lobe would cause which type of field defect:
   a. Pie in sky
   b. Pie if floor
   c. Homonymous hemianopia
   d. Heteronymous hemianopia
9. Which of the following is not a cause of pseudo-disc edema?
   a. Optic disc drusen
   b. Idiopathic intracranial hypertension
   c. Hyperopia
   d. Bergmeister papilla
10. Which is true about RAPD?
    a. A chiasmal lesion may be associated
    b. A patient with optic neuropathy always has RAPD
    c. It is never seen in retinal disease
    d. An RAPD is never seen except in setting of optic neuropathy

ANSWERS

1. c	2. c	3. b	4. c
5. d	6. c	7. d	8. a
9. b	10. c		

SUGGESTED READING

1. Belliveau AP, Somani AN, Dossani RH. Pupillary light reflex; 2019.
2. Bell RA, Waggoner PM, Boyd WM, Akers RE, Yee CE. Clinical grading of relative afferent pupillary defects. Archives of Ophthalmology. 1993;111(7):938-42.
3. Carroll J, Conway BR. Color vision. Handb Clin Neurol. 2021;178:131-53. doi: 10.1016/B978-0-12-821377-3.00005-2. PMID:33832674.
4. Dragoi, Valentin. Chapter 7: Ocular motor system. Neuroscience Online: An Electronic Textbook for the Neurosciences. Department of Neurobiology and Anatomy, The University of Texas Medical School at Houston.
5. Eggers SD. Approach to the examination and classification of nystagmus. Journal of Neurologic Physical Therapy. 2019;43:S20-6.
6. Frisén L. Swelling of the optic nerve head: a staging scheme. J Neurol Neurosurg Psychiatry. 1982;45:13.
7. Gupta M, Bordoni B. Neuroanatomy, visual pathway. 2020.
8. Jong P. A history of visual acuity testing and optotypes. Eye. 2022;10.
9. Kanski JJ, Bowling B. Kanski's clinical ophthalmology e-book: a systematic approach. Elsevier Health Sciences; 2015.
10. Khan Z, Bollu PC. Horner syndrome. In: StatPearls [Internet], StatPearls Publishing; 2022.
11. Leigh RJ, Zee DS. The neurology of eye movements. Contemporary Neurology; 2015.
12. Odom JV, Bach M, Brigell M, Holder GE, McCulloch DL, Mizota A, Tormene AP. International Society for Clinical Electrophysiology of Vision. ISCEV standard for clinical visual evoked potentials: (2016 update). Doc Ophthalmol. 2016;133(1):1-9. doi: 10.1007/s10633-016-9553-y. Epub 2016 Jul 21. PubMed PMID: 27443562.
13. Sekhon RK, Cabrero FR, Deibel JP. Nystagmus types. In: StatPearls [Internet]. StatPearls Publishing; 2021.
14. Shields M, Sinkar S, Chan W, Crompton J. Parinaud syndrome: a 25-year (1991-2016) review of 40 consecutive adult cases. Acta Ophthalmologica. 2017;95(8):e792-3.

CHAPTER 22

Strabismus

Shweta Chaurasia, Shagun Korla, Kiran Kumari

"Better see rightly on a pound a week than squint on a million."
—George Bernard Shaw

LEARNING OBJECTIVES

After going through the chapter, the learner will be able to:

- Understand the relevant physiology of eye movements and related disorders.
- Discuss the sensory aspects of strabismus and relevant motor aspects with regard to strabismus examination.
- Appreciate amblyopia—a preventable cause of blindness in children.
- Discuss common conditions causing strabismus in various age groups.
- Understand the diagnostic criteria of strabismus.
- Discuss the management of different types of strabismus.
- Discuss the geriatric consideration related to strabismus.

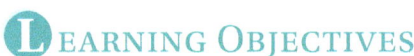

- Amblyopia
- Comitant
- Diplopia/confusion
- Duanes retraction syndrome
- Ductions
- Esotropia/exotropia
- Hypertropia/hypotropia
- Incomitant
- Maddox rod
- Recession-resection
- Suppression
- Vergence
- Versions

INTRODUCTION

Strabismus means misaligned eyes. The term "Strabismus" is derived from a Greek word, which denotes "oblique eyes looking." Often it is referred to as "squint," or "crossed eyes." Both eyes are programmed to fixate binocularly on an object in the straight gaze which transmits two images in the brain where images with slight disparity overlap and fuse and one single image is perceived. In strabismus, one eye gets misaligned or deviated inwards or outwards and a patient with a mature brain experience double vision, and a child with an immature brain suppress one image to avoid confusion and eventually develop amblyopia. Strabismus can develop due to refractive error or binocular fusion or neuromuscular abnormalities. If diagnosed and treated early, it has a very good prognosis. Its prevalence is 2–5% in the general population. Treatment includes refractive error correction, patching therapy, orthoptic exercises, topical drugs, and extraocular muscle surgery.

Etiopathogenesis is unclear. Following two theories regarding cause of strabismus are commonly believed. Claude Worth theory proposes inherent absence of cortical fusional potential as a cause of strabismus whereas according to Chavasse theory motor alignment leads to a poor sensory status and strabismus.

Strabismus or squint is broadly classified as apparent squint or pseudo-strabismus (which includes pseudoesotropia and pseudoexotropia), latent squint (heterophoria) and manifest squint (heterotopia). Manifest strabismus can be concomitant or incomitant.

Causes of Concomitant Squint

Sensory causes: These interfere with a clear image formation in one eye. Refractive errors, anisometropia, media opacities, obstruction of pupillary area, macular and optic nerve diseases, and wrong glass prescription for refractive error.

Strabismus can be the first symptom in certain serious conditions like ocular malignancies like retinoblastoma in children, choroidal melanoma in adults or brain tumors in which fusional mechanism is compromised.

The motor causes: These interfere with ocular alignment, orbital, extraocular muscle, and accommodation abnormalities.

Causes of Incomitant Squint

- **Neurogenic causes:** Hypoplasia of 3rd, 4th, and 6th cranial nerve nuclei, tumors, infections, trauma, toxicity (alcohol, lead, carbon monoxide), vascular (ophthalmoplegic migraine), and demyelinating lesions affecting the third and sixth cranial nerves.
- **Myogenic causes:** Congenital lesions, trauma, muscle incarceration in orbital fractures, post-viral myositis, and chronic progressive external ophthalmoplegia (CPEO).
- **Neuromuscular junction disorders:** Myasthenia gravis.
  - Strabismus is more prevalent with certain syndromes like Down syndrome, cerebral palsy, Apert-Crouzon syndrome, premature infants with low birth weight, and in kids with affected parents or siblings. All siblings of a strabismic child should be screened at an early age for strabismus as sensorimotor anomalies are common in the pedigrees of strabismic probands.
  - Strabismus in immature visual system of children can lead to strabismic amblyopia whereas in mature visual system in adults lead to bothersome diplopia. Cycloplegic refraction should be done in all children. Amblyopia should be corrected before surgery is undertaken in children. Cause of strabismus should always be looked before initiating treatment.
  - Strabismus should be corrected
  - For development or restoration of binocular vision
  - To avoid double vision
  - For increasing visual field
  - Restoration of normal head posture
  - Cosmetic correction for psychological and social reasons.

APPLIED ANATOMY

Extraocular Muscles (Fig. 22.1)

The extraocular muscles are located within the orbit and control the movements of each eye. These extraocular muscles are- Superior rectus, inferior rectus, medial rectus, lateral rectus, inferior oblique, and superior oblique.

Extraocular Movements and Relevant Physiology

The eye movements when tested uniocularly are called ductions and when tested binocularly are called versions.

Ductions

It is checked only monocularly. But it has a disadvantage that in case of paresis normal duction may be seen due to extra innervation achieved on order to compensate for the paresis. Yoke muscles achieve this extra- innervation which demonstrates overaction. Thus, versions pick up paresis which is missed on duction.

Ductions are (Fig. 22.2):
- Adduction
- Abduction
- Circumduction or elevation
- Deo-sursumduction or depression
- Incycloduction
- Excycloduction

Versions

Versions are binocular eye movements that are in the same direction (conjugate eye movements). Versions in three diagnostic planes are (**Table 22.1**):

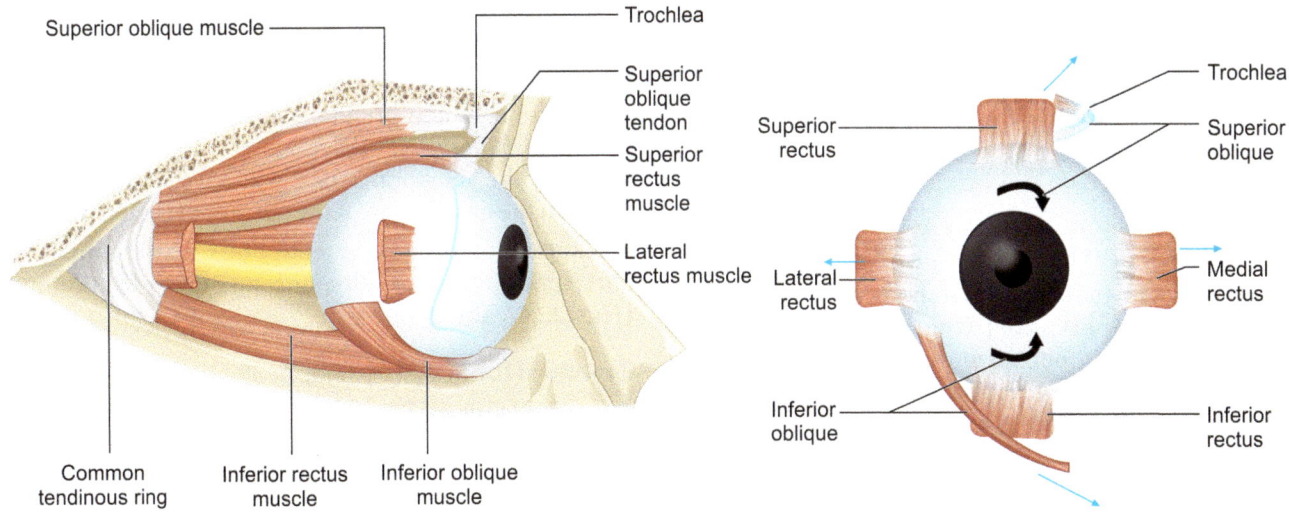

Fig. 22.1: Extraocular muscles.

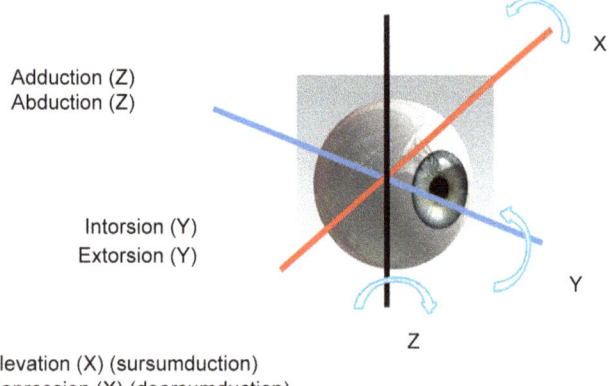

Elevation (X) (sursumduction)
Depression (X) (deorsumduction)

Fig. 22.2: Ductions.

TABLE 22.1: Versions.	
Dextroversion	—
Levoversion	—
Dextroelevation	Dextrocycloversion
Levoelevation	Levocycloversion
Dextro-depression	Depression
Levo-depression	Elevation

TABLE 22.2: Actions of extraocular muscles.			
Extraocular muscles	Primary action	Secondary action	Tertiary action
Superior rectus	Elevation	Intorsion	Adduction
Inferior rectus	Depression	Extorsion	Adduction
Lateral rectus	Abduction	—	—
Medial rectus	Adduction	—	—
Superior oblique	Intorsion	Depression	Adduction
Inferior oblique	Extorsion	Elevation	Adduction

Vergence

Vergence are binocular eye movements that are in the opposite direction (disconjugate eye movements). They help in keeping the squint under control.
- Positive vertical vergence (right eye up, left eye down)
- Negative vertical vergence (right eye down, left eye up).
- Incyclovergence (both eyes intort)
- Excyclovergence (both eyes extort)

Actions of Extraocular Muscles

See **Table 22.2**.

The Rectus-Oblique Intrigue (Fig. 22.3)

It is important to understand that though superior oblique (SO) and inferior oblique (IO) are abductors (tertiary action), but during ocular motility examination their depression and elevation actions respectively are checked in the adducted position as in adducted position. SO is a pure depressor and IO is pure elevator.

Similarly Superior rectus (SR) and inferior rectus (IR) are adductors (tertiary action), but during ocular motility examination their elevation and depression actions are checked respectively in the abducted position as in

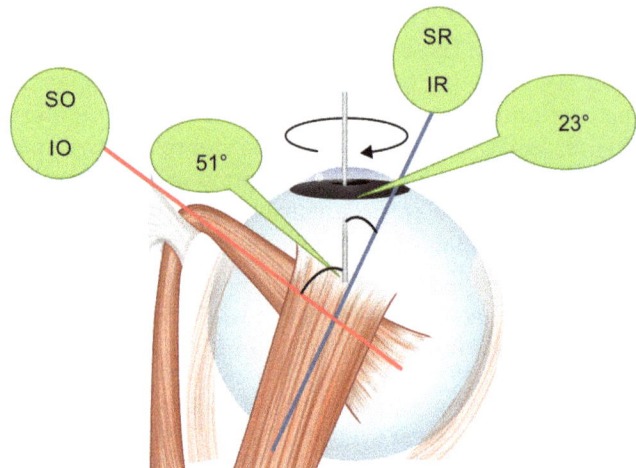

Fig. 22.3: Rectus-oblique intrigue.

abducted position SR is a pure elevator and IR is a pure depressor.

Laws of Muscle Actions

- **Descartes-Sherrington's law of reciprocal innervation:** Describes that agonist and antagonist extraocular muscles share reciprocal innervational relationship.
- **Hering's law:** Describes that pairs of muscles in the two eyes that move them in the same direction are called *yoked muscles,* or synergists.

   Six muscles = Six position = Six cardinal positions (Fig. 22.4)

Key Points

1. Rectii adduct (except LR) and obliques abduct
2. Inferiors extort and superiors intort
3. Rectii act according to their names whereas obliques act opposite to their names.

SENSORY EVALUATION

Physiology of Binocular Vision

We perceive the world as though we have one eye which exists between our two eyes:
1. Primary visual direction
2. Common visual direction

Corresponding retinal points: Every retinal point in one eye shares common primary visual with a retinal point in other eye **(Fig. 22.5)**. These are corresponding points A point on the temporal retina will have a corresponding point on the nasal retina of the other eye **(Fig. 22.5)**.

Horopter: locus of all object points that are imaged in corresponding retinal elements at a given fixation point **(Figs. 22.6A and B)**.

Grades of Binocularity (Fig. 22.7)

Grade 1: Simultaneous macular perception
Grade 2: Fusion
Grade 3: Stereopsis (highest grade of binocularity)

Theory of Correspondence and Disparity

Salient features are:

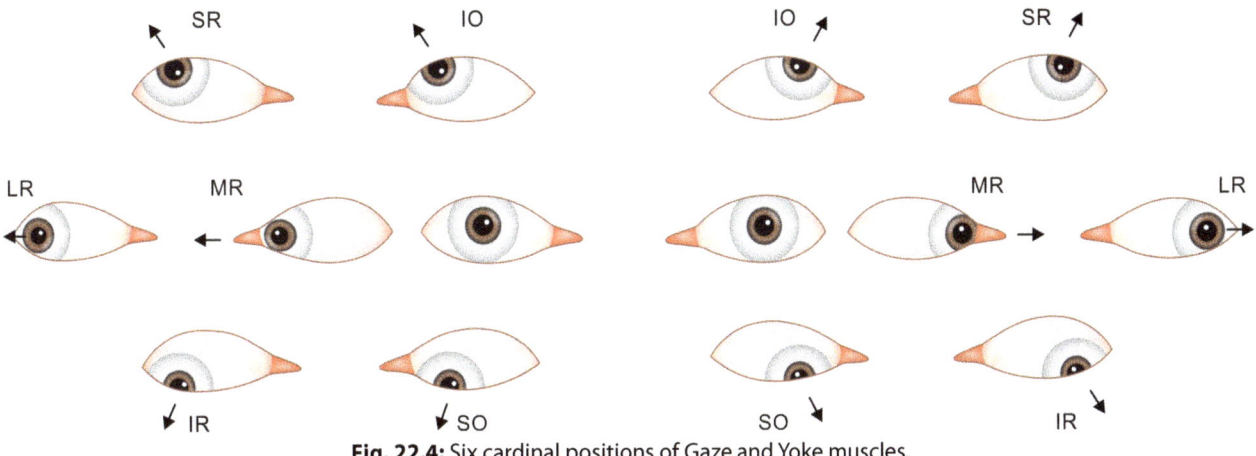

Fig. 22.4: Six cardinal positions of Gaze and Yoke muscles.

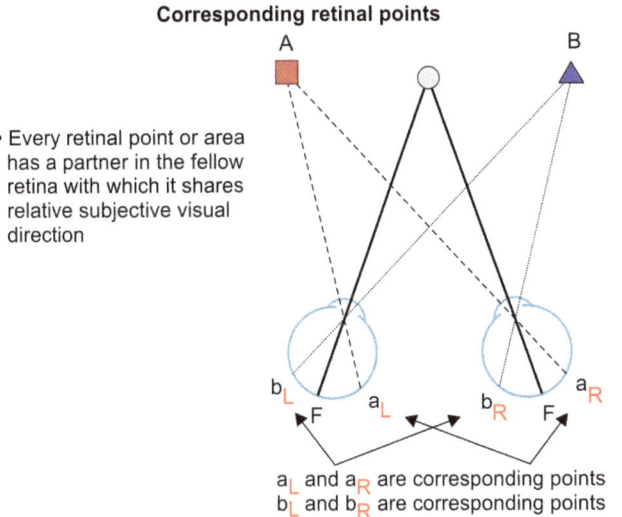

Fig. 22.5: Corresponding retinal points.

- Simultaneous stimulation of corresponding points by one object transmits single visual image without depth.
- **Normal retinal correspondence** results when both foveae share a common primary visual direction.
- **Abnormal retinal correspondence:** The fovea of one eye shares a common primary visual direction with an extrafoveal point on the other eye.
- Binocular single vision with stereopsis results when the horizontal disparity remains within the limits of Panum's area.

Sensory Adaptations to Squint

Mature visual system:
- Occurs after development of bi-foveal fusion.
- Usually after 7–8 years of age
- Includes diplopia and confusion.

Confusion

- Perception of two different objects simultaneously from fixing fovea and deviated fovea result in confusion **(Fig. 22.7)**.
- When fovea of each eye see different objects and patient may see two images superimposed on each other.

Diplopia

- Perception of single object simultaneously at different location in space result in diplopia **(Fig. 22.8)**.

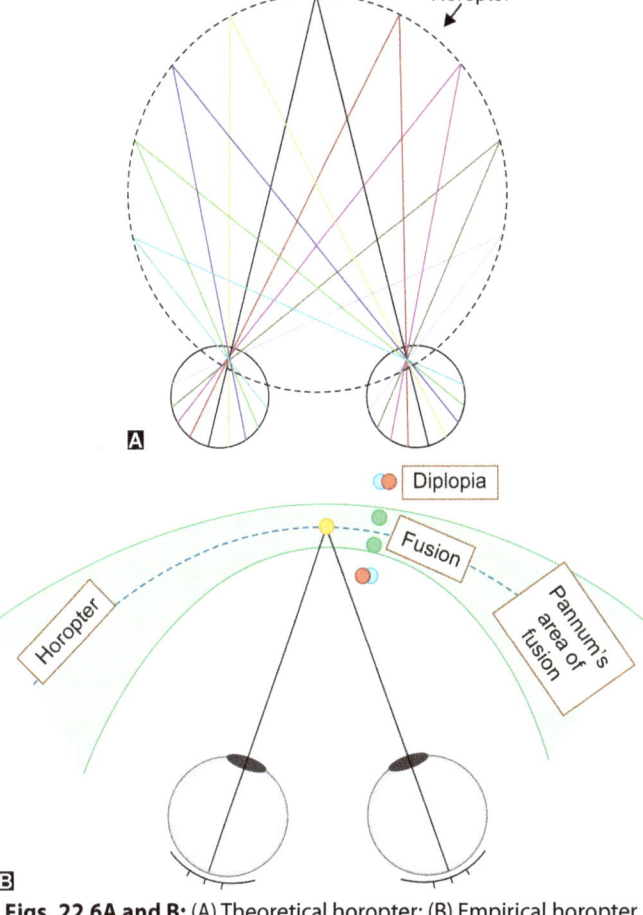

Figs. 22.6A and B: (A) Theoretical horopter; (B) Empirical horopter and Pannum's area of fusion.

- When fovea and extra foveal point of each eye see same object but and hence patient see two images (which are same) but at different locations.
- Usually seen in acquired strabismus in mature visual system over 7–8 years of age.
- Esotropia has uncrossed diplopia and exotropia has crossed diplopia.

Immature Visual System

- Occur when binocularity disrupted before 6 years of age.
- Results in:
  - Cortical suppression
  - Amblyopia
  - Anomalous retinal correspondence (ARC)

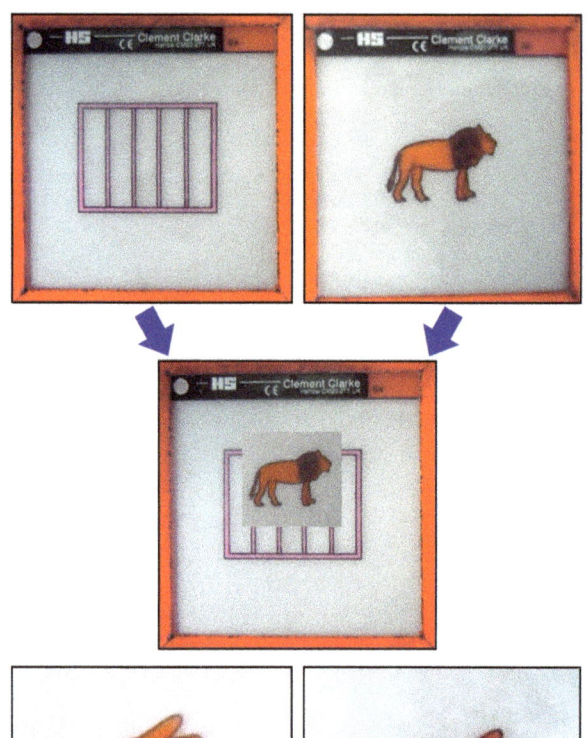

Grade 1
Simultaneous macular perception: When dissimilar objects are seen together, they are perceived together due to simultaneous macular perception
In synoptophore right eye is shown lion and left eye is shown cage. When both viewed together, person see lion in cage due to simultaneous macular perception

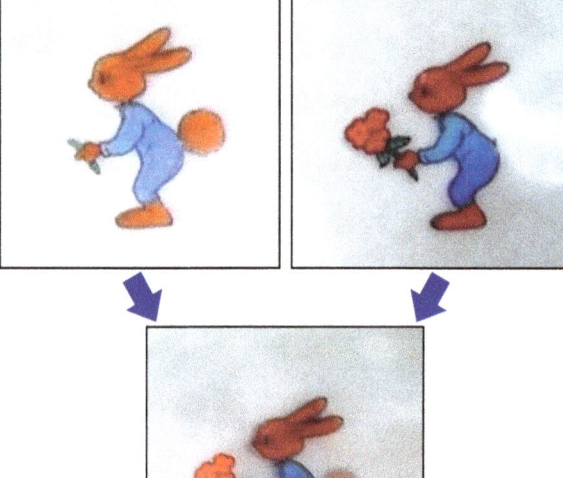

Grade 2
Fusion: When similar objects with small dissimilar parts are seen together, similar images dissimilar parts fuse
In synoptophore right eye is shown rabbit with tail left eye is shown rabbit with flowers. When both viewed together, person rabbit with tail and flowers due to fusion

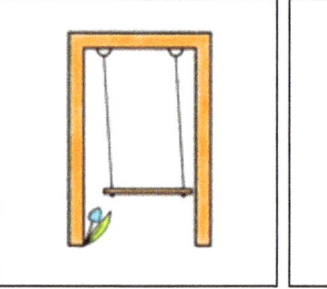 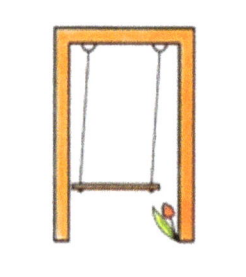

Grade 3
Stereopsis (highest grade of binocularity): When disparate retinal points are fused together within Pannum's area of fusion there is 3-dimensional viewing of object called stereopsis
In synoptophore right eye can be shown swing with nasal/temporal disparity and left eye is also shown nasal/temporal disparity and swing can be seen in 3-dimension with both eyes

Fig. 22.7: Grades of binocularity.

Suppression

- Defined as temporary active cortical inhibition of image formed on retina of the squinting eye.
- Occurs during binocular vision.
- Disappears when squinting eye fixates.

Abnormal Retinal Correspondence

Factors affecting development:

- Age of onset of squint—<6 years
- Patient profile—where single binocular vision previously existed
- Type of squint—more common in isotopes, less common in vertical deviations, in uniocular squint than alternating

Binocular sensory adaptation used to eliminate diplopia by accepting eccentric image location in deviated eye.

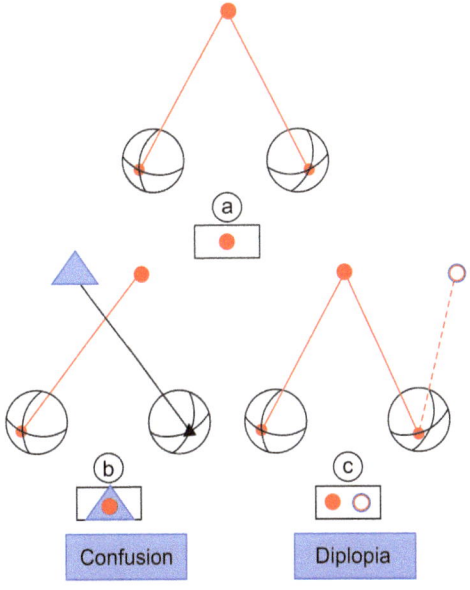

Fig. 22.8: Difference between confusion (two location one localization and diplopia (one location two localization).

Allows brain to accept parafoveal images from deviated eye and superimposes with image from fixing eye. New functional fovea called pseudofovea.

Tests for Sensory Evaluation

WFDT (Worth Four Dot Test)

- Depicts the status of peripheral binocularity.
- Performed in dark, as in brighter illumination patient can see room environment with strong fusion clues, hence testing in dark more dissociating **(Figs. 22.9A to E)**
  - Normal response—is seeing 4 lights, 2 red and 2 green or 1 red, 2 green and 1 light flickering between red and green.
  - Response
    - 4 lights (2 green and 2 red or 2 green, 1 red and 1 yellow)—fusion present.
    - 5 lights (3 green and 2 red)—diplopia (crossed exotropia; uncrossed-esotropia)
    - 3 green or 2 red—cortical suppression

Key Points

- Large scotoma—suppress both distance and near worth 4 dot test.
- Monofixation syndrome—fuse near but suppress distance worth 4 dot test.
- **Large scotoma—suppress both distance and near worth 4 dot test.**
- **Monofixation syndrome—fuse near but suppress distance worth 4 dot test.**
- Worth 4 dots separated by 6° at near (at 1/3 m) and by 1.25° for distance (at 6 m).

Bagolini Striated Glasses Test

- Clear lenses with a linear scratch through center of the lens converting point of light into a streak of light on retina **(Figs. 22.10 and 22.11)**
- Placed obliquely at 45° and 135°
- Provide free binocular view without dissociation

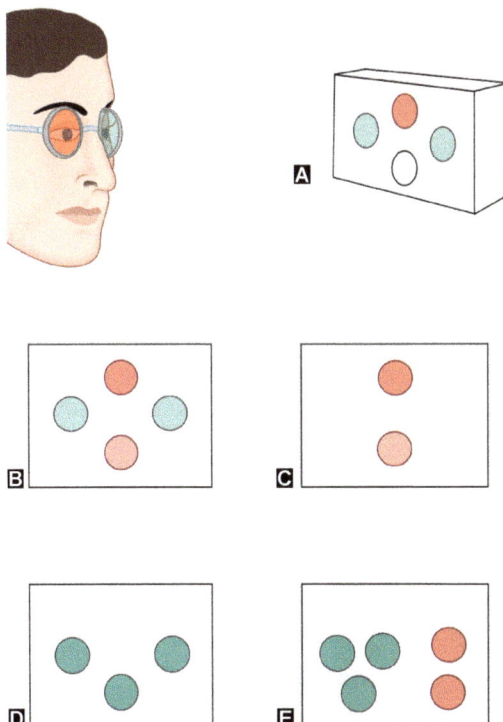

Figs. 22.9A to E: Worth four dot test: (A) 4 lights (2 red and 2 green or 1 red, 2 green and 1 light flickering between red and green)—normal response with NRC or harmonious ARC in presence of small manifest squint; (B) 2 and 2 green or 1 red, 2 green and 1 light flickering between red and green; (C) 2 red—left eye suppression; (D) 3 green—right eye suppression; (E) 5 lights (3 green and 2 red crossed or uncrossed)—diplopia (crossed—exotropia; uncrossed—esotropia).

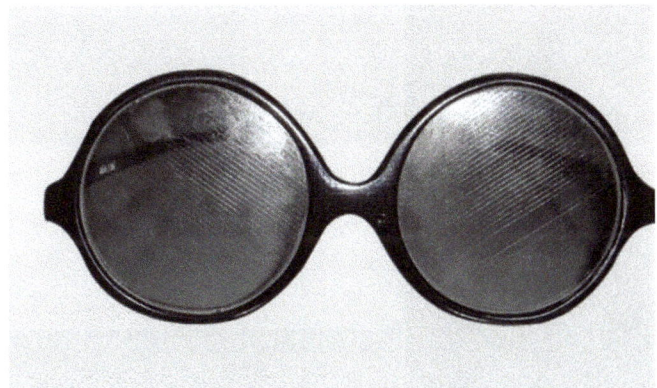

Fig. 22.10: Bagolini striated glass.

Stereopsis Testing

Stereopsis is the ability to fuse horizontally disparate retinal elements within Panum's fusional area resulting in binocular viewing of object in the third dimension (i.e., depth perception). Various tests used are TNO stereo-butterfly test etc. **(Fig. 22.12)**.

MOTOR EVALUATION

Objective tests:
- Head posture
- Hirschberg test
- Cover-uncover test
- Alternate cover test
- Ductions versions; pattern and oblique

- Prism bar cover test (SPCT APCT/PBUCT)
- Krimsky test
- Measurement of vergence
- NPA, NPC, AC/A ratio

Subjective tests:
- Maddox rod
- Maddox tangent scale
- Diplopia test
- Hess/Lee screen test

Head Posture (Figs. 22.13A to C)

It is important to check head posture the moment patient enters the clinic as it may be acquired for different reasons:
- To maintain binocularity as in paralytic squints like opposite side head tilt in 4th nerve palsy **(Fig. 22.13A)**, same side face turn in 6th nerve palsy, or restrictive squints like Duane's retraction syndrome **(Fig. 22.13B)**, Browns syndrome
- To achieve null and improve vision (foveation period) in nystagmus like Infantile nystagmus syndrome or latent nystagmus.
- To keep the diplopic images far if fusion not possible **(Fig. 22.13C)**.

Hirschberg's Test (Figs. 22.14A to E)

- It is a pupillary light reflex test which roughly estimates the type and size of deviation.
    - It is performed by shining a pen torch light and asking the patient to look at the light.
    - If the reflex falls on the If the reflex is at the center in both eyes, it means eyes are aligned and if reflex is not central it means there is presence of squint.
    - Location of reflex with respect to center of pupil tells the type of squint cases of deviated eyes (squint). Reflex always fall opposite to the direction of movement.
        - If reflex nasal cornea it means, there is exotropia.
        - Temporal cornea-esotropia
        - Superior part of cornea-hypotropia
        - Inferior part of cornea-hypertropia
    - Location of reflex with respect to normal pupil estimates the size of deviation.
        - If reflex at pupillary border—15°
        - If reflex midway between pupillary border and limbus—30°
        - If reflex at limbus—45°
        - If reflex far off on sclera—60°
- Hirschberg test should be checked:
    - With glass and without glass to check accommodative squint **(Fig. 22.15)**
    - Distance and near to check convergence excess or insufficiency and divergence excess and divergence insufficiency **(Fig. 22.16)**
    - Right fixing and left fixing to check for comitancy of squint **(Fig. 22.17)**.
        - In comitant squint it is equal.
        - In incomitant squints (paralytic and restrictive) primary deviation is the deviation in affected eye when normal eye takes central fixation and secondary deviation is the deviation in normal eye when affected eye takes or attempts central fixation **(Fig. 22.18)**.
        - Primary deviation is less than secondary in paralytic and restrictive squint.
    - Upgaze and downgaze to look for patterns **(Fig. 22.19)**.

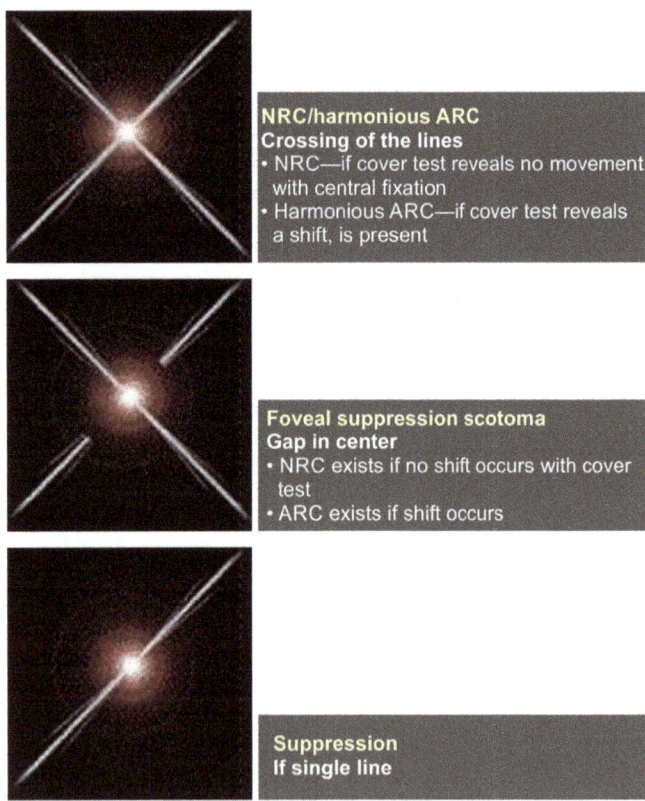

Fig. 22.11: Interpretation of Bagolini striated glasses test.

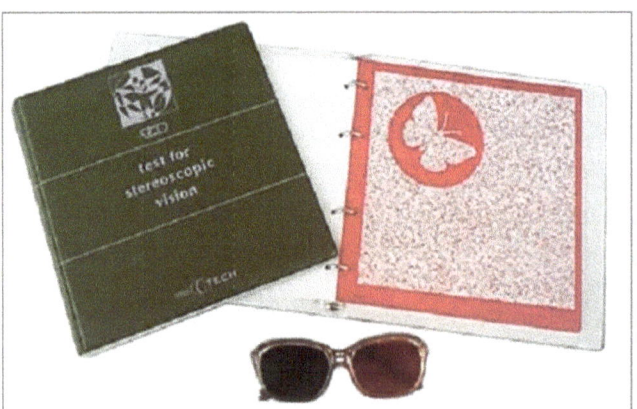
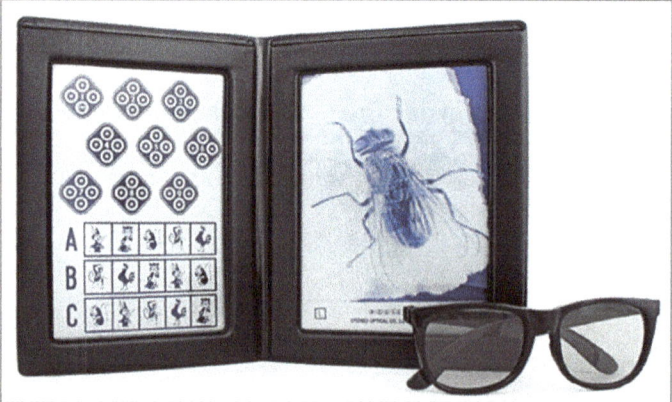

Fig. 22.12: TNO test and stereo-butterfly test.

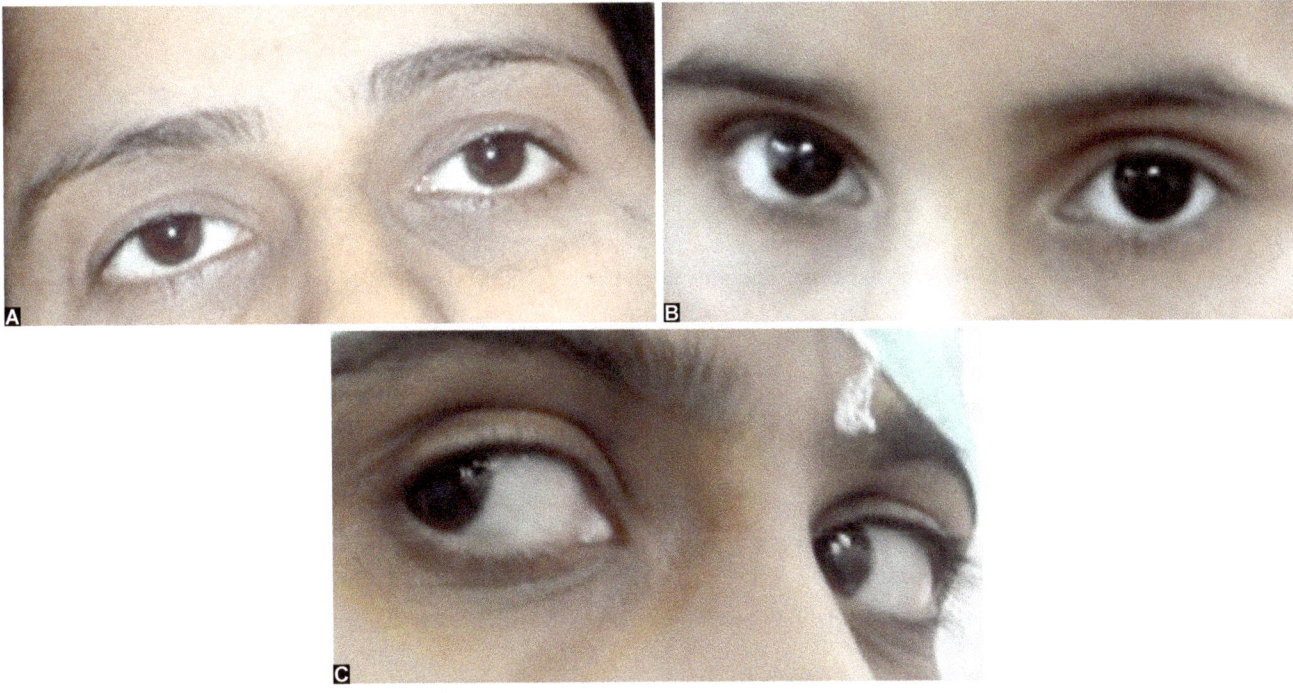

Figs. 22.13A to C: (A) Head tilt in 4th nerve palsy; (B) R face turn in RE ESO DRS; (C) Face turn in manifest nystagmus.

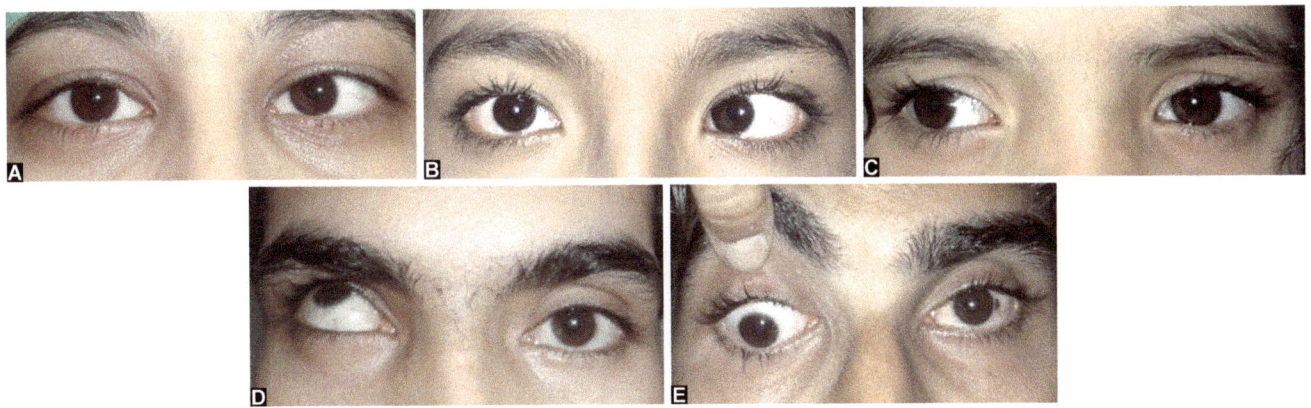

Figs. 22.14A to E: Hirschberg's test: (A) Left eye esotropia 15°; (B) Left eye esotropia 30°; (C) Right eye exotropia 45°; (D) Right eye hypertropia 45°; (E) Right eye hypotropia 45°.

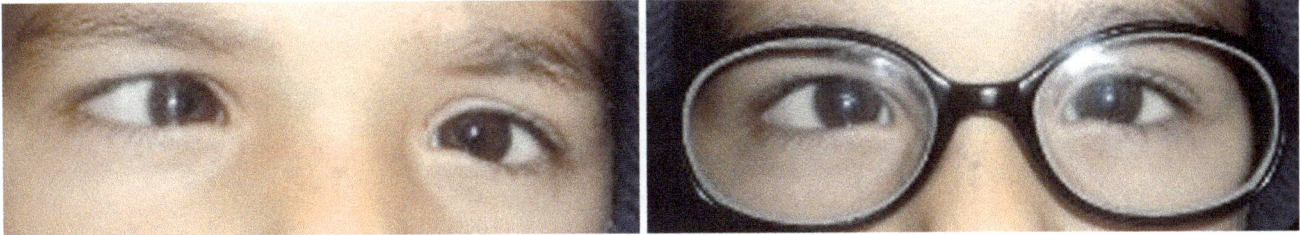

Fig. 22.15: Hirschberg test with glass and without glass to check accommodative squint.

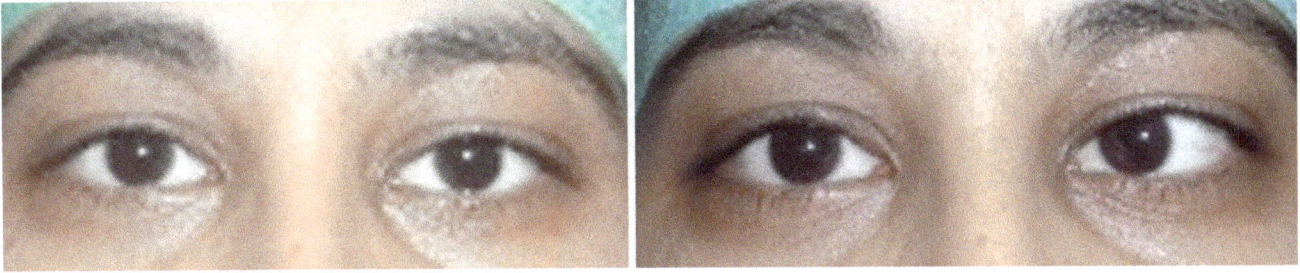

Fig. 22.16: Hirschberg test with distance variation to check convergence excess or divergence excess.

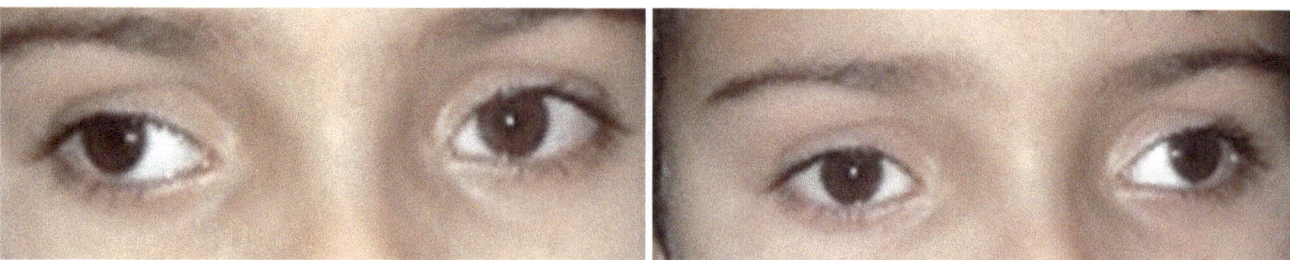

Fig. 22.17: Hirschberg test with right and left fixing to check for comitancy of squint.

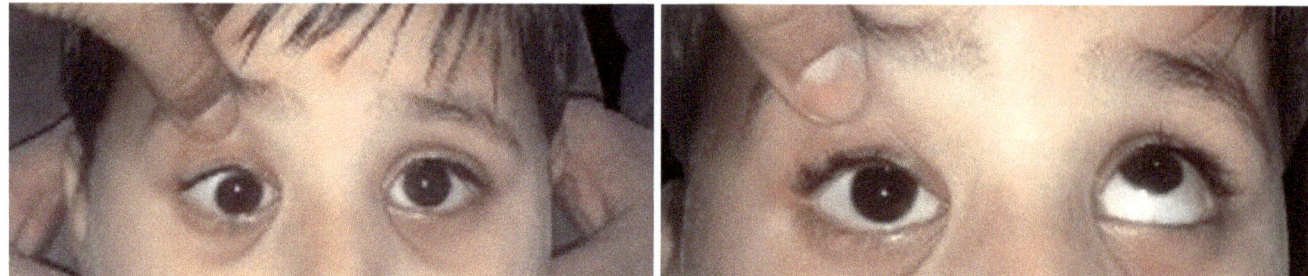

Fig. 22.18: Hirschberg test with primary and secondary deviation.

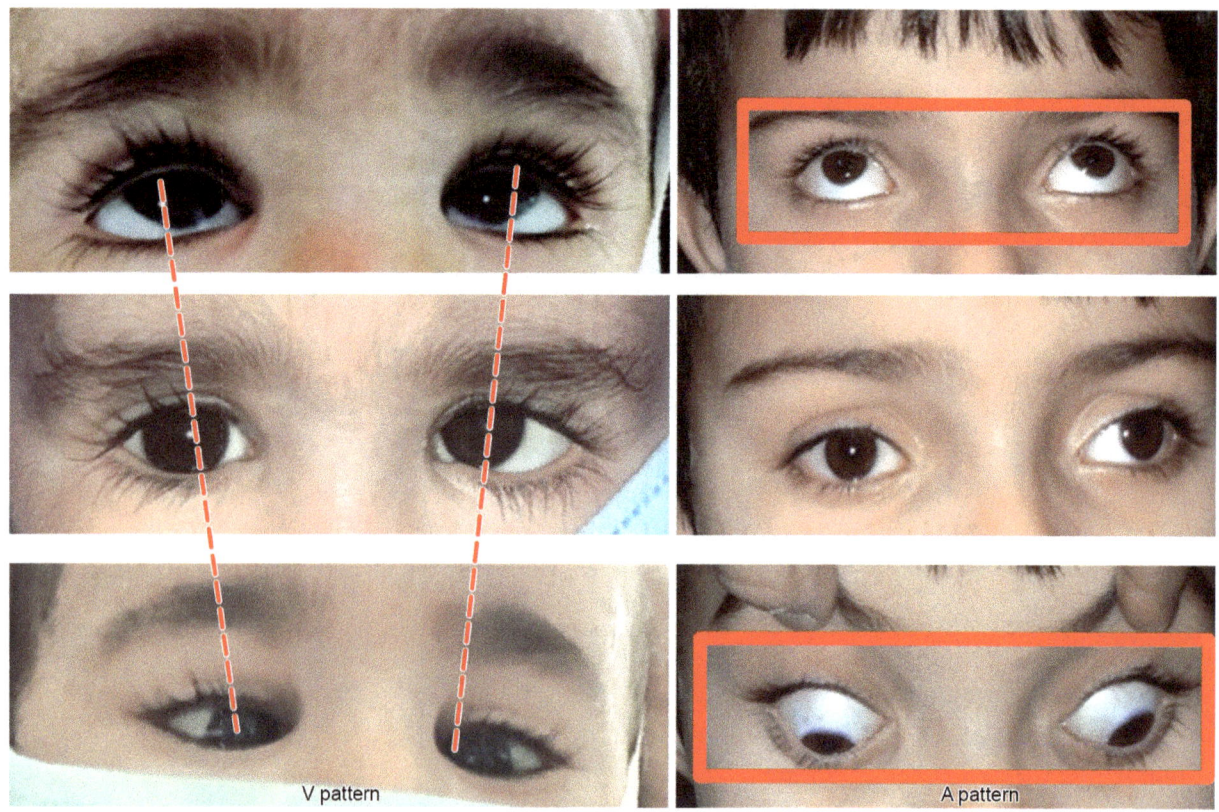

Fig. 22.19: Hirschberg test with upgaze and downgaze.

Cover—Uncover Test

Cover Test
- Detect and confirm heterotropia.
- Reveals type of heterotropia—eso, exo, hyoer, hypo
- **Procedure:** The patient is asked to fixate on a light source. Then, the **normal looking/fixating eye is covered,** and the movement of the other eye is observed.
- In squint is present, the uncovered eye will move in opposite direction to take fixation, while in apparent squint there will be no movement.
- If the eye (without cover) moves inwards (exotropia), outwards (esotropia), upwards (hypotropia), downwards (hypertropia).

Uncover Test
- Detect heterophoria, control of heterophoria (good, fair, or poor), grade of fixation and detects dissociated vertical deviation.
- **Procedure:** It is performed sequentially after cover test. The cover over the eye is removed and eye which was under the cover is observed.

❖ If the eye moves opposite direction to take fixation, it means there is phoria.
  Again, direction of movement of eyes depicts type of heterophoria.

Alternate Cover Test
❖ It is done by alternating patching from one eye to another.
❖ Detects total deviation (both latent along with manifest deviation).

MEASUREMENT OF STRABISMUS

Objective

Prerequisites
❖ Central fixation
❖ Good vision and
❖ No limitation of movement

Limitations
Following deviations are overlooked or cannot be diagnosed:
❖ A small heterophoria
❖ A small angle esotropia
❖ A monofixation syndrome
❖ A cyclodeviation

Assessment of Ocular Movements
❖ Ductions
❖ Versions
❖ Vergence
❖ Duction checked monocularly/Patch test—reveal true versus apparent duction limitation
❖ Duction grading/recording of horizontal muscles
  ➢ 0 to –4:
    • –0 indicating full rotation up to canthus
    • –1 for slight limitation
    • –2 for half the range from the midline to canthus
    • –3 for slight movement from midline but not up to halfway
    • –4 when eye could not cross the midline.

Krimsky Test (Fig. 22.20)
❖ This test utilizes prism and light reflex test to quantify amount of squint.
❖ It is required to put prism on the fixing eye.
❖ This test is useful in children and sensory squints in which one eye has low vision.

Prism Bar Cover Test—Simultaneous/Alternate Test
Apex of prism should point towards deviation (**Fig. 22.21**):
❖ Avoid stacking rather split prism
❖ Large prism for one eye additional prism to the other eye
❖ Relax dynamic factor—accommodation/fusion.

Different Aspects of Measurement of Squint
❖ Distance (9 gaze) and near fixation—basic, excess or insufficiency (**Fig. 22.22**)
❖ With glass without glass accommodative element
❖ Lateral gazes lateral incomitance

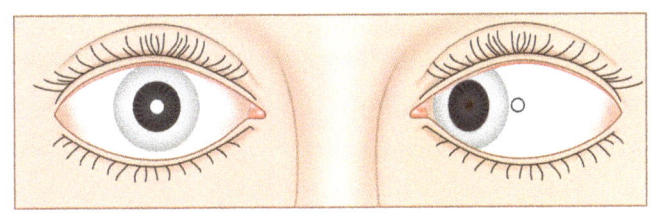
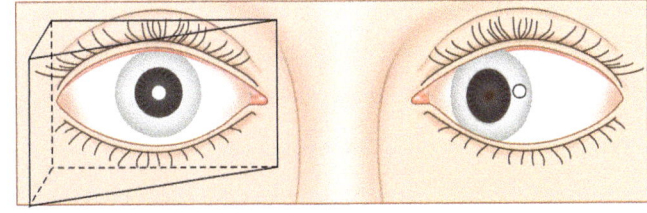
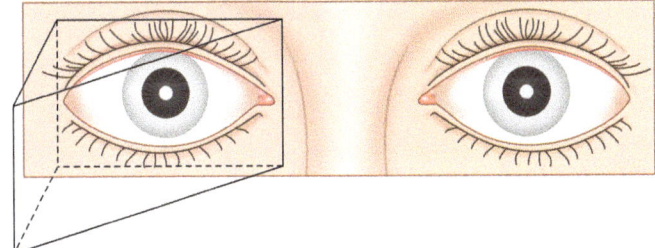

Fig. 22.20: Krimsky test.

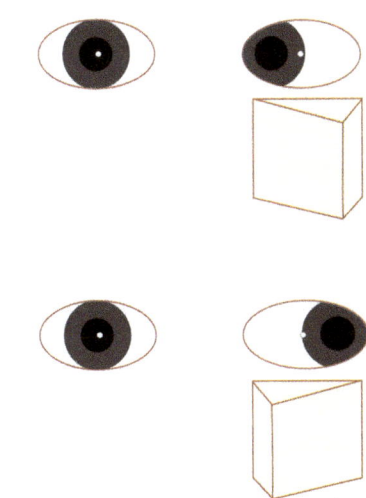

Fig. 22.21: Prism bar test.

❖ Cardinal gazes—incomitance
❖ 25° upgaze and 35° downgaze—pattern
❖ Right fixing and left fixing—primary and secondary deviation
❖ At different times in a day (cyclic presentation)
❖ Objective and subjective angle of deviation—retinal correspondence
❖ Prolonged patch test true/simulated divergence excess; fully dissociated squint
❖ +3D test AC/A ratio

Subjective

Maddox Rod with Maddox Tangent Scale (Figs. 22.23 to 22.25)
❖ Patient is asked to fix on a light source in the center of Maddox tangent scale at 6 meters. A Maddox rod is placed in front of one eye with axis of the rod parallel to the axis of deviation.

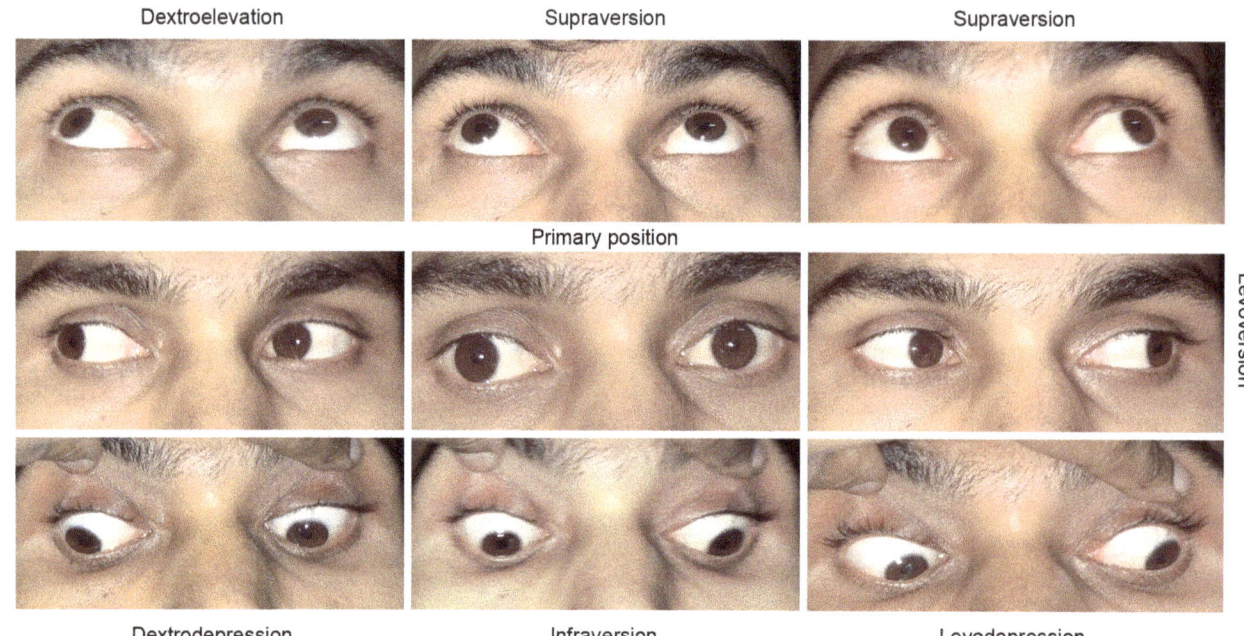

Fig. 22.22: Nine diagnostic positions of gaze.

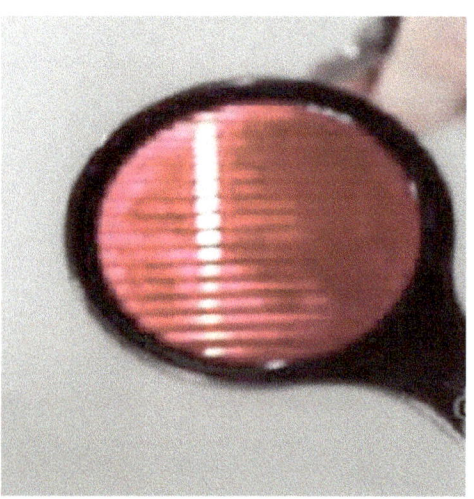

Fig. 22.23: Maddox rod: It converts point source of light into vertical line perpendicular to the grid of cylinders.

❖ The amount of heterophoria in degrees is calculated as number on Maddox tangent scale where the red line falls.

Objective and Objective

Synoptophore (Fig. 21.26): It is based on haploscopic principle which means two locations of object but one localization of image. It can be used diagnostically: (1) to measure horizontal, vertical or torsional deviation, (2) to check sensory binocular status (SMP, fusion and stereopsis), (3) to check subjective and objective deviation, ARC, vergence, etc., and therapeutically to treat, (4) vergence disorders, and (5) amblyopia.

AMBLYOPIA

Amblyopia is clinically defined as "decreased best-corrected visual acuity in one, or less frequently both eyes, in the absence of any obvious organic cause or ocular disease". Amblyopia is among important causes of vision loss in children.

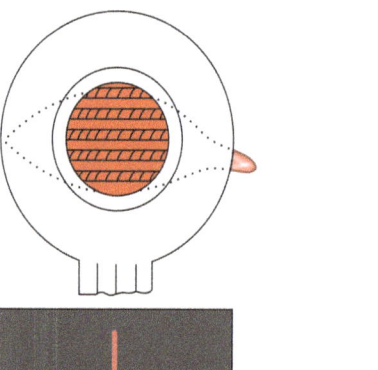
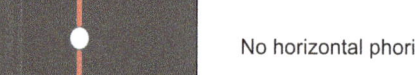
No horizontal phoria

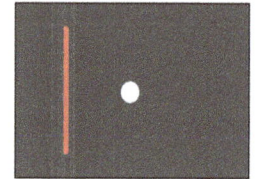
Exophoria

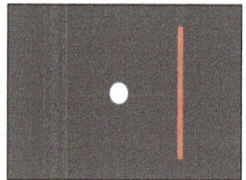
Esophoria

Fig. 22.24: Maddox rod test.

Types of Amblyopia

❖ Sensory deprivation amblyopia—this type occurs when form deprivation occurs due to media opacities like corneal opacity, cataract, vitreous hemorrhage, etc.

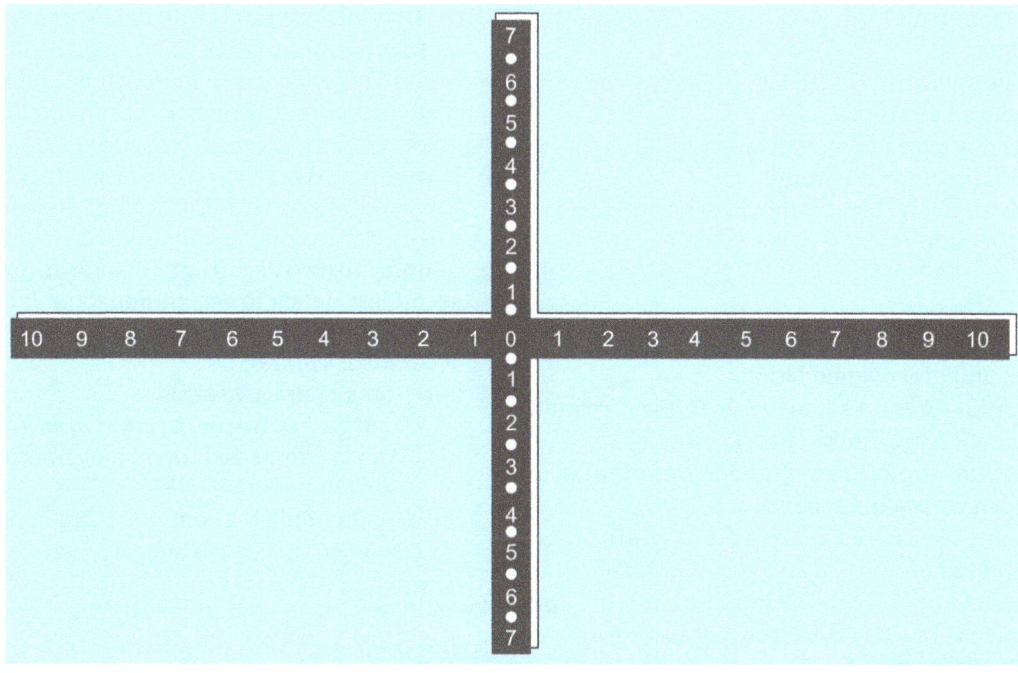

Fig. 22.25: Maddox tangent scale.

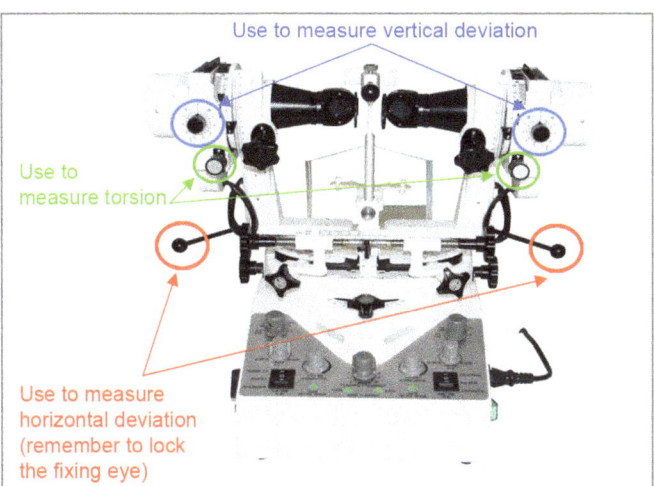

Fig. 22.26: Synoptophore.

- ❖ **Anisometropic amblyopia**
  - ➢ This type of amblyopia occurs when anisometropia (difference of refractive error among both eyes) is present. It can be myopic, hypermetropic or astigmatic.
  - ➢ Hypermetropic anisometropia is the most amblyogenic among all.
- ❖ **Strabismic amblyopia:**
  - ➢ Strabismus in early life inhibits the activation of the retinocortical pathways
  - ➢ Originating from deviating eye which causes loss of connectivity to the cortical spatial information pathways, altering the spatial summation and preventing the integration of contours and shapes which leads to suppression. In strabismus, the different image received by the eyes prevent normal fusion and affect binocular vision and depth of vision with poor or altered stereoacuity. Amblyopia caused by strabismus mainly affects visual acuity and binocular single vision, contrast sensitivity is relatively spared.
- ❖ **Ammetropic amblyopia:** It is caused by large refractive error (without correction) in a child.
- ❖ **Mixed amblyopia:** When amblyopia is caused because of more than one mechanism in presence of more than one amblyogenic factors. Combination of strabismic and anisometropic amblyopia is common, for example, partially accommodative esotropia.

Treatment of Amblyopia

There are different treatment modalities:
- ❖ Optical correction for unilateral amblyopia
- ❖ Optical correction for bilateral refractive amblyopia
- ❖ Occlusion therapy
- ❖ Atropine treatment
- ❖ Bangerter filter treatment

ESOTROPIA

Esotropia is a strabismic condition where one or both eye deviates inwards. This inward deviation can be intermittent or constant, and if only one is deviating eye every time then it is called esotropia of respective eye and if both eye goes in inward deviation alternatively than it is simply called alternating esotropia. If this deviation is same in all gazes it is called comitant, if not, called incomitant. Here we will discuss mainly comitant esotropia. Incomitant exotropia which can be caused paralysis of abducting muscles or restrictive causes like DRS, thyroid orbitopathy, etc.

Various Types of Esotropia
- ❖ **Accommodative**
  - ➢ Refractive
  - ➢ Non-refractive
    - Hyperaccomodative
    - Hypoaccomodative
- ❖ **Partially accommodative**
- ❖ **Non-accommodative**
  - ➢ Infantile esotropia
  - ➢ Essential late onset (basic, convergence excess, divergence insufficiency)

- Acute concomitant
- Microtropia
- Cyclic esotropia
- Stress induced esotropia
- Esotropia due to accommodative spasm
- Nystagmus blockade syndrome

Before discussing this classification in detail, we need to understand AC/A ratio.

AC/A Ratio

It is the amount of accommodative convergence exerted in response to one unit of accommodation.

❖ **High AC/A ratio**—eyes over converge for a given amount of accommodation (eso-shift at near).
❖ **Low AC/A ratio**—under convergence per diopter of accommodation (exo-shift at near).

AC/A can be measured by gradient method or heterophoria method

❖ **Gradient method:** Near deviation at near with and without near add (+3D) is measured and former is substracted from the former and value is divided by near add value (3); normal value by gradient method is 3–5.

$$AC/A = \frac{\text{Near deviation} - \text{near deviation with near add (+3)}}{\text{Near add (+3)}}$$

❖ **Heterophoria method:**

$$\frac{\text{Distance deviation} - \text{near deviation} + \text{IPD (cm)}}{+3}$$

Normal value: 5–7

Accommodative

❖ **Refractive accommodative esotropia (Fig. 22.27):** Refractive accommodative esotropia arises from underlying hypermetropic refractive error (+ 1.5 and +7.0 D), and gets fully corrected with refractive correction at both distance and near and in all gaze positions. Its onset is gradual, intermittent at 2–3 years.
  - It could be normoaccommodative or hyperaccommodative.
  - *Treatment:* Full cycloplegic correction of hypermetropia. Hyperaccommodative esotropia needs bifocals.

❖ **Nonrefractive hyperaccommodative esotropia:** Esotropia is greater for near than at distance, without significant hyperopic refractive error, and caused by high AC/A ratio with normal near point of accommodation (NPA)
  - *Onset:* 6 months to 3 years
  - *Refractive error:* Most common is hypermetropia. Can be emmetropic or myopic
  - *Etiology:* Abnormal synkinesis between accommodation and accommodative convergence
  - *Treatment:* Bifocals with flat top segments that bisect pupil given to relax accommodation thus reducing convergence. Over time can be diminished slowly to promote divergence. Eliminated by 10–12 years of age.

❖ **Nonrefractive hypoaccommodative esotropia:** Esotropia is greater for near than distance fixation and caused by excessive convergence from an increased accommodative effort to overcome primary or secondary deficit in accommodation. It is not related to hypermetropic refractive error
  - *Clinical features:*
    - Small refractive error
    - Large esotropia at near fixation with small deviation at distance and remote near point of accommodation (NPA).
    - Asthenopia is a common complaint.
  - *Treatment:* Executive bifocals

Partially Accommodative Esotropia

Esotropia is partly accommodative which can be corrected with spectacles and partly non-accommodative which will require surgical correction. It can be:

❖ Normoaccommodative
❖ Hyperaccommodative

Non-accommodative Esotropia

❖ Infantile esotropia
❖ Acute onset concomitant esotropia
❖ Microtropia
❖ Cyclic esotropia
❖ Sensory esotropia

Infantile Esotropia (Fig. 22.28)

Clinical features
❖ **Onset:** 4–6 months of age
❖ **Clinical features:** Esotropia >30 prism diopters
❖ No refractive error
❖ No neurological defect
❖ Free alternation or cross fixation with pseudo-abduction deficit
❖ Associated with inferior oblique overactions, nystagmus, dissociated vertical deviations.
❖ Asymmetric optokinetic nystagmus.

Treatment: Surgery should be done before the age of 2 years. Bilateral medial recti recession or unilateral medial rectus recession with lateral rectus resection.

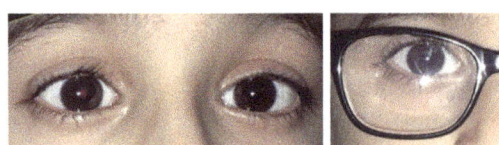

Fig. 22.27: Right eye esotropia full corrected with hyperopic glasses (refractive accommodative esotropia).

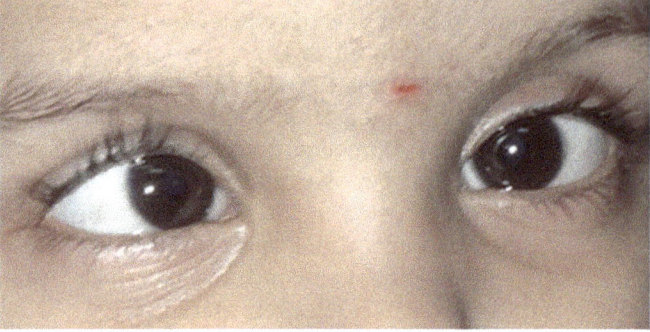

Fig. 22.28: Infantile esotropia.

Microtropia

It is a small angle squint (<10 prism diopters). Its characteristic features includes—amblyopia, anomalous retinal correspondence, relative scotoma on fixation spot, normal or near normal fusional amplitudes, defective stereo-acuity, association with anisometropia.

Acute Concomitant Esotropia

Esotropia acquired in the first or second decade of life with sudden-onset diplopia and minimal refractive error. These patients have good binocular potential. It is of three types:
1. **Swan type:** Due to monocular occlusion or visual loss.
2. **Franceschetti type:** Most common type, due to any physical stress like fever or insufficient divergence reserve.
3. **Bielschowsky type:** This type is associated with high myopia.

Cyclic Esotropia

Has 24-48 hours of large angle esotropia of 40-50 prism diopter squint alternating with similar duration of non-squint with binocular single vision with good fusional amplitudes.

Sensory Esotropia

It is caused by unilateral reduction in visual acuity like cataract, optic atrophy, macular scar which interferes with fusion.

EXOTROPIA

Exotropia is a type of strabismus, where one or both eye deviates outward. Outward deviation can be intermittent or constant, and if only one is deviating eye every time then it is called exotropia of the respective eye, and if both eyes go in outward deviation alternatively then it is simply called alternating exotropia.

Types of Exotropia

- **Physiologic:** Infants in early neonatal age have transient exotropia which resolves with growth by 2-4 months of age. Even a percentage of the normal population also express exophoria but not of any concern.
- **Congenital exotropia:** This is an exodeviation (often constant) with an onset in the first six months of life that does not resolve. There is an increased incidence with cerebral palsy and other neurologic disorders, craniofacial disorders, and ocular albinism.
- **Sensory exotropia:** In this type eye that has poor vision and lacks continuous necessary sensory input deviates outwards with time.
- **Convergence insufficiency:** Eyes diverge due to a lack of appropriate convergence.
- **Consecutive exotropia:** In this type, exotropia is preceded by esotropia. Surgical overcorrection of esotropia also comes under this category.
- **Intermittent exotropia (Fig. 22.29):** It is the most common type. It is commonly found exodeviation, 50-90% of cases of all exotropias, seen in approximately 1% of the general population. Deviation first starts for distance and later also at near fixation. It is more commonly expressed in sunlight so patients complain of "photodiplopia".

Stages of IDS

- Exophoria
- Intermittent exotropia
- Constant exotropia

Types of Intermittent Exotropia

Burian et al., described four types of IDS, which are:
1. Basic—distance and near deviations are equal or difference of each other is less than 10 prism diopters
2. Pseudo-divergence excess—a larger exotropia is present for distance, but this difference is extinguished after the patching of one eye.
3. True divergence excess—a larger exotropia is present for distance, even after 30-60 minutes of monocular occlusion. More than ½ of these patients have a high AC/A ratio and are prone to postoperative overcorrections if operated on for their full distance deviation.
4. Convergence insufficiency—deviation larger for near (>10 prism diopters).

Management

Nonsurgical

- **Spectacle correction of refractive errors:** To improve sensory fusion
- **Observation:** In the absence of reduced visual acuity or amblyopia, a patient with small and stable deviation, can be kept under observation without any intervention
- **Overcorrecting minus lens therapy:** Minus overcorrection induces accommodative convergence and promotes fusion. This can be used only as short-term primary treatment, just to delay surgical correction for some time. In older children, it can cause asthenopia

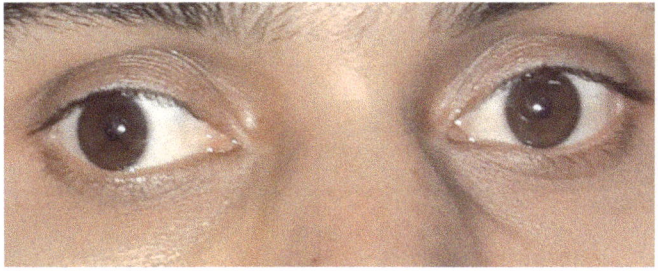
Exotropia for distance

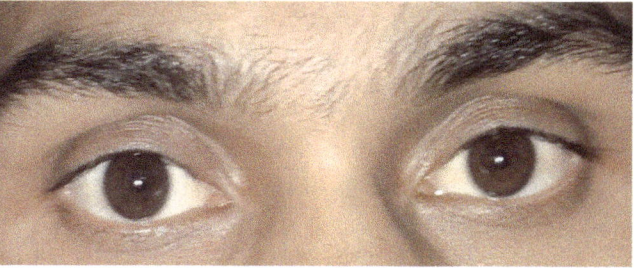
Exophoria with poor control

Fig. 22.29: Intermittent exotropia.

- **Orthoptic therapy:** It is a home-based therapy that includes exercises like pencil push-ups, prism exercises etc., orthoptic therapy improves deviation in basic, divergence excess, convergence insufficiency type
- **Botulinum toxin:** It is proven to be as effective as surgical outcomes, efficacy independent of initial strabismus angle. A toxin is injected to the lateral rectus.
- **Patching:** Not much reliable.

Surgical

Performed to preserve or restore binocular function.

Indications of surgery
- Increasing duration or frequency of manifest squint
- Increase in basic deviation
- Decreased stereoacuity
- Development of suppression
- Asthenopic symptoms
- Confusion and diplopia
- Decreased functioning and performance

Surgical Options
- Bilateral lateral rectus recession (bilateral recession)
- Unilateral lateral rectus recession (unilateral recession)
- Unilateral medial rectus resection (MR resection)
- Unilateral lateral rectus recession combined with medial rectus resection (recession and resection).

INCOMITANT STRABISMUS

- Includes both paralytic and restrictive strabismus (**Table 22.3**).
- Features of incomitant strabismus and difference from comitant squint.
- Paralytic strabismus includes third fourth and sixth nerve palsy.
- Restrictive strabismus includes Duanes retraction strabismus, Browns syndrome, blowout fracture, thyroid orbitopathy.

THIRD NERVE/OCULOMOTOR NERVE PALSY

Cranial third nerve palsy innervates five extraocular muscles—medial rectus (MR), inferior rectus (IR), inferior oblique (IO), superior rectus SR) and levator palpebrae superioris (LPS) and carries parasympathetic outflow to the ciliary ganglion which are responsible for pupillary constriction and accommodation
- Superior branch of third nerve supply SR and LPS
- Inferior branch of third nerve supply MR, IO, IR

Types
- Complete—involves both the superior and inferior branch as well as pupil
- Incomplete—does not involve pupil
- Total—complete paralysis of the extraocular muscles
- Partial—paresis of the extraocular muscles

Clinical Signs and Symptoms
- **Ptosis:** Due to paralysis of levator palpebrae superioris muscle
- **Ocular deviation:** "Down and out" position. In complete palsy, limitation of all ocular movements except abduction and intorsion is seen (intorsion/4th nerve function in third nerve palsy is checked by following conjunctival vessel while patient is asked to look in downgaze). In incomplete palsy may give different clinical signs depending on the superior and inferior branch.
- **Diplopia:** Diplopia may occur in partial palsy but many a times patient do not complain of diplopia due to complete ptosis.
- **Pupil:** In compressive third-nerve palsy, the pupil becomes fixed and dilated due to paralysis of sphincter pupillae.
- Loss of accommodation—ciliary muscle paralysis also leads to loss of accommodation.
- Aberrant regeneration or oculomotor synkinesis. Third nerve palsies (3rd NP) are known to regenerate partially with aberrant innervation known as acquired oculomotor misdirection or synkinesis
- Loss of near reflex

Management

Work-up
- Patients with pupil-sparing third-nerve palsy should be evaluated for any vascular cause.

TABLE 22.3: Difference between paralytic and restrictive strabismus.

	Paralytic	Restrictive
Deviation in primary position	Present and is proportional to the degree of underaction of the affected muscle	Can be present, absent or paradoxical. Disproportionate to the degree of underaction of muscle
Force duction test	Negative, i.e., the eye can easily be moved in the direction of restricted muscle	Positive
Active force generation test	Negative or weak force generation test	Positive
Saccades	Weak/slow in velocity with smaller amplitudes	Normal saccadic velocity till restriction comes into effect
Differential tonometry	No difference in different gaze	High in gaze when muscle acts against tight/restrictive forces
	• Third nerve palsy • Fourth nerve palsy • Sixth nerve palsy • Monocular elevation deficit	• Duane's retraction syndrome • Browns syndrome • Blow out fracture with inferior rectus entrapment • Mobious syndrome • Congenital fibrosis of extraocular muscles

- Ancillary investigations are complete blood count, blood sugar including Hb1AC and erythrocyte sedimentation rate (ESR).
- If the palsy is pupil involving, prompt neuro-ophthalmic evaluation and imaging should be done. MRI is better than CT for intracranial pathology.

Conservative Treatment

Conservative management is advocated as a short-term measure in acute palsy and for patients who are over 50 years of age having a history of diabetes or hypertension. For diplopia, the affected eye can be occluded with the eye patch or fogging lenses. Patients should be followed up every 3 months to check for signs of improvement. If no improvement noted then surgical management is needed after 6 months. Alternate patching should be started in pediatric cases, to prevent amblyopia due to ptosis or squint. Botulinum toxin to lateral rectus causes paralysis of the LR and neutralizes outward deviation.

Surgical Treatment

Patients are observed for at least for 6 months before surgery is planned. Ptosis correction should be done after squint correction only if Bells is good. Surgical options depend on the degree of involvement: complete or partial (extent of involvement of extraocular muscles).

Options for Surgical Management

- Resection of the medial rectus and recession of the lateral rectus muscle.
- Supra-maximal recession of lateral rectus or its periosteal fixation
- Nasal periosteal fixation of globe; LR to MR transposition in complete palsy
- Surgery in normal eye creates fixation duress in aberrant regeneration

FOURTH NERVE/TROCHLEAR NERVE PALSY

It is the most common cyclo-vertical muscle palsy. Most of the palsies are congenital. Causes of acquired palsies include trauma, inflammation, infection, vascular malformation, infarct, tumor or myasthenia gravis as well as iatrogenic causes after sinus, orbital or neurologic surgery.

Clinical Features

- Vertical diplopia—insidious onset or intermittent or acute in acquired
- Hypertropia in affected eye
- Compensatory contralateral head tilt
- Inferior oblique overaction,
- Subjective torsional diplopia in acquired
- Positive Park 3 step test
- Patients with congenital etiology have contralateral head tilt and mid-facial hypoplasia of face **(Figs. 22.30 and 22.31)** and minimal torsional diplopia.

Parks-Bielchowsky Three-Step Test

Helps in identification of a fourth nerve palsy **(Fig. 22.32)**.
- First step—which eye is hypertropic

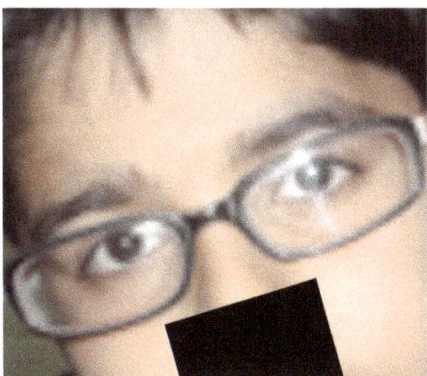
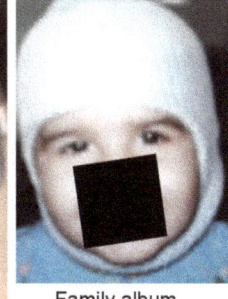

Family album tomography—head posture

Fig. 22.30: Right head tilt in a child in old photograph.

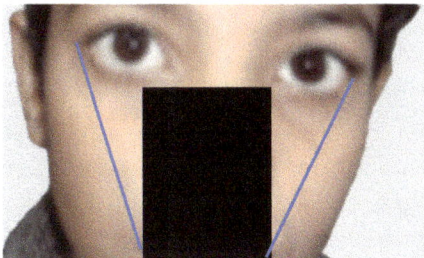

Midfacial hypoplasia

Fig. 22.31: Left sided midfacial hypoplasia in RE SO palsy with left head tilt.

- Second step—which gaze same eye is hypertropic
- Third step—which head tilt eye is hypertropic

The reason that hypertropia is exacerbated in contralateral gaze is that SO palsy causes weakness of depression in adduction. The reason that hypertropia is more with ipsilateral head tilt is that the ocular counter roll reflex stimulates ipsilateral intorters (SO and SR) and contralateral extorters (IO and IR); when the SO is weak, this reflex causes a compensatory increase in ipsilateral SR action, resulting in more hypertropia (as SR is an elevator).

Key Points

The fusional amplitude (increased in congenital cases) is measured by asking the patient to note diplopia when prisms are placed over one eye and progressively increased. A vertical fusional capacity >8–10 diopters points to the presence of compensatory mechanisms that exists with long-standing misalignment, as in congenital cases. Lee charting is useful test during follow up of a newly acquired case of superior oblique palsy to check for improvement over time.

Differential diagnosis:
- Skew deviation
- Thyroid related ophthalmopathy
- Primary inferior oblique overaction

Management

- Occlusion of the affected eye can serve as a temporary measure when recovery is expected.
- Non-surgical treatment include prisms in cases with small comitant hypertropia or in patients not fit for surgery.
- Surgery required for persistent symptomatic fourth nerve palsy when conservative measures fail, when the misalignment has been stable for several months.

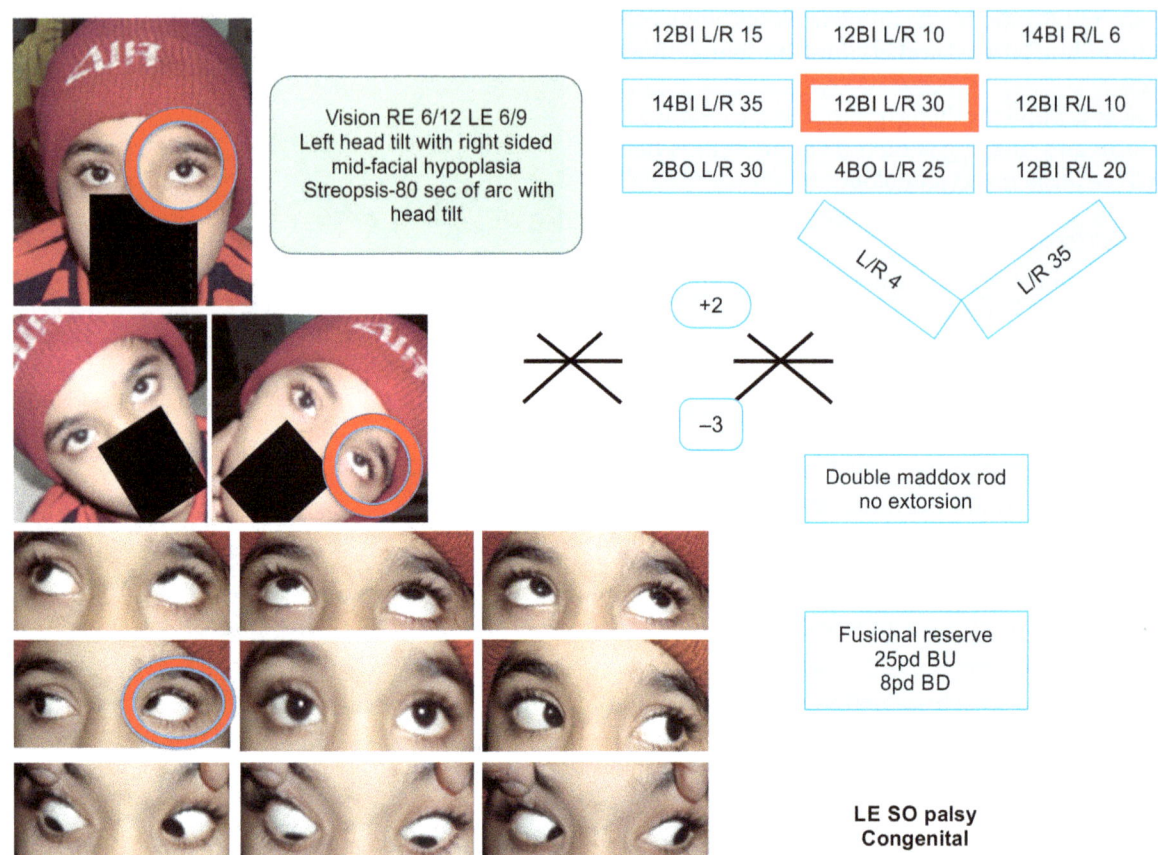

Fig. 22.32: LE SO palsy. Hypertropia of left eye increasing in right gaze and left head tilt.

Surgical Treatment

- Weaken ipsilateral IO
- So underaction—strengthen ipsilateral SO
- Strengthen ipsilateral IR
- Weaken ipsilateral SR

SIXTH OR ABDUCENT NERVE PALSY

Clinical Presentation

- Esotropia
- Abduction deficit/slow abduction saccades
- Ipsilateral face turn
- Diplopia

Differential Diagnosis

- Myasthenia gravis—fluctuating ptosis diplopia that become worse with fatigue. Endorphonium test.
- Restrictive thyroid myopathy—proptosis. Forced duction test reveals restriction.
- Medial orbital wall blowout fracture—neuroimaging, restriction
- Orbital myositis
- Duane syndrome—globe retraction and narrowed lid fissure on adduction, limitation on adduction
- High myopia with compression—restriction on forced duction test
- Divergence paralysis—ductions and versions normal
- Early onset esotropia—abduction is elicited by placing orthoptic patch over one eye

Management

Children

- Observation for 6 months for spontaneous recovery
- Amblyopia treatment—alternate patching
- Fresnel add-on prisms may be given and reduced as the sixth nerve palsy improves.
- If a child loses binocularity and is not recovering sixth nerve function, chemodenervation of the antagonist MR may help to rapidly restore binocularity

Adults

- Observation for 6 months at least
- Fogged glass
- Acute sixth nerve palsy—botulinum toxin of antagonist MR—preventing secondary contracture of the antagonist MR muscle, maintaining binocularity during recovery.
- Surgical indication—if after 6 months of follow up care the remaining deviation is large and in presence of diplopia

Management Options

- If residual function exists:
  - Graded recession/resection
  - Medial rectus (MR) recession
  - Lateral rectus (LR) resection
  - MR recession and LR resection (R & R)
  - R & R and contralateral MR recession (>40 PD)
  - Transposition procedure (weakening of antagonist)
  - Ipsilateral medial rectus in appropriate patients

- If little or no residual function
- Transposition procedures
  - Full-tendon vertical rectus muscle transposition
  - Partial vertical rectus muscle transposition (PVRT)
  - Full tendon vertical rectus muscle transposition with Foster suture
  - **Nishida procedure**—full or partial tendon transposition without tenotomy

MONOCULAR ELEVATION DEFICIT

Paralysis of the superior rectus and inferior oblique of one eye is called double elevator palsy (DEP) or monocular elevation deficit (MED). There is a limitation of elevation of the affected eye which is similar in both abduction and adduction.
- Unilateral defect of upgaze associated with ipsilateral ptosis
- Initially, the upgaze deficiency was attributed to paralysis of both the superior rectus and inferior oblique muscles.
- Term double elevator palsy was later coined by Dunlap in 1952 to describe the weakness affecting both muscles of elevation
- Recently, the SR has been shown to be the muscle mainly responsible for upward rotation of the eye.
- The findings of impaired upgaze can result from SR palsy alone without involvement of the inferior oblique
- Unilaterally impaired upgaze can also be caused by inferior rectus restriction and supranuclear disorders.
- Therefore, the term monocular elevation deficiency (MED) was coined

It can be congenital or acquired.

Causes of Acquired MED

Trauma, hypertension, thromboembolism, sarcoidosis, tumors like acoustic neuroma, pineocytoma, metastasis.

Types
- **Type 1:** Inferior rectus restriction (tight force duction test for IR)
- **Type 2:** Superior rectus palsy
- **Type 3:** Supranuclear type and is usually congenital. It is a combination of both type 1 and 2.

Symptoms
- Inability to elevate the affected eye.
- Double vision
- Abnormal head posture
- Drooping of upper lid
- Decreased vision

Signs
- Ptosis or pseudo-ptosis (improves when hypotropic eye takes up fixation)
- Strabismus (hypotropia of the affected eye and hypertropia of the contralateral eye)
- Bell's phenomenon (poor or absent)
- Amblyopia
- Abnormal head posture (chin elevation)
- Slow saccades

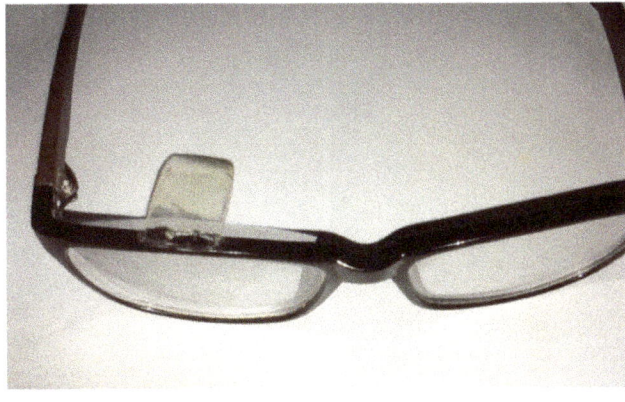

Fig. 22.33: Crutch glass.

Differential Diagnosis
- Thyroid orbitopathy
- Myasthenia gravis
- Orbital floor fractures
- Progressive external ophthalmoplegia
- Third nerve paresis or palsy (superior division)

Management
- Observation for 6 months in acute cases
- Crutch glasses (**Fig. 22.33**) can be given for severe ptosis if ptosis surgery deferred due to poor Bells.

Indications for Surgery
- **Vertical deviation in primary gaze**
- **Deviation causing suppression and amblyopia in children**
- Diplopia in primary gaze (acquired causes)
- Contracted binocular fields
  - *Type 1:* IR recession with conjunctival recession.
  - *Type 2:* Knapp procedure (vertical transposition of the horizontal rectus muscles done) with or without IR recession).

DUANE RETRACTION SYNDROME

Duane retraction syndrome (DRS) is a congenital strabismus that occurs due to abnormal development of the 6th cranial nerve and compensatory mis-innervation from the third cranial nerve. It has characteristic features of difficulty in unilateral or bilateral abduction or adduction, upshoot/downshoot and narrowing of palpebral fissure on adduction.

Types and Pathophysiology

Patients can present with various presentations, but all presentations have caused any insult to the development of the sixth nerve or its nucleus during gestation. So, during development fibers from the oculomotor nerve are redirected to the lateral rectus.
- **Type I (Fig. 22.34):**
  - It is the most common type. The affected eye has poor abduction and good adduction. In these cases, LR receives minimal or absent innervation because of hypoplastic sixth nerve.

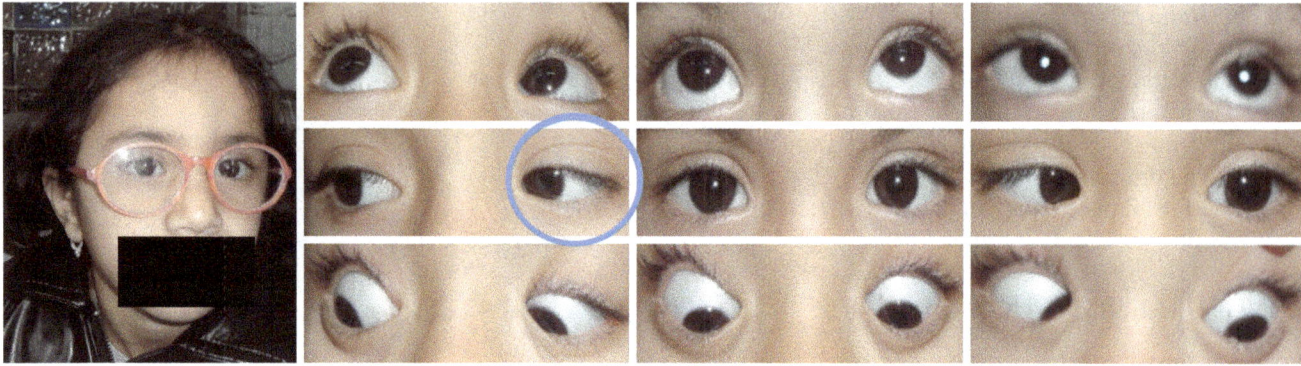

Fig. 22.34: LE esotropic DRS (type1) with left face turn.

- Because of poor abduction of the affected eye, the patient does face turn in the direction of the affected eye for compensation. For example, right face turn for a right type I DRS with esotropia.

❖ **Type II:**
  - Eyes affected with type II DRS have poor adduction and good abduction. As the abducent nerve is intact, so lateral rectus contracts appropriately leading to good abduction.
  - The oculomotor nerve also gives partial innervation to the lateral rectus, splitting of innervation meant to supply only medial rectus into innervation for medial rectus and lateral rectus. So, on attempted abduction, the medial rectus and lateral rectus both get innervation from the third nerve and leads adduction deficit. As paradoxical contraction of lateral rectus on adduction opposes action of medial rectus.

❖ **Type III:** This type is second most common type of DRS. There is the congenital absence of nucleus of abducens nerve and medial rectus and lateral rectus gets equal innervation from oculomotor. Patient have poor adduction and abduction.

Upshoots/Downshoots (Fig. 22.35)

Occurs on attempting adduction, due to inappropriate when strong firing to lateral rectus occurs through aberrant innervation from oculomotor nerve. Due to leash effect horizontal recti pull the eye upward or downward, as the eye rotates up or down past the horizontal plane. These movement in adduction resembles inferior and superior oblique overactions.

DRS classification according to deviation in primary position as esotropic, exotropic or orthotropic is more relevant, and more important in planning surgical management.

Management

Nonsurgical Treatment

Treatment of amblyopia (anisometropic amblyopia).

For small compensatory head position: Prisms to normalize the head posture or to manage intermittent diplopia (though rarely required).

Surgical

Indications for Surgery

- ❖ Significant deviation in primary position
- ❖ Noticeable abnormal head position
- ❖ Significant globe retraction and palpebral fissure narrowing.
- ❖ Significant upshoot or downshoot.

Usually, surgery is electively performed around age 3–8 years, as these patients have stable deviation and excellent fusion. Muscle resections are advices to be avoided in DRS, as resections can make horizontal recti stronger leading to stronger co-contraction and this can worsen the lid fissure narrowing. Before planning the surgery, forced duction test should be performed to detect any restriction of medial rectus and lateral rectus.

Exotropic DRS

- ❖ Ipsilateral lateral rectus recession.
- ❖ LR Y-split procedure for upshoot or downshoot along with the LR recession.

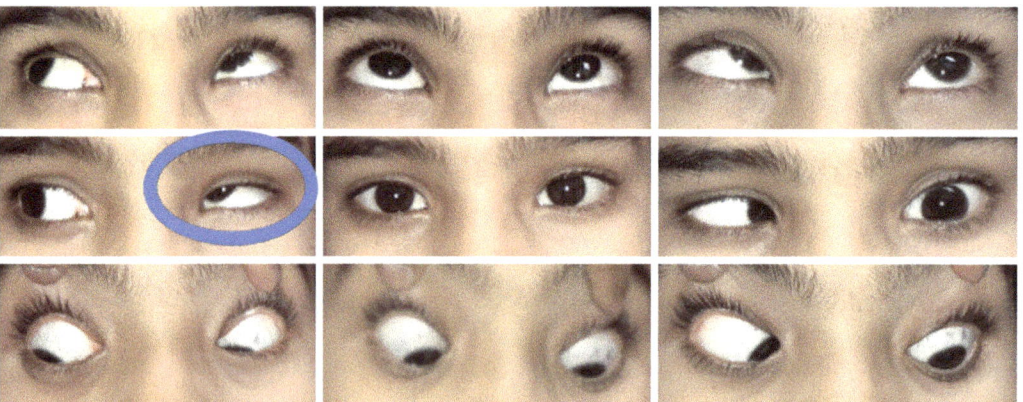

Fig. 22.35: Left eye eso-ortho DRS showing upshoot and retraction of globe on adduction.

Esotropic DRS
- Medial rectus recession should be considered.
- Y-splitting of lateral rectus along with recession improves upshoot and downshoot.
- Vertical rectus transposition for improving abduction.

Limitations of Treatment
- Normal ductions and versions cannot be achieved
- Upshoots, downshoots cannot be completely eliminated

PRINCIPLES OF STRABISMUS SURGERY
- **Cosmetic:** Achieve satisfactory alignment
- **Functional:**
  - Restore and maintain good and equal visual acuity of each eyes
  - Restore binocularity
  - Enlarge field of single binocular vision
  - Correct abnormal head posture

Physiological Basis of Strabismus Surgery
- When a muscle contract, it produces a force that rotates the globe
- Rotation force α length of the moment arm (M) and force of muscle contraction (F)
- Torque generated by muscle depends on:
  - Tautness or laxity of muscle (length tension curve)
  - Arc of contact
  - Strength or power of muscle
  - Length of moment arm
  - It indicates the muscles characteristics, its elasticity and contractility (for horizontal recti)

Choice of Surgery
- Procedure in strabismus surgery on (horizontal, vertical recti or obliques) fall into two categories:
  1. Weakening procedure
  2. Strengthening procedure
- Combination of two, one muscle is weakened and its antagonist is strengthened
- One may choose to do similar weakening procedure on the two eye

Mechanism
Strabismus surgery corrects ocular misalignment by different mechanism:
- Slackening a muscle—recession
- Tightening a muscle—resection, plication
- Reducing moment arm—Faden procedure
  - Changing vector force by transposition
  - Incision types: Fornix, limbal, para-limbal

Recession
Muscle weakening procedure in which muscle is first secured, cut and then sutured away (at measured distance on the sclera) from insertion site along its arc of contact creating new insertion site.

Strengthening Procedures
Resection: Muscle strengthening procedure in which muscle is first marked (a measured value from insertion), sutures are passed from the marked site and muscle secured and then muscle proximal to measured site is cut away after achieving hemostasis and then near muscle end is sutured at original insertion site.

Instruments
See **Figure 22.36**.

NURSING INTERVENTIONS
Nurses can play a very important role in creating awareness about strabismus among parents, educating them about its prognosis, the advantages of early intervention, and the beneficial impact of proper management on the social, physical, and psychological growth of the child. The nurses must inform parents about the need to screen strabismic children and undergo an ophthalmic examination as soon as possible when suspected as strabismus could be the first sign of grave eye disease (like retinoblastoma) and must also educate care providers about systemic and neurological

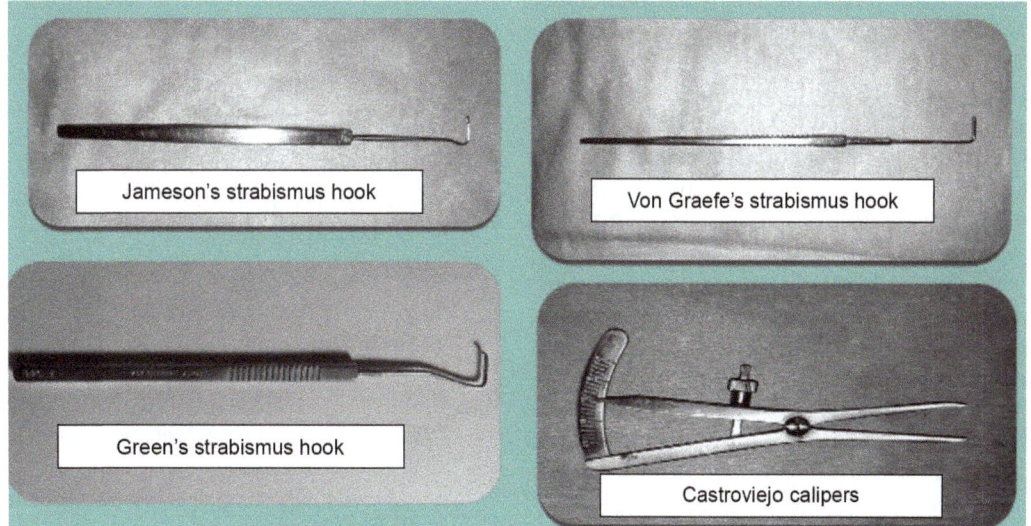

Fig. 22.36: Muscle hooks and caliper for squint surgery.

causes associated with strabismus and need for appropriate referral to a specialist. They should also educate parents about the risks of amblyopia and impaired binocularity if treatment for squint is not adhered. So, nurses can become part of a multidisciplinary team and can play a vital role in patient education, maintaining adherence, and enhancing health care outcome.

GERIATRIC CONSIDERATIONS

Binocular vision problems are common in the elderly, and results in reduced stereopsis, which can lead to functional consequences like falls. It is also reported that binocular vision disorders generally do not get the attention which it deserves.

Generally, geriatric patients present to squint clinic with two type of squint one which was either not treated or neglected in adulthood and other type that is acquired in late age. Acquired strabismus in elderly includes mostly paralytic strabismus due to micro-ischemic events. Others cause include loss of binocular single vision and fusion due to decreased visual acuity due to multiple diseases like cataract, age related macular degeneration, diabetic retinopathy, hypertensive retinopathy, retinal vein occlusion, etc.

Strabismus in elderly can develop due to the worsening of a previously controlled latent deviation. These days incidence of use of antidepressants and antianxiety drugs is increasing. The use of tricyclic antidepressants is associated with decompensation of already existing phoria, and results in diplopia. This disruption of fusion can convert phorias into tropias. Most common symptom is diplopia, for which elderly patients seek the attention of a strabismologist.

Abduction limitation is generally due to sixth nerve paresis or paralysis. Also, a sagging globe can cause abduction limitations which can be overlooked. Gaze palsy, or internuclear ophthalmoplegia are also some of the causes of acquired strabismus. Acquired Brown's syndrome can also be seen in elderly patients due to inflammation near the trochlea or myositis. Chronic progressive ophthalmoplegia may also be seen in the elderly.

Even while doing a squint examination, one needs to be more patient with elderly patients as it is frequent to have age-related hearing disorders, dementia disorders, etc., in late age. Also, while doing a forced duction test thinning of the conjunctiva should be kept in mind.

It is not uncommon for elderly people to develop strabismus and a number of etiologies could be responsible and the most common ones are microvascular causes like diabetes, and hypertension. Other causes could be degenerative, ischemic, metastatic, or less commonly inflammatory and infective. Such patients require for systemic work up. Considering the frequency of cranial nerve palsy as one of the leading causes of ocular misalignment in the geriatric population concurrent with systemic comorbidities, recent-onset strabismus, may be considered as an emergency in this age group. It is important for ophthalmologists and nursing staff to be comfortable handling strabismus in senior citizens. In the elderly, strabismus is treatable, either with vision therapy, prismatic correction, or surgery. Vision training and convergence exercises for convergence insufficiency reduce symptoms and lead to improvement in near points of convergence measurements. The underlying condition of acute strabismus in the elderly may be potentially serious therefore, particularly recent ocular deviations in the geriatric population should be carefully diagnosed and managed and may require collaboration with other departments, such as neurology. Fitness for surgery is also a concern in the elderly. Consideration of anterior segment ischemia and oculocardiac reflex should be considered before surgery. Many a times nonsurgical option, such as prismatic glasses or botulinum toxin injection are recommended in elderly.

SUMMARY

Strabismus is a common childhood disorder that causes deviation or squinting of eyes commonly due to the weakening of extraocular muscles. It is characterized by crossed eyes, i.e., eyes do not look in the same direction at the same time. Strabismus can be treated with eyeglasses, contact lens, prism lens, eye exercises and surgery.

MULTIPLE CHOICE QUESTIONS

1. Strabismus also referred as:
    a. Squinting eyes
    b. Crossed eyes
    c. Wall eyes
    d. All of the above
2. Extraocular muscles are located:
    a. Within the orbit
    b. Behind the orbit
    c. Anterior of retina
    d. Near ciliary bodies
3. What are versions?
    a. Binocular eye movements in the same direction
    b. Binocular eye movements in opposite direction
    c. Uniocular eye movements
    d. Both a and b
4. What does not differentiate a accommodative esotropia from non-accommodative esotropia
    a. Amount of esotropia
    b. High AC/A ratio
    c. High hypermetropia
    d. Far NPA
5. Two non-corresponding retinal points sharing common primary visual direction in a child cause:
    a. Abnormal retinal correspondence
    b. Diplopia
    c. Suppression
    d. Amblyopia
6. For left gaze right medial rectus and left lateral rectus form:
    a. Agonist muscles
    b. Yoke muscles
    c. Synergist muscles
    d. Antagonist muscles
7. Exotropia is greater at distance than near but near becomes equal to distance after applying 3D lens is called:
    a. Simulated divergence excess
    b. High AC/A ratio
    c. Convergence insufficiency
    d. True divergence excess
8. Which of the following is not a weakening surgery?
    a. Recession
    b. Z tenotomy
    c. Inferior oblique modified Elliot and Nankin
    d. Superior oblique tuck
9. Type 1 DRS include all, *except*:
    a. Absent abduction
    b. Narrowing of palpebral fissure on adduction
    c. Upshoot
    d. Absent adduction

10. Which one is correct about monocular elevation deficit:
    a. Tight superior rectus
    b. Tight superior oblique
    c. Paralyzed inferior oblique
    d. Paralyzed superior rectus
11. All are correct about Brown's syndrome, *except*:
    a. Tight elevation in abduction
    b. Deficit elevation in adduction
    c. Y pattern
    d. Overaction superior oblique

ANSWERS

1. d	2. a	3. a	4. a
5. a	6. b	7. b	8. d
9. d	10. d	11. a	

SUGGESTED READING

1. Brodsky MC. Pediatric Neuro-Ophthalmology, 3rd edition. Springer-Verlag; 2016.
2. Brodsky MC. Pediatric Neuro-Ophthalmology. 3rd ed. Springer-Verlag; 2016.
3. Nelson LB, Olitsky SE, (Eds). Harley's Pediatric Ophthalmology, 6th edition. Lippincott Williams and Wilkins; 2014.
4. Parks MM. Atlas of Strabismus Surgery. Harper & Row; 1983.
5. Parks MM. Ocular Motility and Strabismus. Harper & Row; 1975.
6. Pratt-Johnson JA, Tillson G. Management of Strabismus and Amblyopia: A Practical Guide, 2nd edition. Thieme; 2001.
7. Rosenbaum AL, Santiago AP (Eds). Clinical Strabismus Management: Principles and Surgical Techniques. Saunders; 1999.
8. Strabismus Simplified, CBS Publishers, New Delhi, 1999, 2013
9. Strabismus Simplified, CBS Publishers, New Delhi, 1999, 2013.
10. Tasman W, Jaeger EA (Eds). Duane's Ophthalmology on DVD-ROM. Lippincott Williams and Wilkins; 2013.
11. von Noorden GK, Campos EC. Binocular Vision and Ocular Motility. 6th edition. Mosby; 2002.
12. von Noorden GK, Helveston EM. Strabismus: A Decision Making Approach. Mosby; 1994.
13. von Noorden GK. Atlas of Strabismus, 4th edition. Mosby; 1983.
14. Wilson ME, Saunders RA, Trivedi RH (Eds). Pediatric Ophthalmology: Current Thought and A Practical Guide. Springer; 2009.
15. Wright KW, Strube YJ, (Eds). Color Atlas of Strabismus Surgery: Strategies and Techniques, 4th edition. Springer; 2015.
16. Wright KW, Strube YJ, (Eds). Pediatric Ophthalmology and Strabismus, 3rd edition. Oxford University Press; 2012.
17. Wright KW, Strube YJ eds. Color Atlas of Strabismus Surgery: Strategies and Techniques. 4th ed. Springer; 2015.
18. Wright KW, Strube YJ eds. Pediatric Ophthalmology and Strabismus. 3rd ed. Oxford University Press; 2012.

CHAPTER 23

Ocular Injuries

Surbhi Khurana, Parul Chawla Gupta, Ranjan Kumar Behera, Jagat Ram

"An eye for an eye only ends up making the whole world blind."

—Mohandas Gandhi

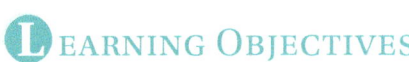 **LEARNING OBJECTIVES**

After going through the chapter, the learner will be able to:
- Define the type of ocular injury.
- Elaborate the mechanism of damage to various parts of eye by injury.
- Discuss the management of ocular injury in emergency.

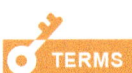 **TERMS**

- **Blunt trauma:** Absence of full-thickness defect in the coats of the eye.
- **Chemical Injury:** Injury by any chemical, acid or alkali.
- **Iridodialysis:** Detachment of the iris from its root.
- **Open globe injury:** Full-thickness defect in the coats of the eye.
- **Symblepharon:** Adhesions between conjunctiva and cornea.
- **Tenonplasty:** Advancement of tenon to the limbus to cover ischemic area.
- **Thermal injury:** Injury by heat.

INTRODUCTION

All ocular structures are susceptible to damage by injuries, but the structure affected depends upon the mechanism of injury. Injury to the eye can be caused by chemicals, heat, radiation or mechanical trauma. Though the eye is protected from injuries by eyelids, cilia and orbital tissue, ocular injuries are relatively common.

CHEMICAL INJURIES

Chemical injuries can be caused by acid or alkali from products like battery acid, lime or fresh mortar. Alkalis cause more damage than acids because of their ability to degrade corneal stroma and affect on the anterior chamber. Acids coagulate and do not penetrate the anterior chamber, hence the decrease in damage.

Clinical Features

- Patients typically present with pain and chemosis.
- Damage to corneal epithelium can be assessed by corneal fluorescein staining.
- Chemical injuries can cause corneal opacity, infection, vascularization, glaucoma, and lid symblepharon.
- Limbal ischemia helps to prognosticate the outcome. It causes persistent epithelial defect and vascularization of the cornea.
- The severity can be graded according to Hughes-Roper-Hall classification **(Table 23.1)**.

Management

- It is essential to explain the prognosis to the patient and the need for frequent follow-ups.
- Such patients usually present in emergencies and require immediate copious irrigation with normal saline, with a thorough cleaning of fornices and debris.

TABLE 23.1: Hughes-Roper-Hall classification.

Grade	Epithelial damage	Stroma	Perilimbal ischemia	Prognosis
I	Present	Minimal haze	None	Good
II	Present	Moderate haze	<1/3	Good
III	Present	Hazy	1/3 to 1/2	Guarded
IV	Present	Opaque cornea	>1/2	Poor

- A steady fluid line to the ocular surface can be achieved using an intravenous infusion set.
- The irrigation is continued till pH returns to normal or for at least 30 minutes.
- Frequent topical antibiotics, steroids and lubricants are required postoperatively. Steroids are essential to decrease inflammation and prevent symblepharon and vascularization.
- Cycloplegics are required to decrease the pain.
- Sweeping of the upper and lower fornices can prevent the formation of symblepharon.
- Topical and systemic vitamin C can help in early healing.
- Tablet doxycycline can decrease the collagenolysis.

Surgical Management

Amniotic membrane transplantation can be beneficial in patients with non-healing defects. Tenonplasty can be beneficial as well. The patients may require surgery for lid abnormalities in later stages.

MECHANICAL INJURIES

- Mechanical injuries can cause a myriad range of damage to the eyes.
- Ocular Trauma Classification Group has classified mechanical injuries into open or closed globe injuries.
  - *Open globe injuries* have a full-thickness defect in the coats of the eye
  - *Closed globe injuries* are devoid of it.
- A sharp object or blunt trauma can cause open globe injuries. Both open and closed globe injuries can affect any or all parts of the eye.
- Injuries can be classified according to the zones involved, presence or absence of pupillary reaction and visual acuity.
- Injuries are divided according to zones from the starting of the anterior segment to backwards, with zone 1 involving the cornea, zone II involving the anterior sclera up to 5 mm from the limbus and zone III involving beyond the 5 mm of the anterior sclera.

Open Globe Injuries

Open globe injuries secondary to blunt trauma are called **rupture of the globe**, where the rupture occurs from inside to outside.

Open globe injuries may be caused by a sharp object, and is called laceration. These can be further classified into penetrating and perforating injuries. Penetrating injuries have just one entry point, and perforating injuries have one entry and one exit point **(Flowchart 23.1)**.

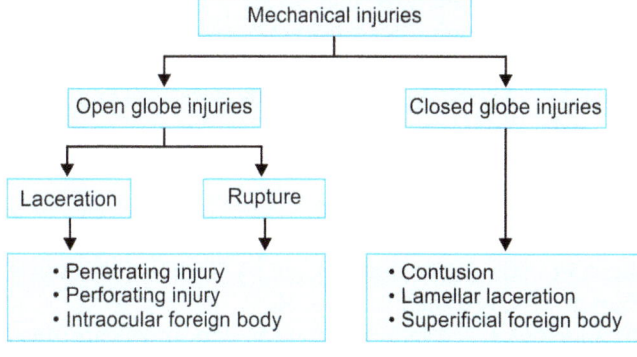

Flowchart 23.1: Classification of mechanical injuries.

Management

- Open globe injuries are ocular emergencies requiring immediate admission and surgical repair, along with antibiotics.
- An eyeshield has to be applied immediately.
- The situation is urgent because of the risk of infection and sympathetic ophthalmia, a dreaded complication.
- Anatomical integrity has to be achieved.
- Corneal sutures are applied using monofilament 10-0 nylon **(Fig. 23.1)**.
- Scleral and conjunctival sutures are applied using absorbable vicryl sutures.

Foreign Body

- Mechanical injury can also be in the form of superficial foreign bodies, like dust, iron, or steel, on the ocular surface; or intraocular foreign bodies (IOFB) after open globe injury.
- These foreign bodies can cause infection and inflammation in the eye if not removed.
- Superficial foreign bodies cause chronic irritation and watering.
- Retained IOFBs can lodge anywhere in the eye.

Management

- Superficial foreign bodies can be removed under topical anesthesia using the slit lamp and 26 gauge needle.

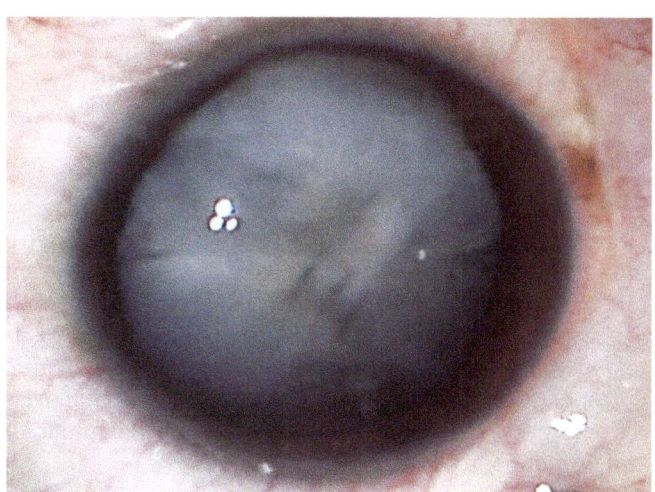

Fig. 23.1: Corneal laceration, repaired using sutures, and traumatic cataract.

Intraocular foreign bodies require removal by surgery and repair of the entry wound.

- ❖ Foreign body injuries are extremely common in industrial workers, hence warranting the need to educate the workers regarding the protective measures and use of goggles during such work.

Closed Globe Injury

Mode of Injury

Direct or coup due to direct effect, and indirect or counter-coup due to the transmitted waves.

- ❖ Injuries caused by blunt trauma can be as minor as a corneal abrasion or as severe as a rupture of the globe.
- ❖ It is important to follow up with the patients of blunt trauma for a long time, as some changes can be progressive.

Mechanism

- ❖ The force is transferred from the cornea to the retina and is then transmitted back from the posterior part to the anterior, causing damage. There is a horizontal transmission of the force as well.
- ❖ Blunt trauma can affect any part of the eye.

Cornea

- ❖ Blunt trauma can cause a corneal abrasion and loss of epithelium.
- ❖ Fluorescein solution can be used to stain the epithelium and assess the defect.

Management

Small abrasion can heal spontaneously, and large abrasion requires antibiotics and lubrication, along with the application of a patch.

Complications

Corneal opacity.

Sclera

- ❖ A contusion can affect all the parts of the eye, from the orbit to the optic nerve.
- ❖ **Globe rupture** can be caused by scleral open globe injury and has a guarded visual prognosis. It occurs due to compression of the globe against the orbital walls. It can cause iris prolapse. Rupture can damage all parts of the eye, including subluxation of the lens, iris damage, vitreous hemorrhage, and retinal detachment.

Management

Urgent repair is required in these cases, along with intravitreal antibiotics to prevent infection. It is important to retain anatomical integrity of the eye by surgery. Sclera is usually repaired by absorbable sutures. Incarcerated iris is removed. Systemic antibiotics are given to prevent infection. Postoperatively, topical antibiotics, steroids and cycloplegics are required to prevent infection and decrease inflammation and formation of granulation tissue.

Iris and Ciliary Body

- ❖ Iridodialysis (tear of iris from the ciliary body) and mydriasis are caused by injury to the iris.

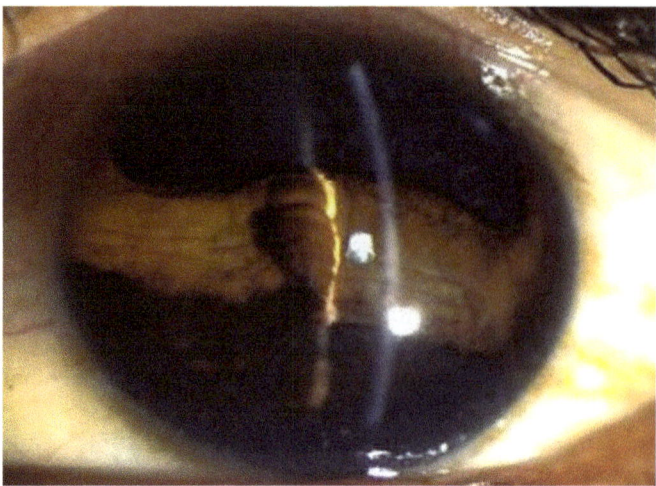

Fig. 23.2: Iridodialysis.

- ❖ Iridodialysis is frequently seen in these cases (**Fig. 23.2**). It can cause a D-shaped pupil.

Management

A large iridodialysis can be repaired using polypropylene sutures.

- ❖ Traumatic mydriasis can be caused due to damage to the sphincter muscle.
- ❖ The ciliary body may be torn from its attachment, causing angle recession, which is seen as a deep anterior chamber and has the propensity to cause glaucoma. It requires a long-term follow-up to look for glaucoma.
- ❖ Tearing of the iris, vessels, or ciliary body can cause hyphema, which is blood in the anterior chamber.

Management

It commonly reabsorbs if it is less than half of the anterior chamber. If more, it can cause a trabecular or pupillary block, causing increased intraocular pressure. Intensive steroid and antiglaucoma therapy are required in such cases. Aspirin is to be avoided because of the risk of rebleeding. If the intraocular pressure is raised persistently or there is the presence of corneal staining, the blood needs immediate drainage from the anterior chamber.

Lens

- ❖ Injury can cause cataracts or dislocation of the lens.
- ❖ Cataracts can be caused after blunt and open globe injury. Rosette cataract is a typical form of traumatic cataract and needs cataract extraction.
- ❖ Sometimes, open globe injury can cause rupture of the anterior lens capsule, causing leakage of lens material in the anterior chamber (**Fig. 23.1**). This can cause increased inflammation and intraocular pressure if the lens material is not aspirated.
- ❖ It is important to assess the integrity of the posterior capsule before surgery.
- ❖ **Vossius ring:** Sometimes pigment deposition can be seen on the lens capsule, caused by the deposition of iris pigments due to the force of the injury.
- ❖ The lens can also dislocate from its usual position after trauma, causing subluxation and hence requiring lens extraction. In dilated pupils, the edge of the lens can

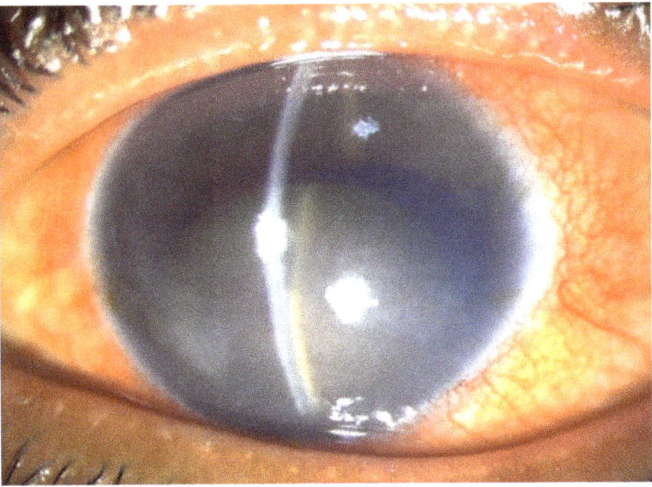

Fig. 23.3: Image showing subluxation of the lens.

be seen in subluxated cases. The depth of the anterior chamber is also irregular, and the iris is also tremulous. Sometimes, the lens may dislocate completely to the anterior or posterior chamber due to trauma **(Fig. 23.3)**. The subluxated lens needs extraction followed by placement of a secondary intraocular lens.

Vitreous

Injury to the vitreous can cause vitreous hemorrhage after both closed and open globe injuries, and might require clearance of the blood.

Choroid

- Choroid can get ruptured due to blunt trauma and can cause decreased vision if the rupture occurs near the macula.
- Choroidal rupture is usually seen as a crescentic scar near the fovea.

Management

Steroids are given to decrease the scarring.

Complication

Choroidal neovascular membrane. Also, choroidal or suprachoroidal hemorrhage can occur after injury.

Retina

- The retina may suffer edematous, or degenerative changes and can be torn or have hemorrhage.
- **Commotio retinae:** A milky white opacity develops on the macula due to the injury and disappears after a few days. The vision may be good in the beginning but usually deteriorates later.
- Macular holes can also occur due to trauma. It is seen as a red punched-out hole at the fovea and requires surgery.
- Post-trauma retinal breaks can lead to retinal detachment, requiring surgery. The retinal breaks are most commonly seen at the superonasal and/or inferotemporal areas. Retinal detachment can occur at the same time, or after days, months or years.

Optic Nerve

- Damage to the optic nerve is rare.
- There can be avulsion of the optic nerve, causing almost nil vision after trauma.

MANAGEMENT OF PENETRATING INJURY

Penetrating injury is an emergency and needs urgent repair to prevent the introduction of any infection.

Wounds of Conjunctiva

Conjunctival lacerations are sutured using absorbable 6-0 or 8-0 vicryl sutures.

Wounds of Cornea

- Corneal lacerations may be linear or stellate.
- The edges of the wound swell up after the injury.
- Small lacerations are usually self-sealing and may or may not require suturing, depending upon the surgeon.
- Large lacerations usually have iris prolapse through them.
- In small recent injuries, the iris can be reposited back using intracameral pilocarpine.
- It is always better to cut the iris to prevent infection in large lacerations with iris incarceration.
- Corneal wounds are repaired using 10-0 nylon, non-absorbable sutures.
- It is always better to suture the anatomical landmarks, like the limbus, first and then proceed accordingly.
- Sutures in the center are usually smaller than the periphery to reduce astigmatism **(Fig. 23.4)**.

Complications

Corneal scarring, decreased vision due to scar, corneal opacity and astigmatism.

Management of Scleral Wounds

- Globe exploration should be done in all cases with scleral wounds to see the extent of the injury.

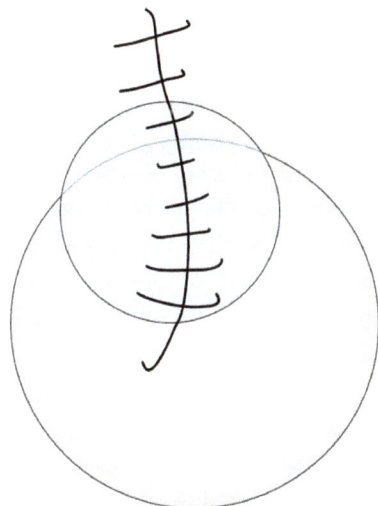

Fig. 23.4: Diagrammatic representation of sutures in open globe injuries, showing small sutures in the center as compared to the periphery.

Management of Lens Injury

- Scleral lacerations should be repaired using absorbable 6-0 or 7-0 vicryl sutures.
- If the wound ruptures the anterior capsule, seepage of the aqueous into the lens causes a swollen cataract.
- In the case of a small wound, localized cloudiness of the lens can produce feathery lines across the posterior cortex, causing a rosette cataract.
- Such changes usually progress to complete cataracts.
- Sometimes, the anterior chamber might be filled with flocculent lens material due to damage to lens capsule. This lens material can cause inflammation and increase intraocular pressure.
- The traumatic cataract may swell, touching the cornea and causing secondary glaucoma.
- Such cataracts need early aspiration. Aspiration can be done in the same sitting at the time of repair or after the repair at a secondary stage.
- These eyes need postoperative antibiotics and steroids to prevent infection and inflammation; otherwise, the eyes may end up in phthisis.

Retained Intraocular Foreign Bodies (IOFBs)

Mechanism

Foreign bodies can cause damage to the eye due to mechanical damage due to the speed by which it enters, infection and chemical effects on the tissues.

- Foreign bodies may pass through the cornea, enter the anterior chamber and get stuck in the iris or angle. It can also pass through the anterior chamber and lens and can damage the retina or lie in the vitreous.
- If it passes through the iris, it can cause an iris hole.
- A foreign body in vitreous can be accessed through the limbal or pars plana route.
- A foreign body in the vitreous can be seen using an indirect ophthalmoscope if the lens is clear and there is no to minimal hemorrhage.
- In cases with hazy media, ultrasonography, CT scan and X-ray be done to identify retained IOFB.
- Sometimes, foreign bodies may pass through the coats of the eye, and lodge in the orbital tissues.
- A foreign body in the retina is usually surrounded by hemorrhage and pigmentation.
- Infections are usually seen in IOFBs consisting of foreign vegetative material.

REACTION TO INTRAOCULAR FOREIGN BODIES

Non-organic Materials

- Glass, plastic, and sand are usually inert materials.
- Gold, platinum and steel are some of the metals which are inert.
- Lead, aluminium and zinc incite some inflammatory responses.
- Iron and copper produce a severe inflammatory reaction, as described below.

Siderosis

The iron foreign body produces an intense inflammatory reaction in the eye, causing siderosis.

Clinical Features

It causes pigmentary changes on the anterior lens capsule with cataract. Iris heterochromia is another feature caused by staining of the anterior capsule. The retina undergoes degenerative pigmentary changes, with attenuation of vessels. Degenerative changes in the lens and retina cause a decrease in vision.

Diagnosis

Foreign body can be seen on ultrasonography, X-ray and CT scan. Electroretinogram shows a decrease in amplitude of 'a' and 'b' waves.

Chalcosis

Deposition of copper due to IOFB causes chalcosis.

Clinical Features

It causes greenish discoloration of the Descemet membrane and lens. A green lustre can also be seen on the retina sometimes. It produces corneal and lens changes similar to Wilson's disease.

Organic Materials

- Vegetative materials may introduce fungal infection into the eye.
- Caterpillar hair can cause intense inflammation in the eye.

DIAGNOSIS OF IOFBs

- Careful slit lamp examination is essential to see the entry wound.
- Ultrasonography can help to assess the posterior segment and identify the foreign body in the posterior segment.
- Magnetic resonance imaging (MRI) is contraindicated in open globe injuries due to the risk of a metallic foreign body.
- CT scan (computerized tomography) and X-ray orbit can also help in the diagnosis.

TREATMENT OF IOFBs

- **Cases where foreign bodies can be left alone:**
  - Inert materials
  - Removal might lead to intensive damage to the globe
- **Foreign body in the vitreous or on the retina:** These foreign bodies can be removed using an intraocular forceps or magnet, which can be introduced through the pars plana or limbal route. Modern vitrectomy instruments help to remove these with caution and minimal damage to the surrounding tissues.
- **Foreign bodies on the iris or lens:** The foreign body over the iris can be removed using intraocular forceps. The foreign body on the lens, can be left alone or removed with the whole lens.

It is important to sensitize people regarding the need to protect themselves from ocular injuries, especially industrial workers and children. Ocular injuries should be treated as an emergency, requiring immediate referral to the specialist.

GERIATRIC CONSIDERATIONS

Although ocular injuries are common among the young population, they can also occur in the elderly due to physical and mental debilitation. Old people may injure their eyes due to falling on the ground and striking surfaces which can occur due to sudden stroke, inability to bear weight, and slipping in the bathroom. This segment of the population needs extra care as they may not be able to address the injury on an urgent basis due to mental debilitation, inability to communicate, and being lonely in the house. They need to be taken immediately to the hospital and given timely ophthalmic care to reduce ocular morbidity and have a better life quality.

NURSING CONSIDERATIONS

Nursing staff should ensure that the patient should receive injection tetanus toxoid and IV antibiotics on presentation to avoid tetanus infection. Patients' eye should be covered with a plastic shield to prevent further trauma and complications. Nursing staff should monitor patients vitals for hemodynamic stability.

> **Case Scenario**
> A factory worker got hit by a nail while working in the factory. He complained of pain and loss of vision after that. On examination in emergency, he had a corneal laceration with iris prolapse. So he had an open globe injury which was repaired in the OT to prevent phthisis bulbi.

SUMMARY

Prevention of ocular injuries is a must to prevent long-term ocular complications like loss of vision which can affect quality of life. Factory workers should wear protective eyegear to prevent ocular injuries. At presentation, patient should receive primary basic treatment followed by ocular management. Proper and timely referral is a must to restore the integrity of eyeball to prevent long-term complications.

MULTIPLE CHOICE QUESTIONS

1. Which of the following is not required in management of hyphema?
   a. Steroids
   b. Antiglaucoma
   c. Aspirin
   d. Cycloplegics
2. All are types of mechanical injuries, *except*:
   a. Open globe injuries
   b. Closed globe injuries
   c. Foreign body
   d. Chemical injuries
3. All of the following are manifestations of posterior segment trauma, *except*:
   a. Retinal detachment
   b. Cataract
   c. Macular hole
   d. Choroidal rupture
4. What is hyphema?
   a. Blood in vitreous
   b. Tear in iris
   c. Blood in anterior chamber
   d. Damage to ciliary body
5. What is the immediate management of chemical injury?
   a. Admission
   b. Repair of injury
   c. Saline wash
   d. IV antibiotics

ANSWERS

1. c   2. d   3. b   4. c
5. c

SUGGESTED READING

1. Cockerham GC. Blunt trauma and nonpenetrating injuries of the anterior segment. Ophthalmol. 1983;90:140-8.
2. Kuckelkorn R, Keller G, Redbrake C, Schrage N. Emertreatment of chemical and thermal eye burns. Acta Ophthalmol Scand. 2002;80(1):4-10.
3. Wagoner MD. Chemical injuries of the eye: current conin pathophysiology and therapy. Surv Ophthalmol. 1997;41(4):275-313.
4. Kuhn F, Morris R, Witherspoon CD, Heimann K, Jeffers JB, Treister G. A standardized classification of ocular trauma. Graefes Arch Clin Exp Ophthalmol. 1996;234(6):399-403.
5. Kuhn F, Pieramici DJ. Ocular trauma: principles and prac New York, Thieme; 2002. pp. 236-46.
6. Kanski JJ. Clinical ophthalmology. A systemic approach. St Louis: Butterworth Heinemann; 2003. pp. 665-80.
7. MacGwin G, Owsley C, Xie A. Rate of eye injury in the United States. Arch Ophthalmol. 2005;123:970-6.
8. Kaushik S, Sukhija J. Blunt ocular trauma. Ann Ophthalmol. 2006;38(3):249-52.
9. McGowan G Jr, Hall TA, Xie A, Owsley C. Trends in eye injury in the United States, 1992-2001. Invest Ophthalmol Vis Sci. 2006;47(2):521-7.
10. Williams DF, Mieler WF, Williams GA. Posterior segment manifestations of ocular trauma. Retina. 1990;109(1):35-44.

CHAPTER 24: Eye Banking, Ocular Prosthesis and Rehabilitation

Ranjan Kumar Behera, Parul Chawla Gupta, Jagat Ram

"Volunteers do not necessarily have the time, they have the heart."
—Elizabeth Andrew

Learning Objectives

After going through the chapter, the learner will be able to:
- Understand the basic structure and functioning of an eye bank.
- Understand the concept, procedure associated with eye donation and its storage and distribution.
- Discuss the importance of an ocular prosthesis, its types, functions and its role in ocular cosmesis.
- Define low vision, its causes and various methods to improve quality of vision in such cases.

Terms

- **Eye banking:** An organization that collects, medically evaluates, and distributes eye tissues for corneal transplant, research, and education.
- **Eye donation:** The process of pledging and donating one's eyes after death for the purpose of corneal transplantations and academic purposes in medical institutes.
- **Ocular prosthesis:** An artificial eye that replaces an absent natural eye due to various causes such as trauma, injury, surgery, etc.
- **Orbital implant:** Artificial spherical structure made up of various materials which are used to replace the lost volume in an orbital cavity in which the eye has been removed surgically.

INTRODUCTION

In this chapter, we will be discussing the basic concepts of eye banking along with the ocular prosthesis which may be used for the damaged eye after injury or a radical eye surgery that results in ocular tissue and volume loss.

EYE BANKING

Eye banks are the institutions which are part of the local health system and are usually attached to a hospital which are responsible for procuring, harvesting and processing of donor corneas. These institutions are regulated by hospitals and are a part of the local health system. Eye banks are registered under a qualified corneal surgeon.

Functions of Eye Bank

- Counseling and motivating family of the deceased for eye donation.
- Proper assessment of medical history, time and cause of death and donor risk factors.
- Safe retrieval and collection of donor corneas along with ophthalmology residents.
- Evaluation, grading and safe storage of donor corneas and ensuring fair and equitable distribution of tissue.
- Prepare and supply donated scleral patches for other eye surgeries and help in preparing amniotic membranes.
- Research activities to find new alternatives or advances in field of corneal transplantation.

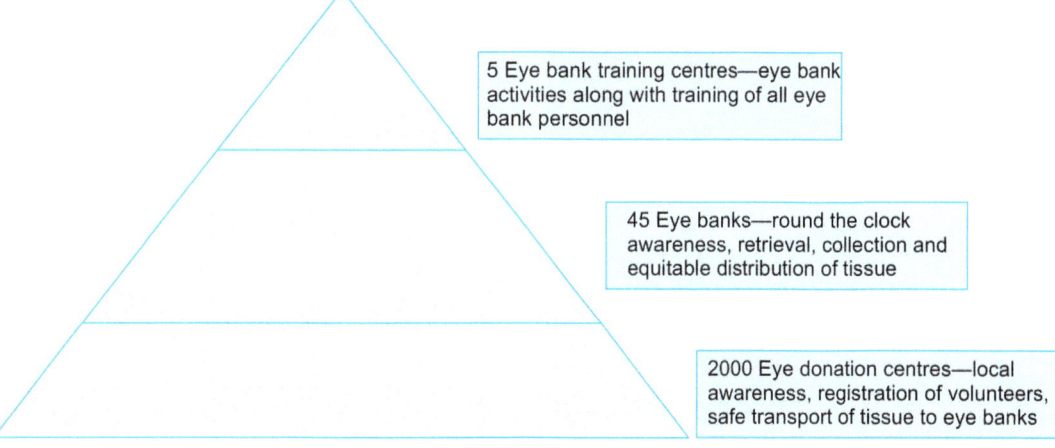

Fig. 24.1: Three tier eye banking system.

Eye Banking System

It is a 3 tier system with each having its own functions and responsibilities **(Fig. 24.1)**.

Basic Infrastructure of an Eye Bank

Basic infrastructure of an eye bank includes:
- A minimum space of 600 sq ft.
- Maintenance of eye bank and regular cleaning.
- Equipment maintenance—a refrigerator to store tissues between temperature between 2-6°C **(Fig. 24.2)**.
- Instrumentation and reagents to remove and store corneas.
- Infection control and waste disposal—all personnel to take proper care and ensure proper disposal of human tissues.

Eye Banking Staff

Eye bank staff includes:
- Eye bank in charge
- Eye bank technician
- Storekeeper
- Social worker

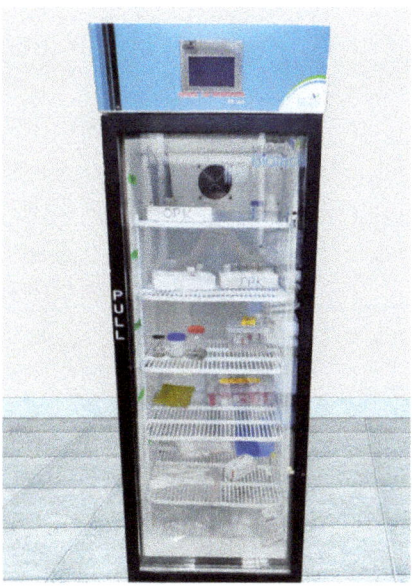

Fig. 24.2: A refrigerator in the eye bank to store various grades of eyes which have been donated and retrieved.

EYE DONATION

Visually impaired account for 285 million people worldwide. About 1,85,000 corneal transplants are done per year worldwide. 87% of the corneas are procured from the donors within the same country. Limited access to viable corneas remains a challenge throughout the world. It can be voluntary eye donation where people realize their social responsibility and inform eye banks to collect eye of their expired relatives or hospital cornea retrieval program where eye banks at hospitals actively motivate relatives of the deceased for eye donation and at the same time being sensitive about their feelings.

Process of Eye Donation

- When a death occurs in the hospital, eye bank staff is informed.
- Eye bank counselor counsels the relatives and if they agree, he ascertains the time, cause and mode of death and ensures that there are no contraindications for donation:
  - Avoid eye donation in cases of death due to septicemia, known case of HIV/hepatitis B or C/cancer/TB/Prion diseases/rabies.
- After taking consent from family members, whole eyeball is retrieved and stored in moist chamber. The blood sample of the deceased is taken. It can be done bedside or after the patient is sent to the mortuary.
  - Ideal time interval between death and eye donation is 6 hours.
- The whole eyeball is examined under microscope and grading of corneal quality is done and cornea is then harvested under aseptic conditions.
- The cornea according to its clarity is stored in specific storage medias in the refrigerator depending upon whether short-term—MK media (1-4 days), intermediate-Optisol (10-14 days) or long-term storage—organ culture/cryopreservation (months to years) is required **(Fig. 24.3)**. Only after serological tests (HIV, HbsAg, HCV, VDRL) of the donors blood comes negative, storing of cornea is done.

  Donor cornea distribution should only be done to registered ophthalmologists, institutions and other eye banks depending upon the indication of the surgical procedure.

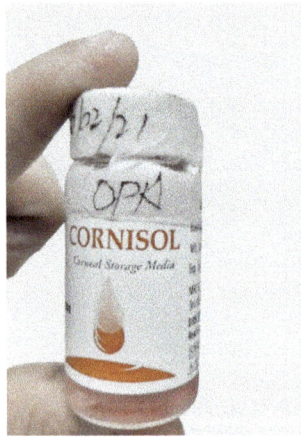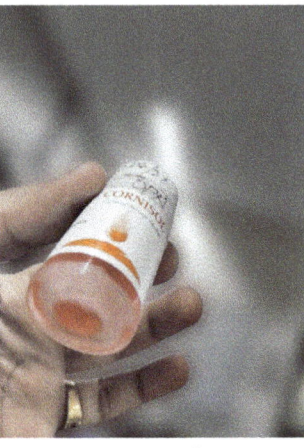

Fig. 24.3: Corneal tissue storage in storage medium.

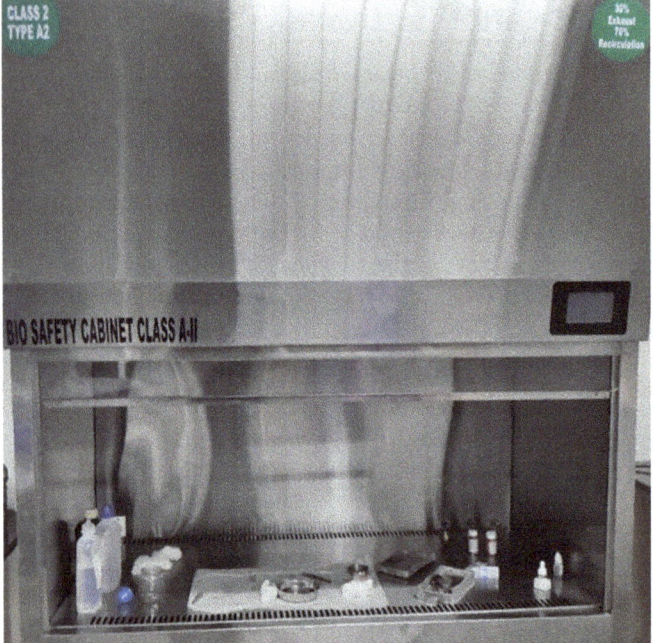

Fig. 24.4: A laminar hood flow biosafety cabin in the eye bank to retrieve and prepare corneal button for examination.

Proper documentation of the recipient should be maintained in the eye bank **(Fig. 24.4)**.

Facts About Eye Donation

- Anyone can pledge for eye donation.
- Eye donation gives sight to two blind people, as one cornea is transplanted to one recipient.
- Eye donation does not disfigure the deceased face.

> **Case Scenario**
>
> The local eye bank of a government hospital received a call from the ICU regarding death of a male. The Eye bank professionals reached the spot and counseled the relatives for eye donation but the cause of death was found to be septicemia. So, should they go ahead with eye donation? Yes, although contraindicated for eye transplantation, these eyes should be retrieved and can be used for research purposes.

SUMMARY

Eye banking has a pivotal role in the ophthalmology department as it caters to the safe, efficient and timely retrieval of the eyes of the deceased which can be evaluated, processed and stored in the eye banks which can be used to provide vision to many patients who are blind due to corneal opacities. Eyes should be used as soon as possible as endothelial health of the cornea gets compromised with time.

OCULAR PROSTHESIS AND REHABILITATION

An ocular prosthesis/artificial eye **(Fig. 24.5)** is a device that replaces the damaged eye caused after injury or a radical eye surgery that results in ocular tissue and volume loss. They look similar to the normal eye. They are made up of biocompatible material, so that the observer is not able to make out whether it is a normal or artificial eye. It is usually placed around 1.5–2 months after radical eye surgeries when inflammation has subsided for better fitting. The material used in these devices can be glass or polymethyl methacrylate (PMMA). These devices can either be readily available in fixed sizes or custom made according to patients' needs and requirements. The artificial eye is in the form of a cup shaped disc that fits behind the eyelids and over the conjunctiva to replace the lost volume with the front surface having normal eye structures to mimic the normal eye. PMMA is usually preferrable due to its more biocompatibility, durability and longer life expectancy.

Orbital Implants

These are special devices used to replace the lost orbital volume and space post radical surgeries. These need to be compatible with the surrounding remaining ocular tissues for better adhesion and preventing rejection and associated inflammation and infection.

These can be either primary implant (placed at time of surgery) or secondary implant (in cases of exposure, migration or extrusion). Implants replace about 70% of orbital volume and enhances the movement of ocular prosthesis and eyelids and also takes care of the cosmetic aspect.

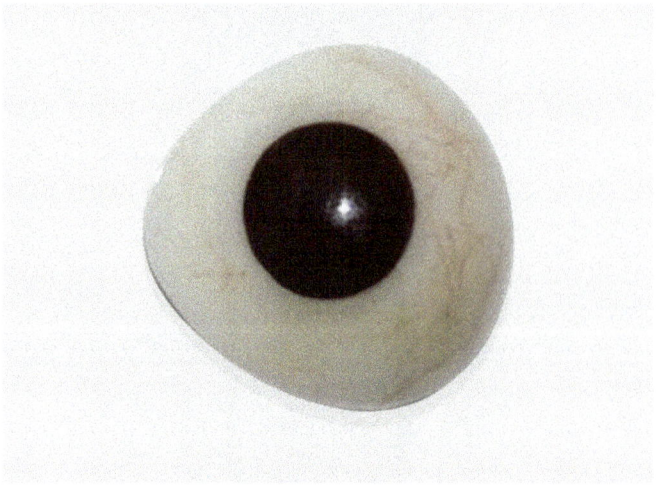

Fig. 24.5: Artificial eye.

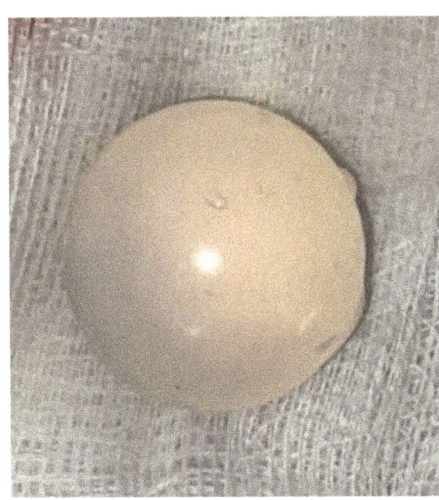

Fig. 24.6: Orbital implant.

The degree of mobility of a normal eye cannot be expected after an orbital implant, although the remaining rectus muscles may be attached to the implant and the remaining surrounding tissues may adhere to the implant surface, but the mobility still remains restricted.

There are various types of orbital implants:
1. **Nonintegrated implants (Fig. 24.6):** Are non-porous materials, i.e., not connected to the orbital tissues. They are easy to insert, cheap and tolerated well and have less complications. They are made up of non-porous silicone act by the forces created between the conjunctiva and the implant.
2. **Integrated implants:** These have porous openings which allows surrounding orbital tissues to grow into the implant which allows better stability and motility. They are expensive and difficult to insert and remove. Examples of integrated implants—hydroxyapatite and porous polyethylene.

Low Vision Aids

A patient with low vision is defined as that as someone who after medical, surgical and/or optical intervention has a corrected visual acuity less than 6/18 to 3/60, or a visual field of less than 20 degrees from point of fixation but uses or is able to potentially use, vision for planning and/or executing a task for which vision is essential. Uncorrected refractive errors account for the major cause of vision impairment about 50%. Other causes:
❖ Cataract
❖ Glaucoma
❖ Trachoma
❖ Diabetic retinopathy
❖ Age related macular degeneration

In a case we encounter a patient with low vision, he should be subjected for refraction for distance and near, visual fields and contrast sensitivity. In case of vitreous/retinal diseases additional tests like color vision, retinal acuity potential, optical coherence tomography, ultrasound and electroretinography are required.

Low Vision Distance Systems

❖ **Spectacles and contact lenses:** To correct high refractive errors with antireflective coatings. Photochromatic filters can be used to reduce glare and photophobia **(Fig. 24.7)**.
❖ **Telescopes:** Used to magnify the apparent size of a distant object. They make distant objects appear closer than they actually are to the subject. They can be handheld telescopes or fixed onto the patients' spectacles **(Figs. 24.8 and 24.9)**.

Low Vision Near Systems

❖ **Magnifying glasses:** High power reading glasses where patient has to focus and read at the focal point. Comfort, free hands during usage and prolonged reading time are its advantages.

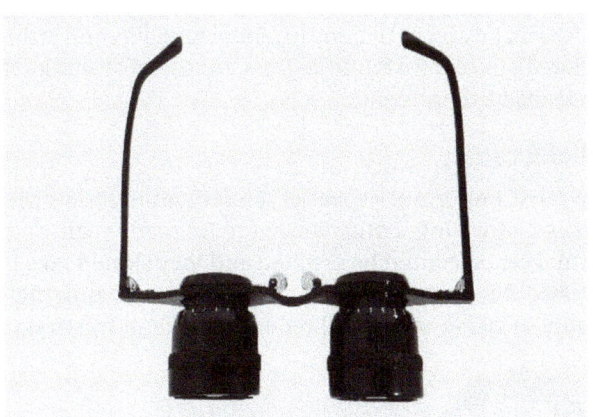

Fig. 24.7: Max TV spectacle.

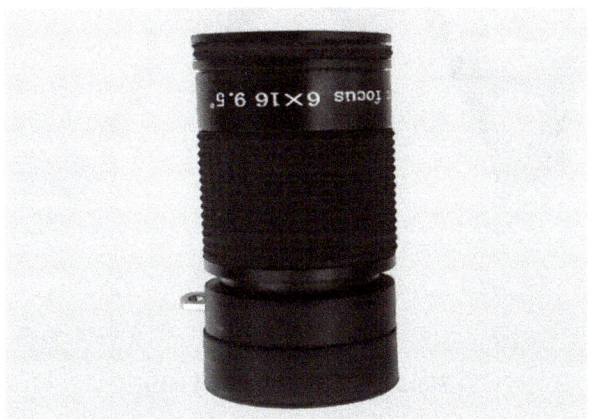

Fig. 24.8: Low vision telescope for distance.

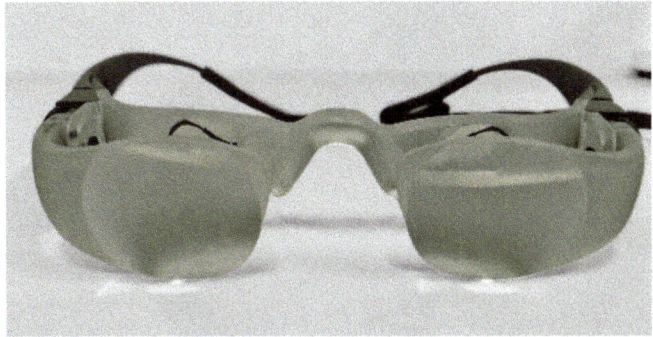

Fig. 24.9: 6X monocular bifocal.

- **Hand magnifiers (Fig. 24.10):** Convex lenses held in front of spectacle plane used for reading signs, price tags, etc.
- **Stand magnifiers (Fig. 24.11):** fixed, focused lenses for old age.
- **Portable video magnifier (Fig. 24.12):** Electronic based optical device used to magnify small letters on a screen in low vision. High cost limits its use.

Non-optical Devices

- **Signature guide:** Used in cases of ARMD to sign documents.
- **Cane stick:** Provides help to low vision patient during movement. High mobility and no maintenance are its advantages.
- **Typoscope:** Improves image quality be reducing glare and enhancing contrast.
- Recent advances relating to retinal implants and artificial intelligence have found success in cases of low vision and needs further research.

Rehabilitation

The most important aspect of rehabilitation in low vision aids is counseling. Patients need to be made realistic that normal vision cannot be restored and they should take help of these devices which may help them in improving the quality of vision which will reduce stress and frustration in

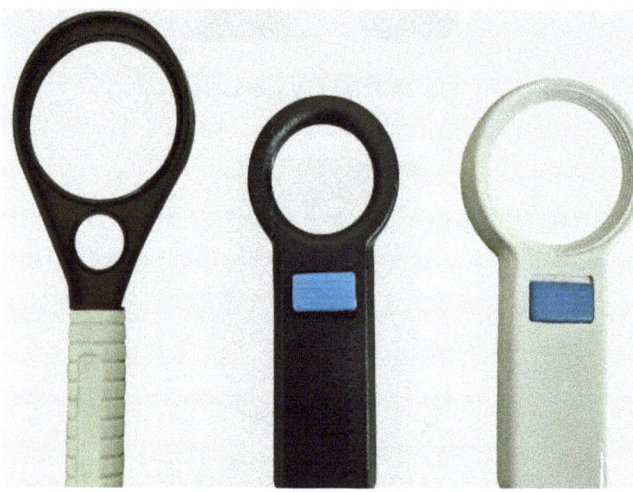

Fig. 24.10: Hand held magnifier.

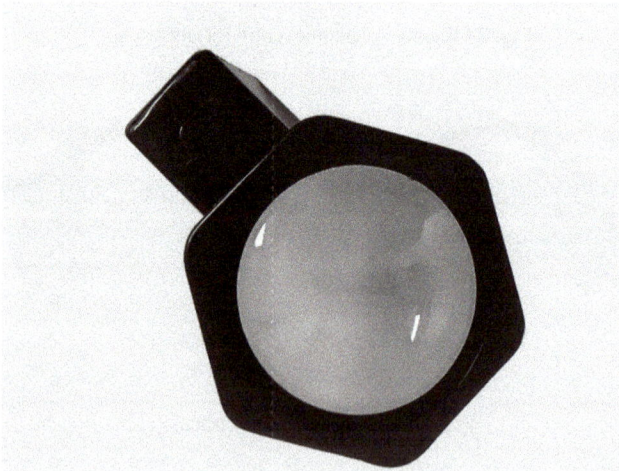

Fig. 24.11: Stand magnifier.

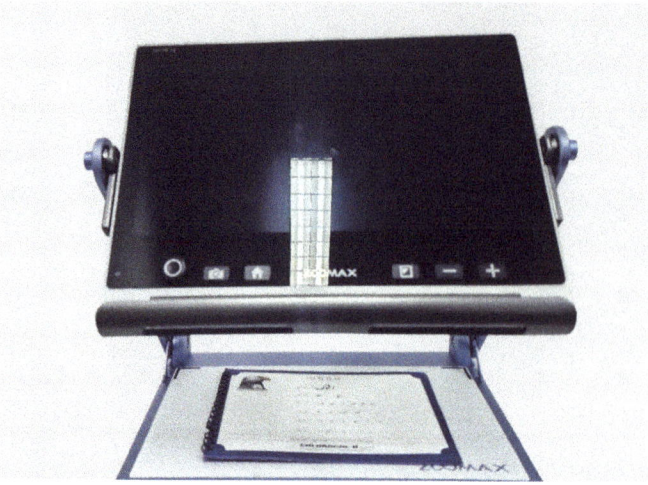

Fig. 24.12: Portable video magnifier.

their lives. Artificial prosthetic devices like artificial eyes need to be kept clean and hygienic by regular washing to prevent development of orbital socket infection.

GERIATRIC CONSIDERATIONS

Corneal transplantation allows a ray of hope for vision which becomes more significant in the elderly populations. Most of the time they have bilateral involvement due to prolonged disease which adds to their morbidity and repetitive corneal transplants make them prone to graft rejections for subsequent corneal transplantations. The older patients who are bilaterally blind should be given priority which can allow them to have some vision to lead a better quality of their remaining life.

NURSING CONSIDERATIONS

Nursing management involves counseling of patients with the help of optometrists about their realistic visual potential and how to use low vision aids. It is important to assess the patient's understanding of the surgical procedure, postoperative care regimen, and the importance of regular follow-up. They can also teach patients how to keep their artificial devices clean, their safe removal and insertion into orbital sockets and to report in cases of development of any infection.

Case Scenario

A 60-year-old male, heavy smoker, came to eye hospital with history of diminution of vision both eyes since 4 years. On examination it was found that he had developed end stage macular scarring both eyes due to age-related macular degeneration. He was counseled about his end stage disease and referred to low vision aid specialist. He advised him to use hand held magnifiers as the patient was having difficulty in near work and was a clerk by profession. Patient came after 2 month follow up and was satisfied with his low vision aid.

SUMMARY

Ocular prosthetic devices and low vision aids help in restoring the orbital volume and help patients to get some amount of functional vision and improved image quality to carry out their daily tasks. Low vison aids should be customized according to the patients' needs and also keeping in mind their cost. Patient counselling is of utmost importance in such cases.

MULTIPLE CHOICE QUESTIONS

1. What is the ideal time of eye donation after death?
   a. 3 hours
   b. 4 hours
   c. 6 hours
   d. 12 hours
2. Intermediate storage using corneal storage media can be done up to what duration?
   a. 1–4 days
   b. 4–7 days
   c. 7–10 days
   d. 10–14 days
3. One eye donation gives vision to how many people?
   a. 1
   b. 2
   c. 3
   d. 4
4. Which of the following is not a contraindication for eye donation?
   a. HIV
   b. Active TB
   c. Septicemia
   d. Road traffic accident
5. Which of the following is not a part of the eye banking system?
   a. Eye camps
   b. Eye bank training centers
   c. Eye banks
   d. Eye donation centers
6. What is the ideal duration of placing an ocular prosthesis post-radical eye surgery?
   a. 1–2 weeks
   b. 2–4 weeks
   c. 4–5 weeks
   d. 6–8 weeks
7. Which material is best suited for an ocular prosthesis?
   a. Plastic
   b. Rubber
   c. HEMA
   d. PMMA
8. What amount of volume is replaced by orbital implants?
   a. 30%
   b. 50%
   c. 70%
   d. 90%
9. Which among these is the major cause of vision impairment in the world?
   a. Cataract
   b. Glaucoma
   c. Retinal disorders
   d. Uncorrected refractive errors
10. Which of the following tests is not done in a case of low vision patient?
    a. Refraction
    b. OCT
    c. Lacrimal syringing
    d. Visual fields

ANSWERS

1. c	2. d	3. b	4. d
5. a	6. d	7. d	8. c
9. d	10. c		

SUGGESTED READING

1. Gain P, Jullienne R, He Z, et al. Global survey of corneal transplantation and eye banking. JAMA Ophthalmol. 2016;134:167-73.
2. Gilbert C, van Djik K. When someone has low vison. Community Eye Health. 2012;25:4-11.
3. Khurana AK, Grover AK, Honavar SG, Khurana BP, Khurana A. Enucleation and evisceration. Disorders of Eyelids, Lacrimal System, Orbit and Oculoplastic Surgery,1st edition. New Delhi: CBS Publishers & Distributors Pvt Ltd; 2017. pp. 440-56.
4. Khurana AK, Sharma N, Sinha R, Khurana A, Khurana BP. Eye banking and eye donation: Retrieval, evaluation, storage and distribution of donor cornea. Disorders of Cornea and Ocular Surface, 1st edition. New Delhi: CBS Publishers and Distributors Pvt Ltd; 2020. pp. 651-64.
5. Kumar A, Ravani R. Low vision management in retinal diseases. Retina: Medical and Surgical Management, 1st edition. New Delhi: Jaypee Brothers Medical Publishers (P) Ltd; 2018. pp. 238-52.
6. Pascolini D, Mariotti SP. Global estimates of visual impairment: 2010. Br J Ophthalmol. 2012;96:614-8.
7. Vajpayee RB, Sharma N, Tabin G, Taylor H. Eye banking—A practical guide. Corneal Transplantation, 2nd edition. New Delhi: Jaypee Brothers Medical Publishers (P) Ltd; 2010. pp. 20-37.

CHAPTER 25

Community Ophthalmology

Mona Duggal, Anshul Chauhan

"I shut my eyes and all the world drops dead; I lift my eyes and all is born again."
—Sylvia Plath

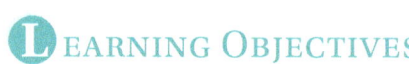

After going through the chapter, the learner will be able to:
- Understand the Indian public health system.
- Describe the main features of primary health system and primary eye care.
- Describe the importance of prevention and screening in primary eye care.
- Understand the application of WHO building blocks in primary care.

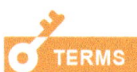

- **Comprehensive primary eye care:** It Includes eye health promotion; prevention, diagnosis, treatment of eye diseases and rehabilitation of those with irreversible blindness and low vision.
- **Community ophthalmology:** It is based on the principles of primary healthcare approach which includes equitable distribution of eye care resources, community engagement in providing eye care, prevention of blindness, use of appropriate technology and multisectoral approach.
- **Primary eye care:** Provision of appropriate, accessible, and affordable care that meets patients' eye care needs in a comprehensive and competent manner.
- **Public health:** The art and science of preventing disease, prolonging life and promoting health through the organized efforts of society.

INTRODUCTION

According to the International Agency for Prevention of Blindness (IAPB), 253 million people worldwide are living with vision impairment and 30% out of which are blind. Globally uncorrected refractive errors and cataract are major cause of blindness and visual impairment and more than 80% of all the visual impairment cases are preventable. A significant percentage of world's blind (20.5%) and (21.9%) of visually impaired population are from India. Whereas, cataract (62.6%), refractive error (19.70%), glaucoma (5.80%) still continues to be main cause of blindness.

Primary health care (PHC) in India is based on the overarching principles of fair distribution of healthcare services, community engagement, disease prevention, use of appropriate technology and multisectoral approach. The PHC is a component of general health system and is provided through a network of Indian public health system (IPHS) in India. It envisages set of uniform standards to strengthen the delivery of quality of health care in the country. Mainly primary eye care (PEC) services in India are provide at three levels: community level, health and wellness centers (HWC), primary health centers (PHCs). The PEC is the essential building block for preventing blindness through preventive activities implemented through community level or at primary level of health care. Community ophthalmology is based on the principles of primary health care approach which includes equitable distribution of eye care resources, community engagement in providing eye care, prevention of blindness, use of appropriate technology and multisectoral approach.

OVERVIEW OF INDIAN PUBLIC HEALTH SYSTEM

The public health system in India is governed by the Union Ministry of Health and Family Welfare (MOHFW) at central level and respective health departments at the state level. In order to provide accessible, affordable, accountable health care services to the vulnerable sections of the population National Health Mission (NHM) under MoHFW was established in 2005. The structure of IPHS is illustrated in **Figure 25.1**.

The eye care services are provided by healthcare cadre working at different levels of care within public health system. Screening and preventive activities to promote eye care is done by Accredited Social Health Activist (ASHA). ASHA is the health staff who belongs to the community and is involved in creating awareness on health and its determinants. She is responsible for mobilizing the community towards better treatment and to promote increased utilization of the existing health services available to the patients. Awareness on common eye diseases, vitamin A prophylaxis from 6 months to 5 years, identification of patients with eye diseases and referral for availability of eye care services are carried out by ASHA. At community level screening of population >30 years of age with presbyopia (poor near vision related to ageing), visual acuity (VA) <6/18 is also done by ASHA. She also undertakes record keeping for referred patients from community and provides follow-up care for postoperative cataract patients. Community screening for the congenital disorders is done for all the children who are born preterm (<32 weeks) within 30 days of their birth. Distribution of spectacles to children and ensuring its regular use is also carried out by ASHA.

At health and wellness center (HWC), the community health officer (CHO) ensures the regular eye screening, management of referral, treatment of refractive errors, ensuring access to free spectacles, and also undertakes home and community based follow up.

Currently, the specialist services are provided at district hospital and above depending upon the availability of ophthalmologist (explained in case scenario).

NATIONAL PROGRAM FOR CONTROL OF BLINDNESS AND VISUAL IMPAIRMENT (NPCBVI)

In India, the National Program for Control of Blindness and Visual Impairment (NPCBVI) was started in the year 1976. The program after its launch aims to reduce prevalence of blindness from 1.4–0.3% by the year 2020 whereby addressing the increasing blindness problem. Health being a state subject, the prerogative of implementation of the national health program remains within the confines of the state government. The ultimate implementation of the program within the state is the collective responsibility of District Health Societies at district level.

HEALTH SYSTEM FRAMEWORK

The health framework attempts to include most important features is the health system which interlinks the healthy system functionality and use. The WHO health system framework provides shorthand for describing health system in a concise manner which is widely used. The WHO health building blocks have become a reference point for all national and global policy makers. However, the role of community in the critical elements is underplayed and not displayed efficiently.

The WHO through its Global Action Plan, 2014–2019 urged its member countries to adapt Universal Eye Health (UEH) Plan to work towards achievement of comprehensive eye care through integration of services. It is also evident that the eye care services need to be stepped up to cater the growing need for services due to increased urbanization

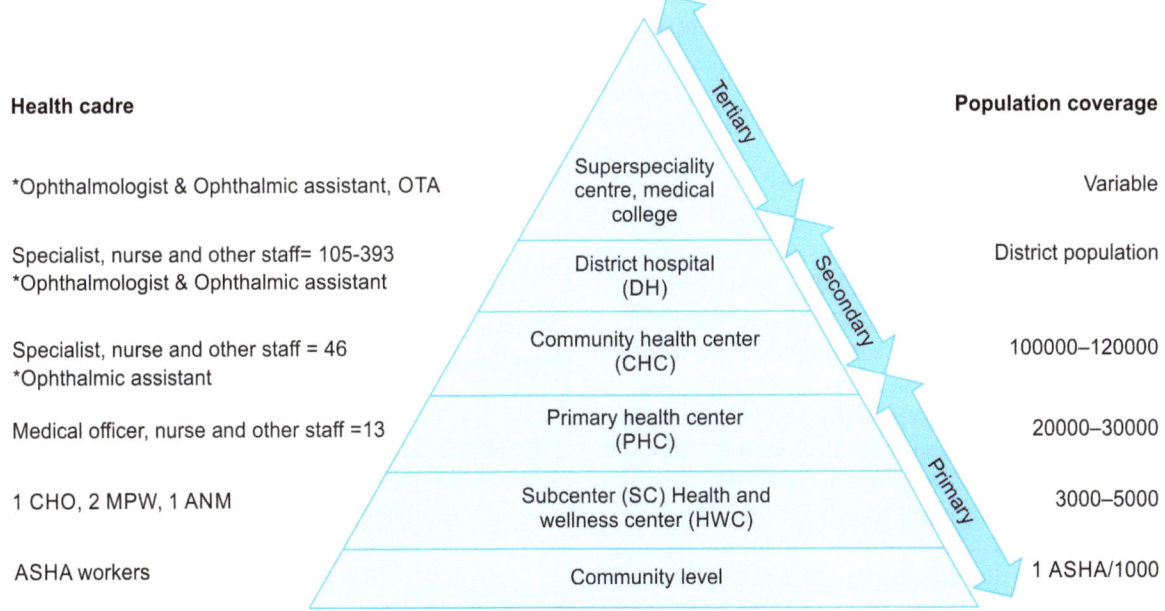

Fig. 25.1: General public health system in India.

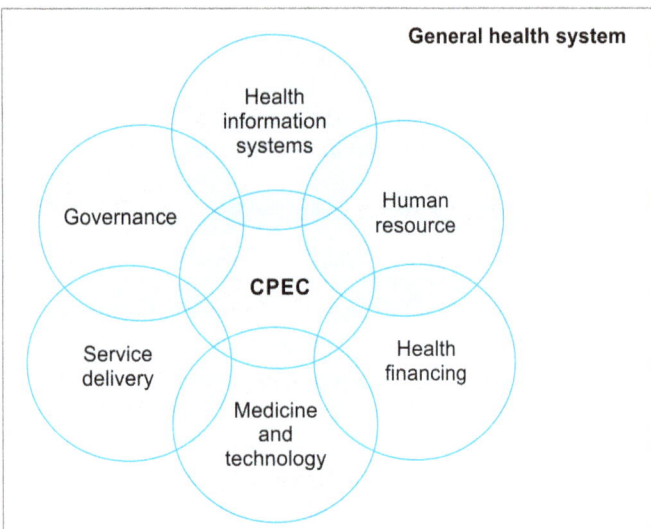

Fig. 25.2: Comprehensive primary eye care (CPEC).

and lifestyle modifications. The Rapid Assessment Survey on Blindness (RAAB) conducted till date in India were mostly conducted in the southern parts of India whereas it does not hold any representativeness from northern and northeastern states. This chapter will focus on India Eye Health system, using eye health system assessment (EHSA) tool (as summarized in **Figure 25.2**).

Governance

In 2015, India took a leap towards development of Eye Health Action Plan with MoHFW and in consultation with WHO, International Agency for Prevention of Blindness (IAPB) and other key stakeholders for adopting WHO Global Action Plan for Universal Eye Care.

The objectives of this plan were to set out comprehensive strategies for eye care services, vision impairment and rehabilitation of the most vulnerable population.

Various international and national organizations are working hand in hand with NBCBVI in providing quality of eye care through providing logistics support, technical support, expanding service delivery to outreach areas and strengthening capacity of the program in terms of infrastructure, manpower and technology.

Various key stakeholders involved in eye care service network in India are enlisted in **Table 25.1**.

Health Management Information System

Health management information system (HMIS) acknowledges the information from various components of health system building blocks and helps in managing the information generated at local, district and national level.

At local level the data is recorded in standard formats which includes the program indicators, budget expenditure, and referrals. Whereas the reporting mechanism may not be uniform throughout so there is a need for efficient management and monitoring of the program through development of HMIS at various levels of care.

The NPCBVI dashboard indicators reflect the patients registered under each disease category, NGOs, public health facilities, private practitioners in each State and Union Territory.

TABLE 25.1: Key stakeholders involved in eye care service network in India.

Stakeholder category	Name of organization
Multilateral and bilateral agencies	• WHO • World Bank • United Nations Children's Fund • Danish Development Assistance Agency • United States Agency for International Development
International NGOs in India	• Sight Savers International • Christoffel Blind Mission • ORBIS International • Operational Eyesight Universal • Rotary International • International Eye Foundation • Lion Club International Foundation • Seva Foundation
National eye care foundation	• All India Institute of Medical Sciences (AIIMS), Delhi • Indian Council of Medical Research (ICMR) • LV Prasad Eye Institute (LVPEI) • Sanakara Nethralaya • Aravind Eye Care System • All India Ophthalmological Society • Eye Bank Association of India • Venu Eye Institute and Charitable Society
Networks and partnership	Vision 2020: Right to Sight India

Eye Care Human Resources and Service Delivery

One of the outlined factors in providing quality eye care services is the availability of trained human resources. In India, range of preventive, promotive, curative services eye care services are delivered through the following cadre **(Table 25.2)**.

The skewed distribution of ophthalmologists in rural and urban areas intensifies the need for accessibility and availability of eye care services to the population.

Whereas it is imperative to say that the precious time of an ophthalmologist is spent on routine service like refraction which affects the overall productivity and while neglecting other critical services.

Noteworthy to say that the focus of NPSBVI on cataract surgical rate (CSR) in past two decades has made a remarkable impact. CSR has increased fourfold presently due to which blindness due to cataract has dropped below 65% as compared to 80% in mid-1980's. Apart from cataract, the program has geared up to tackle other causes of visual impairment viz. glaucoma, diabetic retinopathy (DR), vitreoretinal diseases, corneal blindness, low vision and childhood blindness.

TABLE 25.2: Eye care cadre distribution in India.

Population	Eye health specific cadre	Total number	Per million
1,20,00,00,000	Ophthalmologist	20000	16
	Optometrist	9000	7
	Allied ophthalmic personnel	40000	33

Note: Allied ophthalmic personnel ophthalmic assistant, ophthalmic technician, ophthalmic nurses and opticians

Health Financing

India's public health expenditure was allocated 1.6% of the GDP in the year 2019-2020, which is comparatively low as compared to other countries like Germany (9.4%), USA (8.5%) and China (3.2%).

The eye care budget is allocated to State Health Societies and then distributed to District Health Societies for final implementation of activities. After the financial year 2013-2014 the proportion of the financial allocation to NPCBVI has been changed from 100% centrally funded program to 60:40 ratio (60 centrally funded and 40 state funded) in all states and 90:10 ratio (90 centrally funded and 10 state funded) for North eastern states.

Financial assistance is also given to the NGO's or private practitioner performing cataract surgeries, and dealing with other eye diseases like diabetic retinopathy (DR), glaucoma management, childhood blindness, etc.

Highlights

- To address the unmet the healthcare need of poor and vulnerable population due to catastrophic healthcare expenditure, Pradhan Mantri Jan Arogya Yojna (PMJAY) provides financial cover of up to ₹ 5 lakh per family which also extends to cover 42 eye care packages.
- 13th five-year plan of Government of India has budget provisioned for strengthening existing ophthalmic wing of district/general and taluk hospitals (₹ 300 lakhs for each state)

Medicines and Technologies

- The National List of Essential Medicines (NLEM) proposed a list of medicines that meets the healthcare needs of most of the population. The medicines in the healthcare facilities are made available according to NLEM and dispensed according to the level of services they provide. The list also includes basic essential list of eye medicines available at community level, HWC level, and referral center level for dispensing by Accredited Social Health Activist (ASHA), Community Health Officer (CHO) prophylactically and some medicines to be dispensed only after consultation of the medical practitioner.
- Under one of the principles of the HWC, it is proposed to start telemedicine platform to start screening of diseases at primary level to increase the reach of healthcare services who cannot afford to travel to specialist centers.

Delivering Comprehensive Eye Care through Integration of Services

Various steps have been taken in the past to integrate eye care services into general health system. Recently, launched Ayushman Bharat program under aegis of Government of India aims to provide comprehensive primary health care (CPHC) by the existing health system network through health system strengthening.

The existing staff available at community level, Health and Wellness Center/Primary Health Center (HWC/PHC) level **(Fig. 25.1)** are designated to carry out activities like preventive and curative services (awareness generation on common eye disorders, primary screening for refractive errors, congenital disorder referral). Referral centers are designated to manage/treat the advanced cases like cataract, glaucoma, diabetic retinopathy, corneal blindness, etc. The model will ensure the continuity of services and care through established referral network from peripheral health facilities to district health facility with the help of existing health staff working at each level **(Fig. 25.3)**.

Currently, the activities like early screening of diabetes and other noncommunicable disease program (NCD) are under the ambit of noncommunicable diseases program, Recently, referral of People with Diabetes for DR screening and other eye disease has been mentioned in the HWC guidelines. These are evident steps towards integration of eye health program into general health system.

EQUITY IN ACCESS TO EYE CARE AND COMMUNITY ENGAGEMENT

Equity in eye care means fair distribution of care and resources throughout a group of people without discriminating on the

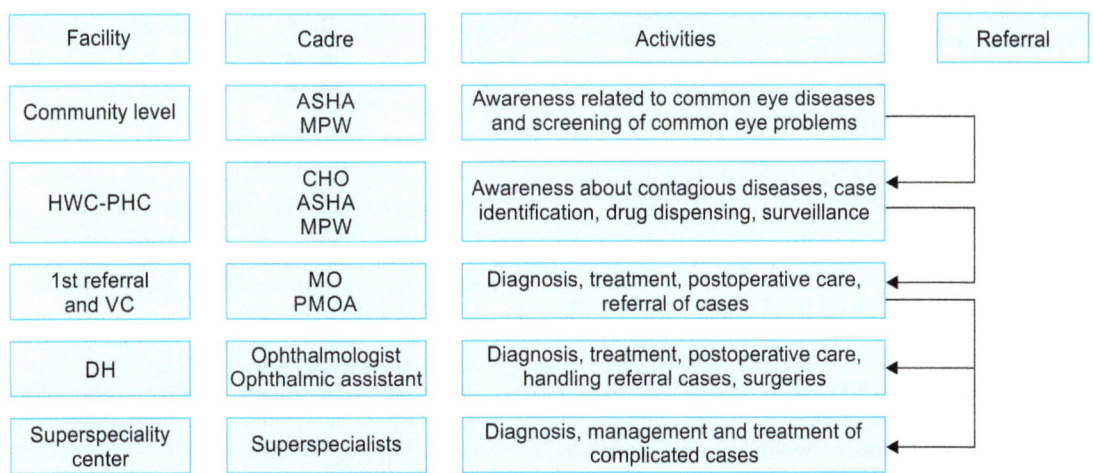

Fig. 25.3: Referral network along public health system involving various healthcare staff.

(ASHA: accredited social health activist; MPW: multipurpose worker; CHO: community health officer; PMOA: paramedical ophthalmic assistant; MO: medical officer; DH: district officer; HWC: health and wellness center; VC: vision center)

basis of ethnicity, gender, age, and social class, although there exist many barriers such as lack of infrastructure, resources, which poses challenges to the service delivery. Number of measures can be taken to address the inequities like providing same quality of eye care services irrespective of gender, age, ethnicity, and geographical distribution. Everyone who reports at the eye clinic or hospital should enjoy same level of care. However, offering equal eye health services to everyone will not lead to equity unless all the persons in the community have a same starting point. To address this, a change in perspective is required and it is important to develop a program revolving around the needing eye care. For example, a clinic or hospital delivering best eye care services is not meeting peoples need unless they have access to them. That is why community engagement is very critical so that the barriers to eye care like lack of awareness, ignorance, cultural factors are effectively addressed.

By addressing eye care needs of specific population who are socially excluded we can plan to extend the implementation of the national programs to these outreach communities.

Case Scenario

Diabetic Retinopathy (DR)
In the rural village Matiana of block Mashobra, district Shimla, ASHA visited households as a part of NCD screening program. While visiting the households she noticed that one male family member aged 56 years have a history of alcohol and smoking consumption since 10 and 12 years respectively. He also had a family history of diabetes and hypertension. ASHA filled CBAC form for him and noticed that the total score is above 7/10 which indicated his risk to NCDs. She immediately refers the patient to auxiliary nurse midwife (ANM) for blood sugar testing and blood pressure (BP) measurement. He was recalled at HWC where his blood sugar readings were taken and blood pressure was measured. His random blood sugar was 136 mg/dL as reported, he was suggested to visit nearest PHC for confirmatory diagnosis. At PHC he was diagnosed with diabetes and was put on diabetic treatment after routine counseling. The patient was then referred to district hospital for DR screening. On dilated fundus examination he was diagnosed with mild nonproliferative diabetic retinopathy (NPDR). He was advised to visit for DR screening after every 1 year so the visible changes if any can be detected early. He was advised to monitor his blood sugar constantly and maintain strict metabolic control.

SUMMARY

India has so far worked towards the integration of the eye care service into general health service in the country. Ayushman Bharat program is one such example which is attempting to layout PEC services at HWC and financial assistance through various eye care packages to extend the services to those in need. Challenges lie in the equitable distribution of manpower in rural and urban areas and data reporting from the states. Further a strong data reporting and recording is required for framing evidence-based policies.

MULTIPLE CHOICE QUESTIONS

1. Uncorrected refractive error and cataract are the major cause of blindness and visual impairment.
    a. True
    b. False
2. Overarching principles of primary healthcare (PHC) in India are:
    a. Fair distribution of healthcare services
    b. Community engagement
    c. Disease prevention
    d. Use of appropriate technology
    e. Multisectoral approach
    f. All of the above
3. Community ophthalmology is based on the principles of primary health care (PHC):
    a. True
    b. False
4. Please select the principles of community ophthalmology:
    a. Equitable distribution of eye care resources
    b. Community engagement in providing eye care
    c. Prevention of blindness
    d. Use of appropriate technology and multisectoral approach
    e. All of the above
5. National Health Mission (NHM) was established in which year?
    a. 2006
    b. 2010
    c. 2005
    d. 2009
6. In which year was National Program for Control of Blindness and Visual Impairment (NPCBVI) started?
    a. 1976
    b. 1979
    c. 1980
    d. 1981
7. Which of the following is not a part of WHO health system framework?
    a. Governance
    b. Health management information system
    c. Human resources
    d. Health financing
    e. Human resources
    f. Service delivery
    g. All of the above
8. Pradhan Mantri Jan Arogya Yojna (PMJAY) provides financial cover of up to ₹ 5 lakh per family?
    a. True
    b. False
9. Health Management Information System (HMIS) helps in managing the information generated at local, district and national level from various components of health system building blocks.
    a. True
    b. False
10. Equity does not mean fair distribution of care and resources throughout a group of people without discriminating on basis of ethnicity, gender, age, and social class?
    a. True
    b. False

ANSWERS			
1. a	2. f	3. a	4. e
5. c	6. a	7. g	8. a
9. a	10. b		

SUGGESTED READING

1. Astbury N. Excellence and equity in eye care. Community Eye Health. 2009;22(69):3. PMID: 19506710; PMCID: PMC2683552.
2. Beyond the building blocks: integrating community roles into health systems frameworks to achieve health for allhttp://orcid.org/0000–0003-0743-7208.
3. Blanchet K, Gilbert C, Lindfield R, Crook S. Eye Health Systems Assessment (EHSA): How To Connect Eye Care With the General Health. IAPB Tech Rep [Internet]. 2012;(April). Available from: http://iceh.lshtm.ac.uk/eye-health-systems-assessment/%0Ahttps://www.iapb.org/wp-content/uploads/Eye-Health-Systems-Assessment.pdf
4. Chokshi M, Patil B, Khanna R, Neogi SB, Sharma J, Paul VK, et al. Health systems in India. J Perinatol. 2016;36(s3):S9-12. Available from: https://www.ncbi.nlm.nih.gov/pmc/articles/PMC5144115/

5. Department of Finance. XIIIth Five Year Plan, 2017–22, Second Year's Programme, 2018–19, Summary Document Schemes And Implementing Agencies [Internet]. India: Department of Finance; 2018 [updated 2018 February].
6. Faal H, Cook C, Thulasiraj RD. Managing information in eye care programmes: The health systems perspective. Community Eye Heal J. 2010;23(74):50-2. Available from: https://www.cehjournal.org/wp-content/uploads/download/ceh_23_74_050.pdf.
7. For ABD, Consultation N. Towards Developing India Eye Health Action Plan a background document for. 2019;(October 2015). Available at: http://www.vision2020india.org/wpcontent/uploads/2016/10/GAP_India_background_document_27102015.pdf.
8. Garg P, Reddy S, Nelluri, C. Training the eye care team: principles and practice. Middle East Afr J Ophthalmol. 2014; 21(2):128-33. https://doi.org/10.4103/0974-9233.129757.
9. Gilbert C. The importance of primary eye care. Community Eye Health. 1998:11(26):17-9.
10. Human resources for health National Rural Health Mission, Ministry of Health and Family Welfare, Government of India. Child Health Division, 2011. Available at: uhc-india.org/reports/hleg_report_chapter_4.Pdf.
11. Johnson GJ. Overview on community ophthalmology. J Indian Med Assoc. 1999;97(8):305-8. PMID: 10643180.
12. Ministry of Finance. Economic Survey 2019 -20 (Vol-II). Econ Surv [Internet]. 2020;2. Available from: https://www.indiabudget.gov.in/economic survey/
13. Ministry of Health and Family Welfare. Ayushman Bharat Pradhan Mantri Jan Arogya Yojana. [Internet]. [cited 2020 Oct 20] Available from: https://pmjay.gov.in/sites/default/files/2020 -09/HBP-2 -0- For-Website.pdf.
14. Ministry of Health and Family Welfare. Pattern of Assistance under the National Programme for Control of Blindness and Visual Impairment (NPCB&VI) during 2017–20. [Internet]. [updated 23 April 2018]. Available from: https://npcbvi.gov.in/writeReadData/mainlinkFile/Patternofass2017 -20.pdf.
15. Misra N, Khanna R. Commentary: Rapid assessment of avoidable blindness and diabetic retinopathy in India. Indian J Ophthalmol. 2020; 68(2): 381-2. DOI:10.4103/ijo.IJO 1133_19. Available from: https://www.ijo.in/ article.asp?issn=03014738;year=2020;volume =68;issue=2;spage =381;epage=382;aulast=Misra
16. National Health Mission, Guidelines on Accredited Social Health Activist https://nhm.gov.in/images/pdf/communitisation/task-group-reports/guidelines-on-asha.pdf
17. National Health Systems Resource Centre. Ayushman Bharat: Comprehensive Primary Health Care through Health and Wellness Centers- Operational Guidelines. 2019;96. Availablefrom:hwc.nhp.gov.in/download/document/45a4ab64b74ab124cfd853ec9a0127e4.pdf.
18. National Health Systems Resource Centre. Eye Care at Health and Wellness Centres: Operational Guidelines. 2020. Available from: https://abhwc.nhp.gov.in/download/document/Operational_Guidelines_for_Primary_Eye_Care_at_HWCs.pdf
19. Npcbvi.gov.in [Internet]. India: National Program for Control of Blindness and Visual Impairment [cited 23 Oct 20]. Available from https://npcvvi.gov.in/Public-DASHBOARD
20. Npcbvi.gov.in [Internet]. India: National Program for Control of Blindness and Visual Impairment http://npcb.nic.in/index1.asp?linkid=29&langid=1
21. Pascolini D, Mariotti SP. Global estimates of visual impairment: 2010. British Journal of Ophthalmology. 2012;96:614-8.
22. Report of the Core-Committee for Revision of National List of Essential Medicines November 2015. Available from:https://main.mohfw.gov.in/sites/default/files/Recommendations.pdf.
23. Sacks E, Swanson RC, Schensul JJ, et al. Community involvement in health systems strengthening to improve global health outcomes: a review of guidelines and potential roles. Int Q Community Health Educ. 2017;37:139-49.doi: 10.1177/0272684X17738089
24. Sapkota YD. Human Resources for eye health in South Asia. Community Eye Health. 2018; 31(102): S1-S2. Available from: https://www.ncbi.nlm.nih.gov/pmc/articles/PMC6134467/.
25. Sight Savers International India. Eye Care in India- A Situational Analysis. 2007;2-18. Availablefrom:http://www.sightsaversindia.in/wpcontent/uploads/2014/06/16482_Eyecare-in-India-A-Situaltion-Analysis.pdf.
26. Trimmel J. Inequality and inequity in eye health. Community Eye Health. 2016;29(93):1-3. PMID: 27601787; PMCID: PMC4995830.
27. Vemparala R. National Programme for Control of Blindness (NPCB) in the 12th Five year plan: An Overview. Delhi J Ophthalmol. 2017;27(4):290-2. Available at: https://www.djo.org.in/articles/27/4/national-programme-for-control.html
28. WHO. Everybody's business: strengthening health systems to improve health outcomes: who's framework for action. Geneva, Switzerland World Health Organization; 2007.B
29. World Health Organization. World report on vision. Vol. 214, World Health Organization; 2019. pp. 1-160. Available: https://www.who.int/publications-detail/world-report-on-vision.
30. World Health Organization. Universal eye health, global action plan 2014-19. Available: https://www.who.int/blindness/AP2014_19_English.pdf

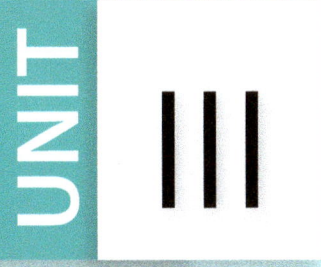

UNIT III: Disorders of Nervous System

OUTLINE

26. **Review of Anatomy and Physiology: Nervous System**
    Daisy Sahni, Richa Gupta

27. **Assessment of Patients with Neurological Disorders**
    Sonali Banerjee

28. **Diagonostic Evaluation in Neurological Disorders**
    Sonali Banerjee

29. **Management of Common Problems in Neuroscience Patients**
    Pooja Thakur

30. **Traumatic Conditions**
    Latika Bajaj

31. **Cerebrovascular Disorders**
    Manisha Nagi, Ashok Kumar, Vivek Kumar Garg, Divesh Kumar Munjal, Kapil Goel

32. **Neoplasms of the Neurological System**
    Manju Dhandapani

33. **Chronic Neurological Problems**
    Vivek Kumar Garg, Manisha Nagi, Ashok Kumar, Jitendra Gairolla, Kapil Goel

34. **Neurological Infections**
    Rakesh Sharma, Deepak Goel, Jitender Chaturvedi

35. **Nerve and Muscle Disorders**
    Priya Baby, Saraswathi Nashi

36. **Movement Disorders**
    Priya Baby, Rohan R Mahale

37. **Cranial Nerve Disorders**
    Rakesh Sharma, Deepak Goel, Jitender Chaturvedi

38. **Neurodegenerative Diseases**
    Monaliza

CHAPTER 26

Review of Anatomy and Physiology: Nervous System

Daisy Sahni, Richa Gupta

"God may forgive your sins, but your nervous system won't."

—Alfred Korzybski

LEARNING OBJECTIVES

After going through the chapter, the learner will be able to:
- Elaborate various subdivisions of nervous system and the functional areas.
- Describe the neuron, action potential and neurotransmitters.
- Describe structure and functions of peripheral and autonomic nervous system.
- Explain in detail manifestations of impaired nervous system.

TERMS

- **Autonomic nervous system:** It includes sympathetic and parasympathetic nervous system.
- **Central nervous system:** It includes brain and spinal cord.
- **Neuron:** Functional unit of nervous system.
- **Peripheral nervous system:** It includes cranial and spinal nerves.

INTRODUCTION

The nervous system (NS) is derived from the ectodermal layer (neuroectoderm). It helps in control and regulation of various body functions. **Flowchart 26.1** depicts the main subdivisions of the nervous system. It can be classified into central nervous system (CNS), which comprises of brain and spinal cord and peripheral nervous system (PNS), which further has two types—somatic and autonomic nervous system (ANS). There are 31 pairs of spinal nerves and 12 pairs of cranial nerves in somatic nervous system. The autonomic nervous system (ANS) has parasympathetic and sympathetic components.

CELLS OF THE NERVOUS SYSTEM

Neurons and neuroglial cells form an important constituent of nervous system.

Neuron: These are excitable cells, which constitute the main structural and functional unit of nervous tissue. These cells are specialized for conduction of nerve impulse, interpretation, and transmission of information.

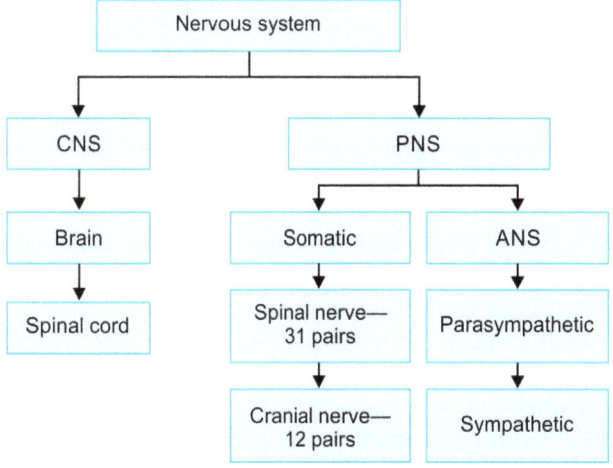

Flowchart 26.1: Subdivisions of the nervous system.

Typical neurons are composed of following parts—cell body (soma, perikaryon) and neurites, which include dendrites and axons **(Flowchart 26.2 and Fig. 26.1)**.

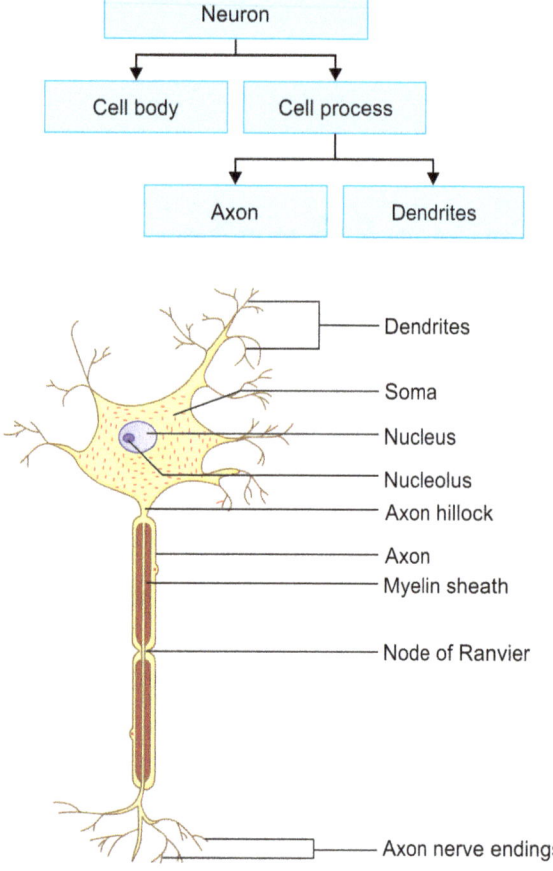

Flowchart 26.2: Different parts of a neuron.

Fig. 26.1: Structure of a neuron.

The cell body contains the central nucleus, and its cytoplasm is rich in Nissl granules. Dendrites are short branching processes which receive signals from other neurons. Each neuron has a single axon. It conducts impulse away from the cell body. The terminal branches of axons are called axon terminals. The axon can extend for several feet. The axon originates from a conical projection. It is hillocks on the body of the neuron. The axon membrane is specialized for the transmission of action potential.

Types of Synapses

Incoming synaptic terminals make contact directly with the dendritic processes. The membrane potential induced in the dendrites spreads passively on the cell body and the rate of neural discharge is controlled through the axon. The gray matter of the CNS is made up of cell bodies and dendrites. Collection of neuronal cell bodies within CNS, are called nuclei and outside CNS are called ganglia. The white matter of the CNS is made up of axons. The axons are surrounded by an insulating sheath of myelin, derived from oligodendrocytes within CNS and Schwann cells outside the CNS. The white appearance of white mater of CNS and of the peripheral nerves is due to the myelin sheath. The myelin sheath is not continuous but is interrupted at intervals by constrictions called nodes of Ranvier **(Fig. 26.1)**. Schwann cells form a delicate sheath which invests the peripheral nerves. It is essential for regeneration of nerve fiber. Damage in the CNS is permanent.

ACTION POTENIAL

Action potential (AP) is defined as a series of electrical changes within the membrane potential of a nerve or muscle fiber. A wave of electrical discharge propagates with rapid movement of charged ions along the cell membrane.

Resting membrane potential (RMP): At resting state of a neuron, the electrical potential of its protoplasm is more negative than compared to that in the extracellular fluid. It depends upon the intracellular and extracellular concentration of sodium (Na^+), potassium (K^+), and chloride (Cl^-) ions. Resting membrane potential of nerve is –70 mV.

Action potential involves two phases, i.e., depolarization and repolarization:

1. **Depolarization:** During depolarization, interior of nerve becomes positive and outside becomes negative and RMP is abolished.
2. **Repolarization:** During repolarization, RMP is restored back, i.e., inside becomes negative and outside gets positively charged.

Transport mechanisms in the cell membrane are:
- ❖ **Sodium potassium pump:** There is active transport of ions against concentration gradient using adenosine triphosphate (ATP)
- ❖ **Selective permeability of cell membrane:** Transport of ions takes place through unequal distribution of 'leak channels' across the cell membrane. In resting condition, almost all potassium leak channels remain open, while sodium leak channels remain closed.

In a normal nerve, no action potential occurs until the membrane of nerve fiber is disturbed. The initial rise in membrane potential is great enough that is threshold stimulus. A minimum of 15–30 mV rise in membrane potential is required to initiate AP. Rising voltage from –70 mV to zero level itself causes many voltages gated sodium channels to open, allowing onset of depolarization with rapid influx of sodium ions. Further rise in membrane potential causes activation of more number of sodium channels and thus more influx of Na^+ ions (overshot). Because of rising membrane potential, more and more sodium ion channels become inactivated. Thus, Na^+ transport is short lived. Simultaneously, there is efflux of K^+ out of nerve fibers causing repolarization. In a myelinated fiber, the nerve conduction is rapid due to saltatory conduction from node to node. The myelin sheath does not allow the exchange of ions (myelin acts as insulator), so action potential occurs only at nodes of Ranvier. This mechanism increases velocity of nerve transmission many folds, with less expenditure of energy.

Neurotransmitters

Impulse transmission occurs at the synapse with the help of neurotransmitters released into the synaptic cleft. These neurotransmitters are stored in synaptic vesicles. When a nerve fiber is depolarized, it generates action potential. Due to the effect of action potential, there occurs influx of calcium ions due to opening of voltage gate calcium channels which lead to a series of chemical changes. As a result, the neurotransmitters are released at the synaptic cleft which binds with the receptor molecules of postsynaptic membrane. This changes the permeability and causes its depolarization.

Following are the major neurotransmitters:

- **Acetylcholine (Ach):** Choline is acetylated by enzyme choline acetyl transferase and stored in synaptic vesicle in presynaptic terminals. It is the transmitter of PNS, neuromuscular junctions and ANS which innervate the sweat glands, etc. Alzheimer's disease is caused due to degeneration of basal nucleus of Meynert, as it is rich in Ach.
- **Catecholamines:** These include norepinephrine, epinephrine and dopamine. In postganglionic sympathetic neurons, norepinephrine is the neurotransmitter. Norepinephrinergic neurons are found in locus ceruleus. In the body, adrenal glands help in secretion of both epinephrine and norepinephrine. Dopamine levels are increased in schizophrenic patients and decreased in Parkinson's patients. It is located in the arcuate nucleus of hypothalamus.
- **Serotonin:** Serotonin is formed from tryptophan and converted into melatonin in the pineal gland and is present in high concentration in raphe nuclei of brainstem.
- **Histamine:** It is formed from histidine and present in neurons of the hypothalamus.
- **Glutamate:** It is most abundant excitatory neurotransmitter. It is present in over 90% of all brain synapses and has a major role in normal functioning of the brain. It is important to note that its levels should be strictly regulated. Its deficiency in the brain causes insomnia, etc.
- **Gamma aminobutyric acid (GABA):** It is an inhibitory neurotransmitter of brain, synthesized from glutamate. Two types of receptors are present in postsynaptic terminal—$GABA_A$, $GABA_B$ to increase conductance of Cl^- and K^+.
- **Glycine:** It is the inhibitory neurotransmitter present within the spinal cord and it helps in increasing Cl^- conductance.
- **Nitric oxide:** It is short-acting inhibitory neurotransmitter in central neurons system and functions as vasodilator in the cardiovascular system. It is also responsible for relaxation of smooth muscles of corpus cavernosum and thus penile erection.

CENTRAL NERVOUS SYSTEM—BRAIN

It comprises of brain and spinal cord. Developmentally, brain can be divided into three parts—prosencephalon, mesencephalon and rhombencephalon. Adult brain can be divided into forebrain, midbrain and hindbrain. **Table 26.1** gives the adult derivatives of brain and **Table 26.2** shows different parts of brain.

Cerebrum

Two cerebral hemispheres together constitute the largest portion of brain. These are divided by a longitudinal fissure and deep down are joined by a mass of white mater called the corpus callosum, whose main function is connection and communication between similar areas of each cerebral hemisphere **(Fig. 26.2)**.

TABLE 26.1: Embryonic subdivisions, adult derivatives and ventricular components of CNS.

Embryonic subdivisions		Adult derivatives	Ventricular compartments
Prosencephalon (forebrain)	Telencephalon	Cerebral hemispheres	Lateral ventricles
	Diencephalon	• Thalamus • Subthalamus • Hypothalamus • Epithalamus	Third ventricle
Rhombencephalon (hindbrain)	Mesencephalon	Midbrain	Cerebral aqueduct
	Metencephalon	• Pons • Cerebellum	Fourth ventricles
	Myelencephalon	Medulla oblongata	
Caudal part of neural tube		Spinal cord	Central canal

TABLE 26.2: Different parts of the brain and their functions.

Parts of brain	Functions
Cerebrum	Conscious perception of sensory and motor functions, cognition, etc.
Basal ganglia	Fine control of movements and inhibition of unintentional movement
Limbic system	Autonomic response to emotion, mood, concerned with recent memory
Diencephalon	
Thalamus	Sensory relay center, influences mood and movement
Hypothalamus	Control center for maintaining homeostasis and regulating endocrine functions of the body
Subthalamus	Associated with basal ganglia and helps in coordination of various motor functions
Epithalamus	Sleep-wake cycle, smell
Brainstem	Contains ascending and descending nerve tracts, houses nuclei of all cranial nerves except Ist and IInd cranial nerve
Midbrain	Visual and auditory reflex centers
Pons	Relay center between cerebrum and cerebellum through middle cerebellar peduncle
Medulla oblongata	Center for several vital autonomic reflexes, e.g., heart rate, breathing, swallowing and vomiting
Cerebellum	Control of muscle movement and tone, regulates extent of intentional movement

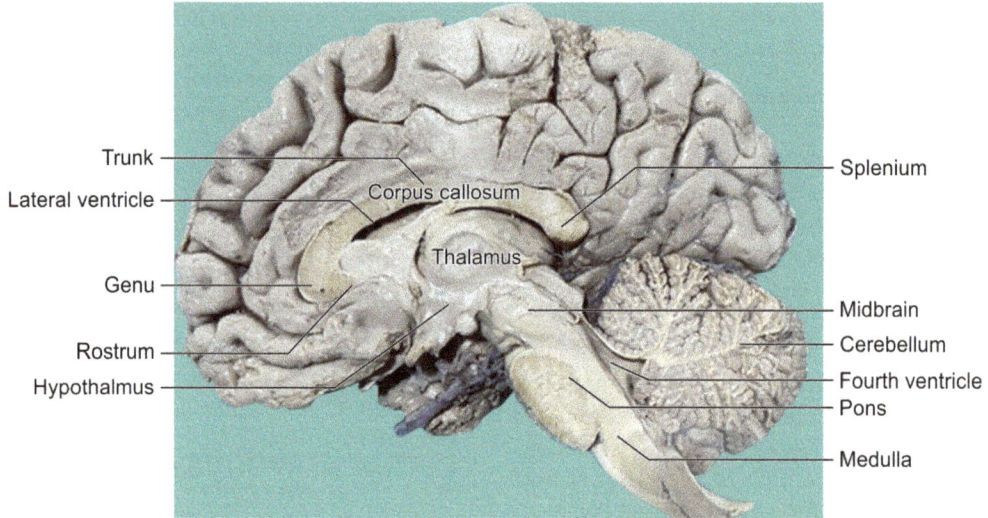

Fig. 26.2: Sagittal section of the brain showing its different parts.

Cerebral cortex composed of nerve cell bodies (gray mater). The deeper part of the cerebrum contains axons (white mater). The cerebral cortex is much folded by gyri (ridges) and sulci (grooves). These infoldings help in increasing the surface area of the cerebrum (**Figs. 26.3 and 26.4**).

Functions of Cerebral Cortex

- **Sensory perception:** Pain, temperature, touch, taste, hearing, sight, smell
- **Higher order functions:** Memory, language, reasoning, learning.
- Initiation and voluntary control of skeletal muscle movement

Each cerebral hemisphere is divided into four lobes by major sulci:
1. Frontal lobe
2. Parietal lobe
3. Temporal lobe
4. Occipital lobe

Functional Areas of Cerebral Cortex (Fig. 26.5)

Major functional areas have been identified in the cerebral cortex. The most used reference map of functional areas is provided by Brodmann, who divided the cortex into 47 areas. Most of the functional areas are active in both hemispheres with some asymmetry which has to do with handedness and language. In right-handed people, the left cerebral hemisphere is dominant for language (writing).

Diencephalon

Diencephalon forms the central core of the cerebrum and is a hidden structure. It lies just above the midbrain. Its main components are the thalamus, epithalamus and hypothalamus. Each represents bilaterally.

Thalamus (Fig. 26.4)

Thalami are two large nuclear masses situated deep in the cerebral cortex. Each thalamus primarily consists of gray matter and subdivided into different groups of nuclei. The neurons in the thalamus are reciprocally connected with cerebral cortex and most nuclei also receive subcortical afferents.

Functions of the Thalamus

- It acts as a relay station for all kinds of sensory information, except olfactory or sense of smell.
- It influences the levels of consciousness and alertness in an individual.
- It helps in emotional tone and recent memory mechanism as it forms a part of the limbic system.

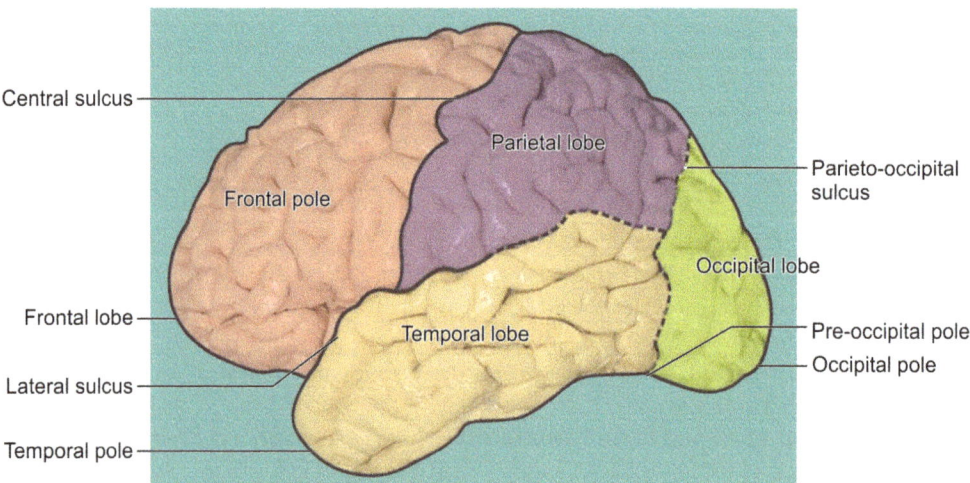

Fig. 26.3: Lateral aspect of a left cerebral hemisphere showing lobes and poles of the brain.

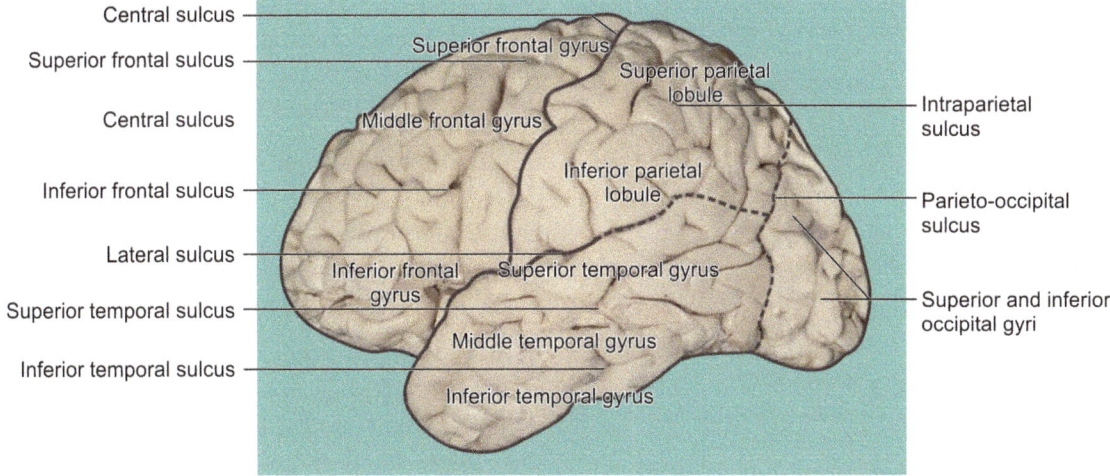

Fig. 26.4: Superolateral surface of left cerebral hemisphere showing sulci and gyri (dotted line depicting parieto-occipital sulcus located on medial surface).

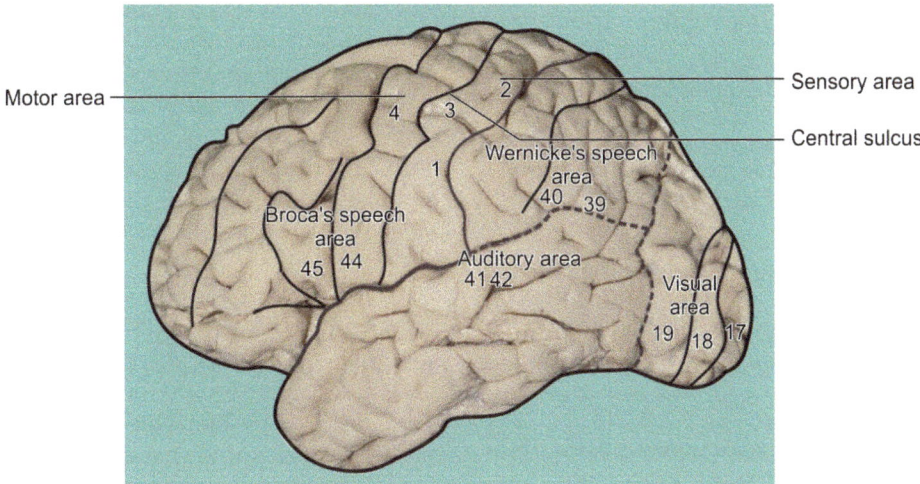

Fig. 26.5: Functional areas of the brain (dotted line depicting parieto-occipital sulcus located on medial surface).

As the thalamus is an important relay and integrative center, a disease/lesion, such as neoplasm or hemorrhage will lead to impairment of all types of senses, proprioception will suffer the most.

Epithalamus

It consists of:

- **Pineal gland:** It is a conical small structure situated in the midline. It is attached to the diencephalon by a pineal stalk. It is also called an endocrine gland on the basis of its structural organization. After the age of 16–17 years, calcium and magnesium salts appear in the pineal gland. With advancing age, concretions of these salts, also called brain sand start accumulating within the pineal gland. In a simple radiograph of the head, the displacement of the pineal gland from midline gives hint to space occupying lesion. The pineal gland maintains circadian rhythm with the help of melatonin hormone. There is popular use of melatonin hormone to treat jet lag and other sleep disorders. Pineal gland disorder may lead to production of less melatonin secretions, which subsequently may result in insomnia, abnormal thyroid function, anxiety, etc. With the onset of puberty, circulating levels of melatonin decrease sharply at the time of ovulation and women experience cyclic variations.

- **Habenular nuclei and their connections:** Habenular nucleus is center for integration of somatic afferent, visceral and olfactory pathways. But there is no clear-cut function attributed to it.
- **Posterior commissure:** It crosses the midline on the dorsal aspect of the cerebral aqueduct. It plays an important role in the bilateral pupillary light reflex.

Hypothalamus

The hypothalamus lies below the thalamus. Anatomically, it is a small structure but physiologically most of the activities in the body are influenced by it. Hypothalamus helps to maintain the homeostasis of the body. It regulates autonomic nervous system, endocrine system and limbic system. The hypothalamic nuclei are divided in four groups, i.e., pre-optic, supraoptic, tuberal and mamillary. Their functions are enumerated in **Table 26.3**.

Major functions of hypothalamus:

- Controls the autonomic nervous system.
- It regulates the endocrine system.
- It secrets (neurosecretions) oxytocin and vasopressin.
- Regulation of food and water intake (by acting on the hunger, satiety and thirst centers of the hypothalamus).
- Regulates the sexual behavior and reproduction.

TABLE 26.3: Nuclei of hypothalamus and their functions.

Hypothalamic nuclei (groups)	No. of nuclei	Functions
Preoptic	1	Regulate release of gonadotropins
Supraoptic	3	• Produces antidiuretic and oxytocin hormone, regulates water balance, circadian rhythm • Regulates body temperature by dissipation of heat and stimulates parasympathetic nervous system
Tuberal	3	• Produces hypothalamic releasing factors • Stimulation of nucleus of thalamus (ventromedial) to inhibit the urge to eat and stimulation of the other nucleus (dorsomedial) which causes obesity
Mammillary	2	• Regulates body temperature by conservation of heat • Stimulates sympathetic nervous system • Receives input from hippocampus

- Regulates the body temperature and the circadian rhythm or biological clock.
- Emotional expressions, such as laughing, crying, sweating, blushing are expressed by integrated activity of ANS and somatic efferent systems.

Lesions in hypothalamic nuclei will clinically present the following:
- Bitemporal hemianopia due to pressure on optic chiasma.
- Hypothalamic syndrome due to pressure on hypothalamus (diabetes, adiposities, weight gain, disturbance in temperature regulation).

Midbrain (Fig. 26.4)

The midbrain is the most cranial and smallest part of the brainstem. It connects hindbrain with the forebrain. Substantia nigra, one of the components of midbrain, is the largest motor nucleus which synthesizes neurotransmitter dopamine. Degeneration of nerve cells in the substantia nigra causes deficiency of dopamine which leads to a condition Parkinsonism.

Pons (Fig. 26.4)

Pons forms a bridge between the cerebellar hemispheres. It is the middle part of the brainstem, situated between midbrain and medulla oblongata. It has two surfaces—ventral and dorsal. A median sulcus on its ventral surface contains the basilar artery. Pontine nuclei (gray matter) relay information from cerebrum to the cerebellum and it houses a sleep center.

Medulla Oblongata (Fig. 26.4)

It is the lowest part of the brainstem, which becomes continuous with the spinal cord below the foramen magnum. Descending fibers of corticospinal tracts produce two large elevations (pyramids) on its ventral surface. These tracts are involved in conscious control of skeletal muscles. Medulla is a center for various vital autonomic reflexes, such as heart rate, breathing, swallowing, vomiting, sneezing and coughing.

Cerebellum (Fig. 26.4)

Cerebellum consists of two cerebellar hemispheres which lie dorsal to the pons and medulla oblongata. It helps in involuntary control of somatic motor activities, which are essential for equilibrium, muscle tone and posture.

Ventricles of the Brain (Fig. 26.4)

The substance of the brain contains four communicating cavities or ventricles. The lateral ventricles are present within the cerebral hemispheres, one on each side of the median plane. They communicate with the third ventricle by interventricular foramen or foramen of Monro.

The third ventricle or cavity lies below the lateral ventricles between the two thalami. It communicates with the fourth ventricle through a small canal, the cerebral aqueduct that runs through the midbrain.

The fourth ventricle, a diamond-shaped cavity, is situated between the cerebellum and pons. It continues below with the central canal of the spinal cord. It communicates with the subarachnoid space through the median aperture (Magendie) and lateral apertures (Luschka) present in the roof of the fourth ventricle.

SECRETION, COMPOSITION AND CIRCULATION OF CEREBROSPINAL FLUID

The ventricles of the brain, the central canal of the spinal cord and the subarachnoid spaces contain cerebrospinal fluid (CSF). CSF acts as a buffer to absorb and distribute external and internal forces endangering the CNS. As there are no lymphatics in the CNS, the CSF functions, such as lymph and also acts as a medium for the transfer of substances between the blood and nervous tissue through a selective exchange (blood brain barrier) as some drugs cannot penetrate the barrier.

Secretion of CSF

The CSF is secreted by the choroid plexuses (CP), located within the ventricles of the brain. Most of the CSF is produced by the choroid plexuses of lateral ventricles. CSF is secreted continuously at about the rate of 0.5 mL per minute, 720 mL per day. However, its volume remains 150 mL, as absorption keeps pace with the secretion.

Circulation of CSF

The secreted CSF in the lateral ventricles, flow through the interventricular foramina (Monro) into the third ventricle which is augmented by the CSF formed in the third ventricle. This fluid passes through the cerebral aqueduct (Sylvian) to the fourth ventricle. The secreted CSF from all the ventricles escapes from the fourth ventricle into the subarachnoid space through one median aperture (foramen of Magendie) and two lateral apertures (foramen of Luschka) and completely surrounds the brain and the spinal cord. Most of the CSF is directed upwards over the cerebral hemispheres, some amount also passes downwards in the spinal subarachnoid space up to the level of second sacral vertebra. For diagnostic purposes, the CSF can be obtained by lumbar puncture from the subarachnoid space above and below the fourth Lumbar vertebra, without damaging the spinal cord.

Absorption of CSF

The CSF is absorbed into the blood through the arachnoid villi, which are tiny finger-like projections of arachnoid mater and they project into the venous sinuses. CSF pressure remains constant at 10 cm H_2O while lying on one side and about 30 cm H_2O when sitting position. In condition of raised intradural pressure, some reabsorption of CSF may also occur through the choroid plexuses.

Functions of CSF

- Protects the brain and spinal cord by maintaining a uniform pressure around them.
- It acts as shock absorber between the skull and the brain.
- Keeps the brain and the spinal cord moist.
- Exchange of nutrients and waste products takes place between CSF and the interstitial fluid of the brain.

Composition of CSF

CSF is a clear, slightly alkaline fluid. Its specific gravity is 1.005. It consists of the following:
- Water
- Mineral salts
- Glucose
- Small amounts of plasma (albumin, globulin), creatinine and urea.
- Few leukocytes.

MENINGES

The brain and the spinal cord are enclosed by three membranes called 'meninges'. They lie between the skull and the brain and between the vertebral foramina and the spinal cord. These are:
1. **Dura mater (outer layer):** A thick, strong, inelastic fibrous membrane.
2. **Arachnoid mater (middle layer):** A delicate, avascular, fibrous membrane.
3. **Pia mater (inner layer):** A thin vascular fibrous membrane. It is closely adherent to the brain and follows its gyri and sulci. Arteries and veins of the brain lie within it.

The main function of meninges is to give support and protection to the brain and the spinal cord. The arachnoid and pia maters are together called leptomeninges. In the CNS, two spaces are associated with the meninges:
- **The subdural space:** It is a potential space between the dura and arachnoid maters. It contains small amount of serous fluid.
- **The subarachnoid space:** This space is between the arachnoid mater and the pia mater. This space contains the CSF.
- **The epidural space:** It is present only in the spinal cord. Dyes used for diagnostic purposes and local anesthetics may be injected into this space.

TABLE 26.4: Differences between spinal and cranial dura.

Spinal dura	Cranial dura
Single meningeal layer only	It consists of an inner meningeal layer and outer endosteal layer
Does not form folds	Forms folds, viz falx cerebri, falx cerebelli, tentorium cerebelli and diaphragma sellae
Epidural space present	Epidural space absent

Cranial Dura Mater

The cranial dura mater consists of two layers: An outer endosteal layer and an inner meningeal layer, with a potential space between the two layers. The meningeal layer is smooth and envelops the brain closely. The cerebral dura becomes continuous with the spinal dura mater.

Dural Infoldings

The dural infoldings sweep towards and divide the cranial cavity into compartments. They also enclose intracranial dural venous sinuses. Following are the folds of the dura mater:
- **The falx cerebri:** Separates the two cerebral hemispheres. It contains two dural venous sinuses viz.
    1. Superior sagittal sinus
    2. Inferior sagittal sinus
- **The falx cerebelli:** Separates the two cerebellar hemispheres.
- **The tentorium cerebelli:** Separates the cerebrum and the cerebellum. It contains the straight and two transverse sinuses.

Spinal Dura Mater

It forms a loose sheath around the spinal cord. It extends from the foramen magnum to the 2nd sacral vertebra. It is an extension of the inner layer of the cranial dura mater, and it is separated from the vertebral periosteum and ligaments within the neural canal by the epidural space. **Table 26.4** enumerates differences between spinal and cranial dura.

BLOOD-BRAIN BARRIER (BBB) AND CEREBRAL CIRCULATION

The CNS needs a stable environment to function properly which is provided by BBB. It protects the CNS (brain + spinal cord) from toxins, etc., and allows the required gases and nutrients to the nervous tissue. BBB structure intervenes between the blood in the capillaries and the extracellular spaces (around the neurons and neuroglia) the most important component of BBB is the tight junctions between the endothelial cells of the blood capillaries. The BBB allows lipids, glucose, some amino acids, water, carbon dioxide and oxygen to pass through it. But substances, such as urea, creatinine, proteins, toxins, and most of the antibiotics cannot pass through BBB. BBB is not fully developed in infants; bilirubin enters the brain tissue if the serum bilirubin is high leading to bilirubin encephalopathy. In case of injury to the brain, toxins or inflammation causes a breakdown of BBB, allowing free diffusion of larger molecules into the nervous tissue.

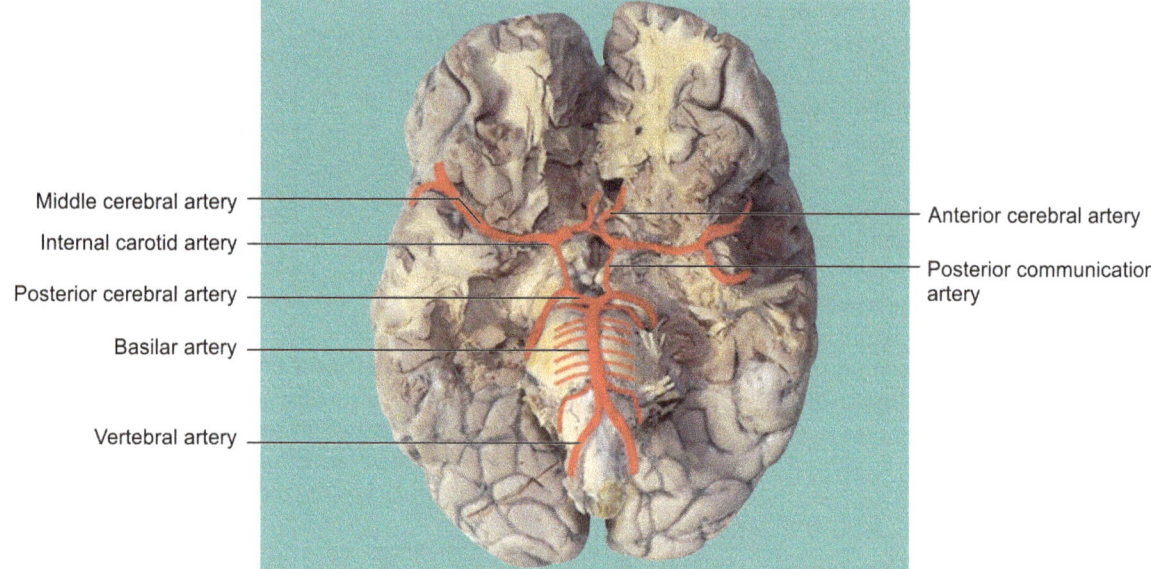

Fig. 26.6: Circle of Willis at the inferior aspect of the brain.

Cerebral Blood Circulation

The brain is dependent on continuous supply of oxygenated blood because of its high metabolic demand of oxygen, glucose, and removal of CO_2, lactic acid and other metabolic products. It is sensitive to hypoxia and hypoglycemia. The brain receives 20% of the total cardiac output, approximately 750 mL of blood per minute. It consumes 20% of the total O_2 used by the body. A person can become unconscious within 10 seconds of stoppage in blood flow to the brain, if this state continues an irreversible brain damage starts in about four minutes. The brain is supplied by two internal carotids and by a pair of two vertebral arteries which join together to form the basilar artery. A circle of Willis is formed (circulus arteriosus) at the base of the brain **(Fig. 26.6)**.

The **circle of Willis** provides collateral circulation if one of its major arteries gets blocked. The important factor which forces the constant blood flow to the brain is the arterial blood pressure. The ability of the brain to maintain constant blood flow is due to its autoregulation despite changes in systemic blood pressure. Autoregulation of the circulation to the brain is accomplished by a compensatory lowering of the cerebral vascular resistance during a decreased arterial pressure and raising of the vascular resistance when the arterial pressure is increased. But autoregulation is not effective when the arterial blood pressure falls very low. The factors which influence vasodilation of the cerebral vessels are an increase in carbon dioxide or hydrogen ion concentration and a reduction in oxygen concentration. A cerebral blood flow of 50–60 mL per 100 g of brain/per minute is considered normal.

Venous Drainage of the Brain

The cerebral hemispheres are drained by superficial and deep cerebral veins, which drain into the dural venous sinuses and open into the internal jugular veins.

RETICULAR FORMATION AND LIMBIC SYSTEM

As the name suggests, the reticular formation is a vague network of nerve cells and nerve fibers. It extends up through the axis of the CNS from the spinal cord to the cerebrum. Reticular formation is located in the central core of the brainstem in which groups of neurons and intersecting bundles of fibers are present in a net like appearance. It receives input from most of the sensory systems and has efferent connections at all levels of CNS. It is involved in sleep and consciousness as well as sensory and motor functions.

Functional divisions of reticular formation: It is divided into two systems.
1. The ascending reticular activating system (ARAS) or reticular activating system (RAS).
2. The descending reticular system (DRS).

Reticular Activating System (RAS)

Most of the ascending tracts (sensory) while passing through the brainstem give collaterals to the reticular formation, which further project to the reticular nuclei of the thalamus and in turn these nuclei project to widespread areas of the cerebral cortex. On stimulation of RAS, the person becomes alert. This is how the RAS is believed to be responsible for maintaining alertness and consciousness. RAS can be stimulated by a sudden bright light and sounds (ringing of alarm clock, etc.) which can arouse consciousness. On the other hand, removal of visual and auditory stimuli will lead to drowsiness and sleep. Certain drugs can affect the functions of RAS, such as tranquilizers, etc. A coma is a state of unconsciousness which may be due to inactivity of RAS.

Descending Reticular System

It consists of descending pathways from reticular formation to the autonomic centers in the brainstem which are critical in controlling the respiratory, cardiac rhythms and other vital functions. Motor nuclei of reticular formation also help to maintain muscle tone and coordinated movements through inter-connections with spinal nerves.

Main functions of reticular formation:
❖ Maintain state of consciousness through its connections by RAS.

- Regulates respiration, heart rate and blood pressure through autonomic centers in the brainstem.

In brief, reticular formation is one of the important regulatory systems in the CNS.

Limbic System

The limbic system (LS) includes those parts of the brain which are concerned with emotional and behavior aspects of the individual, visceral responses associated with emotions and formation of recent memory. It is also known as visceral brain. The structures that form the LS are limbic lobe (cingulated parahippocampal gyri and uncus) and hippocampal formation (hippocampus and dentate gyrus).

Functions of the Limbic System

- Emotional aspects of behavior with visceral responses. Particularly the reactions of fear, anger and emotions associated with sexual behavior.
- Responsible for recent memory
- Integration of olfactory, visceral, somatic impulses reaching the brain.

VERTEBRAL COLUMN

The vertebral (spinal) column is composed of 33 vertebrae. These are cervical 7, thoracic 12, lumbar 5, sacral 5 (fused to form the sacrum) and coccygeal 4 (commonly fused to form coccyx). In between the bodies of vertebrae, there are pads of fibrocartilage called intervertebral discs.

Characteristics of a Typical Vertebra (Fig. 26.7)

All vertebrae possess common features with some regional differences. The body lies anteriorly and a vertebral (neural) arch posteriorly. The lateral and posterior walls of the vertebral arch are formed by a pair of pedicels and a pair of laminae respectively. Transverse processes of a vertebra project where the pedicles meet the laminae. At the back, where two laminae meet is a process called the spinous process. These bony projections can be felt through the skin along the whole length of the spine. The vertebral foramina of all vertebrae form the vertebrae canal which contains the spinal cord. Along the length of the vertebral column, there is an intervertebral foramen on each side formed by a gap between adjacent vertebral pedicles, through which the spinal nerves, blood and lymph vessels pass.

Intervertebral Disc

Intervertebral disc lies between the bodies of adjacent vertebrae. They are thickest in the cervical and lumbar regions, where movement of vertebral column is more. They act as shock absorbers, but with advancing age their resilience decreases. Each disc is composed of a peripheral part, the annulus fibrosis, and a central core by the nucleus pulposus. The annulus fibrosus is made up of fibrocartilage and the nucleus pulposus is a soft gelatinous material. Sometimes when the annulus fibrosus ruptures the nucleus pulposus herniates and protrudes into the vertebral canal, where it may compress the spinal nerves or even the spinal cord.

The Spinal Cord (Fig. 26.8)

The spinal cord extends downwards as a continuation of medulla oblongata from the first cervical vertebra to the lower border of the first lumbar vertebra (L1). Its length is about 43 to 45 cm and weight about 30 g in adults. It occupies the upper two-thirds of the vertebral canal. The spinal cord contains a number of ascending and descending pathways which serve as conduits for nervous information passing to and fro between different parts of the body and the brain. The spinal cord consists of an inner core of gray mater and peripherally white mater, reverse of the arrangement as in the brain. Thirty-one pairs of spinal nerves emerge from the sides of the spinal cord. The part of the spinal cord to which a pair of spinal nerves are attached is known as spinal segment. It is made up of 31 spinal segments—cervical 8, thoracic 12, lumbar 5, sacral 5 and coccygeal 1. The spinal and vertebral segments do not lie at the same level. Their relation helps in understanding and planning for surgical diagnostic and therapeutic purposes.

Major Tracts of the Spinal Cord

- **Medial lemniscus pathway** mediates tactile discrimination, vibration sensation, form recognition and joint and muscle sensation (proprioception)
- **Lateral spinothalamic pathway** mediates pain and temperature sensations.
- **Lateral corticospinal tract** mediates voluntary skilled motor activities.
- **Dorsal and ventral spinocerebellar tracts** transmit information about proprioceptive and muscle reflex activity from the spinal cord to the cerebellum.

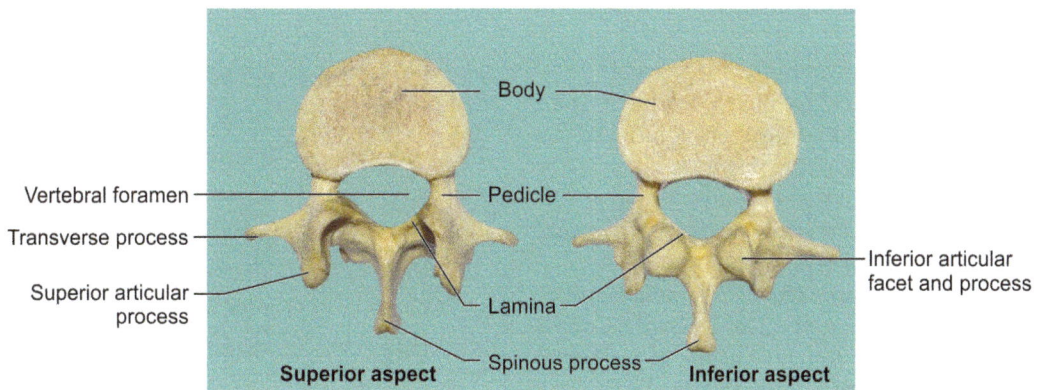

Fig. 26.7: Various parts of a typical vertebra.

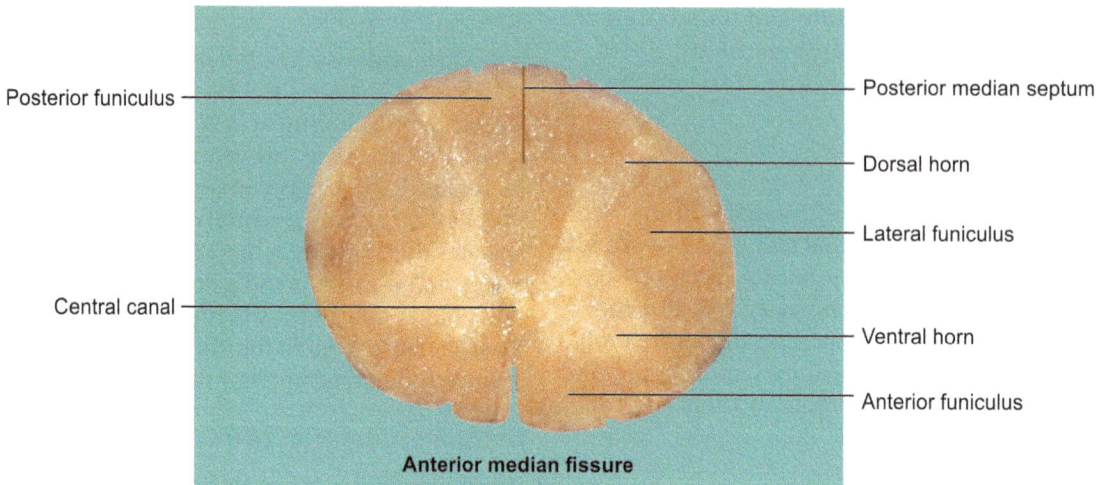

Fig. 26.8: Transverse section of spinal cord.

- **Hypothalamospinal tract** influences preganglionic sympathetic neurons of the intermediolateral horn cells and preganglionic parasympathetic neurons of the sacral parasympathetic nucleus. Interruption of this tract above T1 results in Horner's syndrome.

Spinal Reflexes

A reflex is defined as an involuntary response to a stimulus which is dependent on the integrity of spinal arc. The spinal arch includes a receptor organ, both sensory and motor neurons and an effector organ. In the spinal cord, reflex arcs are important in maintaining muscle tone. The main reflexes are withdrawal reflex, stretch and the Golgi tendon reflex.

Withdrawal Reflex

This reflex is directed towards the preservation of the person. Its example is, if you prick the sole of the sleeping person, the leg will reflex by drawing up.

Stretch Reflex

When the skeletal muscle is stretched, the muscle fibers get elongated, producing stimulation of sensory nerve endings around them. The nerve impulse is carried through sensory neurons to stimulate motor neurons in the anterior horn of the spinal cord causing rapid contraction of the stretch muscle. The stretch reflex is used by clinicians to elicit the tendon jerks. Best example is the knee jerk or ankle jerk.

Important Facts to Remember About the Spinal Cord

- In the neck, the spinal cord segments are cranial to the corresponding vertebrae.
- Spinal cord extends up to lower border of L1 level
- The ascending tracts include the uncrossed fibers from sensory ganglia (gracile and cuneate fasciculi) and the crossed spinothalamic tracts (from posterior horn). They are concerned with different types of sensation.
- The descending tracts are crossed lateral corticospinal tract and uncrossed vestibulospinal tract.
- Lesions in the spinal cord can result from trauma, degenerating and demyelinating disorders, infection or disruption in blood supply. Injury or lesion in the spinal cord will induce motor and sensory problems. The segment of the lesion will be indicated by the affected dermatome (distribution of cutaneous areas supplied by the spinal nerve).

Upper and Lower Motor Neurons

The stimulus to contraction of a skeletal muscle originates at the conscious level in the cerebrum (voluntary joint movement). The motor path ways from the brain to the muscles are two neuron mechanisms. The tracts involved are corticospinal or extrapyramidal.

Upper Motor Neurons (UMN)

The cell bodies are located in the primary motor area of the cerebrum. The axons of these neurons make pyramidal tracts which pass through the internal capsule, pons, medulla and synapse with the cell bodies of lower motor neurons in the anterior horn of gray matter of the spinal cord. The fibers of the pyramidal tract (corticospinal tract) decussate in the medulla oblongata.

Lower Motor Neurons (LMN)

The cell bodies are located in the anterior horn of gray matter in the spinal cord. The fibers emerge from here by the anterior root, join with the incoming sensory fibers to form the mixed spinal nerve; which passes from the intervertebral foramen to transmit the nerve impulses to the skeletal muscles. **Table 26.5** gives the differences in the clinical features of upper and lower motor neuron lesions. Lesion in any area of pyramidal tract is UMN lesion. Hemiplegia is the best example of UMN paralysis.

TABLE 26.5: Clinical differences in the upper and lower motor neuron lesions.

Clinical features	UMN lesion	LMN lesion
Muscle tone	Increased (spasticity)	Decreased (flaccidity)
Muscle wasting	Absent	Present
Extended paralysis	Widespread	Localized
Babinski's signs	Present	Absent
Tendon reflex (Knee or ankle jerk)	Exaggerated	Lost
Muscle clonus	Present	Absent

The LMN paralysis is due to the lesion in anterior horn cells of gray matter in the spinal cord or in the motor fibers of peripheral nerves or in the cranial nerve nuclei. The classical example of LMN paralysis is poliomyelitis (anterior horn cells of spinal cord) and Bell's palsy (involvement of facial nerve).

PERIPHERAL NERVOUS SYSTEM (PNS)

PNS comprises of 31 pairs of spinal nerves and 12 pairs of cranial nerves. Most of the nerves have both motor and sensory components, therefore, are called mixed nerves. Others are either sensory or motor nerves. The impulses enter or exit the CNS through cranial or spinal nerves.

Cranial Nerves (CN)

Twelve pairs of cranial nerves originate on the inferior surface of the brain and come out through foramina at the base of the skull **(Fig. 26.9 and Table 26.6)**.

There are 31 pairs of spinal nerves which arise from both sides of spinal cord and pass through the intervertebral foramina **(Table 26.7)**.

These nerves are grouped according to the associated vertebrae. But in the cervical region there are eight cervical nerves, because the first pair emerges above the first cervical vertebra and the eighth pair leaves the vertebral canal below the seventh (last) cervical vertebra. Near the termination of spinal cord, nerves extend downwards in the subarachnoid space as a sheath of nerves—the cauda equina (horse's tail). The nerves leave the vertebral canal at appropriate levels.

Nerve Roots

Small bundles of nerve rootlets arise from the ventral and dorsal surfaces of the spinal cord. These rootlets converge to form the dorsal and ventral roots. The dorsal root contains sensory (afferent) fibers and ventral root contains motor (afferent) fibers. The ventral and dorsal roots join to form a mixed nerve just before emerging through the intervertebral foramen. Then each spinal nerve divides into dorsal and ventral primary rami. The dorsal primary rami innervate the skin and deep muscles of the back while the ventral primary rami innervate the anterior and lateral aspects of head, neck,

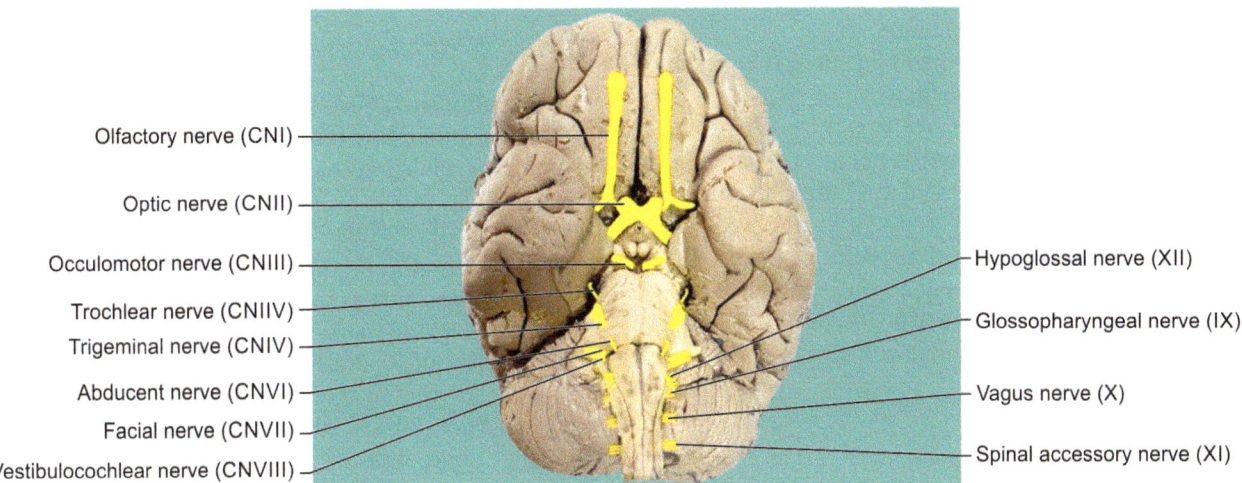

Fig. 26.9: Showing cranial nerves arising from inferior surface of the brain.

TABLE 26.6: Name, type, and functions of cranial nerves along with their roman numbers (RN).

RN	Nerve name	Type	Functions
I	Olfactory	Sensory	Sense of smell
II	Optic	Sensory	Sight (vision)
III	Oculomotor	Motor	Move the eyeball, alter the shape of lens, constrict the pupil, raise the upper eyelid
IV	Trochlear	Motor	Movement of eyeball
V	Trigeminal (3 branches)	Mixed	• Ophthalmic nerve (sensory)—lacrimal gland, conjunctiva, forehead, eyelids, scalp, mucosa of nose • Maxillary nerve (sensory)—cheeks, upper gums and teeth, lower eyelids • Mandibular nerve (mixed)—lower gums and teeth, ear pinnae, lower lip and tongue, chewing
VI	Abducent	Motor	Lateral movement of the eyeballs
VII	Facial	Mixed	Movement of facial expression muscles (motor), sense of taste (anterior 2/3 of tongue), secretion of lacrimal, nasal, submandibular and sublingual glands
VIII	Vestibulocochlear	Sensory	Maintains posture and balance, hearing
IX	Glossopharyngeal	Mixed	Parotid gland secretions, taste (posterior 1/3 of tongue) swallowing and gag reflexes
X	Vagus	Mixed	Swallowing, digestion, regulation of cardiac rate and respiration, sensations of thoracic and abdominal organs, proprioception
XI	Accessory	Motor	Movement of head and neck, proprioception
XII	Hypoglossal	Motor	Swallowing and speech by movement of tongue

TABLE 26.7: Name and number of spinal nerves.

Spinal nerve	Number
Cervical	8
Thoracic	12
Lumbar	5
Sacral	5
Coccygeal	1

trunk and the upper and lower limbs. Spinal nerves from T_1-L_2 have a contribution from preganglionic sympathetic nerve fibers (white communicant).

Plexuses

The ventral/anterior rami of the cervical, lumbar and sacral spinal nerves after their origin intermingle to form nerve plexuses. There are four nerve plexuses on each side of the vertebral column.
1. Cervical plexus is formed by C_1-C_4 spinal nerves—innervate the muscles of neck and diaphragm.
2. Brachial plexus—formed by C_5-T_1 spinal nerves—innervates muscles of upper limb.
3. Lumbosacral plexus—formed by L_2-S_5 spinal nerves—innervates muscles of lower limb.
4. Coccygeal.

The thoracic nerves (12 pairs) do not form plexus. First 11 pairs are the intercostal nerves and the 12th pair is subcostal nerves.

The injuries to peripheral nerves can occur due to compression, trauma, cuts, injections, etc. In case of an injury to the nerve fiber, there will be discontinuity between the axon and the cell body, and then series of degenerative changes take place.

Dermatomes

Dermatomes are strips of skin which extend from the dorsal (back) mid line to a ventral midline. These strips of skin are supplied by sensory branches of the dorsal and ventral rami of a single spinal nerve. Some overlap also occurs between any two adjacent dermatomes. In a clinical setting, a sensory deficit in a particular dermatome will help to assess the damage to a particular spinal nerve or spinal cord segment **(Table 26.8)**.

AUTONOMIC NERVOUS SYSTEM

The autonomic nervous system (ANS) regulates most of the involuntary activities of many organs and tissues including heart muscle, smooth muscle and exocrine glands. ANS consists of both afferent and efferent fibers. The main neurotransmitters of ANS for impulse transmission are norepinephrine and acetylcholine. ANS is divided into two parts—sympathetic and parasympathetic. The division between the two is based on the anatomical and neurotransmitter differences. Both divisions of ANS are physiologically antagonist to each other because they

TABLE 26.8: Body map showing the dermatomes.

Sl. No.	Structures	Dermatomes
1.	Top and back of scalp, lower jaw	C2
2.	Upper neck	C3
3.	Lower neck, upper shoulder	C4
4.	Shoulder, lateral surface of upper limb	C5
5.	Thumb	C6
6.	Posterior surface of upper limb, index and middle fingers	C7
7.	Ring and little fingers	C8
8.	Medial surface of upper limb	T1
9.	Nipples	T4
10.	Xiphoid process	T7
11.	Umbilicus (appendicitis pain)	T10
12.	Inguinal ligament	L1
13.	Medial surface of leg, dorsum of foot	L4
14.	Lateral surface of leg	L5
15.	Posterior surface of lower limb, lateral surface of foot, little toe	L1
16.	Perineum	S2–S4

produce opposite effects but they operate in conjunction with one another. It is the balance in their activities which maintains a stable internal environment of the body.

Sympathetic Nervous System

It is widely distributed throughout the body. It innervates the heart, lungs, muscle in the wall of blood vessels, the hair follicle, sweat glands and viscera of abdomen and pelvis. The sympathetic outflow arises from the preganglionic neurons which are located in the lateral horns (intermediolateral cells) of the first thoracic to second lumbar (T_1-L_2) spinal cord (thoracolumbar outflow). After leaving the spinal cord, the fibers separate and form a chain of ganglia which extend from the neck to pelvis of the person. From the sympathetic chain fibers extend to the affecter organs. The main function of the sympathetic system is to prepare the body for an emergency. **Box 26.1** gives the functions of sympathetic nervous system.

BOX 26.1: Functions of sympathetic nervous system.

- Pupillary dilation
- Increase of heart rate
- Vasoconstriction of blood vessels of the trunk and extremities
- Inhibition of gastric motility
- Vasodilation of coronary arteries
- Dilation of bronchioles
- Decreased urine output
- Increase in blood clotting, metabolic rate and mental alertness

Parasympathetic Nervous System (Craniosacral Outflow)

This system operates in non-stressful situations. Its activation is directed towards conservation and restoration of the body energy. Its primary neurotransmitter is acetylcholine.

SUMMARY

The nervous system helps in control and regulation of various body functions. It can be classified into central nervous system (CNS), which comprises of brain and spinal cord and peripheral nervous system (PNS), which further has two types—somatic and autonomic nervous system (ANS). There are 31 pairs of spinal nerves and 12 pairs of cranial nerves in somatic nervous system. The autonomic nervous system (ANS) has parasympathetic and sympathetic components. Neurons and neuroglial cells form an important constituent of nervous system. The membrane potential induced in the dendrites spreads passively on the cell body and the rate of neural discharge is controlled through the axon.

MULTIPLE CHOICE QUESTIONS

1. All of the following are cells of nervous system, *except*:
   a. Neurons
   b. Astrocytes
   c. Microglia cells
   d. Myocytes
2. All of the following are cranial nerves, *except*:
   a. Trigeminal nerve
   b. Peroneal nerve
   c. Facial nerve
   d. Optic nerve
3. Circle of Willis is formed by all of the following, *except*:
   a. Posterior cerebral artery
   b. Anterior cerebral artery
   c. Middle cerebral artery
   d. Posterior communicating artery
4. One of the following structures is part of brainstem:
   a. Pons
   b. Thalamus
   c. Pineal gland
   d. Hypothalamus
5. Rhombencephalon includes all of the following structures, *except*:
   a. Cerebellum
   b. Diencephalon
   c. Pons
   d. Medulla
6. Visual area is located in which lobe of brain:
   a. Frontal lobe
   b. Parietal lobe
   c. Temporal lobe
   d. Occipital lobe
7. Lateral sulcus separates following lobes of brain:
   a. Frontal lobe from temporal lobe
   b. Parietal lobe from occipital lobe
   c. Occipital lobe from frontal lobe
   d. Frontal and parietal lobe
8. One of the following statements regarding oligodendrocytes is *false*:
   a. One oligodendrocyte myelinates only one axon
   b. Oligodendrocytes form myelin in central nervous system
   c. One oligodendrocyte myelinates many axons
   d. Myelination begins during fourth month of development
9. All of the following are constituent of basal ganglia, *except*:
   a. Caudate
   b. Putamen
   c. Thalamus
   d. Globus pallidus
10. One of the following is NOT an example of commissural fibers:
    a. Corpus callosum
    b. Internal capsule
    c. Anterior commissure
    d. Posterior commissure
11. One of the following statements is *true*:
    a. Trigeminal nerve arises from midbrain
    b. Basilar artery lies in relation to medulla oblongata
    c. Hypoglossal nerve arises from medulla oblongata
    d. Anterior cerebral artery is branch of external carotid artery
12. All of the following are functions of cerebellum, *except*:
    a. Coordination of movements
    b. Maintenance of balance
    c. Function of speech
    d. Regulates intentional movements
13. All of the following are nuclei of hypothalamus, *except*:
    a. Preoptic
    b. Supraoptic
    c. Pulvinar
    d. Tuberal
14. One of the following statements is *false*:
    a. In spinal cord, white matter is located on inner side
    b. In cerebrum, gray matter is located outside
    c. Neuron is functional unit of nervous system
    d. Cranial nerves are part of peripheral nervous system
15. True about sympathetic nervous system is all, *except*:
    a. Pupillary dilation
    b. Increase of heart rate
    c. Vasoconstriction of coronary arteries
    d. Inhibition of gastric motility
16. Which of the following form blood brain barrier?
    a. Neural crest cells
    b. Astrocytes
    c. Microglia
    d. Oligodendrocytes
17. All of the following statements are true, *except*:
    a. Plexuses are formed by ventral rami of spinal nerves
    b. Brachial plexus supplies upper limb
    c. Plexuses are formed by dorsal rami of spinal nerves
    d. Cervical plexus supplies muscles of neck
18. Lateral spinothalamic tract is concerned with one of the following sensations:
    a. Pain and temperature sensation
    b. Sense of vibration
    c. Proprioceptive sensation
    d. Voluntary skilled movements
19. In adults, spinal cord ends at:
    a. L1
    b. L2
    c. L3
    d. T12
20. All of the following form boundaries of fourth ventricle, *except*:
    a. Cerebellum
    b. Pons
    c. Midbrain
    d. Medulla

ANSWERS

1. d	2. b	3. c	4. a
5. b	6. d	7. a	8. a
9. c	10. b	11. c	12. c
13. c	14. a	15. c	16. b
17. c	18. a	19. a	20. c

SUGGESTED READING

1. Barrett KE, Boitano S, Barman SM, Brooks HL. Ganong's review of medical physiology twenty.
2. Inderbir S. Textbook of human histology with color atlas. New Delhi: Jaypee Brithers Medical Publishers; 2006.
3. Kumar V, Abbas AK, Aster JC. Robbins basic pathology e-book. Elsevier Health Sciences; 2017.
4. LeMone PT, Burke KM, Gerene Bauldoff RN, Gubrud P. Medical-surgical nursing: Clinical reasoning in patient care. Pearson; 2014.
5. Ross MH, Pawlina W. Histology. Lippincott Williams and Wilkins; 2006.
6. Standring S (Ed). Gray's anatomy E-Book: the anatomical basis of clinical practice. Elsevier Health Sciences; 2020.
7. Waugh A, Grant A. Ross and Wilson Anatomy and physiology in health and illness E-book. Elsevier Health Sciences; 2014.

CHAPTER 27

Assessment of Patients with Neurological Disorders

Sonali Banerjee

"Nothing has such power to broaden the mind as the ability to investigate systematically and truly all that comes under thy observation in life."

—**Marcus Aurelius**

LEARNING OBJECTIVES

After going through the chapter, the learner will be able to:
- Enlist the purpose of carrying out a neurological examination.
- Obtain history of patients with or without neurological problems.
- Assess the level of consciousness.
- Perform cranial nerve assessment.
- Assess motor and sensory function.
- Assess cerebellar function.

TERMS

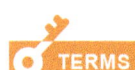

- **Agnosia:** Any damage or compromise to the cerebral lobes leading to failure or inability to recognize, it can be visual, auditory, tactile or autotopagnosia.
- **Apraxia:** Inability to carry out specialized learned skills due to damage of parietal lobe.
- **Aphasia:** Inability of expression and understanding of thoughts in verbal as well as written form.
- **Ataxia:** Inability to coordinate the body movements precisely the gait due to loss of functionality of cerebellum.
- **Amnesia:** Inability to recapitulate information from the past.
- **Cheyne-Stokes respirations:** Periodic, repeated occurrence of breathing between hyperpnea and apnea.
- **Hemiparesis:** Incomplete weakness of one side of body.
- **Papilledema:** Swelling of optic nerve disc due to increase in intracranial pressure.
- **Nystagmus:** Involuntary eye movements.
- **Tandem gait:** Is walking in a straight line with sequence of heel to toe.
- **Reflex:** Immediate/spontaneous, unpredictable, and involuntary response to an external stimulus like striking a tendon by a reflex or knee hammer.

INTRODUCTION

Frequent assessment and monitoring are precedence once a patient is diagnosed with a neurological disorder. Neurological evaluation, is the core of care as it facilitates a thorough understanding to the professional nurses in providing comprehensive and optimal care. The nurses working with the patients are cognizant with quick as well as systematic assessment of the patients seeking treatment. Identification of any abnormal response or dysfunctionality is the prime pursuit in caring for such patients.

NEUROLOGICAL EXAMINATION

Neurological examination is a systematic and comprehensive technique of finding history/data, observing the patient and conducting tests pertinent to the function of a patient's nervous system. The examination is precisely performed in relation to assessments of brain, spinal cord and nerves functionality and also highlighting on level of consciousness, higher mental function, sensory-motor function, and reflexes. The assessment can be used equally efficacious in preliminary patient screening and further for monitoring the progress. Early recognition of neurological damage is beneficial in terms of detection and immediate damage control measures thus accelerating the recovery and reducing the disease related disabilities/complications.

Neurological assessment is obligatory for the patients either as routine procedure or when a patient reaches to the emergency department in a critical condition. Patient centric care is initiated on the basis of history collection which support as the framework. Assessment is done dexterously depending on the situation at the time of admission, but it is always imperative to remember that maximum assessment should be carried out at the first point of contact with the patient. The initial assessment must be a complete examination including all the facets extending from recording or documenting the level of consciousness to assessment of deep tendon reflexes. This preliminary assessment facilitates to generate a baseline data which offers information for comparison in future about the improvement or deterioration of patient's condition. Frequency and the extend of the assessment are determined by the outcomes of the initial assessment and the criticality of the diagnosis.

Purposes

As mentioned above, neurological assessment is performed with dual perspective, first of all it helps to identify neurological problems for the first time, secondly it facilitates in focussed assessment of pre-existing deficits or if identified from the gathered history. Detailed purposes of assessment are enumerated below:

- ❖ To create baseline assessment data.
- ❖ To facilitate in providing database for future comparisons in neurological functionality. It further helps to instantly recognize any improvement or worsening in the patients' health condition.
- ❖ To detect presence of any neurological disorder.
- ❖ To recognize the extent of brain or spine injury.
- ❖ To monitor the status of the patient.
- ❖ To comprehend the progression of the disease.
- ❖ To determine the patient response to treatment and care.
- ❖ To facilitate as routine assessment in outpatient department or before surgery.
- ❖ To provide statistics for research enquiry or educational purpose.

History Taking

Neurological assessment starts with thorough history collection. Initiate the discussion with general information pertinent with patient information and identity.

Present history of manifestations as mentioned below must to asked to the patient pertinent to aspects like onset, duration, severity, frequency, and the precipitating factors.

- ❖ Headache
- ❖ Blurriness of vision
- ❖ Tremors/seizures
- ❖ Numbness/tingling
- ❖ Weakness/paralysis
- ❖ Impaired memory
- ❖ Impaired communication
- ❖ Interference with ADL

Past and family history also plays an important role in understanding the present condition of the patient.

- ❖ **Medical history:** Any major illnesses of the past.
- ❖ **Surgical history:** Specifically related to head or spine.
- ❖ **Accident:** From birth event till date, pertinent to head or spine.
- ❖ Allergies.

Family history related to diabetes, hypertension, stroke, cancer, renal disorders or any bleeding disorders.

Psychosocial history about educational status, occupation—job type, duration, timings, hobbies, social interactions and self-image related facets may be explored by the nurse in detail. Any alteration in level of alertness will eventually lead to restlessness, irritability, personality changes, changes in mental status, mild confusion, agitation.

Equipment

The articles/equipments required for neurological assessment are given in **Box 27.1**.

Prerequisites before Commencement of the Assessment

- ❖ Identification of the patient is foremost essential; it facilitates to perform assessment of the right client. Meticulous precautions are taken for identification of unconscious client.
- ❖ Lucid explanation of the procedure to the client/family irrespective of the level of consciousness of the client. Communication should be continued throughout the procedure.
- ❖ Ensuring patient's privacy to avoid unnecessary discomfort and additional non-cooperation.
- ❖ Washing and drying hands avert cross infection.
- ❖ Sequential arrangement of equipment in a tray facilitates a faster assessment.
- ❖ Place patient in appropriate position. Precaution ought to be taken for comatose patient by avoiding compression of jugular veins thus causing an increase in the intracranial pressure.
- ❖ It is essential to keep in mind and document the patient's gestures, emotions, levels of cooperation throughout the assessment.

BOX 27.1: Articles necessary for assessment.

- Thermometer
- BP apparatus
- Stethoscope
- Vials containing coffee or vanilla extract, sugar, salt
- Alcohol swabs
- Snellen chart
- Cotton applicator
- Needle/pin
- Test tube containing hot and cold water
- Reflex hammer
- Tongue blade
- Penlight
- Tuning fork—128 Hz preferable
- Measuring tape
- Pen and paper.

- ❖ The nurse should also be cognizant with the educational status, cultural background and beliefs of the patients, which might influence the responses.
- ❖ It is essential to understand the following considerations and specifications before commencement of the assessment:
  - ➢ A complete assessment is performed mostly in out-patient department.
  - ➢ A nurse should always be vigilant throughout the assessment in observing any specific changes in behavior, response or alertness.
  - ➢ A nurse should be seated or standing near to the patient in order to prevent any event of injury or fall.
  - ➢ There is minimal or no response from the patient in terms of verbal or tactile stimuli in case the condition is comatose.
  - ➢ Following guidelines are adopted from National Institute of Health and Care Excellence:
    - Minimal components to be documented each time:
      - Vital signs: Respiratory rate, heart rate, temperature, blood pressure, blood oxygen saturation.
      - Scores of Glasgow Coma Scale (GCS)
      - Pupillary size and reactivity to light.
      - Limb movements.
    - Frequency of observation by nurse examiner (Fig. 27.1).

At any point of time if there is any deterioration in score of GCS less than 15, monitoring reverts back to every hour.

Assessment

A. Basic Vital Signs

It is essential to procure details about the vital signs of the patient before proceeding with the assessment. Any abnormality will alert the nurse on various related aspects (Table 27.1).

B. Neurological Assessment

The neurological functions are discussed under assessment of cerebral functions, cranial nerve functions, motor system functions, reflexes, and sensory functions (Fig. 27.2).

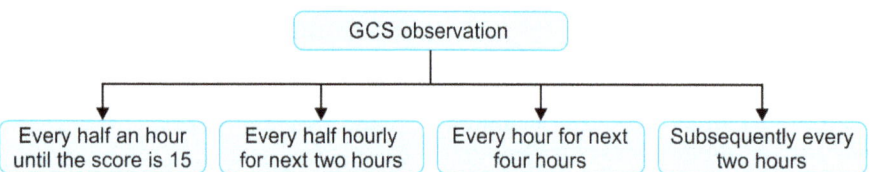

Fig. 27.1: Frequency of GCS assessment.

TABLE 27.1: Vital signs and abnormalities related to neurological disorders.

Vitals	Increase	Decrease
Temperature	Hyperthermia may be indicative of infectious entity—head injury, septicemia, postoperative infection. • Inflammatory conditions like meningitis and encephalitis. • Drug induced	• Spinal shock • Damage to brainstem. • Any alterations may be due to increased ICP or impact on hypothalamus.
Heart rate	Tachycardia—hypoxic conditions, increased ICP, internal hemorrhage.	Bradycardia—injury to cervical spine, advanced stage of increase in ICP
Respiratory rate	It may be altered in neuromuscular disorders like Guillain-Barre syndrome or myasthenia gravis. Increased intracranial pressure will display evidences of irregular, Cheyne–Stokes respiration, later results in respiratory arrest	
Blood pressure	• hypothalamic compromise • Increased systolic blood pressure along with widened pulse pressure and bradycardia is classic triad manifest of increased intracranial pressure.	Injury to cervical spine.
ECG changes	Raised ICP eventually shows Q waves with ST depression, elevated T waves, sinus bradycardia.	

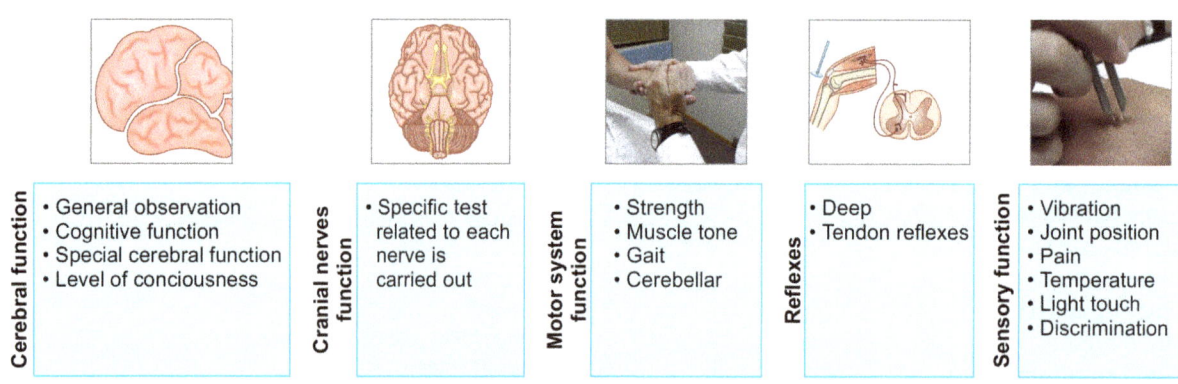

Fig. 27.2: Components of neurological assessment.

I. Cerebral Functions

The cerebrum has two hemispheres with discrete lobes namely frontal, parietal, temporal and occipital lobes. Apart from these lobes, the insula is deep under the sylvian fissure and C-shaped limbic lobe on the most medial aspect of cerebral hemisphere. Each lobe is assigned with specific functionality but most of the activities require coordination of varied cerebral areas in both the halves. It may be assumed that although the occipital lobe is essential for processing of visual images but parts of parietal, frontal and temporal lobes located in both hemispheres also contribute to the processing of complex visual images. Hence it is essential to include every aspect of assessment so as to understand the functionality of the cerebrum.

Before starting discussion regarding the cerebral functions, first we need to have the general observation and cognitive functions of the patients.

General observation

Preliminary assessment after history collection starts with general observation of the patient in the following mentioned facets:

- **Appearance:** It is essential to observe the appearance of the patient, which empowers the nurse to perceive the general condition as well as neurological impairments.
- **Facial expression:** It is part of non-verbal communication, which shows the emotional expression of an individual. The nurse must be vigilant in noting any abnormal facial expression which is divergent.
- **Attitude:** Attitude of the patient towards the treatment often helps the nurse to understand the personality of the patient and also about treatment compliance.
- **Mood:** It is essential to comprehend the mood of the individual and also the appropriateness to the situation.
- **Speech:** Speech can be evaluated on facets of quality, pace, spontaneity, and significance while gathering patient's illness history. The nurse should also notice fluency of dialogues, repetition of words, comprehension and appropriateness of answer. Sometimes the information is counter checked with the significant others (for details regarding speech defects kindly refer to Chapter 6 of Vol II).

Cognitive functions

The cognitive functions comprise of all the mental abilities and functionality like thinking, memory, reasoning, judgement, and also responding to stimuli, attention, perception and processing the information in the cerebral cortex.

- **Orientation:** The nurse firstly evaluates the level of patient's orientation in specifics to self, time, place and person by asking simple questions. Awareness to time is lost preceding to place or person.
- **Memory:** It is essential to elicit the intactness of memory component:
  - *Remote memory:* Childhood events, any surgical history, educational details, etc., are asked by the nurse to the patient so as to elicit the remote memory. For example: What was the name of your primary school teacher?
  - *Recent memory:* The nurse questions the patient to provide specifics of some instructions given earlier while starting the assessment. For example: Can you recollect the names of the three items shown earlier in this tray for your assessment?
  - *Immediate memory:* It may be evaluated by asking the patient to repeat a sequence of numbers or alphabets.
- **Retention and recall:** Patient is asked to repeat after sometime the things or sequence mentioned by the nurse examiner. Recall can be free or serial/sequential. For example: You are expected to repeat the sequence ....15, 29,38,59,21,77.
- **Calculation:** Simple to complex mathematical calculations are given by the nurse as per the educational status of the patient.
- **Abstraction:** It is a suitable explanation of a simple proverb/common saying which will confirm the abstract ideas of the patient to be intact. For example: A bad workman always blames his tools.
- **Similarities/differences:** The nurse queries the patient to recognize resemblances or divergence between concepts, figures, etc. For example: You are expected to identify similarity and difference between a pen and a pencil?
- **Judgement:** Higher level thinking and situations questions are put forward wherein the judgement of the patient is evaluated. For example: Patient is asked to respond about his/her action in case of leaving the house keys inside the locked house?

Special cerebral functions

- **Recognition:** It is considered as one of the specialized cerebral function. Any damage or compromise to the cerebral lobes leads to failure or inability to recognize, which is known as agnosia.
  - Visual agnosia is failure to identify by sight, it occurs when there is the malfunction of the occipital lobe.
  - Auditory agnosia occurs with altered function of the temporal lobe, when patient is unable to identify sounds.
  - In tactile agnosia recognition of touch is failed due to damage of the parietal lobe.
  - Autotopagnosia is characterized by failure to localize or orient the body parts due to damage of the parietal lobe.
- **Execution of skilled activities:** It is another specialized cerebral function. Inability to carry out such function is known as apraxia, occurs due to disfunction of the parietal cerebral lobe. It means the patient is unable to perform simple, familiar, earlier learnt activities like whistling, winking, putting buttons of shirt or shoelace. Apraxia can be dressing inability or constructional incompetence.
- **Communication:** It is yet another function, which is jeopardized. Aphasia impacts an individual's ability of expression and understanding of thoughts in verbal as well as written form. Temporal lobe is involved when it impacts understanding or comprehending, known as receptive aphasia. When the frontal lobe is compromised, there is expressive aphasia.

Fluent aphasia is described as the production of incoherent, jumbled speech, whereas nonfluent aphasia describes an inability to initiate speech or respond to speech with anything other than simple words.

Level of consciousness (LOC)

LOC is determined by using the Glasgow Coma Scale. The scale is globally accepted and in use since 1974, after it was discovered by Dr Brian Jennett and Dr Graham Teasdale. The scale is sub scaled into three—eye opening, best verbal response and best motor response, with further subcategories and scorings. The range of score is between full score of 15 and minimal score of 3 **(Table 27.2)**. A patient obtaining a score of 3 denotes deep comatose state, less than 8 needs immediate attention as the alertness reduces and patient is mostly unconscious. Whereas score of 15 infers a fully alert and conscious state. The scores are graphically documented with display on nurse's chart eventually helps in prompt remedial measures.

Verbal responses cannot be captured in patients who are intubated hence a new coma scale with four points is incorporated for such patients (Wijdicks EF et al).

II. Cranial Nerve Functions

The cranial nerves ascend directly from the central nervous system. The cranial nerves consist of twelve pairs of nerves that branch from the nervous tissue of the brain. Few of the nerves have sensory predominance, whereas few have motor function dominance, rest remaining are mixed type with sensory as well as motor functionality. The sensory branches have main function of transmitting inputs from the sensory organs towards brain, on the other hand the motor branch carries output or impulses from the brain towards visceral organs or glands outside the brain. Defective or dysfunctional cranial nerves are seen in cases with nerve root or nucleus or pathway lesions or injuries or may be due to insult to the various lobes of the brain or evidently a defect or damage to the nerve or the innervating muscle.

Unresponsiveness of comatose patient is the only challenge or limitation for conducting cranial nerve assessment. Assessment of the cranial nerves are tabulated in **Table 27.3**.

TABLE 27.2: Glasgow coma scale.

Component	Response	Score	Nurse action
Eyes response	Spontaneously eye opening	4	Spontaneous
	To speech	3	Calling out came of the patient
	To pain	2	Peripheral pain stimuli
	None	1	
Best verbal response	Oriented	5	Notice and document while communicating with the patient
	Confused	4	
	Inappropriate words	3	
	Incomprehensive sounds	2	
	None	1	
Best motor response	Obeys commands	6	Spontaneously or by verbal instruction
	Localized pain	5	Eliciting movements using **I. Central pain** **Trapezius pinch:** Deep pressure to trapezius muscle **Supraorbital pressure:** Pressure under supraorbital ridge **Sternal pressure:** Knuckle pressure to sternum; **do not rub!** **II. Peripheral pain:** Nail bed pressure
	Withdrawal from pain stimuli	4	
	Abnormal flexion	3	
	Abnormal extension	2	
	Flaccid	1	
Maximum score		15	

TABLE 27.3: Cranial nerves, their functions and abnormal findings in disease conditions.

Cranial nerve	Nerve variant	Functions	Conducting the assessment	Normal findings	Abnormal findings
I. Olfactory nerve	Sensory	Smelling	• Patient is asked to close eyes. • The patient is asked to identify different non-irritating smells (coffee/vanilla/alcohol swab/any other significant smell) through each nostril.	• The patient will be able to identify even when the aromatase item is 3–4 inches away from nostrils. • Common cold should be ruled out before attempting to test.	Anosmia is failure to smell either partial or total loss. Primarily due to damage of olfactory nerve, may also occur in cases of meningitis, damage of temporal or frontal lobe, compressing tumor, hydrocephalus, long-term side effects of antiarrhythmic drugs.

Contd...

Contd...

Cranial nerve	Nerve variant	Functions	Conducting the assessment	Normal findings	Abnormal findings

II. Optic nerve	Sensory	Vision	• For visual acuity (VA) test—the patient is asked to read the Snellen chart.
			• For visual confrontation/field test:
			  – Done with one eye at a time, keeping the other eye closed.
			  – Head is kept in a steady position.
			  – Patient is asked to focus straight.
			  – Patient and nurse sit facing each other at 1 m distance apart.
			  – Nurse examiner moves the finger from outside the patient's visual field towards normal field (vertical/nasal/temporal side).
			  – Patient gestures when he/she can see the finger.
			
			Fundoscopic exam: Mostly conducted by the physician to identify papilledema.
				VA: Normal 20/20 for right eye (OD), as well as left eye (OS).
				
				Visual field test normal
				Nasal aspect: 50–60°
				Upwards: 50–60°
				Downwards: 70°
				Temporal aspect: 80–90°.
				
				Normally the patient will see the finger at same time as the nurse.
					Examiner further moves the finger medially until the patient can see it.

III. Oculomotor nerve	Motor	• Helps to raise upper eyelid • Helps to turn eyeball upward, downward and medial. • Constricts the pupil • Facilitates eye accommodation.	• Observe lids for ptosis • Assess direction of gaze • Eye movements: 9 cardinal positions • Check pupillary size, shape, response and accommodation. (dim the light of the room) • A nurse examiner must check both direct and consensual response. Finally, accommodation of both the pupil is checked. • Documented as PERRLA. • Oculocephalic reflex/doll's eye reflex • The nurse instructs the patient to keep both the eyes open. • The nurse then rapidly turns the head of the patient side to side and later upwards-downwards. • Contraindicated in patients with cervical spine injury.	Normally there is no drooping of eyelids. • Pupil size is 2–4 mm normally. Both pupil size are mostly equal and round in shape. It constricts in response to light. • Both pupils give similar response in the direct and opposite pupil. • Both the pupils accommodate or fix together when object or finger is brought closure to the eyes. • Pupil equal, round, reactive to light and accommodation. • A positive response or intact cranial nerves function is concluded when the eye balls move to opposite direction of the turning of the head.	It can be unilateral or bilateral • **Eyeball:** Exophthalmos/enophthalmos/nystagmus • Nystagmus can be vertical, horizontal or rotatory. • Response may be brisk/sluggish/non-reactive (comatose patients) • **CN III damage:** Loss of consensual response. • The eyeballs or gaze is fixed or mid-position in comatose patient, brain death or damaged cranial nerve III, IV, VI.

Contd...

Contd...

Cranial nerve	Nerve variant	Functions	Conducting the assessment	Normal findings	Abnormal findings
IV. Trochlear nerve	Motor	Facilitate in turning the eyeball in lateral and downward direction.	Same tests as for CN III	Same response as for CN III	Same abnormalities as CN III
V. Abducens nerve	Motor	Facilitate in turning the eyeball in lateral direction.	Same tests as for CN III	Same response as for CN III	Same abnormalities as CN III
VI. Trigeminal nerve Ophthalmic branch	Sensory	Pain, light touch and temperature sensations are perceived in the areas like supraorbital region, upper eyelids, extending up to the head vertex. It also innervates the lacrimal glands, cornea, eyelids, nose and paranasal cavity.	Nurse instructs the patient to close the eyes and inform about the areas being stimulated. Measure bilaterally across both sides, the sensation of: • Pain using pin • Light touch using wisp of cotton • Temperature using cold and hot test tubes. • Assess corneal reflex. • A wisp of cotton is used to gently touch the cornea	In normal response, patient will blink the eyes.	Loss of blinking of both eyes infers that there is unilateral trigeminal nerve lesion.
Maxillary branch	Sensory	Innervates the maxilla area of face, upper jaw, nasal mucosa and maxillary sinus.			
Mandibular branch	Sensory	Innervates the skin over cheek, jaw, lateral aspects of head, lower jaw, oral mucus membrane and frontal aspects of tongue.	• Assess patient's ability to clench teeth. • Jaw reflex—test – Patient is instructed to open the mouth slightly. – Nurse places a finger below the lower lip and taps it gently in a downward direction with the percussion/knee hammer.	Normally an upward jerk is observed.	Clonus may be observed in mandibular branch damage or lesion.
	Motor	Innervates the muscles for mastication.			
VII. Facial nerve	Sensory	Sense of taste	**Taste:** Ask the patient to close eyes and give salt, sugar, coffee, lime to taste.	Taste is predominant as: • Sweet—tip of tongue • Sour/salty—sides • Bitter—back • Face looks symmetrical. • Patient is able to perform: Smiling, frowning, puffing out of cheeks, raising eyebrows, eyelid closure and whistling.	BELL'S PALSY: Paralysis of facial muscle on affected side, loss of taste, dropping of lower eyelids.
	Motor	Facial expression	Ask the patient to smile, forehead wrinkling/frown, puff out cheeks, raise/lower eyebrows, eye lid closure, whistle. Observe for facial asymmetry		
VIII. Vestibulo-cochlear nerve	Sensory	**Vestibular:** Balancing **Cochlear:** Hearing	**Acuity** **Ticking watch test:** Patient is asked to close eyes, a wrist watch is brought close to the ears and asked to identify. **Whisper test:** • Examiner stands out of sight of patient • One ear is covered by palm • Examiner whispers softly 1–2 feet from uncovered ear		

Contd...

Contd...

Cranial nerve	Nerve variant	Functions	Conducting the assessment	Normal findings	Abnormal findings
			Rinne test: • Vibrating tuning fork is placed behind the ear on mastoid process until patient can no longer hear sound. • Then it is placed 2 inches in front of ear. • Same is done for the other ear. **Weber test:** • Vibrating tuning fork is kept on middle of forehead • Ask patient to hear and respond for both the ears.	• Normally air conduction is better than bone conduction which infers that the patient will still hear the sound when the vibrating tuning fork is placed near the external meatus. • Normally the patient will hear equal to both sides.	• In conductive deafness the bone conduction is better than air conduction. • In nerve deafness both air and bone conduction are reduced. But in air conduction sound still heard. • Sound lateralizes to the better functioning ear in Sensorineural hearing loss.
IX. Glossopharangeal nerve	Sensory	Sense of taste and transmits sensory impulse from tongue and pharynx.	• Similar sensory test as CN VII is performed. • While the patient communicates, the nurse notes the pitch and quality of the patient's voice.	Taste is predominant at: • Sweet—tip of tongue • Sour/salty—sides • Bitter—back Normal pitch and tone.	High pitched or hoarse voice infers vocal cord paralysis. A nasal tone may conclude palatal paralysis.
	Motor	Innervates part of the tongue and pharynx and provides motor fibers to the parotid salivary gland.	• Asks the patient to swallow • The patient is instructed to open his mouth wide and say "aahh…." while breathing out followed by "ugh.." while breathing in. • Gag reflex is elicited using a tongue blade.	• The patient is able to swallow the saliva without any difficulty. • While in both instructions: palate of the patient will move symmetrically upward and backward • The uvula will remain in the midline and the two sides of pharynx will contract symmetrically. • Normally narrowing of pharynx with elevation of the roof of tongue and a feeling to vomit is observed.	• If the patient chokes on his saliva while talking, there may be both palatal and pharyngeal weakness. • Absent of gag reflex means loss of sensation due to damage or compression of nerve.

Contd...

Contd...

Cranial nerve	Nerve variant	Functions	Conducting the assessment	Normal findings	Abnormal findings
X. Vagus nerve	Sensory and motor	**Sensory:** Sense of taste **Motor:** Innervates to the heart, lung, and visceral organs as parasympathetic supply.	Same tests as for CN IX	Same response as for CN IX	
XI. Accessory nerve	Motor	• Supplies larynx, pharynx, soft palate. • Innervates the trapezius and sternocleido-mastoid muscles.	The examiner places one hand against the one side of face and ask patient to turn his head against it. **For testing bilateral:** The patient is instructed to force against the hand on the patient forehead. **Trapezius:** Ask the patient to rise his shoulder towards ear. Examiner try to apply pressure on the shoulder when resistance given by patient.	While doing so prominence of sternocleidomastoid muscle on the contra lateral aspect is clearly observed.	Patient is unable to apply pressure against the resistance. **Trapezius weakness:** Shoulder dropping on one side and scapula being displaced downward and laterally.
XII. Hypoglossal nerve	Motor	Supplies the tongue muscles, facilitates speech and swallowing	The nurse examiner inspects the surface, shape, size and position of the tongue. Instructs the patient to hang-out the tongue.	Patient can speak and swallow.	Difficulty in speech, swallowing. Inability to overhang the tongue. Flickering or involuntary movements are noticed when tongue is protruded.

III. Motor System Functions

Motor functions are evaluated in a systematic pattern. Few basic principles are also followed:
- Commences with assessment of upper limbs, then neck and torso lastly the lower limbs are evaluated.
- The concept of near to far i.e., proximal to distal evaluation for the extremities is always followed.
- Furthermore, bilateral comparisons are always done.
- Verification with the baseline findings.
- Functionality levels of the patient and independence of performing ADLs are also taken into consideration.
- Specific methods and observations are incorporated while evaluating comatose patient.

Assessment of motor system initiates with visual examination, wherein the nurse makes a bilateral comparison observation as follows:

1. **Visual examination:**
   - The muscle bulk is noted, measurement of circumference of the muscle mass is done using measuring tape. This helps in determining the presence of muscle wasting/atrophy or hypertrophy.
   - Next in observation will be presence of any abnormal movements like muscular twitching, presence of tremors pertinent during activity or resting tremors as in case of Parkinsonism.
   - Speed of initiating a movement is noticed. Slow initiation of movement is classic feature of Parkinson's disease and it is known as bradykinesia.
   - Muscle tone is detected:
     - Patient is instructed to be calm and relaxed.
     - Next the patient is asked to perform flexion and extension of the joints like wrist, elbow, knees.
     - Following observations are made:
       - Hypotonic response: Decreased resistance or tone
       - Hypertonic response: Increased resistance or rigidity.
       - Spastic response: Spring—like movement.

2. **Muscle strength**: It can be assessed by active and passive resistive movements in an alert and aware patient. It is graded on a scale of 0 to 5 as given in **Table 27.4**.

For an unconscious patient the muscle strength is determined by observing the patient for some time and then in response to painful stimuli. The responses may be categorized as below:
- *Unresponsive:* The patient fails to react to the painful stimuli.
- *Non-purposeful response:* The patient demonstrates no effort for eliminating or pushing the stimuli however there is some response at the stimulated area.

TABLE 27.4: Assessment of muscle strength.	
Muscle Strength	0. No movement/flaccid
	1. Flicker
	2. Movement with gravity removed
	3. Movement against gravity
	4. Movement against resistance
	5. Normal strength

- *Purposeful response:* The patients display efforts to locate the area where the nurse stimulates, and further tries to eliminate or push away.
3. **Gait evaluation:** Gait is an individual's pattern of walking, which requires amalgamation and synchronization of motor, sensory, vestibular functions and essentially requires few components as mentioned below:
   - *Steps:* Features like measurement, swiftness and pace of steps.
   - *Base:* Distance between two feet or legs while walking.
   - *Body posture and position of extremities:* Mannerisms are also noticed while walking.
   - *Swinging upper extremities:* Observe if it is increased or decreased, also if it is one-sided or both sides while walking.
   - *Turning:* Comprises of promptness, steadiness and steps needed to make a turn.
   Examples of abnormal gaits are depicted in **Table 27.5**.
4. **Cerebellar functions:** Coordination and balancing are the two main cerebellar functions. Coordination is evaluated at rest and also while performing activities. Impaired coordination may be observed while an individual performs routine activities of life, like reaching out for objects, walking, climbing etc. Observations are made pertinent to rhythm, speed, and movement accuracy. Specific tests are performed to elicit coordination and balancing as displayed in **Table 27.6**.

TABLE 27.5: Abnormal gaits.	
Abnormal gaits	**Characteristics**
Shuffling/propulsive or Parkinson gait	Recognized by inflexible, stooped posture with neck and head with forward lean. The steps are shorter/closer and faster in pace.
Scissors gait	Patient makes a scissor like pattern while walking. The steps are slow and small. Seen in patients diagnosed with spastic cerebral palsy, upper motor neuron lesion, multiple sclerosis.
High steppage	The leg is raised high with toes directing downwards with foot drop. Seen in patients with confirmation of Multiple sclerosis, Guillain–Barre syndrome, spinal disc herniation.
Hemiparetic/spastic gait	The contralateral side leg is affected and the patient displays a very rigid leg with semi-circular dragging of the foot. Seen in known case of multiple sclerosis and post stroke hemiparesis.
Waddling	Duck-like stride is seen due to increased truncal movements while walking. Significantly detected in patients with progressive muscular dystrophy.

IV. Reflexes

Reflexes are immediate/spontaneous, unpredictable, and involuntary responses to an external stimulus like striking a tendon by a reflex or knee hammer.

Following considerations are invariably followed while a nurse works on the reflexes:
- Minor tension of muscular mass is maintained before testing.
- The nurse strikes the tendon with competence, stability and rapidly.
- Response is detected, graded and compared for both the sides.
- Diversion of attention or isometric contraction done, incase there is reduction or absence of reflex.

Reflex is graded on a scale of 0 to 5
0 – Absent
1 – Hypoactive
2 – Normal
3 – Enhanced/brisk
4 – Unsustained clonus
5 – Sustained clonus

Deep tendon reflexes

Deep tendon reflexes are the specific reflexes elicited by stimulating or tapping the tendons, hence they are also named as muscle stretch reflexes. A soft rubber tipped hammer is used to tap the tendon area to bring about contractions in the muscle fibers. Insult or damage to the nervous impulse pathways may reflect abnormal deep tendon reflexes. The responses may be altered/varied due to electrolyte imbalances precisely calcium and potassium, thyroid hormone abnormalities or due to extremes of age of the patient **(Table 27.7)**.

Pathological reflex

Plantar/Babinski reflex: Extension of the great toe with fanning out of the other toes upon stimulus of the plantar aspect of the foot. It is an explicit indicator of corticospinal tract dysfunction and may be the solitary sign of enduring disease or the only lingering sign of previous disease **(Figs. 27.3 and 27.4)**.

Similar response is seen in case of:
- Chaddock's reflex: Stimulus is given in the lateral malleolus area.
- Oppenheim's sign: Stimulus is given in the medial aspect of the tibia.
- Gordon's sign: Stimulus is provided by squeezing the calf muscles.

V. Sensory Functions

Sensation of pressure, position and vibration are deep sensations, intermediated by longer nerve fibers covered with myelin sheath, through dorsal and lateral columns. Distal joint of the extremity like toes is evaluated for deeper sensations, in case of abnormal response the nurse proceeds with the test on the proximal joins and by increasing the intensity of the stimuli.

Nerve fibers which are non–sheathed with myelin or shorter sheathed fibers passing through the spinothalamic

TABLE 27.6: Cerebellar function testing.

Assessment	Steps	Pictures
1. Stability of the trunk	• The patient is instructed to sit on a chair or side of bed with hands on the lap. • Upright posture is normally seen. • Patients with cerebellar dysfunction will present with frontward/backward/lateral tilting.	
2. Fine finger movements	• Patient is asked to tap thumb with the tip of the index finger as rapid as possible. • Rhythm, rapidity and accuracy of movements are measured. • Same is replicated for the other hand.	
3. Toe tapping	• The patient is instructed to rapidly touch the hand/finger of the nurse or the floor with the front part of the foot. • Observation is made related to rhythm, rapidness and accuracy of the movements and similarly on the other side.	
4. Finger to nose	• Patient is asked to touch the finger of the nurse or own finger with the hand overstretched creating farthest position and later touching his/her own nose tip. • Rhythm, rapidity and accuracy of movements are measured. • Same is replicated for the other hand. • Dysfunctional cerebellum leads to mixing of targets either the nose or the fingertip.	
5. Heel-knee-shin	• Conducted while the patient is on supine position. • Patient is instructed to place the heel of one foot just below the knee of other leg. • Next the patient is asked to move the heel of the foot upwards and downwards along the shin of opposite lower limb. • Observe speed, and correctness of movements. • Any wavering is observed and documented. • Similar test is conducted for the other limb.	
6. Rapid alternating movements	• Have patient alternately tap dorsal and plantar surface of one hand onto other hand, the thigh, or the bed (as fast as possible). • Observe rhythm, speed, and precision of movements.	

Contd...

Assessment	Steps	Pictures
7. Heel walk, toe walk, heel to toe walk	• The patient is expected to walk in a straight line with body weight on the heels of the foot. • The patient is expected to walk in a straight line with body weight on the heels of the foot. • The patient is expected to walk in a straight line with one foot proximately in front of the previous so as the heel touches the toe. • Nurse averts any fall by being near to the patient. • Also known as Tandem gait.	
8. Romberg's test	• Tested to evaluate the balancing function. • Request the patient stand with arms at side and feet together • Start initially with eyes open and then with eyes closed • Nurse must stand close to avoid any fall. • Patient should maintain position with eyes open or closed for 20 seconds with only minimal swaying • Romberg test is positive if patient has tendency to fall.	

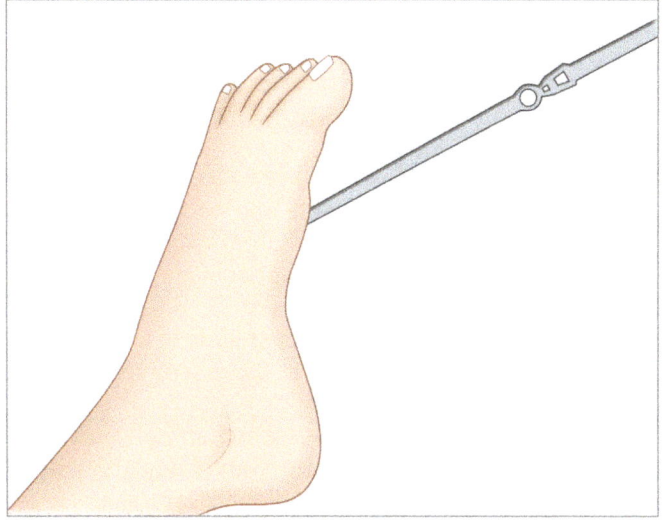

Fig. 27.3: Normal.

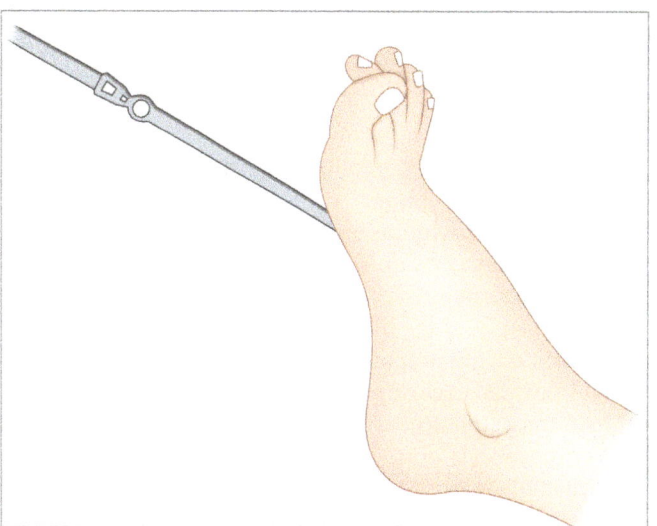

Fig. 27.4: Babinski reflex.

TABLE 27.7: Deep tendon reflexes.

Reflex type	Procedure	Normal reflex	Illustrations
Biceps reflex **C5-C6**	The patient is asked to flex the arm at the elbow with palms down. Nurse places her thumb in the antecubital fossa at base of the biceps tendon. Nurse gently strikes on the thumb with the reflex hammer.	Flexion of arm at elbow.	
Triceps reflex **C7-C8**	Flex patient's elbow holding arm across the chest or hold upper arm horizontally and allow lower arm to go limp. Strike the triceps tendon just above the elbow.	Extension at elbow.	
Brachioradialis reflex (C5-C6)	Strike 1–2 inches above wrist	Supination of hand and flexion of forearm at elbow	
Patellar reflex or knee reflex (L2-L4)	Make the patient sit comfortably with legs hanging freely over side of the bed or chair or have patient lie supine and support the knee in a flexed position. Briskly tap the patellar tendon just below the patella.	Extension of lower leg at knee.	Knee reflex
Achilles reflex (S1)	The patient foot is dorsiflexed at the ankle. Then strike at the Achilles tendon.	Plantar flexion of foot at the ankle.	

tract, are responsible for lighter and superficial sensations like pain and temperature.

Following considerations should constantly be kept in mind by the nurse examiner before commencement of the sensory assessment:

- Patient is:
  - Briefed and prepared about each test beforehand.
  - Informed to close eyes during the sensory assessment.
- Patterns/sequences are avoided while performing the test.
- Comparison is done between right vs left side, distal vs proximal areas.
- Skin markings are done to identify the areas of sensory loss with marker pen or normal pen.

Assessment of sensory functions is depicted in **Table 27.8**.

POST ASSESSMENT

1. Patient is made comfortable and reassured after the assessment is completed.
2. Used items are disposed appropriately.
3. Tray with other items are cleaned.
4. The nurse now washes and dries hands.
5. Meticulous documentation of the assessment is done immediately.
6. Any changes in the findings which are alarming are appropriately informed for necessary action, this is done immediately if the patient condition is critical.

TABLE 27.8: Assessment of sensory functions.

Sensory assessment	Procedure

Vibration	• A low-pitched tuning fork of 128-Hz is used.
	• Tuning fork is lightly tapped on a firm surface.
	• Stem of the fork is placed on the great toe precisely on the distal joint.
	• Ask the patient details about
	  – When sensation was felt?
	  – What is the feel of such sensation?
	  – Where did she/he feel sensation?
	  – Duration of the vibrations (in seconds)?
	• Same steps are replicated for the other side.
	• Proceed proximally for all other joints, one by one and simultaneously note on the other side too.

Sensation of joint positioning	• Examiner holds the big toe of the ailing person and moves it farther from other toes • While moving the toes upward and downward tell the patient to sense the movement. • Move the toe to some extent and ask the person to sense the direction. • If fails to sense, nurse makes the movement intense and furthermore if still not able to sense, evaluation of remaining bigger joints is done. • Analogous test is conducted on the fingers subsequently.

Sensation of pain	• A safety pin or tip of pen is used for eliciting this test.
	• The examiner first shows it to the patient and makes him/her understand the intensity of stimulation which will be eventually used. This is done while patient keeps the eye open.
	• Now the patient is instructed to close eyes.
	• Sensory loss to pain is evaluated from distal end to proximal.
	• Patient is enquired if any changes are perceived as the test is continued with touch points moving upwards.
	• The most commonly tested areas are as below:
	  – Index finger—palm side to elicit sensation of median nerve.
	  – Little finger—palm side to elicit pain sensation innervated by ulnar nerve.
	  – Dorsal aspect of hand, precisely the web space between the index finger and thumb, which briefs about the radial nerve function.
	  – Similarly, dorsal aspect of the foot, specifically the webbed space between great toe and second toe.
	  – Foot is stimulated on the lateral aspect.

Temperature	• This test is specifically done on patients, who experience lesser or loss of pain sensation. Patient is reminded to close the eyes. • The specific areas with evidence of abnormal pain sensation are touched with a cold tuning fork.
Light touch	• Patient is instructed to close eyes. • A random/unpredictable pattern of touch/test is followed. • The skin is stimulated gently with finger or wisp of cotton. • The patient is asked to specify areas touch.
Discrimination	There are two types of test to determine the discrimination as sensory functions. It starts with eye closure by the patient. • Two sharp stimuli are applied on the skin and eventually the distance between the two touch points is reduced. When the patient is able to infer the two stimulation points separately it concludes as intact 2-point discrimination. • When the patient is able to infer two stimuli concurrently, at two opposite sides then it is called double simultaneous stimulation.
Graphesthesia	• The patient is asked to close the eyes. • Then he or she is enquired to recognize the number/alphabet/shape drawn on the palmar aspect using a pen or even fingertip. • Performed on patients with normal light touch sensation.
Stereognosis	• Examination is done for patients with normal light touch and appropriate sense of position. • It is elicited by placing an acquainted thing like coin or cotton wisp on the palm of the patient, which he or she can feel by holding or moving it and recognize it.

Case Scenario

1. Mr S, a 70-year-old male known hypertensive, presents to emergency with a two months history of back pain along with right leg discomfort affecting his thigh and calf muscles. The pain has a burning and cramping quality and sporadically as well impacts the dorsum of his right foot. It is mostly consistent but intensifies when he is walking or lying prone. It was also reported that a forward bend always improved the pain. Walking is limited now and a limp is noticed.
   Vitals: Body temperature is normal, Pulse = 88/min, BP = 168/92 mm Hg, Respiration = 20/min.
   Musculoskeletal: No joint swelling or tenderness. Moderate percussion tenderness noted over lumbar-sacral spine. He is bent forward slightly at the waist and has discomfort with extension of his spine.
   Neurological Assessment
   – *Mental status:* Mr S is alert and fully oriented. Speech is fluent and articulate.
   – *Precise cranial nerve evaluation:* VA = 20/20 OU. PEERLA. EOMI. Face symmetric. SCM and trapezius strength full. Palate and tongue are midline.
   – *Motor system functionality:* Upper extremities—have normal bulk, tone, and strength.

- *Motor:* UE's have normal bulk, tone, and strength.
- Left leg has slightly diminished tone.

Strength

Hip add	Hip abd	Hip flex	Hip ext	Knee ext	Knee flex	DF	PF	Foot inv	Foot ever	Toe ext	Toe flex
5	4+	5	5−	4+	5	4+	5	4	4+	4+	5

Right leg has moderately diminished tone.

Strength

Hip add	Hip abd	Hip flex	Hip ext	Knee ext	Knee flex	DF	PF	Foot inv	Foot ever	Toe ext	Toe flex
4	4−	5−	4	4	5−	4	5−	4−	4+	4+	5−

Deep Tendon Reflexes
Biceps and triceps = 2+ . Patella: L = 1, R = 0. Ankle: L = 2, R = 1.
Plantar responses: Flexor bilaterally.
Sensory Evaluation:
- *Left leg:* Subjective diminished sensation to light touch and sharp over the medial and lateral anterior shin with sparing over the lateral and dorsal foot.
- *Right leg:* Loss of sharp sensation and diminished light touch over the entire leg with sparing of the middle posterior portion of the thigh.
- *Pinprick:* Patchy saddle anesthesia. Vibration sense is mildly diminished bilaterally at the level of the toes.
- *Coordination testing:* No dysmetria or tremor in the arms. Lower extremities have weakness so mild dysmetria on heel-knee-shin may be non-specific.
- *Probable diagnosis:* Cauda equina syndrome

2. A 35-year-old male came to the casualty room with a 3-day history of blurred vision in his left eye. He reports seeing a "dark area" of blurry vision precisely in the center of his vision. Eye movements are difficult too due to pain. There is no diplopia or any previous visual disturbances in the past.

Assessment of Cranial Nerves
- *Mental status:* Patient is fully attentive and willing. He follows commands. His speech is easy and articulate. Concentration and short-term memory intact.
- CN: II:
  - VA = 20/20 OD and 20/200 OS.
  - Pupils OD: 3 mm → 1 mm direct. Fixed at 3 mm indirectly.
  - OS: 3 mm → sluggish to 2 mm direct. 3 mm → 1 mm brisk indirect.
  - Visual fields normal in right eye.
  - Loss of visual field in left eye with some sparing of the peripheral temporal area.
  - Fundoscopic examination: Fundus benign without elevation or erythema of either optic disc.
- *III, IV, VI:* EOMI without nystagmus. + mild pain in the left eye with movement.
- *V/VII:* Sensation and motor strength intact
- *VIII:* Hearing grossly intact
- *IX/X/XII:* Gag intact, palate elevates symmetrically, tongue midline
- *XI:* SCM and trapezius strength full
- *Motor:* Normal bulk, tone, and strength all 4 extremities.
- DTR's symmetric and non-pathological. Plantar responses flexor.
- *Sensory:* Normal light touch vibration and pinprick all four extremities.
- Romberg negative.
- *Coordination:* No dysmetria or tremor. No truncal titubation.
- *Gait:* Narrow-based and steady.

SUMMARY

This chapter dealt in depth about the evaluation of the patients with neurological disorders. Neurological assessment provides a framework for diagnosing the abnormalities and also monitor the progress and compliance with treatment and care. It is obligatory to verify the current findings with the previously documented assessment findings, any deviations from previous parameters should always be attended with utmost priority. Patients are under the nurse's care for longer duration of time, a vigilant recognition of deteriorating responses not only helps saving life but also early recovery. Nurse has a major contribution towards the evaluation of patient's condition. Assessment should be learnt with accuracy and practice of repeated assessments will transform the nurse into further skillful professional.

MULTIPLE CHOICE QUESTIONS

1. One of the most common features of neurological disorders are language deficits and are collectively known as:
   a. Dysphasia
   b. Alogias
   c. Anomia
   d. Aphasia
2. Getting a patient oriented with self, place, and time is as part of the evaluation for:
   a. Long-term memory
   b. Orientation
   c. Function
   d. Short-term memory
3. To test CN _____ patient close one nostril and check each side _____
   a. I, simultaneously
   b. I, individually
   c. II, individually
   d. II, simultaneously
4. A 65-year-old woman has decreased facial expression and is slow in her movements. When she walks, she is hunched over and takes small steps. It does not take much for her to lose her balance. What type of gait abnormality does she have?
   a. Hemiplegic
   b. Spastic diplegic
   c. Parkinsonian
   d. Ataxic
5. If an individual has an inability to initiate speech or respond to speech with anything other than simple words is known as:
   a. Nonfluent aphasia
   b. Fluent aphasia
   c. Disruptive aphasia
   d. Anomic aphasia

6. A 42-year-old woman sustained a road traffic accident and is brought straight to emergency department. On presentation, her eyes are opening to pain. She is making incoherent sounds and localizes to pain. What is the GCS?
   a. 7
   b. 8
   c. 9
   d. 10

ANSWERS

1. d
2. b
3. b
4. c
5. a
6. c

SUGGESTED READING

1. Barker E. Neuroscience Nursing: A Spectrum of Care, 2nd edition. Mosby; 2002. pp. 51-96.
2. Caton-Richards M. Assessing the neurological status of patients with head injuries. Emerg Nurse. 2010;17(10):28-31. doi: 10.7748/en2010.03.17.10.28.c7617. PMID: 20364782.
3. Hickey JV. The Clinical Practice of Neurological and Neurosurgical Nursing, 6th edition. Philadelphia: Lippincott Williams and Wilkins; 2008. pp. 111-53.
4. InformedHealth.org [Internet]. Cologne, Germany: Institute for Quality and Efficiency in Health Care (IQWiG); 2006-. What happens during a neurological examination? 2016 Jan 27 [Updated 2016 Jan 27]. Available from: https://www.ncbi.nlm.nih.gov/books/NBK348940/.
5. Janecek J, Kushlaf H. Gordon Reflex. [Updated 2021 Jan 21]. In: StatPearls [Internet]. Treasure Island (FL): StatPearls Publishing; 2021.
6. Maher AB. Neurological assessment. Int J Orthop Trauma Nurs. 2016;22:44-53. doi: 10.1016/j.ijotn.2016.01.002. Epub 2016 Feb 26. PMID: 27118633.
7. Marsden J, Stevens S, Ebri A. How to measure distance visual acuity. Community Eye Health. 2014;27(85):16. PMID: 24966459; PMCID: PMC4069781.
8. Wijdicks EF, Bamlet WR, Maramattom BV, Manno EM, McClelland RL. Validation of a new coma scale: The FOUR score. Ann Neurol. 2005;58(4):585-93. doi: 10.1002/ana.20611. PMID: 16178024.

CHAPTER 28

Diagnostic Evaluation in Neurological Disorders

Sonali Banerjee

"No man can hope to find out the truth without investigation."

—**George F Richards**

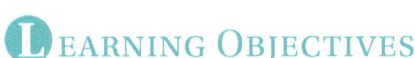 EARNING OBJECTIVES

After going through the chapter, the learner will be able to:
- Enlist the noninvasive and invasive diagnostic evaluation pertinent to neurological disorders.
- List the indications and contraindications for each evaluative procedure.
- Explain each diagnostic procedure.
- Elucidate in detail about pre and post care for the patient undergoing diagnostic procedures.
- List down the complications and related preventive measures.

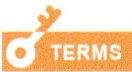

- **Claustrophobia:** An extreme unreasonable or disproportionate fear of being in small or confined places and being unable to escape.
- **Electroencephalogram:** A noninvasive electrophysiological monitoring technique to record electrical activity of the brain and represent it graphically as various wave forms.
- **Electronystagmography:** A noninvasive diagnostic test to monitor involuntary movements of the eye caused by a condition known as nystagmus.
- **Lumbar puncture (spinal tap):** An invasive procedure in which a needle is inserted into the spinal canal, for collecting cerebrospinal fluid (CSF) for diagnostic testing or for therapeutic purposes.
- **Magnetic resonance imaging:** A radiological noninvasive diagnostic technique that utilizes magnetism, radio waves, and a computer to yield real time images of the organs in the body.

INTRODUCTION

Statistics endorsed by World Health Organization that around one billion people across the globe are affected by neurological disorders, and around 68 lakhs of them develop disability or die due to the disease condition. Diagnosing a neurological disorder is a challenging task and eventually is a growing concern. The diagnostics have become innovative and sophisticated with upsurge in the cost. Furthermore, the patient and the family experiences utmost apprehension to understand the intricacies of such advanced tests. Nurses should be well-versed with all the diagnostic test, patient preparation, equipment required etc., pertinent to neurological disorders. The knowledge and the skill of the nurses helps in handling the stressful situation of the patient by enhancing the cognizance related to the specific diagnostic tests.

The neurological diagnostics are broadly classified as noninvasive and invasive as discussed in **Table 28.1**.

Noninvasive Neurological Procedures

These are quick, painless procedures wherein strong magnetic waves or radio waves or simple X-rays are used to visualize the internal environment of the brain or spinal cord and represented in the form of two- or three-dimensional images.

Specific considerations which are essential to be followed while undertaking such procedures are:
- ❖ These are preferred as walk-in or with appointment procedure at the outpatient department.

TABLE 28.1: Neurological diagnostic tests.	
Noninvasive diagnostics	**Invasive diagnostics**
<ul><li>X-rays</li><li>Computer tomography</li><li>Magnetic resonance imaging</li><li>Ultrasonography</li><li>Electroencephalogram</li><li>Electronystagmography</li><li>Cerebral blood flow studies</li><li>Transcranial Doppler</li></ul>	<ul><li>Blood tests</li><li>Lumbar puncture/cerebrospinal fluid analysis</li><li>Myelography</li><li>Positron emission tomography (PET)</li><li>Single proton emission computer tomography (SPECT) scans.</li><li>Electromyography (EMG)</li><li>Nerve conduction velocity (NCV)</li><li>Cerebral angiography</li><li>Biopsy</li></ul>

- Informed written consent is taken from the patients.
- All the jewelry, eyeglasses, and metallic items (watch, hair pins, metallic clips of dentures, etc.) around head and spine should be removed.
- Patient is expected to change into hospital clothing.

Invasive Neurological Procedures

These are performed by accessing the internal environment of the body precisely fluids (blood, CSF) or tissues (brain/spinal cord/muscles) by passing through the skin barrier either piercing through a needle or any other instrument.

Specific considerations which are essential to be followed while undertaking such procedures are:

- Informed written consent is procured from the patients or significant others in case of unconscious/comatose patients or if the patient is minor after apprising the risks or side-effects of the investigative procedure.
- Scan with contrast medium/dye:
  - Blood test like creatinine and blood urea nitrogen (BUN) are done. Nurse should counter check the reports and inform if any abnormality is there.
  - Skin test of the contrast medium is done before the scan.
  - Nil by mouth around 4–6 hours prior to the scan is recommended, only if there is anticipated injection of dye.
  - In such cases allergies need to be checked prior to commencing the test.
  - Patient is informed about sensation of warmth which is experienced when the dye is injected. Subsequently a metallic taste, nausea or vomiting may also be experienced.

NONINVASIVE DIAGNOSTIC PROCEDURES

X-ray

It is the most basic, noninvasive, painless diagnostic procedure undertaken for viewing the skull and spine. The use of X-rays of skull have become now limited with the advancements in the diagnostics still commonly used in primary health care facilities in India. X-rays are films resulted from passing concentrated, low dose-ionized radiation passing through the body. Bones appear white on the film as calcium mineral absorbs the rays very easily.

While performing skull X-ray, precisely anteroposterior and lateral views are recommended which provides views from all aspects. Skull X-ray is recommended to rule out fractures of skull and face, calcifications, and bone erosions, etc. Spinal X-ray is also recommended in both the views, can be done for cervical, thoracic, lumbar or sacral region. Cervical spondylosis, spinal fractures or deformities like scoliosis/kyphosis/lordosis, osteoporosis, vertebral wedging or compression, irregular calcification of bones (osteophytes) can easily be detected from a spinal X-ray.

Specific information which a patient should know before taking an X-ray are enlisted below:
- Other areas like thyroid should be shielded while taking a skull X-ray, and gonadal shielding while taking a sacral X-ray.
- Pregnant woman should not be exposed to the harmful rays. If essential, proper shielding precautions should be taken.

Computer Tomography (CT Scan)

It is the most commonly used noninvasive, pain-free procedure ever since invented by Engineer Godfrey Hounsfield in 1972. CT scan is highly effectual in establishing diagnosis of brain and spinal disorders with precision and promptness. Two-dimensional and multidirectional images are generated by scanning the brain or spine in successive layers. It is mainly used to confirm diagnosis of tumors or space-occupying lesions of brain or spinal cord, inflammation of cerebral tissues, insufficiencies in cerebral circulation, clotting of blood (cerebral thrombosis, hematoma) or bleeding generally seen in cases of stroke, head injury, aneurysm, hydrocephalus, intervertebral disc herniation, stenosis in the spine, etc. Duration of the procedure may be around 20–40 minutes. The CT scan can be suggested by injecting fluoroscopic dye for few specific conditions. The patient is advised to be relaxed during the procedure. CT scan has advantage of imaging even in unconscious patient and also imaging patients who are contraindicated for MRI procedure.

Magnetic Resonance Imaging (MRI Scan)

In late seventies, Sir Peter Mansfield along with Paul Lauterbur and Raymond Vahan Damadian were acknowledged for the invention of MRI scan, which was a breakthrough in neurodiagnostic with various benefits over CT scan. MRI basically applies the sequencing of mechanism of the strong magnetic field and radio waves. The strong magnetic field initially rearranges the water molecules of the tissues, subsequently the radio waves are passed through tissue which aid to identify the shifting of the water molecules and bring them back to previous state. A three-dimensional or a two-dimensional image is then generated by the computer. Brain injury/tumor/stroke/infection/inflammation/vascular insufficiencies and spinal disorders like tumors/disc prolapse/injury can easily be detected. Apart from this epilepsy related brain damage or multiple sclerosis can easily be diagnosed with MRI imaging **(Fig. 28.1)**.

Patients with implanted metallic devises like cochlear implants, pacemaker, pins and plates of internal stabilization of fractures, aneurysm clips, knee/hip replacement items are strictly prohibited from doing MRI scan. It is also contraindicated for patients with obesity, extreme claustrophobia, back pain, movement disorders, uncooperative restless patients.

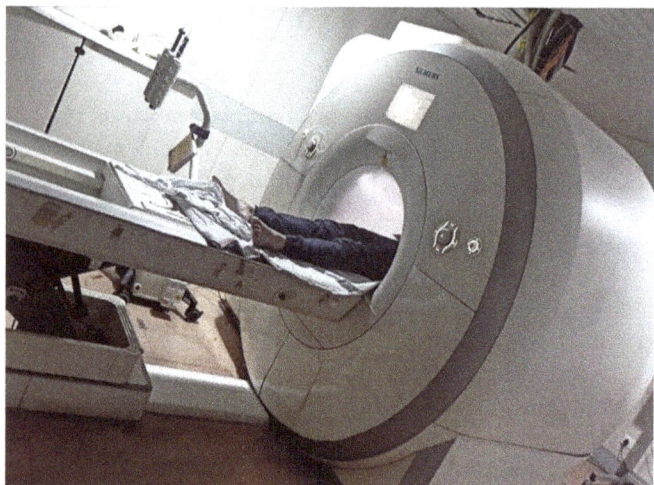

Fig. 28.1: MRI scanner with imaging in progress.

Functional MRI (fMRI) is further more advanced MRI which helps to capture magnetic properties of blood so as to create real-time imaging of cerebral circulation to a specific part of the brain. Its usability is seen in identifying intricate lesions of head injury, degenerative disorders like Alzheimer's disease, and preoperative diagnostics for epilepsy. It is also beneficial for identifying the eye gaze. It has further added value in diagnosing multiple sclerosis. Its applicability is seen in social science research too.

Important Considerations

Before CT Scan/MRI

- For CT scan/MRI/the patient is advised to lie down on a sliding table, with adjustment of the posture to procure an accurate image.
- The scanner is facilitated with communication system and monitoring for any inconvenience of the patient during the procedure.
- Patient should not move while the X-ray/CT scan/MRI/ is taken.
- Images are taken from various views/angles, later on processed and displayed on the films imaging the brain or the spinal cord.
- A very mild dose of tranquilizer or sedation is occasionally given to patients who are very agitated, restless, children or elderly, so as to keep them still during the procedure, with the view to avoid artifacts and enhance quality of the images.
- Patients may experience **claustrophobic** inside the narrow chamber. Nurses should explain in simple language that it's a normal phenomenon experienced by almost everyone and it is essential to remain motionless during the scan.
- Loud knocking noises are heard precisely during the MRI scan; this aspect should also be informed prior start of the procedure for better cooperation by the patient. Ear plugs or head phones may be used to lessen the perception.

After CT Scan/MRI

Scan with contrast medium/dye:

- Patient is checked for any allergic response to the iodine-based contrast, and treated immediately with antihistamines if such is identified.
- Patient is advised to drink plenty of fluids so as to eliminate the dye out of the body as quicky as possible.
- Special observations are essential for children or elderly patients.

Ultrasonography

In ultrasonography, high-frequency sound waves are used to develop images. The transducer leads obtain such waves, which are further captured and displayed by the computer into real-time images. It takes around 20–30 minutes for the test to be performed.

Following are the diagnostic usability of ultrasonography:

- The usage in neurodiagnostic is mostly seen in diagnosing hydrocephalus or cerebral hemorrhage among the new born babies, who sustain birth injuries.
- Cerebral blood vessels are visualized by performing transcranial Doppler, which is helpful in identifying the stroke risk.
- It is helpful in monitoring the fluctuations in ICP among adults.
- High-resolution transbulbar optic sonography is helpful in identifying increased ICP among neonates and children.
- Brain parenchyma sonography is done to differentiate between idiopathic PD (IPD) and atypical parkinsonian syndromes (APS).
- It helps in establishing diagnosis of movement disorders.

Electroencephalogram (EEG)

Hans Berger in 1924 for the first-time recorder the human EEG, representing one of the oldest noninvasive diagnostics to capture brain activity in real-time wave images. EEG mainly captures summed electrical field activity (measured in voltage) formed by pyramidal cortical neurons that are aligned corresponding to the scalp.

Before EEG Procedure

Patient is instructed for hair wash/shampoo before coming for the test. Sometimes nil by mouth is expected when sedatives/tranquilizers are injected for inducing sleep. NPO is significantly essential in triggered seizure activities, wherein the patient might aspirate during convulsion, hence NPO is always preferred. Strict instructions are given to avoid caffeinated drinks and beverages, tea, and chocolates, etc. Also sometimes they are instructed to withhold their regular medications.

Procedure

The patient is reclined on a chair or bed during the test. Numerous electrodes are attached to the scalp after applying the conductive gel. The electrodes are further attached to the leads which facilitate in transferring the electrical impulses/signals from the surface of cerebral cortex to the EEG machine **(Fig. 28.2)**, the impulses are then plotted graphically on a paper after they are amplified. EEG records brain waves in terms of its frequency, amplitude and characteristics.

Duration of the test may span from one to three hours as sometimes brain activities are monitored in the form of waves during sleep, which may produce 100 pages of recorded graph papers.

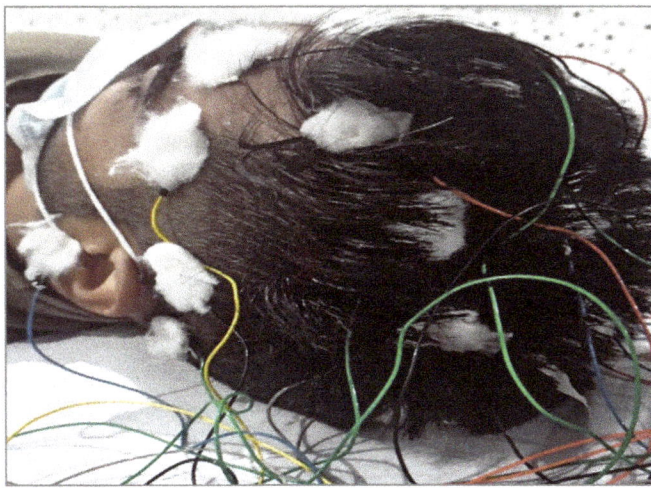

Fig. 28.2: Electrodes and lead of an electroencephalogram.

Sequence of EEG test may is shown in **Figure 28.3**. **Types of brain waves** are discussed in **Table 28.2**.

Apart from diagnosing seizure disorders, EEG helps also to diagnose metabolic/inflammatory and infective entities of the brain. It also aids in evaluating sleep disorders, also emotions, monitoring brain activity when in phase of unconsciousness and brain death. It also helps in evaluation of hearing by using cochlear implants electrodes as sensors. EEG is mostly done to detect seizure activities, various stimuli-like flashing of bright flickering lights, noise are exposed and simultaneously brain impulses are monitored. Various instructions are given to the patient during the test like opening and closure of eyes, inhalation, and exhalation. Hyperventilation upsurges the serum pH, which can activate seizure activity.

Post EEG

- ❖ Patient is asked to wash hair after reaching home to remove the sticky gel.
- ❖ The withheld medications should be taken subsequently.

Advancement in EEG

See **Figure 28.4**.

Intracranial EEG

Electrodes are inserted directly into the brain parenchyma through burr holes in the skull with the view to abate the signal intrusions. This helps to locate the foci of origin of seizure activity, it is highly effective for patients planned for epilepsy surgery. Further to these, patients are instructed to perform cognitive activities like reading, speaking or performing motor activities which aid to identify the involvement of brain areas and impacts.

TABLE 28.2: Types of brain waves and characteristics.

Wave type	Characteristics
1. Alpha waves	• **Frequency:** 8–12 Hz • Occipital leads reflect dominant waves • **Obliteration of the wave:** Eye movements, anxiousness, sudden noise or touch sensation. Prominent when relaxed.
2. Beta waves	• **Frequency:** 13–30 Hz • Frontal and central leads reflect dominant waves • **Triggered by:** Movement of eyes like opening eyelids, anxiety, active thinking and alertness.
3. Theta wave	• **Frequency:** 4–7 Hz • Temporal leads reflect dominant waves
4. Delta wave	• **Frequency:** 0.5–4 Hz • Captured during sleep activity precisely sleep stage 3 and 4.

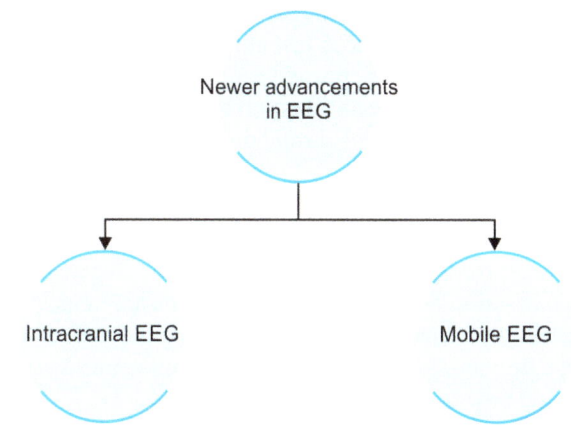

Fig. 28.4: Advancements in EEG.

Mobile EEG

Recent experimentations are being undertaken to enhance the portability and reducing the bulky features by making it more compact, user friendly, less expensive and facilitating recording the EEG from home settings by creating mobile EEG. These gadgets received satisfactory responses but the only challenge was that patients verbalized discomfort wearing it in the public.

Electronystagmography (ENG)

It involves a series of tests to diagnose nystagmus, i.e., disorder of involuntary eye movements, dizziness and balance

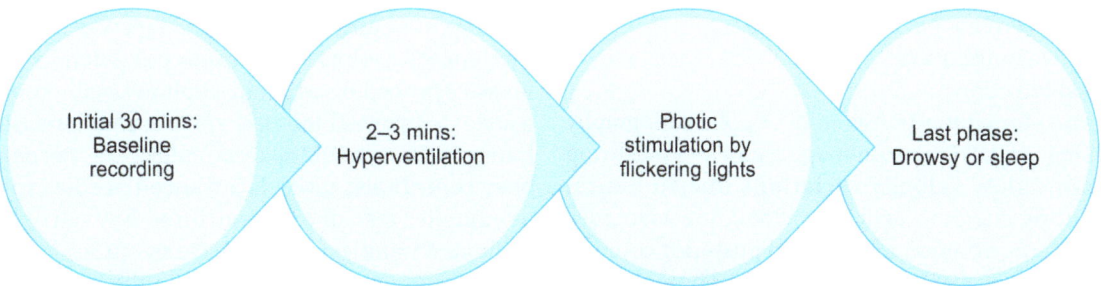

Fig. 28.3: Sequence/duration of EEG test.

disorders especially due to dysfunctional vestibular system. Hence, it facilitates in the evaluation of the oculomotor and vestibular cranial nerves with objectivity. It is a noninvasive, OPD procedure wherein, small electrodes are placed around/encircling eyes so as to capture the activities of eye movement. Further to this, sometimes patient is instructed to wear special eyewear when electrodes are replaced by infrared images.

Transcranial Doppler (TCD) and Transcranial Color Doppler (TCCD)

These are the two variants of Doppler ultrasonography that quantify the blood flow velocity through the cerebral blood vessels. It is achieved by measuring the resonances of ultrasound waves moving transcranially (through the cranium). They are also categorized as one of the methods of acoustocerebrography as spectral analysis of the acoustic signals are done. These diagnostic tests are gaining momentum in use by most of the diagnostic centers as they are low-priced and fast analysis in nature and the equipment/machine are portable and light weight. The tests are frequently used in combination with other tests such as CT scans, MRI, MRA, and carotid ultrasound.

Functionality

High-frequency sound waves (usually a multiple of 2 MHz) are emitted by ultrasound probe which resonates with other body parts and subsequently these echoes are sensed by a sensor in the probe. For cerebral arteries, the echoes have diverse frequencies depending on the course and speed of the blood flow because of the Doppler effect.

The frequency of the echo is lower than the emitted frequency when the blood flow is away from the probe and vice versa. The echoes are analyzed and converted into velocities that are displayed on the computer display. Skull bones block most of the ultrasound waves transmission. Hence waves are captured from areas with thinner walls, leading to least distortion to the sound waves known as insonation windows, e.g., the temporal region just above the cheekbone/zygomatic arch, over the eyes, beneath the jaw, and from the backside of the head.

Indications

- Cerebral emboli
- Stenosis
- Vasospasm from a subarachnoid hemorrhage
- Bleeding from a ruptured aneurysm
- Ischemic cerebrovascular disease
- Subarachnoid hemorrhage
- Arteriovenous malformations
- Arrest in the cerebral circulatory system
- Perioperative monitoring
- Meningeal infection

Recent times functional transcranial Doppler sonography (fTCD) is being used. It is a neuroimaging tool for measuring cerebral blood flow velocity variations due to neural activation during cognitive activities. Blood flow velocities are recorded in the anterior, middle, and posterior cerebral arteries using pulse-wave Doppler technology. The technique is noninvasive and easy procedure. This procedure has facilitated to the explication of cognitive (language, color processing, intelligence), motor, and sensory functions in both the hemispheres. Its usability is beneficial among adults as well as children.

Cerebral Blood Flow Studies

Cerebral blood flow (CBF) is quantified as volume of blood delivered to a well-defined mass of tissue per unit time. It is otherwise also defined as the volume of blood that passes through a specific quantity of brain tissue during a particular period of time. Typically, CBF is measured in units of mL of blood per 100 g of tissue per minute. Significant evidence for clinical management of neurocritical care patients is accessed by the cerebral blood flow. Larger blood supply, oxygen and glucose usage are observed to the cerebral areas that are very active. Trailing these increases can display the active areas of the brain.

CT and MR perfusion techniques measure the quantity of blood that flows through a particular volume of brain tissue. Sometimes Xenon-133, a radioactive substance/tracing material is used either intranasal or injected intra-arterial to determine the cerebral perfusion. It is not very a popular/common test as it is an expensive test and there is exposure to radioactive substance. It has a nonportable machine, consequently it stances challenge of shifting out the critically ill patients from the neuro-ICU. CT scan, MRI, PET, ultrasonography and transcranial Doppler are preferred over this test.

INVASIVE NEURODIAGNOSTIC TESTS

Specific Blood Tests for Neurological Disorders

Patients attending neurological OPD or those undergoing surgeries are recommended to get the routine blood tests like complete blood counts which includes RBC, hemoglobin, hematocrit, WBC, neutrophils, lymphocytes, platelets, urea and electrolytes like sodium, potassium and bicarbonate. Liver function tests would include: alanine aminotransferase (ALT), aspartate aminotransferase (AST), alkaline phosphatase (ALP), gamma-glutamyl transferase (Gamma GT), and A/G ratio (albumin/globulin ratio). Some neurologists also advise the patient to do blood glucose, precisely fasting and postprandial or sometimes even glycosylated blood glucose is advised. Hormones like thyroid assay, cortisol, antidiuretic hormone, etc., are also tested. Specific blood tests and their potential disorders are depicted in **Table 28.3**.

Lumbar Puncture and Analysis of Cerebrospinal Fluid

Lumbar puncture (LP) or spinal tap, was first familiarized by Heinrich Quincke a German physician in 1891. It is an invasive procedure wherein a hollow needle supported with a stylet is inserted into the spinal canal, precisely into the lumbar subarachnoid space to collect CSF. Recent inventions have contributed towards advanced needles with attached manometer, test tube fitment, three-way valves, ergonomics facilitated handles/grips to ease the procedure. The site of insertion of needle is preferred in the interspace between 3rd and 4th lumbar or between 4th and 5th lumbar spine to

TABLE 28.3: Specific blood tests and their probable/potential disorders.

Tests	Disorders
1. Serum procalcitonin	• Helps to differentiate between bacterial and viral meningitis • Higher values of procalcitonin confirms a bacterial entity
2. Blood glucose, protein, CBC	• Always compared with CSF values of glucose, proteins and blood cells in conditions where infection of brain or meninges is doubtful • Combination of blood glucose levels and WBC values can predict outcomes of recovery from acute ischemic stroke
3. Serum lactate, serum ferritin, C-reactive protein, absolute neutrophil count (ANC), erythrocyte sedimentation rate (ESR)	• These are inflammatory mediators. • Higher levels of these markers help in diagnosis of early meningitis among children. • A low CSF lactate, ANC, ESR, and serum—CRP in combination could rationally rule out the bacterial meningitis.
4. Blood cultures	Helpful to identify the bacteria involved in causing the infection of brain parenchyma or meninges.
5. Genetic testing	It is essential to rule out high-risk cases, i.e., those who already have family history of neurological genetic disorders. Such patients are addressed with genetic counseling. Tests are done to identify following disorders: • Cell-free DNA from the mother's blood: Down syndrome • Blood test for alpha-fetoprotein, human chorionic gonadotropin, and estriol (2nd trimester): Spina bifida • Amniocentesis • Chorionic villi sampling
6. Biomarkers: Neurofilament light chain Blood amyloid-β Additional Biomarkers	• Protein called neurofilament light chain (NfL) detects Alzheimer's disease before onset of symptoms. Parkinson's disease • Blood amyloid-β: Values should always be linked with CSF values. • Additional biomarkers: BACE1, BIN1, α-synuclein, neurofilaments, sNRG-1, YKL-40, acylcarnitines, 24-hydroxycholesterol, 27-hydroxycholesterol, autoantibodies against Aβ42, autoantibodies to anti-CAPS, and certain microRNA types. • Dementia and Alzheimer's disease)
7. Specific autoantibodies (anti-AChR, anti-MuSK or anti-LRP4)	Blood test is done to detect autoantibodies for: • Acetylcholine receptor (AChR) • MuSK protein (muscle-specific kinase) • LRP4 (lipoprotein related protein 4)

keep it safe without touching the spinal cord which ends at the level of 1st lumbar **(Fig. 28.5)**.

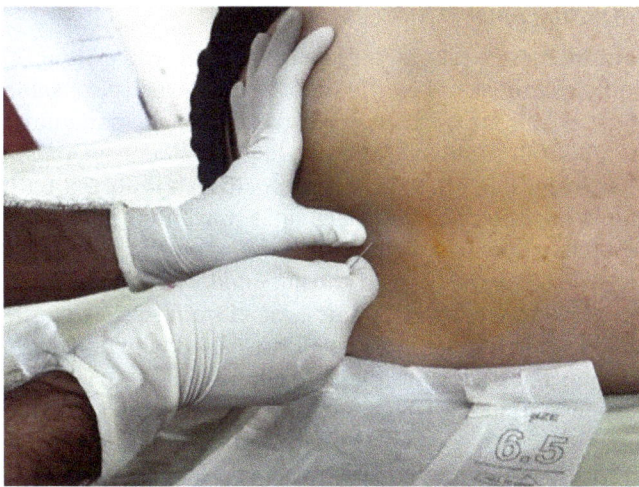

Fig. 28.5: Insertion of LP needle between L3 and L4 interspace.

Indications for Lumbar Puncture

❖ **Evaluative/diagnostic:**
  ➢ CSF pressure measurement
  ➢ CSF analysis for diagnosis of disease
  ➢ *Meningitis:* Bacterial/viral/fungal
  ➢ *Alzheimer's disease:* CSF biomarkers like amyloid-β (Aβ42), total tau (T-tau), and phosphorylated tau (P-tau).
  ➢ Intrathecal radio-opaque dye
❖ **Therapeutic/treatment related:**
  ➢ Spinal anesthesia
  ➢ Intrathecal antibiotics
  ➢ Intrathecal chemotherapy
  ➢ CSF aspiration/removal to release the benign ICP

Contraindications of LP

❖ Idiopathic increased ICP
❖ Bleeding disorders
❖ On antiplatelet or anticoagulant therapy
❖ Dermal infections at LP site
❖ Scoliosis or kyphosis

A CT scan is recommended to rule out following high-risk patients before taking them up for LP:
❖ Head trauma
❖ Elderly client, more than 60 years.
❖ Papilledema (or other signs of increased ICP)
❖ Altered mental status/Glasgow coma scale
❖ Convulsions

Preparation of the Patient Before LP

No dietary or fluid restrictions before the commencement of the test are required. Patient is instructed to avoid smoking, alcohol consumption, anticoagulants as there is a chance of bleeding. Patient is expected to change into hospital clothing and empty the bladder prior to the test. Young children may be sedated for better cooperation. Usually, patient is released from OPD after 1 to 2 hours. The family is advised to take the patient home in supine position as driving is not allowed immediately after the procedure.

Procedure of LP

Equipment: A sterile LP set consists of sterile gloves, drapes, sterile test tubes or vials, LP needle with stylet (disposable preferred), dressing material is required. Other items required are antiseptic solutions, saline, sealing with tincture benzoin.

Position: Knee chest in lateral position supported with pillow or sitting position (facilitates maximum interspace separation).

At all times a sterile field is maintained, which is facilitated by following aseptic techniques, use of sterile gloves, sterile drapes. Then the lumbar region is cleaned with antiseptic solution. Local anesthesia is generally administered to numb the pain sensations. A hollow needle is then introduced in the subarachnoid space between two lumbar vertebrae, stylet is removed, penetrated further to collect the CSF in a sterile container **(Figs. 28.6A and B)**.

The easy way to recognize CSF, it looks colorless and falls in thread-like strings. Analysis of CSF is depicted in **Table 28.4**. Once the procedure is done, the needle is gently removed, pressure is applied on to the puncture site and then sealed **(Fig. 28.6B)**. Simultaneously peripheral blood sample is collected for comparison of components like sugar, protein, etc.

Postprocedural Care

- ❖ Patient should be in supine position and should be provided bed rest for 6 to 8 hours after the test. Sitting upright immediately after the test may aggravates the pain.
- ❖ The site of puncture is sealed, any leakage or bleeding should be reported.
- ❖ Analgesics and antibiotics are taken as advised.

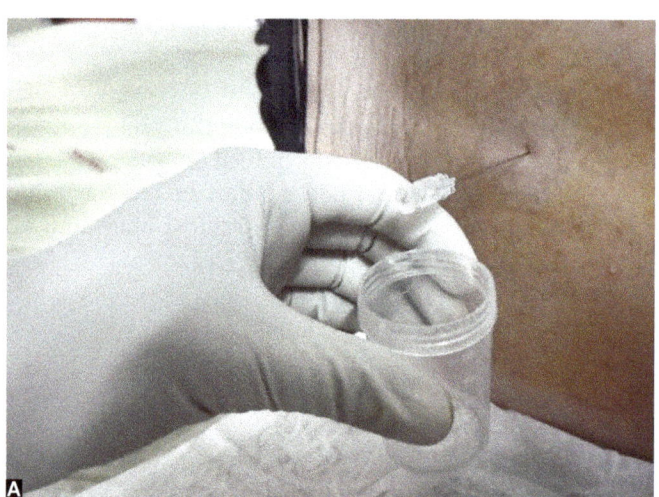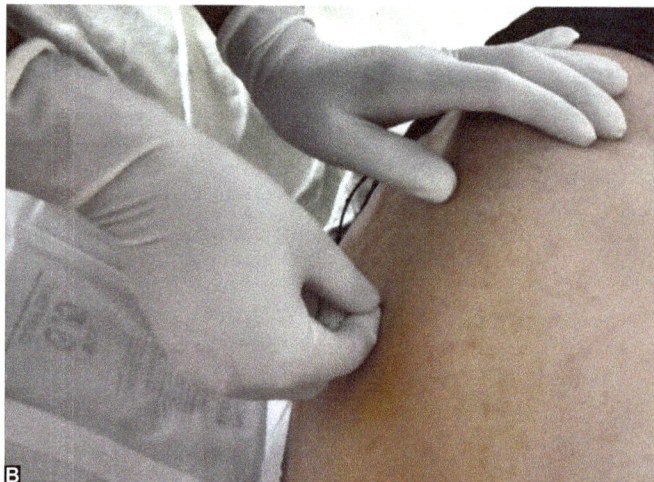

Figs. 28.6A and B: CSF collection and pressure application after LP needle is removed.

TABLE 28.4: Cerebrospinal fluid analysis.

Characteristics	Normal	Abnormal findings
1. Physical characteristics	• Clear and colorless • Volume: Around 150 mL • Specific gravity: 1.007 • Pressure: 76–200 mm H_2O	• Cloudy (presence of WBC/dead cells/microorganisms) when infected as in meningitis or encephalitis • **Xanthochromia:** Previous ICH • Increased in hydrocephalus • Increased in SAH, infection • **Increased ICP:** Meningitis, SAH, GBS • **Decreased ICP:** Abscess, tumor
2. CSF Proteins	16–45 mg/dL	Increased in meningitis, brain abscess, brain/spinal tumor, stroke neurosyphilis
3. WBC	0–5 cells/mm^3	• Increased in meningitis, multiple sclerosis, tumors • Neutrophils increased in bacterial infection • Lymphocytes increased in viral infection • Eosinophils increased in parasitic infection
4. Glucose	40–80 mg/dL (2/3rd concentration of blood glucose)	Deceased in inflammation, increased in SAH
5. Lactate	10–20 mg/dL	Increased in bacterial or fungal meningitis
6. CSF culture and sensitivity	Sterile	• Bacterial/viral/fungal infection • CSF AFB smear positive for TB meningitis
7. CSF VDRL	Absent	Positive with neurosyphilis
8. CSF CRP	Normal	Increased in bacterial meningitis

(CSF: cerebrospinal fluid; ICH: intracranial hemorrhage; ICP: intracranial pressure; SAH: subarachnoid hemorrhage; WBC: white blood cell; CRP: C-reactive protein; VDRL: venereal disease research laboratory; SAH: subarachnoid hemorrhage; GBS: Guillain-Barré syndrome; AFB: acid-fast bacteria)

- Avoid strenuous exercise for a day or two depending upon general condition of the patient.
- Advised to drink plenty of fluids for next two days.
- Headache is a common side effect after the procedure, with varying intensity due to leakage of CSF from the site of puncture or mainly pertinent to spinal root irritation.

Complications

- **Trauma** is one of the initials occurring complication as the procedure starts.
- Next, we see the presence of **bleeding** evident in the CSF sample itself when the test is initially starts to commence, subsequently the CSF sample becomes clear. If it is persistent then there might be chances of SAH.
- Patient commonly experience **postdural puncture headache (PDPH) after** the procedure is over. It is identified by the manifestation of a headache in combination with substantial orthostatic component within five days of a lumbar puncture. Few of the nursing interventions are discussed in the section of postprocedure care. Atraumatic needles are recommended to avoid or minimize the PDPH.

Myelography

It is also an invasive investigative procedure to visualize the spinal canal precisely from the cervical subarachnoid space to lumbar with the view to identify the following:
- Spinal cord lesions: Tumor/abscess/vascular abnormalities
- Displacement of the vertebral bone/bones
- Prolapsed intervertebral disc or herniation
  - Intervertebral disc extrusion (IVDE)
  - Intervertebral disc protrusion (IVDP)
  - Acute noncompressive nucleus pulposus extrusion (ANNPE)
  - Hydrated nucleus pulposus extrusion (HNPE)
  - Intradural/intramedullary intervertebral disc extrusion (IIVDE)

With advancements in MRI, the use of myelography has become limited. Only done for the patients for whom MRI is contraindicated and the thecal sac visualization is essential. It is primarily done to visualize any partial or complete obstruction of CSF flow or the contrast medium. The procedure takes 60–90 minutes and can be done in the neurological OPD.

Before Myelography

Patient is advised NPO/skip the meal previous to the procedure. Educate the patient to drink around 3,000 mL water or fluids for next 24 hours. Patient is also informed to keep the head end elevated after the procedure as diffusion of contrast should not reach the cranial vault which may lead to seizures.

Procedure

Usually a lateral knee-chest position is recommended. The surface markings are done and cleaned with antiseptic agents. Aseptic technique is strictly maintained at all times. Lumbar puncture set and contrast medium are essential equipment for the procedure.

Starts with giving local anesthesia and then a lumbar puncture (refer to the procedure discussed earlier), approximately 10 mL of CSF is removed after the LP needle is placed in the correct intervertebral space. Subsequently 10 mL of water-soluble contrast medium is slowly injected. This enhances the imaging of the spine when seen on CT/X-ray when taken in series. Once the dye is injected, it disperses upward through CSF and uptakes into nerve roots.

After Myelography

- Neurological assessment and monitoring of vital signs are continued till patient is discharged.
- Head end elevation of 30° and stringently following bed rest for six to eight hours is expected from the patient.
- The room is kept less noisy, without bright lights and temperature regulated.
- Patient is expected to avoid rigorous activities or walking.
- Head end is kept elevated for nearly half a day after myelography.
- Fluid intake should be increased to 3,000 mL/day for next 48 hours.
- In absence of nausea or vomiting and after 3–4 hours, patient can start taking orally.
- Patient is advised to report for abnormalities like increased in temperature, signs of meningeal irritation (nausea, vomiting, nuchal rigidity, pain or spasm of back, irritability), difficulty in urination.
- Symptomatic treatment of nausea, vomiting, headache should be done on priority.

Side effects of contrast medium: Elderly patients are more at the risk.
- Seizures
- Delirium, confusion, hallucinations
- Chest pain
- Obstruction of VP shunt

Positron Emission Tomography (PET)

Two- or three-dimensional images of brain activity are captured after injecting low molecular weight radioactive isotopes (tracer) with shorter half-life, into the circulation. It uses dual annihilation/extinction photons for image creation. The test is mostly conducted at tertiary or quaternary healthcare facilities, with the help of specialized technicians. After injecting the tracer, the patient should be lying inside a scanner, sensor perceives the emitted gamma rays. Precisely the tracer uptake by the brain parenchyma is measured and data processing is done by computer and results are displayed to make predictions of disorders as follows:
- Measure the metabolism level of cells or tissues
- Detect brain parenchymal tumors/lesions
- Convulsion disorders
- Memory disorders
- Changes in the brain after occurrence of an injury
- Motor neuron disorder
- Parkinson's disease
- Alzheimer's disease
- Stroke
- Epilepsy
- Neuropsychiatric disorders

It takes lengthier time for the procedure to be conducted; the patient has to wait for 45 minutes to one hour for uptake of the tracer. Then the scan begins and continues for 45 minutes to one hour. As it involves injection of radioactive substances and special scanning machines like linear accelerator, hence it is expensive and rare diagnostic.

Single Photon Emission Computed Tomography (SPECT) Scan

It is a nuclear medicine imaging modality which helps in additional estimation of certain brain functionality by more advanced nuclear imaging test. It uses radiopharmaceuticals for localization of lesions and mostly similar to PET scan in terms of the procedure. It is recommended as an additional test after the MRI is done for more accuracy and precision for complex diagnosis.

Following diagnosis can be done:
- Brain tumors
- Seizure impact on various brain parts. It helps to localization the area of epileptic seizure origin before the surgery.
- Degenerative spinal disorders
- Stress fractures
- Neuropsychiatric disorders
- Staging of Parkinson's disease

A dopamine transporter imaging with single-photon emission computed tomography (DaT-SPECT) scan may be recommended to aid in diagnosing Parkinson disease. During a SPECT scan, the patient lies on a sliding table of a scanner while a gamma camera rotates around the head and captures the images where the radioisotope has traveled. That information is converted by computer into cross-sections that are stacked to produce a detailed three-dimensional image of tracer within the brain. SPECT is very comparable to PET in its use of radioactive tracer and detection of γ-rays. The differences in both the diagnostic tests are depicted in **Table 28.5**.

Before PET/SPECT Scan

Instruct patient to fast overnight before the test, though water intake is allowed. Avoid dextrose saline as intravenous infusion as results may show discrepancy.

After a PET/SPECT Scan

The patient is instructed to drink ample number of glasses of water and fluids to flush the radioactive substances out of the body. Also instruct to double flush the toilets after use until 48 hours have passed after the test.

Electromyography (EMG)

It is a diagnostic test which records the electrical activity in the skeletal muscles.

Indications

- Disorders of nerve (carpel tunnel syndrome)
- Disorders of muscle (muscular dystrophy)
- Spinal nerve root compression (herniated interverbal disc)
- Motor neuron disorder (amyotrophic lateral sclerosis)
- Peripheral nerve damage (motor neuronopathy, sensory ganglionopathy or neuropathy)
- Demyelinating neuropathies

In the above-mentioned disorders, eventually there is damage in the muscle or the motor nerves which supply the muscles leading to development of abnormal electrical impulses.

Before Electromyography

- No NPO is required, only patient is asked to withhold anticoagulants as there are chances of some bruising or fine bleeding.
- Patient is also informed that they might experience slight discomfort or pain.
- Physician should be informed by patient about the implanted pacemaker before the test is scheduled.

Procedure

Insertion of very fine needles or wires are done into the muscles to capture the electrical impulses during resting phase or active movement phase. The needles are connected to the wires and on the other side connected to the EMG machine which records the impulses and generates graphical representation. Duration of the study is approximately 60–90 minutes depending on the number of nerves or muscles involved.

After Procedure

The needles are gently removed. Observations are made for bruising or bleeding. Patient is informed to report back in case of continued bleeding or pain.

Nerve Conduction Velocity (NCV)

The test helps to gauze:
- The nerve's capacity to send a signal
- Speed at which the nerve sends the signal
- Size of the nerve signal.
- It helps to detect similar disorders as done by EMG.

Before Nerve Conduction Velocity

Patient is instructed not to apply any moisturizer (lotion, cream or oil) over the skin surface after bath on the day of the procedure. Instruct to avoid consumption of sweetened beverages or caffeine, smoking, at least two to three hours prior to test. Physician should be informed by patient about the implanted pacemaker before the test is planned.

TABLE 28.5: Difference between SPECT and PET scans.

SPECT scan	PET scan
• Less expensive, affordable	• More expensive
• SPECT emit only a single γ-ray during decay that is measured directly	• PET emit dual/multiple γ-ray during decay
• Nuclides used in SPECT have a longer half-life	• Nuclides/isotopes used in PET scan have shorter half-life
• Easily available in most of the hospitals	• Few hospitals have the PET scan facility as it requires advanced machines, setup, and skillful technicians

Procedure

A set of recording electrodes is attached over the skin just above the muscles. Wires connect the electrodes to an EMG machine. A small electrical pulse (similar to the sensation of static electricity) is discharged on the skin so as to stimulate the nerve to the muscle or skin. The electrical signal is viewed on the EMG machine. Reports are then verified for the presence of any nerve damage or muscle disease. This test has advantage over EMG as it does not cause any discomfort/pain/bleeding. Mostly it in done in conjunction with EMG.

Cerebral Angiography

Cerebral angiography is an invasive, routine, neurodiagnostic procedure which offers high-resolution, three-dimensional, pathoanatomical data about the cerebral vasculature and also facilitates real-time analysis of cerebral circulation. It is recognized as the gold standard for outlining vascular lesions of the brain (or sometimes for spine). Angiograms are regularly executed in a hospital outpatient or inpatient setting and may take up to 3 hours, followed by a 6- to 8-hour resting period. A spinal angiogram is used to detect blockage of arteries or blood vessels malformations in the vessels to the spinal cord.

Indications

- Cerebral aneurysms
- Basilar occlusion
- Carotid stenosis
- Arteriovenous malformation

Prior to Procedure

- Nil by mouth for 8–12 hours
- Informed written consent
- Removal of dentures, glasses
- Hospital gown to be worn
- **Insertion site preparation:** Shaving, antiseptic treatment
- Nurse evaluates baseline vitals and neurological status
- Distal pulses are marked

Procedure

The patient is expected to wear a hospital gown. In this procedure, patient is sedated and also given local anesthesia prior commencing. Once the patient is settled, a catheter is inserted into the venous circulation following aseptic precautions. Traditionally, a transfemoral access is performed but recent days the neuro interventionalists are accessing left-sided transradial approach, as it is more precisely possible, safe with minimal complications and an effective substitute. Once the catheter is stabilized into the blood access, dye is slowly injected into cerebral circulation and multiple images are taken for diagnosing the following:

- Detect blockage or narrowing/stenosis of cerebral blood vessels
- Determine the location and size of an aneurysm
- Thrombosis
- Vasospasm
- Stroke
- Arteriovenous malformations
- Show the blood supply of a tumor prior to surgery or embolectomy

After the Procedure

- Once the procedure is completed, the catheter sheath is removed and direct manual pressure or by mechanical pressure (sand bag) is applied on the needle insertion site. This prevents bleeding. Ice packs are also effective in controlling bleeding by vasoconstriction.
- Patient is advised bed rest for 8–12 hours.
- Vitals signs are evaluated frequently for initial half an hour.
- Monitor for the neurovascular status of the distal extremities: Sensation, warmth, color, pedal pulse, capillary refill.
- Observe puncture site for bleeding or bruises.
- Patient is also advised to flush the contrast medium out of body by increasing the water or fluid intake to around 3–4 L. Simultaneously a stringent intake and output record should be maintained.

Complications

- Allergic response to contrast medium
- Embolic stroke
- Hematoma at the catheter insertion site
- Pulmonary embolism
- Contrast medium induced:
  - Nephropathy
  - *Encephalopathy:* Tonic-clonic seizures
  - Transient hemiparesis and aphasia

Some of the advanced neurological centers have facility of digital subtraction angiography (DSA) which helps to identify occlusions, stenosis or plaques of the cerebral blood vessels, vascular defects, postoperative assessment of anastomosis of cerebral vessels, and clipping of aneurysms.

Biopsy

Biopsy comprises the removal and investigation of a small piece of tissue from the body. Muscle/nerve biopsies are used to diagnose neuromuscular disorders. A small sample of muscle or nerve is removed under local anesthetic (pain-relieving medication) and studied under a microscope. The muscle sample may be removed either surgically, through a slit made in the skin, or by needle biopsy, in which a thin hollow needle is inserted through the skin and into the muscle. A piece of the nerve may be removed through a small surgical incision in proximity to the ankle, or occasionally close the wrist. Muscle and nerve biopsies are usually executed in an outpatient testing facility. A skin biopsy can be used to measure small nerve fibers or to test for certain metabolic disorders. A small piece of skin is removed under local anesthesia, generally in an OPD. A brain biopsy, used to determine tumor type or certain infections, requires surgery to remove a small piece of the brain or tumor. A brain biopsy is an invasive procedure that carries its own risks.

Case Scenario

1. A 64-year-old man, known case of uncontrolled type 2 diabetes mellitus, hypertension, and hyperlipidemia.
   Presented with:
   – Right upper and lower extremity weakness, accompanying with facial drop and slurred speech starting nearly 2.5 hours prior to the presentation.
   – No reporting/evidence of visual disturbance, headache, chest pain, palpitations, dyspnea, dysphagia, fever, dizziness, loss of consciousness, bowel or urinary incontinence, or trauma.
   – Significant history of cigarette smoking (1 pack per day for 15 years).
   – No significant family history. In the emergency department, his vital signs were stable.
   Assessment:
   – Right-sided facial droop
   – Dysarthria
   – Right-sided hemiplegia
   – National Institutes of Health Stroke Scale (NIHSS) score was calculated as 7
   Recommended diagnostic: Routine blood test and MRI head.
   Findings: MRI of the head revealed an acute 1.7 cm infarct of the left periventricular white matter and posterior left basal ganglia.
   Diagnosis: Acute ischemic cerebrovascular accident (CVA).
   Plan for treatment: Patient is suitable for thrombolytics as symptoms started within 4.5 hours of presentation.

2. A 19-year-old college student, came to the emergency department with chief complains of severe headache and skin rash.
   History of present illness
   – She had sore throat in the previous week and experienced nausea and vomiting since last two days.
   – She noticed "spots" on his arms, legs, trunk, and abdomen.
   – Just before her presentation to the emergency department, she developed fatigue, headache, neck pain, and photophobia.
   Past medical history: No significant illness/surgery.
   Family history: Non-contributory.
   Physical exam:
   Vital signs: Temperature, 36.8°C; **heart rate:** 112/minute; **respiratory rate:** 24/minute; **blood pressure:** 90/40 mm Hg.
   Pertinent physical exam findings included: Tachycardia, hypotension, and purpuric lesions on his arms, legs, trunk.
   Neurological assessment:
   – *Appearance:* Ill looking
   – Oriented
   – Presence of nuchal rigidity, positive, Brudzinski and Kernig signs
   Recommended diagnostics:
   – *Blood tests:* CBC, blood culture
   – Lumbar puncture was contraindicated due to purpura rashes.
   – Echocardiography
   – Chest X-ray
   Findings
   – *Blood test:*
     ♦ Platelets: 87×10^9/L
     ♦ PTT: 84.1
     ♦ PT: 20
     ♦ INR: 1.8
     ♦ D-dimer: 23.4 (High)
     ♦ Fibrinogen :107 (Low)
     ♦ Blood culture: Positive, presence of *Neisseria meningitidis*
   – *Echocardiography:* Mild left ventricular enlargement with decreased EF of 30%
   – *A chest X-ray:* Pulmonary edema.
   Diagnosis: Meningitis and disseminated intravascular coagulation (DIC)

SUMMARY

The chapter dealt in detail about commonly done diagnostic tests for validating the findings of neurological assessment and confirmation of the neurological disorders. All the diagnostic tests were discussed under two broad headings, namely noninvasive and invasive diagnostics. The chapter has also covered specific blood or spinal fluid test to endorse the findings. Main emphasis is extended to enhance the cognizance of the nurses pertinent to patient preparation, after-procedure care, complications and its care and patient-family education. Once the nurse is skilful in performing the patient assessment, knowing aptly about diagnostic findings and monitoring, it facilitates early stabilization in acute/emergency condition, providing comprehensive and subsequently fastens rehabilitation.

MULTIPLE CHOICE QUESTIONS

1. Absolute contraindication for proceeding with lumbar puncture:
   a. Papilledema
   b. Severe neck stiffness
   c. Age >65 years
   d. Large cerebellar tumor with surround edema

2. Diagnostic tests for epilepsy include all of the following, *except*:
   a. Simple blood tests   b. EEG
   c. Brain scan   d. Wada test

3. A 24-year-old woman is admitted to hospital having experienced a fit. Her mother states it lasted for around 90 secs, during which she fell to the ground and had involuntary 'jerking' movements of her arms and legs. She was unconscious during this time. She does not take regular medication, however states that this kind of episode has been happening to her once every 6 to 8 months, for the past 2.5 years. The last episode was similar, though accompanied by incontinence of urine. How will be the diagnosis confirmed?
   a. Clinical diagnosis
   b. CT head
   c. MRI head
   d. Standard EEG

4. A 69-year-old woman presents with 'a terrible headache'. It has been going on for about two or three days now. She has been feeling generally unwell alongside this, with fever. She noticed increased pain when brushing her hair this morning. What would be the most appropriate initial investigation?
   a. CT head   b. C-reactive protein
   c. ESR   d. Lumbar puncture

5. A 42-year-old lady who has presented with headache. He describes it as 'thumping' all over and the worst headache he has ever had. He has occasional migraines but is normally fit and well. He drinks 10 units a week and has smoked 10 cigarettes a day for 20 years. Neurological examination is normal. What is the most appropriate initial investigation?
   a. CT head scan with contrast
   b. CT head scan without contrast
   c. Lumbar puncture
   d. MRI head

ANSWERS

1. a   2. a   3. a   4. c
5. b

SUGGESTED READING

1. Abbasi Gharibkandi N, Hosseinimehr SJ. Radiotracers for imaging of Parkinson's disease. Eur J Med Chem. 2019;15;166:75-89. doi: 10.1016/j.ejmech.2019.01.029. Epub 2019 Jan 14. PMID: 30685535.
2. Alakbarzade V, Pereira AC. Cerebral catheter angiography and its complications. Pract Neurol. 2018;18(5):393-8. doi: 10.1136/practneurol-2018-001986. Epub 2018 Jul 18. PMID: 30021800.
3. Alstadhaug KB, Odeh F, Baloch FK, Berg DH, Salvesen R. Post-lumbar puncture headache. Tidsskr Nor Laegeforen. 2012;132(7):818-21. English, Norwegian. doi: 10.4045/tidsskr.11.0832. PMID: 22511093.
4. Askamp J, van Putten MJ. Mobile EEG in epilepsy. Int J Psychophysiol. 2014;91(1):30-5. doi: 10.1016/j.ijpsycho.2013.09.002. Epub 2013 Sep 20. PMID: 24060755.
5. Barros G, Bass DI, Osbun JW, Chen SH, Brunet MC, Peterson EC, et al. Left transradial access for cerebral angiography. J Neurointerv Surg. 2020;12(4):427-30. doi: 10.1136/neurintsurg-2019-015386. Epub 2019 Oct 24. PMID: 31649205.
6. Berrih-Aknin S, Frenkian-Cuvelier M, Eymard B. Diagnostic and clinical classification of autoimmune myasthenia gravis. J Autoimmun. 2014;48-49:143-8. doi: 10.1016/j.jaut.2014.01.003. Epub 2014 Feb 13. PMID: 24530233.
7. Blennow K, Zetterberg H. Biomarkers for Alzheimer's disease: current status and prospects for the future. J Intern Med. 2018;284(6):643-63. doi: 10.1111/joim.12816. Epub 2018 Aug 19. PMID: 30051512.
8. Bot JC, Barkhof F, Polman CH, Lycklama à Nijeholt GJ, de Groot V, Bergers E, et al. Spinal cord abnormalities in recently diagnosed MS patients: added value of spinal MRI examination. Neurology. 2004;62(2):226-33. doi: 10.1212/ wnl.62.2.226. PMID: 14745058.
9. da Costa RC, De Decker S, Lewis MJ, Volk H; Canine Spinal Cord Injury Consortium (CANSORT-SCI). Diagnostic imaging in intervertebral disc disease. Front Vet Sci. 2020;7:588338. doi: 10.3389/fvets.2020.588338. PMID: 33195623; PMCID: PMC7642913.
10. Davis A, Dobson R, Kaninia S, Giovannoni G, Schmierer K. Atraumatic needles for lumbar puncture: why haven't neurologists changed? Pract Neurol. 2016;16(1):18-22. doi: 10.1136/practneurol-2014-001055. Epub 2015 Sep 8. PMID: 26349834.
11. Dimoka A. How to Conduct a Functional Magnetic Resonance (fMRI) Study in Social Science Research. MIS Quarterly. 2012; 36(3)3:811-40. Accessed March 29, 2021. http://www.jstor.org/stable/41703482.
12. EurekAlert!. Blood test detects Alzheimer's damage before symptoms. 2019.https://www.eurekalert.org/pub_releases/2019-01/ wuso-btd011719.php
13. Haas D, Biomarker for Alzheimer's Disease, Ch15, Hans-Peter Deigner, Matthias Kohl,pg 333-49. https://doi.org/10.1016/B978-0-12-805364-5.00015-9
14. Hsu SY, Yeh LR, Chen TB, Du WC, Huang YH, Twan WH. Classification of the multiple stages of Parkinson's disease by a deep convolution neural network based on 99mTc-TRODAT-1 SPECT images. Molecules. 2020;19;25(20):4792. doi: 10.3390/ molecules25204792. PMID: 33086589; PMCID: PMC7587595.
15. https://www.gwengagedesign.com/portfolio/lumbar-puncture-device-2/
16. Julián-Jiménez A, Morales-Casado MI. Usefulness of blood and cerebrospinal fluid laboratory testing to predict bacterial meningitis in the emergency department. Neurologia. 2019;34(2):105-13. English, Spanish. doi: 10.1016/j.nrl.2016.05.009. Epub 2016 Jul 26. PMID: 27469578.
17. Kane NM, Oware A. Nerve conduction and electromyography studies. J Neurol. 2012;259(7):1502-8. doi: 10.1007/s00415- 012-6497-3. Epub 2012 May 22. PMID: 22614870.
18. Kishk NA, Ebraheim AM, Ashour AS, Badr NM, Eshra MA. Optic nerve sonographic examination to predict raised intracranial pressure in idiopathic intracranial hypertension: The cut-off points. Neuroradiol J. 2018;31(5):490-5. doi: 10.1177/1971400918789385. Epub 2018 Jul 19. PMID: 30024291; PMCID: PMC6136137.
19. Lin CH, Li CH, Yang KC, Lin FJ, Wu CC, Chieh JJ. A biomarker for disease severity and progression in Parkinson disease. Neurology. 2019;93(11):e1104-e1111. doi: 10.1212/WNL.0000000000008088. Epub 2019 Aug 16. PMID: 31420461.
20. Lu FM, Yuan Z. PET/SPECT molecular imaging in clinical neuroscience: recent advances in the investigation of CNS diseases. Quant Imaging Med Surg. 2015;5(3):433-47. doi: 10.3978/j.issn.2223-4292.2015.03.16. PMID: 26029646; PMCID: PMC4426104.
21. Lutters B, Groen RJM, Koehler PJ. Myelography and the 20th Century Localization of Spinal Cord Lesions. Eur Neurol. 2020;83(4):447-52. doi: 10.1159/000509863. Epub 2020 Sep 1. PMID: 32871581; PMCID: PMC7592936.
22. Masjedi M, Khosravi A, Sabetian G, Rahmanian MR. Incidental intrathecal injection of meglumine diatrizoate. Iran Red Crescent Med J. 2014;16(5):e9661. doi: 10.5812/ircmj.9661. Epub 2014 May 5. PMID: 25031869; PMCID: PMC4082529.
23. Mheich A, Dufor O, Yassine S, Kabbara A, Biraben A, Wendling F, et al. HD-EEG for tracking sub-second brain dynamics during cognitive tasks. Sci Data. 2021;8:32. https://doi.org/10.1038/s41597-021-00821-1
24. Nayak CS, Anilkumar AC. EEG Normal waveforms. [Updated 2020 Jul 31]. In: StatPearls [Internet]. Treasure Island (FL): StatPearls Publishing; 2021.
25. Onishi S, Sakamoto S, Okazaki T, Kurisu K. Iodinated contrast encephalopathy after coil embolization of unruptured aneurysms. Asian J Neurosurg. 2018;13(3):858-60. doi: 10.4103/ajns.AJNS_334_16. PMID: 30283566; PMCID: PMC6159015.
26. Patel DM, Weinberg BD, Hoch MJ. CT myelography: clinical indications and imaging findings. Radiographics. 2020;40(2):470-84. doi: 10.1148/rg.2020190135. Epub 2020 Feb 14. PMID: 32058837.
27. Ridler C. Alzheimer disease: Blood amyloid-β successfully signals AD. Nat Rev Neurol. 2018;14(4):195. doi: 10.1038/ nrneurol.2018.19. Epub 2018 Feb 16. PMID: 29449699.
28. Sanaei Dashti A, Alizadeh S, Karimi A, Khalifeh M, Shoja SA. Diagnostic value of lactate, procalcitonin, ferritin, serum-C-reactive protein, and other biomarkers in bacterial and viral meningitis: A cross-sectional study. Medicine (Baltimore). 2017;96(35):e7637. doi: 10.1097/MD.0000000000007637. PMID: 28858084; PMCID: PMC5585478.
29. Shen LH, Liao MH, Tseng YC. Recent advances in imaging of dopaminergic neurons for evaluation of neuropsychiatric disorders. J Biomed Biotechnol. 2012:2593-49. doi: 10.1155/2012/259349. Epub 2012 Apr 10. PMID: 22570524; PMCID: PMC3335602.
30. Shokrollahi MR, Shabanzadeh K, Noorbakhsh S, Tabatabaei A, Movahedi Z, Shamshiri AR. Diagnostic value of CRP, procalcitonin, and ferritin levels in cerebrospinal fluid of children with meningitis. Cent Nerv Syst Agents Med Chem. 2018;18(1):58-62. doi: 10.2174/1871524916666160302103223. PMID: 26931764.)
31. Silva NA, Goldstein IM. Obstruction of ventriculoperitoneal shunt after myelography-report of a unique case and its treatment. World Neurosurg. 2020;134:443-7. doi: 10.1016/j. wneu.2019.11.067. Epub 2019 Nov 20. PMID: 31756508.
32. Siuly S, Zhang Y. Medical big data: neurological diseases diagnosis through medical data analysis. Data Sci Eng. 2016;1:54-64. https://doi.org/10.1007/s41019-016-0011-3
33. Somers B, Long CJ, Francart T. EEG-based diagnostics of the auditory system using cochlear implant electrodes as sensors.

Scientific Reports. 2021;11(1):5383. DOI: 10.1038/s41598-021-84829-y.
34. Steinborn M, Friedmann M, Makowski C, Hahn H, Hapfelmeier A, Juenger H. High resolution transbulbar sonography in children with suspicion of increased intracranial pressure. Childs Nerv Syst. 2016;32(4):655-60. doi: 10.1007/s00381-015-3001-2. Epub 2016 Jan 13. PMID: 26759020.
35. The Clinical Practice of Neurological and Neurosurgical Nursing. Joanne V. Hickey. Lippincott Williams & Wilkins. 6th edition pp.93-115.
36. Tripathi M, Kumar A, Bal C. Neuroimaging in Parkinsonian Disorders. Neurol India. 2018;66 (Supplement):S68-S78. doi: 10.4103/0028-3886.226460. PMID: 29503329.
37. Walter U, Niehaus L, Probst T, Benecke R, Meyer BU, Dressler D. Brain parenchyma sonography discriminates Parkinson's disease and atypical parkinsonian syndromes. Neurology. 2003;60(1):74-7. doi: 10.1212/WNL.60.1.74
38. You S, Ou Z, Zhang W, Zheng D, Zhong C, Dong. Combined utility of white blood cell count and blood glucose for predicting in-hospital outcomes in acute ischemic stroke. J Neuroinflammation. 2019;16(1):37. doi: 10.1186/s12974-019-1422-7. PMID: 30764852; PMCID: PMC6375165.
39. Yıldırım N, Varol A. A research on estimation of emotion using EEG signals and brain computer interfaces 2017 International Conference on Computer Science and Engineering (UBMK), Antalya, Turkey; 2017. pp. 1132-36, doi: 10.1109/UBMK.2017.8093523.

CHAPTER 29

Management of Common Problems in Neuroscience Patients

Pooja Thakur

"The human brain is probably one of the most complex single objects on the face of the earth; I think it is, quite honestly."
—**Bill Viola**

Learning Objectives

After going through the chapter, the learner will be able to:
- Define the altered level of consciousness and increased intracranial pressure.
- Describe the etiology of the altered level of consciousness and increased intracranial pressure.
- Identify the stages of the altered level of consciousness.
- Describe the pathophysiology of altered level of consciousness and increased intracranial pressure.
- Enumerate the clinical manifestations and complications of patients with altered consciousness level and increased intracranial pressure.
- Discuss the medical management for patients with altered level of consciousness and increased intracranial pressure.
- Explain the surgical management of patients with increased intracranial pressure.
- Discuss the nursing management of patients with altered level of consciousness and increased intracranial pressure.
- Understand various types of intracranial surgeries.
- Discuss the nursing management of the patients undergoing intracranial surgeries.

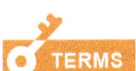

TERMS

- **Altered levels of consciousness:** Decreased wakefulness, awareness, or alertness.
- **Aneurysm:** Weakening of an artery wall leading to a bulge, or distention of the artery.
- **Arrhythmia:** Problem with the rate or rhythm of the heartbeat.
- **Benzodiazepines:** Drugs primarily used for treating anxiety, but may also be used in treating several other conditions.
- **Brain herniation:** Displacement of a portion of the brain because of increased pressure inside the skull.
- **Capsulotomy:** A psychosurgical intervention for anxiety disorders and obsessive–compulsive disorders that are resistant to conventional treatments.
- **Cingulotomy:** A procedure in which tissue in the anterior cingulate region is targeted and altered in a very focused manner.
- **Coma:** A state of prolonged unconsciousness wherein a person cannot be woken up even to painful stimuli, light, or sound.
- **Craniectomy:** Removal of a part of the skull to relieve pressure in the brain.
- **Hydrocephalus:** Imbalance between the production and absorption of CSF leading to enlarged ventricles.
- **Intraventricular pressure:** One of the most important measurements for evaluating cardiac function.
- **Reticular activating system:** A component of the reticular formation in vertebrate brains located throughout the brainstem.
- **Transcranial doppler flow tests:** A diagnostic procedure using sound waves to detect medical problems that affect blood flow in the brain. It can detect stroke caused by blood clots, narrowed sections of blood vessels, vasospasm due to a subarachnoid hemorrhage, tiny blood clots, and more.
- **Urinary retention:** Inability to voluntarily void urine.

ALTERED LEVEL OF CONSCIOUSNESS (ALOC)

Normal brain activity needs a continual supply of oxygen and glucose. If this supply is disrupted, the person will lose consciousness in a matter of seconds and may suffer lasting brain damage. ALOC is a state of diminished attentiveness or inability to arouse and a lack of awareness of one's surroundings. Alteration in one's state of awareness could be the outcome of several pathophysiologic events. Changes in the brain's chemical environment (for example, exposure to toxins or intoxicants), insufficient oxygen or blood flow in the brain, and excessive pressure within the skull can all result in altered levels of consciousness. Prolonged unconsciousness is recognized as an indicator of a medical emergency. A decrease in awareness indicates that both cerebral hemispheres or the reticular activating system have been affected. A lower state of consciousness is associated with greater morbidity and mortality. Consciousness is a vital indicator of a patient's medical and neurological health.

CONCEPT AND DEFINITION

The normal state of consciousness includes either the level of wakefulness, awareness, or alertness in which most people function when they are awake or one of the known stages of normal sleep from which the individual may be easily woken. Level of consciousness is a measurement of a person's sensitivity to environmental stimuli. Any measure of arousal or alertness that is not normal is considered an altered level of awareness. A moderately reduced degree of awareness is categorized as lethargy, a state in which a person may be awakened easily. Obtunded people are sad and cannot be completely aroused. Stuporous people are those who cannot be awakened from a deep slumber. Coma is the incapacity to respond purposefully. The Glasgow coma scale and other scales have been developed to assess the state of consciousness.

EPIDEMIOLOGY

Patients with impaired consciousness continue to provide a diagnostic problem in both the prehospital and emergency settings (ER). ER hospitalizations for unconscious patients account for 0.4–1% of total admissions. In Japan, a prevalence rate of around 18.8 persons/per million population at the moment has been reported. The crude prevalence rate ranged from 967–4,070 per 100,000 people, with an average of 2394 per 100,000 population. In India, where there are currently 1.27 billion people, it is believed that 30 million of them experience neurological problems.

ETIOLOGY

Systemic infection, which encompassed infectious disorders but excluded CNS infection by CSF study, was the most common cause of the altered level of consciousness (e.g., septic shock and sepsis). Examples of metabolic causes include hypoglycemia, DKA, hyponatremia, uremic encephalopathy, and hyperammonemia. Except for TBI, the causes of stroke include cerebral infarction and intracranial hemorrhage. Myocardial infarction, ventricular tachycardia, aortic dissection, impending rupture of an aortic aneurysm, and cardiac tamponade are examples of cardiogenic and vascular causes. Seizures, including epileptic and psychogenic non-epileptic seizures, may also cause an altered level of consciousness. Hazardous substances that cause toxicity include pesticides, anaphylaxis, carbon monoxide, chemical agents, sedative overdoses, and adverse drug reactions (e.g., antiepileptic drugs). **Tables 29.1 and 29.2** depict various causes of altered level of consciousness.

TABLE 29.1: Causes of altered level of consciousness.

1. Neurogenic	2. Toxins	3. Drugs
• Unilateral hemispheric disease and brainstem herniation • Closed head injury (concussion or contusion) • Meningitis or encephalitis • Hypertensive encephalopathy • SAH, epidural hematoma, subdural hematoma, etc. • Ventriculoperitoneal shunt malfunction • CVA • Parkinsonism • Myasthenia gravis • Intracranial mass • Demyelinating disease (e.g., multiple sclerosis) • Seizure • Post-ictal state • Status epilepticus • Basilar artery occlusion • Brainstem tumor • Cerebellar hemorrhage • Pontine hemorrhage	• Carbon monoxide poisoning • Toxic alcohol ingestion (e.g., ethylene glycol, methanol) • Alcohol intoxication or alcohol withdrawal syndrome • Chronic salicylate toxicity • Anticholinergic drug toxicity • Neuroleptic malignant syndrome • Serotonin syndrome • Envenomation • Excited delirium (cocaine, methamphetamine, PCP, or other psychostimulant induced) • Opioid overdose • Benzodiazepine overdose	• Amphetamines • Anticholinergics • Anticonvulsants • Barbiturates • Benzodiazepines • Clonidine • Cocaine • Ethanol • Haloperidol • Narcotics • Phenothiazines • Salicylates • Selective serotonin uptake inhibitors (SSRIs) • Tricyclic antidepressants

Contd...

Contd...

4. **Gastrointestinal and renal** • Hepatic encephalopathy • Wernicke's encephalopathy • Uremic encephalopathy • Peritonitis	5. **Electrolyte disturbance** • Hypercalcemia • Hypermagnesemia • Hyponatremia • Hypernatremia • Hypophosphatemia	6. **Cardiopulmonary** • Hypoxia • Hypercarbia • Congestive heart failure (CHF) • Pulmonary embolus • Hypertensive encephalopathy

7. **Infectious**
• Meningitis or encephalitis
• Sepsis
• Urinary tract infection
• Pneumonia
• Severe viral infection (e.g., COVID-19)
	8. **Miscellaneous**
	• Heat stroke or malignant hyperthermia
	• Hypothermia
	• Vasculitis
	• Hyperviscosity syndromes (e.g., thrombotic thrombocytopenic purpura)
		9. **Endocrine**
		• Adrenal insufficiency (Addisonian crisis)
		• Diabetes mellitus
		  – hypoglycemia
		  – Diabetic ketoacidosis
		  – Hyperosmolar hyperglycemic nonketotic coma
		• Thyroid disease
		  – Myxedema coma (severe hypothyroidism)
		  – Thyroid storm

TABLE 29.2: Various mnemonics depicting causes of altered level of consciousness.

| A. **Mnemonic: AEIOU TIPS**
• **A**lcohol (or toxic alcohols) or abdominal aortic aneurysm
• **E**pilepsy (status epilepticus), electrolytes, hepatic encephalopathy, endocrine problems
• **I**nsulin (hypoglycemia), intussusception, or inborn errors of metabolism
• **O**piates or overdose
• **U**remia
• **T**rauma (head injury), temperature (hypothermia, hyperthermia), toxemia, brain tumor
• **I**nfections (sepsis, meningitis, encephalitis)
• **P**sychogenic, pulmonary embolism, poisoning (toxin ingestion)
• **S**pace occupying lesions, stroke, shock, seizure, shunt (ventriculoperitoneal) | B. **Mnemonic: I WATCH DEATH**
• **I**nfection
• **W**ithdrawal
• **A**cute metabolic causes
• **T**rauma
• **C**NS causes
• **H**ypoxia
• **D**eficiencies (nutritional)
• **E**ndocrinopathies (adrenal insufficiency, myxedema, hyperthyroidism)
• **A**cute vascular causes
• **T**oxins or drugs
• **H**eavy metals | C. **Mnemonic: SMASHED**
• **S**epsis or substrates (abnormal glucose, thiamine deficiency)
• **M**eningitis or mental illness (acute psychosis)
• **A**ccident (head trauma, CVA) or alcohol intoxication or withdrawal
• **S**eizing or stimulants
• **H**ypertension, hyperthyroidism, Hypercarbia, hypoxia or hypotension, hypothyroidism
• **E**lectrolytes (sodium, hypercalcemia) or encephalopathy
• **D**rugs (drug withdrawal, carbon monoxide, lithium, steroids, salicylates.) |

PATHOPHYSIOLOGY

❖ Normal awareness is maintained by certain regions of the cerebral cortex, thalamus, and brainstem. The role of the reticular formation in these is well established. Theoretically, a network of neural connections called the ascending reticular activating system receives sensory data from the reticular formation and sends it to the cerebral cortex through the thalamus and midbrain. This system is known to control wakefulness and sleep, therefore any disruptions to it from illness, injury, or metabolic changes may result in a change in consciousness.

❖ Diffuse insult to both cerebral hemispheres (metabolic/toxic/hypoxic/ischemic) or focal lesion affecting ascending reticular activating system (ARAS) located in the upper pons, midbrain, and diencephalon.

Disruption in the cells of the nervous system, neurotransmitters, or brain anatomy

Faulty impulse transmission, impeding communication within the brain or from the brain to other parts of the body

STAGES OF ALTERED LEVEL OF CONSCIOUSNESS

The abnormal state of consciousness is more difficult to define and characterize, as evidenced by many terms applied to altered states of consciousness by various observers. ***Clouding of consciousness*** is a very mild form of altered mental status in which the patient has inattention and reduced wakefulness **(Table 29.3)**.

CLINICAL MANIFESTATIONS

Symptoms that may be associated with decreased consciousness include:
❖ Loss of bowel or bladder function
❖ Poor balance and difficulty walking
❖ Dizziness
❖ Lightheadedness
❖ Irregular heartbeat
❖ Tachycardia
❖ Hypotension
❖ Sweating
❖ Generalized weakness

TABLE 29.3: Stages of altered level of consciousness.

Stages	Summary	Description
Conscious	Normal	People who can quickly state their name, location, date, or time are self-oriented
Confused	Disoriented; impaired thinking and responses	People are labeled as "obtuse" or, "confused" if they do not respond instantly with their name, location, and time. A puzzled individual may be confused, bewildered, and have difficulty following directions. Individuals with delayed thinking and memory loss are at risk. Sleep deprivation, hunger, allergies, environmental contaminants, prescription and nonprescription medications, and disease might all have a role
Delirious	Disoriented; restlessness, hallucinations, sometimes delusions	Delirious denotes a person who is agitated or restless and has a substantial lack of concentration
Somnolent	Sleepy	A somnolent person only makes chaotic motions or nonsensical mumbles as responses to stimuli
Obtunded	Decreased alertness; slowed psychomotor responses	Obtundation is characterized by fatigue, a loss of interest in one's surroundings, and slow reactions
Stuporous	Sleep-like state (not unconscious); little/no spontaneous activity	Stupor is a state of awareness where the sole reaction to painful stimuli is grimacing or pulling away
Comatose	Cannot be aroused; no response to stimuli	Comatose people do not react to stimuli; they do not gag or have corneal reactions, and they may not even have pupillary responses to light

DIAGNOSTIC EVALUATION

A thorough medical history and physical examination, including a detailed neurological evaluation, are required to diagnose and treat reduced consciousness. Level of consciousness (LOC) is also assessed using cough and gag reflexes.

Assessment

Examine the look, behavior, and any signs of trauma or chemical exposure. Check the posture, gait, and motor activity for the appropriateness of movement). Assess the patients for the baseline level of awareness and confirm the family members who are aware of it. Make use of various scales, such as AVPU (Alert, Verbal, Painful, Unresponsive) and/or the Glasgow Coma Scale to assess LOC. Common mnemonics used to help physicians construct a differential diagnosis and treatment plan for a patient are depicted in **Table 29.2**. These may not include all the reasons for the altered LOC but include a majority of the most prevalent ones.

The following information should also be gathered while collecting history from a patient with altered LOC:
- History of any trauma.
- When was the patient last seen normal?
- What is the patient's usual state of LOC?
- Was there a gradual or abrupt change in LOC?
- Any preceding symptoms, such as headache, seizure-like activity, aura, or depression?
- Any relevant environmental factors, such as exposure to extreme heat or cold or toxins etc.
- Evidence of any drug and use of alcohol.
- Inquire about patients' use of illicit substances, prescription medicines, or alcohol.
- History of any recent illness or preexisting conditions (e.g., diabetes, seizure disorder). Inform the doctor about any drugs the patient is taking, such as insulin or anticonvulsants.
- History of any mental illness.

A thorough physical examination can help rule out some of the causes, such as diabetic crises or arrhythmias, that can be treated right away. The following components should be included in the physical examination:
- **Look for a compromised airway:** It is reasonable to assume that every patient with an altered LOC has or will have a compromised airway.
- **Examine respiration:** Changes in respiration might show the source of the problem. Acidosis and other brain disorders can cause Cheyne-Stokes respirations. Hypoxia, pneumothorax, acidosis, drug toxicity, and midbrain lesions can all induce hyperventilation. Apneustic breathing has been associated with pons lesions caused by stroke, meningitis, hypoglycemia, or hypoxia. Ataxic breathing shows damage to the medulla and lower pons. Toxins or a chemical overdose might result in bradypnea or hypoventilation.
- **Assess pupils:** Check whether both pupils are equal and receptive to light. Dilated pupils, as well as pinpoint pupils, can be signs of certain toxidromes. Increased ICP and brain herniation can also alter pupil size and response.
- Conduct a thorough neurological examination, looking for alterations in motor or sensory function as well as speech anomalies.
- **Check blood glucose level:** Hypoglycemia especially in the elderly is one of the commonest causes of altered LOC.
- Look for incontinence.
- **Check the patient's temperature:** Both hypo- and hyperthermia may lead to altered LOC.
- Perform a full head-to-toe examination to look for any signs of trauma or any other abnormal findings.
- **Neurological evaluation:** Strength, sensation, balance, reflexes, and memory all need to be tested (Refer Chapter 27).

Various Diagnostics Tests

In addition to comprehensive medical history and physical examination, the following tests should be carried out:

- **Complete blood count (CBC):** This is done to determine whether the patient is anemic. An increased WBC count implies some infection or inflammation in the body.
- **Toxicology screen:** In this, a blood or urine sample is used to identify the presence and amounts of pharmaceuticals, illicit substances, and toxins in the system.
- Blood tests to evaluate sodium, potassium, chloride, and bicarbonate levels.
- **Liver function tests (LFT):** To assess the liver's health by evaluating levels of proteins, liver enzymes, or bilirubin in the blood.
- Electroencephalogram (EEG) to assess brain activity.
- Electrocardiogram (EKG) to evaluate the heart's electrical activity (heart rate and rhythm).
- **Chest X-ray:** To evaluate the heart and lungs.
- CT scan of the head for high-resolution images of the brain.
- MRI of the head to look for brain injuries or other brain disorders.

Various Scales Used to Assess LOC

Various scales used to assess LOC are the Glasgow coma scale; awake, receptive to verbal stimulation, sensitive to painful stimuli, or unresponsive (AVPU) scale; Grady Coma Scale (GDS); and Full Outline of Unresponsiveness (FOUR) scale.

- **Glasgow coma scale:** This is the most extensively used test for measuring LOC objectively. It is now widely used to assess people with brain injuries or altered degrees of consciousness. Responses to stimuli are analyzed, scored, and totaled to yield a total score on a scale of 3–15, with a lower score suggesting a lower degree of consciousness.
- **AVPU Scale:** This scale determines whether a person is awake, receptive to verbal stimulation, sensitive to painful stimuli, or unresponsive. A carer talks to or screams at the individual to assess voice response. A little painful stimulus, such as a pinch, is used to assess pain responsiveness; pain responses include groaning or withdrawing from the stimulus. Like the AVPU, the ACDU scale is simpler to use and has comparable accuracy. ACDU assesses alertness, disorientation, sleepiness, and unresponsiveness in patients.
- **Grady Coma Scale:** The Grady Coma Scale ranks persons from I to V according to their level of confusion, stupor, profound stupor, abnormal posture, and coma respectively.
- **Full Outline of Unresponsiveness (FOUR):** This scale was developed to assess consciousness in intubated trauma patients in whom all components of GCS cannot be assessed. It consists of four subscales, namely ocular, motor, brainstem reflex, and breathing pattern, with scores ranging from 0 to 4, and a total score ranging from 0 to 16.

MEDICAL MANAGEMENT

The initial line of treatment for patients with a changed LOC is to stabilize ABCs, protect the patient from additional injury (e.g., immobilizing the C-spine, if necessary), and address reversible causes as soon as feasible. Reversible causes include hypoglycemia, hypo-/hyperthermia, seizures, certain arrhythmias, opioid overdose, hypoxemia, and other shock states. In the absence of a reversible etiology, management should include cardiac monitoring, periodic review, and supportive therapy (e.g., oxygen, intravenous access, temperature control).

If the altered conscious level is determined to be caused by arrhythmia, a compromised airway, respiratory distress, shock, stroke, sepsis, an environmental or behavioral emergency, toxic substances, or trauma, it should be treated as per the respective Clinical Practice Guideline **(Box 29.1)**.

Management of Syncope

It is characterized as a momentary loss of consciousness followed by a near-immediate recovery of awareness when the patient lies down. The underlying cause, which might be arrhythmia, stroke, drunkenness, hypoglycemia, vagal stimulation, or pulmonary embolism, must be discovered.

If a cause is discovered, follow the Clinical Practice Guidelines to treat it. A 12-lead ECG should be performed on all persons suffering syncope. Benzodiazepines should be administered to patients who are suffering from seizures. Monitor blood glucose levels. Dextrose should be administered if the patient has hypoglycemia. If IV access is not accessible, glucagon should be given. During and after a seizure, patients are typically hypoxic. They may require supplemental oxygen or ventilatory support. Seizures can be caused by conditions, such as stroke, trauma, toxins, infection, and hypoxia. Treat these diseases in accordance with the Clinical Practice Guideline in effect.

It should be mentioned that seizures caused by alcohol withdrawal are potentially lethal. If the patient has recovered to their normal state, demonstrates capability, has someone to accompany them, has access to medical follow-up, and there is no sign of underlying trauma or infection, they may be permitted to go home. Discharge instructions should be provided clearly and patients should be motivated for regular follow-up.

BOX 29.1: The guidelines include the following treatment and interventions.

- **Airway:** Maintain the airway patent. Reposition the patient as per requirement.
- **Breathing:** Look for respiratory depression; check SPO_2, $ETCO_2$, and CO readings
- **Circulation:** Assess for signs of shock
- Assess LOC by making use of Glasgow coma score AVPU/FOUR
- Check pupils
- Look for neck rigidity or pain with range of motion
- Monitor blood glucose level
- EKG for arrhythmias
- **Assess breath odor:** Possible unusual odors include alcohol, acidosis, ammonia
- **Extremities/skin:** Hydration, edema, temperature

Management of Hypoglycemia

Hypoglycemia can occur as a result of several disorders (for example, sepsis, intoxication, or toxic exposure) and can mimic any other cause of altered LOC. Hypoglycemia should be treated as needed with dextrose, glucagon, or oral glucose. Patients with diabetes who return to normal may want to remain at home. These persons may do so as long as they realize the risks of staying at home and the hypoglycemia is caused by dietary changes or insulin doses that can be controlled at home.

Management of Hyperglycemia

Patients with hyperglycemia who have a changed LOC require hydration, insulin, and maybe vasopressors to be started in the hospital. The patients may exhibit the symptoms, such as weakness, nausea, vomiting, stomach pain, tachypnea, tachycardia, hypotension, indications of dehydration, and/or impaired mental status. These patients with hyperglycemia should get aggressive fluid resuscitation.

To achieve a SpO_2 greater than 92%, high-flow oxygen should also be supplied.

NURSING MANAGEMENT OF THE PATIENTS

Assessment

Start by analyzing the verbal response while assessing a patient who has an altered LOC. By figuring out the patient's orientation to time, people, and place, the verbal response is assessed. The patient is questioned about the time of day, the season of the year, where they are, and whether there are any visitors, family members, or medical professionals present. Other questions, such as "When is the next holiday?" might reveal more about the patient's cognitive processes. If the patient is intubated or has a tracheostomy, it should be carefully recorded.

The degree of consciousness of a patient is determined by their ability to open their eyes spontaneously or in response to a stimulus. Patients cannot do this task because of significant brain impairment. The nurse should look out for any injuries or periorbital edema that could prevent the patient from opening his/her eyes and should also record whether this interferes with eye-opening.

Motor responses include spontaneous, intentional movement (for instance, the aware patient can move all four extremities with equal force), movement only in response to noxious stimuli (for instance, pressure/pain), and abnormal posture. If the patient does not comply with instructions, the motor response is assessed by applying a painful stimulus to the nail bed or squeezing a muscle. Intentional or appropriate behavior is recognized patient pushes away or withdraws ("patient withdraws to unpleasant stimuli").

An intentional reaction occurs when the patient can switch their body's sides in response to unpleasant stimuli. An inappropriate or unintentional response is haphazard and purposeless. Deliberate or decorous postures are both acceptable. Flaccidity is a symptom of the most serious neurologic disability. Sometimes, if the patient has been administered pharmacological paralyzing medications, posturing cannot be induced.

In addition to LOC, the nurse continuously evaluates measures such as respiratory state, ocular signs, and reflexes.

Nursing Diagnoses

Based on the assessment data of a patient with altered LOC, following nursing diagnoses may be formulated:
- ❖ Ineffective airway clearance related to altered LOC
- ❖ Risk of injury related to altered LOC
- ❖ Deficient fluid volume related to alteration in oral intake
- ❖ Impaired oral mucous membranes related to mouth-breathing, absence of pharyngeal reflex, and altered fluid intake
- ❖ Risk for impaired skin integrity related to immobility
- ❖ Impaired tissue integrity of cornea related to diminished or absent corneal reflex
- ❖ Ineffective thermoregulation related to damage to the hypothalamic center
- ❖ Impaired urinary elimination (incontinence or retention) related to impairment in neurologic sensing and control
- ❖ Bowel incontinence related to impairment in neurologic sensing and control and also related to impaired nutrition
- ❖ Disturbed sensory perception related to neurologic impairment

Planning and Goals

Maintaining a clear airway, preventing injury, achieving fluid volume balance, maintaining intact oral mucous membranes, maintaining normal skin integrity, preventing corneal irritation, achieving effective thermoregulation, and achieving effective urinary elimination are the objectives of care for the patient with altered LOC. Maintaining bowel continence, correctly interpreting environmental cues, keeping a healthy family or support system, and averting issues are other goals.

The nursing care given might mean the difference between life and death since the unconscious patient's defense reflexes are compromised. Until the patient's basic reflexes—coughing, blinking, and swallowing—return and they become conscious and oriented, the nurse must be in charge of the patient to maintain continuity of care. Therefore, the main goal of nursing is to make up for the absence of these protective reactions.

Nursing Interventions

Maintaining the Airway

The provision of a proper airway and breathing is the most important element of treating a patient with altered LOC. There is a danger of airway blockage if the patient aspirates vomit or nasopharyngeal secretions or if the tongue and epiglottis relax, occluding the oropharynx.

A serious issue is created by the build-up of secretions in the throat. The risk of aspiration must be eliminated by removing these secretions since the patient cannot swallow and has no pharyngeal reflexes. Aspiration can be avoided by 30° elevating the head end side of the bed. It will also be beneficial to place the patient in a lateral or semi-prone posture, which allows the jaw and tongue to go forward and encourage secretion outflow.

Positioning on its own is not always sufficient. Suctioning and dental care may be crucial for the patient. Suction is used to remove secretions from the posterior pharynx and upper trachea. The thumb and fingers are rotated while being continuously suctioned to remove the catheter. By rotating the catheter, the suctioning end does not rub against the skin, which would otherwise cause damage to the mucosa, and bleeding. The patient is hyperoxygenated and hyperventilated both before and after suctioning to prevent hypoxia. In addition to these treatments, postural drainage and chest physiotherapy may be used to improve pulmonary hygiene, unless the patient's underlying condition forbids them. Additionally, the chest should be palpated at least once every eight hours to listen for breath sounds or the absence of them. Patients with impaired LOC typically need to be intubated and given mechanical respiration, regardless of these precautions or the severity of the impairment. Nursing interventions for patients who are mechanically ventilated include maintaining the patency of the endotracheal tube or tracheostomy, giving frequent oral care, watching arterial blood gas values, and maintaining ventilator settings.

Protecting the Patient

The patients should be provided with padded side rails. These should be raised at all times for the patient's safety. Priorities should include preventing harm from intrusive wires and equipment, as well as eliminating other possible causes of risk (e.g., restraints, tight dressings, environmental irritants, damp bedding or dressings, tubes, and drains). Appropriate precautions must be taken to prevent Medical Device-Related Pressure Injury (MDRPI). Protecting the patient's dignity throughout LOC changes is another aspect of protection. Simple gestures like providing isolation and conversing with the patient while providing nursing care assist to preserve the patient's humanity. Additionally, it is important to refrain from making negative remarks regarding the patient's health or outlook because people in mild comas could still be able to hear. The nurse must make sure that the comatose patient's needs are met since they require greater advocacy.

Maintaining Fluid Balance and Managing Nutritional Needs

The state of hydration is assessed by assessing intake and output patterns, examining mucous membrane turgor, and analyzing laboratory results. Initial hydration requirements are provided by intravenously administering the necessary fluids. Blood transfusions must be done as per the requirements of the patients. Signs and symptoms of fluid overload and increased ICP should be assessed periodically. Tube feeding should be started to maintain the nutritional status of the patients.

Providing Mouth Care

The mouth is examined for pain, dryness, and crusting. The unconscious patient needs meticulous dental care since parotitis is a risk if the mouth is not maintained clean. To get rid of crusts and secretions and keep the mucous membranes moist, the mouth is gently cleaned and washed. Petroleum jelly applied in a thin layer to the lips shields them against encrustations, dryness, and cracking. The patient's endotracheal tube needs to be moved often to the opposite side of the mouth to prevent mouth and lip ulcers.

Maintaining Skin and Joint Integrity

Continual examination and care of the skin are important to maintain skin integrity. Unconscious patients cannot react to outside stimuli, thus they need extra attention. The examination includes a regular rotation plan to avoid pressure, which can cause skin necrosis and collapse. Additionally, turning stimulates the proprioceptive (position awareness), vestibular (equilibrium), and kinesthetic (movement feeling) systems. After rotating, the patient is carefully adjusted to avoid ischemic necrosis over pressure points. Since, it shears and rubs the skin's surface, dragging the patient up in bed must be avoided. To prevent injuries, maintaining correct body posture and passive movement of the extremities are crucial. Splints or foam boots can be used to reduce footdrop and ease pressure on the toes while sleeping. The legs are kept straight by the trochanter rolls that support the hip joints. Hands should be held slightly supinated, with the fingers softly flexed. It is important to locate the pressure points on the heels. Specialty beds, such as fluidized or alternating air mattresses, may be used to relieve pressure on bony prominences.

Preserving Corneal Integrity

Some unconscious individuals have open eyes and inadequate or absent corneal responses. If the cornea is irritated or scraped, keratitis and corneal ulcers are more prevalent. Wipe the eyes with cotton balls soaked in sterile normal saline to remove dirt and discharge. If necessary, artificial tears may be administered every two hours. One typical adverse effect of cranial surgery is periocular edema (swelling around the eyes). It may be advised to apply cold compresses, but care must be taken to prevent contact with the cornea. Eye patches should only be used under strict supervision due to the possibility of corneal damage from contact with the patch.

Achieving Thermoregulation

A respiratory or urinary tract infection, a drug reaction, or damage to the part of the hypothalamus that controls body temperature can all result in a high fever in a patient. Unconscious patients frequently have very high body temperatures due to damage to the brain's heat-regulating center or serious intracranial infections. Such temperature increases need to be controlled since the increased metabolic needs of the brain might overwhelm cerebral circulation and oxygenation, leading to the degeneration of the brain. A poor prognosis and brainstem injury are indicated by persistent heat without a confirmed clinical cause of infection. A little temperature rise might result in dehydration. The surroundings may need to be changed based on the patient's condition to promote a normal body temperature.

Strategies for reducing fever include:
- Cover the patient with a light sheet only.
- Giving acetaminophen as directed.
- Covering up with a hypothermia blanket.
- To improve surface cooling, provide a cold sponge bath and let an electric fan be on over the patient.

❖ Monitor the temperature frequently to assess the response to the therapy and to prevent an excessive decrease in temperature and shivering.

Preventing Urinary Retention

A patient with an altered LOC is commonly incontinent or has urine retention. The bladder should be palpated or inspected at regular intervals to identify pee retention, as a full bladder may be an undiagnosed cause of overflow incontinence. Portable bladder ultrasound equipment can aid in bladder control and retraining programs. If urine retention is detected, an indwelling urinary catheter coupled to a closed drainage system is first inserted. A catheter may be inserted to monitor urine production during the acute phase of illness. Because catheters are a major source of infection in the urinary system, the patient is examined for fever and cloudy urine. The discharge from the urethral orifice is monitored. When the patient's circulatory system is stable and no diuresis, sepsis, or voiding dysfunction occurred, the urinary catheter may be removed. Although many unconscious patients urinate spontaneously after catheter removal, the bladder should be palpated or evaluated for urine retention frequently with a portable ultrasonography tool. If necessary, an intermittent catheterization regimen might be started to guarantee complete bladder emptying at regular intervals.

An external catheter (condom catheter) for the male patient and absorbent pads for the female patient may be used for the patients passing urine involuntarily. As soon as the patient regains consciousness, a bladder-training should be initiated. Skin irritation and skin disintegration in the incontinent patient are regularly monitored. Proper skin care is required to avoid these concerns.

Promoting Bowel Function

The abdomen is evaluated for distention by listening for bowel sounds and using a tape measure to measure the girth of the belly. Infection, medications, and hyperosmolar fluids can all cause diarrhea. Frequent loose stools might be caused by fecal impaction. Commercial feces collection bags are available for people suffering from fecal incontinence.

Constipation

It can be caused by immobility and a lack of dietary fiber. Monitor the frequency and consistency of bowel movements. Examines the patient's rectal cavity for evidence of fecal impaction. Stool softeners may be recommended. A glycerine suppository may be prescribed to help in bowel emptying. Enema may be administered every other day or as per need of the patients.

Providing Sensory Stimulation

Sensory stimulation assists the unconscious patient in overcoming excessive sensory deprivation. The normal day and night activity and sleep routines are followed in an attempt to maintain a sense of daily rhythm. The nurse speaks to and touches the patient, and she encourages family and friends to do the same. Touching the patients and spending enough time with them are also important modes of communication. It is also vital to avoid making any disparaging remarks about the patient's health or prognosis in his/her presence.

At least once every 8 hours, the nurse orients the patient to time and location. A tape recorder can be used to add sounds from the patient's home and job. As a way of enhancing the surroundings and offering familiar input, family members might read to the patient from a beloved book and propose radio and television shows that the patient previously appreciated. When a patient is out of coma, she/he may experience agitation, indicating that they are becoming more aware of their surroundings but are still unable to react or talk effectively. While this is distressing for many family members, it is a favorable clinical sign. It is critical at this phase to limit the patient's stimulation by minimizing background sounds, having just one person speak to the patient at a time, giving the patient more time to respond, and allowing for periodic rest or quiet times. When the patient regains awareness, filmed family or social activities may help him/her recognize relatives and friends and relive missing moments.

Meeting Family's Needs

The family members of the patients may be in a state of crisis and experience significant anxiety, denial, rage, regret, sadness, and reconciliation. If the patient has considerable residual impairments, the family may require a large amount of time, assistance, and support to adjust to these changes. To assist family members in mobilizing their adaptive capacities, the nurse can reinforce and clarify information about the patient's condition, allow the family to be involved in care, and listen to and encourage venting of feelings and concerns while supporting them in their decision-making process about post-hospitalization management and placement. Participation in support groups established by the hospital, rehabilitation center, or community organizations may be beneficial to families.

Monitoring and Managing Potential Complications

When a patient has a low LOC and is unable to turn, cough, or take deep breaths, problems including pneumonia, aspiration, and respiratory failure are possible. Patients are more prone to suffer lung problems the longer they remain asleep. Vital signs and respiratory function are continuously examined for signals of respiratory failure or distress. Chest physiotherapy and suctioning are started to avoid respiratory complications, such as pneumonia. If pneumonia develops, cultures are taken to identify the infection and provide the appropriate treatments.

Skin breakdown and pressure ulcer prevention measures are employed throughout all phases of therapy, including hospital, rehabilitation, and home care, and the patient with altered LOC is regularly examined for indicators of decreasing skin integrity. The factors that contribute to impaired skin integrity are addressed (for example, incontinence, insufficient nutritional intake, pressure on bony prominences, edema, etc.). If pressure ulcers develop, appropriate dressing material should be used. Bacterial contamination, which can cause sepsis and septic shock, is prevented in pressure ulcers.

Furthermore, the patient should be closely monitored for signs and symptoms of deep vein thrombosis.

Patients suffering from deep vein thrombosis are at risk of developing pulmonary embolism. Prophylactic subcutaneous heparin or low-molecular-weight heparin should be given. Thigh-high elastic compression stockings or pneumatic compression stockings should be used to reduce the risk of clot formation. The nurse should watch for redness and swelling in the lower limbs.

Expected Patient Outcomes

Following all the above said interventions, various expected outcomes may include that the patient:

- Maintains clear airway and demonstrates appropriate breath sounds
- Experiences no injuries
- **Attains/maintains the adequate fluid status:**
  - Has no clinical signs or symptoms of dehydration
  - Demonstrates a normal range of serum electrolytes
  - Has no clinical signs or symptoms of overhydration
- Attains/maintains healthy oral mucous membranes
- Maintains normal skin integrity
- Has no corneal irritation
- Attains or maintains thermoregulation
- Has no urinary retention
- Has no diarrhea or fecal impaction
- Receives appropriate sensory stimulation
- **Caregivers cope with the crisis by:**
  - Verbalizing fears and concerns
  - Participating in patient's care and providing sensory stimulation by talking and touching
- **Is free of complications:**
  - Has arterial blood gas values within normal range
  - Displays no signs or symptoms of pneumonia
  - Exhibits intact skin over pressure areas
  - Does not develop deep vein thrombosis

GERIATRIC CONSIDERATIONS

Altered LOC is one of the main complaints among elderly patients. They are more likely to present with changed mental status as a result of a stroke, any illness, drug-drug interactions, or any changes in their living environment. delirium, dementia, depression, etc., are quite prevalent in the elderly. Patients with dementia, severe sickness, physical fragility, infection or dehydration, visual impairment, recent surgery, heavy alcohol intake, and renal impairment are all at higher risk of developing delirium. Acute mental status changes are more serious and are frequently the result of delirium, stupor, or coma. Individuals may exhibit signs of motor abnormalities in addition to cognitive alterations, since many vascular events have a cumulative effect on the patient's function. It is important to recognize the signs of altered mental status at its earliest, identify the underlying causes, and provide appropriate care to reduce morbidity and mortality in the patients. Acute alteration in mental status can be caused by several significant medical illnesses and need immediate detection and treatment for best results. The nurses should assess the patient's mental status and cognitive skills regularly. An altered level of consciousness in elderly patients also affects other important issues like the accuracy of patients' history, knowledge of their diagnosis, and discharge instruction.

Case Scenario

1. A 60-year-old male was found unresponsive by his wife while he was sitting in a chair watching TV. His eyes appeared to be partially open. He did not respond to shaking even. She immediately called for an ambulance. At the time of the arrival of the ambulance, he was awake and alert. His blood pressure was 160/90 and he had a regular pulse of 75 bpm. He was transported to the emergency department. What should be the line of treatment in an emergency.
2. A 65-year-old man is brought to the emergency department. The history is given by his relative, who stated that they were called to a store for this person. At the store, they found him lying on the ground unconscious but breathing normally. After their arrival, the patient awoke but was unable to give coherent responses to questions or commands. What should be the next step in his management?

SUMMARY

Levels of consciousness range from normal alertness and attention to many altered states. It starts with confusion and delirium to stupor and coma. Sometimes, it may start with a mild state and rapidly progress through to a higher stage. Meticulous nursing care is required to prevent further complications in the unconscious patients.

MULTIPLE CHOICE QUESTIONS

1. **Which test is extensively used to assess the level of consciousness?**
   a. Glasgow coma scale
   b. AVPU scale
   c. Full outline of unresponsiveness
   d. Grady coma scale
2. **In the scale AVPU, the letter V stands for?**
   a. Vision
   b. Verbal
   c. Velocity
   d. Vicarious
3. **Symptoms of altered mental status may include:**
   a. Confusion, coughing, and inattentiveness
   b. Intense concentration, coughing, confusion
   c. Difficulty concentrating, communicating, singing
   d. Confusion, inability to focus, indecisiveness
4. **Which stage of altered level of consciousness a person is agitated or restless and has a substantial lack of concentration?**
   a. Confused
   b. Obtunded
   c. Delirious
   d. Somnolent
5. **Proprioceptive is connected with:**
   a. Equilibrium
   b. Positioning
   c. Hearing
   a. Walking

ANSWERS

1. a   2. b   3. d   4. c
5. b

SUGGESTED READING

1. Cecil, RL, Goldman, L, Schafer Al. Goldman's Cecil medicine. 24th ed. Philadelphia: Elsevier/Saunders; 2012.
2. Cooksley T, Rose S, Holland M. A systematic approach to the unconscious patient. Clin Med. 2018;18(1):88. doi:10.7861/clinmedicine.18–1-88
3. Daroff R, Fenichel G, Jankovic J, Mazziotta J. Bradley's neurology in clinical practice. 6th edition; 2012. Available from http://www.clinicalkey.com

4. Kim KT, Jeon JC, Jung CG, et al. Aetiologies of altered level of consciousness in the emergency room. Scientific Reports 12.2022: 4972. https://doi.org/10.1038/s41598-022-09110-2.
5. Kondziella D, Bender A, Diserens K, et al. European Academy of Neurology guideline on the diagnosis of coma and other disorders of consciousness. Eur J Neurol. 2020;27(5):741-56. doi:10.1111/ene.14151
6. McNarry AF, Goldhill DR. Simple bedside assessment of the level of consciousness: comparison of two simple assessment scales with the Glasgow Coma scale. Anaesthesia. 2004;59(1):34-7. doi:10.1111/j.1365-2044.2004.03526.x
7. Moses S. Altered level of consciousness.2012. Available from http://www.fpnotebook.com/neuro/LOC/AltrdLvlOfCnscsns.htm
8. Nasution AH, Prima A. Incidence of loss of consciousness in critically ill patients referred to the anesthesiologist in the emergency department. Asian J Infect Dis. 1979;3(1):41-4.
9. Obiako OR, Oparah S, Ogunniyi A. Causes of medical coma in adult patients at the University College Hospital, Ibadan Nigeria. Niger Postgrad Med J. 2011;18(1):1-7.
10. Rakel RE, Rakel D. Textbook of family medicine. 8th ed. Philadelphia: Elsevier/Saunders. 2011.
11. Reichhart MD, Meuli R. Alterations of the level of consciousness related to stroke. Behav Cognitive Neurol Stroke. 2013;4:312.
12. Reichhart MD, Meuli R. Alterations of the level of consciousness related to stroke. Behav Cognitive Neurol Stroke. 2013 Feb 28;4:312.
13. US Department of Health and Human Services. National and regional estimates on hospital use for all patients from the HCUP nationwide inpatient sample. Agency for healthcare research and quality website. 2011 Available from http://hcupnet.ahrq.gov/HCUPnet.jsp
14. Veauthier B, Hornecker JR, Thrasher T. Recent-onset altered mental status: Evaluation and management. Am Fam Physician. 2021;104: 461-70.
15. Völk S, Koedel U, Pfister HW, Schwankhart R. Impaired consciousness in the emergency department. Eur Neurol. 2018;80(3-4):179-86. doi:10.1159/000495363.
16. Wang J, Li Z, Yu Y, Li B, Shao G, Wang Q. Risk factors contributing to postoperative delirium in geriatric patients post orthopedic surgery. Asia Pacific Psychiatry. 2015;7(4):375-82. doi:10.1111/appy.12193

INCREASED INTRACRANIAL PRESSURE

CONCEPT AND DEFINITION

Intracranial pressure (ICP) elevation is a frequently occurring complication in neurosurgical and neurological conditions. The patients exhibit a wide variety of clinical signs and symptoms because of increased intracranial pressure. Various causes may include any cerebral mass, issues with cerebrospinal fluid (CSF) circulation, or intracranial degenerative processes. Its onset might be abrupt or gradual. Measurement, continuous monitoring, and treatment of increased ICP are all well-established processes. Intracranial hypertension (IH) is a clinical condition characterized by increased intracranial pressures. The normal ICP value is shown in **Table 29.4**.

TABLE 29.4: Normal intracranial pressure values.

Age group	Normal range (mm Hg)
Adults	<10 to 15
Children	3–7
Infant	1.5–6

EPIDEMIOLOGY

The real prevalence of cerebral hypertension is unknown. The Centers for Disease Control and Prevention (CDC) estimates that 2.5 million persons had a traumatic brain injury (TBI) in 2010. TBI is linked with elevated ICP. Thus, its monitoring is suggested for all patients with severe TBI. According to studies of American-based populations, the incidence of idiopathic intracranial hypertension (IIH) in the general population varies from 0.9 to 1.0 per 100,000 with the prevalence rising in overweight women.

ETIOLOGY

Table 29.5 depicts the various causes along with the pathophysiological process of increased ICP.

PATHOPHYSIOLOGY

Cerebrospinal fluid (CSF) a clear fluid found in the brain and spinal cord subarachnoid spaces and ventricles acts as a cushion for the brain and spinal cord. The choroid plexus secretes it in the lateral ventricles, and it travels to the third ventricle via the foramen of Monro. The Sylvius aqueduct transfers CSF from the third to the fourth ventricle. It then drains into the subarachnoid space via the foramina of Magendie and Luschka before being reabsorbed into the dural venous sinuses by arachnoid granulation.

Cerebral blood flow (CBF) is regulated and maintained by a homeostatic process called cerebral autoregulation maintaining CBF between 50- and 150-mm Hg mean arterial pressure. Cerebral perfusion pressure (CPP) is the net pressure gradient causing blood flow to the brain. So, CPP is the force driving blood into the brain. Thus, it is the primary determinant of cerebral blood flow. CPP is a calculated measure, so, mean arterial pressure (MAP) and ICP must be measured simultaneously by making use of invasive means. The formula to calculate CPP is MAP-ICP. This homeostatic mechanism ensures that as MAP or CPP

TABLE 29.5: Causes of increased intracranial pressure.

Pathophysiology process	Causes
Focal brain edema (localized mass lesion)	Traumatic hematomas (extradural, subdural, intracerebral); neoplasms (gliomas, meningiomas, metastasis); ischemic or hemorrhagic stroke, abscess
Diffuse brain edema	Encephalitis, meningitis, diffuse head injury, seizures, encephalopathy (hepatic, toxic, uremic, or septic), hypoxemic ischemic encephalopathy, water intoxication, Reye's syndrome, subarachnoid hemorrhage, lead encephalopathy, near drowning
Disturbance of CSF circulation	Obstructive hydrocephalus, Communicating hydrocephalus, Subarachnoid hemorrhage
Obstruction to major venous sinuses	Depressed fractures overlying major venous sinuses. Cerebral venous thrombosis
Vascular malformations	Arteriovenous malformation
Idiopathic	Benign intracranial hypertension

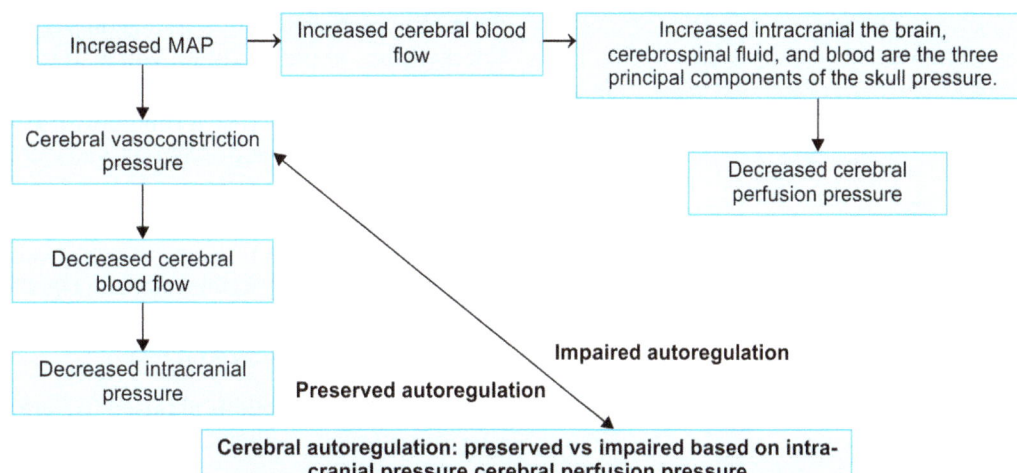

Fig. 29.1: Effect of cerebral autoregulation on intracranial pressure.

increases, resistance increases (vasoconstriction) in the small cerebral arteries. Conversely, this process maintains constant CBF by decreasing cerebrovascular resistance or vasodilation when MAP or CPP decreases. Lower blood pressure may result in lower CPP and CBF in patients with impaired autoregulation. A decrease in MAP results in cerebral vasodilation, an increase in cerebral blood volume, and, as a result, an increase in ICP **(Fig. 29.1)**.

The Monro-Kellie Concept of ICP

The brain, cerebrospinal fluid, and blood are the three principal components of the skull. As per the Monroe-Kellie principle, the contents of the skull have a constant volume.

The Monro-Kellie concept arose from the first description of ICP in 1783 by Scottish anatomist Alexander Monro. Later, he was helped by his colleague George Kellie. In 1926, Harvey Cushing, an American neurosurgeon, developed the theory as we know it today. He maintained that the volume of the brain, blood, and CSF is constant with an undamaged skull. When one component increases, one or both of the other components decrease. Thus, when there is an increasing mass lesion of the brain parenchyma, the CSF or blood (mostly venous) will decrease until the compensatory limit is reached, at which time, we will have a raised ICP. Various factors, as enlisted in **Table 29.5**, raise ICP by increasing one or more of the three components.

The intracranial volume-pressure curve in **Figure 29.2** shows how a small increase in the volume of one of the intracranial components can be compensated by a decrease in another component. However, once these compensatory measures are exhausted, an increase in the volume will lead to an increase in ICP. If there is an increase in the volume during the compensation phase more rapidly than the ICP, this should be an indication of impending volume decompensation.

Cushing Triad

It involves three clinical symptoms happening together signaling increased intracranial pressure. These are bradycardia, widened pulse pressure (the increasing gap between systolic and diastolic blood pressure) and irregular respiration. When the ICP is too high the elevation of blood pressure is a reflex mechanism to maintain CPP. High BP

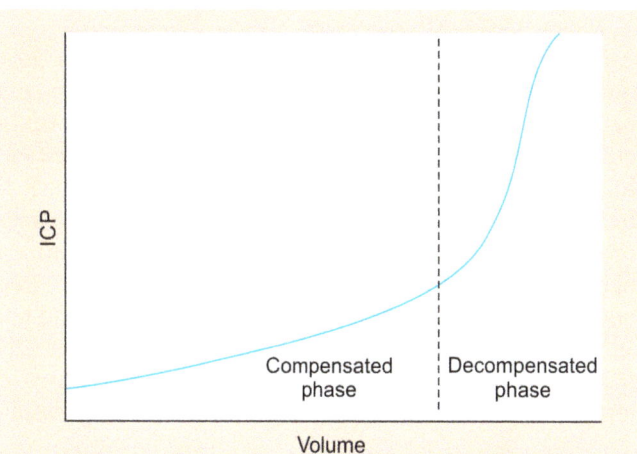

Fig. 29.2: Cerebral volume–pressure curve depicting the relationship between ICP and an increase in the intracranial component volume.

leads to reflex bradycardia and compromised brainstem affecting respiration. Because of high ICP, ultimately the contents of the cranium will be displaced downwards. This will lead to a life-threatening event, i.e., brain herniation requiring urgent attention. Various sites of brain herniation are shown in **Figure 29.3**. **Cingulate herniation** is the most common type. In this, the innermost part of the frontal lobe is scraped under part of the falx cerebri, the dura mater at the top of the head between the two hemispheres of the brain. **Central trans herniation** is the subtype of downward transtentorial herniation of the brain. It involves descent of the diencephalon and midbrain. **Lateral trans herniation** occurs due to unilateral or asymmetric mass effects. The medial parts of the temporal lobe are pushed into the ambient cistern and up against the brainstem. In **tonsillar herniation**, the cerebellar tonsils move downward through the foramen magnum possibly causing compression of the lower brainstem and upper cervical spinal cord as they pass through the foramen magnum. In transcalvarial **herniation**, the brain squeezes through a fracture or a surgical site in the skull.

As discussed above, alteration in ICP can result from various conditions affecting the brain tissue, CSF, and blood volume. It is also true that its maintenance depends on several physiological factors, such as autoregulation, vessel

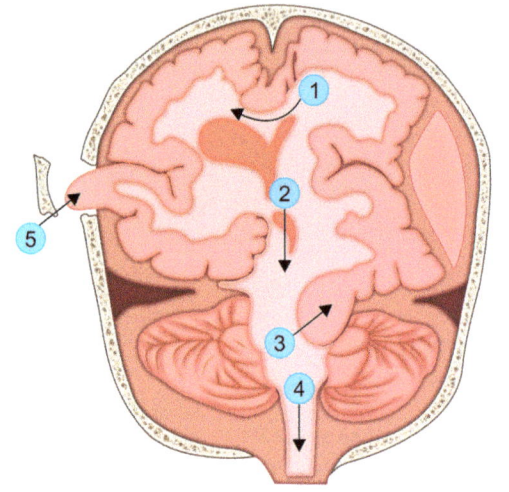

Fig. 29.3: Various sites of herniation: (1) Cingulate; (2) Central transtentorial; (3) Lateral transtentorial; (4) Tonsillar; (5) Transcalvarial.

the midbrain, reticular formation, and periaqueductal gray. Compression of the midbrain will lead to compression of the reticular formation and the periaqueductal gray. When the compressions activate the central triggering zone, symptoms, such as diplopia, nausea, and vomiting will occur. Accumulation of blood, tissue, and CSF may also produce optic nerve compression obstructing the axoplasmic flow inside the optic nerve, resulting in axon swelling, which will affect the visual acuity in the patients **(Fig. 29.4)**.

CLINICAL MANIFESTATIONS

The clinical manifestations of raised ICP are generally non-specific and even insidious in onset **(Box 29.2)**.

DIAGNOSTIC EVALUATION

Assessment

Although there is no clear relationship between the intensity of symptoms and the degree of hypertension, the combination of headache, papilledema, and vomiting is typically regarded as symptomatic of increased ICP. If a patient exhibits the signs and symptoms, such as headaches, vomiting, and altered mental state ranging from sleepiness to coma then clinical suspicion for intracranial hypertension should be raised. Blurred vision, double vision due to cranial nerve abnormalities, photophobia, optic disc edema, and finally optic atrophy are all examples of visual alterations. Infants with an open anterior fontanelle may have a bulge overlaying the region.

compliance, and mean arterial pressure (MAP) **(Figs. 29.1 and 29.2)**. The volume of the brain is characteristically fixed. The two most important components contributing to ICP are the cerebral blood flow and the balance between the production and absorption or outflow of the CSF. If the volume of either of these two components increases for example because of intracranial hemorrhage or an inability to effectively absorb or drain CSF, and the buffering mechanisms are already exhausted, then the resulting net volume expansion will lead to increased ICP and eventually intracranial hypertension (ICH) as well as downward herniation of the uncus via the tentorial notch, compressing

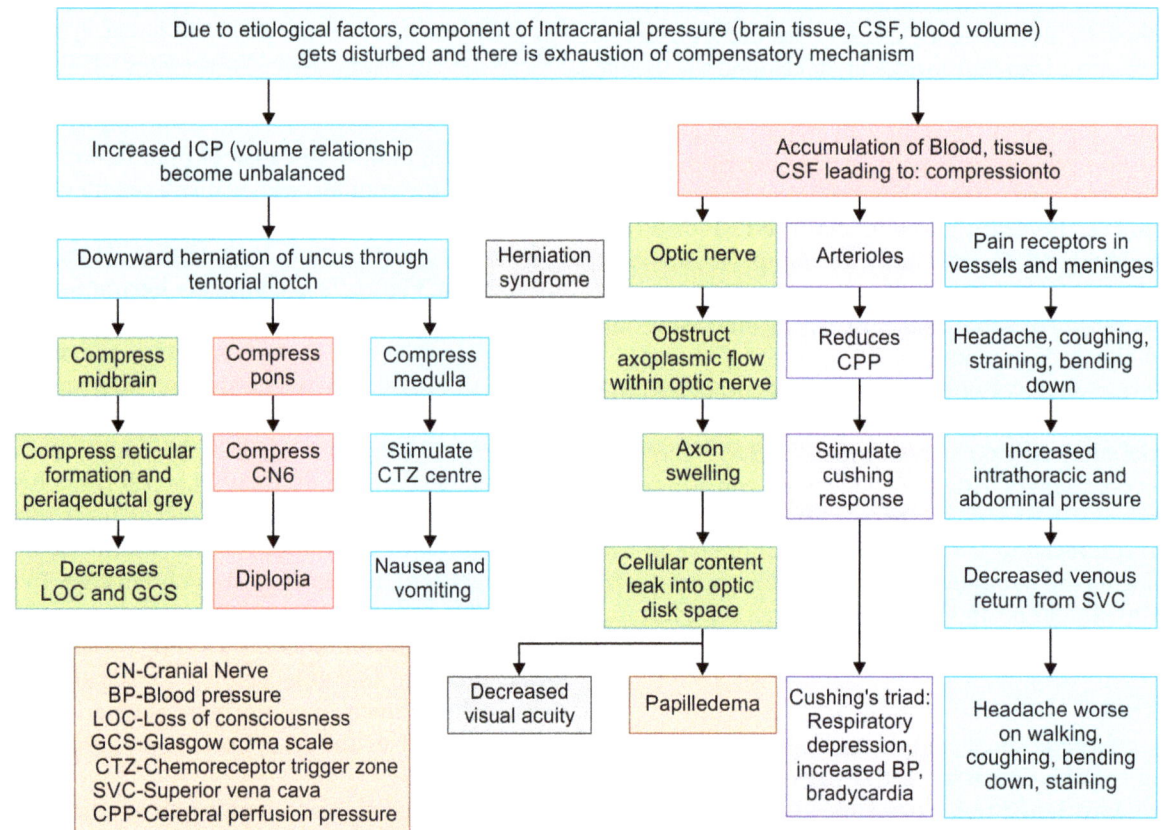

Fig. 29.4: Pathophysiology of increased intracranial pressure.

BOX 29.2: Manifestations of increased ICP.

- Headache
- Nausea and vomiting
- Systolic hypertension
- Bradycardia
- Cushing's triad
- Cheyne-Stokes respiration
- Confusion
- Loss of consciousness and finally coma as the pressure worsens
- Drowsiness
- Anorexia
- **Visual disturbances:**
  - *Blurred vision:* Often the first manifestation noted by the patients
  - *Visual field loss:* Early finding
  - Visual acuity is usually preserved
- Double vision
- Pupils not reacting to light and unequal pupils
- Papilledema
- Neck/back pain
- Convulsions
- Pulsatile tinnitus
- Blackouts
- Decreased GCS/coma

TABLE 29.6: Indications for intracranial pressure (ICP) monitoring.

Condition	Comments
Subarachnoid hemorrhage	With associated hydrocephalus—ventriculostomy allows therapeutic drainage and ICP monitoring
Spontaneous intracerebral hemorrhage	There is no solid clinical evidence that monitoring patients in this category is beneficial
Reye's syndrome	Active treatment of elevated ICP reduces mortality. Serum ammonia levels of more than 300 mg/100 mL and a worsening conscious state are typically regarded as reasons for monitoring
Brain tumors	Not recommended generally, but may be beneficial in certain individuals who are at high risk of swelling or obstructive hydrocephalus, such as after posterior fossa surgery
Normal pressure hydrocephalus	A positive response to CSF diversion is predicted by an increase in spontaneous nocturnal "B" waves
Decompensated hydrocephalus	Can be a valuable diagnostic tool in complex cases
Benign intracranial hypertension	A lumbar subarachnoid catheter is often used for both diagnostic testing and therapy response monitoring
Other potential indications	Meningitis, encephalitis, venous sinus thrombosis, hypoxic brain swelling following drowning, and hepatic encephalopathy

Evaluation

Increased ICP should be evaluated with a complete history, physical examination, and supporting investigations. To avoid herniation and mortality, it is vital to recognize increased ICP as soon as feasible. As an example, consider a malignant middle cerebral artery stroke with high ICP. Younger persons are more prone to have a malignant middle cerebral artery stroke. Typically, these patients are admitted to the critical care unit. The neurological examination must be done regularly. A shift in mental state is typical, as is the creation of a fixed and dilated pupil. Patients presenting with symptoms suggestive of a cerebral insult should undergo computed tomography (CT) scan of the brain, which can indicate edema as low-density areas and a lack of gray/white matter separation on an unenhanced image. Cisterns and sulcal regions may also be destroyed.

In some circumstances, a CT scan can also indicate the reason. Increased ICP is indicated by flattened gyri, narrower sulci, or ventricular compression. Serial CT scans are utilized to track the development or improvement of edema.

A funduscopic exam can reveal papilledema, a marker of elevated ICP because the cerebrospinal fluid is in continuous contact with the fluid surrounding the optic nerve.

Measurement of Opening Pressure with a Lumbar Puncture (LP)

During this procedure, a needle is introduced into the subarachnoid space. In order to note CSF pressure before drainage, this may be connected to a manometer. A high ICP is indicated by a value greater than 20 mm Hg. Brain imaging should be done before the surgery since LP might induce a sudden shift in volume that could result in herniation and a quick decline in ICP.

ICP Monitoring

ICP monitoring can be employed as a diagnostic tool or as therapeutic guidance. The most typical application of continuous ICP monitoring is in the management of severe closed-head injuries. Several devices can be used for ICP monitoring. The procedure involves the placement of a fiberoptic catheter into the brain parenchyma to measure the pressure transmitted to the brain tissues. Various indications of ICP monitoring are shown in **Table 29.6**.

External Ventricular Drain (EVD)

The pressure in the lateral ventricles can be measured using a manometer coupled to a drain inserted directly into the ventricles.

Optic Nerve Sheath Diameter (ONSD)

ICP elevation may be identified by using ultrasonography to measure the diameter of the optic nerve sheath. Usually, 2–3 measurements are taken in each eye at a distance of 3 mm behind the globe. 0.48–0.63 cm is considered the usual range for detecting elevated ICP.

MEDICAL MANAGEMENT

If possible, primary management concentrates on the specific process that is contributing to the rise in ICP (such as surgical removal of mass lesions, dexamethasone treatment for edema associated with intracranial tumors, control of hydrocephalus, etc.).

Management of Raised ICP

Elevated ICP eventually will aggravate brain damage. Secondary brain damage occurs hours to days after the first injury. Cerebral ischemia, cerebral edema, and the neurochemical interplay of excitatory neurotransmitters, free radical generation, and high intracellular calcium and potassium levels are all detrimental processes. Various therapeutic strategies for lowering the ICP should be started concurrently along with treatment of the underlying cause. Secondary brain injury is exacerbated by hypoxia and hypotension. Majority of the treatments aim to lower cerebral blood volume and the fluid component of brain tissue. CSF drainage or surgical removal of brain tissue is undertaken in some cases.

General Management

- **Airway:** Hypoxia raises ICP through vasodilation and cerebral edema. Coughing or bucking during laryngoscopy and intubation might cause the ICP to rise further. As a result, even if the patient is unconscious, sedatives should always be administered prior to intubation. Esmolol, labetalol, and lignocaine can all be administered to reduce the hemodynamic effects of laryngoscopy.
- **Ventilation:** Hypercarbia is a potent cerebral vasodilator causing an increase in cerebral blood volume and ICP. Hence, hypoventilation should be avoided and normocapnia maintained.
- **Blood pressure:**
  - In a brain with inadequate autoregulation, hypotension reduces cerebral perfusion pressure. For better outcomes, Brain Trauma Foundation (BTF) recommendations propose maintaining systolic blood pressure at 100 mm Hg for patients 50-69 years old, or at 110 mm Hg or higher for those 15-49 or >70 years old (Level III). Elevated blood pressure is prevalent in raised ICP patients. This is a compensating mechanism to keep the CPP in place. When autoregulation is compromised, as in traumatic brain injury (TBI), ICP may rise.
  - It also has the potential to cause cerebral bleeding in specific scenarios, such as hemorrhagic stroke or postoperative neurosurgery patients. Antihypertensive medicines, such as sympatholytic blockers (labetalol, esmolol) or centrally acting-agonists (clonidine) can be used for therapy. Vasodilators such as nitroprusside and nitroglycerine should be avoided since they raise ICP.
- **CPP:** It is recommended a target CPP value of 50-70 mm Hg for survival and better results, depending on the patient's autoregulatory condition. A value of 70 or above increases the risk of acute respiratory distress syndrome.
- **Fluids:** Fluid therapy should be initiated with saline. Albumin should be avoided. Hypo-osmolar fluids should be avoided. Hyponatremia should be corrected since it increases cerebral edema.
- **Sedation and analgesia:** In patients with elevated ICP, sedation, and analgesia help with mechanical breathing, suctioning, and seizure management while also preventing coughing, bucking, and agitation. It primarily has protective effects on the brain by lowering the cerebral metabolic rate of oxygen consumption and the closely related cerebral blood flow (CBF). Analgesics should be used as a proper complement to sedatives. The main analgesics are more recent opioids like fentanyl. Opioids given in large bolus doses, however, may have negative effects on ICP and CPP.
- **Facilitation of cerebral venous drainage:** To stimulate CSF circulation from the intracranial to the spinal compartment and to improve cerebral venous drainage, the head end of the bed should be kept raised at 15-30° with the head in a neutral posture. To avoid internal jugular vein compression, ties around the tracheostomy, endotracheal tube, or cervical collar should be adjusted. Any increase in intra-abdominal or intrathoracic pressures might potentially obstruct venous drainage.
- **Fever control:** Fever is a powerful vasodilator and boosts metabolic rate by 10-13% per degree Celsius. It raises ICP. Antipyretics and hydrotherapy should be used to treat fever.
- **Glucocorticoids:** Steroid administration as a temporizing strategy works effectively for the neurological deficiency attributable to vasogenic edema caused by brain tumors, abscesses, or non-infectious neuroinflammation. When present, rICP may be decreased during the next 2-5 days. Dexamethasone is frequently administered intravenously at a dosage of 4 mg every 6 hours.

  Steroids should not be used to treat elevated ICP, improve outcomes following a TBI, or stop spontaneous bleeding (Level I Evidence). In the CRASH experiment, using methylprednisolone for 48 hours increased the chance of mortality significantly.

  After Tier zero treatment, which involves carrying out all the basic interventions for all the neurocritical care patients irrespective of increased ICP, a non-contrast CT scan should be done when the patient may be transferred without risk.

First-tier Treatment

Significant deviations from the normal physiological condition in general physiologic balance can have a deleterious effect on ICP and/or cerebral perfusion. Attention is thus focused on maintaining appropriate arterial oxygen tension and keeping the patient euvolemic and euosmotic. Fever should be avoided because it raises ICP, which is an independent predictor of poor prognosis following a serious head injury. Seizures lead to elevated ICP and should be treated promptly with conventional anticonvulsant loading regimens.

- **CSF drainage:** CSF drainage is an efficient means of reducing ICP when an intraventricular catheter is used to monitor it. This can be performed by performing intermittent drainage for brief durations in response to increased ICP. Infection and bleeding are the most serious dangers of ventriculostomy. Most studies show bacterial colonization rates ranging from 0 to 19% rather than symptomatic infection rates. The prevalence of ventriculostomy-related hematoma is around 2%.
- **Elevation of the head of the bed:** Elevating the head of the bed to 30° increases jugular venous outflow and decreases ICP. In hypovolemic individuals, this may be linked with a drop in blood pressure and an overall drop in cerebral perfusion pressure. So, hypovolemia must be ruled out.

- **Analgesia and sedation:** This is often performed with the administration of intravenous propofol, etomidate, or midazolam for sedation, and morphine or alfentanil for analgesia and antitussive action.
- **Neuromuscular blockade:** Any muscular activity may further elevate ICP by raising intrathoracic pressure and blocking cerebral venous outflow. If analgesia and sedation do not relieve the pain, neuromuscular blocking is explored. However, preventive use of neuromuscular blockade in individuals without confirmed intracranial hypertension has not been found to enhance prognosis. It is connected with an increased risk of consequences such as pneumonia and sepsis, and it might hide seizure activity.
- **Diuretics:** Mannitol, an intravascular osmotic agent that may pull fluid from both the normal and pathological brain, is the most widely utilized agent. Furthermore, it raises cardiac preload and CPP, lowering ICP via cerebral autoregulation. Mannitol reduces blood viscosity, which causes reflex vasoconstriction and a reduction in cerebrovascular volume. The most serious side effects of mannitol administration include hypovolemia and the creation of a hyperosmotic condition. The serum osmolality level should not exceed 320 mOsm/kg.
- **Hyperventilation:** Hyperventilation reduces ICP by causing hypocapnic vasoconstriction, which is mediated by metabolic autoregulation. However, in certain cases, hyperventilation causes or worsens cerebral ischemia. Another issue is the development of tachyphylaxis as a result of compensating for systemic alkalosis. As a result of the rebound CSF acidosis and vasodilatation that occurs when eucapnia is restored, the effect of the set level of hypocapnia is diminished, making weaning more difficult.
- **Antiseizure therapy:** Seizure activity raises the cerebral metabolic rate (CMR) and cerebral blood flow (CBF). Increased ICP is caused by CBF that exceeds tissue demand. According to the most recent BTF guidelines, phenytoin should be used to reduce the occurrence of early posttraumatic seizures (PTS) within 7 days of injury.

Second-tier Treatments

- **Barbiturate coma therapy:** Barbiturates at large dosages are beneficial in treating refractory intracranial hypertension; however, they are inefficient or potentially harmful as a first-line or prophylactic therapy in patients with head trauma. High-dose barbiturate therapy reduces brain metabolic activity. This causes a decrease in cerebral blood flow, which is linked to metabolism, and a drop in ICP. The use of barbiturates in the treatment of refractory intracranial hypertension necessitates close monitoring and has a high risk of consequences, the most frequent of which is hypotension. This might explain why there is no established benefit on outcome in brain injuries. Cerebral electrical activity should ideally be monitored continuously throughout high-dosage barbiturate therapy, with burst suppression activity providing a physiologic endpoint for dose titration. To avoid rebound intracranial hypertension, therapy should be tapered off gradually.
- **Optimized hyperventilation:** To prevent hyperventilation-induced ischemia, more vigorous hyperventilation is used, along with concurrent assessment of jugular venous saturation. It is based on the notion that following a head injury, there is an uncoupling of cerebral blood flow and metabolism. Relative cerebral hyperemia develops and manifests as a low cerebral arterial-venous oxygen differential. Hyperventilation would not result in cerebral ischemia in such individuals by lowering cerebral blood volume and hence ICP. The extent, to which samples collected from one jugular bulb are indicative of the oxygen saturation of blood in the contralateral hemisphere, or even of fluctuations within the ipsilateral hemisphere, is a key problem with this approach. As a result, even when global measurements indicate sufficient oxygen delivery, localized regions of cerebral ischemia may develop.
- **Therapeutic hypothermia:** Hypothermia has been studied in brain injury as a method of reducing ICP and as a potential neuroprotective technique. Although cooling to 34°C can be beneficial in decreasing resistant intracranial hypertension, it is linked with a high risk of consequences, such as respiratory, viral, coagulation, and electrolyte issues. When induced hypothermia is reversed, there appears to be a large recovery in ICP. Despite an imbalance in treatment groups, a randomized controlled study of mild hypothermia following severe closed head injury failed to reveal any advantage on the outcome.

SURGICAL MANAGEMENT

If ICP cannot be managed medically, decompressive surgical methods should be tried. If the patient is not fit for surgery, then additional Tier Two therapies should be done. The degree of sedation can be enhanced by utilizing drugs, such as propofol.

1. **Resection of mass lesions:** These are done to decrease the ICP and as a definitive therapy for the lesions. Acute epidural and subdural hematoma must be evacuated, and abscesses must be drained. Decompression is also aided by the resection of intracranial lesions, such as lobar/cerebellar bleeding or brain parenchyma (such as contusion). Pneumo-encephalus tension has to be released.
2. **Decompressive craniectomy (DC):** A piece of the skull vault is removed during DC, which immediately lowers the ICP. Patients who have diffuse cerebral swelling from a TBI, meningoencephalitis, a stroke with brain edema, or non-infectious neuroinflammatory disorders are treated with it (e.g., acute demyelinating encephalopathy). A decompressive hemicraniectomy (DHC) is typically performed.

Decompressive craniectomy has been associated with subdural hygroma, hemorrhagic swelling ipsilateral to the craniectomy site, and hydrocephalus. In patients with severe TBI, a large frontotemporoparietal DC (not less than 12 × 15 cm or 15 cm diameter) is preferred to a small one since it reduces mortality and improves neurologic outcomes.

NURSING MANAGEMENT OF PATIENTS

Assessment and management of the airway, breathing, and circulation should always be the priority. The management of the patients should be targeted toward:
- ❖ Maintenance of cerebral perfusion pressure by raising MAP
- ❖ Treatment of the underlying cause.
- ❖ Lowering of ICP.

Various nursing interventions to be carried out for patients with increased ICP are discussed as follows.

- ❖ **Monitor neurological status:** Assessment of consciousness level using the Glasgow coma scale, and motor and sensory assessment should be done at least once in each shift for all the patients. Patients with acute neurological problems should be evaluated every 1 hour including pupil examination and the findings should be documented in the flow sheet. Any change in neurological status should be reported to the doctor immediately.
- ❖ **Prevent increase in ICP:** For acute patients with/at risk for raised intracranial pressure, care should be provided in such a manner that prevents elevations in ICP. Nursing care should include measures for lowering/preventing intrathoracic and intraabdominal pressure increases, as well as lowering metabolic rate. So,
  - ➢ Maintain good head and neck alignment.
  - ➢ Insert oral gastric drainage tube to maintain gastric decompression (nasal tubes contraindicated).
  - ➢ Maintain HOB elevation at 30° to increase jugular venous drainage (to reduce cerebral blood volume). Higher increases may cause an increase in stomach pressure or an obstruction in cerebral blood flow.
  - ➢ Good head and neck alignment preserves jugular venous drainage. The outflow of blood and CSF from the cerebral compartment is aided by jugular venous drainage.
  - ➢ Avoid hip flexion >30°.
  - ➢ Avoid positions that may increase abdominal or intrathoracic pressures, such as prone or semi-prone.
  - ➢ Space nursing care activities to avoid prolonged periods of stimulation to the patient.
  - ➢ Use sedatives/narcotics as ordered to minimize cough/gag; suction only when needed.
  - ➢ If sedatives/narcotics fail to control cough in patients with severe brain injury, review with the physician other options, such as neuromuscular blockade. If neuromuscular blocking agents (NMBs) are used to control ICP, continuous EEG monitoring should be implemented as NMBs can mask seizure activity.
  - ➢ Hourly temperature monitoring is required.
- ❖ **Monitor patients with increased ICP:** Additional monitoring is essential for acute patients with/at risk of elevated intracranial pressure. Report changes quickly to physician:
  - ➢ Monitor core temperature q 1 h. If cooling blankets and/or neuromuscular blockers are used, continuous monitoring should be considered.
  - ➢ Lower temperature with the use of a cooling blanket gradually to avoid shivering.
  - ➢ Neuromuscular blockers may help to reduce temperature, but may cause a rapid drop in temperature.
  - ➢ As long as it is not contraindicated, the usual temperature goal is set to 32–34°C. The goal is to get the temperature in target as rapidly as possible after the return of spontaneous circulation (ROSC). The temperature should not exceed 34°C.
  - ➢ Monitor vital signs very carefully. Treat hypotension and hypovolemia promptly.
  - ➢ During the acute phase, blood gases should be checked every 6 hours and as per requirement. Keep $PaCO_2$ 35–40 (or lower if ordered) and PaO_2 >80–90 unless otherwise ordered. Unlike other ventilated patients, $PaCO_2$ is the target, not the pH.
  - ➢ If mannitol is prescribed or hypertonic saline is used, serum electrolytes and osmolality should be measured every 6 hours or as directed. Notify the neurosurgeon if serum osmolality is more than 320 (mannitol) or hypertonic saline (greater than 340), or if blood sodium is greater than 156 with hypertonic saline.
  - ➢ Keep an eye on increased/diluted urine production.
  - ➢ Correct hyper-/hyponatremia slowly (0.5–1 mmol/L/hr of change in either direction)
  - ➢ Monitor blood sugar closely. Avoid hyper- or hypoglycemia.
  - ➢ Neurogenic fever and/or diabetes insipidus can be caused by hypothalamic dysfunction (DI). Fever is related to a worse neurological result and increases oxygen consumption in the brain. Shivering increases metabolic rate and heat generation while also promoting vasoconstriction, which lowers heat loss. Sedation and neuromuscular blockade can reduce body temperature by reducing heat generation (due to muscle activity).
  - ➢ Polyuria, low urine osmolality, high serum osmolality, and hypernatremia are all symptoms of DI. It can result in severe and fatal dehydration. Acute DI after serious brain damage has a very dismal result.
  - ➢ A sympathetic increase in cerebral blood flow can be triggered by hypercarbia, acidosis, hypoxemia, or hypotension. Increased cerebral blood volume might raise ICP. Patient-induced hyperventilation might be a symptom of elevated ICP.
  - ➢ Hypotension and/or hypovolemia can decrease cerebral blood flow. A rise in BP may be a sign of increased ICP as the body attempts to maintain cerebral perfusion pressure (CPP). Hypertension with widening pulse pressure, bradycardia, and irregular respirations suggests brainstem herniation (Cushing's Triad). Urgent intervention is needed in such patients.
  - ➢ The brain is completely reliant on glucose for energy. Hypoglycemia depletes the brain's energy reserves. Hyperglycemia has been linked to poor neurological outcomes. Thus, careful monitoring is important.
- ❖ **Monitor intraventricular pressure:**
  - ➢ The nurse is in charge of establishing, zeroing, leveling, and maintaining an ICP monitoring circuit.

- Continuously monitor the waveform. Record mean ICP on the flow sheet's neuro section, q 1 h, and prn. Place the ICP drain at the level specified by the neurosurgeon (e.g., 15 cm above the external auditory meatus). CPP should be calculated for each measured ICP.
- ICP drainage goal is ~ <20 mL per hour. If drainage exceeds this volume, or ICP is > ordered goal, or drainage abruptly stops, contact the neurosurgeon immediately.
- Normal ICP <10 mm Hg. Normal CPP = 60–80 mm Hg. CPP <50 mm Hg may indicate a significant reduction in cerebral blood flow.

GERIATRIC CONSIDERATIONS

Increased intracranial pressure (ICP) is a dangerous and often lethal condition. Increased ICP can cause brain damage, seizures, coma, stroke, or death. While trauma is still a prominent cause of morbidity and mortality in people of all ages, elderly patients because of multimorbidity status are at a higher risk of severe disability or death. In the presence of any intracranial masses (tumors, cysts, or hydrocephalus), the ICP can increase rapidly. During physical assessment, older patients should be closely monitored for all the bodily systems but with particular attention to areas of concern identified during their history. All older patients are checked for orthostatic hypotension. The deep tendon (muscle stretch) reflex must be evaluated. Diagnosis, prognosis and goal of treatment need to be discussed with family members.

Case Scenario

1. A 22-year-old male patient with a head injury, transferred to an intensive care unit had elevated intracranial pressure when he arrived at the emergency room. The doctor prescribed a diuretic to be administered to the patient to reduce ICP. The nurse anticipates which diuretic will be ordered, and why?
2. A 19-year-old boy met with an accident while returning from work. The vital signs at admission in the emergency room are Temperature: 97.1°F, HR: 65/min, BP: 102/70, RR: 16, and 96% oxygen saturation. Eyes open to painful stimuli, equal but slow to react to light, does not seem to recognize his family. As per Glasgow coma scale, what score would you give him upon admission?

SUMMARY

When conducted in a stepwise, timely assessment, continuous monitoring, and treatment of rising ICP may improve the patients' outcomes. Benefits on functional outcomes may be more visible when treatment is done in a more personalized manner. Recent research and efforts are being made toward precision management of acute brain injury, with ICP being an important component.

MULTIPLE CHOICE QUESTIONS

1. In a patient with acute head injury who is at risk for raised intracranial pressure. Which of the following nursing intervention will help in easy facilitation of cerebral venous drainage?
   a. Maintain HOB elevation at 30°
   b. Antiseizure medication
   c. Maintain euvolemia
   d. Monitor core temperature
2. Which of the following is contraindicated in a patient with increased ICP?
   a. Lumbar puncture
   b. Midline position of the head
   c. Hyperosmotic diuretics
   d. Barbiturates medications
3. Which of the following readings in a patient with head trauma depicts Cushing's triad:
   a. BP 150/112, HR 110, RR
   b. BP 90/60, HR 80, RR 22
   c. BP 190/50, HR 48, RR 8
   d. BP 80/40, HR 49, RR 12
4. The target CPP in a patient with severe TBI as per Brain Trauma Foundation:
   a. 10–30 mm Hg
   b. 30–50 mm Hg
   c. 50–70 mm Hg
   d. 70–90 mm Hg
5. Which of the following sedative medications is preferred for use before intubation in a patient with raised ICP?
   a. Esmolol
   b. Zolpidem
   c. Eszopiclone
   d. Alprazolam

ANSWERS

1. a   2. a   3. c   4. c
5. a

SUGGESTED READING

1. Asgeirsson B, Grande PO, Nordstrom CH. A new therapy of post-trauma brain edema based on haemodynamic principles for brain volume regulation. Intensive Care Medicine. 1994;20:260-7.
2. Bernard S, et al. Treatment of comatose survivors of out-of-hospital cardiac arrest with induced hypothermia. NEJM. 2002;346.
3. Carney N, Totten AM, O'Reilly C, Ullman JS, Hawryluk GWJ. Guidelines for the Management of Severe Traumatic Brain Injury, 4th edition.
4. Changa AR, Czeisler BM, Lord AS. Management of Elevated Intracranial Pressure: a Review. Curr Neurol Neurosci Rep. 2019;19(12):99.
5. Cooper DJ, Myburgh J, Heritier S, Finfer S, Bellomo R, Billot L, et al. SAFE-TBI Investigators; Australian and New Zealand Intensive Care Society Clinical Trials Group. Albumin resuscitation for traumatic brain injury: is intracranial hypertension the cause of increased mortality? J Neurotrauma. 2013;30(7):512-8.
6. Dunn LT. Raised Intracranial Pressure. Neurol Neurosurg Psychiatry 2002;73(I):23-i27.
7. Eisenberg HM, Frankowski RF, Contant CF, et al. High dose barbiturate control of elevated intracranial pressure in patients with a severe head injury. J Neurosurg. 1988;69:15-23.
8. Friedman DI, Jacobson DM. Idiopathic intracranial hypertension. J Neuroophthalmol. 2004;24(2):138-45.
9. Godoy DA, Seifi A, Garza D, Lubillo-Montenegro S, Murillo-Cabezas F. Hyperventilation Therapy for Control of Posttraumatic Intracranial Hypertension. Front Neurol. 2017;8:250.
10. Gu J, Huang H, Huang Y, Sun H, Xu H. Hypertonic saline or mannitol for treating elevated intracranial pressure in traumatic brain injury: a meta-analysis of randomized controlled trials. Neurosurg Rev. 2018.
11. Haddad SH, Arabi YM. Critical care management of severe traumatic brain injury in adults. Scand J Trauma Resusc Emerg Med. 2012;20:12.
12. Hays AN, Lazaridis C, Neyens R, Nicholas J, Gay S, Chalela JA. Osmotherapy: use among neurointensivists. Neurocrit Care. 2011;14(2):222-8.
13. Holzer M, et al. Mild therapeutic hypothermia to improve the neurologic outcome after cardiac arrest. NEJM. 2002;346.

14. Joseph M. Intracranial Pressure Monitoring: Vital Information Ignored. Indian J of Crit Care Med. 2005;09(1):35-41.
15. Kilgore KP, Lee MS, Leavitt JA, Mokri B, Hodge DO, Frank RD, et al. Re-evaluating the Incidence of Idiopathic Intracranial Hypertension in an Era of Increasing Obesity. Ophthalmology. 2017;124(5):697-700.
16. Lundberg N. Continuous recording and control of ventricular fluid pressure in neurosurgical practice. Acta Psychiat Neurol Scand. 1960;36(suppl 149):1-193.
17. Marehbian J, Muehlschlegel S, Edlow BL, Hinson HE, Hwang DY. Medical Management of the Severe Traumatic Brain Injury Patient. Neurocrit Care. 2017;27(3):430-446. 32.Knapp JM. Hyperosmolar therapy in the treatment of severe head injury in children: mannitol and hypertonic saline. AACN Clin Issues. 2005;16(2):199-211.
18. Miller JD, Piper IR, Dearden NM. Management of intracranial hypertension in head injury: matching treatment with cause. Acta Neurochirurgica Supplementum 1993;57:152-9.
19. Monro A. Observations on Structure and Functions of the Nervous System, Creech, and Johnson, Edinburgh, UK; 1783.
20. Muizelaar JP, Marmarou A, Ward JD, et al. Adverse effects of prolonged hyperventilation in patients with severe head injury: a randomized clinical trial. J Neurosurg. 1991;75:731-9.
21. Munakomi S, M Das J. Intracranial Pressure Monitoring. StatPearls Publishing; Treasure Island (FL); 2022.
22. Myburgh J, Cooper DJ, Finfer S, Bellomo R, Norton R, Bishop N, et al. The SAFE Study Investigators. Saline or Albumin for Fluid Resuscitation in Patients with Traumatic Brain Injury. N Engl J Med. 2007;357:874-884.
23. Nehring SM, Tadi P, Tenny S. Cerebral Edema. StatPearls Publishing; Treasure Island (FL); 2021.
24. Neilsen, N. et al. Targeted Temperature Management at 33C versus 36C after cardiac arrest. NEJM; 2013.
25. Raboel PH, Bartek Jr J, Andresen M, Bellander BM, Romner B, Intracranial Pressure Monitoring: Invasive versus Non-Invasive Methods—A Review. Crit Care Res Pract. 2012, Article ID 950393, 14 pages, 2012. https://doi.org/10.1155/2012/950393
26. Roberts DJ, Hall RI, Kramer AH, Robertson HL, Gallagher CN, Zygun DA. Sedation for critically ill adults with severe traumatic brain injury: A systematic review of randomized controlled trials. Crit Care Med. 2011;39:2743-51.
27. Rosner MJ, Daughton S. Cerebral perfusion pressure management in head injury. J Trauma. 1990;30:933-41.
28. Shrestha G, Pradhan S. Management of intracranial hypertension: Recent advances and future directions. Bangladesh Crit Care J. 2017; 5(1):53-62.
29. Singhi SC, Tiwari L. Management of Intracranial Hypertension. Indian J Pediatr. 2009;76(5):519-29.
30. Skoglund K, Enblad P, Hillered L, Marklund N. The neurological wake-up test increases stress hormone levels in patients with severe traumatic brain injury. Crit Care Med. 2012;40:216-22.
31. Smith, J. Tjandra JJ, Clunie GJA, Andrew HK. (2006). Textbook of Surgery. Wiley-Blackwell. 446. ISBN 1-4051-2627-2.
32. Smith M. Refractory Intracranial Hypertension: The Role of Decompressive Craniectomy. Anesth Analg. 2017;125(6):1999-2008.
33. Stevens RD, Shoykhet M, Cadena R. Emergency Neurological Life Support: Intracranial Hypertension and Herniation. Neurocrit Care. 2015;23(2):S76-S82.
34. Tripathy S, Mahapatra AK. Targeted temperature management in brain protection: An evidence-based review. Indian J Anaesth. 2015;59(1):9-14.
35. Upadhyay P, Tripathi VN, Singh RP, Sachan D. Role of hypertonic saline and mannitol in the management of raised intracranial pressure in children: A randomized comparative study. J Pediatr Neurosci. 2010;5(1):18-21.
36. Velle F, Lewén A, Howells T, Nilsson P, Enblad P. Temporal effects of barbiturate coma on intracranial pressure and compensatory reserve in children with traumatic brain injury. Acta Neurochir (Wien). 2021;163(2):489-98.
37. Weed LH, McKibben PS. Pressure changes in the cerebrospinal fluid following intravenous injection of solutions of various concentrations. Am J Physiol. 1919;48:512-30.
38. Worthley LI, Cooper DJ, Jones N. Treatment of resistant intracranial hypertension with hypertonic saline. Report of two cases. J Neurosurg. 1988;68:478-81.

INTRACRANIAL SURGERY

The phrase "brain surgery" refers to several medical operations that entail correcting the structural problem in the brain. There are several types of brain surgeries. Medical advances have enabled surgeons to operate on regions of the brain without making a single incision in or near the head. Brain surgery is a delicate and difficult procedure. The kind of brain surgery performed greatly depends on the problem being treated. For example, a brain aneurysm can be repaired using a catheter which is introduced into an artery in the groin. However, if the aneurysm gets ruptured, an open surgery called craniotomy may have to be performed. It is essential to treat life-threatening brain illnesses and disorders, as well as those that have the potential to cause lasting brain damage. Surgery may be considered for conditions causing:

- Brain tissue changes, such as benign or malignant tumors, infections, injury, etc.
- Impaired or abnormal blood flow in the brain, such as cerebral aneurysms, subdural hematomas, and subarachnoid or intraventricular hemorrhages.
- Cerebrospinal fluid changes, such as infection or hydrocephalus.
- Changes in brain function, such as epilepsy or Parkinson's disease.

Though all the surgical procedures carry some risk post-operatively, intracranial surgeries being a major medical event, may involve extra risk. The particular potential risks may include impairment in speech, vision, coordination, balance, cognition, etc.

Cranial surgical approaches: Table 29.7 shows three different surgical approaches—supratentorial, infratentorial, and transsphenoidal. Burr holes may be used in neurosurgical procedures to make a bone flap in the skull, to aspirate a brain abscess, or to evacuate a hematoma **(Fig. 29.5)**.

TYPES OF INTRACRANIAL SURGERIES

Craniotomy

A craniotomy is a surgical technique that involves removing a portion of the skull to expose the brain and execute surgery. Brain tumors, aneurysms, arteriovenous malformations, subdural empyemas, subdural hematomas, and intracerebral hematomas are among the most frequent disorders that may be treated using this method. Specialized instruments and equipment are used to remove the bone flap, which is a portion of bone. The bone flap is removed temporarily, held at the surgical instrument table, and then replaced after the surgery is completed. The bone can be discarded, kept in the abdomen subcutaneous area, or cryopreserved under cold

TABLE 29.7: Cranial surgical approaches.

Approaches	Site location and nursing intervention	
Supratentorial	**Site of surgery:** Above the tentorium **Incision location** An incision is created above the region to be operated on, which is normally behind the hairline. **Nursing interventions** • Maintain head of bed elevation 45°, with the neck in neutral alignment. • Avoid positioning the patient on the operative side if a large tumor has been removed.	
Infratentorial	**Site of surgery:** Below the tentorium, brainstem. **Incision location** The incision is made at the nape of the neck, around the occipital lobe. **Nursing interventions** Maintain proper neck alignment. Avoid flexion of the neck to prevent possible tearing of the suture line.	
Transsphenoidal	**Site of surgery:** Sella turcica **Incision location** • The incision is made beneath the upper lip to gain access into the nasal cavity. • Continue to use nasal packing and reinforce as required. Instruct the patient to avoid blowing his/her nose. • Maintain a raised head of the bed to improve venous drainage and drainage from the surgical site. • Provide frequent oral care	

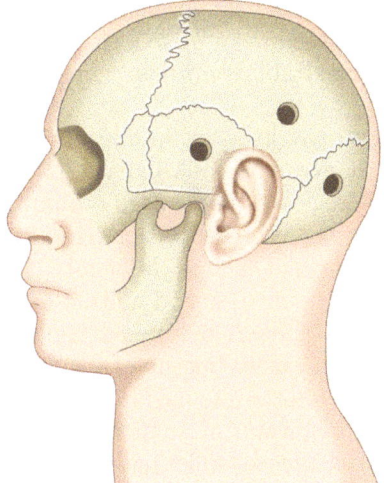

Fig. 29.5: Burr holes.

storage conditions in some situations, depending on the etiology and rationale for the treatment. Cranioplasty is the surgical method used to rebuild and put the bone flap back into the skull during a second intervention. The open brain surgery is performed to:
❖ Remove tumors
❖ Clip off an aneurysm
❖ Drain blood or fluid from an infection
❖ Remove abnormal brain tissue

After the surgery, the bone flap is frequently secured in place using plates, sutures, or wires. In the case of malignancies, infection, or brain edema, the hole may be left open.

Types of Craniotomy

Craniotomies are classified into several categories. Each type is called by the operation technique or site.

- ❖ **Stereotactic craniotomy:** A stereotactic craniotomy employs use of previously obtained images (MRI or CT scan) to guide the surgeon to the exact location of the lesion. It enables them to differentiate between healthy and diseased tissue. Stereotactic procedures can also assist the surgeon in determining the optimal location for a scalp incision. This makes it simpler to undertake minimally invasive operations and create smaller incisions.
- ❖ **Endoscopic craniotomy:** A small incision is made in the skull by the surgeon during an endoscopic craniotomy. They insert an endoscope, a tiny illuminated instrument equipped with a camera. This procedure is typically utilized with keyhole craniotomies.
- ❖ **Awake craniotomy:** Awake craniotomy is performed when the patient is awake. The surgeons will ask questions while monitoring the brain activity during the procedure. Cortical mapping is done by the surgeon using a small electrical stimulation device. The patient is observed for movement or some ability, e.g., speech when a particular area is stimulated. This helps them to avoid removing vital areas. The surgical team speaks to the patient regularly, the patient is observed for his ability to name objects and also is asked to report any abnormal sensations.
- ❖ **Keyhole craniotomy:** Brain tumors are removed with a keyhole craniotomy. It is a less invasive operation with fewer scars and a faster recovery period. The surgeon creates a tiny incision behind the ear. This incision is used to remove the brain tumor.
- ❖ **Supraorbital 'eyebrow' craniotomy:** It is a minimally invasive surgical procedure that results in little scarring. It is used to remove certain brain tumors which are located in or under the frontal lobes and around the area of the optic nerves and above the pituitary gland. The surgeon creates a tiny incision in the brow.
- ❖ **Pterional (frontotemporal) craniotomy:** This is a unique approach that provides wide access to the skull base. The pterion is the junction point of the frontal, temporal, sphenoid, and parietal bones of the skull. A pterional craniotomy, also known as a frontotemporal craniotomy, is performed around the pterional and includes the removal of a portion of the pterion. The surgeon creates an incision beneath the hairline to gain access to various sections of the brain. It is considered a fundamental tool in the armamentarium of the neurosurgeon.
- ❖ **Orbitozygomatic craniotomy:** An orbitozygomatic craniotomy can be used to treat difficult tumors and aneurysms. It provides access to the anterior and middle cranial fossae as well as the deep sellar and basilar apex regions. The surgeon temporarily removes a portion of the bone that forms the orbit, eye socket, and cheek curve. This allows the surgeon to access deeper areas of the brain while lowering the danger of brain injury.
- ❖ **Posterior fossa craniotomy:** The lowest region of the skull is known as the posterior fossa. It is close to the brainstem and cerebellum, which are in charge of balance and coordination. A tumor in the posterior fossa can put strain on the cerebellum, brainstem, and spinal cord. A posterior fossa craniotomy can be used to remove the tumor and relieve the pressure. This is accomplished by making an incision at the base of the skull.
- ❖ **Translabyrinthine craniotomy:** It is a procedure that involves creating an incision in the scalp behind the ear. Then a portion of the mastoid bone as well as the semicircular canals, which aid in balance are removed. It is used to remove a vestibular schwannoma, commonly known as an auditory neuroma. An acoustic neuroma is a benign tumor that develops on the nerve that links the inner ear to the brain. It leads to hearing loss and balance problems. Hearing loss arises from the removal of the semicircular canals. The procedure, on the other hand, reduces the chance of facial nerve injury.
- ❖ **Bifrontal craniotomy:** A bifrontal craniotomy, or extended bifrontal craniotomy, is used to remove tough tumors near the front of the brain. It is a traditional skull base procedure that is generally performed if the tumor is too complicated for minimally invasive surgery. The surgeon makes an incision behind the front hairline. They remove a section of the bone that defines the curvature of the brow, allowing them access to the front of the brain. The procedure is also used to implant devices for movement disorders, such as Parkinson's disease.

Procedure of Craniotomy

Depending on the method being used, the right head position is fixed after the patient has fallen asleep. It is crucial to provide appropriate cushioning throughout to prevent pressure points on delicate body parts. The area of the skull where the craniotomy will be performed will determine where the incision will be made. Anatomical points are verified at this stage before the incision if neuronavigation is being used to help the surgical craniotomy.

The incision is often made across the frontal, temporal, parietal, or occipital bones, or over a combination of bones while performing surgery in the supratentorial region. The incision is often made on the back of the head beneath the transverse sinus for infratentorial surgery. The hair in the region may be shaved off once the appropriate position for the incision on the skin has been selected. For aesthetic purposes, the incision should ideally be made beneath the hairline. The surgical region is cleansed with the appropriate antiseptic agent once the incision has been verified, and then standard sterile draping procedures are used. To aid in haemostasis, a local anesthetic with epinephrine is often given on the visible skin incision.

Following the skin incision, the muscles behind the scalp are cut apart to reveal the skull. To have sufficient exposure to the surgical region to be focused on, retractors can be applied to the margins of the incision. The scalp flap can be secured with sutures or fishhook retractors. If necessary, the pericranium can be divided and utilized in place of dural during the closure. The craniotome, also known as the cranial drill, is used to create many burr holes in the skull. To prevent inserting the craniotome into the brain tissue, caution must be used. A Freer elevator or Penfield dissector is used to separate the dura after the holes have been cleansed of any remaining bone fragments.

A craniotome saw is used to join the burr holes, and after gently separating the bone flap from the dura below, it is elevated. The surgical instrument table holds the bone flap until the procedure's closing phase. The dura is sliced and retracted during the intradural operation to reveal the brain.

After the brain operation is finished, plates and screws are used to restore the bone to its original location. Before sealing the scalp, it is important to achieve sufficient hemostasis. Following the reattachment of the covering tissues, the anatomical layers of the scalp are sutured. A subdural or subgaleal drain can be left in place to drain the collected blood products, depending on the surgeon's preferences.

Craniectomy

Craniectomy is a neurosurgical procedure that involves removing a part of the skull to relieve pressure on the underlying brain. This operation is often carried out when a patient has suffered a very serious brain injury with considerable quantities of blood or brain swelling all over the place.

Procedure

Patients who have suffered brain damage serious enough to require a craniectomy are often already in the hospital and under careful observation. The anesthesia team transports patients to the operation room, where they will be closely monitored while under anesthesia. On the side of the skull where the most compression is occurring, normally, the neurosurgeons will create an incision in the scalp during this time (especially in cases where the compression is caused by a blood clot). A drill is used to drill holes into the skull once the skin and supporting tissues have been removed and moved out of the way.

The bone is cut out once the holes are joined together using a saw. The bone is often kept in a freezer in the hopes that it can be reinserted once the patient's brain swelling has reduced and their condition is more stable. Patients are given a custom-fit helmet to wear throughout the bone removal procedure to avoid further brain damage. After the bone has been removed and any bleeding surrounding the brain has been stopped, sutures are used to seal the skin and connective tissue around the brain.

Resective Surgery

The most popular kind of surgery used to treat epilepsy. MRI is used to pinpoint the part of the brain where seizures take place. The surgeons can surgically remove the area of the brain that is causing seizures using resective surgery.

Multiple Subpial Transection

It is a surgical technique by which connections of the epileptic focus are partially cut without resection. It is used for seizure foci in nonresectable articulate areas. If the seizures do not usually begin in the same region of your brain, it could be more helpful than resective surgery.

Hemispherectomy

"The most extreme form of epilepsy surgery" is hemispherectomy. A surgeon performs this treatment by completely, partially, or fully disconnecting the diseased part of the brain from the normal hemisphere. It is applied when epileptic episodes have completely affected one side of the brain. Younger infants, newborns with brain injury, and older children with severe seizures are the most frequent candidates for this type of surgery. This is one of the most successful operations at stopping seizures in carefully selected patients.

Lobotomy

A lobotomy, also known as leucotomy, is a form of psychosurgery that has been used to treat mental health issues, such as schizophrenia and mood disorders. Psychosurgeries are operations in which a portion of the brain is physically removed or altered. There are two main approaches to separate the tissue in the prefrontal cortex during lobotomies:

1. **Frontal lobotomy:** A leucotome, a surgical tool that resembles an ice pick, was used by the surgeon to cut through the brain tissue after drilling holes into the sides of the skull.
2. **Transorbital lobotomy:** To access the brain, a surgeon inserts a leucotome into the eye socket and pound it with a hammer through a thin layer of bone.

With advances in medicine, psychosurgeries are no longer commonly carried out. The only time surgery is often done is when all other forms of therapy have failed. Surgical procedures that are still used today include:

Cingulotomy

Cingulotomies are the most often performed psychosurgical procedure. Anterior cingulate tissue, which is linked to the perception of chronic pain, is altered with this particular type of surgery. It is occasionally applied to treat signs of chronic and severe anxiety disorders, such as obsessive-compulsive disorder (OCD), severe mood disorders, such as treatment-resistance depression or bipolar disorder, Heroin addiction, Chronic pain syndromes that do not respond to other treatments, and severe schizophrenia with aggressive behavior.

- **Anterior capsulotomy:** Severe OCD that is resistant to medication and therapy may benefit from an anterior capsulotomy. It entails changing the area of the brain that transmits information to the prefrontal region from the thalamus and brainstem.
- **Subcaudate tractotomy:** A subcaudate tractotomy may be used to treat delusions and hallucinations. It involves cutting connections between the limbic system and a part of the prefrontal lobe called the orbitofrontal cortex.
- **Limbic leucotomy:** It combines a cingulotomy and a subcaudate tractotomy. Since the 1970s, it has been used to treat OCD and mood disorders.

Corpus Callosotomy

The corpus callosum, a network of nerves that connects the left and right hemispheres of the brain, is severed during a corpus callosotomy. Researchers discovered in a 2017 study that corpus callosotomy may be a useful therapy for generalized epilepsy in patients with drug-resistant epilepsy. It prevents seizures by interrupting the spread of seizures from hemisphere to hemisphere. Corpus callosotomy is most often used in children who have bad seizures that start in one half of their brain and spread to the other.

Biopsy

Use of this treatment allows for the microscopic examination of a tiny portion of the tumor or brain tissue. This requires a little skull incision and perforation.

Minimally Invasive Endonasal Endoscopic Surgery

Through the nose and sinuses, the surgeon can perform this kind of surgery to remove tumors or lesions. It enables them to enter specific areas of the brain without cutting. An endoscope, a telescopic tool with lights and a camera so the surgeon can see where they are operating, is used throughout the surgery. The pituitary gland, the base of the skull, and tumors developing in the lower portion of the brain can all be treated with this.

Minimally Invasive Neuroendoscopy

Neuroendoscopy is a minimally invasive procedure that employs endoscopes to remove brain tumors. During this procedure, the surgeon may drill tiny holes the size of a dime in the skull to gain access to certain areas of the brain.

Procedure

A narrow tube called an endoscope is inserted through the mouth, nose, or tiny incisions in the skull during this minimally invasive procedure to access or remove brain tissue. Tools are inserted via the endoscope, which has a light and camera on the end, to do the operation. One kind of neuroendoscopy is endoscopic transsphenoidal surgery, commonly known as endoscopic pituitary surgery. In order to remove brain tumors and lesions close to the pituitary gland, which is directly behind the bridge of the nose, the endoscope must be inserted through the nose.

Deep Brain Stimulation

A battery-operated medical device called an implantable pulse generator is implanted to deliver electrical stimulation to specific areas in the brain.

Procedure

Similar to a biopsy, this surgery includes cutting a small hole in the skull, but the surgeon will introduce a small electrode into a deep region of the brain rather than removing tissue. Electrical impulses will be transferred from the electrode to the battery near the heart to assist treat Parkinson's disease symptoms, among other conditions.

Posterior Fossa Decompression

This treatment involves parts of the brain called the cerebellum and brainstem. For example, to treat a Chiari malformation, the surgeon creates an incision behind the patient's head and removes a tiny part of the bone at the base of the skull. This removal gives the cerebellum more room and relieves strain on the spinal cord.

Thrombectomy and Cerebral Aneurysm Repair

The surgeon directs surgical devices, such as a catheter or small metal wires via a big blood artery into the patient's groin to reach the brain vessels, using contrast dye to locate the troublesome blood vessel without having to open up the patient's skull. Patients with a blood clot in a brain artery, a cerebral aneurysm (a weakened and bulging region in an arterial wall), or a burst aneurysm that causes bleeding into the brain are the most common candidates for the treatment.

Stereotactic Radiosurgery

Some patients with brain cancer are treated with stereotactic radiosurgery, which may involve the use of a Gamma Knife, although this is not surgery in the traditional sense, and the "knife" is not truly a knife. Radiosurgery is a type of external radiation therapy that does not need an incision. Specialized equipment, such as the Gamma Knife brand, carefully administers a high dosage of radiation that targets tumors or other lesions while causing minimal harm to surrounding healthy tissue.

NURSING MANAGEMENT FOR THE PATIENTS WITH INTRACRANIAL SURGERIES

Preoperative Management

CT scanning may be used as a preoperative diagnostic tool to show the lesion and the degree of surrounding cerebral edema, ventricular size, and displacement. MRI delivers information comparable to a CT scan and evaluates the lesion in different planes. Cerebral angiography can be done to evaluate the blood supply of a tumor or to provide information about vascular abnormalities. Transcranial Doppler flow tests are performed to assess intracranial blood vessel blood flow.

To lessen the risk of postoperative seizures, most patients are given an antiseizure medicine, such as phenytoin (Dilantin) or a phenytoin metabolite (Cerebyx) before surgery (paroxysmal transient disturbances of the brain resulting from a discharge of abnormal electrical activity)

Corticosteroids, such as dexamethasone (Decadron), may be given preoperatively to minimize cerebral edema. Fluids can be restricted again. If the patient has cerebral dysfunction and tends to retain fluid, a hyperosmotic agent (mannitol) plus a diuretic agent, such as furosemide (Lasix) may be administered intravenously immediately before and occasionally during surgery. If there is a risk of brain contamination, the patient may be given antibiotics; and diazepam may be provided before surgery to reduce anxiety.

Preoperative Nursing Management

The preoperative evaluation acts as a benchmark against which postoperative condition and recovery are evaluated. This evaluation includes assessing LOC and response to stimuli as well as recognizing any neurologic abnormalities, such as paralysis, visual dysfunction, personality or speech changes, and bladder and bowel issues. The 5-point scale is used to assess distal and proximal motor strength in both the upper and lower limbs.

The comprehension and responses of the patient and family to the expected surgical operation and its probable sequelae are evaluated, as is the availability of support networks for the patient and family. Adequate surgical preparation, including consideration of the patient's physical and mental status, can lower the risk of anxiety, fear, and postoperative problems. The patient's neurologic impairments and their possible consequences following surgery are evaluated. Trochanter rolls are placed on the extremities and the feet are positioned against a footboard if there are motor deficiencies, weakness, or paralysis of the arms or legs. A patient who can ambulate is encouraged to do so. If the patient is aphasic, writing materials or images and word cards depicting the bedpan, glass of water, blanket, and other commonly used things may aid enhance communication.

Patient and family preparation involves providing information about what to expect during and after surgery. The surgical site is shaved soon before surgery (typically in the operating room) to prevent any superficial abrasions from becoming infected. In the operating room, an indwelling urinary catheter is implanted to empty the bladder and monitor urine output while diuretics are administered.

Following surgery, the patient may have a central and arterial line put in for fluid administration and pressure monitoring. The thick head dressing used after surgery may temporarily impede hearing. If the eyes are swollen shut, vision may be limited. If the patient has a tracheostomy or endotracheal tube, he/she will be unable to talk until the tube is withdrawn, thus an alternate form of communication should be arranged.

Because of the changed cognitive status, the patient may be ignorant of the approaching procedure. However, encouragement and attention to the patient's requirements are required. Whatever the patient's level of awareness, the family requires comfort and support since they recognize the importance of brain surgery.

Postoperative Management

Assessment

The frequency of postoperative surveillance is determined by the patient's clinical status. Assessing respiratory function is critical since even mild hypoxia might worsen cerebral ischemia. The breathing rate and pattern are constantly monitored, as are the arterial blood gas readings. Vital sign fluctuations are carefully observed and documented since they suggest a rise in ICP. The patient's temperature is taken at regular intervals to check for hyperthermia caused by hypothalamic injury. Neurologic examinations are performed regularly to detect elevated ICP caused by cerebral edema or hemorrhage. A change in LOC or reaction to stimuli might be the first indication of rising ICP.

The surgical dressing is examined for signs of bleeding or CSF leaking. The nurse must be on the lookout for the emergence of complications; all evaluations are conducted with these issues in mind. Seizures are a possible complication, and any seizure activity is meticulously documented and reported. Restlessness might develop as the patient gets more responsive, or it can be caused by pain, disorientation, hypoxia, or other stimuli. The goal of ongoing postoperative care is to identify and reduce cerebral edema, relieve pain and avoid seizures, and monitor ICP.

Postoperative Nursing Management

Nursing Diagnoses

Based on the assessment data, major nursing diagnoses after intracranial surgery may include the following:

❖ Ineffective cerebral tissue perfusion related to cerebral edema
❖ Potential for ineffective thermoregulation related to damage to the hypothalamus, dehydration, and infection
❖ Potential for impaired gas exchange related to hypoventilation, aspiration, and immobility
❖ Disturbed sensory perception related to periorbital edema, head dressing, endotracheal tube, and effect of ICP
❖ Body image disturbance related to changes in appearance or physical disabilities

Other nursing diagnoses may include poor communication (aphasia) due to brain tissue injury and a greater risk of impaired skin integrity due to immobility, pressure, and incontinence. Physical mobility may be compromised as a result of a neurologic impairment caused by neurosurgical surgery or the underlying condition.

Goals

These include maintaining neurologic homeostasis to increase cerebral tissue perfusion, appropriate thermoregulation, normal breathing and gas exchange, the capacity to cope with sensory deprivation, adaptability to changes in body image, and preventing any potential complications.

Nursing Interventions

Maintaining Cerebral Tissue Perfusion

It is critical to monitor the patient's respiratory status since even little declines in oxygen levels (hypoxia) can cause cerebral ischemia and alter the clinical course and prognosis. The endotracheal tube is retained in place until the patient displays clinical indications of waking and has sufficient spontaneous breathing, as determined by arterial blood gas analysis and clinical examination. Impaired cerebral oxygenation can cause secondary brain injury.

After brain surgery, some degree of cerebral edema develops; it tends to peak 24-36 hours after surgery, resulting in reduced responsiveness on the second postoperative day. Controlling cerebral edema is covered in the prior section in the management of elevated ICP. When any portion of the system is treated, strict asepsis is used to monitor intraventricular drainage.

Mannitol, which raises serum osmolality and pulls free water from parts of the brain, is used to treat cerebral edema (with an intact blood-brain barrier). Osmotic diuresis then excretes the fluid. Dexamethasone (Decadron) is given intravenously every 6 hours for 24-72 hours; the route is changed to oral as soon as practicable, and the dosage is decreased over 5-7 days.

Every 15-60 minutes/as per requirement, vital signs and neurologic status (LOC and responsiveness, pupillary and motor responses) are evaluated. The ICP rises, hence extreme head rotation should be avoided. The patient is positioned on his/her back or side with one pillow under the head following supratentorial surgery. Depending on the ICP level and the neurosurgeon's discretion, the head of the bed may be raised 30°. The patient is maintained on one side (off the back) following posterior fossa (infratentorial) surgery, with the head supported by a tiny, hard cushion. In order to keep the neck in a neutral posture, the patient may be rotated to either side. While turning, the body should be turned as a unit to prevent placing strain on the incision and possibly tearing the sutures. The head of the bed may be elevated slowly as tolerated by the patient.

The patient's posture is changed every 2 hours, and skin care is provided regularly. While changing positions, care is taken to avoid interrupting the ICP monitoring system.

Regulating Temperature

There could be a moderate temperature increase following brain surgery. Surgery can harm the hypothalamus regions of the brain that control body temperature. High temperature should be treated promptly to combat its effect on brain metabolism and function.

Nursing interventions involve maintaining a close watch on the patient's body temperature and taking the following steps to lower it—removing blankets/extra clothing, cold sponging, and administering the prescribed drugs to lower fever.

On the other hand, prolonged neurosurgery operations may also result in hypothermia. Rewarm the patient. Shivering, which raises cellular oxygen requirements should be avoided.

Improving Gas Exchange

Due to immobilization, immunosuppression, reduced LOC, and hydration restriction, the patient undergoing neurosurgery is at risk for lung infections and poor gas exchange. Atelectasis and secretions accumulating in dependent regions are two effects of immobility that damage the respiratory system. Due to their inability to expectorate thicker secretions, patients with limited fluid intake may be more susceptible to atelectasis. The occurrence of pneumonia in neurosurgical patients may be due to aspiration and immobility.

The nurse examines the patient for indications of a respiratory infection, such as a rise in body temperature, a rapid heartbeat, and changes in breathing, and also auscultates the lungs for abnormal sounds.

Every two hours, the change position of patient to promote clear pulmonary secretions and avoid stasis. Other techniques to expand compressed alveoli can be implemented once the patient regains awareness, including yawning, sighing, deep breathing, incentive spirometry, and coughing (unless contraindicated). Coughing and suctioning both elevate ICP, thus, if necessary, the oropharynx and trachea are suctioned to eliminate secretions. Suctioning should be handled with caution. The oxygen delivery system's increased humidity may aid in liquifying secretions. The nurse and respiratory therapist collaborate to assess the effectiveness of chest physical therapy.

Relieving Pain

Acetaminophen is typically used for pain and fevers over 99.6°F (37.5°C). Headache is common following a craniotomy, which is caused by the scalp nerves being stretched and inflamed during surgery. Codeine taken orally is frequently adequate to alleviate headache. Morphine sulphate can also be utilized to treat postoperative pain in craniotomy patients. Because of the significant risk of seizures following supratentorial neurosurgical operations, antiseizure medication (phenytoin, diazepam) is indicated for patients who have had a supratentorial craniotomy. To maintain the drugs within the therapeutic range, serum levels are checked.

Managing Sensory Deprivation

Periorbital edema is a typical side effect of intracranial surgery because fluid drains into the dependent periorbital regions when the patient is positioned prone during the procedure. Hematoma can form under the scalp and migrate to the orbit, causing ecchymosis (black eye).

Before surgery, the patient and family should be informed that one or both eyes may become edematous for a short period. After surgery, elevating the patient's head (if not contraindicated) and administering cold compresses to the eyes will help in minimizing edema. If periorbital edema worsens, the surgeon should be informed because it may suggest the development of a postoperative clot or that there is increased ICP and inadequate venous drainage.

Additional factors that can affect sensation include a bulky head dressing, the presence of an endotracheal tube, and the effects of increased ICP. In the absence of bleeding or a CSF leak, every effort is made to keep the head dressing as small as possible. If the patient requires mechanical breathing using an endotracheal tube, every attempt is made to extubate the patient as soon as clinical indicators indicate it is possible. The consequences of increased ICP are continuously evaluated in the patient.

Enhancing Self-image

The patient is encouraged to express his/her sentiments and frustrations with any change in look. Nursing care is provided in response to the patient's emotions and feelings. If the patient has misunderstandings concerning puffiness around the eyes, periorbital bruises, or hair loss, accurate information may be required. Grooming, wearing the patient's own clothes, and covering the head with a turban (and, eventually, a wig until hair growth begins) are all encouraged. Social connections with close friends, relatives, and medical employees may boost a patient's self-esteem.

Monitoring ICP and Managing Potential Complications

In patients having intracranial surgery, a ventricular catheter or another form of drain is commonly implanted. The catheter is linked to an outside drainage system. The pulsations of the fluid in the tube indicate the catheter's patency. A stopcock connected to the pressure tube and transducer can be used to measure the ICP.

Turning the three-way stop-cock to the appropriate position determines the ICP (Hickey, 2003). To avoid CSF drainage, verify that the system is tight at all connections and that the stopcock is in the right position; if fluid is withdrawn too quickly, the collapse of the ventricles and brain herniation may occur (Hickey, 2003). When the ventricular pressure is normal and steady, the catheter is withdrawn. If the catheter looks to be occluded, the neurosurgeon must be contacted.

The potential complications that can occur within hours of surgery may include increased ICP, bleeding and hypovolemic shock, altered fluid and electrolyte balance, infection, and seizures. These complications require close communication between the nurse and the surgeon.

Monitoring for Increased ICP and Bleeding

Elevated ICP and hemorrhage are both potentially fatal for patients who have had intracranial neurosurgery. Following points must be kept in mind while caring for such type of patients.

- ❖ An increase in blood pressure and a reduction in pulse with respiratory failure may suggest elevated ICP.
- ❖ An accumulation of blood under the bone flap (extradural, subdural, or intracerebral) may endanger life. Every patient who does not awaken as expected or whose health worsens should be suspected of having a clot. If the patient develops any new postoperative neurologic impairments, an intracranial hematoma is suspected (especially a dilated pupil on the operative side). In these cases, the patient is quickly returned to the operating room for clot extraction, if necessary.
- ❖ Conditions, such as cerebral edema, infarction, metabolic abnormalities, and hydrocephalus can all resemble the clinical signs of a clot.
- ❖ Early symptoms and changes in clinical status are reported to the surgeon, and the patient is continuously watched for indicators of problems. Therapies are started as soon as possible, and the nurse supports in assessing therapy response. The nurse also offers assistance to the patient and his or her family.
- ❖ If signs and symptoms of increased ICP appear, head of the patient should be aligned in a neutral position without flexion to promote venous drainage, head of the bed should be elevated to 30°, and administer mannitol (an osmotic diuretic).

Managing Fluid and Electrolyte Disturbances

Fluid and electrolyte imbalances may develop because of the patient's underlying disease or as consequence of surgery. Disturbances in fluid and electrolytes can lead to the development of cerebral edema.

The postoperative hydration regimen is developed on an individual basis and is dependent on the kind of neurosurgical surgery. Fluid volume and composition are changed based on daily blood electrolyte readings, as well as fluid intake and outflow.

Sodium retention can develop immediately after surgery. Electrolytes should be monitored regularly. Intake and output are calculated using losses from temperature, respiration, and CSF drainage. Fluid restriction may be required in individuals with cerebral edema.

After the first 24 hours, oral fluids are often resumed (Hickey, 2003). Before starting oral fluids, the existence of gag and swallowing reflexes must be confirmed. Fluids may need to be delivered via alternate ways in certain individuals with posterior fossa tumors due to difficulty swallowing. After resuming the diet orally, the patient should be monitored for signs and symptoms of nausea and vomiting (Hickey, 2003).

Patients having brain tumor surgery are frequently given high dosages of corticosteroids, which causes hyperglycemia. As a result, serum glucose levels are monitored every four hours. Because these individuals are prone to stomach ulcers, histamine-2 receptor antagonists (H2 blockers) are administered to reduce gastric acid output. The patient should be evaluated for gastrointestinal discomfort.

The patient may also develop diabetes insipidus, which is characterized by excessive urine output. The specific gravity of the urine is tested hourly, and fluid intake and output are recorded.

Syndrome of inappropriate antidiuretic hormone (SIADH), which causes water retention with hyponatremia and serum hypo-osmolality, occurs in a wide range of central nervous system illnesses that cause fluid abnormalities (brain tumor, head trauma). Nursing management includes a meticulous recording of intake and output, urine specific gravity tests, and monitoring of serum and urine electrolyte studies while adhering to fluid restriction instructions.

Preventing Infection

Infections may be associated with the neurosurgical operation. The presence of intravenous and arterial lines for fluid administration and monitoring may further increase the risk of infection. Patients who have extensive intracranial procedures and those who have external ventricular drains in situ for more than 48–72 hours are at a higher risk of infection.

The incision site is checked for any signs of redness, pain, swelling, separation, or foul odor. In the initial postoperative phase, the dressing is frequently stained with blood. It is critical to strengthen the dressing using sterile pads to minimize contamination and infection. If the dressing is badly soiled or displaced, it should be notified as soon as possible.

CSF may flow through the wound after suboccipital surgery. Because of the risk of meningitis, this complication is hazardous. Any unexpected flow of fluid from a cranial wound is immediately reported since a significant leak necessitates immediate surgical correction. Pay close attention to the patient who complains of a salty taste, since this might be caused by CSF trickling down the throat. Coughing, sneezing, or nose blowing should be avoided since they might induce CSF leakage by putting pressure on the operation site.

While handling dressings, drainage systems, and intravenous and arterial lines, aseptic procedure should be employed. The patient is closely followed for signs and symptoms of infection, and cultures are taken from patients who have a suspected infection. Adequate antibiotics are given as directed.

Monitoring for Seizure Activity

Seizures and epilepsy can occur as a result of any intracranial operation. To minimize additional cerebral edema, seizures must be avoided. Administering the recommended antiseizure medicine before and soon after surgery may help to avoid seizures in the months and years to come.

Monitoring and Managing other Potential Complications

Additional issues may emerge within the first two weeks or afterward, affecting the patient's recovery. These may include deep vein thrombosis, pulmonary embolism, pulmonary and urinary tract infections, pressure ulcers, etc. Most of these issues may be prevented by regular position changes, sufficient suctioning of secretions, screening for pulmonary difficulties, surveillance for urine complications, and skin care.

PROMOTING HOME AND COMMUNITY-BASED CARE

A neurosurgical patient's recovery at home is determined by the extent of the surgical treatment and its success. The patient's strengths and limits, as well as their role in aiding recovery, are discussed with the family. The nurse participating in patients' home and ongoing care after cranial surgery must remind patients and family members of the importance of health promotion and prescribed health screening. Unless another health concern necessitates a specific diet, no dietary restrictions are usually necessary. While showering or taking a bath is permissible, the scalp should be kept dry until all sutures have been removed. If the skull bone has been removed, a protective helmet may be recommended by the neurosurgeon.

Patients are discharged from the hospital as quickly as possible unless complications arise. Individuals with significant motor impairments require considerable physical treatment and rehabilitation. Individuals who have post-operative cognitive and verbal problems require psychological assessment, speech therapy, and rehabilitation. Throughout hospitalization and home care, the nurse collaborates with the physician and other healthcare specialists to provide the most comprehensive rehabilitation possible. Other potential outcomes include paralysis, blindness, and convulsions.

When a tumor, accident, or disease reduces the patient's prognosis, care is focused on keeping the patient as comfortable as possible. The home care nurse, hospice nurse, and social worker collaborate with the family to arrange for extra home health care or hospice services, as well as the patient's placement in an extended-care facility.

GERIATRIC CONSIDERATIONS

The geriatric population may be at a higher mortality and worse functional outcomes compared with younger groups despite neurosurgical procedures. These procedures may do more harm than good and are possibly performed less frequently on elderly patients with altered LOC, because of the perception of poor prognosis in them. However, significant proof that intracranial surgeries in old age would have a deleterious effect on outcome in elderly patients are lacking. In addition, hospitalization of the older population may be connected with numerous other medical issues.

SUMMARY

Brain surgery is a complex and difficult procedure. It encompasses a wide range of medical operations aimed at treating structural issues in the brain. The kind of brain surgery performed is significantly dependent on the problem being treated. Patients can develop a wide range of complications postoperatively. Meticulous nursing care is required to identify and treat the problems among these patients.

MULTIPLE CHOICE QUESTIONS

1. A surgical procedure in which a portion of the skull is temporarily removed to reveal the brain and carry out an intracranial procedure?
   a. Craniectomy
   b. Craniotomy
   c. Lobectomy
   d. Lobotomy

2. A surgical procedure in which the nerve pathways in a lobe or lobes of the brain are severed from those in other areas?
   a. Psychoanalysis
   b. Prefrontal lobotomy
   c. Transorbital lobotomy
   d. Thrombectomy

3. A type of external radiation therapy that uses special equipment to position the patient and precisely give a single large dose of radiation to a tumor?
   a. Endoscopic surgery
   b. Psychosurgery
   c. Stereotactic surgery
   d. Neuroendoscopy surgery

4. In which position the infratentorial craniotomy should be performed?
   a. Left lateral
   b. Right lateral
   c. Prone
   d. Supine

5. Which of the following is a loop diuretic?
   a. Mannitol
   b. Glycerin
   c. Isosorbide
   d. Furosemide

ANSWERS

1. b   2. b   3. c   4. c
5. d

SUGGESTED READING

1. Alkhaibary A, Alharbi A, Alnefaie N, Oqalaa Almubarak A, Aloraidi A, Khairy S. Cranioplasty: A Comprehensive Review of the History, Materials, Surgical Aspects, and Complications. World Neurosurg. 2020;139:445-52.
2. Beniwal M, Shukla D. Management of Perforator Plunge in the Transverse Sinus. Pediatr Neurosurg. 2016;51(5):273-5.
3. Bhaskar IP, Zaw NN, Zheng M, Lee GY. Bone flap storage following craniectomy: a survey of practices in major Australian neurosurgical centers. ANZ J Surg. 2011;81(3):137-41.
4. Britannica, T. Editors of Encyclopaedia. lobotomy. Encyclopedia Britannica; 2022.
5. González-Darder JM. History of the craniotomy. Neurocirugia (Astur). 2016;27(5):245-57.
6. https://www.britannica.com/science/lobotomy
7. Sahuquillo J, Dennis JA. Decompressive craniectomy for the treatment of high intracranial pressure in closed traumatic brain injury. Cochrane Database Syst Rev. 2019;12(12):CD003983.
8. Schizodimos T, Soulountsi V, Iasonidou C, Kapravelos N. An overview of management of intracranial hypertension in the intensive care unit. J Anesth. 2020;34(5):741-57.
9. Subbarao BS, Fernández-de Thomas RJ, Eapen BC. Post Craniotomy Headache. StatPearls Publishing; Treasure Island (FL): 2022.

CHAPTER 30

Traumatic Conditions

Latika Bajaj

"Head and spinal injuries even once in a lifetime will change your view of your life and yourself. You may not get a chance for resentment."

—Sukhpal

LEARNING OBJECTIVES

After going through the chapter, the learner will be able to:
- Define and classify types of head and spinal cord injuries.
- Recognize clinical signs and symptoms of head and spinal cord injuries.
- Describe the pathophysiology and diagnostic evaluation related to head and spinal cord injuries.
- Outline the emergency management and treatment options for head and spinal cord injuries.
- Elaborate on the nursing management of patients with head and spinal cord injuries.
- Understand the need for injury prevention.

TERMS

- **Anterior cord syndrome:** The anterior 2/3 of the spinal cord is primarily affected; also referred to as incomplete cord syndrome.
- **Brown-Séquard syndrome:** Hemisection of the spinal cord, or damage to one-half of the spinal cord, causes paralysis and a loss of proprioception.
- **Cauda equina syndrome:** Leg paralysis, bowel incontinence, urine retention, and sexual dysfunction caused by damage to the nerve roots below L2.
- **Central cord syndrome:** The most typical type of cervical spinal cord injury that causes severe damage to the spinal cord's core corticospinal tract.
- **Cerebral perfusion pressure (CPP):** The difference between mean intracranial pressure (ICP) and mean arterial pressure (MAP). 60–80 mm Hg is considered normal.
- **Closed brain injury:** Any harm to the brain caused by an external force that does not fracture the skull.
- **Coma:** Glasgow coma scale score of 8 or less; a state from which the person cannot be awakened.
- **Concussion:** An abrupt and transitory impairment of brain function brought on by a head injury or violent shaking, such as a momentary loss of consciousness or change in vision and balance.
- **Contusion:** An impact-induced bruise to a particular region of the brain, brought on by ruptured blood vessels.
- **Craniotomy:** A surgical procedure that entails drilling a hole through the skull to remove a bone flap and gain access to the brain.
- **Craniectomy:** A procedure that involves removing an extensive piece of the skull and subsequently restoring it.
- **Complete spinal cord injury:** Complete loss of function below the damage level. No expected functional recovery exists.
- **Conus medullaris:** Injury or illness damaging the nerve roots' central nervous system.
- **Cord concussion:** Transient paraplegia, also known as neurapraxia, is a mild spinal cord injury that is characterized by varying degrees of sensory impairment and motor paralysis.
- **Diffuse axonal injury (DAI):** The brain parenchyma experiences a broad insult to the nerve cell axons that results in scattered lesions.
- **Hematoma:** Blood clotting.

- **Intracranial pressure (ICP):** Pressure inside the skull that is created by brain tissue, blood, and CSF.
- **Ischemia:** A low oxygen level frequently caused by an arterial blood flow restriction or inadequate blood flow to the tissue.
- **Incomplete spinal cord injury:** Mild damage to the spinal cord. It gets recovered with time.
- **Laminectomy:** A surgery that involves the removal of tiny bones from the spine's lamina that expands the spinal canal to release pressure from the nerves or spinal cord.
- **Neurogenic shock:** This condition arises as a result of the lack of autonomic nervous system function below the lesion. The clinical effects of this loss of sympathetic innervation include a decline in cardiac output, venous pooling in the extremities, and peripheral vasodilation.
- **Open head injury:** A wound that pushes objects or pieces of the skull into the brain.
- **Primary brain injury:** The harm sustained immediately following impact.
- **Paraplegia:** Due to an injury below the neck, the lower half of the body is paralyzed.
- **Posterior cord syndrome:** A rare kind of partial spinal cord damage that impacts the dorsal columns.
- **Spinal shock:** A rapid decrease in reflex activity in the spinal cord below the site of injury (areflexia).
- **Secondary brain injury:** Changes that develop over time (from a few hours to many days) after the initial brain damage.
- **Tetraplegia:** A neck injury that results in complete paralysis of all four limbs, called quadriplegia as well.

INTRODUCTION

Traumatic conditions refer to physical injuries that develop suddenly, are severe, and necessitate rapid medical attention. Several causes include car accidents, sports-related injuries, falls, natural disasters, and a wide range of other physical injuries that can occur at home, in the workplace, or even while walking the streets.

The current chapter elaborates on traumatic brain injury and spinal cord injury.

TRAUMATIC BRAIN INJURY

DEFINITION

Traumatic brain injury (TBI), often referred to as craniocerebral trauma, neurotrauma, is a disturbance in the brain's regular function that is caused by an outside force. It is the main global cause of mortality and disability. TBIs are described as "a disruption in the normal operation of the brain that can be caused by a bump, blow, or jolt to the head, or by a penetrating head injury," according to the Centre for Disease Control and Prevention (CDC).

EPIDEMIOLOGY

The annual incidence of TBI is 69 million (95% CI 64–74 million), with the Southeast Asian and Western Pacific regions bearing the greatest burden of the disease's overall impact. According to the CDC, there were 2.87 million TBI cases in the US in 2014, with more than 837,000 of those cases involving children. An estimated 13.5 million people in the United States struggle with a disability brought on by traumatic brain injury. In India, it is believed that every year, between 1.5 million and 2 million people suffer injuries and 1 million people die due to TBI.

ETIOLOGY AND TYPES

The most common reasons for traumatic brain injury (TBI) include automobile accidents, slips and falls, assaults, violence, crimes, gunshot wounds, and collisions with objects. TBI affects men more frequently than it does women. Brain injury can be classified into a number of different categories. Depending on the timing of the onset of injury it can be primary or secondary; as per the cause it can be closed or penetrating; depending on the morphology it can be focal or widespread fractures; and as per severity, it can be mild, moderate, and severe.

I. According to the Time of Onset

Primary injury: It is the primary damage caused by the initial trauma. It involves contusion, blood vessel damage, and axonal shearing, in which the axons of neurons are stretched and ripped, and it happens at the time of trauma. The main injury may result in damage to the meninges and blood-brain barrier, as well as possible neuronal death. Cells are destroyed in an unspecific way.

Secondary injury: An indirect effect of the primary injury is secondary injury. It happens as a result of trauma-related processes after hours and even days following an initial brain injury and contributes significantly to the death and brain damage brought in by TBI. It encompasses a wide range of cellular, chemical, tissue, or blood vessel changes in the brain that promote continuous brain tissue deterioration.

II. Based on the Mechanism of Injury

❖ **Closed/non-penetrating brain injury:** It is characterized by obvious brain injury that is caused by an external impact without the entry of any foreign items into the brain. The meninges have not been punctured, regardless of whether the skull has been damaged. Children under the age of four suffer many of their fatalities from closed-head injuries, while adolescents suffer the majority of their physical and cognitive impairments from them. It has two types:
  1. *Acceleration injuries:* These occur by the brain's free movement inside an unconstrained head (e.g., whiplash injury). The place of the hit (coup injury) can sustain a contusion and the opposite side of the skull may also sustain a contusion if the force striking the head is sufficient (coup-contrecoup injury).
  2. *Non-acceleration injuries:* These are brought on by a head injury while the head is constrained; as a result, the brain does not accelerate or slow down inside the skull (e.g., blow to the head). These typically cause the skull to distort (crack), damaging the brain and meninges in a concentrated area.

- **Open/penetrating brain injury:** An open or penetrating brain injury can result from a bullet, knife, or other sharp object striking the brain. This rupture in the dura mater allows hair, skin, bone, and other debris to enter the brain. The damage may be contained in the region where the foreign object was located. However, the total harm may also result in other severe problems, such as brain edema. The symptoms may vary depending on the extent of brain damage.

III. Based on Morphology

- **Skull fractures:**
  - *Linear:* A thin-line-like break in the skull that does not result in bone splintering, depression, or distortion.
  - *Depressed:* Inward folding (depression) of the skull vault into the cerebral parenchyma.
  - *Compound:* Involves a splintering of the bone as well as a break-in, or loss of skin.
  - *Basilar:* A condition that occurs near the base of the brain and can lead to CSF leaking.
- **Focal injuries (Fig. 30.1):**
  - *Epidural hematoma (EDH):* Blood that has accumulated between the dura and the skull's interior surface.
  - *Subdural hematoma (SDH):* A buildup of blood in the subdural area.
  - *Subarachnoid hemorrhage (SAH):* Bleeding under the arachnoid layer, specifically inside the layers of the dura.
  - *Intracerebral hematoma or contusion (ICH):* The tissue or ventricles of the brain accumulate blood.
  - *Intraventricular hemorrhage:* Bleeding into the brain's ventricles.
- **Diffuse injuries:**
  - *Concussion:* A mild brain injury that typically does not cause permanent brain damage and may cause a brief loss of consciousness.
  - *Multiple dot contusions:* Brain tissue has numerous minute blood vessel breaches or microhemorrhages.

- *Hypoxic ischemic injury:* Brain damage caused by hypoxia, ischemia, or a combination of these conditions.
- *Axonal Injury:* The brain parenchyma experiences scattered lesions over a large area.

IV. Based on the Degree of Severity (Glasgow Coma Scale)

- **Mild (13–15):** Eyes are open, and the patient is awake. Some symptoms include headaches, memory loss, confusion, dizziness, and a 30-minute period of unconsciousness.
- **Moderate (9–12):** The person is drowsy and their eyes are wide open to stimuli; 20 minutes to 6-hour-long periods of unconsciousness. Although there may be some brain hemorrhage or edema, the patient is arousable.
- **Severe (≤8):** The person is unconscious and his eyes would not get open despite stimulation. A more than 6-hour period of unconsciousness can be there.

PATHOPHYSIOLOGY

Traumatic brain injury can cause primary or secondary brain damage. Primary injury is the term used to describe the early brain damage brought on by trauma. Secondary injury develops a few hours to days after the initial injury and is mainly brought on by persistent bleeding or brain edema.

The skull is a fixed, tightly confined space that prevents the expansion of the cranium's contents. Due to the increased volume of the cranium's contents caused by any bleeding or swelling inside the skull, there is an increase in intracranial pressure (ICP). As a result, the brain's blood flow is reduced, which reduces the quantity of oxygen available and makes it difficult to discharge waste. Anoxia of brain tissue results in incorrect metabolism, which causes brain tissue ischemia and infarction, resulting in the death of brain tissue and cells **(Flowchart 30.1)**.

CLINICAL MANIFESTATIONS

Traumatic brain injury can have a wide range of immediate or delayed physical, cognitive, psychological, and physiological symptoms. The symptoms may vary depending on the extent of the TBI, but some may not be injury-specific **(Tables 30.1 and 30.2)**.

DIAGNOSTIC EVALUATION

1. **Primary survey:** Evaluation and stabilization of A, B, C, D, and E stands for airway, breathing, circulation, disability (neurologic state), exposure, and environmental control.
2. **Complete clinical assessment:**
   - As soon as the patient is stable enough, a comprehensive neurologic examination is carried out. Children and newborns should have thorough exams for retinal hemorrhage.
   - A funduscopic examination may reveal traumatic retinal detachment and the absence of retinal venous pulsations due to elevated intracranial pressure (ICP).

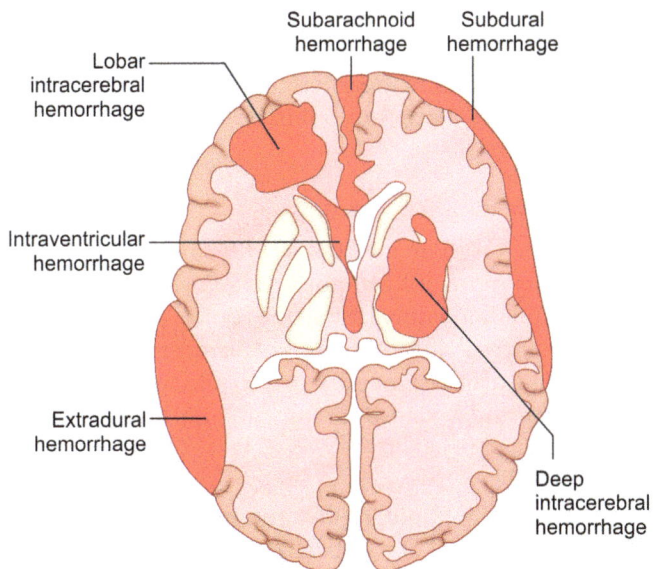

Fig. 30.1: Types of focal injuries.

Flowchart 30.1: Pathophysiology of traumatic brain injury.

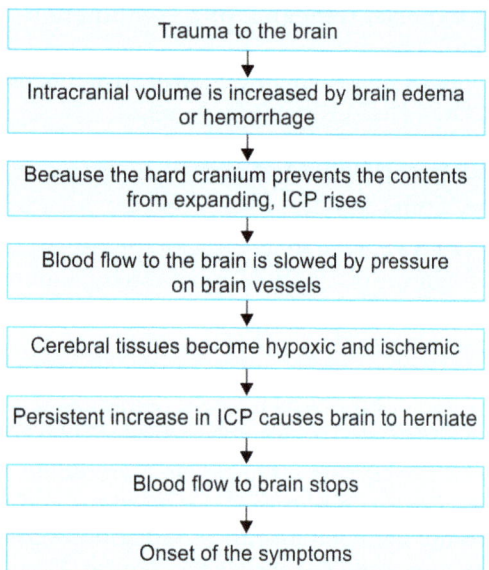

3. **Neuroimaging:** Imaging should always be done on patients who have focal neurologic symptoms, protracted vomiting, seizures, a history of loss of consciousness, or clinically suspected fractures. Imaging should also always be considered for patients with GCS scores under 15.
   X-ray: Plain X-rays can detect some skull fractures, but they do not give a complete picture of brain injury, therefore they are usually avoided.
   Computed tomography (CT): CT is the ideal choice for early imaging.
   ➢ Compared to brain tissue, acute bleeding, and contusions have an opaque (dense) appearance.
   ➢ Arterial epidural hematomas typically appear as lenticular-shaped opacities enclosing brain tissue around the primary meningeal artery.

TABLE 30.1: Mild traumatic brain injury.

Physical symptoms	Sensory symptoms	Cognitive symptoms
Either with or without unconsciousness if unconsciousness occurs, may be for a few seconds and a few minutes	Blurred vision	Confusion or disorientation
Headache	Tinnitus	Impairments in concentration or memory
Nausea or vomiting	Changes in the sense of smell or an unpleasant aftertaste	Mood swings or fluctuations in mood
Drowsiness or fatigue	Sensitive to light or sound	
Speech difficulties		Experiencing anxiety or depression
Sleeplessness or excessive sleeping		
Dizziness or loss of balance		

TABLE 30.2: Moderate to severe traumatic brain injury.

Physical symptoms	Sensory symptoms	Cognitive symptoms
Loss of consciousness that lasts for numerous minutes, hours, or days	Blurred vision	Comatose and other abnormalities in consciousness
Chronic headaches or headaches that get worse	Diplopia	Deeply confused
Nausea or vomiting that occurs repeatedly	Tinnitus	
Seizures or convulsions	Changes in the sense of smell or an unpleasant aftertaste	Agitation, or any other abnormal behavior
Dilation of pupils in one or both eyes	Sensitive to light or sound	Feeling down or sad
Halo sign: Bleeding or clear fluid leaking from the ears or nose		
Battle's sign (acute bruising/swelling behind the ears or around the eyes)		
Having trouble waking up from sleep		
Numbness/weakness		
Lack of balance or coordination		
Breathing difficulty		
Speech problems		

➢ Subdural hematomas are often observed as crescent-shaped opacities enveloping brain tissue.
➢ While a chronic subdural hematoma seems hypodense in comparison to brain tissue, a subacute subdural hematoma may have a radiopacity similar to brain tissue (isodense).
➢ Midline displacement, ventricular and cisternal compression, and sulcal effacement are signs of a mass effect.
➢ The hematoma should normally be surgically removed if it moves more than 5 mm from the midline (**Figs. 30.2A to C**).

Magnetic Resonance Imaging

❖ Magnetic resonance imaging (MRI) may be useful for detecting more mild contusions, diffuse axonal injury, and brain stem injury later in the clinical course.
❖ Magnetic resonance imaging is often more sensitive than CT for the diagnosis of extremely small acute or isodense subacute and isodense chronic subdural hematomas.

Angiography

Angiography, CT angiography, and magnetic resonance angiography (MRA) are all useful for evaluating vascular damage.

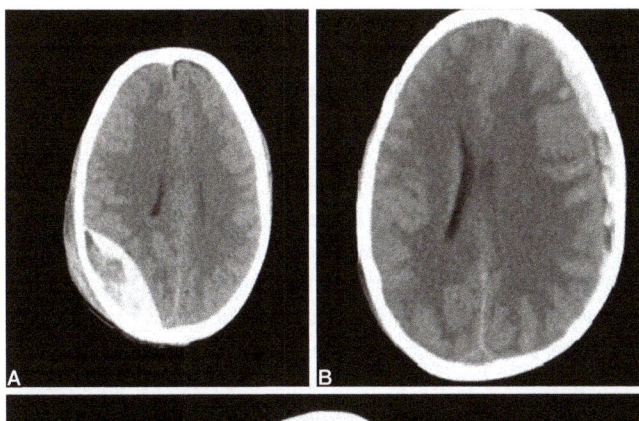
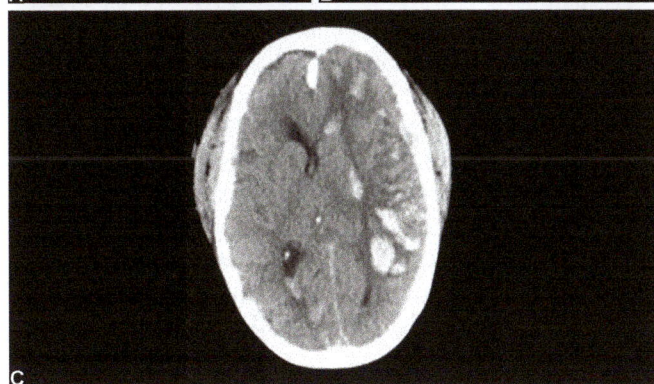

Figs. 30.2A to C: CT scans of intracranial hematomas: (A) Epidural hematoma; (B) Subdural hematoma; (C) Right intraparenchymal hemorrhage.

EMERGENCY MANAGEMENT

Airway

- Airway compromises can result from blood clots, teeth, foreign objects in the oropharynx, soft-tissue laxity, posterior tongue retraction brought on by obtundation following head trauma, and edema or hematoma brought on by direct neck trauma.
- If the patient talks, it is instantly confirmed that the airway is patent.
- Endotracheal intubation is required for patients whose airway patency, airway protection mechanisms, oxygenation, or ventilation are in question or who have a significant oropharyngeal injury.
- Blood and foreign material are removed by suction or manually. Ideally, capnography would be used to confirm proper endotracheal tube placement, but carbon dioxide colorimetry is also a viable option.
- When a patient requires an artificial airway and endotracheal intubation is either inappropriate or impracticable (for example, due to airway edema), a surgical or percutaneous cricothyrotomy is necessary (due to severe craniofacial injury, for example).

Note: Cervical spine immobilization should always be on priority while evaluating or modifying a patient's airway until cervical spine injury has been ruled out by examination, imaging, or both. Examples include the use of MILS or a rigid collar (manual in-line immobilization techniques).

Breathing

- The entire chest wall is checked for any chest damage, visible symptoms of trauma, and adequate expansion of the chest wall.
- Auscultation usually reveals whether or not the air exchange is adequate.
- Endotracheal intubation and mechanical ventilation are used to address any kind of insufficiency.

Circulation

- The heart rate and blood pressure are checked, and symptoms of shock are noted (e.g., tachypnea, dusky color, diaphoresis, altered mental status, poor capillary refill).
- Direct pressure is used to stop external bleeding.
- Isotonic saline (0.9% normal saline) is used to start in two large-bore (14- or 16-gauge) IVs.
- Consideration should be given to administering blood component therapy.
- Patients who have substantial intra-abdominal hemorrhage are evaluated by focused assessment with sonography for trauma (FAST), which may determine that they need an emergency laparotomy.
- Lactate or arterial blood gases are measured at the bedside (along with the calculation of base excess).

Disability (Neurologic Dysfunction)

- The initial assessment also includes a quick, focused neurologic evaluation.
- The patient's degree of consciousness and the extent of intracranial injury are assessed using the Glasgow coma scale (GCS) and pupillary sensitivity to light, respectively.
- Gross motor activity and sensation in each extremity can be used to identify serious spinal cord injuries.
- Before giving out sedatives and paralytics, patients are evaluated.
- Patient reevaluations should be done regularly (e.g., every 15–30 minutes initially, then every 1 hour after stabilization).
- Post-injury improvement or deterioration may help to assess the injury's severity and prognosis.

Exposure/Environmental Control

- To ensure that no injuries are missed, the clothes of patients are completely removed (by cutting off clothing) and the entire body surface is examined for signs of occult trauma.
- The patient is kept warm to avoid hypothermia (e.g., using heated blankets and heated IV fluids).

MEDICAL MANAGEMENT

Mild Injury

- Patients with mild injuries who did not lose consciousness or just briefly had, having stable vital signs, a normal head CT scan, and normal mental and neurologic function may be discharged home with the requirement that their family can keep a careful eye on them for additional 24 hours.

- They are informed that if any of the following occur, patients should be brought back to the hospital:
  - Worsening of mental function (e.g., disoriented/confused, unable to recognize people, behaves inappropriately)
  - Seizures
  - Focal neurologic impairments
  - Worsening headache
  - Vomiting
- Patients who could not be closely monitored after being discharged due to loss of consciousness or abnormalities in their neurological or mental function are usually kept overnight in the hospital or under close observation in the emergency room. If symptoms persist, a follow-up CT scan could be done in 8–12 hours.
- Those who exhibit modest abnormalities on a head CT but may not exhibit any neurologic changes (such as minor contusions, subdural hematomas without a mass effect, or subarachnoid hemorrhages), may only require a follow-up CT within 24 hours. These individuals might be sent home if their CT scan is stable and their neurologic exam results are unremarkable.

Moderate and Severe Injury

- Unless additional injuries are present, patients with moderate injuries frequently do not need mechanical ventilation, intubation, ICP monitoring, or other interventions. Although the head CT results are normal, these individuals should still be hospitalized and monitored because worsening is a possibility.
- Patients with severe injuries are admitted to a critical care unit. Due to the fact that airway protective reflexes are frequently impaired and may cause ICP to rise, patients are intubated endotracheally while efforts are taken to avoid this from happening.
- Another procedure that can be used to reduce post-injury mortality is cerebral perfusion pressure (CPP) monitoring.
- A repeat CT should be performed, especially if the ICP has increased unexplainably. It is also important to conduct close monitoring using the GCS and pupillary response.
- Proactively treating hypoxia, hypercapnia, hypotension, and elevated ICP in the early stages will help prevent further consequences.

Other Management Measures

- **Intravenous fluids**: Isotonic crystalloids or blood and blood products, when necessary, are used to maintain normovolemia. Hypovolemia is dangerous. As cerebral edema can be exacerbated, hypotonic fluids should be avoided. Fluids containing glucose have been linked to both hyperglycemia and brain ischemia. The best fluids to use during resuscitation are isotonic solutions like ringer lactate and normal saline.
- **Diuretics like mannitol or hypertonic saline:** If the patient is hemodynamically stable, a quick intravenous bolus of mannitol 20% can be administered (within 5 minutes). In place of mannitol, hypertonic saline 3% NS (2–5 mL/kg) IV over 10 minutes can be given if there are signs of elevated ICP and hypotension. Mannitol should not be given to patients who have hypotension because it will make their hypovolemia worse through osmotic diuresis.
- **Transient hyperventilation:** Hyperventilation works by lowering $PaCO_2$ and constricting cerebral blood vessels. If there are herniation symptoms, hyperventilation with a target $PaCO_2$ of 28–35 mm Hg can be utilized for a brief period while awaiting final treatment. Cerebral ischemia can result from aggressive and sustained hyperventilation.
- **Barbiturates:** Barbiturates may be effective in treating elevated ICP that is resistant to standard treatments. They work by lowering cerebral metabolism and cerebral vasoconstriction, which lowers ICP. When the patient is already hypotensive, they should not be used. This could make hypotension worse.
- **Coagulopathy:** Patients with severe TBI have a high incidence of coagulopathy (40–50%), which might increase secondary brain injury by causing more hematoma and obstructing hemostasis. In the initial care of TBI, coagulopathy must be identified and corrected. Prothrombin time (PT), INR, partial thromboplastin time (aPTT), platelet counts, and fibrinogen levels should all be regularly checked as part of routine coagulation testing. Vitamin K, platelet concentrates, and fresh frozen plasma (FFP) are frequently used. More effectively than FFP and vitamin K, prothrombin complex concentrate (PCC) has been proven to treat warfarin-induced coagulopathy. Patients with renal failure can receive desmopressin (0.3 µg/kg IV) to momentarily enhance uremic platelet function.
- **Seizure prophylaxis:** Post-traumatic seizures (PTS) must be avoided in the acute stage otherwise they may worsen the secondary brain injury. The significant brain damage might occasionally result from prolonged seizures lasting longer than 30 minutes. There are two types of seizures: early (occurring within 7 days of a TBI) and late (occurring more than 7 days after a head injury). In TBI patients, phenytoin has demonstrated effectiveness in preventing early PTS. Thus, phenytoin (or fosphenytoin) is advised as a seizure preventative in all patients admitted to the hospital with moderate or severe TBI and an abnormal head CT scan. If there are no seizures after 7 days, the seizure prophylaxis is discontinued. Another widely used AED is levetiracetam. Muscle relaxants do not stop seizures; instead, they only hide the clinical symptoms while underlying brain damage continues. The treatment of seizures using muscle relaxants is prohibited.
- **Sedation:** For the protection of the airway, patients with severe TBI frequently need to be intubated. To ensure that pain is alleviated and that patients are not disturbed, analgesia and sedation are necessary. Select quick-acting drugs with less hemodynamic impact. This will enable frequent neurological assessment as needed. Midazolam and quick-acting opioids are both options. Dexmedetomidine infusion is another potential medication that permits sedation, analgesia, and patient arousal for examination as required.

Fluid Therapy

The fluids recommended are shown in **Box 30.1**.

> **BOX 30.1:** Fluid therapy.
>
> **0.9% Normal saline (isotonic saline)**
> - First preference
> - Very little risk of causing brain edema
> - Accessible and affordable
>
> **3% Normal saline (hypertonic saline)**
> - Effective resuscitation fluid
> - Lower ICP and prevent brain edema with a higher osmolality
> - Increases the cardiac output and improves cerebral perfusion
> - Enhances microcirculation and modulates immunological response
> - Used as a single bolus treatment.
> - Safe in patients with ongoing volume loss and hypotension.
>
> **Mannitol 20%**
> - If the patient is hemodynamically stable, a fast bolus of 0.25–1 g/kg IV is administered because it improves microcirculation
> - Not administered to individuals with hypotension, but rather worsens hypovolemia by osmotic diuresis
>
> **Blood**
> - Ideal replacement for blood loss
> - Its availability takes some time.
> - To enhance the flow of oxygen to the brain, blood volume loss of more than 20% must be reversed.
>
> The fluids that are **NOT** advised are:
> **Ringer's lactate:** Slightly hypoosmolar (270 mOsmol/L) in head injury patients, which could exacerbate cerebral edema
>
> **Isotonic glucose (5% glucose)**
> - Exacerbate cerebral edema, elevating ICP; quickly turns hypoosmolar following the use of glucose
> - In a patient with a severe brain injury, adverse effects of hyperglycemia are evident.
>
> **Colloids**
> - Large size of their molecules prevents them from leaving the intravascular compartment and aids in stabilizing systolic blood pressure
> - Does not make cerebral edema worse
> - Little volume is needed (1:1)
> - Costs 40–80 times as much as crystalloids
> - May cause allergic responses or anticoagulation side effects.

SURGICAL MANAGEMENT

- ❖ The need for surgery is indicated by the presence of a >5 mm midline shift in the brain, compression of the basal cisterns, and deteriorating neurologic examination findings.
- ❖ Although not all cerebral hematomas require prompt surgical evacuation, doing so may be necessary to prevent or treat brain shift, compression, and herniation. Small intracerebral hematomas rarely require surgery. Patients with small subdural hematomas can frequently be treated without surgery.
- ❖ Although less urgent than acute subdural hematomas, chronic subdural hematomas may necessitate surgical drainage.
- ❖ Decompressive craniectomy is advised when increased ICP is unresponsive to prior treatments, and is occasionally used as a first line of treatment.
- ❖ Large or arterial epidural hematomas are treated surgically but repeated CT scans can be used to track smaller epidural hematomas thought to have venous origins (e.g., at the time of surgery to drain a significant hematoma). During this procedure, a sizable piece of the skull is removed, and duraplasty is performed to make way for restoration in the future. The amount and location of bone removal may vary depending on the damage, but the opening that is made needs to be sizable enough to prevent brain tissue from being forced up against the edges of the defect because of swelling.

NUTRITIONAL MANAGEMENT

- ❖ Patients with head injuries often have hypermetabolism and hypercatabolism, which results in a negative nitrogen balance that can surpass 30 g per day. Measurements such as body weight, height, body mass index (BMI), and physical characteristics should be taken. Blood markers such as serum albumin, transferrin, and lymphocyte count can be used to assess nutritional status.
- ❖ Once the patient is hemodynamically stable, early enteral feeding should be started. Protein consumption should be 1.5–2.5 g/kg/body weight and caloric intake should be 30–35 kcal/kg/wt.
- ❖ These requirements should be regularly reevaluated and appropriately adjusted on the basis of the determined nitrogen balance.
- ❖ Enteral nutrition should be preferred over parenteral feeding because the latter is linked to significantly increased infection morbidity.
- ❖ Nutrition therapy should begin as soon as possible after admission between 24 and 48 hours and complete nutritional assistance should be achieved no later than 7 days after the injury.

NURSING MANAGEMENT (FIG. 30.3)

Emergency Room Management

- ❖ Assess the level of consciousness. Patients with a Glasgow coma scale (GCS) score of 8 need to be intubated. Nurses should assist with the placement of an endotracheal tube to secure the airway, ensure adequate oxygenation (PaO_2 >60 mm Hg), regularly monitor blood pressure, cardiac function, and blood saturation and continuous waveform capnography (if available) and initiate peripheral intravenous (IV) therapy.
- ❖ A complete blood count, electrolytes, glucose, coagulation parameters, blood alcohol level, urine toxicology, and a thorough neurologic examination all should be assessed as soon as possible.

Ongoing Management

- ❖ **Positioning:** The patient should be positioned correctly with their neck in a neutral position and the head end of the bed elevated to 30°. This promotes cerebral venous outflow. Rigid cervical collars should be loosened or removed to lower ICP.
- ❖ **Temperature control:** In addition to improving brain metabolism and the prognosis after an injury, hypothermia also reduces ICP by 40% and cerebral blood flow by 60%. It thereby decreases the chance of further brain damage. To sustain normothermia, antipyretic medications, sponging, etc., should be employed.

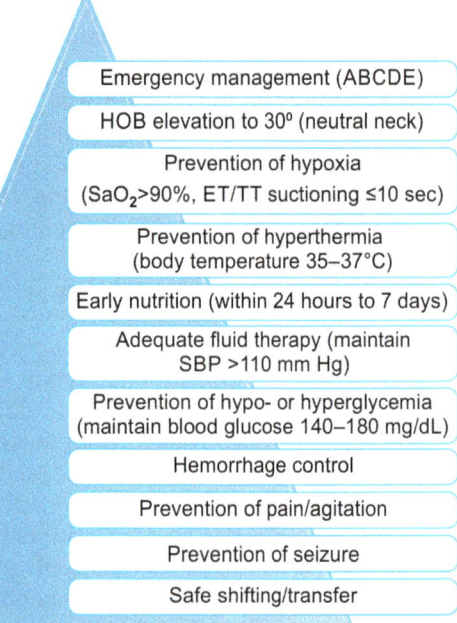

Fig. 30.3: Nursing interventions for the patient with TBI.

- **Prophylaxis for stress ulcers:** Stress ulcers, also known as Cushing's ulcers, commonly cause death in intensive care unit patients. Early enteral feeding, H2-blockers, proton-pump inhibitors, and sucralfate all are used as stress ulcer preventative measures.
- **Nutrition:** The recommendations state that feeding should begin within 24 hours of injury. Accounting for more than 50% of total caloric expenditure, and providing 1–1.5 g of protein per kg of body weight for the first two weeks after the injury, has been demonstrated to provide better outcomes. Compared to parenteral nutrition, enteral nutrition is better.
- **Fluid therapy:** Fluid management helps to recover heart rate, tissue perfusion, and vascular capacity. Hypertonic saline may be used in patients with STBI and systemic shock. To keep euvolemia stable, isotonic fluids such as normal saline can be given.
- **Hyperventilation:** The cerebral autoregulation caused by hyperventilation decreases $PaCO_2$, cerebral blood flow, and ICP. It is used if the ICP and CPP both are more than 30 mm Hg.
- **Glucose management:** Extreme blood glucose levels, whether very high or very low, need to be handled appropriately. A target range of up to 140 mg/dL or even 180 mg/dL would be suitable. If a patient has hyperglycemia and their blood sugar level is more than 200 mg/dL, insulin therapy should be initiated.
- **Drug administration:** An increase in ICP can be avoided by administering sedatives. ICP is also decreased by using mannitol or a sodium chloride hypertonic solution. Propofol, injectable dexmedetomidine, and fentanyl are frequently given in patients who are being ventilated mechanically. The use of steroids in TBI is not advised. To treat post-traumatic seizures, phenytoin is recommended. Levetiracetam is another option that is available.
- **Shifting of patients:** TBI patients are transferred safely and with great care, and the proper transferring equipment should be available. It should be done by trained experts under close supervision, with support for vital organs, continuous observation, protection of the spine, and meticulous documentation.
- **Postoperative care:** After surgery, patients should be admitted to the neurocritical care ICU for additional monitoring and care. Humidified mechanical breathing is used to preserve normothermia, maximize CPP, and prevent subsequent brain injury. Patients with severe TBI are at risk for developing deep vein thrombosis (DVT), particularly if they were intubated. To lower this risk, use range-of-motion exercises, intermittent pneumatic compression devices, and medication prophylaxis as necessary.

SPINAL CORD INJURIES

DEFINITION

A spinal cord injury (SCI) is an insult to the spinal cord that results in a temporary or permanent disruption of the cord's motor, sensory, or autonomic functions. Patients with SCI often suffer from severe, lifelong brain abnormalities and disabilities.

EPIDEMIOLOGY

- The National Spinal Cord Injury Association estimates that up to 4,50,000 Americans are affected by spinal cord injuries (SCI). Other groups place the number at a modest 2,50,000. In the United States, an estimated 17,000 new SCIs occur annually.
- The prevalence of SCI in India is 0.15 million, with an average yearly incidence of 15,000 cases.
- According to the World Health Organization (WHO), SCI is becoming more common in developing countries like India, and it is anticipated that the expense of medical care for SCI will be comparable to that in industrialized countries.
- The incidence in men is five times higher than in women.
- The majority of spinal cord injuries affect young, healthy people.
- Men between the ages of 15 and 35 are most frequently afflicted.
- In young children with spinal injuries, the fatality rate is typically higher.
- The cervical cord continues to be the most often affected area.

RISK FACTORS

It includes factors including age, gender, drug and alcohol misuse, engaging in dangerous physical activity, forgoing protective gear when working or playing, and diving into shallow water.

CAUSES

SCI may occur because of:
- **Trauma:** This category includes assaults, gunshot wounds, falls, sports injuries (particularly when diving into shallow water), industrial accidents, and car accidents.

- Illnesses like rheumatoid arthritis, transverse myelitis, spinal stenosis, multiple sclerosis, and Friedreich's ataxia.
- Spina bifida, kyphosis, scoliosis, and other developmental abnormalities.

TYPES

There are two types of spinal cord injuries: total (complete) and partial (incomplete) **(Fig. 30.4)**.

1. **Complete:** Complete paralysis (loss of function) occur below the level of injury. The body is affected on both sides. It involves:
   - Tetraplegia/quadriplegia
   - Paraplegia
   - Triplegia

   Tetraplegia is the most severe form of total spinal cord paralysis. Every limb may become paralyzed as a result of this. The severity of the damage depends on where it occurs in the cervical spine. In paraplegia, the afflicted person loses all sensation and movement in their body. Triplegia often occurs from the consequences of an incomplete spinal cord injury.

2. **Incomplete:** Compared to complete injuries, incomplete spinal cord injuries are more frequent. The spinal cord is damaged in about 60% of cases. One or both sides of the body still have some function after incomplete damage. There are still some channels of communication between the body and the brain. There are five common types of incomplete spinal injuries:
   a. Brown-Séquard syndrome
   b. Anterior cord syndrome
   c. Central cord syndrome
   d. Cauda equina lesions
   e. Conus medullaris syndrome

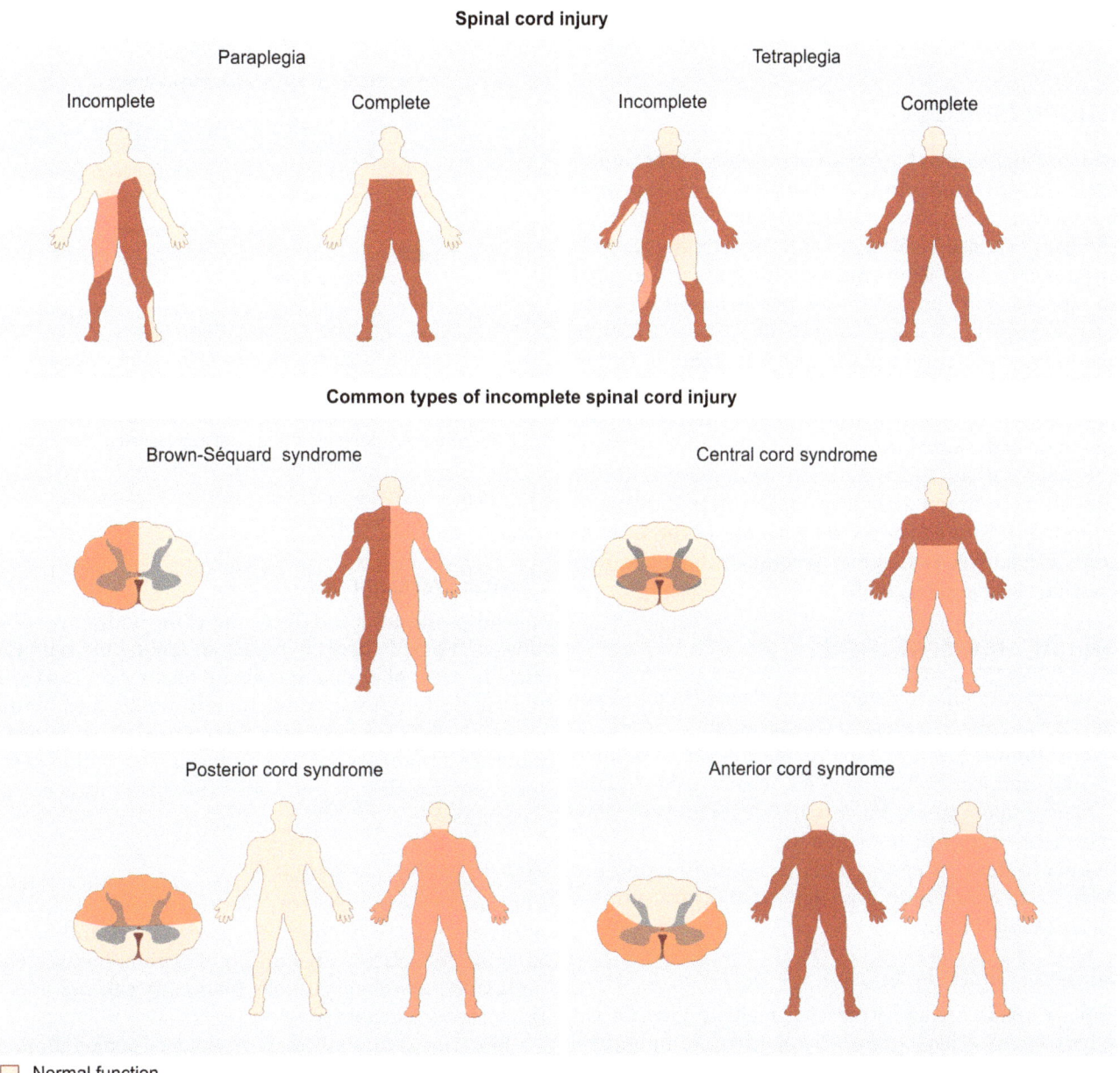

Fig. 30.4: Types of spinal cord injury.

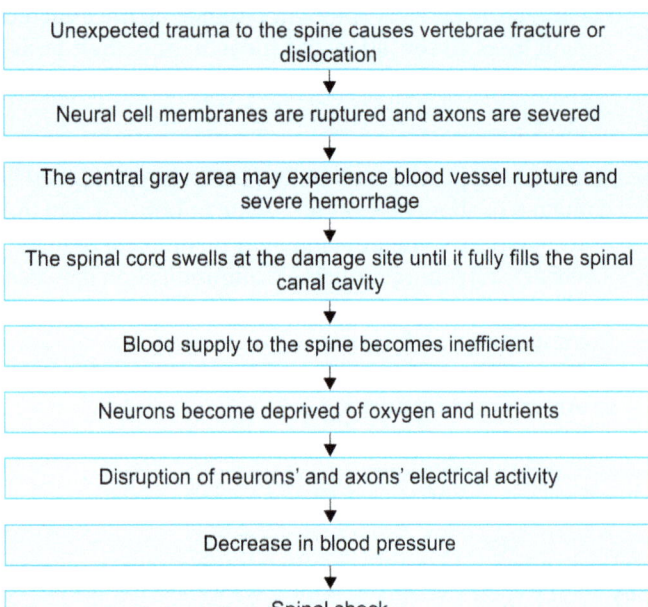

Flowchart 30.2: Pathophysiology of spinal cord injury.

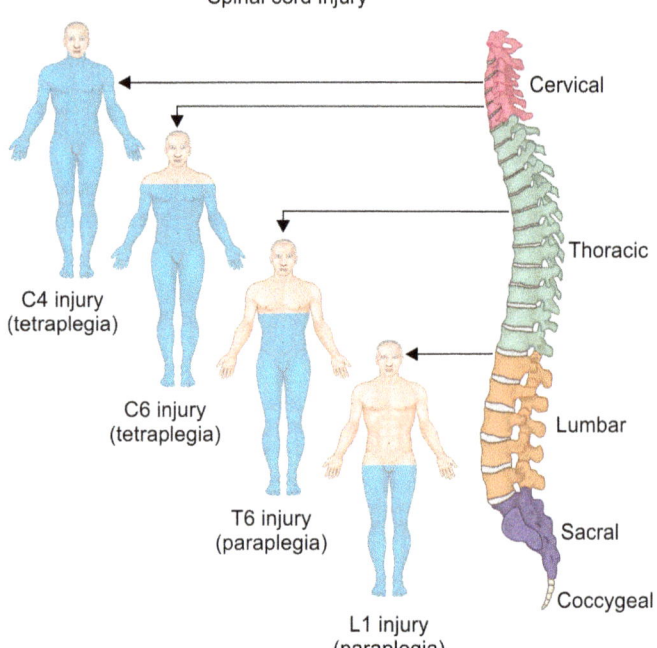

Fig. 30.5: Spinal injuries and its effects.

PATHOPHYSIOLOGY

Spinal cord injuries may be primary or secondary. Mechanical interference, transaction, or distraction of neuronal components cause primary spinal cord injury. Primary spinal cord injury can also be brought on by penetrating wounds from guns or bullets. When a mass fills the space in the spinal cord after an acute impact injury, parenchymal pressure rises, resulting in spinal cord compression. The venous side of the microvasculature will collapse with rapid or severe compression, resulting in vasogenic edema. Vasogenic edema increases parenchymal pressure and may hasten the progression of dysfunction.

Even parts of the spinal cord that are unharmed during spinal shock momentarily lose their functionality and are unable to interact normally with the brain. Loss of reflexes and limb sensation may accompany total paralysis **(Flowchart 30.2 and Fig. 30.5)**.

CLINICAL MANIFESTATIONS

The severity of a spinal cord injury is determined by the extent of damage and the neurological classification.
- ❖ **Neurological level:** The neurological level, as defined by the American Spinal Injury Association (ASIA), is the lowest spinal segment where both sides of the body have normal sensory and motor function.
- ❖ **Neurological category**: This is assessed using the American Spinal Injury Association (ASIA) impairment scale **(Table 30.3)**.

Complete Spinal Cord Injury

Complete spinal cord injury causes immediate, total, flaccid paralysis, loss of all feeling and reflex activity, and autonomic dysfunction below the level of the injury (including loss of anal sphincter tone).

TABLE 30.3: ASIA impairment scale.		
A	Complete	All motor and sensory capabilities are lost from the sacral S4 to S5
B	Sensory incomplete	S4–S5 of the sacrum are included, while sensory and motor functions are still present below the neurologic level.
C	Motor incomplete	More than half of the major muscles have a muscle grade of less than three, and motor function is still present below the neurologic level.
D	Motor incomplete	Motor function is unaffected below the neurologic level, and at least half of the major muscles have a muscle grade of 3 or higher.
E	Normal	Both the sensory and motor systems are functioning normally.

Cervical (Neck) Injuries

It involves the arms and the center of the body; one or both sides of the body may be impacted. Among the symptoms include a loss of normal bowel and bladder control (which may include constipation, incontinence, and bladder spasms); difficulty breathing due to respiratory muscular paralysis; numbness; sensory abnormalities; stiffness (from increased muscle tone); and others like paralysis, aches, and weakness.

Thoracic (Chest Level) Injuries

The following symptoms may also occur: numbness; sensory abnormalities; a decline in regular bowel and bladder function (which may include constipation, incontinence, and bladder spasms); spasticity, pain, and weakened muscles (increased muscular tone).

Blood pressure abnormalities, unusual perspiration, and difficulty maintaining a normal body temperature are further symptoms of cervical or upper thoracic spinal cord injuries.

Lumbar Sacral (Lower Back) Injuries

Lower back spinal injuries may have varying degrees of impact on one or both legs as well as the muscles that regulate bowel and bladder function. Reduced bowel and bladder control, sensory changes, discomfort, and numbness, stiffness (increased muscular tone), weakness, and numbness are a few symptoms.

Incomplete Cord Injury

- Incomplete spinal cord injuries can cause hyperactive deep tendon reflexes as well as motor and sensory deficits.
- Depending on the cause, motor, and sensory loss may be permanent or temporary; for example, a concussion may cause functional loss temporarily, whereas a contusion or laceration may cause functional loss more permanently.
- Spinal shock is a condition when the cord swells quickly, resulting in total neurologic disability that resembles a complete cord injury.
- The symptoms go away in one to several days, but the residual impairments frequently persist.

Depending on which part of the cord is affected, there are various distinct symptoms that can be present.

- **Brown-Séquard syndrome:**
  - The cause is unilateral hemisection of the cord.
  - Patients also develop ipsilateral spastic paralysis and loss of position perception below the lesion in addition to the contralateral loss of pain and warmth sensation.
- **Anterior cord syndrome:**
  - Patients experience bilateral loss of motor and pain feeling below the lesion, which is caused by direct injury to the anterior spinal cord or to the anterior spinal artery.
  - Proprioception and vibration in the posterior cord are unaltered.
- **Central cord syndrome:**
  - After a hyperextension injury, it typically happens in patients with a congenitally or degeneratively constricted cervical spinal canal.
  - Compared to the legs, the arms have a larger impairment of motor function. Loss of posture, vibration, and light touch are all symptoms of damaged posterior columns.
  - If the spinothalamic circuits are disrupted, sensations of pain, temperature, and usually light or deep touch are lost.
  - Hematomyelia, a spinal cord hemorrhage brought on by trauma and usually confined to the cervical central gray matter, is what causes the symptoms of lower motor neuron injury (muscle weakness and atrophy, fasciculations, and reduced tendon reflexes in the arms). Damage to the lower motor neurons is usually irreversible.
  - Localized loss of pain and temperature perception typically coexists with proximal motor weakness.
- **Cauda equina lesions:**
  - The distal legs typically suffer partial motor or sensory loss, or both.
  - Sensory problems typically affect one side more than the other and are typically bilateral but asymmetric.
  - The perineal area typically has less sensation (saddle anesthesia). Incontinence or retention-related bowel and bladder problems may happen.
  - Women may have a decreased sexual response, while men may have erectile problems.
  - The bulbocavernosus and anal wink reflexes are aberrant, and the anal sphincter tone decreases.
- **Conus medullaris syndrome:** Damage to the lumbar nerve roots and sacral cord causes the bladder, colon, and lower limbs to become areflexic, while the sacral segments themselves may still have some residual reflexes (e.g., bulbocavernosus and micturition reflexes).

DIAGNOSTIC EVALUATION

- A comprehensive medical check-up that includes a complete neurological assessment.
- Patients who have the following conditions must be evaluated for spinal cord and spine injuries: head injuries, pelvic fractures, penetrating injuries to the area of the spine, serious blunt injuries, injuries sustained in falls from heights, and injuries sustained when diving into the water, other injuries that should also be considered in elderly patients after minor falls.
- Injury to the spine and spinal cord should also be considered in individuals who have altered sensorium, localized spinal discomfort, unpleasant distracting injuries, or compatible neurologic abnormalities.
- Imaging is used to detect lesions in the spinal column and spine as well as to assess nerve function, including reflex, motor, and sensory function.
- Injury manifestations can be categorized using the ASIA (American Spinal Injury Association) Impairment Scale.

Nerve Studies

The ability to move each extremity is evaluated. During the sensory evaluation, it is important to examine the following senses: light touch (posterior column function), pinprick (anterior spinothalamic tract), and location sense. The thoracic roots should also be tested on the back while determining the sensory level in order to prevent being fooled by the cervical cap. Priapism is a sign of spinal cord damage. Rectal tone may be diminished, and deep tendon reflexes may be exaggerated or non-existent.

Imaging

- **Plain X-rays:** They were utilized traditionally.
- **CT:** Conducted for locations that appear aberrant on X-rays and for areas that, according to clinical results, are at risk of harm. Due to its higher diagnostic accuracy and ease of acquisition, it is widely employed as the major imaging investigation for spinal trauma today.
- **MRI:** Although it might not be available at once, it is the most accurate examination for observing the spinal cord and other soft tissues. It aids in identifying the kind and site of cord injury.
- **CT angiography:** It is done to rule out dissection of the vertebral artery

MANAGEMENT

Immediate Phase

- A spinal cord injury requires immediate medical attention since it is an emergency. The length of time between the injury and rehabilitation has a significant impact on the outcome.
- Preventing subsequent spinal cord or spine damage is a key objective.

Immobilization

- The spine should be completely immobilized as soon as it is possible to stabilize the position without exerting undue pressure.
- The cervical spine should be immobilized using a rigid collar. The neck is manually maintained straight (inline stabilization) during endotracheal intubation. Patients with thoracic or lumbar spine injuries can be transferred prone or supine.

Acute Phase

The goals of management include:
- To stop the further spread of SCI
- To look out for signs of developing neurological impairments.
- To preserve oxygenation and cardiovascular stability

Respiratory Therapy

- Upper cervical spine injuries result in the loss of spinal cord innervation of the phrenic nerve. Due to the possibility that hypoxemia would impair spinal cord function; oxygen is administered to maintain a high arterial PO_2.
- If endotracheal intubation is necessary, diaphragmatic pacing might be a possibility for patients with high cervical lesions; however, extreme attention must be used to avoid flexing or stretching the patient's neck, as this could exacerbate the damage. By electrically stimulating the phrenic nerve, diaphragmatic pacing aims to assist the patient's breathing.
- The perfusion of the spinal cord is increased and the frequency of hypotensive episodes is decreased when the mean arterial pressure (MAP) is maintained at least 85 mm Hg.

Pharmacologic Therapy

There are currently no generally accepted pharmaceutical therapies for this condition. Useful drugs include the ones listed below.

- **Corticosteroids:** To improve the outcome after spinal cord damage, substantial doses of corticosteroids have long been administered within 8 hours of the lesion. There is, however, a higher chance of wound infection, pulmonary embolism, sepsis, and death. Thus, it is not recommended to use corticosteroids and their use has reduced.
- **Thyrotropin-releasing hormone:** Helps in reducing mediators of secondary damage.
- **Baclofen:** In order to lessen spasticity. Administered 3 times a day, 5 mg of baclofen (maximum, 80 mg during a 24-hour period) or each day, three 4 mg doses of tizanidine orally (maximum, 36 mg during a 24-hour period).
- Patients who are not responding to oral medicines may be considered for intrathecal baclofen administration of 50–100 µg once a day.

Skeletal Fracture Reduction and Traction

- It involves stabilizing the spinal column as well as immobilization, reduction, and dislocations (restoration of normal position).
- Traction is applied to the tongs using weights; the amount utilized is based on the size of the patient and the degree of fracture-dislocation. This may help to restrict spine mobility.
- The skull can be secured with tongs (metal braces inserted in the head and fastened to body weights or a harness for traction).
- Wearing the spine braces for a prolonged amount of time may be necessary.
- Numerous types of cervical tongs are available, including Crutchfield, Gardner-Wells, and Vinke tongs.

There are numerous skeletal tongs that all entail some sort of fixation in the cranium.

The Gardner-Wells tongs: The most popular and easily accessible tongs are Gardner-Wells tongs. They are made up of stainless steel and have two 30-degree angled pins and a hoop **(Fig. 30.6)**.

Precautions:
- The best way to prevent iatrogenic harm is to put pins carefully.
- The external auditory meatus is aligned with the pin site entrance, which is 1 cm above the pinna (earlobe).
- Check the pin's pressure-sensitive spring-loaded indication, which should protrude 1–2 mm to indicate 30 inches/pounds of pressure, is functioning properly.
- The pins need to be tightened all at once.
- Traction weights should be introduced gradually and in order, e.g., starting with 10 pounds, increase to 5 pounds per level. A C5-C6 injury, for instance, requires 35 lb of traction weight.
- After 24 hours, Gardner-Wells tongs must be retightened.

Crutchfield and Vinke tongs: They are used to treat cervical spine fractures. After inserting the tong points just into the outer layers of the bone in the parietal region of the skull, the tong is connected to the pulling mechanism. This treatment can be carried out under local anesthesia in the operating room or in the ward **(Figs. 30.7A and B)**.

Halo device: The halo device **(Fig. 30.8)** consists of a stabilizing bar, a halo vest, and a metal ring that wraps around the patient's head and is pinned to the skull. The metal pins pierce the skull but do not go inside it. They are positioned opposite one another, providing opposing force that causes the cranium to be firmly fixed. To prevent the pin sites from becoming superficially infected, frequent cleaning is necessary.

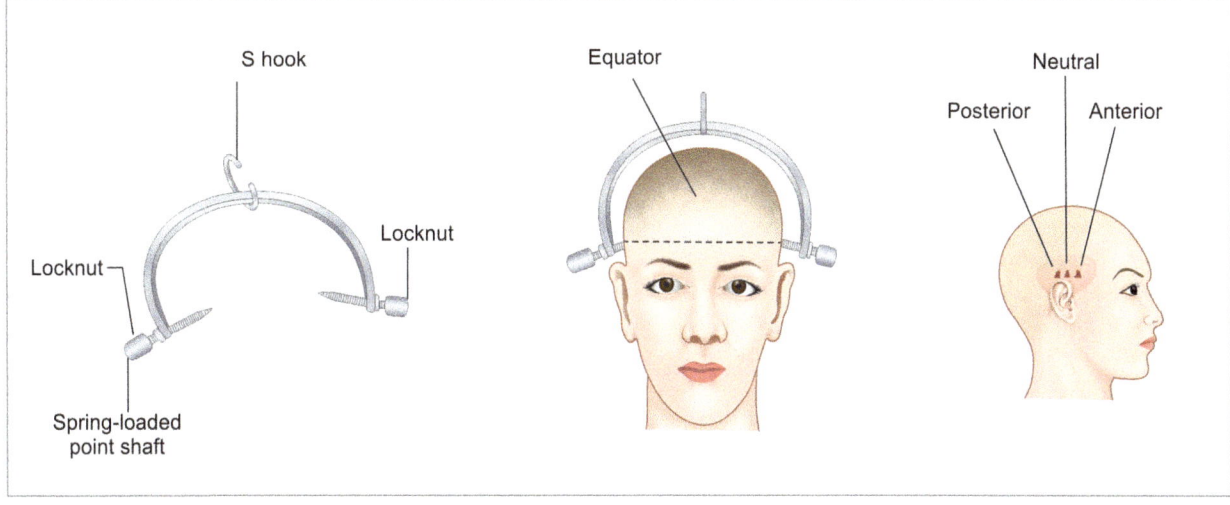

Fig. 30.6: The Gardner-Wells tongs.

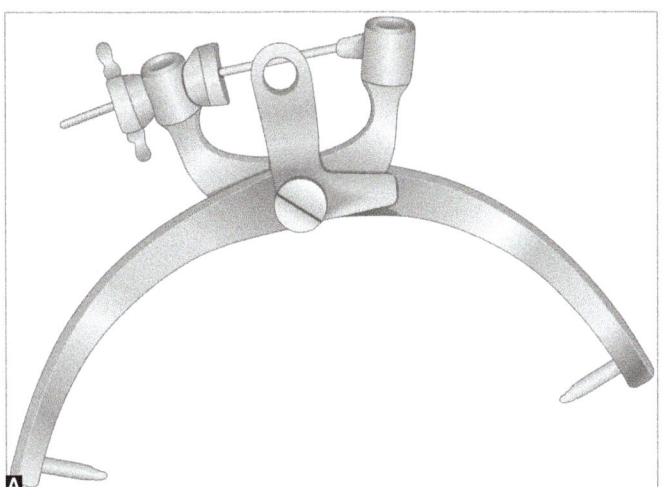

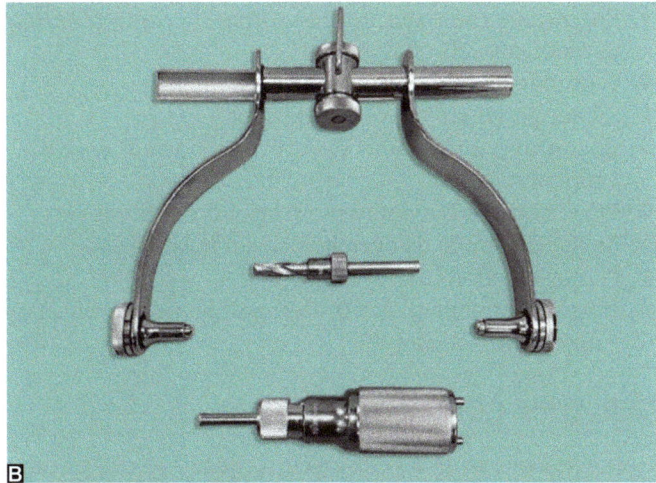

Figs. 30.7A and B: (A) Crutchfield tongs; (B) Vinke tongs.

Thoracic and lumbar injuries are frequently treated surgically, and this is followed by immobilization with a custom brace. Traction is not recommended for these patients before, during, or after surgery.

SURGICAL MANAGEMENT

A spinal cord injury (SCI) can be surgically treated either right away or later. Patients with partial SCI require urgent surgical

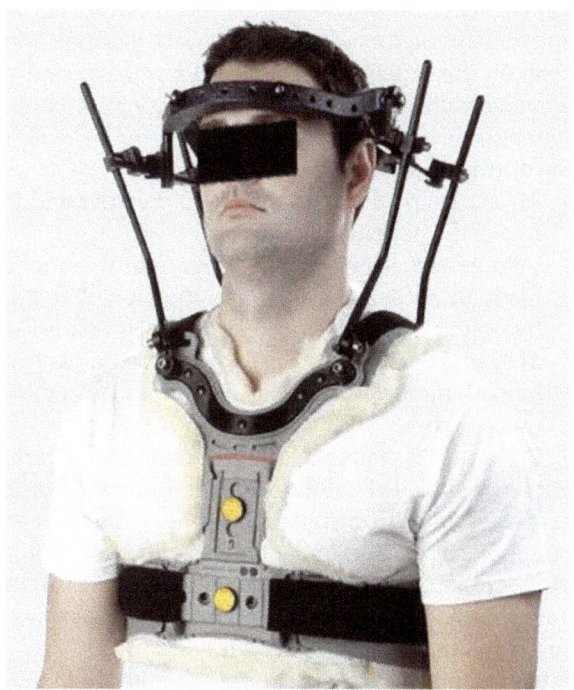

Fig. 30.8: Halo device.

intervention more frequently. If neurologic impairment worsens, urgent surgical intervention is also carried out. The nature and extent of the injury, as well as any issues with spinal stability, all have an impact on the decision to have surgery.

Spine surgery for SCI mostly entails:
❖ Vertebral decompression (i.e., spinal cord)
❖ Spine's stability

Vertebral Decompression

If the spinal cord or nerves are compressed, surgery may help relieve the symptoms.
❖ **Diskectomy:** This involves removing a part of the disc to release pressure on the nerves.
❖ **Laminotomy or laminectomy:** To enlarge the spinal canal and relieve pressure, a small piece of bone is removed, either a segment of the bony arch or the entire bony arch.

- **Foraminotomy or foraminectomy:** This involves enlargement of the apertures for the nerve roots by removing bone and other tissue.
- **Corpectomy:** The vertebral body and the discs between the vertebrae are removed.

NURSING MANAGEMENT

- **Respiratory management:**
  - Keep a close eye on the patient's breathing pattern, depth, and rate.
  - Assist the patient in measuring inspiratory lung volumes with incentive spirometry.
  - Adjunctive therapies, such as CPT and postural drainage, suctioning, bronchoscopy, and mechanical cough assistance, should be given when required and directed in order to help mobilize and clear secretions.
- **Positioning:** Assist in keeping the C-spine immobilized until the cervical spine injury has been completely ruled out. Attach a rigid or semirigid cervical collar, position the head on the trolley using tape and sandbags, and align the neck with the body (unless the patient is extremely agitated).
- **Cardiovascular management:**
  - Always keep an eye on the blood pressure and heart rate of the patients.
  - Volume resuscitation and vasopressor treatment are likely to be used to treat hypotension. The aim of treatment is to maintain mean arterial pressure (MAP) of 85 mm Hg or above for 7 days (a method known as hemodynamic push), which may enhance neurologic outcomes.
  - Euvolemia is maintained with the aid of isotonic fluids.
- **Musculoskeletal management:** Range-of-motion exercises, positioning techniques, weight-bearing exercises, electrical stimulation, and orthoses or splinting to avoid loss of muscle length and contractures are a few non-pharmacologic management methods for spasticity and to maintain muscle strength.
- **Integumentary system:** The cornerstones of managing pressure ulcers are prevention and early identification. Utilize a skin risk assessment instrument, such as the Braden scale, and routinely examine the patient's skin. The risk-reduction measures are:
  - At least once every two hours, turn the patient
  - Prevent the patient from being placed on bone prominences like the trochanters, sacrum, and heels
  - Reduce moisture
  - Routinely examine the skin behind splints and braces
  - Use a wheelchair with pressure-relieving cushions
  - Educate patients and offer nutritional guidance
- **Genitourinary management:**
  - Provide adequate catheter care
  - Ensure routine bladder emptying, between every 4 to 6 hours.
  - Educate self-catheterization and bladder retraining if applicable

REHABILITATION

Continued rehabilitation is necessary for patients recovering from neurotrauma after they are discharged from the hospital. The objective is to increase independence.

- **Physiotherapists (PTs)** work to increase a patient's mobility and address their strength, endurance, balance, and sensation while also educating the patient's family.
- **Occupational therapists (OTs)** assist in enhancing independence in daily living activities like cooking, bathing, using the restroom, and other. OTs assist patients with regaining the coordinated use of their limbs as well as the cognitive abilities required to carry out daily duties.
- **Speech and language pathologists (SLPs)** aid with speaking abilities, swallowing, language, and cognition.
- **Therapeutic recreation specialists (TRs)** talk to patients about their interests and hobbies and try to include those pursuits in a treatment plan.
- **Dieticians** make sure that a person is receiving enough nourishment and assist with any problems brought on by a lack of appetite or difficulties eating.
- **Neuropsychologists** assess the effects of TBI on thinking, behavior, and emotions. Utilize this knowledge to create a treatment and discharge plan, educate the patient and their family, engage in cognitive retraining, put behavior management techniques into place after an accident, and more.

Airway function is improved by **respiratory therapists**.

HOME CARE

- Encourage patient and family to continue with the well-defined short-term goals
- Teach patient and family about self-care management
- Encourage the patient to continue the rehabilitation program after discharge
- Take medications as prescribed
- Advice patient to take a healthy diet
- Encourage the patient to return to normal activities gradually
- Encourage the patient to use relaxation techniques
- Advise patient to do exercises on a regular basis.
- Plan rest period between activities
- Instruct patient and family to report if any side effect or complication occurs

GERIATRIC CONSIDERATIONS

Geriatric trauma is a term used to describe the trauma that occurs to an elderly person. The ability of the elderly population to recover from damage is often lower, and they are more vulnerable to trauma from very minor types of harm. The physiological responses of older people to serious injuries may be significantly impacted by medications used to address pre-existing chronic illnesses and comorbidities which increases the likelihood of future problems.

Case Scenario

1. A 29-year-old man who had fallen from the third level arrived at a trauma center. He was vomiting and bleeding from his nose when he arrived. Simple airway procedures were used to maintain his airway. His secretions were suctioned while he was in the lateral position. He had a Glasgow coma scale (GCS) score of 8 (eye 1; verbal 3; motor 4) and the bilateral pupillary reaction was (2+/2+). Preoxygenation was done and an endotracheal tube of size 8 was inserted and secured. He was shifted for CT scanning.
2. A 19-year-old boy was injured after he fell into the water while on vacation with his friends. He was pulled from the water. He was placed on his back, supported at the neck, and covered with a blanket. Within 15 minutes, paramedics arrived on the scene. The injured boy reported having excruciating neck discomfort and being unable to move his arms or legs. He had equal, light-responsive pupils. His vital signs showed a heart rate of 82 beats per minute, a blood pressure of 100/72, and 22 breaths per minute. He was given a cervical collar, placed on a stretcher, with his head immobilized, given 100% oxygen, and was shifted to the trauma hospital.

SUMMARY

The most frequent cause of death worldwide is neurotrauma. It is a medical emergency that needs to be attended in a right away. Patients who have only minor wounds may be kept under observation and discharged from the hospital. Patients who have sustained moderate to severe wounds require more intensive care, assisted breathing, surgery, drugs, and continued observation. In order to resume their regular lives, these individuals must undergo physical and mental rehabilitation and rely on their families. While some individuals may eventually regain some function, others may continue to have ongoing problems.

MULTIPLE CHOICE QUESTIONS

1. **What of the following step should be taken if a patient is suspected of having spinal damage?**
   a. Provide routine care
   b. Apply cervical collar of appropriate size
   c. HOB elevated to 30°
   d. Head tilted to one side
2. **Leakage of CSF from the ears and nose after a TBI is known as:**
   a. Racoon sign
   b. Battle sign
   c. Halo sign
   d. Murphy sign
3. **How would you interpret a patient's GCS of E2, V3, and M5?**
   a. Capable of obeying orders and having their eyes open to commands
   b. Eyes alert to discomfort, inappropriate words, and ability to localize trapezius pinch
   c. Open eyes on their own, oriented, and can follow directions
   d. Confusion and withdrawal in response to pain, with closed eyes
4. **After a head injury, the advised position:**
   a. Supine
   b. Left lateral
   c. HOB elevated at 30°
   d. Prone
5. **The recommended mannitol dosage is:**
   a. 0.25–1 g/kg
   b. 1.25–2 g/kg
   c. 2.25–3 g/kg
   d. 3.25–4 g/kg
6. **What is the appropriate body temperature to maintain in head injury patients?**
   a. 32–35°C
   b. 35–37°C
   c. 37–39°C
   d. >40°C
7. **Early management of spinal cord injury is:**
   a. Ice application
   b. Exercise
   c. Psychological support
   d. Immobilization
8. **The standard method to diagnose spinal cord injury is:**
   a. Ultrasonography
   b. MRI
   c. Blood tests
   d. Urine routine examination
9. **Central cord syndrome is:**
   a. A result of forces causing damage to the periphery of the spinal cord
   b. Most frequently affects elderly people with cervical spine degenerative changes
   c. Characterized by a disproportionate loss of lower extremities function compared to upper extremity function
   d. Frequently linked to penetrating wounds
10. **In cases of acute spinal cord damage, regular respiratory assessment is crucial, because:**
    a. They are at a higher risk of respiratory failure due to the loss of their protective respiratory muscles.
    b. These patients usually have phrenic innervation, which can be made worse by the use of steroids.
    c. Arterial blood gas readings in these patients can be erroneous.
    d. In quadriplegic patients, it is the third most common cause of death.

ANSWERS

1. b	2. c	3. b	4. c
5. a	6. b	7. d	8. b
9. a	10. a		

SUGGESTED READING

1. Anjum A, Yazid MD, Daud MF, Idris J, Hwei Ng AM, Naicker AS, et al. Spinal Cord Injury: Pathophysiology, Multimolecular Interactions, and Underlying Recovery Mechanisms. J Mol Sci. 2020;21(20):7533. Available from: https://www.mdpi.com/1422-0067/21/20/7533/htm
2. Brazier Y, Han S. Causes and effects of traumatic brain injury (TBI) 2018. Retrieved from https://www.medicalnewstoday.com/articles/179837.
3. Carney N, Totten AM, Reilly CO, Ullman JS, Bell MJ, Bratton SL. Brain Trauma Foundation TBI Guidelines, 4th edition. 2016. Guidelines for the Management of Severe Traumatic Brain Injury; pp. 1–10. Retrieved from https://www.ncbi.nlm.nih.gov/pmc/articles/PMC5672675/#ref38
4. Centers for Disease Control and Prevention (CDC), Traumatic Brain Injury (TBI): Incidence and Distribution, 2014. Introduction to Brain Injury—Facts and Stats, February 2000. Retrieved from https://www.aans.org/Patients/Neurosurgical-Conditions-and-Treatments/Traumatic-Brain-Injury
5. Dewan MC, Rattani A. Estimating the global incidence of traumatic brain injury JNS 2018 Retrieved from https://thejns.org/view/journals/j-neurosurg/130/4/article-p1080.xml.

6. Gururaj G. Epidemiology of traumatic brain injuries: Indian scenario. Neurol Res. 2002;24(1):24-8. Retrieved from https://pubmed.ncbi.nlm.nih.gov/11783750/#:~: text=It%20is%20estimated%20that%20nearly,at%20the%20time%20of%20injury.
7. Hadley MN, Walters BC, Aarabi A. Guidelines for the management of acute cervical spine and spinal cord injuries. Neurosurgery. 2013;72(Suppl 3):1-259. Available from https://www.msdmanuals.com/en-in/professional/injuries-poisoning/spinal-trauma/spinal-trauma#v16881392
8. Liao KH, Chang CK, Chang HC, Chang KC, Chen CF, Chen TY, et al. Clinical practice guidelines in severe traumatic brain injury in Taiwan. Surg Neurol. 2009;72(Suppl 2):S66-73. Retrieved from https://www.ncbi.nlm.nih.gov/pmc/articles/PMC5672675/#ref14
9. Rehabilitation Council of India. Spinal Cord Injury. Available from: http://www.rehabcouncil.nic.in/writereaddata/spinal.pdf.
10. Spinal Cord Injury. 2021 American Association of Neurological Surgeons. 2021 Retrieved from https://www.aans.org/en/Patients/Neurosurgical-Conditions-and-Treatments/Spinal-Cord-Injury.
11. Wilberger JE, Mao G. Spinal Trauma. MSD MANUAL Professional Version. 2019 Available from https://www.msdmanuals.com/en-in/professional/injuries-poisoning/spinal-trauma/spinal-trauma.
12. Wilberger JE. Traumatic Brain Injury (TBI). Johns Hopkins University MSD MANUAL 2019 Retrieved from https://www.msdmanuals.com/en-in/professional/injuries-poisoning/traumatic-brain-injury-tbi/traumatic-brain-injury-tbi.
13. Woolf AD, Pfleger B. Burden of major musculoskeletal conditions. Bull World Health Organ. 2003;81:646–56. Retrieved from https://www.marinemedicalsociety.in/article .asp?issn=09753605;year=2019;volume=21;issue=1;spage=46;epage=50;aulast=Sing#ref7
14. Yılmaz T, Kaptanoğlu E. Current and future medical therapeutic strategies for the functional repair of spinal cord injury. World J Orthop. 2015;6(1):42-55. Retrieved from doi: 10.5312/wjo.v6.i1.42.
15. Ziemer A. Classification of Traumatic Brain Injury Retrieved from 2021 https://www.physio-pedia.com/Classification_of_Traumatic_Brain_Injury.

CHAPTER 31

Cerebrovascular Disorders

Manisha Nagi, Ashok Kumar, Vivek Kumar Garg, Divesh Kumar Munjal, Kapil Goel

"Strokes do not discriminate…It can happen to anyone."

—Linda Steuer

LEARNING OBJECTIVES

After going through the chapter, the learner will be able to:
- Define the key terms related to various cerebrovascular disorders (stroke and aneurysm).
- Describe the epidemiology of various cerebrovascular disorders.
- Elaborate pathophysiology of various cerebrovascular disorders.
- Explain the medical and nursing management of these diseases.
- Discuss the geriatric considerations of various cerebrovascular disorders.

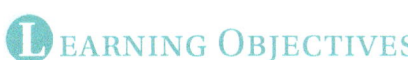

- **Cerebral aneurysm:** Outpouching of the cerebral artery.
- **Cerebrovascular Accident (CVA):** Stroke is also named as cerebrovascular accident and brain attack.
- **Coiling and clipping:** The interventions done for the treatment of various types of aneurysms.
- **rtPA:** Recombinant tissue plasminogen activator, intravenous thrombolysis.
- **Stroke:** Sudden loss of brain function resulting from disruption of blood supply to a part of the brain.
- **Subarachnoid hemorrhage (SAH):** Bleeding into subarachnoid space.
- **Transient ischemic attack:** A "mini stroke" wherein the blood clot blocks an artery for a short time.

INTRODUCTION

The cerebrovascular refers to the blood flow inside the brain. In cerebrovascular disorders, the blood flow to an area of the brain is permanently or temporarily affected by bleeding or ischemia. One or more cerebral blood vessels are involved in the pathological process. The signs and symptoms depend on which part and how much area of the brain is affected. The current chapter details two common cerebrovascular disorders i.e. stroke and aneurysm.

STROKE

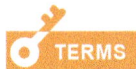

In Stroke, Time is equal to Brain. Time Lost is Brain Lost.

"Stroke, or cerebrovascular accident (CVA) is defined as a sudden loss of brain function resulting from disruption of blood supply to a part of the brain, which results in infarction or death of brain tissue."
—WHO.

Sometimes a stroke is referred to as a "brain attack." Similar to how a heart attack can harm the heart, a stroke can also harm the brain. A stroke happens when a portion of the brain does not receive the blood it requires because a blood vessel bursts or the brain's blood supply is interrupted. Brain cells start to die without oxygen, which can cause death or lasting damage **(Fig. 31.1)**.

A stroke is a brain injury caused by the sudden interruption of the blood flow to the brain. Remember, when dealing with stroke, TIME is BRAIN.

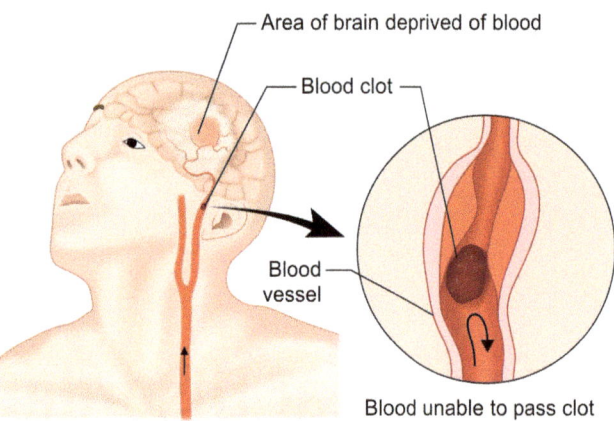

Fig. 31.1: Stroke due to blockage of blood vessels of brain.

TYPES OF STROKE

There are two major types of stroke:
1. Ischemic stroke
2. Hemorrhagic stroke

In addition of major types of stroke, there is one more type of stroke called '**transient ischemic attack (TIA)**'

Ischemic Stroke

A clot (thrombus) plugs a blood vessel in an ischemic stroke, preventing flow of blood to the brain and causing damage. 80–85% of those who have strokes experience this type of stroke, making it the most prevalent **(Fig. 31.2)**. The clot may develop in a variety of locations, including the heart, the neck's larger blood vessels, or the brain's main blood vessels (thrombosis). This type of ischemic stroke is called thrombotic stroke. An embolic stroke is another type of ischemic stroke in which a small traveling clot, i.e., an emboli travels to the brain and block blood vessel. Brain tissue may get injured when one part of the brain is deprived of oxygen resulting in loss of the body's functions that were regulated by that damaged brain region. Moreover, clots may stop up small blood veins deep inside the brain (lacuna stroke).

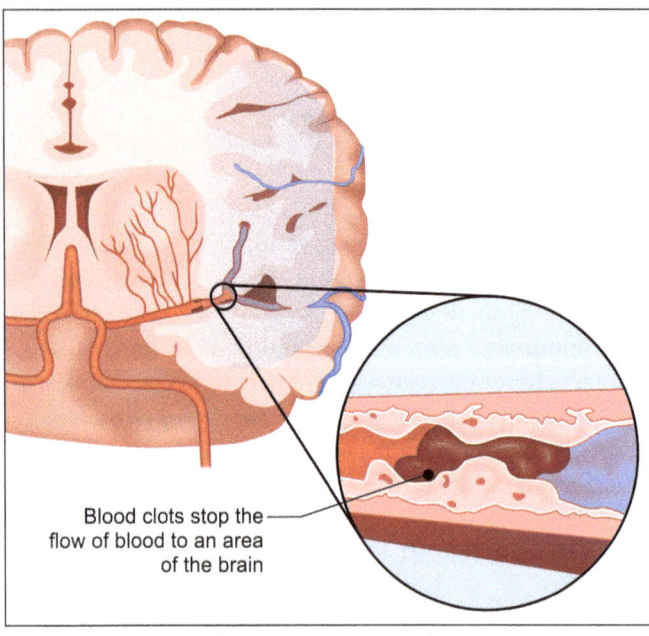

Fig. 31.2: Ischemic stroke.

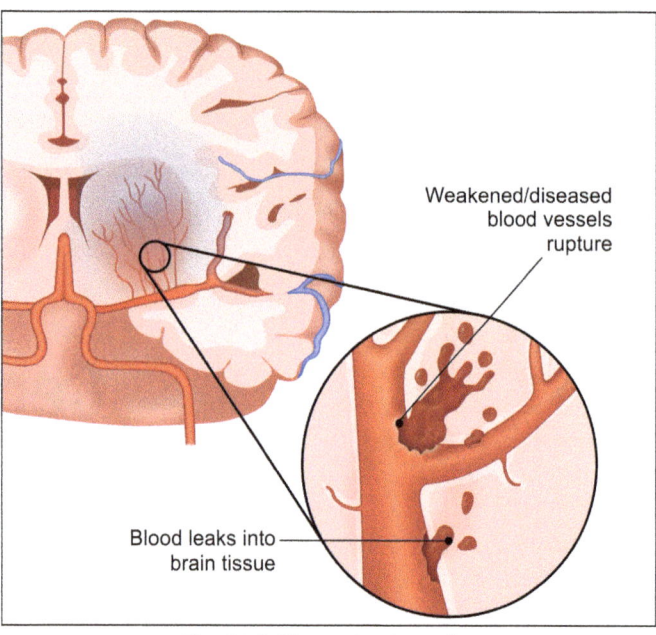

Fig. 31.3: Hemorrhagic stroke.

Hemorrhagic Stroke

This form of stroke, which affects 15–20% of patients with stroke, is brought on by increased blood pressure in a blood vessel, which causes it to rupture and flow into the brain **(Fig. 31.3)**. In this instance, the pressure caused by the bleeding affects brain cells. An aneurysm is a thin or weak area in an artery that can bulge out and burst, resulting in a stroke. Bleeding occurs from vessels within the brain parenchyma mainly due to:

❖ Hypertensive bleed
❖ Arteriovenous malformations (AVM) bleed
❖ Aneurysm rupture

Types of Hemorrhagic Stroke

❖ **Intracerebral hemorrhage (ICH):** Bleed in brain parenchyma.
❖ **Subarachnoid hemorrhage (SAH):** Bleed in subarachnoid space of the brain.

Transient Ischemic Attack (TIA)

It is a "mini stroke" that occurs when a blood clot blocks an artery for a short time. The symptoms of a TIA which are very similar to those of a stroke, are like the warning signs of a stroke, but they usually last only a few minutes to several hours but disappear completely. About 10 percent of strokes are preceded by TIA's.

Significance of a Mini-Stroke

A mini-stroke is a warning of a more severe stroke. About 10% of those who have a mini stroke develops a bigger stroke over the next three months. However, if treatment is sought after a mini stroke, the risk of a major, disabling, or fatal stroke can be minimized.

EPIDEMIOLOGY OF STROKE

Stroke is a frequent yet deadly condition that can leave a person permanently incapacitated or result in death.

> **BOX 31.1:** According to World Stroke Organization.
>
> - Worldwide one person every two seconds suffers a stroke
> - 16% of the population worldwide will suffer a stroke in their lifetime
> - Every four seconds in the world someone dies as a result of a stroke
> - Up to 90% of strokes are preventable if the risk factors are managed appropriately

One in every six people will experience a stroke at some point in their lifetime, making it the third greatest cause of mortality worldwide **(Box 31.1)**. Young and old people alike are susceptible. Worldwide, more than 15 million individuals have a stroke every year; 5.5 million pass away and 5 million are left permanently disabled. Stroke incidence is rising in India and other emerging nations. More than 80% of stroke cases take place in developing and poor nations. For the first stroke, the yearly crude incidence rate is 145 per 100,000 people

ETIOLOGY

Figure 31.4 illustrates some of the important risk factors of stroke that an individual can alter or address. *"An ounce of prevention is better than a pound of cure,"* the ancient saying goes. The secret to prevention may lie in understanding the risk factors. Reduce the chance of having a stroke by concentrating on the variables that can control.

PATHOPHYSIOLOGY (FLOWCHART 31.1)

A stroke is described as a short neurological episode resulting from impaired brain blood flow. Blood flow to the brain is regulated by two vertebral arteries posteriorly positioned and two internal carotid arteries located anteriorly. In contrast to ischemic stroke, which is caused by insufficient blood and oxygen delivery to the brain, hemorrhagic stroke is caused by bleeding of blood vessels. Thrombotic and embolic disorders can occur from ischemic occlusion in the brain. Vascular atherosclerosis-induced arterial constriction affects blood flow in thrombosis. Eventually, plaque accumulation causes the arterial chamber to narrow and clot, which causes thrombotic stroke. A reduction in blood flow to the brain during an embolic stroke result in an embolism, acute stress, and early cell death (necrosis). During necrosis and the loss of neuronal function, plasma membrane rupture, organelle expansion, and the leakage of cellular contents into extracellular space all take place. Additional significant events that contribute to stroke pathology include elevated excitotoxicity, inflammation, energy failure, oxidative stress, free radical-mediated toxicity, acidosis, complement activation, activation of glial cells, cytokine-mediated cytotoxicity, intracellular Ca^{2+} levels, loss of homeostasis, deterioration of the blood-brain barrier, and leukocyte infiltration. Hemorrhagic stroke causes internal damage and stress to the internal structure of the brain, which causes blood vessels to burst. Its detrimental effects on the circulatory system lead to infarction. There are two distinct types of bleeding: subarachnoid and intracerebral. Blood builds up unusually inside the brain as a result of blood vessels bursting in ICH. The main causes of ICH are excessive anticoagulant use, hypertension (HTN), abnormal vasculature, and thrombolytic medications. As a result of a brain injury or cerebral aneurysm in subarachnoid hemorrhage (SAH), blood accumulates in the subarachnoid space of the brain.

CLINICAL MANIFESTATIONS

A stroke occurs suddenly. Most people display two or more symptoms. A sign or symptom could appear out of nowhere and become worse soon. According to National Institute of Neurological Disorders and Stroke (NINDS)-2002, after

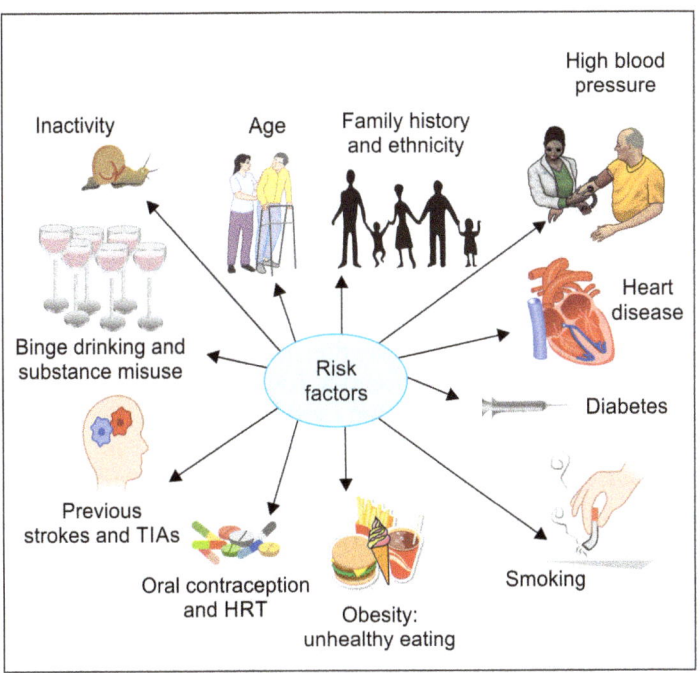
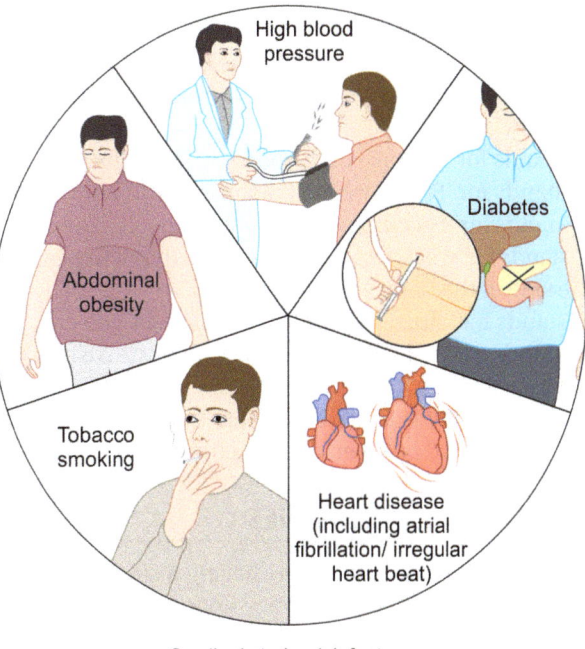

Fig. 31.4: Risk factors of stroke.

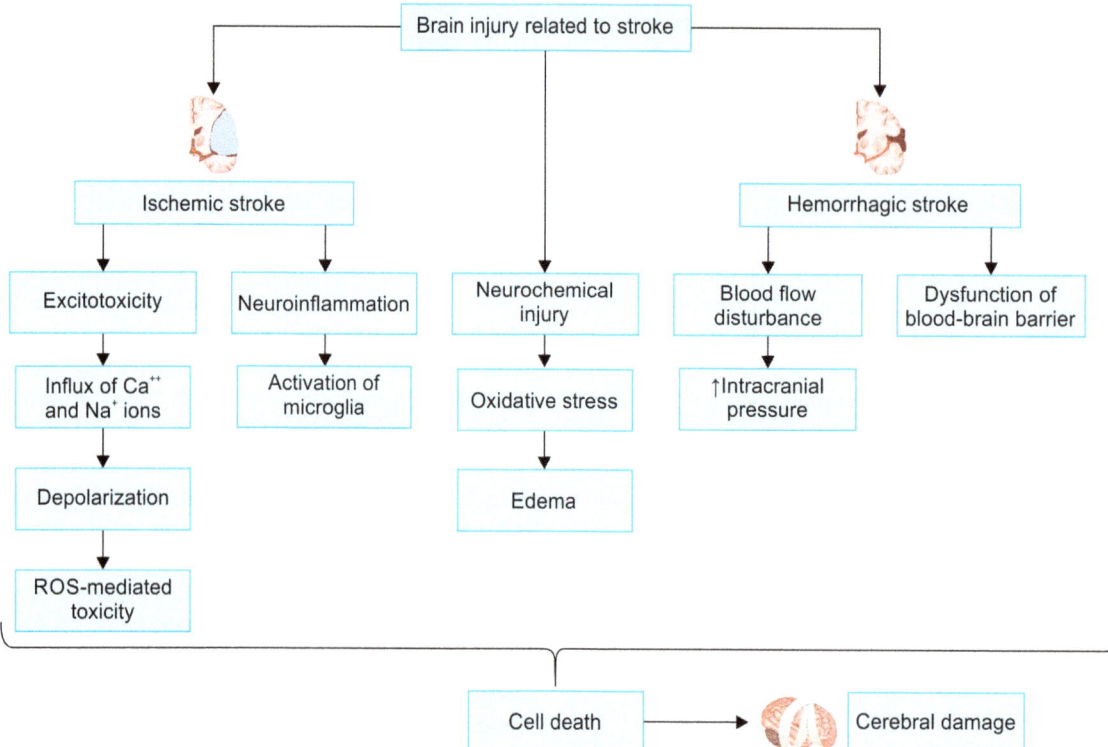

Flowchart 31.1: Pathophysiology of stroke.

a stroke, one or more of the following symptoms may arise minutes or hours later and quickly get worse.
- Sudden blindness or difficulty seeing in one or both eyes
- Sudden difficulty walking, lightheadedness, or losing balance
- Sudden disorientation or difficulty speaking or understanding speech
- Sudden severe headache with no apparent reason.
- Sudden weakness of numbness of face, upper limb or lower limb (mainly on left or right side of the body).

Mnemonics to identify 'Stroke': It is very essential to identify the stroke patients as quickly as possible so that appropriate treatment can be commenced timely to save the victim. For this there in Mnemonics to identify Stroke which is **"BE FAST"** Here;
'B' stands for 'Balance of the body of the victim
'E' stands for 'Eye problem like slurred vision or vision loss
'F' stands for 'Facial Deviation to one side'
'A' stands for 'weakness in Arm or Leg of the victim, preferably one side of the body'
'S' stands for 'Slurred speech or problem in speech'
'T' stands for 'Time, in case of any of the stroke symptoms, don't waste time, rush to the nearest hospital where 24 × 7 CT scan facility is available so that quick and appropriate treatment could be given to the victim (Fig. 31.5).

DIAGNOSTIC MODALITIES

A patient who is thought to be having a stroke is evaluated by physicians in the emergency department (ED) using a variety of techniques. Physicians can identify the type and site of a stroke as well as the reason it occurred with the aid of a physical examination, medical history, family history,

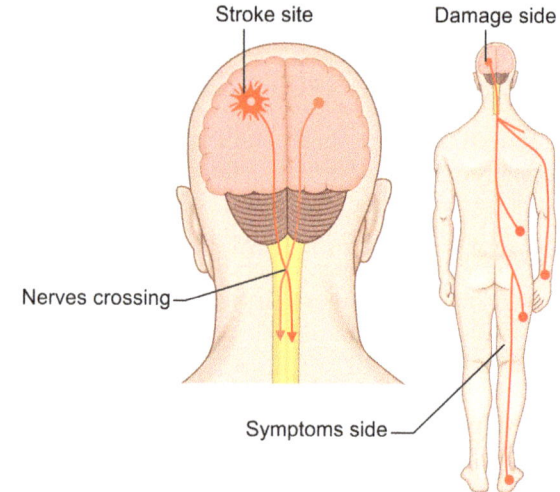

Fig. 31.5: Stroke site versus damage site.

blood tests, risk factors and various imaging like non-contrast computed tomography (NCCT) Head, magnetic resonance imaging (MRI) of Brain, CT, or MR angiography (**Figs. 31.6A to D**).

To preserve brain function after a stroke, an immediate, precise diagnosis is essential. The type of stroke determines the type of treatment, and for the majority of treatments to be effective, they must be initiated within 4.5 hours of the onset of symptoms.

MEDICAL MANAGEMENT

Stroke Unit and Stroke Team

- Ideally, people who have a stroke are admitted to a "stroke unit", a ward or dedicated area in hospital staffed by nurses and therapists with experience in stroke treatment.

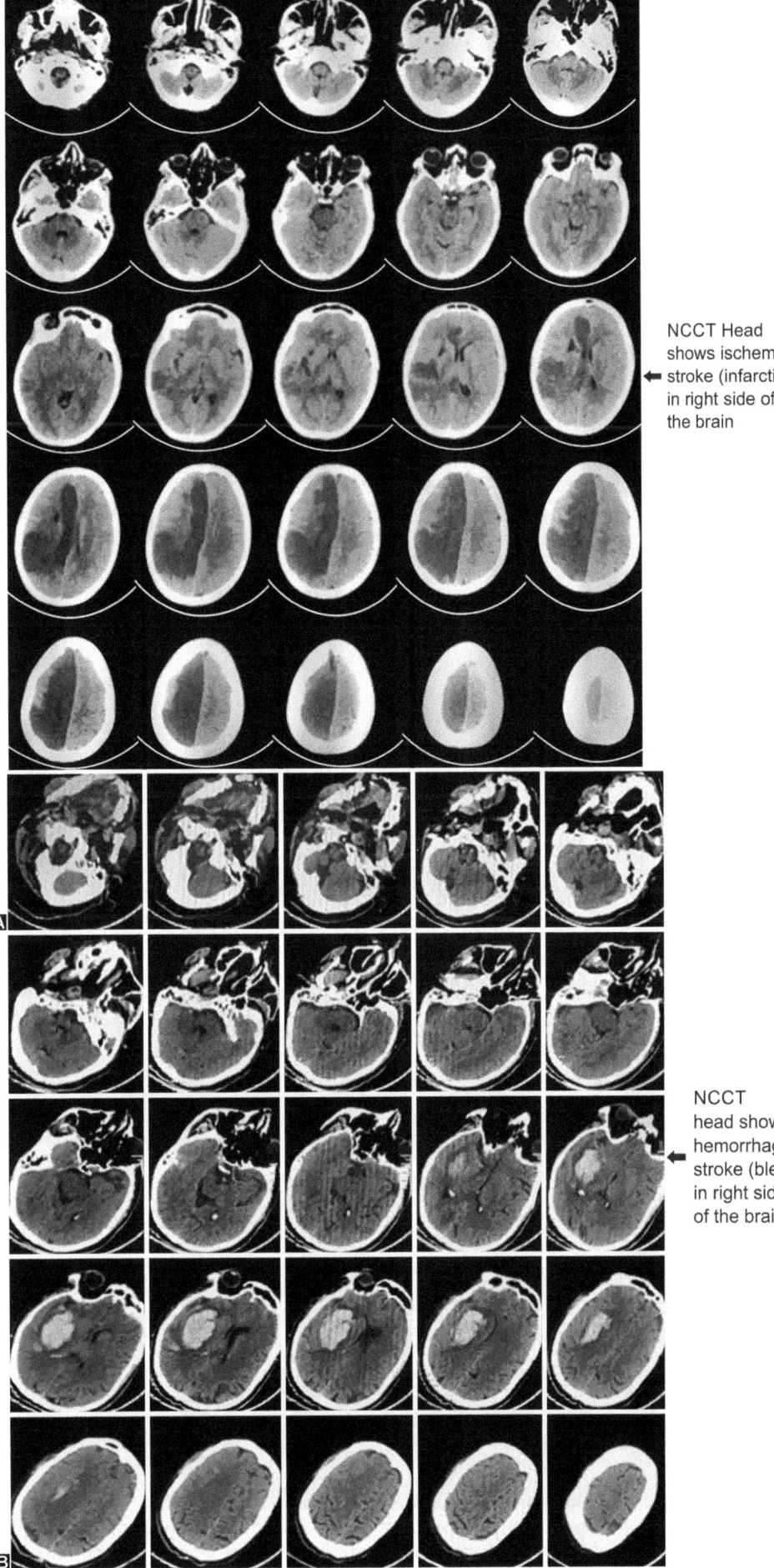

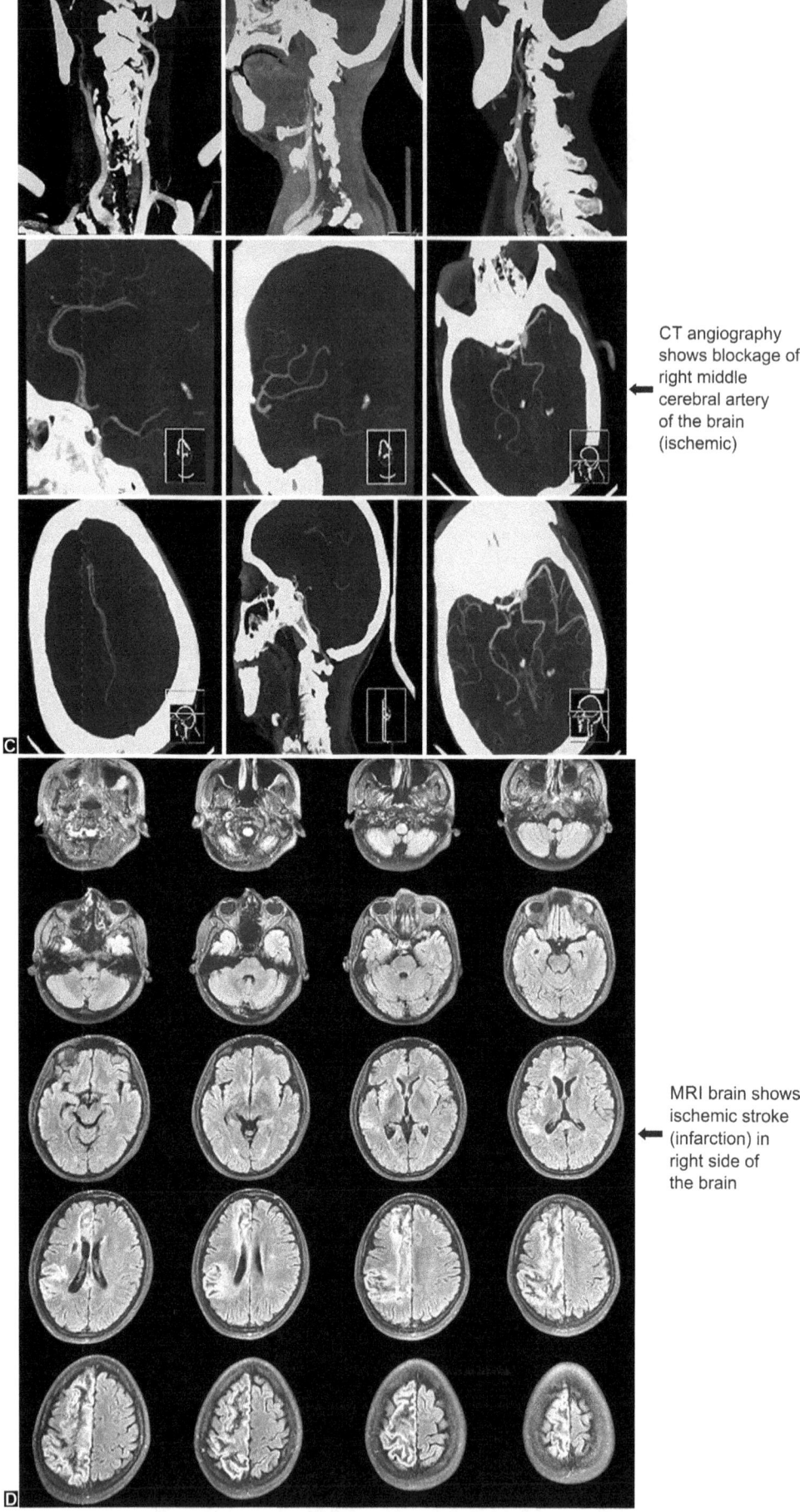

Figs. 31.6A to D: Diagnostic evaluation of stroke: (A) Noncontrast computed tomography (NCCT) head shows ischemic stroke (infarction) in right side of the brain; (B) NCCT head shows hemorrhagic stroke (bleed) in right side of the brain; (C) CT angiography shows blockage of right middle cerebral artery of the brain (ischemic stroke); (D) MRI brain shows ischemic stroke (infarction) in right side of the brain.

- It has been shown that people admitted to a stroke unit have a higher chance of surviving than those admitted elsewhere in hospital, even if they are being cared for by doctors without experience in stroke.

In Stroke, around 2 millions neurons permanently die within 1 minute. Thus, in stroke 1 minute = 2 millions! So in stroke Every Minute Matter! We have to Act FAST to save life of the stroke patients.

Anyone suspected of having a stroke should be admitted right away to a hospital with the best resources available, as stroke is an emergency. The modality of treatment depends on the window period (duration from onset of first symptoms of stroke to treatment) in case of acute ischemic stroke:

- **≤4.5 hours:** Intravenous thrombolysis (IVT) with injection rtPA (recombinant tissue plasminogen activator)
- **>4.5 to 6 hours:** Intra-arterial thrombolysis (IAT) with injection rtPA
- **>6 to 8 hours:** Device or mechanical thrombectomy (MT).

Pharmacological Management

Clot-busting medications like rtPA can be used to treat a stroke brought on by blood artery blockage (recombinant tissue Plasminogen Activator). To prevent lasting brain damage and consequent impairment, the clot should be removed as soon as possible. As soon as the first symptom is noticed, the patient must be transported to the hospital. For the best outcome, rtPA should be administered as an injection as soon as possible after such a stroke and no later than four and a half hours. Patients with stroke receive a variety of additional medications to stop recurrent strokes. The blood-thinning medication, aspirin, especially in patients with thickened blood arteries brought on by smoking, high blood pressure, diabetes, and high cholesterol levels, lowers the risk of a recurrence of stroke. Patients with heart illness, especially those with an irregular heartbeat (atrial fibrillation) or damaged heart valves, benefit from the stronger blood-thinning medication, warfarin, which reduces the risk of stroke. Don't give the person anything to drink if they are unresponsive or drowsy to prevent risk of aspiration.

NINDS Recommended Timeframe for Acute Ischemic Stroke Treatment (Fig. 31.7)

- **Time of patient arrives in medical emergency outpatient department (EMOPD):** When stroke patient arrives at emergency department (ED).
- **Evaluation by EMOPD Doctor/Registered Nurse (RN) within 10 minutes of arrival of patient:** This includes
  - History of the event:
  - Vitals
  - *Time of the onset:* Accurate, e.g., 3:19 PM.
  - Initiate laboratory work which includes complete hemogram, coagulogram [international normalized ratio (INR)/prothrombin time (PT)/percutaneous thrombin injection (PTI)], complete biochemistry, stat blood sugar.
  - Neurological assessment using NIHSS (National Institutes of Health Stroke Scale). NIHSS is a 42 points scale with 13 domains.
  - It identifies stroke severity. NIHSS <6 = Mild stroke, 6–12 = Moderate stroke, >12 = Severe stroke. It is useful in determining suitability for thrombolysis and also for post thrombolysis monitoring.
- Inform to stroke team members (includes neurologist, radiologist, stroke nurse) within 15 minutes.
- Initiate NCCT Head and CT angio of cerebral and neck vessels within 25 minutes and their interpretation within 45 minutes **(Fig. 31.8)**.
- **Thrombolysis in golden hour:** Eligible patients should get bolus dose of clot busting drug within 60 minutes of arrival in ED followed by its infusion **(Box 31.2)**.

Other Medications

- **Anti-platelets:** Tablet ecosprin and tablet clopivas (clopidogril) used to prevent platelet aggregation in patients with stroke to prevent recurrence by averting thrombosis.
- **Anti-coagulants:** Oral anticoagulant (e.g., tablet warfarin) and parenteral anticoagulant e.g., injection heparin used to prevent thrombus formation in patients who are susceptible to have stroke in future or to prevent recurrence.
- **Atorvastatin or rosuvastatin drug** used to prevent hypercholestremia which leads to antherosclerotic

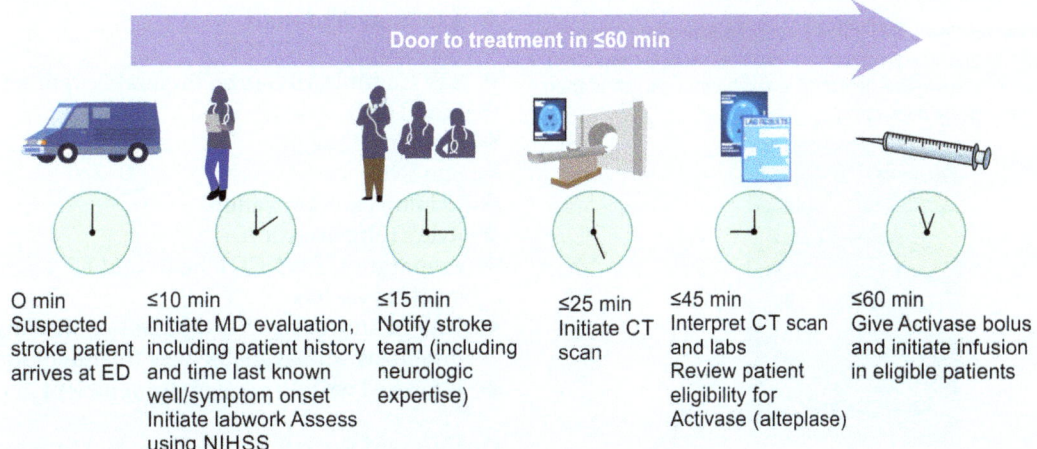

Fig. 31.7: National Institute of Neurological Disorders and Stroke (NINDS) recommended time-frame for acute ischemic stroke treatment.

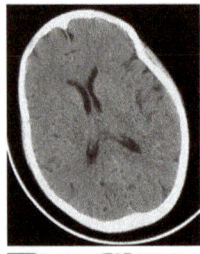
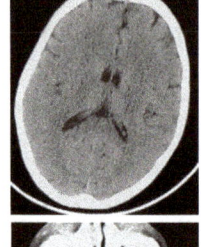

NCCT

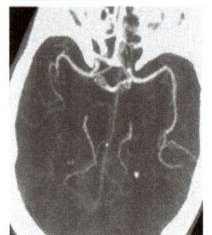
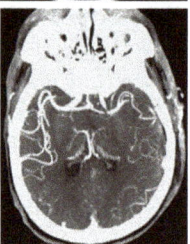

CT angiography

Fig. 31.8: NCCT head and CT angiography of brain vessel.

> **BOX 31.2:** How to administer intravenous thrombolytic therapy: Inj. tPA (clot busting drug).

Dosages: 0.9 mg/kg (maximum dose 90 mg) over 60 minutes with 10% of the dose given as a bolus over 1 minute
e.g., patient weight 70 kg
Total dose = 70 × 0.9 = 63 mg
10% bolus over 1 min = 6.3 mg
Then infusion for 1 hour = 56.7 mg.

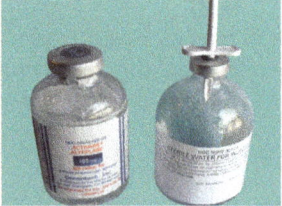

rtPA injection with its solvent

Intra-arterial thrombolysis (IAT): Injection tPA, maximum dose 22 mg infused over 1 hour directly on clot.

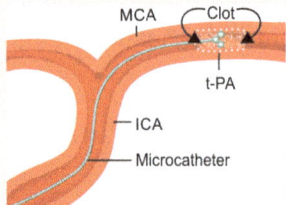

Intra-arterial thrombolysis (IAT)

Mechanical thrombectomy (MT): This is accomplished by inserting a catheter into the femoral artery, directing it into the cerebral circulation, and deploying a corkscrew-like device to trap the clot, which is then withdrawn from the body by suction.

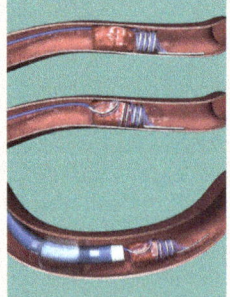

Mechanical thrombectomy

Injection tenecteplase: It is a new clot busting drug used for thrombolysis in acute ischemic stroke.

disease of blood vessels of brain to prevent stroke in future.
- ❖ **Anti-hypertensive** to control hypertension and anti-diabetic drugs to control diabetic mellitus plays important role to prevent stroke in majority of patients.

Note: Dosage of the medications depends on the patient's condition.

SURGICAL MANAGEMENT

Rarely are strokes treated or prevented with surgery. A neurosurgeon may aspirate the blood clot if the stroke was brought on by a significant amount of brain bleeding. Surgery might be helpful in patients who occasionally have abnormal blood vessels due to birth, as it could stop further bleeding. In the meanwhile, vascular surgeons conduct carotid endarterectomy to clear a blockage caused by fatty deposits in the carotid artery in the neck, the primary blood channel transporting blood from the heart to the brain, to stop a stroke from happening again. A surgeon may perform surgery to insert a metal clip at the base of an aneurysm (a thin or weak area in an artery that swells out and may burst) or remove aberrant blood vessels in order to treat hemorrhagic stroke. Decompressive hemicraniectomy is done by neurosurgeons to reduce increased ICP in case of malignant infarct or massive ICH.

DIETETICS

A balanced diet that includes whole grains, veggies, and fruits is crucial. The patient should be provided with dietary instructions at the time of discharge from the hospital. The patients need to keep an eye on their food due to health issues like excessive cholesterol or diabetes.

NURSING MANAGEMENT OF PATIENTS

Nurses have an important role to play in the prevention and management of stroke. Stroke nurses play a pivotal role in providing care to the acute stroke patients. The role of stroke nurses is highlighted in the following points.

Pre-thrombolysis Nursing Management
- ❖ Assessment of vitals
- ❖ Assessment of NIHSS
- ❖ 2 IV Cannula 18 Gauze. Preferably in brachial veins.
- ❖ Blood tests
- ❖ Stat blood sugar
- ❖ Stat INR
- ❖ Urinary catheterization.
- ❖ Ryle's tube insertion.
- ❖ Preparation for NCCT head and CT angio of neck and cerebral vessels
- ❖ Patient and/or his/her relatives counseling for event, its prognosis, and available best treatment modalities.
- ❖ Informed written consent from patient or close relative.

During and Post-thrombolysis Nursing Management
- ❖ BP monitoring every 15 min × first 2 hours
- ❖ Then every 30 min × 6 hours
- ❖ And after that every 1 hour × 24 hours

- **NIHSS Assessment:** At 2 hours, 6 hours and 24 hours
- **Blood Sugar:** At 2 hours, 6 hours and 24 hours.
- Pulse, respiration, temperature.

Note: If there is worsening of 4 points in NIHSS: Stop tPA infusion and shift patient for stat NCCT head to rule out intra cranial hemorrhage (ICH).

Complications of Thrombolysis
- Anaphylaxis
- Intracranial hemorrhage (ICH)
- Systemic bleeding

Post-thrombolysis Attention for Doctors and Nurses
- No anti-platelets e.g., ecospirin or clopivas for the next 24 hours.
- No anticoagulants e.g., injection heparin or injection clexan for the next 24 hours.

Strictly Avoid for 6 Hours after Thrombolysis
- IM injections
- Urinary catheterization
- RT insertion
- Oral care with toothbrush
- Blood samples
- Mobilization of operated leg (preferably right leg) in case of IAT or Device.

Management for Hemorrhagic Stroke
- Main goal is to maintain systolic BP 140–160 mm of Hg.
- Treat increased ICP.
- **Surgical intervention:** Decompressive hemicraniectomy to reduce increased ICP.

A big responsibility for nurses: BP control
- If Systolic BP is >180 mm of Hg or diastolic BP is >110 mm of Hg.
- Confirm with 2 readings 5–10 minutes apart
- If persistent, injection labetolol 10–20 mg IV over 1–2 mins.
- Repeat every 10–20 mins to a total dose of 300 mg or bradycardia.

For all acute strokes: Nurses' responsibility
- Gugging Swallowing Screening (GUSS) test to prevent aspiration pneumonia.
- Coordinate for physiotherapy/occupation therapy/speech therapy to start early rehabilitation.
- Coordinate for all required investigations e.g., 2D echo, MRI/MRA etc.
- Stroke education to whole family members.
- Discharge planning.
- Follow-up planning.

GERIATRIC CONSIDERATIONS

One of the main causes of disability and death worldwide is stroke. Age significantly raises the risk of stroke. The chances of stroke increases almost double after 55 years of age in both men and women. In USA, a stroke occurred at an average age of 69.2 years in 2005. Recent studies indicate that the risk of stroke is rising in persons between the ages of 20 and 54, most likely due to secondary factors that are already present. Age is a significant factor that determines stroke outcome and is connected with stroke prevalence. The number of stroke patients will climb as the percentage of the old rises, resulting in an ever-increasing percentage of stroke-related deaths. We need to learn more about stroke in this population since effective therapy of older stroke patients has been linked to better outcomes.

Case Scenario

1. A primary stroke center received a presentation from a 20-year-old male with acute left sided weakness and imbalance, decreased level of consciousness, and no prior medical history. A hyperdense basilar artery and no bleeding were seen on head CT scan. A mid-basilar occlusion was detected by CT angiography. A hyperdense basilar artery and no bleeding were seen on a head CT scan. A mid-basilar occlusion was detected by CT angiography. His mid-basilar blockage was established by an angiography at a comprehensive stroke center after he had received Alteplase intravenous tPA. He had mechanical thrombectomy along with basilar artery recanalization. After two days, his neurological examination showed improvement, and he was sent home. He was back to normal and working when he had a three-month follow-up.
2. Suddenly developing right-side weakness, a 65-year-old female with a history of HTN and hyperlipidemia visited a primary stroke clinic. She was found to have a right hemiplegia, dysarthria, right facial droop, right homonymous hemianopsia, global aphasia, and left gaze preference (NIH stroke scale = 22). Just ambiguous hypodensity was seen on a head CT scan in the left middle cerebral artery (MCA) area. A left middle cerebral artery blockage was detected by CT angiography. After being moved to a comprehensive stroke center, where digital subtraction angiography revealed left middle cerebral artery blockage, she was administered alteplase intravenous tPA at two hours after the onset of her symptoms. She had a mechanical thrombectomy and MCA recanalization. She just experienced a very slight expressive aphasia and right facial droop the following day (NIHSS = 2). She had no neurological impairments three months later (NIHSS = 0).
3.
   - HK, 19-year-old female residence of Ropar (PB)
   - Cause of sudden onset of right UL/LL weakness
   - Deviation of face to the Lt. side
   - Inability to speak
   - Time of onset: Since 10:15 AM on 12/7/14
   - Time of reaching ED at 11:50 AM on same day
   - Vitals parameters: BP = 90/60 mm of Hg, Pulse: 78/min
   - Temp. afebrile, Resp = 22/min
   - Blood Sugar: 129 mg/dL
   - INR = 1.5
   - History of RHD x 4 years.
   - NIHSS at admission = 21 (major stroke)
   - NCCT head (time 11:54 AM) = grossly normal
   - CT angio neck and cerebral vessels = Left M1 MCA occlusion.

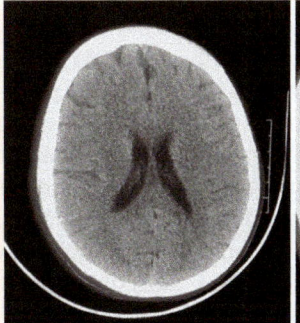 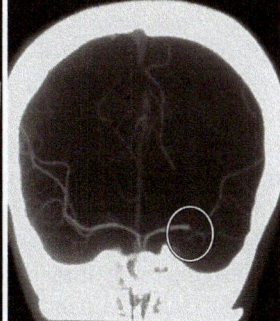

Fig. 31.9: Prethrombolysis NCCT head and CT angio of HK.

- After informed written consent IVT was started at 12:50 PM followed by mechanical thrombectomy at 2:25 PM.
  - Complete recanalization occurred (vessel completely opened)
  - Patient shifted to NSW at bed no. 34.
  - 6 hours NIHSS was = 13, 24 hours NIHSS was = 8
- Door to CT time: 4 minutes
- Door to needle time: 60 minutes

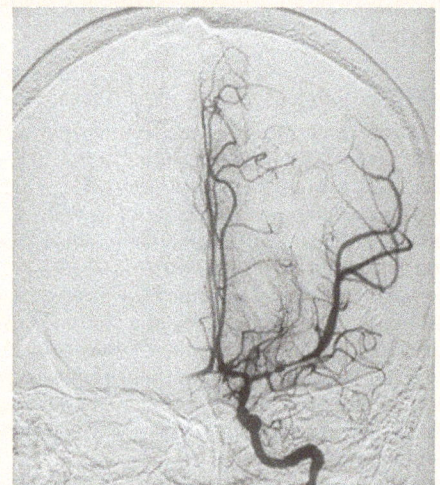

Fig. 31.10: Post thrombolysis DSA (complete recanalization of blocked vessel) of HK.

CEREBRAL ANEURYSM AND SUBARACHNOID HEMORRHAGE

A cerebral aneurysm is the saccular outpouching of a cerebral artery. These out pouching commonly occurs at the site of arterial bifurcation in the circle of Willis, with many shapes like pedunculated, sessile, and occasionally multi-lobulated aneurysms. Cerebral aneurysm rupture usually results in a subarachnoid hemorrhage (SAH), defined as bleeding into the subarachnoid space.

EPIDEMIOLOGY

The crude global incidence of SAH has declined by 40% between 1980 and 2010, but there is a significant variation in SAH incidence according to age, sex, region, and the prevalence of blood pressure, and smoking. Between 1980 and 2020, SAH incidence declined by 40.6% in Europe, 46.2% in Asia, and 14.0% in North America. Intracranial saccular aneurysms or berry aneurysms account for approximately 80–90% of all intracranial aneurysms.

ETIOLOGY

The etiology of cerebral aneurysms remains unclear. Many extrinsic, congenital, and genetic factors have been implicated in forming various aneurysms. According to degenerative theory, the intima covered by adventitia bulges from a local weakness. Forbus suggested aneurysms were acquired lesions resulting from degeneration of the elastic membranes due to continued overstretching, combined with an underlying congenital defect in the muscular portion of the arterial wall. Glynn proposed that the degeneration of the internal elastic lamina, possibly caused by atherosclerosis, was the leading cause of the formation of a saccular aneurysm.

He also proposed that both acquired and congenital defects are responsible for the internal elastic defects. Research has demonstrated an association between the presence of specific human leukocyte antigen alleles and the genetic role they may play in aneurysm formation. The mean age of rupture of an aneurism is between 50–55 years. While most aneurysmal SAH occurs in the range of 40 to 60 years of age, young children and older adults can also be affected. Black Americans are at higher risk than White Americans. There is a higher incidence of aneurysmal SAH in females, which may relate to hormonal status. Although the etiology of most aneurysms is yet unknown, bacterial, and fungal infections have also been known to cause an infectious aneurysm.

CLASSIFICATION OF ANEURYSM

As per size, aneurysms can be classified as small, large, and giant and as per shape these can be classified as Berry or saccular, giant or fusiform; mycotic; dissecting; and traumatic/charcot **(Table 31.1)**.
- **Small aneurysms** are <11 millimeters in diameter.
- **Large aneurysms** are 11–25 millimeters.
- **Giant aneurysms** are >25 millimeters in diameter.

RISK FACTORS

Numerous nonmodifiable (age, gender, ethnicity, family history, aneurysm location, size) and modifiable (hypertension, body mass index, tobacco, and illicit drug use) risk factors are there. Not all the aneurysms will rupture. Aneurysm characteristics like location, size and growth during follow-up evaluation period may affect the risk that an aneurysm can rupture. In addition, medical conditions may also influence aneurysm rupture.
- **Smoking:** Smoking is linked to the development and rupture of cerebral aneurysms. Smoking may cause multiple aneurysms to form in the brain.
- **High blood pressure:** High blood pressure weakens and damages arteries, making them more likely to rupture.
- **Size:** The big aneurysms are the ones which are most likely to get rupture in a person who previously did not show any symptoms.
- **Location:** Aneurysms located on the posterior communicating arteries and possibly those on the anterior communicating artery have a higher risk of getting ruptured than those at other locations in the brain.
- **Growth:** Aneurysms which grow, even if they are small, are at increased risk of getting ruptured.
- **Family history:** A family history of rupture of aneurysm suggests an increased risk of rupture for aneurysms detected in family members. The incidence of familial aneurysms among SAH is 6–20%.

The greatest risk of aneurysm include obesity, tobacco use, alcoholism, high cholesterol, copper deficiency and increasing age. Studies show that there is a reduced occurrence of SAH in some premenopausal women, especially those without a history of smoking. Hormone Replacement reduced the risk in postmenopausal women who had never smoked.

TABLE 31.1: Classification of aneurysm.

Type of aneurysm	Characteristics
Berry or saccular	The most common type, usually congenital, appears as a bifurcation in the anterior circulation, primarily at the base of the brain or circle of Willis and its branches, grows from the base of the arterial wall with a neck or stem, contains blood, the thinned dome is usually the site of rupture.
Giant or fusiform	It can be irregular in shape and larger than 2.5 cm. Atherosclerotic involves mainly the internal carotid, or vertebrobasilar artery rarely ruptures, has no stem, can act like a space-occupying lesion in the brain, and is difficult to manage.
Mycotic	It can be irregular in shape and larger than 2.5 cm, and atherosclerosis involves mainly the internal carotid, or vertebrobasilar artery, rarely ruptures, has no stem, can act like a space-occupying lesion in the brain, and is difficult to manage.
Dissecting	It may occur during angiography, secondary to trauma, syphilis, or arteriosclerosis, or when blood is forced between layers of the arterial wall, the intima is pulled away from the medial layer, allowing blood to enter.
Traumatic/Charcot-Bouchard 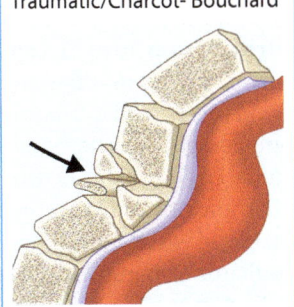	Sometimes called a "pseudo aneurysm," which may occur following trauma. A small aneurysm that can be seen in the area of the basal ganglia and/or the brainstem in individuals with a history of hypertension, chronic hypertension causes fibroid necrosis in the penetrating and subcortical arteries, weakening the arterial walls and causing the formation of small aneurysmal outpouching.

PATHOPHYSIOLOGY

Aneurysm formation is initiated by hemodynamically triggered endothelial dysfunction. An inflammatory response implicating several cytokines and inflammatory mediators as well as macrophages, T cells, and mast cells ensues. Concurrently, smooth muscle cells (SMCs) undergo phenotypic modulation to a proinflammatory phenotype. The inflammatory response in vessel wall leads to disruption of internal elastic lamina, extracellular matrix digestion, and aneurysm formation. Loss of mural cells and further inflammation and vessel wall degeneration ultimately lead to rupture of aneurysm **(Fig. 31.11)**.

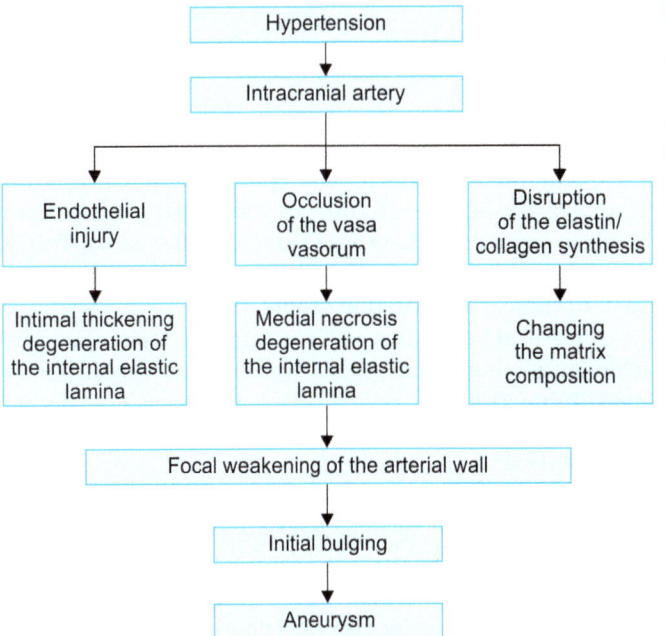

Fig. 31.11: Pathophysiology of aneurysm.

CLINICAL MANIFESTATIONS

Unruptured Aneurysm

Most of cerebral aneurysms do not show symptoms until they become very large, or they get ruptured. Small unchanging aneurysms generally will not produce any symptoms.

A larger aneurysm that is slowly growing may press on the tissues and nerves causing:

- Pain above and behind the eye
- Weakness
- Numbness
- Paralysis on one side of the face
- Vision changes or double vision.
- Dilated pupil

Ruptured Aneurysm

When an aneurysm gets rupture, one always experiences a sudden and extremely severe headache (e.g., worst headache in one's life) and may also develop:

- Nausea
- Vomiting
- Double vision
- Sensitivity to light
- Stiff neck
- Seizures
- Loss of consciousness (this may happen for short or may be prolonged)
- Cardiac arrest.

DIAGNOSIS

History and Physical Examination

If the symptoms are present, apply Hunt and Hess scale. Most warning headaches are indications of unrecognized subarachnoid hemorrhage. If the patient shows symptoms of an aneurysm, then to rule out the disease, the patient needs to be assessed based on Hunt and Hess scale. This is the scale used to assess the severity of an aneurysm on the basis of clinical presentation **(Table 31.2)**.

The World Federation of Neurosurgical Society (WFNS) scale for grading the aneurysm was originally published in 1988 **(Table 31.3)**.

Specific Test

- **Computerized tomography (CT):** A CT scan is always the first test used to determine if someone has bleeding in the brain. The test produces images which are 2D "slices" of the brain. CT can be plain or contrast; a contrast is found to be easier to observe the blood flow in the brain and may indicate the presence of an aneurysm **(Figs. 31.12 and 31.13)**. This test is known as a CT angiogram.
- **Cerebrospinal fluid test:** It is done to check for the presence of red blood cells in fluid surrounding the brain and spine. If a patient has symptoms of a ruptured aneurysm, but the neurosurgeon is not able to diagnose with the help of CT, cerebrospinal fluid testing can help.
- **Magnetic resonance imaging (MRI):** 2D or 3D MRI is used for the aneurysm. MRI done to collect a detailed view of arteries is called MR angiography **(Figs. 31.14A to C)**.

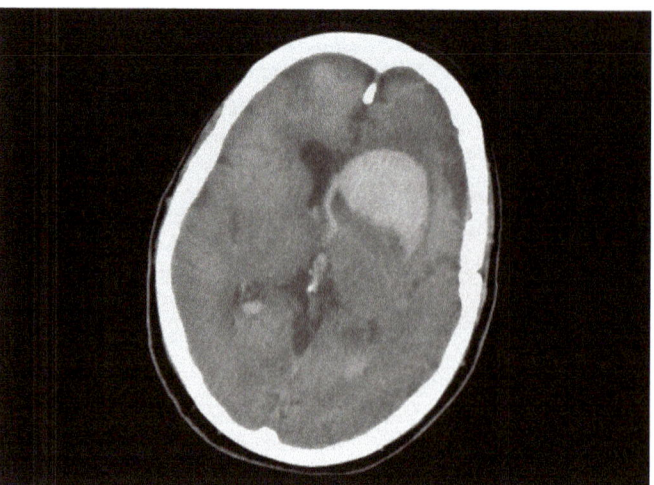

Fig. 31.12: NCCT head subarachnoid hemorrhage, frontal intraparenchymal hematoma with rupture into ventricular system.

- **Cerebral angiogram:** A thin and flexible tube (catheter) is inserted into a large artery, which is in the groin or the wrist. The catheter threads pass the heart to the arteries in the brain. A special dye is injected into the catheter traveling to the arteries throughout the brain. This test is usually used when other diagnostic tests do not provide enough information.

MEDICAL MANAGEMENT

The goal of treatment for both ruptured and unruptured aneurysms is to decrease the risk of blood flow from an aneurysm and into the brain. Not all aneurysms which are not ruptured require treatment. For a ruptured brain aneurysm, initially, the patient is put on nimodipine to decrease the risk of blood supply to the brain becoming severely disrupted (cerebral ischemia).

- **Pain relievers,** such as acetaminophen (Tylenol, etc.), may be used to treat headache.
- **Calcium-channel blockers** prevent calcium from entering into cells of the blood vessel walls. These medications may lessen the risk of having severe symptoms from the erratic narrowing of blood vessels (vasospasm) that may be a complication of a ruptured aneurysm. One of these medications, nimodipine (Nymalize), has shown to decrease the risk of delayed brain injury which is caused by insufficient blood flow after a subarachnoid hemorrhage from a ruptured aneurysm.
- **Interventions to prevent a stroke from insufficient blood flow** include IV injections of a drug to dilate the blood vessels, which elevates blood pressure to overcome the resistance of narrowed blood vessels. An alternative intervention to prevent stroke is angioplasty. In this procedure, a surgeon uses a catheter to inflate a tiny balloon that expands a narrowed blood vessel in the brain caused due to vasospasm. Vasodilator also may be used to expand blood vessels in the affected area.
- **Anti-seizure medications** may be used to treat seizures related to a ruptured aneurysm. These medications include levetiracetam (Keppra), phenytoin (Phenytek, Dilantin), valproic acid, and others. Their use is debated by several experts and is generally subject to caregiver discretion based on the medical needs of each individual.

TABLE 31.2: SAH clinical grading scale.

Grade	Hunt and Hess criteria	Mortality rate (%)
0	Unruptured aneurysm without symptoms	0
1	Asymptomatic or minimal headache and slight nuchal rigidity.	1–3
1a	No acute meningeal or brain reaction but with fixed neurological deficit	1–3
2	Moderate to severe headache, nuchal rigidity, no neurological deficit other than cranial nerve palsy.	3–5
3	Drowsy, confused, or mild focal deficit	9–19
4	Stupor, moderate to severe hemiparesis possible early decerebrate rigidity, and vegetative disturbances	23–42
5	Deep coma, decerebrate rigidity, moribund	70–77

TABLE 31.3: WFNS grading scale.

Grade	GCS score	Presence of motor deficit
1.	15	No motor deficit
2.	13–14	No motor deficit
3.	13–14	Motor deficit present
4.	7–12	Motor deficit present or absent
5.	3–6	Motor deficit present or absent

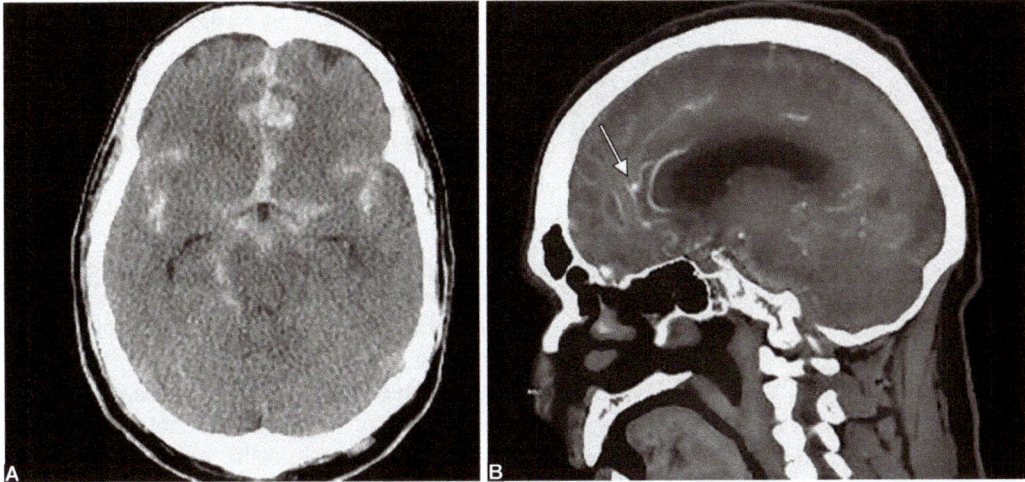

Figs. 31.13A and B: Head CT: (A) Demonstrates diffuse subarachnoid hemorrhage at the time of hospital admission with CT angiogram; (B) Showing a 5-mm ruptured pericallosal artery aneurysm (arrow).

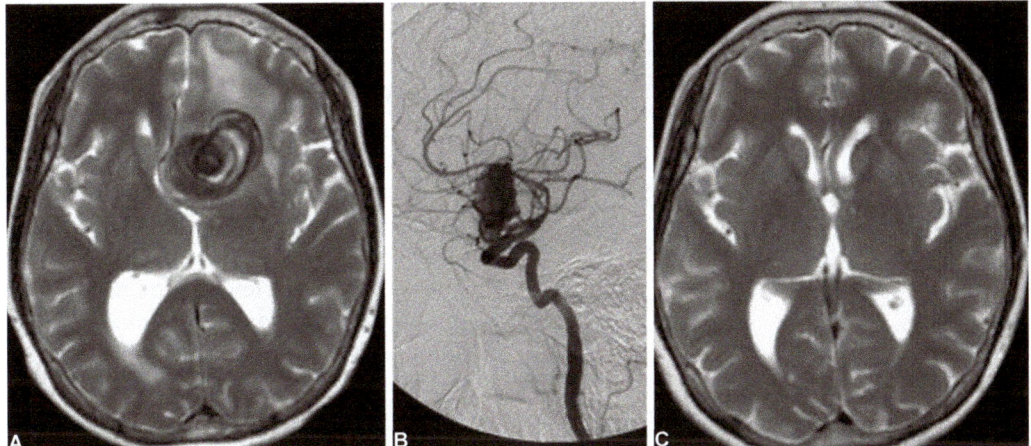

Figs. 31.14A to C: A 73-year-old female with severe frontal headache and cognitive decline. (A) T2-weighted MRI demonstrates a giant aneurysm which is projecting into the inferior left frontal lobe. There is a laminated appearance to the aneurysm wall consistent with thrombus. There is also a substantial amount of vasogenic edema; (B) Left ICA cerebral angiogram shows a large paraophthalmic aneurysm; however, the aneurysm size on luminal imaging is substantially smaller than that on cross-sectional imaging; (C) Following flow diversion treatment, MRI performed 30 months later demonstrates resolution of the edema and mass effect. The patient's symptoms improved.

SURGICAL MANAGEMENT

Here are two common treatment options for a ruptured brain aneurysm.

- ❖ **Clipping by surgery is a procedure to close off the aneurysm:** The surgeon removes a section of skull to access the aneurysm and locates the blood vessel that feeds the aneurysm. Then the neurosurgeon places a small metal clip on the neck of the aneurysm to stop blood flow into it **(Fig. 31.15)**.
- ❖ **Endovascular treatment** is a less invasive procedure than surgical clipping. It is usually preferred in the posterior aneurysm. The surgeon inserts a catheter into the artery, usually in the wrist or groin, and threads it through the body to the aneurysm. The surgeon then uses a device—a flow diverter, an intraluminal flow disrupter, a stent or coils—or different combinations of various devices to destroy the aneurysm from inside the blood vessel **(Fig 31.16)**.

Both procedures pose potential risks, particularly bleeding in brain or loss of blood flow to the brain. The endovascular coil is less invasive and may be initially safer, but it may carry a slightly higher risk of necessitating a repeat procedure in the future due to the aneurysm reopening.

- ❖ **Flow diverters:** Newer treatments available for brain aneurysms include tubular stent-like implants (flow diverters) that work by diverting blood flow away from an aneurysm sac. The diversion stops blood movement within the aneurysm and stimulates the body to heal the site, encouraging reconstruction of the parent artery.

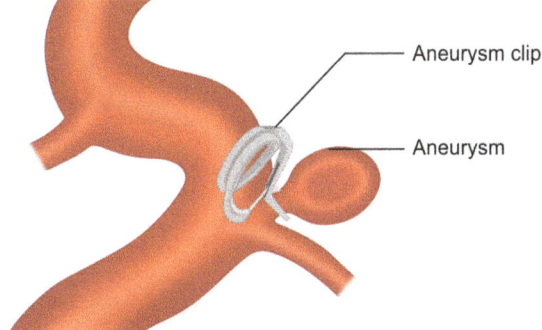

Fig. 31.15: Clipping of aneurysm.

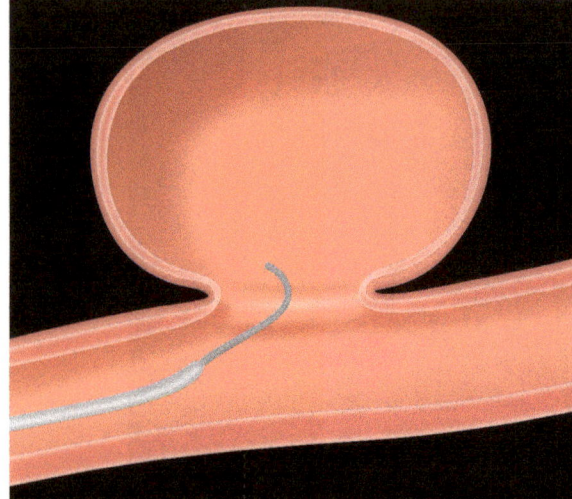
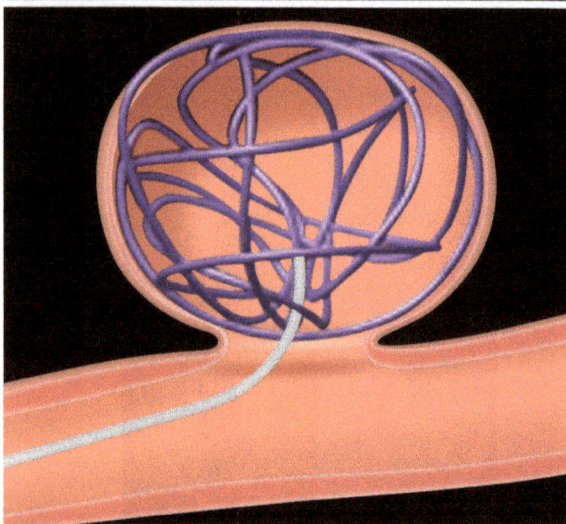
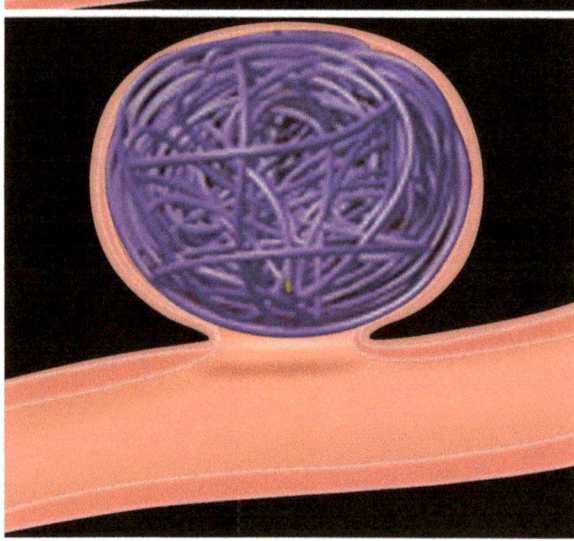

Fig. 31.16: Endovascular coiling.

Flow diverters may be particularly useful in larger aneurysms that cannot be safely treated with other options.

Lifestyle changes to lower the risk: If a person has an unruptured brain aneurysm, he may lower the risk of its rupture by making these lifestyle changes:

❖ **Do not smoke or use recreational drugs:** If one smokes or uses recreational drugs, talk to the health care provider about strategies or an appropriate treatment program to help quit.

❖ **Control the blood pressure if one has high blood pressure** will help preventing aneurysm.

❖ **Eat a healthy diet and exercise:** Changes in diet and exercise can help lower blood pressure. Talk to the health care provider about changes that are appropriate.

COMPLICATIONS OF ANEURYSM

Complications that can further develop after the rupture of an aneurysm include:

❖ **Re-bleeding:** An aneurysm that has leaked or ruptured is at risk of bleeding again. Re-bleeding can further cause damage to brain cells.

❖ **Narrowed blood vessels in the brain:** After a brain aneurysm ruptures, the blood vessels in the brain may contract and become narrower (vasospasm). This condition can lead to an ischemic stroke, in which there is limited blood flow to the brain cells, causing additional cell damage and loss.

❖ **A buildup of fluid within the brain (hydrocephalus):** A ruptured brain aneurysm often occurs in space between the brain and thin tissues covering the brain. The blood can block fluid movement surrounding the brain and spinal cord. As a result, excess fluid puts pressure on the brain and can damage the tissues.

❖ **Change in sodium level:** Bleeding in the brain can disrupt the balance of sodium in blood. This may occur from damage to the hypothalamus, an area near the base of the brain. A decline in blood sodium levels can lead to swelling of the brain cells and permanent damage.

POST-TREATMENT CLINICAL MANAGEMENT

Potential post-treatment changes to monitor.

❖ **Change in level of consciousness (LOC):** It may include confusion or agitation that waxes and wanes.

❖ **Motor deficits:** May include pronator drift weakness, hemiparesis.

❖ **Cardiac changes:** May include hypertension, dysrhythmias, congestive heart failure (CHF) and pulmonary edema from fluid therapy, and "sympathetic storms" from increases in intracranial pressure (ICP).

❖ **Increased ICP:** May require ventriculostomy with ICP monitoring for elevated ICP that may respond to drainage of cerebrospinal fluid (CSF) or mannitol administration.

❖ **Edema:** It may occur with cranial nerve deficits in relation to the affected artery; may involve visual, motor, and sensory dysfunctions.

❖ **Decreased oxygenation:** May require intubation and controlled ventilation.

❖ **Meningeal irritation:** May occur as head, neck, or back pain: (primary components to assess).

❖ **Ischemic injury:** May occur from prolonged temporary arterial occlusion or intraoperative hypotension, injury to surrounding or intraoperative aneurysm rupture, Pain, and headache. Require pain assessment and interventions.

❖ **Loss of appetite:** May signal vasospasm or deterioration in the LOC.

- **Infection:** Fever may be a warning signal of infection.
- **CSF drainage:** Occurs from a dural leak.
- **Electrolyte imbalance (hyponatremia):** Occurs in 10% to 34% of patients and can cause confusion and lead to seizures or progress to coma in patients not treated appropriately. Cerebral salt wasting (CSW) versus the syndrome of inappropriate antidiuretic hormone (SIADH) must be determined. If the cause is CSW with failure of the central nervous system to regulate sodium absorption, the treatment is to increase fluid intake. For SIADH, the intervention is to restrict fluids, which allows the serum sodium level to rise, or in severe cases, volume replacement may be needed.
- **Fluid imbalance:** Crystalloid and colloid solutions are used to counter vasospasm; imbalances can result in diabetes insipidus (DI), SIADH, or CSW (described above).
- **Seizures:** Occur in approximately 25% of patients because of the disruption in blood flow and irritation of the brain from the blood. Administration of anticonvulsants is recommended.
- **Increased ICP:** This can occur immediately following the aneurysm rupture and fluctuates as the patient's condition waxes and wanes, resulting in cerebral ischemia.
- **Deep vein thromboses (DVTs) and pulmonary embolism (PE):** Risk requires close monitoring and early detection.
- **Rebleeding:** This occurs if the aneurysmal clip is not occlusive or is improperly placed.
- **Severe onset of neurologic deficits:** This may occur if an adjoining cerebral vessel was inadvertently clipped during the placement of the aneurysmal clip. Requires immediate notification of the surgeon and immediate imaging with a possible return to the operating room (OR) and re-clipping of the aneurysm.
- **Vocal cord swelling:** This may occur from prolonged surgery.

NURSING MANAGEMENT

Nursing Diagnosis

- Pain (headache) related to cerebral irritation from intracerebral bleeding and irritation of cerebral tissue.
- Decreased adaptive capacity (intracranial) or ineffective tissue perfusion related to obstruction of CSF circulation or decreased absorption of CSF.
- Decreased cardiac output related to hypertensive-hypervolemia therapy and volume expanders.
- Ineffective cerebral tissue perfusion related to constriction and narrowing of arteries and re-bleeding.
- Electrolyte imbalance related to salt wasting, fluid overload, and polyuria.
- Risk for injury (seizures) related to cerebral irritation.
- Risk for injury (falls) related to confusion/disorientation.
- Deficient knowledge related to SAH, its cause, treatment, potential complications, and outcomes.
- Altered cerebral tissue perfusion related to edema, increased ICP or decreased cerebral perfusion pressure (CPP).
- Fear (of the unknown) related to the life-threatening event and future well-being.

Acute/Post-acute Care

- SAH carries a high risk of death and mortality. Admission to a neuroscience critical care unit (NCCU) for acute critical care is important for serial neurologic assessments and hemodynamic monitoring to prevent potential complications (e.g., vasospasm or rebleeding).
- Patients are initially maintained on bed rest with the HOB elevated in a quiet environment. Routine monitoring of neurologic status and vital signs with cardiac monitoring is maintained until the patient is stable and free of complications.
- Keeping the patient well-hydrated decreases the impact of the spasmodic vessels.
- In anticipation of postoperative arterial vasospasm and ischemia, volume expanders can be used to counter the effects of vessel narrowing.
- Hypertension, hypervolemia and hemodilution therapy, or triple-H therapy (HITE therapy), is frequently used. Agents used include plasma protein fraction, saline, 3% saline, albumin, and starch.
- Ideally, hematocrit is maintained in the range of 30% to 40%. Blood volume is measured using central venous pressure (CVP) and pulmonary capillary wedge pressure (PCWP) using a triple lumen catheter.
- IV normal saline or colloids are infused at 100–400 mL/hour.
- Plasma 250 mL is administered over 15–30 minutes. Some clinicians prefer 3% saline.
- Presser agents (dopamine or phenylephrine) are used to elevate systolic blood pressure and to maintain mean arterial pressure (MAP) in the range of 100–110 mm Hg.
- Improvement is usually observed as cerebral perfusion improves hour by hour under the skilled eyes of the neuroscience clinician, who balances blood pressure and MAP with the volume expanders and observes for complications (e.g., fluid overload, electrolyte imbalances, cerebral edema, congestive heart failure (CHF), and rebleeding), cardiac output should be kept in the range of 6.5–8 L/min.
- In addition to the routine post procedure care discussed in previous sections, there are special considerations for postoperative aneurysmal surgery, requiring monitoring for neurologic changes (e.g., LOC) that might indicate increased ICP related to bleeding caused by problems with the aneurysm clip. These intraoperative mechanical problems involve occlusion of adjacent vessels, vasospasm, and evolving edema.

GERIATRIC CONSIDERATIONS

The prevalence of unruptured cerebral aneurysms (UCAs) in elderly patients is increasing in the ageing population. UCA management in elderly patients may have challenges because of decreased life expectancy, increased comorbidities and treatment risks, and poor prognosis in case of rupture. Elderly patients present with unique considerations including frailty, cognitive dysfunction, etc.

Case Scenario

Mrs Reena is a 38-year-old female who reported to the hospital's emergency department with intermittent right-side headache for 5 years, and left lower limb numbness for 3 months. The MRI head and digital subtraction angiography confirmed the diagnosis of right middle cerebral artery (MCA) aneurysm. What will the surgical and nursing management of this patient?

SUMMARY

Cerebrovascular disorders are the acute medical emergencies characterized by compromised cerebral perfusion or problem in the vasculature leading to rapid onset of neurological symptoms. Stroke is the sixth leading cause of death in USA. The most important controllable risk factors include HTN, hyperlipidemia, diabetes mellitus (DM), and smoking, in addition to lifestyle factors such as poor diet/nutrition, obesity, and physical inactivity. People who have had their first stroke or TIA may experience a cumulative relative risk reduction of vascular events of 80% if they implement five proven prevention strategies, including diet changes, exercise, statins, aspirin, and use of antihypertensive drugs. Awareness of the public is very important to prevent the occurrence of these problems.

MULTIPLE CHOICE QUESTIONS

1. An ischemic stroke occurs due to:
   a. Block in a blood vessel supplying to the brain
   b. Bleed in the brain
   c. Block in a vein
   d. Block in a nerve
2. All of the following general symptoms might be suggestive of a stroke, except?
   a. Sudden hunger   b. Sudden numbness
   c. Sudden blurring   d. Sudden slurring
3. What is the term used for paralysis of the arm, leg, and trunk on the same side of the body due to stroke?
   a. Hemophilia   b. Akinesia
   c. Aphagia   d. Hemiplegia
4. Which type of a stroke that involves bleeding into the brain?
   a. Ischemic   b. Hemorrhagic
   c. Transient   d. Aneurismic
5. Which of the following is the number one reason for the intracerebral hemorrhagic stroke?
   a. Heparin overdose   b. Tachycardia
   c. Chronic blood pressure d. Fall
6. Which of the following instrument may be used to assess the likelihood of a stroke patient being able to manage at home subsequent to hospital discharge?
   a. Glasgow coma scale   b. APGAR score
   c. Braden scale   d. Barthel scale
7. Which term is used for mini-stroke:
   a. MND   b. ALS
   c. HCV   d. TIA
8. What is known as a blood clot, fat globule or gas bubble created in one part of body that circulates in the blood stream?
   a. Embolism   b. Thrombus
   c. Infarction   d. Necrosis
9. Which of the following is not a modifiable risk factors for ischemic and hemorrhagic stroke?
   a. Drug abuse   b. Blood pressure
   c. Obesity   d. Hypotension
10. Which of the following drug may help to prevent an ischemic stroke in future?
    a. Warfarin   b. Clopidogrel
    c. Statins   d. Zoloft
11. Paraplegia means:
    a. Paralysis of one side of the body
    b. Paralysis of one side both upper limbs
    c. Paralysis of both lower limbs
    d. Paralysis of all the limbs
12. Quadriplegia means:
    a. Paralysis of one side of the body
    b. Paralysis of one side both upper limbs
    c. Paralysis of both lower limbs
    d. Paralysis of all the limbs
13. Chances of stroke can be decreased by, except:
    a. Diabetes   b. Hypertension
    c. Hypotension   d. High cholesterol
14. Difference between embolus and thrombus is:
    a. An embolus is usually a detached part of thrombus
    b. A thrombus is usually a detached part of embolus
    c. Thrombus can block bold vessels but embolus does not
    d. Both embolus and thrombus are same
15. What is another name for a stroke?
    a. Brain stroke   b. Heart attack
    c. Myocardial infarction d. CKD
16. Which of these lifestyle factors plays the biggest role in increasing the risk for stroke in younger adults?
    a. Obesity   b. High BP
    c. No exercise   d. Alcohol
17. If a person has an ischemic stroke, how quickly should the person be treated to minimize long-term problems?
    a. Within 24 hours   b. With 1 hour
    c. Within 30 minutes   d. Within 4.5 hours
18. Which type of medicine is given to help prevent a stroke?
    a. Medicine to prevent clots from forming and blood-thinning medicines
    b. Clot busting medicine
    c. Hypoglycemic drugs
    d. Hypotensive drugs
19. Condition that may mimic stroke include:
    a. Hypoglycemia   b. Hypertensive encephalopathy
    c. Migraine   d. Neuropathy
20. Surgery is an option in which condition:
    a. Ischemia   b. Myocardial infarction
    c. Hemorrhagic   d. Diabetic neuropathy
21. What is the term for a weakening of an arterial wall inside the brain, such that the artery balloons outward?
    a. Embolism   b. Aneurysm
    c. Stroke   d. MI
22. What is a brain aneurysm?
    a. Out pouching of blood vessel in brain
    b. Collapsing of artery in the brain
    c. Narrowing of artery in the brain
    d. Knot in the brain
23. The local dilatation of an artery is called a(n):
    a. Infarct   b. Ischemia
    c. Stroke   d. Aneurysm
24. A classic diagnostic system of intracranial aneurysm is the patient's complaint of:
    a. Numbness of an arm or leg
    b. Double vision
    c. Severe headache
    d. Dizziness and tinnitus
25. Which of the following are possible complications of a patient with intracranial aneurysm?
    a. Cerebral hypoxia   b. Vasospasm
    c. Increased ICP   d. All of the above

26. Most patients with hemorrhagic strokes are placed in bed in which position?
    a. High-Fowler's
    b. Prone
    c. Supine
    d. Semi-Fowler's (head of bed at 15–30°)

ANSWERS

1. a	2. a	3. d	4. b
5. c	6. d	7. d	8. a
9. d	10. a	11. c	12. d
13. c	14. a	15. a	16. a
17. d	18. a	19. c	20. c
21. b	22. a	23. d	24. c
25. d	26. d		

SUGGESTED READING

1. Blanco M, Castillo J. Major advances in the treatment of stroke. Nat Rev Neurol. 2013;9(2):68-70.
2. Boehme AK, Esenwa C, Elkind MSV. Stroke Risk Factors, Genetics, and Prevention. Circ Res. 2017;120(3):472-95.
3. Brown R. Natural history of intracranial aneurysms. Neurovascular update: present practices and future directions.
4. Buonacera A, Stancanelli B, Malatino L. Stroke and Hypertension: An Appraisal from Pathophysiology to Clinical Practice. Curr Vasc Pharmacol [Internet]. 2017 [cited 2023];17(1):72-84. Available from: https://pubmed.ncbi.nlm.nih.gov/29149815/
5. Campbell BCV, De Silva DA, Macleod MR, Coutts SB, Schwamm LH, Davis SM, et al. Ischaemic stroke. Nat Rev Dis Prim [Internet]. 2019 Dec 1 [cited 2023];5(1). Available from: https://pubmed.ncbi.nlm.nih.gov/31601801/
6. Campbell BCV, Khatri P. Stroke. Lancet. 2020;396(10244):129-42.
7. Campbell BCV. Advances in stroke medicine. Med J Aust. 2019;210(8):367-74.
8. Cerebral Aneurysms Fact Sheet National Institute of Neurological Disorders and Stroke (nih.gov) accessed on 28/8/22).
9. Cheng W, Zhao Q, Li C, Xu Y. Neuroinflammation and brain–peripheral interaction in ischemic stroke: A narrative review. Front Immunol. 2023;13.
10. Lee M, Huang WY, Weng HH, Lee J Der, Lee TH. First-ever ischemic stroke in very old Asians: Clinical features, stroke subtypes, risk factors and outcome. Eur Neurol. 2007;58(1):44-8.
11. N, Hoh BL, Hasan D. Review of Cerebral Aneurysm Formation, Growth, and Rupture. Stroke. 2013;44:3613-22. https://doi.org/10.1161/STROKEAHA.113.002390
12. Pandian JD, Sudhan P. Stroke epidemiology and stroke care services in India. J Stroke. 2013;15(3):128-34. doi: 10.5853/jos.2013.15.3.128. Epub 2013 Sep 27. PMID: 24396806; PMCID: PMC3859004.
13. Pistoia F, Sacco S, Degan D, Tiseo C, Ornello R, Carolei A. Hypertension and Stroke: Epidemiological Aspects and Clinical Evaluation. High Blood Press Cardiovasc Prev. 2016;23(1):9-18.
14. Puy L, Parry-Jones AR, Sandset EC, Dowlatshahi D, Ziai W, Cordonnier C. Intracerebral haemorrhage. Nat Rev Dis Prim [Internet]. 2023 Mar 16 [cited 2023];9(1):14. Available from: http://www.ncbi.nlm.nih.gov/pubmed/36928219
15. Ryba M, Grieb P, Podobińska I, Iwańska K, Pastuszko M, Górski A. HLA antigens and intracranial aneurysms. Acta Neurochir (Wien). 1992;116(1):1-5. doi: 10.1007/BF01541246. PMID: 1615764.
16. Sadasivan C, Fiorella DJ, Woo HH, Lieber BB. Physical factors effecting cerebral aneurysm pathophysiology. Ann Biomed Eng. 2013;41(7):1347-65. doi: 10.1007/s10439–013-0800-z. Epub 2013. PMID: 23549899; PMCID: PMC3679262.
17. Singh TP, Weinstein JR, Murphy SP. Stroke: Basic and clinical. In: Advances in Neurobiology. Springer New York LLC; 2017. pp. 281-93.
18. Vermeulen M, van Gijn J. The diagnosis of subarachnoid haemorrhage. J Neurol Neurosurg Psychiatry. 1990;53(5):365-72. doi: 10.1136/jnnp.53.5.365. PMID: 2191083; PMCID: PMC488050.
19. Zacharia BE, Hickman ZL, Grobelny BT, DeRosa P, Kotchetkov I, Ducruet AF. Epidemiology of aneurysmal subarachnoid hemorrhage. Neurosurg Clin N Am. 2010;21(2):221-33. doi: 10.1016/j.nec.2009.10.002. PMID: 20380965.

CHAPTER 32

Neoplasms of the Neurological System

Manju Dhandapani

"Second and third opinions can be valuable, but don't spin your wheels and lose time by getting ten opinions."
—Peter Black, Living with a Brain Tumor

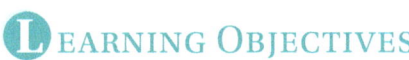

After going through the chapter, the learner will be able to:
- Define brain tumors.
- Classify the types of brain tumors.
- Discuss the pathophysiology and clinical manifestations of brain tumors.
- Elaborate on the treatment strategies and nursing management of patients with brain tumors.
- Discuss the geriatric considerations pertaining to brain tumors.

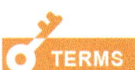

- **Axial tumor:** Tumor within the brain.
- **Brachytherapy:** A technique of delivering radiation internally, directly into the tumor.
- **Extra-axial tumor:** Tumor outside the brain.
- **Infratentorial:** Below tentorium cerebelli.
- **Stereotactic:** A technique used for precisely directing the tip of a delicate instrument or radio beams to a specific location.
- **Supratentorial:** Above tentorium cerebelli.
- **Tumor:** A group of abnormal cells or mass that form in any part of the body.

INTRODUCTION

Intracranial tumors are the growth or mass located in the brain or other tissues within the cranial cavity. Majority of the intracranial tumors are brain tumors. Knowing the types and exact location of the tumor aids in the right treatment choice. The clinical manifestations and disability can be the results of the tumor or complications of its treatment modalities. Hence, long-term care may be required in patients with metastatic and recurrent tumors and also for patients with disabilities. Palliative care including comprehensive nursing care and rehabilitation is the mainstay of management along with surgery, chemotherapy, or radiotherapy. The outcome may depend on many factors such as type, location, response to treatment, and compliance with the therapeutic regimen.

BRAIN TUMOR

"Every year World Brain Tumor Day is celebrated on 8 June. It is celebrated to make the public aware of this deadly disease. It is an opportunity to make people realize that we need to eat healthy and maintain a healthy lifestyle if we want to reduce the risk of any disease".

DEFINITION

A brain or intracranial tumor is an abnormal growth of cells within or surrounding the brain within the intracranial cavity. They can be benign or malignant.

TYPES OF BRAIN TUMORS (TABLE 32.1)

The classification based on the location within the cranial cavity such as supra tentorial or infratentorial tumors is important to comprehensively understand the symptomatology and surgical approach. Based on the tissue from which the tumor originated, brain tumors can be histologically classified into various types such as astrocytoma, oligodendroglioma, ependymoma, meningiomas (29%), nerve sheath tumors such as vestibular schwannomas, posterior fossa or infratentorial tumors such as cerebellar tumors and tumors of glands including pituitary tumors. etc. **(Table 32.1)**.

The commonest cancer that metastasizes to the brain in males is lung cancer. Other cancers that metastasize include breast cancer, colon cancer, renal cancer, prostate cancer, melanoma, and cancers of the uterus, rectum, etc.

TABLE 32.1: Types of brain tumors.

Characteristic	Types
Based on the location within the cranial cavity	**Axial tumors:** Tumors are within the brain.
	Extra-axial tumors: Tumors are in the surrounding tissues such as meninges, nerves pituitary glands, etc.
Based on location within the brain	**Supratentorial tumors:** Tumors are located above the tentorium cerebelli.
	Infratentorial tumors: Tumors are located inferior to tentorium cerebelli in the posterior fossa. They are also known as posterior fossa tumors.
Based on the tissue involved within the intracranial cavity	**Gliomas:** Tumors are originated within the brain: There are three types of gliomas depending on the glial cells involved. 1. **Astrocytoma:** Tumors arise from the astrocytes. 2. **Oligodendrogliomas:** Tumors arise from oligodendrocytes. 3. **Ependymomas:** Tumors originate from ependymal cells of the lining of the ventricles.
	Meningioma: The tumor originates in the meninges, the most common type of primary brain tumor
	Medulloblastoma: The tumor originates within the brain stem. Most of them are grade IV malignant tumors.
	Pituitary tumors: Tumors arise from the pituitary gland where most of them are adenomas.
	Craniopharyngioma: Tumors in supra-sellar space originated from remnants of epithelium derived from Rathke's pouch during the embryonic development.
	Schwannoma: Benign tumors of the 8th cranial nerve.
Based on the spread of the tumor	**Benign:** Tumors are non-cancerous.
	Malignant: Tumors are cancerous.
Based on the origin	**Primary:** Tumors are originated from the brain.
	Metastatic: Tumors are metastasized from other parts of the body to the brain or intracranial cavity.

GRADING OF BRAIN TUMOR

Based on the WHO classification, there are four grades of intracranial tumors depending on the characteristics of the tumor. Grades I and II are considered as benign and grade III and IV are considered as malignant tumors **(Table 32.2)**.

TABLE 32.2: Grading of intracranial tumors.

Grade I	Slow-growing tumor, long-term survival, postoperative opportunity of heal after resection
Grade II	Comparatively slow growing, often recurs, sometimes tends to progress to higher grades of malignancy
Grade III	High proliferative potential, histologically malignant tumor, most patients receive adjuvant radiation and/or chemotherapy
Grade VI	Rapid proliferation, cytologically malignant tumor, very aggressive

EPIDEMIOLOGY

Central nervous system tumors include tumors of the brain, other intracranial tissues, cranial nerves, spinal nerves, spinal cord, and the meninges. Brain and central nervous system (CNS) tumors represent approximately 1% of all newly diagnosed cancers and about 2% of cancer deaths. The overall age-adjusted incidence of brain and CNS tumors was 22.64 per one lakh population in the United States and 5-10 in one lakh population in India. Most brain and CNS tumors that are diagnosed are nonmalignant and the most common type of nonmalignant brain and CNS tumors are meningioma. The most common type of malignant tumors are gliomas and the majority of diagnosed gliomas are glioblastomas (Stage IV gliomas). About 60% of all primary brain tumors are malignant gliomas. Out of these, about 40–50% are glioblastoma multiforme (Stage IV gliomas) followed by 30–35% anaplastic astrocytoma (stage III). The highest percentage of all brain tumors that originate in the intracranial cavity are benign growth such as meningiomas. Most of the primary malignant cerebral tumors occur in the cerebral cortex with the highest percentage developing in the frontal lobe (26%) followed by temporal (19%), parietal lobe (12%), cerebellum (5%), brainstem (4%), occipital lobe (3%) and 2% in cerebral ventricles **(Fig. 32.1)**.

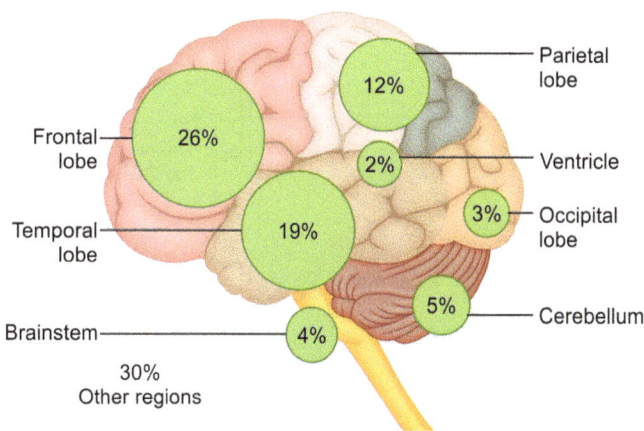

Fig. 32.1: Distribution of intracranial tumors based on location.

Intracranial tumors are one of the common causes of mortality and morbidity worldwide and occur in people of all ages. Brain tumors are reported more commonly in children and older adults. But metastatic brain tumors are more common in adults. Incidence of all brain and intracranial tumors is highest in adults greater than 40 years old with a median age of 59 years. The incidence of nonmalignant brain and CNS tumors increases with increasing age. Among children, zero to 14 years old, astrocytic tumors and medulloblastoma are the most common malignant brain and CNS tumors globally.

The overall incidence of brain and CNS tumors is higher among female patients compared with male patients. The incidence of malignant brain tumors is higher in males (incidence ratio (IR): 8.39 vs 6.06 for male vs female]), whereas nonmalignant brains are more common in female patients (IR:18.72 vs 11.95 for female vs male). Gliomas, glioblastoma multiforme (GBM), medulloblastoma, and CNS lymphoma occur more commonly in male patients than in females. However, malignant meningioma is more common among females. Most nonmalignant tumors occur more often in female patients compared in males.

The incidence of malignant brain tumors varies significantly by region of the globe. The incidence of malignant tumors is lowest in Southeast Asia, east Asia, and India as compared to the United States, Canada, Europe, and Australia. However, East Asia and Southern Europe have reported a higher incidence of malignant meningioma.

There is a global variation in mortality reported by malignant brain and CNS tumors. Mortality is highest in areas with the highest brain and CNS tumor incidence, with the highest rates in northern Europe. Survival after diagnosis with a nonmalignant brain tumor is significantly higher, with 1-year relative survival of 94.5% and 5-year relative survival of 90.8%. Survival is poorest after diagnosis with GBM, for which 1-year survival is 37.4% and 5-year survival is 4.9%.

ETIOLOGY

Though there are numerous potential risk factors reported across the studies, only a few of them are found to have associations with the occurrence of brain tumors. They include exposure to ionizing radiation, genetic association, and a history of allergies. Genetics play a role in the occurrence of glioma, meningioma, pituitary adenoma, and CNS lymphoma.

- ❖ **Age:** Though all age groups are affected by brain tumors, children and old age have a high risk where malignant tumors are found to be more common in older adults.
- ❖ **Race:** The incidence of malignant tumors is lowest in Southeast Asia, east Asia, and India as compared to the United States, Canada, Europe, and Australia. However, East Asia and Southern Europe have reported a higher incidence of malignant meningioma.
- ❖ **Radiation exposure**: Exposure to ionizing radiation results in DNA changes/mutation and initiates the carcinogenic process. The duration and intensity of radiation exposure also may be a concern in relation to the incidence of brain tumors.

PATHOPHYSIOLOGY

As the tumor develops and progresses, inflammation along with edema may be settled in the brain and surrounding tissues. The tumor along with edema may compress and exert pressure on the nerves, CSF pathway, or brain stem resulting in pain and neurological deficits with sensory and motor deficits. The presence of tumor mass and edema results in intracranial hypertension which produces the initial and many of the later symptoms. The rise in ICP reduces the cerebral perfusion pressure and hence cerebral blood flow which in turn can result in ischemia. This ischemic part of the brain is highly vulnerable to edema. The compression of brain tissue due to tumors and associated ischemia can act as epileptogenic foci and result in seizures in these patients **(Flowchart 32.1)**.

CLINICAL MANIFESTATIONS

Depending on the type, location, and speed at which it grows, the clinical manifestations of patients with brain tumors may have slow onset with timely progression or rapid onset with fast progression. The symptoms associated with benign tumors are subtle in nature, while that of malignant gliomas

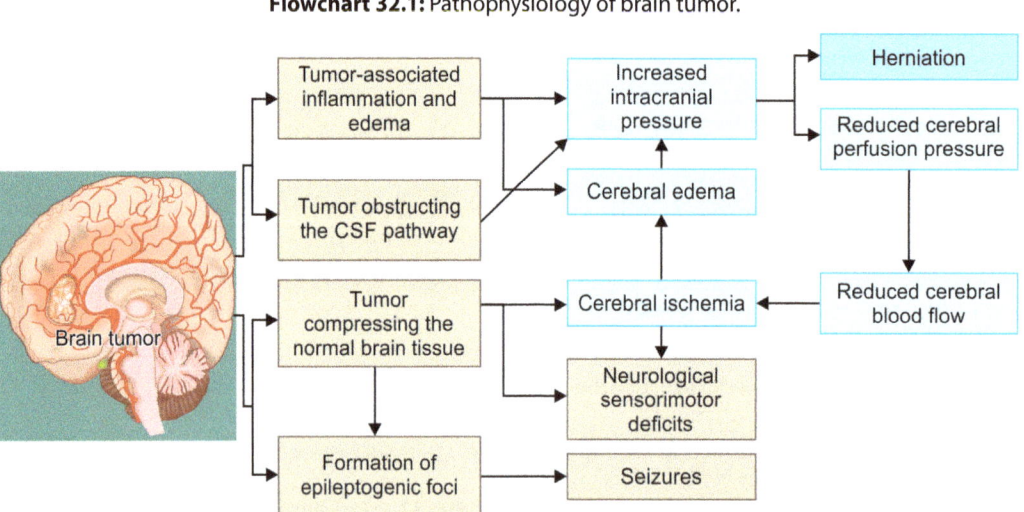

Flowchart 32.1: Pathophysiology of brain tumor.

and other intracranial malignant tumors, the symptoms progress very fast. However, the symptoms experienced by the patients depend on several factors such as location, type, size, and tumor spread. Very small tumors may not cause symptoms as they are not large enough to compress or irritate the brain or the surrounding tissues, glands, ventricles, blood vessels, or brain stem. As evident in pathophysiology, most of the patients would report symptoms related to increased intracranial pressure (ICP) such as headache, nausea, vomiting, and focal neurological deficits such as hemiparesis or aphasia.

The most common symptom is headache, for most types of tumors which can raise the ICP. The headache with tumors mostly occurs in the morning and is associated with nausea, vomiting, or blurring of vision. The other common symptoms reported by the patients include headache, vomiting, blurred vision, extremity weakness, and sensory alterations. Other symptoms are due to focal neurological deficits or cognitive-behavioral impairment. The common symptoms reported in various tumors include the following:

* Headache that worsens in the morning
* Nausea or vomiting
* Visual impairment: Double vision, blurred vision, or loss of vision which can be unilateral or bilateral depending on the location of the tumor
* Hemiparesis
* Problems in balance: Gait ataxia or truncal ataxia, common in cerebellar/posterior fossa tumors
* Speech problems: aphasia, dysarthria
* Fatigue
* Cognitive deficits such as impairment in short-term and recent memory, lack of attention/concentration, poor problem-solving or judgment
* Confusion
* Restlessness
* Vertigo
* Dizziness, or syncope
* Inability to follow commands and impairment in consciousness as the ICP continues to rise
* Personality and behavior changes
* Newly onset seizures
* Hearing impairment
* Other sensory impairments such as loss of smell and taste.

Depending on the location of the tumor the symptoms may vary and may aid in localizing the tumor. Frontal lobe tumors result in cognitive deficits, and personality changes along with focal neurological deficit (FND) such as hemiparesis or aphasia. Tumors in the parietal lobe can lead to impairment in processing of the sensory information and result in loss of smell, taste, vision, or hearing. Tumors in the occipital lobes can cause vision loss. The temporal lobe tumors can result in hearing loss and receptive aphasia. The posterior fossa or cerebellar tumors are associated with problems in balance and coordination. Tumors of the sellar or suprasellar region can result in vision impairment due to optic chiasm compression. The pituitary region tumors can lead to symptoms related to hormonal imbalances. Among all brain tumors, vestibular schwannomas are the commonest cause of unilateral hearing loss.

DIAGNOSTIC MODALITIES

Many conditions such as infection (meningitis, encephalitis, tuberculomas, or abscess), degeneration, and vascular conditions can mimic brain tumors. Hence, a comprehensive diagnostic approach is necessary not only to diagnose but also for aiding the treatment. Primary brain tumors which are small and slow in progress are often diagnosed incidentally as they mostly remain asymptomatic. It is advisable to suspect the possibility of a brain tumor when the patient experiences frequent headaches with or without FNDs and pressure symptoms. Patients who are known cases of cancer are often suspected to have metastasis when they report headaches, FNDs, or cognitive-behavioral changes. A complete history and thorough physical and neurological examination along with appropriate diagnostic investigations would aid in an accurate diagnosis. Though a thorough neurological examination may not confirm the presence of a brain tumor, it can help to locate the location and spread.

The following investigations are done in addition to ***history and neurological examination***:

* **Brain computed tomography (CT scan):** CT scan of the brain would help in most intracranial tumors. CT chest, abdomen, and pelvis are done to look for other lesions of primary.
* **Magnetic resonance imaging (MRI):** MRI helps in providing more accurate details of the tumor which is already confirmed in the CT scan or may identify the tumors which are not identified in the CT image. It helps in a comprehensive evaluation of the brain and other intracranial structures. It uses magnetic field energy to create images and delivers accurate information about the soft tissues and the tumor. An intravenous contrast agent may be used to highlight various tissues. MRI with contrast may help in identifying the invasion of the tumor, functional MRI helps in identifying the areas of the brain responsible for main functions, perfusion MRI will aid in identifying the vascularity of the tumor and MR spectroscopy identify the biochemical nature of the tumor or the biochemical changes that have occurred in the brain. All of these can aid the surgeon in planning the treatment modality for the patient.
* **Positron emission tomography (PET):** A PET scan may be done to detect some types of fast-growing tumors; it is less useful in slow-growing tumors. A whole-body PET scan may be considered to identify the location of cancerous lesions elsewhere in the body where the tumor would have primarily originated.
* **Biopsy:** A biopsy is obtained for diagnosing the exact histological type of the tumor. The biopsy can lead to injury to different parts of the brain with or without significant bleeding. In patients with brain tumors, excisional biopsy is often done where the surgeon collects the biopsy specimen at the time of surgical removal of the tumor. Chemotherapy or radiotherapy is often planned based on the biopsy report. A frozen section biopsy is often done during the surgery to identify the type and nature of the tumor which aids in surgical decision-making on the extent of tumor excision. An image-guided stereotactic

needle biopsy is done when the tumor is located in some important location that is difficult to remove.
- ❖ **Lumbar puncture and cerebrospinal fluid analysis:** It helps to identify the presence and type of tumor cells in CSF. It helps in identifying the tumor type even without a biopsy. It can detect tumors such as CNS lymphomas.

MANAGEMENT

Treatment of brain tumors is highly individualized and depends on the location, size, and type of tumor. The goals of metastatic brain tumor treatment are to relieve pain and to improve neurological function and quality of life. Monitoring the patient along with surgery, chemotherapy or radiotherapy is the mainstay of treatment modalities. A collaborative model of care is required including neurosurgeons, radiation oncologists, nurses, and physiotherapists.
- ❖ **Monitoring:** The progress of the symptoms must be monitored to plan the timing of surgery. Tumors that are small and not increasing in size may not be operated on but will be monitored through periodic imaging studies.
- ❖ **Surgical management:** Surgery is the treatment of choice for brain tumors, though there can be a certain risk of injury to the brain and hemorrhage. The main goal of surgery is to remove the tumor completely or to debulk the tumor to reduce ICP, the compressive effect of the tumor, and the chance for recurrence. However, the risks are minimized with intraoperative monitoring and imaging as well as minimally invasive and endoscopic surgical techniques with the help of a high-powered microscope. Even the advanced technologies do not guarantee the complete removal of all tumors where the surgery may be accompanied by chemotherapy, radiotherapy, or both. Using an appropriate surgical approach depending on its location, tumor resection or decompression is performed.
  - ➢ *Surgical approach:* A craniotomy is performed to approach most of the tumor, where the location of the craniotomy approach will depend on the tumor location. Many of the skull base tumors, especially sellar/suprasellar tumors are removed through the trans-nasal and trans-sphenoidal approaches. With the advancement in technology, endoscopic techniques are getting more attention for both transcranial and transsphenoidal approaches.
    - Resection: A gross total or subtotal tumor resection is done depending on the type and spread of the tumor. The goal of surgery in the primary brain tumor is to remove the entire tumor along with its capsule which is known as gross total excision. Gross total resection is done mostly for primary benign tumors where the entire tumor or 98% of the tumor is removed. A subtotal resection is done where the tumor is invaded to important structures; removing the entire tumor may have life risk to the patient. Ultrasonic aspiration of the tumor may also be done where the tumor is aspirated after breaking it down into small pieces using a small ultrasonic probe. The goal of surgery in metastatic brain tumors is to decompress the brain to reduce pain and improve neurological function. An open biopsy is also performed along with the surgery. Rapid deterioration of neurological function warrants an emergency decompression. The removal of the tumor will reduce intracranial pressure and its compression effect on the brain and adjacent structures.

    If the patient is having hydrocephalus, a shunt, mostly ventricular-peritoneal shunt may be done before surgery or after surgery. The shunt helps in reducing the ICP while maintaining the optimal drainage of CSF.

    During the operation, if needed, a neurosurgeon places some tabs into the affected region. The purpose is to release chemotherapeutic agents to destroy the remaining abnormal cells.
    - Stereotactic Radiosurgery (SRS): This technique is a nonsurgical, minimally invasive procedure done to deliver precise narrow beams of radiation to a tumor using a Gamma Knife, Cyber Knife, or linear accelerators (photon therapy). It is a precise, high-dose form of image-guided radiation therapy. It is done for tumors that are resistant to conventional treatment and is performed using techniques to minimize damage to the surrounding healthy tissues.
- ❖ **Radiation therapy:** The goal of radiotherapy is to destroy the remaining part of tumors that persist after surgery, to manage patients with inoperable tumors, or to treat tumors with high surgical risk. It helps to eliminate malignant tumors, to prevent/reduce recurrence, and to shrink tumors for easier removal. Most brain tumors can be partially or completely resected. Radiation therapy is done for incompletely resected low-grade tumors, malignant tumors, and recurrent tumors. The dose of radiation therapy may be adjusted to preserve the surrounding healthy tissue. Two types of radiation therapy can be used for brain tumors: Both external and internal radiation therapy can be used for patients with brain tumors. Most of the patients are treated with external radiation therapy. Brachytherapy or internal radiation delivers high doses of radiation into the tumor for a short duration of time. It reduces the damage to nearby tissues. Radiation can be delivered using silicon plaques coated with a radioactive isotope placed inside the tumor or through brachytherapy catheters connected to an Omaya reservoir placed under the scalp. Patients undergoing radiation therapy can develop some side effects such as sore throat, skin redness, etc. Radiation therapy is provided in multiple cycles to permit the normal tissue to replenish and is given either as an alternative to surgical resection or in conjunction with surgery.
- ❖ **Chemotherapy:** Chemotherapy is prescribed depending on a patient's needs such as to reduce the size of the tumor before surgery, to remove any remaining part of the tumor after surgery, to treat metastasis, and to reduce symptoms as a part of palliative care. Chemotherapy can be used as adjuvant therapy for secondary brain tumors, including breast, prostate, and myeloma metastatic to the brain. The drugs may be given orally, intravenously,

or intrathecally where they are injected into the CSF through a lumbar puncture or a device placed under the scalp. Steroids are the mainstay of chemotherapy. Chemotherapy may be done alone or in combination with radiation therapy. Patients undergoing chemotherapy may develop side effects such as fatigue, nausea, vomiting, alopecia, steroid-induced myopathy, and infection. The most efficient and effective chemotherapy drugs used in treating brain tumors include temozolomide, carmustine, and lomustine. Chemotherapy is administered in cycles, as it affects the normal cells also. The gap given in between the cycle gives time for the healthy cells to regenerate.

- **Other drugs:** Corticosteroids mainly dexamethasone are given to patients with brain tumors to reduce the inflammation that can be developed due to tumors, surgery, or radiation therapy. It reduces perilesional inflammation and edema. They are started once the tumor diagnosis is made and continued during the postoperative period but later tapered and stopped. Although they reduce inflammation, they are generally given only for a short duration to prevent any serious side effects such as high blood pressure, diabetes, muscle weakness, osteoporosis, and infection. Medications are given to reduce the side effects of radiation therapy and chemotherapy such as nausea and vomiting. Non-steroidal anti-inflammatories can be given to reduce headaches during the pre-operative period and postoperative periods. Anti-convulsants are given to prevent seizures, especially in patients with supratentorial tumors.

NURSING MANAGEMENT

Comprehensive and collaborative nursing care is mandatory for patients with brain tumors. Respiratory and hemodynamic dysfunction can be in patients with brain tumors, especially in the case of brain stem tumors, cerebellopontine angle tumors, or posterior fossa tumors. The nurse needs to ensure that the patient maintains stable respiratory and hemodynamic status as these vital dynamics are affected by worsening neurological function or vice versa. The main goal of nursing management are:

- To maintain the optimal respiratory and hemodynamic status
- To maintain neurological functions by preventing increased ICP, and maintaining cerebral blood flow and perfusion
- To reduce the pain
- To maintain nutritional status
- To maintain bowel and bladder elimination
- To minimize or manage the disability associated with neurological deficits, and treatment modalities
- To assist maintain activities and enhancing the independence
- To prevent infection and other complications related to surgery and hospital stay
- To prevent complications associated with neurological deficits and treatment regimen
- To educate patients and family caregivers

Assessment and Nursing Interventions

- **To maintain the optimal respiratory and hemodynamic status:**
  - Monitor respiratory and hemodynamic status frequently, maybe every half an hour or preferably to have continuous monitoring in patients who are at risk of respiratory or hemodynamic dysfunction
  - Provide ventilator support for the patients who require and maintain the support based on the respiratory assessment
  - Assess cough reflex and other respiratory parameters such as SpO_2, respiratory rate, and arterial blood gas analysis during the weaning process
  - Initiate and continue respiratory rehabilitation to facilitate lung function
  - Perform nebulization, chest physiotherapy, need-based tracheal toileting, and postural drainage
  - Monitor and maintain circulatory status (blood pressure and pulse rate) with adequate fluid and dietary support or pharmacological support if required

- **To maintain neurological functions by preventing increased ICP, and maintaining cerebral blood flow and perfusion:**
  - Monitor symptoms of raised ICP such as headache, blurred vision, pupillary changes, or deterioration in the level of consciousness (GCS score)
  - Inform any changes related to raised ICP and get investigated to avoid any impending harm to the patient
  - Elevate the head of bed 30^0 to enhance optimum venous drainage
  - Prevent flexion of the neck and keep the neck straight
  - Provide adequate comfort and rest to the patients
  - Manage pain using appropriate pharmacological and non-pharmacological measures
  - Monitor and manage body temperature to keep the metabolism optimum
  - Ensure clubbing of activity to enhance the period of rest

- **To reduce the pain (headache):**
  - Monitor the location, severity, fluctuation, and progress of pain.
  - Report headache immediately as it can indicate raised ICP due to an increase in edema or post-operative bleeding.
  - Administer prescribed analgesics and other drugs to relieve pain as continuous pain can increase restlessness and ICP.
  - Provide appropriate non-pharmacological modalities to alleviate pain such as deep breathing exercises or progressive muscle relaxation.
  - Utilize diversion therapy by engaging the patient in interesting activities, guided imagery, etc.
  - Evaluate the effectiveness of the pain management modalities and modify them accordingly.
  - Report any sudden increase in pain along with increasing neurological deficits as it may warrant emergency surgery.
  - Monitor sleep and take measures to facilitate sleep.

- ❖ **To maintain nutritional status:**
  - ➢ Monitor the consciousness level and gag reflex of the patient before initiating oral feed, especially in patients who have CP angle tumors, posterior fossa tumors, or patients who have lower cranial nerve involvement.
  - ➢ Choose the appropriate route of feeding depending on the ability of the patient to swallow and based on the consciousness.
  - ➢ Ensure early feeding to compensate for the nutritional requirements of these patients.
  - ➢ Ensure adequate dietary intake to compensate for the side effects of nausea and vomiting associated with radiotherapy or chemotherapy.
  - ➢ Preset diet in a pleasant manner especially for patients with anorexia, nausea, and vomiting.
  - ➢ Provide a high-protein diet to enhance post-operative recovery.
  - ➢ Provide small-frequent diet.
  - ➢ Maintain intake and output.
  - ➢ Inform the gastrointestinal symptoms to the physician and manage them with appropriate medications such as antiemetics.
  - ➢ Prevent/manage oral mucositis associated with chemotherapy or radiotherapy with oral care and cryo/ice-chip therapy.
  - ➢ Provide diet counseling by emphasizing the importance of nutrition in recovery.
  - ➢ Monitor nutritional status using appropriate techniques.
- ❖ **To maintain bowel elimination:**
  - ➢ Monitor bowel dysfunction symptoms such as constipation, impaction, inadequate emptying, or incontinence.
  - ➢ Assess for constipation in bedridden patients.
  - ➢ Administer laxatives or suppositories.
  - ➢ Perform digital stimulation if required after proper lubrication, with special caution in patients with neutropenia and thrombocytopenia.
  - ➢ Plan and implement a bowel program to prevent incontinence and facilitate evacuation. It may be performed every 2 days after 30 mts of a major meal (to get the benefit of gastrocolic reflex).
- ❖ **To maintain bladder elimination:**
  - ➢ Monitor for bladder dysfunction such as urgency, frequency, retention, incontinence, and frequent urinary tract infections.
  - ➢ Assess for symptoms or signs of bladder retention in self-voiding patients .
  - ➢ Perform intermediate catheterization or indwelling catheterization depending on the patient's requirement.
  - ➢ Take measures to prevent UTI; implement CAUTI (Catheter-associated UTI) bundle and monitor signs and symptoms of UTI.
  - ➢ Treat UTI with appropriate antibiotics based on culture and sensitivity report of urine.
- ❖ **To minimize or manage the disability associated with neurological deficits, and treatment modalities to assist maintain activities of daily living and enhancing the independence:**
  - ➢ Assess the sensory and motor neurological deficits of the patient and monitor their severity.
  - ➢ Assess the dependency level using appropriate tools.
  - ➢ Initiate sensory and motor rehabilitation as early as possible.
  - ➢ Take measures to reduce pain before performing rehabilitation.
  - ➢ Assist in necessary activities of daily living depending on the deficits while encouraging the patient to perform independently.
- ❖ **To prevent complications associated with neurological deficits and treatment regimen and to prevent infection and other complications related to surgery and hospital stay:**
  - ➢ Assess the patient's risk for developing complications such as pressure sore, deep vein thrombosis (DVT), UTI, contractures, infection, etc.
  - ➢ Take measures to prevent complications in all the patients.
  - ➢ Range of motion exercise to prevent DVT and contractures.
  - ➢ Pneumatic compression devices and anticoagulant therapy to prevent DVT.
  - ➢ Enhancing mobility, changing the position and pressure-eliminating devices to prevent pressure sore.
  - ➢ Appropriate catheter care to prevent UTI.
  - ➢ Wound care, drain care, prophylactic antibiotics, and aseptic techniques to prevent infection in post-operative patients.
  - ➢ Monitor symptoms of any infection, send appropriate samples for culture and sensitivity, and initiate treatment as early as indicated.
  - ➢ Monitor for CSF leak in case of a patient with trans-sphenoidal surgery.
  - ➢ Monito and manage diabetes insipidus and electrolyte imbalance in patients of sellar/suprasellar tumors.
  - ➢ Monitor gag/cough reflex where the lower cranial nerves are involved.
  - ➢ Identify complications early, report to the treating team, and document.
  - ➢ Ensure appropriate management if a patient develops any complication.
- ❖ **To educate patients and family caregivers:**
  - ➢ Educate the patient and caregivers depending on the medications and other therapeutic requirements during home care such as catheter care, pressure sore/UTI/DVT/contracture prevention strategies.
  - ➢ Inform about the timely follow-up and investigations.
  - ➢ Encourage them to continue home-based or institutionalized rehabilitation.
  - ➢ Inform about the symptoms that need emergency attention and require hospital visits such as emerging neurological deficits, severe pain, signs of infection, and other complications associated with tumor or treatment.
  - ➢ Inform the caregivers about the neuropsychological symptoms that can be expected in the patients and get a consultation if required.

- Involve the patient in day-to-day activities as the patient's condition is improving.
- Assess the risk of falls at discharge and teach about measures to prevent fall.
- Encourage the patient to consider consultation and counseling for sexual dysfunction.
- Monitor quality of life during follow-up and take appropriate measures to enhance the quality of life.

The comprehensive care must continue through the entire continuum of treatment. Nurses also must ensure that the essential assessment and interventions are performed during the perioperative period, during chemotherapy and radiation therapy cycles. The patients and family caregivers must be educated about homecare and maintaining compliance with the entire treatment modalities and follow-up.

Rehabilitation

The rehabilitative process should be initiated soon after the diagnosis, to maintain neurological function and prevent or reduce associated complications, especially in patients with hemiparesis. A complete rehabilitation may not be possible preoperatively due to headaches and raised ICP. However, comprehensive rehabilitation must be initiated during the post-operative period and must be continued even after discharge depending on the deficits or symptoms that the patient continues to suffer. It can be provided as home-based or institution-based therapy. Patients must be assessed for the need for physical rehabilitation, both motor and sensory rehabilitation, and neuropsychological rehabilitation and it must be initiated depending on the requirement. Respiratory rehabilitation is mandatory in patients who suffer from respiratory dysfunction. Gradual weaning from respiratory support is obtained while providing respiratory rehabilitation.

GERIATRIC CONSIDERATIONS

The geriatric population is at high risk of developing brain tumors, especially malignant tumors such as glioblastoma. Age-related changes along with the aggressive nature of the tumor make the prognosis worsen. The associated neurological deficits may increase the risk of falls and injury in the elderly. Hence, appropriate fall and injury prevention strategies must be advised while ensuring to have caregivers stay with the patient. The tolerance and effectiveness of treatment modalities may be reduced during old age. Hence, collaborative strategies best for the patient must be implemented to enhance their quality of life.

Case Scenario

Mr X, 65-year-old is admitted to the neurosurgery ward with an early morning headache and is associated with vomiting that started since 5 months. He was on treatment for pain and vomiting without much relief. He developed blurred vision and right hemiparesis a week ago. On imaging, he was diagnosed to have left frontal glioblastoma multiforme. He was operated on and shifted to the neurosurgery ICU. On examination, he is E2VETM5 and is on ventilator support. Bilateral pupils are equal and sluggishly reacting to light. He is having right hemiparesis with muscle power of 3/5 in the right upper and lower extremities.

1. Discuss the preoperative management for Mrs Y.
2. Discuss postoperative nursing management and transition to home care for this patient.
3. Discuss the measures to improve cerebral blood flow in Mr X.

SUMMARY

Patients with brain tumors require individualized and comprehensive treatment strategies. While gross total tumor resection is the mainstay of treatment for primary tumors, sub-total resection along with adjuvant radiotherapy or chemotherapy is preferred for malignant tumors. Comprehensive nursing care, rehabilitation, and timely follow-up are essential components of a treatment strategy to improve the quality of life of the patients. Hospital-to-home transition care must be provided to the family caregivers and they must be empowered with adequate knowledge in homecare. The nurse must possess competency in neurological assessment and must be a keen observer to identify and manage the subtle changes in the patient during the entire treatment process.

MULTIPLE CHOICE QUESTIONS

1. Which of the following is a malignant brain tumor?
   a. Pituitary tumor
   b. Craniopharyngioma
   c. Glioblastoma
   d. Schwannoma
2. Which of the following tumor is associated with lower cranial nerve dysfunction?
   a. Pituitary tumor   b. Craniopharyngioma
   c. Glioblastoma   d. Schwannoma
3. The common choice of chemotherapy drugs for patients with brain tumors is_____
   a. Prednisolone   b. Dexamethasone
   c. Temozolomide   d. Hydrocortisone
4. The most common site of the primary tumor that metastasizes to the brain in females is_____
   a. Breast   b. Esophagus lungs
   c. Cervix   d. Ovary
5. The most common site of the primary tumor that metastasizes to the brain in males is_____
   a. Breast   b. Esophagus
   c. Lungs   d. Prostate
6. Which of the following is the top priority while caring for a postoperative patient who underwent resection of a brain tumor?
   a. Maintaining cerebral tissue perfusion
   b. Maintaining ABC
   c. Performing a neurological assessment
   d. Administering anticonvulsant
7. World Brain tumor day is celebrated on:
   a. 8th June   b. 8th July
   c. 1st Oct   d. 16th Sept
8. Tumor originates within the brainstem:
   a. Medulloblastoma   b. Astrocytoma
   c. Oligodendrogliomas d. Ependymomas
9. The drug of choice to reduce ICP by reducing cerebral edema is:
   a. Mannitol   b. Hydrocortisone
   c. Dexamethasone   d. Prednisolone
10. The common surgical approach for pituitary tumors:
    a. Transcranial   b. Transsphenoidal
    c. Suboccipital   d. Retro-mastoid

ANSWERS

1. c   2. d   3. c   4. a
5. c   6. b   7. a   8. a
9. c   10. b

SUGGESTED READING

1. Adhikari S, Walker BC, Mittal S. Pathogenesis and Management of Brain Tumor-Related Epilepsy. In: Debinski W(Ed). Gliomas [Internet]. Brisbane (AU): Exon Publications; 2021 Apr 30. Chapter 12. Available from: https://www.ncbi.nlm.nih.gov/books/NBK570699/ doi: 10.36255/exonpublications.gliomas.2021.chapter12.
2. Barnholtz-Sloan JS, Ostrom QT, Cote D. Epidemiology of Brain Tumors. Neurol Clin. 2018;36(3):395-419. doi 10.1016/j.ncl.2018.04.001. Epub 2018 Jun 15. PMID: 30072062.
3. Dasgupta A, Gupta T, Jalali R. Indian data on central nervous tumors: A summary of published work. South Asian J Cancer. 2016;5(3):147-53. doi: 10.4103/2278-330X.187589. PMID: 27606302; PMCID: PMC4991137.
4. Das S, Mishra RK, Agrawal A. Prognostic factors affecting outcome of multifocal or multicentric glioblastoma: A scoping review. J Neurosci Rural Pract. 2023;14(2):199-209. doi: 10.25259/JNRP_41_2022. Epub 2022 Dec 15. PMID: 37181186; PMCID: PMC10174113.
5. Drappatz J. Medical care of patients with brain tumors. Continuum (Minneap Minn). 2012 ApBatchelor TT, Byrne TN. Supportive care of brain tumor patients. Hematol Oncol Clin North Am. 2006;20(6):1337-61. doi: 10.1016/j.hoc.2006.09.013. PMID: 17113467.r;18(2):275–94. doi: 10.1212/01.CON.0000413658.04680.74. PMID: 22810127.
6. Kreatsoulas D, Damante M, Gruber M, Duru O, Elder JB. Supratotal Surgical Resection for Low-Grade Glioma: A Systematic Review. Cancers (Basel). 2023;15(9):2493. doi: 10.3390/cancers15092493. PMID: 37173957; PMCID: PMC10177219.
7. Mezzacappa FM, Thorell W. Neuronal Brain Tumors. [Updated 2022 Nov 21]. In: StatPearls [Internet]. Treasure Island (FL): StatPearls Publishing; 2023 Jan-. Available from: https://www.ncbi.nlm.nih.gov/books/NBK576406/
8. Miller KD, Ostrom QT, Kruchko C, Patil N, Tihan T, Cioffi G, Fuchs HE, Waite KA, Jemal A, Siegel RL, Barnholtz-Sloan JS. Brain and other central nervous system tumor statistics, 2021. CA Cancer J Clin. 2021;71(5):381-406. doi: 10.3322/caac.21693. Epub 2021. PMID: 34427324.
9. Phillips KA, Fadul CE, Schiff D. Neurologic and Medical Management of Brain Tumors. Neurol Clin. 2018;36(3):449-66. doi: 10.1016/j.ncl.2018.04.004. Epub 2018. PMID: 30072065.
10. Pruitt AA. Medical management of patients with brain tumors. Continuum (Minneap Minn). 2015;21(2 Neuro-oncology):314-31. doi: 10.1212/01.CON.0000464172.50638.21. PMID: 25837898.
11. Schiff D, Lee EQ, Nayak L, Norden AD, Reardon DA, Wen PY. Medical management of brain tumors and the sequelae of treatment. Neuro Oncol. 2015;17(4):488-504. doi: 10.1093/neuonc/nou304. Epub 2014 Oct 30. PMID: 25358508; PMCID: PMC4483077.
12. Shah U, Morrison T. A review of the symptomatic management of malignant gliomas in adults. J Natl Compr Canc Netw. 2013;11(4):424-9. doi: 10.6004/jnccn.2013.0057. PMID: 23584345.
13. Wen PY, Schiff D, Kesari S, Drappatz J, Gigas DC, Doherty L. Medical management of patients with brain tumors. J Neurooncol. 2006;80(3):313-32. doi: 10.1007/s11060–006-9193–2. Epub 2006. PMID: 16807780.
14. Yeole BB. Trends in the brain cancer incidence in India. Asian Pac J Cancer Prev. 2008;9(2):267-70. PMID: 18712971.
15. Zarnett OJ, Sahgal A, Gosio J, Perry J, Berger MS, Chang S, Das S. Treatment of elderly patients with glioblastoma: a systematic evidence-based analysis. JAMA Neurol. 2015;72(5):589-96. doi: 10.1001/jamaneurol.2014.3739. PMID: 25822375.

SPINAL TUMORS

Manju Dhandapani

"You only worry about your head or spinal column. Everything else, some way or another, will repair in time."
—Tony McCoy

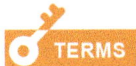 EARNING OBJECTIVES

After going through the chapter, the learner will be able to:
- Define spinal tumors.
- Classify the types of spinal tumors.
- Discuss the pathophysiology and clinical manifestations of spinal tumors.
- Elaborate on the treatment strategies and nursing management of patients with spine tumor.
- Discuss the geriatric considerations in spinal tumors.

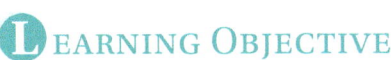 TERMS

- **Brachytherapy:** A technique of delivering radiation internally, directly into the tumor.
- **Extra medullary:** Inside dura mater, the outermost layer of meninges covering the spinal cord.
- **En bloc resection:** It is the surgical removal of the entire organ or tissue as a whole.
- **Intradural:** Outside medulla, here it is outside the spinal cord.
- **Intramedullary:** Within the medulla, here it is within the spinal cord.
- **Radiosurgery:** A form of radiation therapy in which a high dose of radiation is delivered to a very small, precisely selected area.
- **Stereotactic:** A technique used for precisely directing the tip of a delicate instrument or radio beam to a specific location.
- **Tumor:** A group of abnormal cells or mass that form in any part of the body.

INTRODUCTION

Spinal tumors are the growth or mass located in either the vertebral column or the spinal cord that results in pain, neurological deficits, and disability. Knowing the types and exact location of the tumor aids in the right treatment choice. The clinical manifestations and disability can be the results of the tumor or complications of its treatment modalities. Hence, long-term care may be required in patients with metastatic and recurrent tumors. Palliative care including comprehensive nursing care and rehabilitation is the mainstay of management along with surgery, chemotherapy, or radiotherapy. The outcome may depend on many factors such as type, location, response to treatment, and compliance with the therapeutic regimen.

CONCEPT AND DEFINITION

A spinal tumor is an abnormal growth of cells within or surrounding the spinal cord and/or spinal column. They can be benign or malignant.

TYPES OF SPINAL TUMORS

Various types of spinal tumors are shown in **Table 32.3** and **Figure 32.2**. Based on the tissue from which the tumor is originated, spinal tumors can be histologically classified into various types such as meningiomas (29%), nerve sheath tumors (24%), and ependymomas (23%), astrocytoma, chordoma, neurofibroma, and osteosarcoma, etc.

TABLE 32.3: Types of spinal tumors

Characteristic	Types
Based on the location along the spinal column	**Cervical:** Tumors are in the region of the cervical vertebra
	Thoracic: Tumors are in the region of thoracic vertebra
	Lumbar: Tumors are in the region of lumbar vertebra
	Sacral: Tumors are in the region of the sacrum
Based on location in relation to the spinal cord and spinal column (Fig. 1)	**Intramedullary:** Tumors are located inside the spinal cord
	Intradural-extramedullary: Tumors are located outside the spinal cord but within the dura matter. They are usually developed from nerve roots, blood vessels, or the meningeal layers
	Extradural: Tumors are located outside the dura matter but within the vertebral/spinal column
Based on the spread of the tumor	**Benign:** Tumors are non-cancerous
	Malignant: Tumors are cancerous
Based on the origin	**Primary:** Tumors are originated from the spine or spinal cord
	Metastatic: Tumors are metastasized from other parts of the body

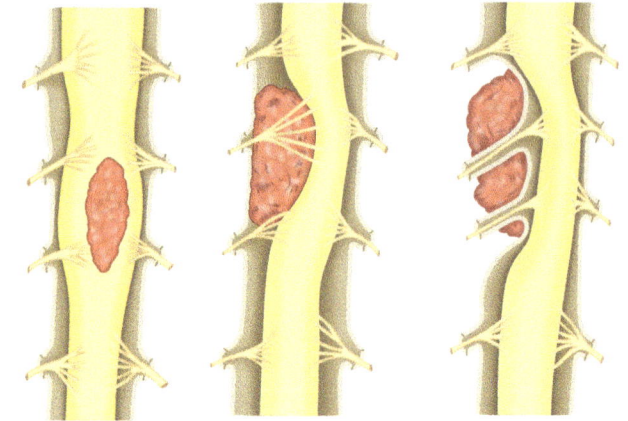

Fig. 32.2: Types of spinal tumors in relation to the spinal cord and spinal column.

The commonest cancer that metastasizes to the spine in males is lung cancer, while in female are breast cancer. Other cancers that metastasize include prostate cancer, leukemia, lymphoma, multiple myeloma, melanoma, sarcoma, and cancers of the kidney, thyroid, and gastrointestinal tract.

EPIDEMIOLOGY

The global incidence of spinal cord tumors is 0.74 per one lakh population with 0.77 in females and 0.7 in males. The incidence is found to be lowest in the children with the peak incidence above 70 years of age. The five years survival rate is 75%- and 10-year survival rate is 64% with a mortality rate of 3.20% and a recurrence rate of 4.90%. The incidence rate of malignant tumors is considerably low as compared to benign tumors (0.22 vs 0.69-0.76). Secondary (metastatic) spinal tumors are common as compared to primary tumors. They comprise more than 90% of the spine tumors. It is reported that 30–70% of the patients with cancer develop metastasis to the spine. The commonest types of intramedullary tumors are astrocytomas and ependymomas, intradural extramedullary are meningiomas and nerve sheath tumors and extradural are osteosarcomas and vertebral metastatic tumors. A similar pattern of incidence is reported in India where the hospital-based yearly incidence for all spinal tumors was 0.24 in one lakh persons. The malignant and benign spinal cord and vertebral tumors encompassed 32.58% and 67.42% respectively of all tumors.

ETIOLOGY

The risk factors for spinal cord tumors are majorly unidentified. However, the role of lifestyle, dietary patterns, sedentary lifestyle, obesity, and consumption of tobacco are well known in the development of many cancers, including those that originate in or metastasize to the spine. Although there are no risk factors that are reported to be associated with spine tumors, the following factors may increase its risk:
- Exposure to high levels of electromagnetic radiation, especially during childhood
- Hereditary cancers, for instance, neurofibromatosis, Turcot syndrome, tuberous sclerosis, von Hippel-Lindau disease, Li-Fraumeni syndrome, Gorlin syndrome, and Cowden syndrome
- Weakened immune function, may be due to acquired or congenital conditions, treatment with immunosuppressants for autoimmune diseases or organ transplantation, treatments for other cancers or HIV/acquired immunodeficiency syndrome (AIDS).

PATHOPHYSIOLOGY

As the tumor develops and progresses, inflammation along with edema may be settled in the spinal cord and surrounding tissues at the level of the tumor and one or two levels above and below. The tumor along with edema may compress and exert pressure on the spinal cord, sensory and motor nerves, nerve roots, and ganglion resulting in pain and neurological deficits with sensory and motor deficits along with bladder-bowel dysfunction. Invasion of the tumor to the vertebra will result in vertebral instability and mechanical dysfunction in the spine disturbing its mobility **(Fig. 32.3)**.

CLINICAL MANIFESTATIONS

The clinical manifestations of patients with spinal tumors have slow onset with timely progression. However, the symptoms experienced by the patients depend on several factors such as location, type, size, and tumor spread. Very small tumors may not cause symptoms as they are not large enough to compress or irritate the spinal cord or the surrounding tissues, nerve roots, blood vessels, or bony structures. The commonest symptoms reported by the patients include back pain, extremity weakness, sensory alterations, and bowel or bladder incontinence. The most common symptom is back pain, for all types of tumors.

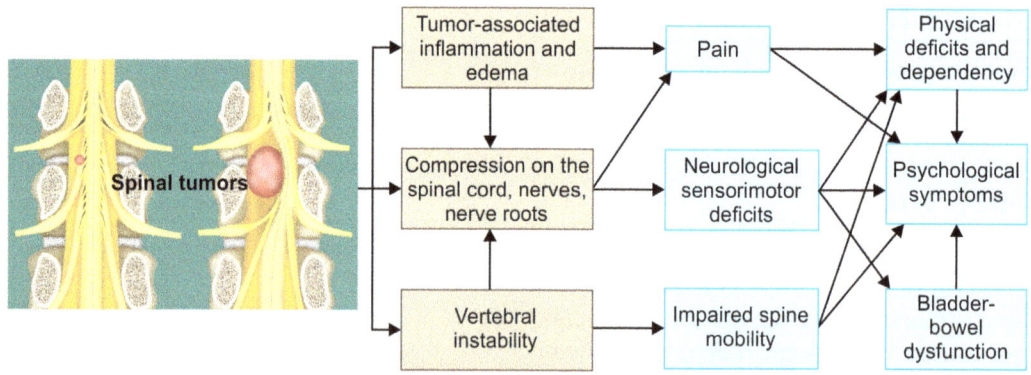

Fig. 32.3: Pathophysiology of spinal cord tumor.

The pain associated with tumors is mostly reported in the middle and lower back due to the high incidence of tumors at these levels.

Back pain is the most common symptom of both benign (noncancerous) and malignant (cancerous) spinal tumors. A spinal tumor is suspected when the patient experiences back pain without any specific injury, stress, or physical activity but can get worse with strain, such as from exercise, sneezing, or coughing. The pain is of dull and persistent in nature and has slow onset with a gradual increase. Over the time, pain can be severe to the extent of sleep disturbance and impairment in activities of daily living. Pain may become radicular in nature due to nerve root involvement and may radiate to hips, legs, feet, or arms. The pain can be sharp and shooting during this phase.

Other symptoms of spinal tumors include:
- **Sensory symptoms:** Numbness, tingling, or loss of sensation in extremities or chest, loss of temperature sensation
- **Motor symptoms:** Varying degree of muscle weakness resulting in paralysis in the extremities or chest, muscle twitches or spasms, loss of bowel and/or bladder control (bowel incontinence and urinary incontinence)
- Abnormal reflexes
- Stiffness in the back or neck
- Tenderness in the spine
- Difficulty walking with risk for falls
- Impaired sleep
- Impaired activities of daily living
- Mild depression and other psychological symptoms
- Scoliosis or other spinal deformity resulting from a large metastatic or invasive tumor.

DIAGNOSTIC EVALUATION

Many conditions such as infection (tuberculosis, and fungal infections), degeneration, metabolic and various medical conditions can mimic spinal tumors. Hence, a comprehensive diagnostic approach is necessary not only to diagnose but also for aiding the treatment. Primary spinal cord tumors are often diagnosed incidentally as they are small and mostly remain asymptomatic. It is advisable to suspect the possibility of a spine tumor as the patients would often try to associate the back pain with any previous stress or mild mechanical injury. Patients who are known cases of cancer are often suspected to have metastasis when they report back pain. A complete history and thorough physical and neurological examination including sensorimotor evaluation and reflexes would aid in early diagnosis.

The following investigations are done in addition to history and neurological examination:
- **Spine X-rays:** They are helpful in detecting secondary tumors as most of the metastatic tumors are located in bony parts of the spinal column. They also give a good overall view of the alignment of the spine and allow the surgeon to plan for the correct interpretation of the intraoperative images.
- **Magnetic resonance imaging (MRI):** It is the most useful screening test for the diagnosis of spinal cord tumors and is the preferred test to diagnose tumors of the spinal cord and surrounding tissues. It helps in a comprehensive evaluation of the spinal cord, nerves, and surrounding spine (bony and soft tissue). An intravenous contrast agent may be used to highlight various tissues. It uses magnetic field energy to create images and delivers accurate information about the soft tissues and bony structures of the spine. The patients who are contraindicated for an MRI are prescribed a CT scan with myelogram instead. A whole spine MRI with and without contrast must be obtained for a new spinal lesion to identify skip lesions existing in the spine.
- **Computed tomography (CT scan):** CT scan of the spine would help in defining the boney architecture of the lesion and aid in surgical planning. CT chest, abdomen, and pelvis are done to look for other lesions of primary origin.
- **Positron emission tomography:** A whole-body PET scan may be considered to identify the location of cancerous lesions elsewhere in the body where the tumor would have primarily originated.
- **Biopsy:** A biopsy is obtained for diagnosis and should always be done before surgery except in rare circumstances. A biopsy will help in identifying the type of tumor which is detrimental to aiding the treatment strategies.
- **Bone scan:** It helps in detecting the bony architecture which is vital to make the surgical decision and instrumentation.
- **Blood tests:** Laboratory tests should include serum protein electrophoresis/urine protein electrophoresis, complete blood count, basic metabolic panel, and erythrocyte sedimentation rate/C-reactive protein, calcium, and alkaline phosphatase. These investigations help to rule out the possibilities of multiple myeloma, leukemia, and infection and to identify the bone breakdown products released into the blood.

TREATMENT

Treatment of spinal tumors is highly individualized. It depends on the location, size, and type of tumor. The main goals of treatment of metastatic spinal tumors are to relieve pain and to improve neurological function and quality of life. Monitoring the patient along with surgery, chemotherapy or radiotherapy is the mainstay of treatment modalities. A collaborative model of care is required including medical and surgical oncologists, neurosurgeons, radiation oncologists, nurses, and physiotherapists.

Monitoring

The progress of the symptoms must be monitored to plan the timing of surgery. Tumors that are small and not increasing in size may not be operated on but will be monitored through periodic imaging studies.

Surgical Management

Surgery is the treatment of choice for spinal tumors, though there can be a certain risk of injury to the spinal cord, nerves, or nerve roots. However, the risks are minimized with intraoperative monitoring and imaging as well as minimally invasive and endoscopic surgical techniques with the help of a high-powered microscope. Even the advanced technologies do not guarantee the complete removal of all tumors where the surgery may be accompanied by chemotherapy, radiotherapy, or both. Using an appropriate surgical approach, tumor resection or decompression is performed which is followed by spine stabilization.

Surgical Approach

A laminectomy at the level of the tumor is performed to approach the tumor. Sometimes the tumors are approached from the anterior aspect by dissecting the ribs.

Resection

Tumor resection is done as en bloc resection in primary tumors and as gross total or intralesional resection in metastatic tumor. The removal of the tumor will reduce its pressure on spine structures and thus pain and other symptoms.

The goal of surgery in the primary spinal tumor is to remove the entire tumor along with the vertebral body known as en bloc excision. Hence, this technique is performed for tumors such as chordomas, osteosarcomas, etc. Surgical intervention for a primary tumor of the spine should typically proceed only once a tissue diagnosis is made and appropriate preoperative staging and planning have been completed. A marginal en bloc resection removes only the tumor and a wide en bloc resection removes the tumor along with a layer of healthy tissue around the tumor.

The goal of surgery in metastatic spinal tumors is to decompress the spinal cord and nerve roots or to alleviate spinal instability or imminent instability with the aim of reducing pain and improving mechanical and neurological function. An open biopsy is also performed along with the surgery. Rapid deterioration of neurological function warrants an emergency decompression. A gross total excision is performed in secondary/metastatic tumors while preserving or sacrificing nerve roots and blood vessels depending on the tumor invasion. Intralesional or gross total resection is done for tumors such as osteoblastoma and other metastatic lesions.

Spine Stabilization

Spine stabilization using appropriate techniques may be required after the resection of the tumor to preserve maximum mechanical and neurological function and it depends on the extent of surgical approach and vertebral resection. Spine stabilization can be done by vertebroplasty or kyphoplasty, with or without other techniques such as the insertion of rods, pins, or wires. The patient needs complete bed rest with special braces if there is a delay in fixation devices.

Stereotactic Radiosurgery (SRS)

This technique is a nonsurgical, minimally invasive procedure done to deliver precise narrow beams of radiation to a tumor using a gamma knife, cyberknife, or linear accelerators (photon therapy). It is a precise, high-dose form of image-guided radiation therapy. It is done for tumors that are resistant to conventional treatment and is performed using techniques to minimize damage to the surrounding healthy tissues.

Radiation Therapy

The goal of radiotherapy is to destroy the remaining part of tumors that persist after surgery, to manage patients with inoperable tumors, or to treat the tumors with high surgical risk. It helps to eliminate malignant tumors, to prevent/reduce recurrence, and to shrink tumors for easier removal. The majority of spinal tumors respond to surgery and can be partially or completely resected. Radiation therapy is done for incompletely resected low-grade tumors, malignant tumors, and recurrent tumors. The dose of radiation therapy may be adjusted so as to preserve the surrounding healthy tissue.

There are two types of radiation therapy that can be used for spine tumors: Both external and internal radiation therapy can be used for patients with spine tumors. Most of the patients are treated with external radiation therapy. Brachytherapy or internal radiation delivers high doses of radiation into the tumor for a short duration of time. It reduces the damage to nearby tissues. Radiation can be delivered using silicon plaques coated with a radioactive isotope placed inside the tumor or through brachytherapy catheters. Patients undergoing radiation therapy can develop some side effects such as sore throat, skin redness, etc. Kindly see Chapter 41 for the care of the patients undergoing radiotherapy.

Chemotherapy

Chemotherapy is prescribed depending on a patient's needs such as to reduce the size of the tumor prior to surgery, to remove any remaining part of the tumor after surgery, to treat metastasis, and to reduce symptoms as a part of palliative care. Chemotherapy is used to treat primary spinal cancers, such as neuroblastoma, lymphoma, and germ cell tumors. Chemotherapy can also be used as adjuvant therapy for secondary spinal tumors, including breast, prostate, and myeloma metastatic to the spine. The drugs may be given orally, intravenously, or intrathecally where they are injected into the tumor through a lumbar puncture or a device placed under the scalp. Steroids are the mainstay of chemotherapy. Chemotherapy may be done alone or in combination with radiation therapy. Patients undergoing chemotherapy may develop side effects such as fatigue, nausea, vomiting, alopecia, steroid-induced myopathy, and infection. Kindly see Chapter 41 for the care of the patients undergoing chemotherapy.

Other Drugs

Non-steroidal anti-inflammatories, anti-convulsant, tricyclic antidepressants, steroids, and opioids can be used for pain management. Both gabapentin and pregabalin can be used to reduce pain. Corticosteroids are given to patients with spinal tumors to reduce the inflammation that can be developed due to tumors, surgery, or radiation therapy. Although they reduce inflammation, they are generally given only for a short duration to prevent any serious side effects such as high blood pressure, diabetes, muscle weakness, osteoporosis, and infection. Medications are given to reduce the side effects of radiation therapy and chemotherapy. These may help ease some of the side effects of radiation, such as nausea and vomiting.

NURSING MANAGEMENT

Comprehensive and collaborative nursing care is mandatory for patients with spinal tumors. Respiratory and hemodynamic dysfunction in patients with spine tumors are not very common. However, the nurse should ensure that the patient maintains stable respiratory and hemodynamic status. The main goals of nursing management are:
- To reduce the pain
- To maintain nutritional status
- To maintain bowel and bladder elimination
- To minimize or manage the disability associated with neurological deficits, and treatment modalities
- To assist in maintaining activities and enhancing the independence
- To prevent complications associated with neurological deficits and treatment regimen
- To educate patients and family caregivers

Assessment and Nursing Interventions

The assessment and nursing interventions for each of the above-listed goals are as follows:
- **To reduce the pain:**
  - Monitor the location, severity, fluctuation, and progress of pain. The pain may be throbbing in case of vertebral invasion of the tumor while radiating in case of nerve root compression.
  - Administer prescribed analgesics and other drugs to relieve pain
  - Provide appropriate non-pharmacological modalities to alleviate pain such as cold or hot compression or ultrasound or electrical stimulation
  - Utilize diversion therapy by engaging the patient in interesting activities, guided imagery, etc.
  - Evaluate the effectiveness of the pain management modalities and modify them accordingly
  - Report any sudden increase in pain along with increasing neurological deficits as it may warrant emergency surgery
  - Monitor sleep and take measures to facilitate sleep
- **To maintain nutritional status:**
  - Ensure adequate dietary intake to compensate for side effects of nausea and vomiting associated with radiotherapy or chemotherapy
  - Preset diet in a pleasant manner especially for patients with anorexia, nausea, and vomiting
  - Provide high protein diet to enhance post-operative recovery
  - Provide small-frequent diet
  - Maintain intake and output
  - Inform the gastrointestinal symptoms to the physician and manage them with appropriate medications such as antiemetics
  - Prevent/manage oral mucositis associated with chemotherapy or radiotherapy with oral care and cryo/ice-chip therapy
  - Provide diet counseling by emphasizing the importance of nutrition in recovery
  - Monitor nutritional status using appropriate techniques
- **To maintain bowel elimination:**
  - Monitor bowel dysfunction symptoms such as constipation, impaction, inadequate emptying, or incontinence
  - Assess for constipation in patients receiving opioids for pain management, paralysis
  - Administer laxatives or suppositories
  - Perform digital stimulation if required after proper lubrication, with special caution in patients with neutropenia and thrombocytopenia
  - Plan and implement a bowel program to prevent incontinence and facilitate evacuation. It may be performed every 2 days after 30 minutes of a major meal (to get the benefit of gastro-colic reflex)
- **To maintain bladder elimination:**
  - Monitor for bladder dysfunction such as urgency, frequency, retention, incontinence, and frequent urinary tract infections
  - Assess for symptoms or signs of bladder retention in self-voiding patients
  - Perform intermediate catheterization or indwelling catheterization depending on the patient's requirement
  - Take measures to prevent UTI; implement CAUTI (Catheter-associated UTI) bundle and monitor signs and symptoms of UTI
  - Treat UTI with appropriate antibiotics based on culture and sensitivity report of urine
- **To minimize or manage the disability associated with neurological deficits, and treatment modalities so as to assist maintain activities of daily living and enhancing the independence:**
  - Assess the sensory and motor neurological deficits of the patient, and monitor their severity
  - Assess the dependency level using appropriate tools
  - Initiate sensory and motor rehabilitation as early as possible
  - Use devices to stabilize the spine
  - Take measures to reduce pain before performing rehabilitation
  - Assist in necessary activities of daily living depending on the deficits while encouraging the patient to perform independently
- **To prevent complications associated with neurological deficits and treatment regimen:**
  - Assess the patient's risk for developing complications such as pressure sore, deep vein thrombosis (DVT), UTI, contractures, infection, etc
  - Take measures to prevent complications in all patients
    - Range of motion exercise to prevent DVT and contractures
    - Pneumatic compression devices and anticoagulant therapy to prevent DVT
    - Enhancing mobility, changing the position and pressure-eliminating devices to prevent pressure sore
    - Appropriate catheter care to prevent UTI
    - Wound care, drain care, prophylactic antibiotics, and aseptic techniques to prevent infection in post-operative patients

- Identify complications early, report to the treating team, and document
- Ensure appropriate management if a patient develops any complication

❖ **To educate patients and family caregivers:**
- Educate the patient and caregivers depending on the medications and other therapeutic requirement during home care such as catheter care, pressure sore/UTI/DVT/contracture prevention strategies
- Inform about the timely follow-up and investigations
- Encourage to continue home-based or institutionalized rehabilitation
- Inform about the symptoms that need emergency attention and require hospital visits such as emerging neurological deficits, severe pain, signs of infection, and other complications associated with tumor or treatment
- Assess the risk of falls at discharge and teach about measures to prevent fall
- Encourage the patient to consider consultation and counseling for sexual dysfunction
- Monitor quality of life during follow-up and take appropriate measures to enhance the quality of life

The comprehensive care must continue through the entire continuum of treatment. Nurses also must ensure that the essential assessment and interventions are performed during the perioperative period, during chemotherapy and radiation therapy cycles. The patients and family caregivers must be educated about homecare and maintaining compliance with the entire treatment modalities and follow-up.

Rehabilitation

The rehabilitative process should be initiated soon after the diagnosis to maintain spinal function and prevent or reduce associated complications. A complete rehabilitation may not be possible preoperatively due to pain and spine instability. Bracing using appropriate devices to maintain vertebral stability and pain management using appropriate modalities including heat, cold, ultrasound, and electrical stimulation must be performed preoperatively to prevent further damage and to preserve or improve current function. However, comprehensive rehabilitation must be initiated during the post-operative period and must be continued even after discharge depending on the deficits or symptoms that the patient continues to suffer.

GERIATRIC CONSIDERATIONS

The geriatric population is at high risk of developing spinal tumors. The associated neurological deficits may increase the risk of falls and injury in the elderly. Hence, appropriate fall and injury prevention strategies must be advised while ensuring to have caregivers stay with the patient. The tolerance and effectiveness of treatment modalities may be reduced during old age. Hence, collaborative strategies best for the patient must be implemented to enhance their quality of life.

Case Scenario

Mrs Y, 55-year-old is a known case of breast cancer for 5 years. She is brought to the hospital due to a fall. On examination, she is conscious, and her vitals are stable. Muscle strength in lower limbs is 3/5 bilaterally with loss of sensation in both the limbs. She has been suffering from back pain for 4–5 months. On the MRI image, she was found to have metastasis to T6 vertebrae with spinal cord compression. She is now operated for surgical excision of the tumor with spine stabilization and is in neurosurgical ICU.
1. Discuss the preoperative management for Mrs Y
2. Discuss the post-operative nursing management and transition to home care for this patient.

SUMMARY

Patients with spinal tumors require individualized and comprehensive treatment strategies. En bloc surgical excision is the common choice for primary tumor and gross total excision along with adjuvant radiotherapy chemotherapy is preferred. Comprehensive nursing care, rehabilitation, and timely follow-up are essential components of a treatment strategy to improve the quality of life of the patients. Hospital-to-home transition care must be provided to the family caregivers and they must be empowered with adequate knowledge in homecare.

MULTIPLE CHOICE QUESTIONS

1. A tumor that is formed within the spinal cord is known as:
   a. Leptomeningeal tumor
   b. Intramedullary tumor
   c. Intradural extramedullary
   d. Intramedullary extradural tumor
2. Radiating pain reported by the patients of spinal tumors is due to:
   a. Invasion of tumor to vertebra
   b. Cord compression
   c. Nerve root compression
   d. Meningeal layer involvement
3. Which of the following is the commonest type of spinal tumors:
   a. Meningioma
   b. Ependymoma
   c. Schwannoma
   d. Nerve sheath tumors
4. The most common site of the primary tumor that metastasizes to spine in females is_____
   a. Breast
   b. Lungs
   c. Cervix
   d. Ovary
5. The most common site of the primary tumor that metastasize to spine in males is_____
   a. Prostate
   b. Bladder
   c. Lungs
   d. Rectus

ANSWERS

1. b   2. c   3. a   4. a
5. c

SUGGESTED READING

1. Bhat AR, Kirmani AR, Wani MA, Bhat MH. Incidence, histopathology, and surgical outcome of tumors of spinal cord, nerve roots, meninges, and vertebral column - Data based on single institutional (Sher-i-Kashmir Institute of Medical Sciences) experience. J Neurosci Rural Pract. 2016;7(3):381-91.
2. Goodarzi A, Clouse J, Capizzano T, Kim KD, Panchal R. The Optimal Surgical Approach to Intradural Spinal Tumors: Laminectomy or Hemilaminectomy? Cureus. 2020;12(2):e7084.
3. Kumar N, Tan WLB, Wei W, Vellayappan BA. An overview of the tumors affecting the spine-inside to out. Neurooncol Pract. 2020;7(Suppl 1):i10-i17.
4. Kurisunkal V, Gulia A, Gupta S. Principles of Management of Spine Metastasis. Indian J Orthop. 2020;54(2):181-93.
5. Lawton AJ, Lee KA, Cheville AL, Ferrone ML, Rades D, Balboni TA, Abrahm JL. Assessment and Management of Patients With Metastatic Spinal Cord Compression: A Multidisciplinary Review. J Clin Oncol. 2019;37(1):61-71.
6. Metastatic Spinal Cord Compression: Diagnosis and Management of Patients at Risk of or with Metastatic Spinal Cord Compression. Cardiff (UK): National Collaborating Centre for Cancer (UK); 2008 Nov. PMID: 22171401.
7. New PW, Marshall R, Stubblefield MD, Scivoletto G. Rehabilitation of people with spinal cord damage due to tumor: literature review, international survey and practical recommendations for optimizing their rehabilitation. J Spinal Cord Med. 2017;40(2):213-21.
8. Ottenhausen M, Ntoulias G, Bodhinayake I, et al. Intradural spinal tumors in adults—update on management and outcome. Neurosurg Rev. 2019;42:371-88.
9. Raj VS, Lofton L. Rehabilitation and treatment of spinal cord tumors. J Spinal Cord Med. 2013;36(1):4-11.
10. Takami T, Naito K, Yamagata T, Ohata K. Surgical management of spinal intramedullary tumors: a radical and safe strategy for benign tumors. Neurol Med Chir (Tokyo). 2015;55(4):317-27.
11. Wagner A, Haag E, Joerger AK, et al. Comprehensive surgical treatment strategy for spinal metastases. 2021;7988:11.
12. Welch WC, Frederick A, Schiff D. Spinal cord tumors. https://www.uptodate.com/contents/spinal-cord-tumors.
13. Wewel JT, O'Toole JE. Epidemiology of spinal cord and column tumors. Neurooncol Pract. 2020;7(Suppl 1):i5-i9.
14. Zaveri GR, Jain R, Mehta N, Garg B. An Overview of Decision Making in the Management of Metastatic Spinal Tumors. Indian J Orthop. 2021;55(4):799-814.
15. Ziu E, Viswanathan VK, Mesfin FB. Spinal Metastasis. StatPearls. https://www.ncbi.nlm.nih.gov/books/NBK441950/

CHAPTER 33

Chronic Neurological Problems

Vivek Kumar Garg, Manisha Nagi, Ashok Kumar, Jitendra Gairolla, Kapil Goel

*"The brain is the organ of destiny. It holds within its humming mechanism.
Secrets that will determine the future of the human race."*

—**Wilder Penfield**

LEARNING OBJECTIVES

After going through the chapter, the learner will be able to:
- Define various chronic neurological problems, e.g., headaches, migraine, seizures and epilepsy, and restless leg syndrome.
- Describe the epidemiology of chronic neurological problems.
- Elaborate pathophysiology of various chronic neurological problems.
- Explain the medical and nursing management of these disease conditions.
- Discuss the geriatric considerations related to each chronic neurological disorder.

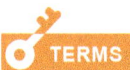

TERMS

- **Chronic:** The conditions persisting for a long time.
- **Epilepsy:** It is characterized by recurrent, unprovoked seizures.
- **Migraine:** It is a type of headache.
- **Restless leg syndrome:** It is a condition in which there is an irreversible compulsion to move the legs.
- **Secondary headache:** It is the headache that occurs as a complication of other diseases.
- **Status migrainosus:** Severe intractable migraine attack a debilitating attack, lasting for more than 72 hours.

INTRODUCTION

Neurological disorders include a wide range of disorders and can affect a large number of people. In the current chapter, the common neurological disorders discussed are headache, migraine, seizures, and epilepsy. Restless leg syndrome is also touched upon at the end of the chapter.

HEADACHE

Headache also called cephalalgia, is one of the most common chronic pain syndromes. It is one of the most commonest reported symptoms of patients approaching for the medical treatment. The direct and indirect socioeconomic costs of headaches to society are around $14 billion per year. It is a symptom rather than a disease entity, it may indicate organic disease (neurological or other), a stress response, vasodilation, skeleton muscle tension, or a combination of factors. Headaches are the most common form of pain and are a major reason cited for days missed by a client from his/her work or school, as well as visits to healthcare providers. While most headaches are not dangerous, certain types can be a sign of the more serious disease condition.

DEFINITION

Headache is the pain in any part of the head, including the inside of the head, scalp, upper neck, face, etc.

EPIDEMIOLOGY

- Lifelong prevalence of headache is 96%.

- It is more common in females. The headaches are burdensome in women between the ages of 15 and 49 years.
- Worldwide, an active headache disorder of any type is present in 52% of the population studied (males 44.4%, females 57.8%), migraine in 10% (males 8.6%, females 17.0%).
- Each day, 15.8% of the world's population had a headache.
- Headache for 10 or more days every month affects 2–4% of the world's adult population.

CLASSIFICATION OF HEADACHE

The International Classification of Headache Disorders (ICHD) was first time published in the year 1988 and till date, this has undergone two revisions, the most recent being in 2013. By convention, the headache classification is based on the characteristics of each individual headache. The detailed features are specific to the individuals and may be used to differentiate between the primary and secondary headaches.

1. **Primary headache:** It is the one for which no organic cause can be identified. It is thought to occur because of any dysfunction or any over-activity of pain-sensitive features in the head. This is not caused by any underlying medical condition. Some people may be genetically more likely to develop primary headaches. As per the International Classification of the Headache Disorders, 3rd Edition (Beta Version), primary headache includes migraine, tension-type, cluster headaches, and other primary disorders.
2. **Secondary headache:** In this, the symptoms are associated with another organic cause, such as a brain tumor or an aneurysm. They are considered a symptom or sign of a condition. Although most headaches do not indicate serious disease, persistent headaches require further investigation. Serious disorders related to headaches include brain tumors, subarachnoid hemorrhage, stroke, severe hypertension, and meningitis, etc. Types of secondary headaches that are not necessarily dangerous and resolve once the underlying condition is treated include:
   - Cranial or cervical vascular disease or injuries.
   - Disorder of the cranium, neck, eyes, nose, sinuses, teeth, mouth, or other facial or cervical structure
   - Nonvascular intracranial disorder
   - A substance or its withdrawal
   - Infection
   - Psychiatric disorders
   - Disorder of homeostasis
   - Dehydration headache.

Various potential precipitating factors of headache may include a change in eating pattern (not eating, excessive eating, certain dietary substances), relationship to the menstrual cycle, sexual intercourse, pregnancy, menopause, psychosocial stressors, changes in sleep pattern, weather changes, hot or cold wind, excessive exposure to lights, excessive exercising, consumption of alcohol, smoking, etc.

Migraine

Migraine is a familial disorder characterized by recurrent attacks of headache widely variable in intensity, duration, and frequency. Attacks are commonly unilateral and are usually associated with anorexia, nausea, and vomiting.

Triggers of Migraine

Various triggering factors of migraine may include:
- Disturbed sleep pattern
- Drugs
- Physical exertion
- Hormonal changes
- Visual, olfactory, and auditory stimuli
- Weather changes
- Hunger
- Psychological factors

Phases of Migraine

The migraine with aura can be divided into four phases **(Fig. 33.1)**:

1. **Prodromal phase:** Noticed in approximately 60% of patients, these symptoms occur hours to days before a migraine headache. Symptoms may include depression, irritability, feeling cold, food cravings, increased urination, diarrhea or constipation, anorexia, and change in activity level. Patients usually experience the same prodromal with each migraine headache.
2. **Aura phase:** Aura occurs in a minority of patients who experience migraines. This phase usually lasts for less than an hour, and it provides enough time for the patient to take the prescribed medication to avert an attack. This period is characterized by focal neurologic symptoms. Visual disturbances (i.e., light flashes and bright spots) are most common and may be hemianopia (affecting only half of the visual field). Other symptoms that may follow include slight weakness of an extremity, drowsiness, dizziness, numbness, and tingling of the lips, face, or hands; mild confusion.

   This period of aura corresponds to the phenomenon of cortical spreading depression (CSD) which is associated with reduced metabolic demand in abnormally functioning neurons. This can be associated with decreased blood flow; however, cerebral blood flow studies performed during migraine headaches demonstrate that although changes in blood vessels occur during phases of migraine, cerebral blood flow is not the main abnormality.
3. **Headache phase:** As a decline in serotonin levels occurs, a throbbing headache (unilateral in 60% of patients)

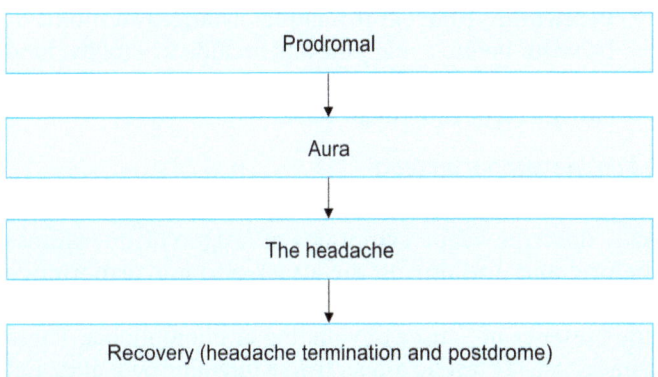

Fig. 33.1: Phases of migraine.

intensifies over several hours. This headache is severe and incapacitating and is often associated with photophobia (light and/or sound sensitivity), nausea, and vomiting; irritability; and fatigue. Its duration varies, ranging from 4 to 72 hours.

4. **Recovery phase:** In the recovery phase (termination and postdrome), the pain gradually subsides and can even last up to 24 hours. Muscle contraction in the neck and scalp is common, with associated muscle aches and localized tenderness, exhaustion, and mood changes. Any physical exertion exacerbates the headache pain. During this post-headache phase, patients may sleep for extended periods.

Classification of Migraine

Migraine headache is the most common type of vascular headache. It is generally subclassified into two types:
1. Migraine, which is of an idiopathic nature
2. Non-migraine, which arises from an identifiable etiology (see later discussion). Migraine headaches are a biological disease of the CNS in which nerve cells and chemical messengers in the brain malfunction.

Migraine headaches are also classified according to the following clinical symptoms:
- Unilateral versus bilateral presentation;
- Variances in intensity, duration, and frequency of attacks
- Associated sensory, motor, or mood disturbances.

According to the headache classification committee of the International Headache Society, migraine has been classified as:
- Migraine with an aura (formerly known as classical migraine)
- Migraine without an aura (formerly known as common migraine)

Migraine with an Aura

Migraine with aura occurs only in about 10% of those with migraine. Neurological symptoms known as an aura may present 10–30 minutes before the migraine.
- **Auras** mainly include visual disturbances (for e.g., scintillating scotomas flashing lights or zigzag lines, speech difficulty, sensory disturbances with paresis of the arms or legs, anorexia, change in activity level, motor changes with weakness paralysis, and mental confusion, dizziness, or loss of consciousness, throbbing pain over the eye, and forehead. At around the face beginning unilaterally and spreading bilaterally, usually peaks in an hour but it may last for hours or even days.
- **Prodromal phases:** It includes changes in mood or behavior before a migraine and include irritability, food cravings, or other behaviors that occur with migraine either with or without an aura.

Migraine without an Aura

These headaches are not starting with an aura. Patients may describe vague symptoms of fatigue or uneasiness beforehand and during the attack and may experience diarrhea, nausea, and vomiting. The diagnosis requires the presence of nausea or vomiting or photophobia. These attacks usually last no longer than a migraine with aura and may continue for several days.

Pathophysiology

The cause of migraine headaches is unknown, and the pathophysiology is not fully understood. The traditional theory that migraine auras are associated with intracerebral vasoconstriction of the cerebral arteries and that the actual headache is caused by vasodilation fails to account for the prodromal symptoms and has not been satisfactorily demonstrated by cerebral blood flow (CBF) studies **(Fig. 33.2)**.

Assessment: The assessment for headaches is described in health history guidelines include the following:
- **Headache characteristics:** Age and time of onset, location, frequency (initial and present), severity, duration, quality (deep, superficial, steady, throbbing, stabbing, or burning); situations or activities that make the headache better or worse.
- **Presence of an aura:** Duration and relationship to the onset of pain.
- **Associated symptoms** occurring before, during, or after a headache: Nausea, vomiting, photophobia, phonophobia, visual disturbances, lightheadedness, dizziness, vertigo, incoordination, redness of the eye, facial symptoms (sweating, paleness, flushing), fatigue or sleepiness, mood swings, motor or sensory changes in the extremities, weakness, paresthesia.

Migraine Diagnostic Criteria

1. *Migraine with an aura (classic):*
   - Reversible visual disturbance or sensory symptoms are present
   - There is a gradual presentation (4 minutes) of at least one aura symptom
   - Aura symptoms usually resolve within 60 minutes.
   - Headache usually follows the aura but can precede it or begin simultaneously with it.
2. *Migraine without an aura (common):* Pain is characterized by at least two of the following features:
   - Unilateral location
   - Pulsating quality
   - Moderate to severe intensity
   - Increase with routine physical activity
   - Headache lasts anywhere from 4 to 72 hours.
   - Headache is associated with at least one of the following features:
     - Nausea
     - Vomiting
     - Photophobia

Neurodiagnostic: The differential diagnosis of headaches is:

1. *Acute single headache:* This can be caused by:
   - Subarachnoid hemorrhage
   - Encephalitis
   - Meningitis
   - Post-concussion syndrome
   - Autonomic hyperreflexia
   - Caffeine withdrawal hypoglycemia
   - Optic neuritis glaucoma
   - First migraine sinusitis/otitis systemic infection
   - "Hangover" reaction hypoxia/hypercapnia

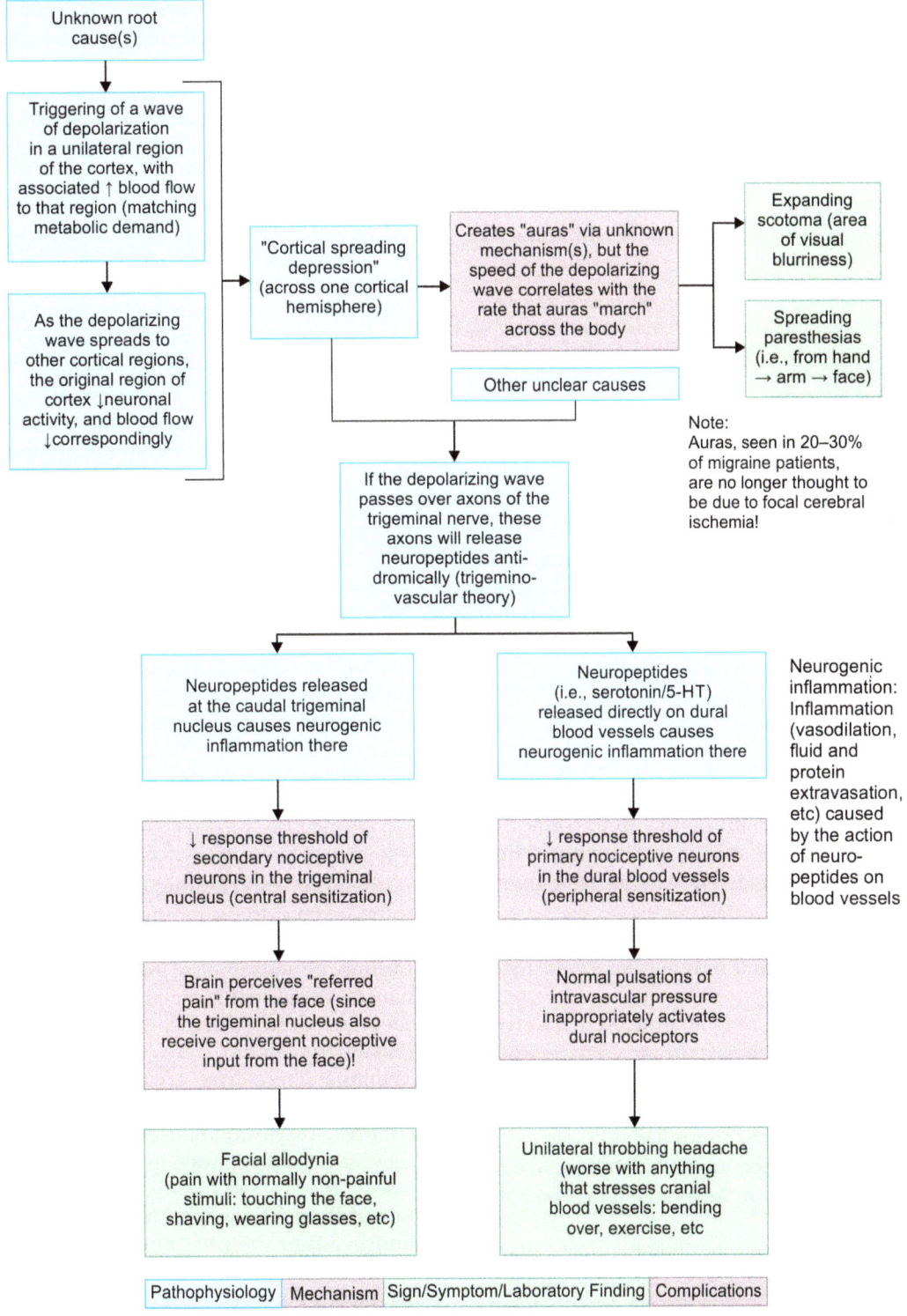

Fig. 33.2: Migraine and auras—pathogenesis and clinical findings.

2. ***Acute recurrent headache:*** This can be caused by:
   - Subarachnoid hemorrhage
   - Hydrocephalus cerebral tumors
   - Intracranial hypertension
   - Systemic hypertension
   - Cluster headache
   - Migraine
   - Tic douloureux
   - Pheochromocytoma

3. ***Subacute headache (days to week):*** This can be caused by:
   - Subdural hematoma
   - Cerebral tumor
   - Brain abscess
   - Sinus thrombosis
   - Pseudotumor cerebri
   - CSF leak
   - Temporal arteritis tooth/gum disease

4. ***Chronic daily headache (months or years):*** This can be caused by:
   - Cerebral tumor
   - Tension headache
   - Analgesic rebound
   - Pseudotumor cerebri
   - Eye strain
   - Cervical spondylosis

   The diagnosis of idiopathic headache often becomes one of exclusion.

> **CT/MRI:** Should be obtained with the acute presentation of a new-onset severe headache or in patients with a nonacute headache presentation accompanied by at least one abnormal finding on the neurologic examination. Scans may be ordered as part of a complete neurodiagnostic workup.
>
> **EEG:** Depending on the patient's presentation, may be obtained if there is a history of a recent head injury or a pattern of focal neurologic deficits associated with the headache.

Treatment

Although a majority of the patients with migraine attacks can be managed properly, there is currently no complete cure as such. Treatment generally focuses on three specific goals:
1. Removal or modification of any precipitating factors
2. Controlling the severity and duration of attacks
3. Prevention of recurring attacks

Medical Management

a. Outpatient or Home Care

- Patients often visit the emergency department for headache relief (e.g., status migrainosus). These patients may require IV fluids, antiemetics, steroids, and dihydroergotamine (DHE).
- Rarely is a patient admitted to the hospital unless the headache is severe and unrelenting, requiring IV medications.
- Patients are usually managed in the OPD setting only, which may include collaborative care with a multidisciplinary team.
- The earlier a migraine is treated, the more likely it is that it can be contained and controlled. Although some precipitating factors, such as menstruation, are not easily controlled, others can be modified or eliminated altogether.
- The controllable factors may include dental problems, refractive errors in eyeglasses, irregular sleeping patterns, diet, excessive caffeine intake, skipping meals, exposure to oscillating lights, fluorescent lighting, use of OTC medications, and side effects from prescription medications.
- Reclining in a cool, dark room with a cool pack applied to the forehead or temples is recommended as an adjunct therapy.
- Patients can be counseled in behaviors that may help prevent or relieve headaches, including the following:
  - Regular sleep patterns
  - Exercise at least three times per week
  - Avoidance of foods that contain tyramine and monosodium glutamate (MSG) and caffeine.
  - Stress management
  - Limitation of medications and compliance with a prescribed headache regimen, including those listed in the following discussion.
- An analgesic should be administered immediately at the onset of symptoms since research indicates that drug absorption is slowed during a migraine attack.
- Oral nonsteroidal anti-inflammatory drugs (NSAIDs), such as aspirin, ibuprofen, and naproxen sodium, are particularly effective in managing pain. Prevention of recurrent attacks is the goal of headache treatment.
- Since many headaches can be linked to specific triggers. Thus identification, elimination, or minimization of the responsible triggers should be the main objective.
- Relaxation training, cognitive/behavioral therapy, and biofeedback could also be tried as alternative therapies.
- Other adjunctive therapies such as acupuncture and hypnosis may provide additional long-term relief, but there is still little empirical evidence to support their effectiveness.

b. Pharmacological Treatment

Medicines used to treat headaches are:
- **Non-specific medication:** There are a number of medicines that we use to treat headaches either prescribed or over-the-counter, for example, ibuprofen or aspirin, etc. If these drugs are taken for a long period of time, they can lead to many side effects like injuries to the liver, nausea, ulcer or bleeding, etc. Aspirin, caffeine, and acetaminophen (excedrin migraine) may also be helpful.
- **Dihydroergotamine (DHE 45, migraine):** These drugs are available as a nasal spray as well in injectable form. These work by stopping the release of natural substances in the brain contributing to the headache. These are to be taken if the symptoms of migraine tend to last longer than 24 hours. The side effects of this drug may include the worsening of migraine-related vomiting and nausea. People with coronary artery disease, high blood pressure, kidney disease, or liver disease should avoid dihydroergotamine.
- **Triptans:** These drugs are normally medically advised. Rizatriptan (Maxalt, Maxalt-MLT) and sumatriptan (Imitrex, Tosymra) are used to treat migraine because they block pain pathways in the brain. They might not be safe for those at risk of stroke or heart attack.
- **Lasmiditan (Reyvow):** This newer oral tablet is now approved for the treatment of all types of migraine. Lasmiditan significantly improves headache pain. Lasmiditan can have sedative effects which cause dizziness, so the people taking it are advised not to drive or operate any machinery for at least 6–8 hours.
- **Opioid medications:** Many people who are not tolerating or able to take above discussed medicines, narcotic, and opioid medications might help. Because these drugs can lead to addiction, so, they are usually used only if no other treatments are effective.
- **Anti-nausea drugs:** These can help if migraine with aura is accompanied by nausea and vomiting. Anti-nausea drugs include chlorpromazine, and metoclopramide. These drugs are usually taken with pain medications. Many of these medications are not safe to take during pregnancy. If one is pregnant or trying to get pregnant, consult the doctor before using these medications.

Preventive medications

These medications can help to prevent frequent episodes of migraines. These are recommended in case of frequent, long-lasting, or severe headaches which are not responding well to treatment.

Preventive medication helps in reducing how often one gets the migraine, how severe the attacks are as well how long they last. Options include:

- **Blood pressure-lowering medications:** These include beta-blockers such as propranolol (Inderal, InnoPran XL, and others) and metoprolol tartrate (Lopressor). Calcium channel blockers such as verapamil (Verelan) can be helpful in preventing migraines with aura.
- **Antidepressants:** These include tricyclic antidepressants (amitriptyline) which can prevent migraines.
- **Anti-seizure drugs:** Topiramate and valproate (Topamax, etc.) might help in case of less frequent migraines. These medications lead to various side effects such as weight changes, dizziness, nausea, etc. These medications are not generally recommended for pregnant women or women planning to conceive.
- **Botox injections:** Injections of Ona botulinum toxin A (Botox) about every 12 weeks may help prevent migraines in some adults.
- **CGRP monoclonal antibodies** are newer drugs approved by the FDA to treat migraines. They are given monthly or quarterly by injection. The most common side effect is the reaction at the injection site.

c. Nutritional Considerations

Avoidance of certain foods and beverages has been effective for preventive and abortive therapy for headaches. Often trial and error results in eliminating foods and commercial additives that are headache triggers. A diary is useful in the elimination of foods and beverages that trigger headaches and to establish a healthy diet.

d. Psychosocial Considerations

- It is not surprising that individuals with a history of recurring headaches, which frequently disrupt their lives with pain, discomfort, and disability, often develop anxiety and depression.
- The holistic management of headaches includes assessment of individuals' ability to cope and effectively deal with the psychosocial implications.
- Antidepressants [e.g., tricyclic antidepressants and selective serotonin reuptake inhibitors (SSRIs)] are often part of the overall medication management.

Cluster Headache

Cluster headaches are a distinct clinical and epidemiologic type. They are also vascular but occur less frequently than migraine headaches. Cluster headaches have been described as one of the most severe forms of headache and occur predominantly in young men. They are often triggered by alcohol intake.

The typical age of onset is between the ages of 30 and 60 years. On the basis of their duration, cluster headaches are divided into two clinical types:

1. **Episodic cluster:** Occurs in cycles that may last 7 days to 12 months and are usually separated by a remission that may last 2 weeks.
2. **Chronic cluster:** Occurs in attacks that last approximately a year and have no remission, or a remission of less than 2 weeks
   - The onset is sudden, and the pain usually reaches a crescendo within 2–15 minutes.
   - These headaches are uncommon. Often the individual complains of extreme pain centered on or near one eye.
   - The pain is usually unilateral and occurs primarily in the ocular, frontal, or temporal areas.
   - With the activation of the autonomic nervous system, there is the occurrence of associated symptoms of conjunctival infection, photophobia, nasal stuffiness and/or rhinorrhea, forehead and facial sweating, and ipsilateral lacrimation, miosis, ptosis, or edema of the eyelid.
   - There is no nausea and vomiting. Instead, the symptoms may begin during sleep, with the individual awakening or crying out with complaints of a deep, penetrating steady pain.

Etiology/Pathophysiology

The pathophysiology is unknown but may be similar to that of migraine headaches (discussed earlier). The trigeminal nerve (CNV) is implicated in the production of pain. This activates the release of substance P and vasoactive substances.

Medical Management

The use of prophylactic, abortive, or analgesic therapy is appropriate. In addition, the calcium channel blocker (verapamil) and the serotonin antagonist methysergide, and other headache remedies may be used.

Tension Headache

Although typically not as severe as migraine, tension-type headaches are far commonest, with a lifetime prevalence in the general population of up to 80%. There is often a degree of associated disability, and this, combined with the high frequency, produces a significant socioeconomic impact. Tension-type headache is a dull, bilateral, mild-to-moderate intensity pressure—pain without striking associated features that may be categorized as infrequent, frequent, or chronic and are easily distinguished from migraine.

They are usually bilateral and last 30 minutes to 7 days. Patients complain of a dull, non-pulsatile, persistent pain in the back of the neck. Some individuals describe the experience as feeling as if their head were in a vise, squeezing without letup.

Tension headaches may be related to mood disorders, anxiety, or sleep problems. A combination of migraine and tension headache is not uncommon.

For tension headaches, pharmacotherapy is the mainstay of treatment. Monoamine oxidase inhibitor drugs have shown efficacy but are used only infrequently owing to the potential side effects. Nonmedication management techniques, including physical therapy and other manual therapies, various local injections, and counseling including cognitive behavior therapy, relaxation techniques, and biofeedback, may have limited benefit but have not been shown to be not equivocally effective in the treatment of headaches. Although acupuncture does not have proven efficacy in the treatment of tension-type headaches, a 2016 Cochrane analysis for migraine prevention found it to be effective in reducing the frequency of attacks.

Secondary Headache

Numerous secondary headaches are cataloged by ICHD. These include headaches attributed to infection, trauma, vascular disease, or homeostatic disorders, toxic or withdrawal headaches, and headaches due to nonvascular intracranial conditions.

Inclusion in the list of secondary headaches is based solely on the rigorous scientific literature support of the headache as having a secondary cause, and the headaches are viewed as secondary if headache begins or worsens in relation to the development of a pathologic condition and, further, if they clear or improve with the amelioration of the condition. Types include:

1. **Giant cell arteritis:** Giant cell arteritis is a granulomatous inflammatory vasculopathy affecting the medium and large-sized arteries, usually including the superficial temporal artery.
   - The disorder affects older individuals, especially women, with the mean age of 70 years. The most prominent clinical feature, occurring in a majority (90%) of patients, is the new-onset but fairly nonspecific headache.
   - Other symptoms include scalp tenderness and jaw claudication, and the condition may be associated with polymyalgia rheumatica in 50% of the patients.
   - Loss of vision can occur in up to 20% of patients.
   - The sedimentation rate and the C-reactive protein are usually raised, with a reported mean sedimentation rate of 70 mm/hour.
   - It is highly recommended that the high-dose steroid treatment is to be initiated immediately, followed by an early temporal artery biopsy. Newer noninvasive diagnostic modalities, such as the temporal artery ultrasound, that could simplify the diagnosis, are under review.

2. **Medication overuse headache:** Medication overuse headache involves the tendency among some to overuse abortive or analgesic medications in the management of migraine, leading ultimately not to the expected improvement but to the development of a more refractory headache pattern. With discontinuance, and after a latency, clinical improvement is described in approximately half of the patients. The mechanism is unclear, and the evidence for both the existence of and management of this often stigmatizing diagnosis is not rigorous, thus the value of sudden and complete removal of purportedly overused symptomatic medications is unclear and may produce unanticipated negative outcomes.

NURSING MANAGEMENT OF HEADACHE

Nursing Assessment

Thorough assessment of the patient complaining of headache is very important in order to diagnose a specific type for its appropriate management. Certain specific questions may include:

1. What is the location of the headache? Is it unilateral or bilateral? Does it radiate?
2. What is the quality? Is it dull, aching, steady, boring, burning, intermittent, continuous, and paroxysmal? How many headaches occur during a given period of time?
3. What are the precipitating factors, if any-environmental (e.g., sunlight, weather change), foods, exertion, etc.?
4. What makes the headache worse (e.g., coughing, straining)?
5. What time (day or night) does it occur?
6. How long does a typical headache last?
7. Are there any associated symptoms, such as facial lacrimation (excessive tearing), or scotomas (blind spots in the field of vision)?
8. What usually relieves the headache (aspirin, nonsteroidal anti-inflammatory drugs, ergot preparation, food, heat, rest, neck massage)?
9. Does nausea, vomiting, weakness, or numbness in the extremities accompany the headache? Does the headache interfere with daily activities?
10. Do you have any allergies?
11. Do you have insomnia, poor appetite, or loss of energy?
12. Is there a family history of headaches?
13. What is the relationship of the headache to your lifestyle? Is there any physical or emotional stress?

Nursing Diagnosis

Based on the assessment certain nursing diagnoses could be:

1. Acute pain/chronic pain (headache) related to intercerebral arterial vasoconstriction manifested by subjective complaints.
2. Disturbed sleep pattern related to pain and discomfort secondary to headache.
3. Anxiety related to the inability to predict the onset, duration, and outcome.
4. Hopelessness related to loss of control of headache symptoms and elimination of aggravating factors.
5. Deficient knowledge related to etiology, prevention, and treatment.

Nursing Interventions

- **Assess and monitor vital signs:** Vital signs may be altered during a patient's pain episode. Fluctuations can indicate whether a patient's condition is improving or worsening.
- **Teach patients nonpharmacologic pain management:** Nonpharmacologic pain management techniques like relaxation, darkness, cool compresses, and massage can help with pain relief.
- **Schedule activities during the peak effects of pain relievers:** The headache pain can be debilitating and prevent the patient from working, caring for family, and performing ADLs. Schedule nursing tasks and patient care when pain is most controlled.
- **Identify precipitating factors**: Migraine headaches can have triggers such as stress, too much caffeine or caffeine withdrawal, missed meals, weather changes, exhaustion, exposure to smoke or strong odors, and many more factors. Helping the patient identify the specific

instances of migraine occurrences can decrease episodes of headache.

- ❖ **Administer pain medications as indicated:** Over-the-counter (OTC) medications specific to migraines are available. Medications should be administered before the onset of the pain or during the prodrome phase when symptoms such as irritability or difficulty concentrating begin.
- ❖ **Patient teaching guide:** It is important to teach individuals how to self-manage their headaches.
- ❖ A headache diary is useful to help patients identify possible triggers, headache trends, and the efficacy of therapy for prevention and relief.
- ❖ Patients should understand how their diet could affect their headaches as well as be aware of potential environmental triggers for their headaches.
- ❖ Teaching the patient how and when to take the prescribed medication appropriately should not be overlooked.
- ❖ Patients with chronic headaches can become anxious over the anticipation of a potentially incapacitating headache.
- ❖ Overreliance on analgesic medication can then become an issue, especially since it can give rise to rebound headaches.
- ❖ Patterns of disability and pain behaviors may emerge, resulting in a significant impact on the patient's quality of life.
- ❖ Avoid factors that can trigger a headache:
  - ➢ Foods containing amines (cheese, chocolate), nitrites, vinegar, onions, fermented or marinated foods, monosodium glutamate, caffeine, nicotine, ice cream, alcohol, emotional stress, fatigue and medications such as ergot-containing and monoamine oxidase inhibitors.
- ❖ Use stress reduction techniques such as relaxation
- ❖ Participate in regular exercise
- ❖ Contact health care providers immediately if the following occur:
  - ➢ Symptoms become more severe, last longer than usual, or are resistant to medication
  - ➢ Nausea, vomiting, change in vision, or fever occur with the headache
  - ➢ Problems with medications

GERIATRIC CONSIDERATIONS

In elderly individuals, 2/3 of the headaches are the primary, such as tension-type headache or migraine; however, there is a 2 times higher risk of secondary causes, such as giant cell arteritis or intracranial lesions, than in younger adults. Management in older adults can be challenging because of the many multiple medical comorbidities as well as differences in drug metabolism and clearance.

> **Case Scenario**
>
> Seema reported in medical OPD that for the last few weeks, she is experiencing severe throbbing pain on the right side of her forehead above the ear level. After the headache begins, she feels nauseous and occasionally gets dizzy. When asked about the nature of dizziness, she reports that it lasts only as long as the headache, and does not increase with changes in position. What management should be done?

SUMMARY

Headache is the most common symptom of any disease. It may indicate a neurological disease or stress or combination of multiple factors. Its life long prevalence is 96% and is most common between ages of 15–49 years. Some headaches are familial. Headaches are broadly divided into primary and secondary headaches. It is important to identify the cause of headache in order to manage it properly.

MULTIPLE CHOICE QUESTIONS

1. Which of the following is not a primary headache?
   a. Migraine   b. Tension headache
   c. Cluster headache d. Meningitis
2. Which headache is life-threatening?
   a. Hypertension associated
   b. Meningitis
   c. Stroke-associated headache
   d. All the above
3. Which form of headache has features such as a rigid neck, high fever and altered mental status?
   a. Migraine   b. Tension headache
   c. Cluster headache d. Meningitis
4. Which of the following foods is a potential "trigger" for a migraine attack?
   a. Coffee, alcohol   b. Chocolate cheese
   c. MSG processed foods   d. All the above
5. Which type of headache is generally described as "a tight band-like discomfort involving the whole head"?
   a. Migraine   b. Tension headache
   c. Cluster headache d. Temporal arteritis
6. Cluster headache affects more men as compared to women. What is more common with cluster headaches?
   a. Pain can be eased with aspirin or ibuprofen
   b. Pain is severe around the eyes
   c. You see flashing lights
   d. Headache ends quickly

ANSWERS

| 1. d | 2. d | 3. d | 4. d |
| 5. b | 6. b | | |

SUGGESTED READING

1. Ellen B. Neuroscience nursing "spectrum of care", 2nd edition. Published by Mosby; 2002.
2. https://calgaryguide.ucalgary.ca/migraines-and-auras-pathogenesis-and-clinical-findings/
3. https://my.clevelandclinic.org/health/diseases/9639-headaches
4. https://thejournalofheadacheandpain.biomedcentral.com/articles/10.1186/s10194-022-01402-2/tables/1
5. https://www.mayoclinic.org/diseases-conditions/migraine-headache/diagnosis-treatment/drc-20360207
6. https://www.msdmanuals.com/en-in/home/brain,-spinal-cord,-and-nerve-disorders/headaches/overview-of-headache
7. https://www.nursetogether.com/headache-migraine-nursing-diagnosis-care-plan/#:~:text=The%20Nursing%20Process&text=Treatment%20usually%20includes%20medications%20like,and%20disability%20of%20the%20condition.
8. Johnn HV. The clinical practice of neurological and neurosurgical nursing, 7th edition. Published by Wolter Kluwer; 2013.
9. Sudddarth S and Brunner. A Textbook of Medical-Surgical-Nursing, 11th edition. Published by Lippincott Williams and Wilkins; 2008. pp. 1147-9.

EPILEPSY

One of the most prevalent, persistent, and diverse neurological illnesses, epilepsy is characterized by recurrent, unprovoked seizures. Generally speaking, there are three types of epilepsy: idiopathic, symptomatic, and cryptogenic. When there is a potential genetic predisposition but no known underlying cause, epilepsy is referred to as idiopathic. A known or suspected central nervous system (CNS) illness is thought to be the cause of symptomatic epilepsies and syndromes. A condition whose cause is masked is referred to as cryptogenic. The etiology of cryptogenic epilepsies is unknown.

A seizure is a single episode of jerky movements and epilepsy is the occurrence of two or more than two unprovoked jerky movements or seizures in an individual, irrespective of the duration of seizures and or the gap between two seizure episodes.

TYPES OR CLASSIFICATION OF SEIZURES

Typically, seizures are classified as focal or generalized.

Focal Seizures

Electrical activity in one part of the brain causes focal seizures. This kind of seizure may cause loss of consciousness

- ❖ **Focal seizures with loss of awareness or consciousness**: These seizures cause a shift in consciousness or loss of awareness that feels like a dream. Even though they may appear conscious, people experiencing these seizures simply stare off into space and are unresponsive to their surroundings. They might make repetitive mouth movements, hand rubbing motions, word repetitions, or circular walking. They might not even be aware of having had a seizure or remembering it.
- ❖ **Focal seizures without loss of consciousness:** These type of seizures might alter how things sound, feel, appear, smell, and taste. But there is no loss of consciousness as a result of the seizures and it lasts for a minute or even less than one minute.
  People experiencing these seizures may find themselves suddenly feeling angry, happy, or depressed. Some people experience nausea or other strange, difficult-to-explain sensations. Speaking difficulties and uncontrollable jerking of a bodily part, like an arm or a leg, might be symptoms of these seizures. Additionally, they could result in acute sensory sensations as tingling, vertigo, and seeing flashing lights.

Generalized Seizures

These types of seizures are defined as seizures that appear to affect all parts of the brain from the moment they begin. Generalized seizures come in various forms, including:

Absence Seizure (Formerly known as Petit Mal Seizure)

This type of seizure is usually found in children. A person experiencing an absence seizure will generally stare out into space or make small, non-verbal motions like blinking their eyes or smacking their lips. They normally last between five and ten seconds. The frequency of these seizures can reach hundreds each day. They might appear in groups and bring on a momentary loss of consciousness.

Tonic Seizures

The muscles become tight during tonic seizures. Typically, the back, arms, and legs muscles are impacted by these seizures. These seizures can cause people to lose consciousness and drop to the ground.

Atonic Seizures

Muscle control is lost during atonic seizures, commonly referred to as drop seizures. People experiencing this kind of seizure may drop their heads or suddenly fall to the ground.

Clonic Seizures (Seizures with Clonus)

Muscle jerks that are repeated during clonic seizures are common. The neck, face, and arms on both sides of the body are typically affected by these seizures.

Myoclonic Seizures (Seizures with Myoclonus)

Typical symptoms of myoclonic seizures are quick, short jerks or twitches in the arms and legs. In many cases, there is no loss of consciousness.

Tonic-clonic Seizures (Seizures with Tonic Clonus)

The most severe kind of epileptic seizures are tonic-clonic seizures, also referred to as grand mal seizures. They may result in an abrupt loss of consciousness, rigidity, and trembling. Sometimes they make patients bite their tongues or lose control of their bladder. They might go on for a while. Additionally, tonic-clonic seizures can begin as focal seizures before spreading to affect most or all of the brain.

EPIDEMIOLOGY

Epilepsy is the 4th most common neurological disorders. It affects 1-2% of the population globally. Approximately 50 million people are affected from it worldwide. The prevalence rate of epilepsy is 0.5-1% in India. The rate of prevalence is greater in rural areas than urban areas.

ETIOLOGY

The etiology of epilepsy depends on the type of seizure and age of patient. In infants, the causes of epilepsy are intracranial insult during birth, hypoxia, febrile, inherited malformation of the brain, metabolic disorders and sometimes infections. In adolescent and adults, other than trauma and infection, idiopathic epilepsy is also the main cause of epilepsy.

PATHOPHYSIOLOGY

The imbalance between the release of excitatory and inhibitory neurotransmitters—more release of excitatory neurotransmitters and less release of inhibitory neurotransmitters—is what causes epilepsy. Glutamate (Glu), for example, is the primary excitatory neurotransmitter of the CNS. Glu is linked to a number of receptors. Each of these exerts an excitatory impact over the postsynaptic neuron.

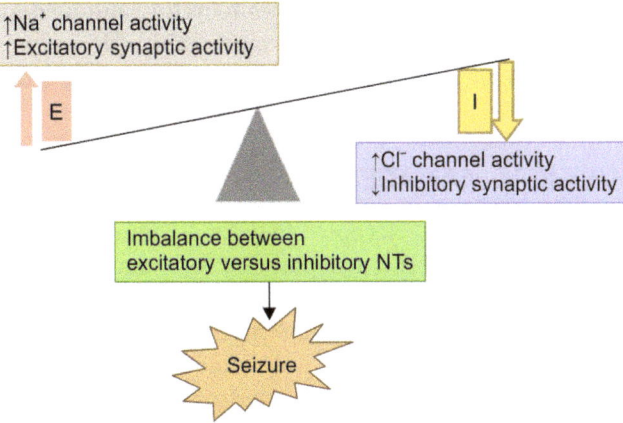

E: Excitatory, I: Inhibitory, NTs: Neurotransmitters
Fig. 33.3: Pathophysiology of epilepsy.

NMDA receptors, for example, are ligand-operated cation channels, and attachment of Glu causes the channel to open. The inflow of Na⁺ depolarizes the neuron's membrane, increasing the likelihood that it will reach fire threshold. Similarly, Inhibitory neurotransmitters, such as GABA, which is the primary CNS equivalent of glu, work by activating Cl channels linked with the GABA-A receptor. The inflow of negative charge hyperpolarizes the neuron, raising the firing threshold and causing the postsynaptic neuron to fire less frequently as shown in **Figure 33.3**.

CLINICAL MANIFESTATIONS

Clinical signs and symptoms of the seizures depend on the site of the focus and its spreading to other body parts. If the discharges initiate in one part of hemisphere, then it is known as partial or focused seizures, when it originates from both hemispheres simultaneously then the condition is known as generalized and sometimes it originates from one side and spread to other part then it is known as partial seizure with generalized epilepsy. During the tonic phase, which lasts 20–30 seconds and is followed by a momentary stoppage of respiratory movements and central cyanosis, there is a sudden loss of consciousness. The clonic phase follows, with jerky movements of the limbs and face. The movements gradually cease, and the individual may fall asleep for a while before waking up disoriented and irritated. This is also called seizure semiology.

The type of seizure (focused or generalized) affects the symptoms differently. Additionally, they might be minor to severe. Seizure signs and symptoms may include:
- Temporary confusion.
- Staring.
- Uncontrollable jerking movements of the arms and legs.
- Loss of awareness or consciousness (in moderate to severe seizures).
- Alterations in emotions or cognition. Deja vu, often known as the fear or worry of living this situation again, is also experienced by the patients.

DIAGNOSTIC MODALITIES

Epilepsy can be diagnosed by taking the patient's history (like age, native place, symptoms experienced by the patients, any family history of epilepsy, any insult to the brain, any history of epilepsy, duration of the seizure, frothing, defecation or micturition during the seizure, etc.). After that, imaging techniques like CT scan, MRI and EEG can also help in the diagnosis of epilepsy.

EEG

The most efficient method for diagnosing epilepsy is electroencephalography (EEG). When an abnormal EEG is noticed, it aids in determining if the seizure is focal or generalized, and it might additionally rule out the patient's epilepsy syndrome. The seizure is focused when the EEG shows a localization of the electrical discharge. Pathologic high frequency oscillations (pHFOs), which are short EEG occurrences in the range of 100 to 600 Hertz, are detected in generalized epilepsy. On the other hand, MRI helps in detecting tumors (mostly present in frontal or temporal region of the brain with little or no swelling or fluid around the tumors), structural abnormalities of the brain during the delivery time, mesial temporal sclerosis, vascular malformations like arteriovenous malformation or cavernous hemangioma, gliosis, neurocysticercosis, etc., as all these changes in the brain contributes in generating seizures in epileptic patients.

Magnetic Resonance Imaging (MRI)

Strong magnets and radiowaves are used in an MRI scan to produce a detailed image of your brain. A brain MRI may reveal alterations that could cause seizures.

Computed Tomography (CT)

A CT scan produces cross-sectional images of brain using X-rays. Brain's alterations that could lead to a seizure can be seen during a CT scan. Tumors, bleeding, and cysts are some examples of these changes.

Positron Emission Tomography (PET)

A small quantity of low-dose radioactive material is injected into a vein for a PET scan. The information aids in identifying the brain's active regions and spotting changes.

Single-Photon Emission Computed Tomography (SPECT)

A small quantity of low-dose radioactive material is injected into a vein during a SPECT exam. A thorough 3D map of the blood flow in brain that takes place during a seizure is produced by the test.

MEDICAL MANAGEMENT

Antiepileptic drugs (AEDs) are still the mainstay of epilepsy treatment. Based on the type of epilepsy being diagnosed, antiepileptic medications are chosen. Antiepileptic medications work to reduce neuronal hyperexcitability, but they can also have unintended side effects. AEDs are used to treat epilepsy depending on a number of variables, including seizure type, concurrent medication therapy, and efficacy of AEDs, ADR prevention, and environmental factors. The main challenge in optimizing AED therapy is managing, preventing, and treating side effects. No AED has been proven to be particularly successful in treating epilepsy, and most AEDs have well-known adverse effects. Patients who have just been diagnosed with epilepsy can be given first-line, conventional AEDs such as phenytoin (PHT) (dosage: 4–8 mg/kg), carbamazepine (CBZ) (dosage: 15–30 mg/kg), phenobarbital (PB) (dosage: 4–6 mg/kg), or valproic acid (VPA) (dosage: 15–50 mg/kg), and the dose of the drugs depend on the body weight of the patients. However, a lot of newer AEDs have been developed over the past ten years, including lamotrigine, levetiracetam, oxcarbazepine, zonisamide, topiramate, and gabapentin. They all perform the same functions, which include preventing neuronal excitement or increasing neuronal inhibition by pharmacological processes that alter voltage-gated cation channels, block glutamatergic processes, enhance GABAergic activity, and change the neurotransmitters release. A number of AEDs attach to the sodium channel when it is inactive, aiding in the voltage- and frequency-dependent decline of conduction. With the exception of lacosamide, which is a slow inactivator of sodium channels, CBZ, PHT, LTG (lamotrigine), and OXC (oxcarbazepine) affect fast sodium channel inactivation. If necessary, these AEDs can be administered concurrently because they each have a unique mode of action. AEDs with comparable mechanisms of action, however, may cause neurological adverse effects such as dizziness, diplopia, sleepiness, headache, ataxia, and nystagmus when taken simultaneously. Some AEDs, including zonisamide, felbamate, rufinamide, and topiramate, also have an effect on sodium channels; however, it is not yet known whether this binding is connected to these drugs' pharmacological effects or not. Rufinamide, which is recommended for partial seizures but has only little effectiveness, is more successful in treating children who have generalized seizures associated with Lennox-Gastaut syndrome (LGS). Some AEDs inhibit calcium channels that are triggered at low or high voltages, preventing depolarization and the release of neurotransmitters, such as ethosuximide, which only affects T-type calcium channels. Pregabalin and gabapentin bind to the high voltage-activated calcium channels' $\alpha 2\delta$ subunit and reduce anxiety, neuropathic pain, and epileptic seizures. Numerous broad-spectrum AEDs, including zonisamide, topiramate, lamotrigine, and levetiracetam bind to voltage-activated calcium channels in various ways. A few AEDs affect the GABA-A receptor, either by increasing their sensitivity to synaptically released GABA (benzodiazepines, barbiturates), or by altering the synthesis (sodium valproate), re-uptake (tiagabine), or metabolism (vigabatrin) of GABA at the synapses. Topiramate, levetiracetam, and felbamate all control GABA-A receptor responses. Numerous AEDs with a broad spectrum of efficacy in a variety of seizure types, including sodium valproate, felbamate, topiramate, zonisamide, and likely rufinamide, have numerous mechanisms of action (MOA). Some of these AEDs, including felbamate, zonisamide, and topiramate, block particular glutamate receptor subtypes, which decreases rapid excitatory neurotransmission. When levetiracetam binds to synaptic vesicle protein 2A (SV 2A), it interferes with synaptic vesicles recycling and prevents the release of several neurotransmitters. The action of these drugs on various neurotransmitters is shown in **Figures 33.4A and B**.

SURGICAL MANAGEMENT

This is the generally accepted benchmark for determining refractoriness and the acceptability for consideration of resective epilepsy surgery given the poor likelihood of response to medical therapy following the failure of two AEDs. Although the percentage of individuals who may benefit from surgery is unclear, it is assumed to be no more than 2% of the entire cohort. With a 0.5% incidence and a 7,50,000 prevalence in the USA, there could be up to 3,500 incident cases and 15,000 prevalent cases when surgery is an option. For more than 20 years, the number of epilepsy surgeries has remained constant at about 1,500 cases annually.

Surgery could be an option if at least two anti-seizure medications are ineffective. Surgery aims to prevent seizures from occurring. The best candidates for surgery are those whose seizures always start in the same region of the brain. The different types of epilepsy surgeries are temporal lobe surgery, other areas of the brain like frontal, occipital or parietal, removal of corpus callosum, lesionectomy, hemispherectomy, etc. These procedures can reduce the frequency of seizures for many years, but physicians recommend these types of crucial surgeries in those patients only in which the patients are expected to get benefit.

- ❖ **Lobectomy:** Generally, neurosurgeons remove the small portion (lobe) of brain from where seizures originate.
- ❖ **Laser interstitial thermal treatment, commonly known as thermal ablation:** With this less intrusive technique, a precise region in the brain where seizures start is targeted with highly concentrated energy. This kills the seizure-causing brain cells.
- ❖ **Multiple subpial transection (MST):** In order to stop seizures, this kind of surgery requires numerous cuts being made in the brain. When the part of the brain where seizures begin cannot be safely removed, it is typically done.
- ❖ **Corpus callosotomy:** The network of connections between the neurons in the right and left sides of the brain is severed during this procedure. Seizures that originate in one half of the brain and spread to the other are treated with this. However, seizures may continue to happen on the side of the brain where they first occurred even after surgery.
- ❖ **Hemispherotomy:** One side of the brain is completely cut off from the other side and the body after this surgery. Only when medication fails to control seizures or when seizures only affect half the brain is this sort of surgery utilized. Following this procedure, many daily functional abilities could be lost. But with therapy, youngsters can frequently regain such skills.
- ❖ **Electrical stimulation or arousal:** Devices that give electrical stimulation may be helpful if the part of the brain where seizures begin cannot be removed or detached. Together with ongoing anti-seizure medication use, they

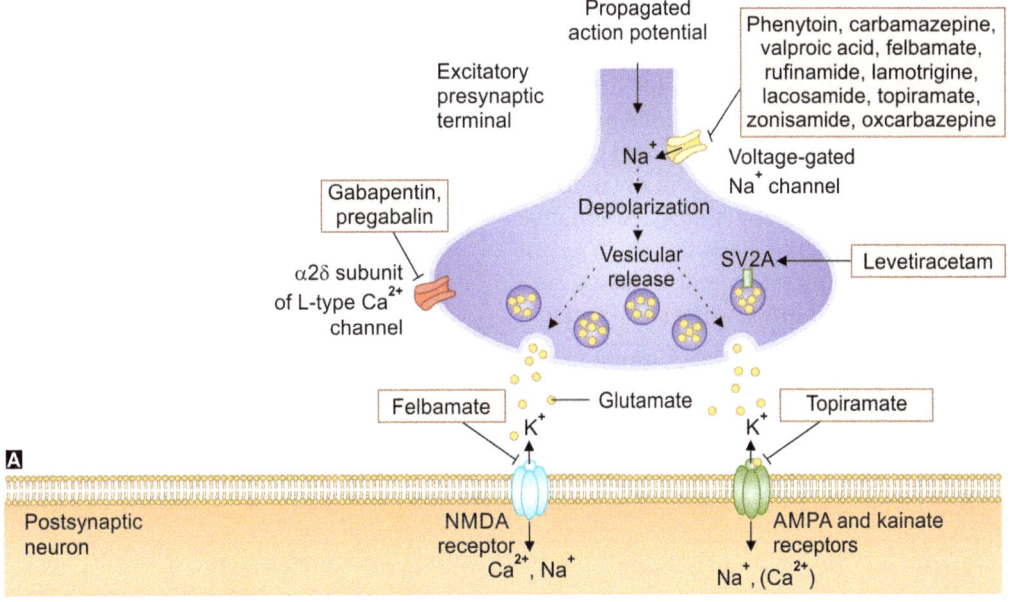

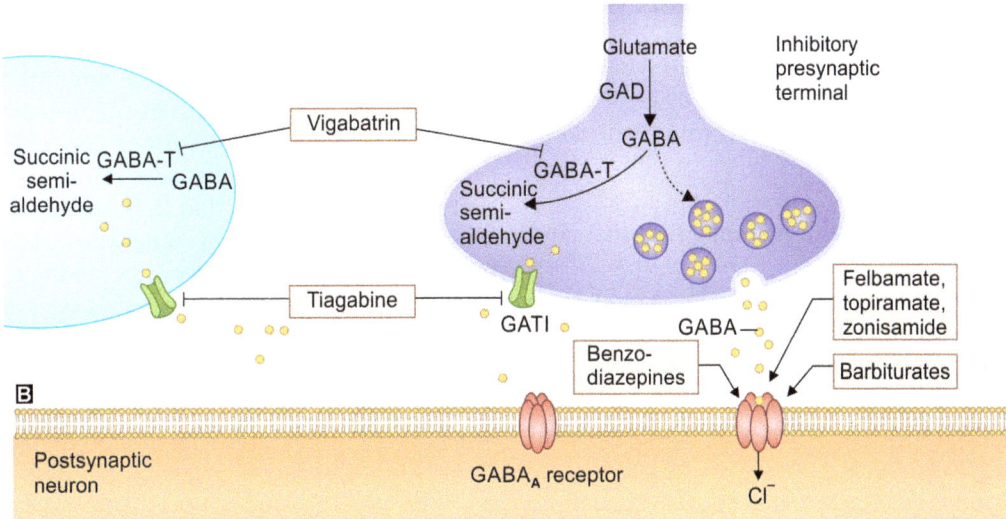

Figs. 33.4A and B: Proposed mechanisms of action of currently available antiepileptic drugs (AEDs) at excitatory and inhibitory synapses: (A) Excitatory synapse; (B) Inhibitory synapse.
(*Courtesy:* Liefferinge J V et al, 2013)

can lessen seizures. The following are stimulation tools that could reduce seizure frequency.

- ❖ **Vagus nerve stimulation (VNS):** The vagus nerve in the neck is stimulated by a device inserted beneath the skin of the chest, which causes the brain to receive messages that prevent seizures.
- ❖ **Responsive neurostimulation:** On the outside of the brain or inside brain tissue, a device is implanted. When a seizure is detected, the gadget can give electrical stimulation to stop it.
- ❖ **Deep brain stimulation (DBS):** To generate electrical impulses, surgeons implant tiny wires called electrodes inside specific regions of the brain. The brain activity that results in seizures is controlled by the impulses. Under the skin of the chest, a pacemaker-like device with electrodes is positioned. This regulates the level of stimulation generated **(Fig. 33.5)**.

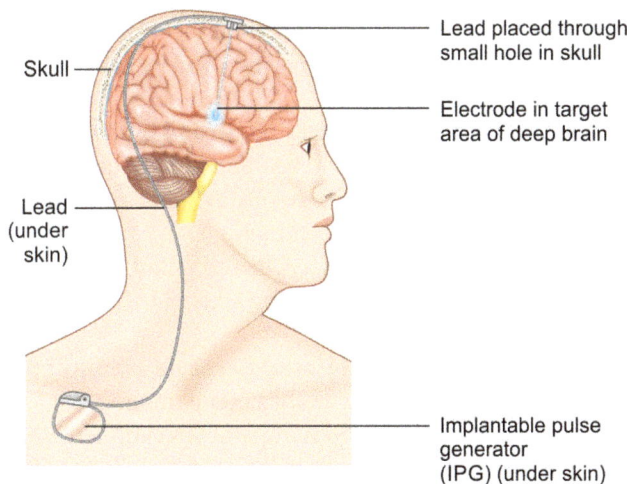

Fig. 33.5: Deep brain stimulation (DBS).

DIETETICS

The ketogenic diet (KD), which consists of a low-carb, high-fat, and adequate protein diet, is a recognized, efficient nonpharmacologic therapy option for intractable pediatric epilepsy. Although KD was introduced in 1921 and has had an increase in usage over the past ten years, many medical experts are not familiar with this therapy strategy. Alternative and more adaptable KD versions have been created in recent years to make the medication more acceptable, lessen side effects, and make it more accessible to a wider set of patients with refractory epilepsy.

NURSING MANAGEMENT

The main aim of the nursing management is to minimize the adverse effects associated with AEDs. Following are the various management parameters:
- The seizures must be stopped as soon as feasible.
- Maintain the patient's seizure-free condition and ensure adequate brain oxygenation.
- The establishment of an airway and appropriate oxygenation.
- If the patient does not wake up or respond, an endotracheal tube with a cuff should be introduced.
- Monitoring and evaluation of heart and respiratory function.
- Sedatives and various AEDs.
- Observing and recording the patient's response and seizure activity.
- If at all possible, the patient is shifted to a side-lying position to aid in the drainage of pharyngeal secretions.
- The IV line should be carefully observed.
- Drug compliance
- **Patient education:** The following actions can be taken to aid in seizure control:
  - Use medication as directed. Without first consulting your healthcare practitioner, do not change the dosage. Discuss with your provider any changes you think should be made to your medication.
  - Get adequate rest. Sleep deprivation can cause seizures. Make sure you get enough sleep every night.
  - Don a bracelet with a medical alert. If you suffer another seizure, emergency responders will be better equipped to treat you.
  - **Exercise:** Being physically active and exercising may help you maintain good health and fight depression. If you get fatigued while exercising, make sure to drink enough water and take a break.
  - Lead a healthy lifestyle. A healthy lifestyle includes controlling stress, consuming alcohol in moderation, and quitting smoking.
  - Use caution around water. Never go swimming or boating by yourself without a companion.
  - Protect yourself by donning a helmet when riding a bike and engaging in sports.

First Aid Management of Fit

Take the following actions to assist someone having a seizure:
- Gently roll the person to one side.
- Put a soft object beneath the person's head.
- If wearing tight neckwear, loosen it.
- Avoid putting anything in the person's mouth, even your fingers.
- Avoid attempting to stop someone from having a seizure.
- Remove potentially hazardous items if the victim is moving.
- Remain with the person until assistance from a doctor arrives.
- Keep a careful eye on the individual in order to describe the seizure in detail.
- Note down the time of onset and duration of seizure.
- Stay calm.

STATUS EPILEPTICUS

Status epilepticus is characterized by prolonged or recurrent seizures that, if untreated, can result in brain injury, severe impairment, coma, and death in both children and adults. While convulsive status epilepticus is often diagnosed clinically, nonconvulsive status epilepticus needs EEG confirmation. Early control of seizures remains critical in preventing status epilepticus consequences. This is especially true with convulsive status epilepticus, when there is more evidence that therapy improves outcomes. When status epilepticus becomes resistant, frequently as a result of GABA and NMDA receptor modification, anesthetic medications are required to suppress seizure activity. It can be treated with a continuous intramuscular midazolam or intravenous lorazepam, thiopental or pentobarbital, but there is limited information on the selection, dose, and duration of their usage. Thus, the treatment objectives and severity of therapy are still being debated, particularly in the case of nonconvulsive status epilepticus, when prolonged therapeutic coma might lead to severe consequences.

GERIATRIC CONSIDERATIONS

The prevalence of epilepsy rises with age. These age groups have particular treatment challenges like recurrent comorbidities and, by extension, numerous comedications are added to physiological ageing, which affects the metabolism of many medicines. Comorbidities include cardiovascular, renal, hepatic, neurological, mental, and degenerative conditions. In comparison to the old AEDs, the many new ones that are now available have not been very effective. According to studies, new compounds are more well-tolerated and have higher compliance rates. They also have less interactions with comedications than previous AEDs, some just require a single daily dose, and rigorous biological control is not required. Thus, at the moment, these developments has increased the complexity of managing epilepsy while simultaneously enabling better individualized care for elderly patients.

Case Scenario

1. A female patient, 24 years old, resident of rural, Punjab came to the Neurology Department, PGIMER, Chandigarh, with past history of generalized tonic-clonic seizures. She was started on phenytoin (PHT) 300 mg BD for last one year. She was showing the signs of gum hyperplasia, hirsutism, ataxia, nystagmus, tremors. So, she was having signs of phenytoin induced toxicity. Her MRI brain was normal and EEG showed abnormal and suggestive of diffuse epileptiform discharges. Her PHT levels were more than 30 µg/mL. Normal range is 10–20 µg/mL. The neurologists then decreased the PHT dosage from 300 mg BD to 200 mg BD. After few days, PHT-induced toxicity was reversed.
2. A male patient, 22 years old, resident of urban, Haryana came to Neurology Department, PGIMER, Chandigarh, with past history of simple partial with secondary generalization. He was started on carbamazepine 200 mg BD, but after a few days of initiating of therapy, he came to OPD with skin rash. The neurologist then tapered the medicine and started levetiracetam 250 mg BD, and gradually increasing up to 500 mg BD. The skin rash after few says subsided.

SUMMARY

Epilepsy's effects might last far longer than just the brief intervals when seizures happen. The quality of life and "wellness" of the person with epilepsy, as well as that of their family members can be considerably negatively impacted by negative effects on mental, physical, and social health, which has a large cost to society. The healthcare professionals need to be well-versed with the hazards associated with epilepsy. Early detection, treatment, and counselling is required. Additional research and data to inform management are desperately needed in several fields, such as the treatment of depression associated with epilepsy, side effects of AEDs, etc.

MULTIPLE CHOICE QUESTIONS

1. Which of the following is false about epilepsy?
    a. Single seizure
    b. Chronic
    c. Unavoidable circumstance
    d. Heterogenous
2. Main difference between simple partial and complex partial seizure is:
    a. Acute or chronic
    b. Less or more time
    c. Consciousness or unconsciousness
    d. Absence or presence of aura
3. All are excitatory neurotransmitters, *except*:
    a. AMPA
    b. NMDA
    c. GABA
    d. Glutamate
4. Choose the most important reason for the precipitation of seizure.
    a. Increased glutamate, increased GABA
    b. Increased AMPA, increased GABA
    c. Increased glutamate, decreased GABA
    d. Decreased glutamate, increased GABA
5. Which of these AEDs is a newer AED?
    a. Carbamazepine
    b. Lamotrigine
    c. Phenytoin
    d. Valproate
6. Epilepsy is a disorder of:
    a. Cardiovascular
    b. Central nervous system
    c. Reproductive
    d. Urology
7. Spina bifida can be caused by long-term use of which drug?
    a. Carbamazepine
    b. Phenytoin
    c. Lamotrigine
    d. Sodium valproate
8. Keto diet is:
    a. High carbohydrates, low fat, high protein
    b. Low fat, low carbohydrates, high protein
    c. Low protein, low fat, low carbohydrates
    d. High protein, low carbohydrates, high fat
9. Which of these AEDs is a conventional AED?
    a. Zonisamide
    b. Lamotrigine
    c. Levetiracetam
    d. Carbamazepine
10. Which of the following AED is a slow inactivator of sodium channel?
    a. Oxcarbazepine
    b. Lacosamide
    c. Phenytoin
    d. Carbamazepine
11. Which of the following AED is more useful in treating Lennox-Gastaut syndrome?
    a. Zonisamide
    b. Rufinamide
    c. Oxcarbazepine
    d. Gabapentin
12. Which of the following AED affects T-type calcium channels?
    a. Rufinamide
    b. Oxcarbazepine
    c. Pregabalin
    d. Ethosuximide
13. Which of the following drug is used to treat neuropathic pain also?
    a. Pregabalin
    b. Levetiracetam
    c. Lamotrigine
    d. Topiramate
14. Levetiracetam acts via receptor:
    a. SV2A
    b. GABA-A
    c. T-Type calcium channels
    d. Na channel
15. What is the prevalence of epilepsy globally?
    a. 1–2%
    b. 5–10%
    c. 10–20%
    d. 6–7%
16. Incidence of seizure is high in which age group?
    a. Infants
    b. Early childhood and late adulthood
    c. Middle age
    d. Old age
17. Epilepsy is caused by:
    a. Increase in excitatory neurotransmitters
    b. Decrease in inhibitory neurotransmitters
    c. Both A and B
    d. There is no role of neurotransmitters in epilepsy
18. A 22 years old male patient came to OPD with a history of seizures. His EEG and MRI were normal. Which type of epilepsy he has?
    a. Idiopathic
    b. Symptomatic
    c. Cryptogenic
    d. Both B and C
19. A 30 years old male patient came to OPD. His mother told the doctor that last night he had seizures. The patient's right hand had tonic-clonic movements, then the whole body had tonic-clonic seizures. He also fell down and became unconscious for 40–60 seconds. The probable type of seizure is:
    a. Partial seizure
    b. Generalized tonic-clonic seizure
    c. Partial seizure with secondary generalization
    d. Myoclonic
20. Refractory epilepsy is:
    a. When patients are on monotherapy and seizures are under control
    b. When patients are on polytherapy and seizures are under control

c. When patients are on monotherapy and seizures are uncontrolled
d. When patients are on polytherapy and seizures are uncontrolled

ANSWERS			
1. a	2. c	3. c	4. c
5. b	6. b	7. d	8. d
9. d	10. b	11. b	12. d
13. a	14. a	15. a	16. b
17. c	18. a	19. c	20. d

SUGGESTED READING

1. Aggarwal R, Sharma M, Modi M, Kumar GV, Salaria M. HLA-B × 1502 is associated with carbamazepine induced Stevens-Johnson syndrome in North Indian population. Hum Immunol [Internet]. 2014;75(11):1120-2. Available from: http://dx.doi.org/10.1016/j.humimm.2014.09.022
2. Bhathena A, Spear BB. Pharmacogenetics: improving drug and dose selection. Curr Opin Pharmacol. 2008;8(5):639-46.
3. Brodie MJ. Antiepileptic drug therapy the story so far. Seizure [Internet]. 2010;19(10):650-5. Available from: http://dx.doi.org/10.1016/j.seizure.2010.10.027
4. deShazo RD, Kemp MSF. Allergic reactions to drugs and biological agents. JAMA [Internet]. 1997;278(22):1895-906. Available from: http://www.ncbi.nlm.nih.gov/pubmed/1433700
5. Garg V, Goyal M, Khullar M, Saikia B, Medhi B, Prakash A, et al. Presence of allele CYP3A4 × 16 does not have any bearing on carbamazepine-induced adverse drug reactions in North Indian people with epilepsy. Indian J Pharmacol [Internet]. 2020 [cited 2021 Feb 6];52(5):378. Available from: https://pubmed.ncbi.nlm.nih.gov/33283769/
6. Garg VK, Goel N, Singh S, Kashyap D. Phenytoin in Personalized Medicine. EC Neurol. 2018;10(8):727-8.
7. Manford M. Recent advances in epilepsy. J Neurol [Internet]. 2017;264(8):1811-24. Available from:pmc/articles/PMC5533817/
8. Modi M, Singh R, Goyal M, Gairolla J, Singh G, Rishi V, et al. Prevalence of epilepsy and its association with exposure to Toxocara canis: A community-based, case-control study from rural Northern India [Internet]. Vol. 22, Annals of Indian Academy of Neurology. Wolters Kluwer Medknow Publications; 2019 [cited 2021 Feb 6]. p. 533. Available from: https://pubmed.ncbi.nlm.nih.gov/31736600/
9. Modi M, Singh R, Goyal MK, Gairolla J, Singh G, Rishi V, et al. Prevalence of Epilepsy and its Association with Exposure to Toxocara canis: A Community Based, Case-control Study from Rural Northern India. Ann Indian Acad Neurol [Internet]. 2018 [cited 2021 Feb 6];21(4):263-9. Available from: http://www.ncbi.nlm.nih.gov/pubmed/30532354
10. Pamplona MM, Paris CM, Bethesda RJP, Shizuoka MS, Wolf P, Angeles EL, et al. Proposal for Revised Classification of Epilepsies and Epileptic Syndromes. 1989;30(389).
11. Potschka H. Pharmacological treatment strategies: Mechanisms of antiepileptic drugs. Epileptology [Internet]. 2013;1(1):31-7. Available from: http://dx.doi.org/10.1016/j.epilep.2012.11.004
12. Schachter SC. Seizure disorders. Med Clin North Am. 2009;93(2):343-51. 2009;93(2):343-51.
13. Sirot E, Baumann, P. Therapeutic Drug Monitoring and Pharmacogenetic Tests in Pharmacovigilance—When and What? European Psychiatry 2009;24(S1):1-1. doi:10.1016/S0924-9338(09)70340-2.
14. Sridharan R, Murthy BN. Prevalence and pattern of epilepsy in India. Epilepsia. 1999;40(5):631-6.
15. Van Liefferinge J, Massie A, Portelli J, Di Giovanni G, Smolders I. Are vesicular neurotransmitter transporters potential treatment targets for temporal lobe epilepsy? Front Cell Neurosci. 2013; 7:1-24.

RESTLESS LEG SYNDROME

Restless legs syndrome (RLS) is also known as Willis-Ekbom disease. In this there is a strong urge to move the lower extremity. The patient experiences uncontrolled sensation like itching, pulling, moving, crawling, burning, etc. It is a genetic and also associated with many conditions, diseases, and medications.

This sensation usually occurs in an individual when lying down in bed or while sitting for a long period of time like while long drives, watching a movie in the theater, etc. Symptoms usually occur in the evening. Some time it makes patient difficult to fall asleep.

ETIOLOGY

Genetics: RLS has been found to be a genetic syndrome in some cases. So, there is chance of disease transfer from parent to their children. Around 92% of the patients have their first degree relative with the same history.

Age: People of any age can have RLS. It may begin in childhood or adulthood. But chances of having this problem increase with the age.

Gender: It is more common in women as compared to the men.

In addition, there are many medical conditions which are also associated with the development of RLS, including anemia, uremia, hypothyroidism, depression, fibromyalgia, Parkinson's disease, kidney disease, diabetes, rheumatoid arthritis, Peripheral neuropathy, Pregnancy, Dialysis, medications like antidepressants, anti-allergy drugs, anti-nausea medication, etc. Caffeine, nicotine and alcohol can also make the symptoms worse.

Clinical Manifestations

Leg discomfort: These usually describe by the patients as creeping, burning, itching, crawling, tugging, pulling, throbbing, etc., invariably occurring at inactivity time, mostly at night bed time.

Urge to move leg: Uncontrolled impulse to move limb during prolonged resting time.

Sleep disruption:
- Bedtime behavior problems
- Day time sleepiness
- Behavior and work performance problems due to sleeplessness.

Diagnostic Test

There is no specific test for restless syndrome. The diagnosis is made based on the symptoms. A complete medical history, physical, neurological examination, blood test may be conducted to rule out any other possible health problems associated with RLS. An overnight sleep study may be recommended to evaluate for sleep disorders.

For diagnosis of RLS the five criteria as shown in **Figure 33.6** need to be met.

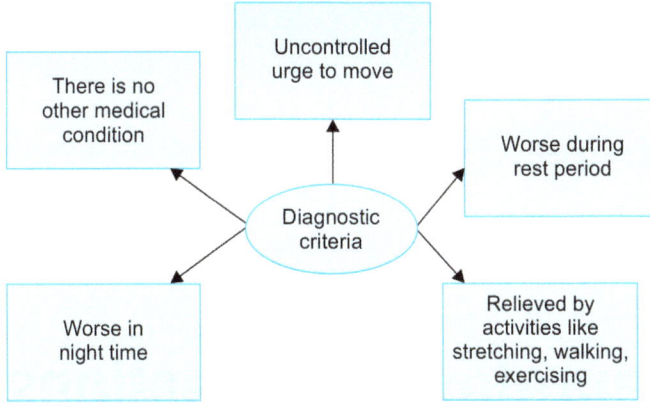

Fig. 33.6: Diagnosis of RLS.

MANAGEMENT

Treatment of RLS depends on the intensity of symptoms. Treatment should be taken only if quality of life is affected by insomnia, excessive day time drowsiness.

Non-pharmacological interventions: Non-drug treatments are tried first, if symptoms are mild. These include:
- Getting regular exercise, such as riding a bike, physical exercises within a few hours of bedtime.
- Follow good sleep habits. Avoid reading, watching TV before sleep.
- Avoiding or limiting caffeine containing foods
- Apply heating pad, cold compressor rubbing your legs to provide temporary relief.
- Soak in a warm tub

Medical Management
- Magnesium supplements.
- Iron supplement.
- In severe symptoms can give:
  - Dopamine agonists which can control the urge to move, sensory symptoms in the legs, e.g., ropinirole patch, pramipexole, etc., are FDA approved dopamine agonist.
  - Antiseizure medications can slow or block signals from nerves in the legs.
  - Benzodiazepine can be given in very severe symptoms.
  - Opioids like methadone, oxycodone can also be used only in severe cases, these drugs have very severe addiction properties.

GERIATRIC CONSIDERATIONS

Chances of restless leg syndrome increases with the increase in the age of the person. As it may disturb the sleep pattern, so the elderly persons need to be observed very carefully.

SUGGESTED READING

1. American Academy of Sleep Medicine Clinical Practice Guideline. The Treatment of Restless Legs Syndrome and Periodic Limb Movement Disorder in Adults—An Update for 2012: Practice Parameters with an Evidence-Based Systematic Review and Meta-Analyses. (https://j2vjt3dnbra3ps7ll1clb4q2-wpengine.netdna-ssl.com/wp-content/uploads/2017/07/TreatmentRLS.pdf) Accessed 8/4/23
2. American Sleep Association. About Restless Legs Syndrome (https://www.sleepassociation.org/patients-general-public/restless-legs-syndrome/) Accessed 8/4/23
3. Avecillas JF, Golish JA, Giannini C, Yataco JC. Restless legs syndrome: Keys to recognition and treatment. Cleve Clinic J Med. 2005;72(9):769-87. Accessed 8/4/23.
4. National Sleep Foundation. Restless Legs Syndrome Diagnosis. (https://www.sleepfoundation.org/articles/restless-legs-syndrome-diagnosis) Accessed 8/4/23.
5. Restless Legs Syndrome Foundation. Understanding RLS. (https://www.rls.org/understanding-rls) Accessed 8/4/23.
6. Restless syndrome. https://my.clevelandclinic.org/health/diseases/9497-restless-legs-syndrome accessed 8/4/23.

CHAPTER 34

Neurological Infections

Rakesh Sharma, Deepak Goel, Jitender Chaturvedi

"It is a war of nerves and there will be casualties."

—David Peace

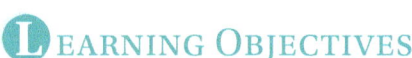

After going through the chapter, the learner will be able to:
- Enumerate various neurological infections.
- Describe the epidemiology and etiopathogenesis of meningitis, encephalitis, brain abscess, and neurocysticercosis.
- Recognize the clinical presentation of various neurological infections.
- Understand the diagnostic modalities of the neurological infections.
- Discuss the medical and nursing management of various neurological infections.
- Appreciate the collaborative care of various neurological infections.

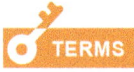

- **Brain abscess:** Formation of pus, that encapsulate and remain in the brain parenchyma.
- **Encephalitis:** Inflammation of cerebral tissue.
- **Meningitis:** Inflammation of the layers of brain and spinal cord.
- **Neurocysticercosis:** Pork tapeworm infestation in the brain, these worms make cysts in the brain parenchyma.
- **Nuchal rigidity:** Stiffness or tightness of the neck, patient feel pain on movement of the neck.

INTRODUCTION

The neural tissues are protected from various invading pathogens by virtue of different in-built protective mechanisms. The most important of this is blood–brain barrier (BBB) along with humoral and cellular immunity. Neurological infections come into clinical existence when pathogens invade neural tissues or their coverings (meninges). These infections includes meningitis, encephalitis, and brain abscesses. Globally, these infections continue to cause significant mortality and morbidity. In this chapter, details regarding pathological changes, manifestations, diagnostic procedures, assessment of patients, and collaborative management of each neurological infection are discussed.

MENINGITIS

CONCEPT AND DEFINITION

Meningitis is inflammation of the three layers (dura mater, arachnoid mater and pia mater) which covers brain and spinal cord.

EPIDEMIOLOGY

Worldwide, the mortality rate secondary to meningitis has been reduced by 21% from 1990 (4,03,012) to 2016 (3,18,400). Whereas the number of cases has increased from 2.50 million (1990) to 2.82 million (2016). The overall incidence range from 207.4/100,000 population in South Sudan to 0.5/100,000 population in India. A high burden of meningitis has been reported in central and western sub-Saharan African continues. In India, age-standardized mortality secondary to meningitis has dropped at least 50% from 1990 to 2016. However, the actual incidence is reported very low due to imprecise surveillance system.

ETIOLOGY

Various pathogens causing meningitis are depicted in **Box 34.1**.

BOX 34.1: Various pathogens causing meningitis.

Bacteria
- *Streptococcus pneumonia*: Located in the respiratory tract, sinuses, and nasal cavity. It is the *leading cause of bacterial meningitis*. Mainly occurs in older adults.
- *Neisseria meningitis*: Transmitted via saliva and respiratory fluid (coughing, kissing). The most common age group are teens, young adults, and older adults.
- *Haemophilus influenzae*: It used to be the most common cause among children, however, a significant reduction is noted after vaccination.
- *Staphylococcus aureus*: Usually present on the skin and in the respiratory tract. Primarily infect older age groups.
- *Group B streptococcus*: Commonly present in gastrointestinal and genital tracts, mainly transmitted during vaginal delivery. The most common age group infected by this are newborns, older adults, and children.
- *E. coli*: Transmitted by eating food prepared by infected people with poor hand hygiene. This organism mainly infects newborns.
- *Hospital-acquired meningitis*: Primarily caused by gram-negative bacilli among post-craniotomy patients. *Staph. aureus* is the usual organism.
- *Tubercular meningitis*: Is caused by *Mycobacterium tuberculosis*, which is a acid-fast bacillus.

Viruses
- *Non-polio enteroviruses*: Usually occur in late spring. More common in the younger age group, risk drops as age advances.
- *Other viruses are*: Mumps virus, herpes viruses, Epstein-barr Virus, varicella-zoster virus, herpes simplex viruses, measles virus, influenza virus, arboviruses, and lymphocytic choriomeningitis virus. People with poor immunity and on chemotherapy drugs are susceptible populations for viral meningitis.

Fungus
- Fungal meningitis may result from the entry of fungi into CNS during a neurosurgical procedure or even during an epidural injection.
- *Cryptococcus neoformans* is the most common cause of fungal meningitis. It affects immunocompromised population, such as HIV-positive, those who are on chemotherapy for leukemia or lymphoma, and prolonged steroid therapy for various reasons. *C. neoformans* are found in the soil, decaying wood, and is transmitted via pigeons and chickens. Other fungi that may cause meningitis are *Histoplasma, Blastomyces, Coccidioides*.

RISK FACTORS

- **Age:** Extremes of age is a risk factor for developing bacterial meningitis, i.e., children, and elderly with comorbidities, such as diabetes mellitus, etc.
- **Community:** People living in crowded places such as hostels, swimming in infected water, institutions where people are in very close contact are at high risk to *Neisseria meningitis*.
- **Traveling:** Traveling to meningitis belt areas, such as sub-Saharan Africa, Sudan, and Niger during summer.
- **Healthcare professionals**: Those who are routinely exposed to pathogens causing meningitis are at risk for meningitis.
- **Weather**: Meningitis commonly occurs during early spring, winter and mostly secondary to respiratory viral infection.

PATHOPHYSIOLOGY

Meningitis generally results either through inoculation of pathogens from the bloodstream from existing infection or by direct entry of pathogens followed by traumatic brain injury or invasive procedure. Once the pathogen enters the body; they attach to the mucous epithelium and start circulating within bloodstream.

The causative organism gradually breaks the blood-brain barrier (BBB) and starts proliferation in the cerebrospinal fluid (CSF) in SAS. Once the pathogen enters into the subarachnoid space (SAS), they start proliferation, and further inflammation.

Many defense cells play an essential role in the immune response, especially endothelial cells, perivascular macrophages, and mast cells. Also, release of inflammatory mediators, such as interleukin-1 (IL-1), tumor necrosis factor (TNF), and prostaglandins (PG). As a result of an inflammatory process, blood-brain barrier permeability gets impaired, and the formation of purulent exudates that causes cerebral edema and increased intracranial pressure **(Flowchart 34.1)**.

CLINICAL MANIFESTATIONS

- The typical triad of clinical symptoms of meningitis are headache, fever, and nuchal rigidity.
- A high fever present throughout the illness.
- The headache is usually of severe in intensity which is due to meningeal irritation.
- **Nuchal rigidity:** Patients usually complain of a stiff neck while flexing the head, which is an early sign.
- **Positive Brudzinski's sign:** The method of checking the Brudzinski's signs is to keep the patient in the supine position. Slowly flex the head of the patient; this will

Flowchart 34.1: Pathophysiology of meningitis.

Entry of pathogens via endogenous or exogenous rout
↓
Pathogen attach to the mucous epithelium and start circulation within bloodstream
↓
Pathogen gradually breaks the BBB and starts proliferation in the cerebrospinal fluid (CSF) in subarachnoid space (SAS)
↓
Further proliferation and inflammation into the subarachnoid space
↓
Inflammatroy response by the body's defense mechanism
↓
Formation of purulent exudates, cerebral edema and increased ICP

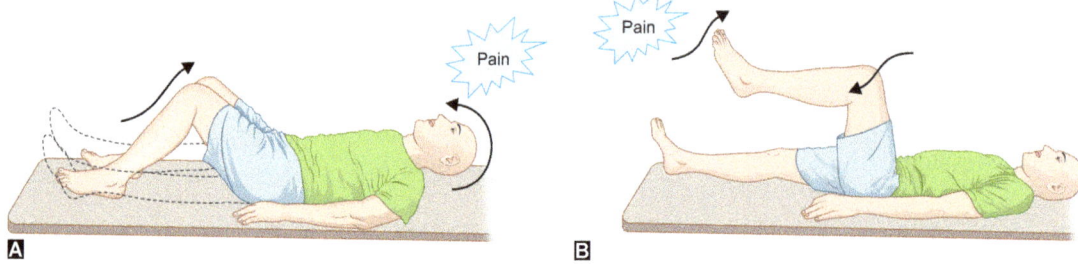

Figs. 34.1A and B: Signs of meningeal irritation: (A) Brudzinski's signs; (B) Kernig's sign.

result in flexion of ankles, knees and hips, which indicates meningeal irritation **(Fig. 34.1A)**.
- **Positive Kernig's sign:** To check the Kernig's sign, keep the patient in a supine position, flex one hip and knee joint to make 90° angle. Gradually extend the thigh; at this point, the patient will experience pain and spasm in the thigh, and a resistance will be felt by the examiner **(Fig. 34.1B)**.
- Photophobia, behavior change, a decreased level of consciousness (LOC), lethargy or confusion.
- Skin rash and petechiae may be seen
- Almost one-third of patients may develop seizures
- Gradually headache becomes more progressive and accompanied by vomiting, which indicates increased intracranial pressure (ICP).

COMPLICATIONS

The patient suffering with meningitis is prone to develop many complications. These may include:
- Increased ICP, which is the most common cause of unconsciousness.
- Long-term residual neurological dysfunctions.
- Cranial nerve III, IV, VI, VII, VIII dysfunction may occur in bacterial meningitis, which usually resolves within a few weeks after recovery from meningitis.
- Hearing impairment, deafness, tinnitus, blindness, ptosis, diplopia, facial paresis, vertigo.
- Some patients may develop hemiparesis, dysphasia, and hemianopsia; these can resolve after several weeks.
- In acute cerebral edema, patients may develop seizures, cranial nerve oculomotor palsy, bradycardia, increased ICP, coma and death.
- The exudate forms and causes adhesions that block the normal flow of CSF, and non-communicating hydrocephalus may occur.
- **Waterhouse-Friderichsen syndrome:** Signs and symptoms are petechiae, disseminated intravascular coagulation (DIC).

DIAGNOSTIC EVALUATION

A patient showing the signs and symptoms of meningitis as has been discussed earlier, along with detailed physical examination, need to undergo the following investigation:
- **Complete blood count:** Elevated WBCs counts in bacterial meningitis and viral meningitis.
- Blood cultures are collected to identify the organism.
- **CSF examination:** CSF is evaluated for pressure, protein, glucose, leukocytes.
  - *Bacterial meningitis:* CSF opening pressure is elevated from 200–500 mm H_2O; WBC count elevated to >1000 cells/µL; protein level increased to >500 mg/dL; glucose level decreased by <45 mg/dL.
  - *Viral meningitis:* CSF opening pressure is normal to slightly elevated; WBC count elevated to 500–1000 cells/µL; protein level increased 50–500 mg/dL; glucose level in normal 45–75 mg/dL.
  - *Fungal meningitis:* CSF opening pressure is >200 mm H_2O; WBC count elevated to >20 cells/µL; protein level increased >45 mg/dL; glucose level in normal or decreased.
- **Radiological investigations:**
  - *X-ray:* To identify infected sinuses.
  - *CT and MRI:* With/without contrast scan will help to rule out other disorders. CT scan may show evidence of elevated ICP or the presence of hydrocephalus.
- Changes in personality and bizarre behavior may be seen at the onset.

MEDICAL MANAGEMENT

The medical management should be initiated soon after the provisional diagnosis based on the clinical examination and diagnostic results.
- IV antibiotic therapy is administered based on the culture report (e.g., bacterial or tuberculous meningitis).
- **Antifungal drugs:** Amphotericin B and the triazoles, fluconazole and itraconazole are for cryptococcal meningitis.
- **Antiviral drugs:** Acyclovir, IV, for 10 to 21 days.
- **Note:** before administration of antibiotics, CSF samples should be taken for culture and sensitivity.
- Dexamethasone or other corticosteroids, through IV, to minimize meningeal inflammation. The steroid may be administered before or along with the 1st dose of antibiotic and it should be given for the next 4 days at an interval of 6 hours, for adults. These patients should be observed for gastrointestinal bleeding.
- Symptomatic management for shock, seizures, with fluid volume expander and anticonvulsant medications.
- Standard measures to be taken in managing and preventing increased ICP, e.g., head end elevation, mannitol, and frusemide.

NURSING MANAGEMENT

Nursing Assessment

- History collection, such as recent travel from sub-Saharan Africa, Sudan, and Niger, health care professionals working in infectious wards/units, residence of rural or slum, family history.

- Assess vital signs and perform a detailed physical examination (baseline and at frequent intervals) to record baseline and ongoing interventions.
- **Neurological examination:** Assess for the signs of meningeal irritation, such as nuchal rigidity, hyper-irritability, hyperalgesia, photophobia.
- Assess respiratory status to begin respiratory support if necessary.

Nursing Diagnoses

- Acute pain (headache, neck pain, body-ache) related to meningeal irritation, swelling of intracranial pressure.
- Hyperthermia related to infection or inflammation.
- Ineffective cerebral tissue perfusion related to cerebral edema, inflammation.
- Risk for imbalanced fluid volume related to hyperthermia and decreased fluid intake.
- Sleep pattern disturbance related to agitation or increased sensitivity to environmental stimuli.
- Impaired physical mobility related to complete bed rest.
- High risk for injury related to seizure potential, impaired consciousness, cognitive impairment.

Nursing Interventions

- Maintain patent airway, perform suction if necessary.
- Administer oxygen
- Monitor oxygen saturation, blood gases; assess signs and symptoms of respiratory distress.
- Monitor sign and symptoms of increased ICP (decreased level of consciousness, dilated pupils, widened pulse pressure).
- Provide or assist in personal hygiene activities (especially two-hourly oral care).
- **Take measures to prevent injury:** Keeping side rails up, bed at low when the patient is alone, and other necessary precautions.
- **Hyperthermia management:** Administering antipyretic drugs (e.g., paracetamol 650 mg orally in adult patients), keeping the room temperature at 20–20°C, giving tepid baths, applying hypothermia blankets.
- **Pain in the head (headache) management:** Raise the head 30°, applying an ice cap if needed, maintaining a quiet and dark environment, administer analgesics (e.g., paracetamol or acetaminophen 650 mg or codeine 15–30 mg q 4 h) orally in the adult patient.

Prevent Complications

- Skin care, every 2–4 hourly.
- Assess bony prominence areas and special care to prevent pressure sore.
- Assist and teach deep breathing exercises if the patient is conscious and follows instructions. This intervention has the potential to reduce lung atelectasis in bed-ridden patients.
- To prevent thrombophlebitis, apply elastic stocking to the bed-ridden patient.
- **Special monitoring in meningococcal meningitis:** Monitor signs of adrenal insufficiency (hypotension, respiratory collapse, petechiae) in the patient diagnosed with meningococcal meningitis.

FUNGAL MENINGITIS/MENINGOENCEPHALITIS

Fungal meningitis is a rare infection of the central nervous system. It occurs in immunocompromised people, e.g., HIV-positive patients, immune suppressive medications, and organ transplants, etc.

The most common causes are:
- *Aspergillus fumigatus* (mold)
- *Cryptococcus neoformans* (yeasts)
- *Histoplasma capsulatum* (dimorphic fungi)
- *Blastomyces dermatitidis* (dimorphic fungi)
- *Candida* (yeasts)
- *Coccidioides immitis* (dimorphic fungi).

People in digging work, like farmers, coal miners, and construction workers, are at high risk of fungal encephalitis.

Pathophysiology

Fungal meningitis develops from either direct invasion or through the existing fungal infection in the body (hematogenous spread). Typically, the fungal spores from the environment enter the body via inhalation and infect the lungs, resulting in respiratory symptoms of pneumonitis. As infection progresses; the fungi enter the bloodstream (fungemia) and then the central nervous system.

Clinical Manifestations

The following are the symptoms of fungal meningitis:
- Fever
- Weakness/malaise
- Body aches, headache
- **Meningeal irritation:** Positive Brudzinski and Kernig sign
- **Symptoms of increased ICP:** Headache, vomiting, decreased LOC
- Behavior changes
- Hydrocephalus
- Seizures

Diagnostic Modalities

- A history of organ transplantation, immunomodulatory drugs, HIV infection, occupation, and travel.
- A detailed neurological assessment.
- Serologic test for fungal antibodies.
- Lumbar puncture for CSF analysis. Cerebrospinal fluid (CSF) pleocytosis (≥5 nucleated cells/mL)
- Neuroimaging studies.
- MRI to identify any hemorrhage, or meningeal inflammation.

Complications

- Stroke (*Aspergillus fumigatus* may have a hemorrhagic or ischemic stroke)
- Focal neurologic signs based on the affected brain areas.

Medical Management

- **Anti-fungal therapy:**
  - Amphotericin B, usually administered IV.
  - Patients have to be explained about side effects such as nausea, vomiting, fever, decreased Hb level, uremia, electrolytes (potassium and magnesium) imbalance, and renal toxicity.
  - Fluconazole, flucytosine can be given orally.

- ICP management by lumbar puncture and or CSF shunting.
- Prophylactic anticonvulsant drugs can be administered to manage seizures.

Nursing Management

Nursing Assessment

Similar to arthropod-borne viral encephalitis.

Nursing Diagnoses

Similar to arthropod-borne viral encephalitis.

Nursing Interventions

- Assess for signs and symptoms of increased ICP and initiation of appropriate measures to control and manage ICP.
- Manage fever by non-pharmacological measures, such as cold sponging, loose cotton cloths; if unable to control fever, initiate pharmacological actions.
- Administer analgesics to control and manage the pain.
- Ensure fluid intake to prevent dehydration.
- Initiate preventive strategies for injury prevention from seizures or potential falls.
- Monitor side effects of anti-fungal therapy and need to address the renal status of patients.

Case Scenario

A male patient, 70-year-old, resident of rural slum from a low socioeconomic family, who came to the emergency department with a 3-day history of **worsening confusion and somnolence.** He also complained of **headache and stiff neck.**
His 10-year-old grand son who visited last week was recently diagnosed with pneumonia.
He has a history of seizure disorder.
Type-II DM diagnosed 2 years ago.

On physical examination, patient was confused, unresponsive, patient is in distress.
Vital signs: BP 80/60 mm Hg, P 124, RR 22, T 39.8°C
Nuchal rigidity—positive
Kernig's sign—positive
Brudzinski's sign—negative

Laboratory investigations
Cultures CSF; Gram stain: Gram-positive diplococci; CT scan—no abnormalities

Management
- IV antibiotic therapy—Claforan (cefotaxime) and Rocephin (ceftriaxone)
- Dexamethasone or other corticosteroids
- Anticonvulsant drugs
- Standard measures to be taken in managing and preventing increased ICP, e.g., head end elevation, Mannitol, and Frusemide.

ENCEPHALITIS

CONCEPT AND DEFINITION

Encephalitis is the inflammation of the brain tissue, caused most commonly by viruses, but also can be by bacteria, fungi or parasites. Based on the causative organism, encephalitis is classified as follows:
A. Arthropod-borne viral encephalitis
B. Herpes simplex encephalitis (HSV encephalitis)

Arthropod-borne Viral Encephalitis

Arthropod-borne viruses, also known as arboviruses, are transmitted by arthropod (mosquitoes, psychosis, ticks, and ceratopogonids). An arbovirus is replicated inside the arthropod vector-before transmission to a susceptible host. The virus is disseminated through the saliva of the vector and transmitted into the host during the blood-feeding process. Arthropod-borne viruses cause epidemic encephalitis, such as Japanese encephalitis, Eastern equine, Western equine, Venezuelan, St Louis, West Nile Virus and spreads by mosquitoes. The occurrence of the cases are in the late summer and early fall season.

Pathophysiology

The natural reservoir of most of the viruses are birds, and mosquitoes and transmit the virus into the human body. Most of the viruses are unable to develop sufficient numbers in the blood to re-infect a mosquito. Viruses circulate in the blood and enter the central nervous system through the olfactory tract, and lodges in different parts of the brain (cortical gray matter, brainstem, thalamus). Activation of the inflammatory process and formation of exudate results in meningeal irritation and elevated intracranial pressure leading to altered sensorium.

Clinical Manifestations

- A patient infected with arthropod-borne viruses experiences signs and symptoms, such as headache, fever, listlessness, weakness, drowsiness, nausea, and vomiting. The severity of clinical manifestation depends on the type of virus. The neurological symptoms are a stiff neck, confusion, seizure, stupor, ataxia, tremors, and photophobia. St Louis encephalitis has a unique clinical manifestation, SIADH, with a lower level of sodium concentration in the blood.
- In the Asian region, Japanese encephalitis is the most common viral encephalitis caused by a mosquito-borne flavivirus.
- Long-term clinical manifestation includes mental retardation, change in personality, psychosis, dementia, deafness, blindness, paralysis or weakness, and epilepsy.
- Patients infected with the West-Nile virus can cause acute flaccid paralysis. Symptoms of poliomyelitis result from West Nile virus infection to motor neurons of anterior horns in the spinal cord.

Diagnostic Evaluation

- A detailed history taking and physical examination are paramount in diagnosing viral encephalitis
- CSF evaluation, neuroimaging (MRI) (St. Louis: Inflammation in the basal ganglia; West Nile encephalitis: Inflammation in the periventricular areas; Japanese encephalitis: Thalamus).
- The presence of IgM antibodies in the CSF and blood indicated West Nile encephalitis and Japanese encephalitis.

Medical Management

There is no specific treatment for arthropod-borne viruses encephalitis. The patient, is given symptomatic treatment, including management of increased ICP, fever, pain and seizures.

Nursing Management

Nursing Assessment

- History collection related to environment, presence of mosquito, psychosis, ticks, and ceratopogonids.
- Physical examination-specifically stiff neck, changes in personality, confusion, paralysis or muscle weakness.
- Symptoms of increased ICP, such as headache, photophobia.
- CSF analysis-presence of IgM antibodies.
- CT Scan and MRI.

Nursing Diagnoses

1. Impaired cerebral tissue perfusion, related to cerebral edema and increased ICP.
2. Pain related to swelling of intracranial contents.
3. Hyperthermia related to infection, inflammation and pressure on hypothalamus.
4. Sleep pattern disturbance related to agitation or increased sensitivity to environmental stimuli.
5. Risk for injury related to agitation, seizure potential or altered consciousness.

Nursing Interventions

- Most of the patients are treated based on symptoms, and the nurse needs to plan and deliver nursing care to the patient for fever and headache on an outpatient basis. If a patient is severely sick, they need to be hospitalized.
- The primary goal is to evaluate a patient's neurological status and record the findings to evaluate and compare in the future. Along with the nursing management of fever, headache, and body pain, nurse initiates preventive strategies for injury prevention from seizure or potential fall.
- In some cases, death or a lifelong neurological deficit may develop. The patient and family will require rehabilitation support and education to manage and cope with the situation.
  It is also necessary to educate the family and society to take precautionary measures to reduce the mosquito population near residency areas.

Herpes Simplex Encephalitis

Herpes simplex encephalitis is inflammation of the brain parenchyma with neurologic dysfunction caused by the Herpes simplex virus type-1 or type-2.

HSV-1 is 1 of 8 human herpes viruses and is the most common sporadic virus causing herpes simplex encephalitis in all age groups. It is more prevalent in developed countries.

The infection rate is high among very young (up to 3 years of age) and adults aged more than 50-years, almost equally distributed in both genders.

Pathophysiology

The etiology of herpes simplex encephalitis is unknown. Infection depends upon the immunity status of a particular person.

After the entry of the virus into the body, it remains dormant for a long time until reactivated based on the immunity level. Once the virus finds a suitable condition, HSV enters into the central nervous system (CNS) by retrograde transport through the olfactory nerves or trigeminal nerves or by way of the bloodstream.

The virus lodges in the frontal and temporal lobes and initiates host immune response and inflammatory cascades results in brain tissue destruction, edema, and consequent neurological sequelae.

Clinical Manifestations

Followings are some of the important symptoms of herpes simplex encephalitis:

- Fever
- New onset seizures
- Hallucination
- Focal neurologic signs based on the affected brain areas

Diagnostic Evaluation

- A detailed history taking and physical examination
- CSF evaluation to identify—leukocytosis; increased mononuclear cell pleocytosis; elevated proteins level; normal or slightly decreased glucose level.
- Polymerase chain reaction (PCR) test—to identify DNA (deoxyribonucleic acid) of virus and viral antibodies.
- MRI with gadolinium is preferred to distinguish between post-infection encephalomyelitis and acute viral encephalitis.
- EEG may show slow, diffuse brain wave complexes in the temporal lobe.

Complications

- Edema in the temporal lobe can result in compression of the brainstem
- Motor and sensory deficit
- Aphasia

Medical Management

- Once the patient is diagnosed with herpes simplex encephalitis, antiviral therapy (acyclovir or ganciclovir) should be started. Early initiation of antiviral drugs has a good prognosis. Treatment for 10–21 days is indicated for the herpes simplex virus. To prevent crystallization of the drug in the urine, a slow intravenous administration of the drug for 1 hour is recommended.
- Prophylactic anticonvulsant drugs are administered to manage seizures.

Nursing Management

Nursing assessment—similar to arthropod-borne viral encephalitis.

Nursing diagnoses—similar to arthropod-borne viral encephalitis.

Nursing Interventions

- The nurse must periodically perform a neurological evaluation to evaluate the progress of the patients' health status.
- Pharmacological (analgesics, e.g., opioids) and non-pharmacological (reduce the light, maintain a quiet environment in the patient unit, limit visitors, cluster the nursing care) measures to be taken to reduce the bodyache, headache.

- Opioids must be used cautiously; they may mask the neurological symptoms.
- Initiate injury preventive measures due to seizure or fall.
- Monitor urine output; antiviral therapy can affect normal renal functions.
- Encourage the patient's family members to participate in nursing care while the patient is in the coma stage.
- Provide supportive care to the family members, addressing their issues and psychological concerns.
- Most of the patients are treated based on symptoms, and the nurse needs to plan and deliver nursing care to the patient for fever and headache on an outpatient basis. If a patient is severely sick, they need to be hospitalized.
- The primary goal is to assess a patient's neurological status and record them to evaluate and compare in the future. Along with the nursing management of fever, headache, and body pain, nurse initiates preventive strategies for injury prevention from seizure or potential fall.
- In some cases, death or a lifelong neurological deficit may develop. The patient and family will require rehabilitation support and education to manage and cope with the situation.
- It is also necessary to educate the family and society to take precautionary measures to reduce the mosquito population near residency areas.

Case Scenario

A 65-year-old female from the hilly areas arrives to the emergency department in August by her family for **increasing confusion and altered mental status.** The patient's attendants stated that the patient was in her usual state of good health until she developed **fever and fatigue** 5 days back.
Over the next 3 days, she developed **nausea, vomiting, and diarrhea** associated with increasing headache.
On examination: Fever—103.5°F; breathing—rapid, shallow, and labored.
Investigations: Blood cultures; CT head—negative

Lumbar puncture:
- Opening pressure of 16 cm H_2O
- Pleocytosis of 625 cells/μL (56% neutrophils, 41% lymphocytes
- Glucose concentration—43 mg/dL
- Protein concentration of 116 mg/dL
- The CSF Gram stain was negative
- CSF testing for West Nile virus IgM was positive

Treatment:
- Amphotericin B
- ICP management
- Prophylactic anticonvulsant drugs

BRAIN ABSCESS

CONCEPT AND DEFINITION

Brain abscess is a pathological condition of pus collection within brain parenchyma. It accounts for 8% of intracranial masses in developing countries and 1–2% in Western countries. The incidence of the intracranial abscess has been reported highest (49/100,000) in Southeast Asia, whereas, in the Western population, it is approximately 1500–2500 cases per year. It is found to be more common in males than females (1.3:1). It affects in all age groups but more prevalent in the first two decades.

ETIOLOGY

The most common causes of brain abscess are:
- Complications of infections within paranasal sinuses—10% of all brain abscess
- Otogenic infections (otitis media)—40% of all brain abscess
- Intracranial surgery, skull fracture or even after oral surgery.
- Infection carried by the blood from other remote areas, such as generalized lung disease, bronchiectasis, empyema, lung abscess, acute bacterial endocarditis, congenital heart diseases and skin infections.

PATHOPHYSIOLOGY

Mostly, bacteria (*Streptococci, Staphylococci aureus*) are the cause of brain abscesses. The pathogen may enter into the brain parenchymal tissues directly through cranial surgery or trauma to the skull or extension from the ear, mouth, sinus, and mastoid infection.

There are four stages in the development of brain abscess:
1. Early cerebritis (1–4 days)—inflammation of the brain
2. Late cerebritis/(4–10 days); formation of pus
3. Early capsule formation (11–14 days); formation of capsule
4. Late capsule formation: (>14 days)—formation of hard capsulation/granuloma

In the initial phase of infection, the brain tissue is soft, edematous, and infiltrated with polymorphonuclear leukocytes. Gradually necrotic tissue liquefies; and formation of abscess, which becomes encapsulated by fibroblasts. This fibroblast zone is replaced by collagenous connective tissue, which is not equal in thickness at all places; thinner part in the deepest portion. This thin part of the brain abscess wall towards the ventricular region is responsible for intraventricular rupture, an independent risk factor for poor outcomes in patients with brain abscesses. The abscess may be of various sizes and shapes, usually lies in the white matter and rupture from the thinner side into the ventricles and show various signs and symptoms **(Flowchart 34.2)**.

CLINICAL MANIFESTATIONS

- Severe headache, chills, fever, malaise.
- Elevated leukocyte counts

Flowchart 34.2: Pathophysiology of brain abscess.

In the initial phase of infection, the brain tissue is soft, edematous, and infiltrated with polymorphonuclear leukocytes
↓
Liquefication of tissues
Formation of abscess, which becomes encapsulated by fibroblasts
↓
This fibroblast zone is replaced by collagenous connective tissue
↓
The abscess may be of various sizes and shapes, and show various signs and symptoms

- **Neurological symptoms:** Confusion, drowsiness, generalized or focal seizures, sensory or motor deficits, aphasia, ataxia, meningeal irritation, hemiparesis, signs of increased ICP (headache, vomiting, decreased LOC).
- **Abrupt rupture of abscess:** Coma, possible brain herniation syndrome, >50,000 WBCs counts in the CSF.
- Signs and symptoms may vary according to the location of the abscess.

DIAGNOSTIC EVALUATION

- A detailed history taking about recent infection of the middle ear, sinus, lung, any ear, nose, oral, skull surgery, skull trauma, and physical examination.
- Lumbar puncture: Elevated CSF pressure, elevated WBCs counts, high protein, and normal glucose level.
- Electroencephalography (EEG), CT scan-to localize the lesion.
- CT or MRI guided aspiration of an abscess to find the pathogens.

MEDICAL MANAGEMENT

- **Antimicrobial therapy:** For anaerobic bacterial infections, penicillin G (20 million U) and chloramphenicol (4–6 g/daily via IV in divided doses) are given. A specific antibiotic should be given as per culture and sensitivity test
- To control and manage increased ICP, mannitol, with dexamethasone, is administered.
- **Surgical drainage of abscess:** CT or MRI-guided aspiration of abscess is used to drain the abscess. This will also help reduce ICP. A sample of pus for culture and sensitivity should be taken.
- **Surgical excision:** If the abscess is well encapsulated, then a surgical attempt is tried to remove the abscess along with its wall or membrane.
- The patient is given symptomatic treatment for fever (antipyretics), pain (analgesics), seizures (anticonvulsant).

NURSING MANAGEMENT

Nursing Assessment

- History collection about recent upper respiratory infection, ear infection, recent surgery (intracranial, oral, ENT)
- **Physical examination:**
  - Cranial nerve assessment, third and sixth cranial nerve deficits.
  - The triad of fever, headache, and the focal neurologic deficit is observed.
  - Pain, grand mal seizures, nausea and vomiting, nuchal rigidity
- Rupture of abscess is usually presented with suddenly worsening headache followed by emerging signs of meningismus.
- **Lumbar puncture:** Rarely required and only should be performed with a prior CT and MRI scan after ruling out increased intracranial pressure because of the potential for cerebrospinal fluid (CSF) herniation and death.

Nursing Diagnoses

1. Impaired cerebral tissue perfusion, related to seizures activity.
2. Pain related to accumulation of pus in intracranial cavity.
3. Risk of fall related to loss of body balance during seizures.

Nursing Interventions

- The key important role of the nurse is to perform a neurologic assessment, administer prescribed drugs, monitor the response of treatment, and execute collaborative care to the patient and family members.
- Management of increased ICP is by providing a noise-free environment, limiting visitors and clustering of care, head-end elevation up to 30°.
- Monitor and document the response of drugs.
- Initiate injury prevention strategy from seizure, such as raise up the side rails and pad them with cloth, keep any object that may cause injury to the patient.
- Record the electrolyte levels and initiate necessary action if abnormal findings are reported in results.
- Nursing interventions should be planned based on the sign and symptoms of a particular patient.
- The nurse should evaluate the distress level of the family, explain the patient's status and support them to cope up with the situation.

Case Scenario

A 80-year-old male patient with chief complaints, 1-week history of left hemiparesis, ataxia, dysphagia, dysarthria, and facial droop. On admission, he denied nausea, vomiting, abdominal pain, or respiratory distress.

Medical history
He had been receiving prednisone (40 mg/day) as immunosuppressive therapy for glomerulonephritis and chronic obstructive pulmonary disease for 3 months.

Surgical history
A craniectomy was performed, and drainage from the abscess was sent to the microbiology laboratory for bacterial, fungal, and mycobacterial culture.

Neuroimaging
Magnetic resonance imaging (MRI) of the brain revealed a right frontal lobe multiloculated lesion with significant ring enhancement and marked diffusion restriction, indicating an abscess with surrounding edema. A midline shift due to mass compression of the right ventricle was also noted.

Treatment
The patient was treated empirically with metronidazole and ceftriaxone.

NEUROCYSTICERCOSIS

CONCEPT AND DEFINITION

Neurocysticercosis (NCC) is a parasitic infection caused by larvae of the pork tapeworm (*Taenia solium*) in the central nervous system (CNS).

ETIOLOGY

Neurocysticercos mainly affects the farming communities from Africa, Asia, and Latin America. It is commonly found in animal husbandry practice areas where pigs and cattles

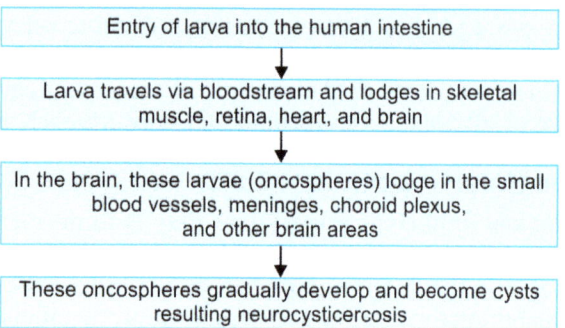

Flowchart 34.3: Pathophysiology of NCC.

come in contact with the human feces. Worldwide, NCC is the most common cause of epilepsy; approximately 30% of total epilepsy cases are developed by parasites. Almost one million in India, 0.31–4.6 million in Africa, and 0.45–1.35 million in Latin America, people suffer from epilepsy due to NCC. In India, incidences of NCC are more in meat-eating states, such as Uttar Pradesh, Maharashtra, Telangana, Andhra Pradesh.

PATHOPHYSIOLOGY

Humans are definitive or primary, and pigs are intermediate or secondary hosts harboring the pork tapeworm's larva stage (*Taenia solium*). A segment of tapeworm, known as proglottid, is excreted into the feces. These proglottids consist thousands of eggs can survive in the environment and infect human and pig. Once the egg enters the pig, it becomes larva form and gets attached to many muscles. When a human eats undercooked meat of an infected pig, these larva enters into the human intestine and via bloodstream lodges in skeletal muscle, retina, heart, and brain. In the brain, these larvae (oncospheres) lodge in the small blood vessels, meninges, choroid plexus, and other brain areas. These oncospheres gradually develop and become cysts resulting Neurocysticercosis (**Flowchart 34.3**).

CLINICAL MANIFESTATIONS

- Seizures
- Hydrocephalus
- Headaches
- Nausea
- Other neurological signs and symptoms are based on the location and number of parasites within the brain.

DIAGNOSTIC EVALUATION

- History taking and physical examination.
- CT or MRI-CT will be helpful to identify small, homogenous, ill-defined lesions.
- CBC including eosinophils count.
- EEG (electroencephalograms)—it will show abnormal waves.
- CSF analysis: Increased opening pressure, presence of eosinophils, increased protein, and decreased glucose value.
- Serological test for cysticercosis—ELIZA test.

MANAGEMENT

- **Anthelmintic drugs:** Praziquantel* (50 mg/kg/day in three divided doses for one day) and albendazole* (15 mg/kg, twice daily) are preferred drugs for CNS cysticerci and *T. solium*.
- **Anticonvulsant therapy:** Dose, duration, and type of drug depend the upon the patient's clinical presentation. (e.g. Phenytoin*, 100 mg orally)
- **Anti-inflammatory drugs**—e.g., ibuprofen* 200–400 mg orally, every 6–8 hours with meal, in adult patients.
- **Corticosteroids**—to suppress inflammation which is developed during treatment.
- **Shunting (ventriculoperitoneal shunt):** If the blockage in the CSF flow, the patient show symptoms of hydrocephalous.

NURSING MANAGEMENT

Nursing Assessment

- History collection about non-vegetarian diet especially pork or meat eating, use of uncooked meat, etc.
- Physical signs on neurological examination are highly variable and depend on the number, site, and size of the lesions.
- Cranial nerve assessment
- CT and MRI provide objective evidence on the number and topography of lesions and their stage of involution; contrast medium administration.
- MRA is a valuable non-invasive imaging method to demonstrate segmental narrowing or occlusion of intracranial arteries in patients with subarachnoid neurocysticercosis.

Nursing Diagnoses

1. Impaired cerebral tissue perfusion, related to cerebral infection and increased ICP.
2. Pain related to disturbance in the balance of intracranial content and increased ICP.
3. Sleep pattern disturbance related to agitation and pain.
4. Risk for injury related to seizure potential and altered consciousness.

Nursing Interventions

- Most neurocysticercosis patients do not require hospitalization. They are advised to follow the drug regimen and be educated about lifestyle modification, especially about seizures. Nurses' responsibility is to explain to the patient and family about the treatment, diet, and changes in the daily living activities.
- Most of the patients are treated based on symptoms, and the nurse needs to plan and deliver nursing care to the patient for nausea, vomiting, and headache on an outpatient basis.
- Explain about the home or work environmental safety. Family members/co-workers/teachers must know about patients' disease condition and support during seizure activities if it occurs.

---

*Check contraindications before administration.

- The patient must have to wear a medical alert tag, must have an emergency contact number with him/her.
- Educate family members about the causes and how Neurocysticercosis can be prevented, such as hand washing after toilet use, before eating, cook properly, wash vegetables and fruits. Those who eat pig meat (pork) need to cook properly.

GERIATRIC CONSIDERATIONS FOR NEUROLOGICAL INFECTIONS

Screening of older persons with a history of CNS infection with symptoms like acute/chronic headache, high blood pressure, fever, seizures, rigidity of neck and spine, muscle weakness, and symptoms of dementia needs special attention.

Many times, comorbid conditions and CNS infections are intertwined; in addition to that, age-related changes make it much more difficult to make a correct diagnosis of such patients. Old-age populations are more at risk for fall injury, nutritional deficit, treatment compliance, etc. The elderly clients require not only physical care but also psychological care and support.

Case Scenario

A 35-year-old female, arrives to emergency with the chief complaints of dizziness and mild seizures for the past 3 months.
She also suffers from dyspepsia, nausea with scanty non-bilious vomiting for last 10 days.
Her family noticed an increase in the frequency of her intermittent syncopal attacks within the past 5 days.
The patient was transported to a nearby hospital in the emergency department. Her body weight is 55 kg.

Investigations
CT of the brain showed multilobulated cystic mass in the posteromedial left temporal/occipital region with surrounding edema.
MRI of the head without contrast reveled a nodular focus of enhancement within the multilobulated cystic mass in the brain with the suspicion of NCC.

Treatment
Levetiracetam 500 mg once a day.
Albendazole 400 mg twice a day and is seizure free.

SUMMARY

In this chapter, neuroinfectious diseases are discussed and elaborated with respect to their causes, pathophysiology, clinical presentation and management. Nursing management has been explained based on the signs and symptoms of various conditions. Also, home management and education to family members is discussed. Nurses must consider the age of patients, especially old age as there could be variation in their responses towards the neuroinfection management. Lots of antibiotic therapy may have multiple effects on the body organs helping in metabolism and excretion of drugs.

MULTIPLE CHOICE QUESTIONS

1. A client, age 21, is admitted with bacterial meningitis. Which hospital room would be the best choice for this client?
   a. A private room down the hall from the "nurses' station
   b. An isolation room three doors from the "nurses' station
   c. A semiprivate room with a 32-year-old client who has viral meningitis
   d. A two-bedroom with a client who previously had bacterial meningitis

2. Mr Akshay was suffering from diabetes, he decided to travel to Saharan Africa. He stayed in dormitories, and after return back to India, he developed otitis media and complained of neck stiffness and fever. On CSF examination, it was purulent in appearance. What must have been the cause of such complaints?
   a. Viral meningitis
   b. Otitis interna
   c. Bacterial meningitis
   d. Tubercular meningitis

3. A patient has classical symptoms, fever, headache and nuchal rigidity. In which condition these classical symptoms are found?
   a. Brain tumor
   b. Alzheimer's disease
   c. Meningitis
   d. Myasthenia gravis

4. What investigations would you undertake to establish the diagnosis of meningitis?
   a. CSF analysis
   b. Blood culture
   c. Sputum culture
   d. CT scan

5. Positive Kernig's sign and Brudzinski's sign are observed in:
   a. Meningitis
   b. Multiple sclerosis
   c. Appendicitis
   d. Stroke

6. _____ is a type of encephalitis, commonly occure in immunocompromised people?
   a. Arthropod-borne viral encephalitis
   a. Fungal encephalitis
   b. Herpes simplex encephalitis
   c. St Louis encephalitis

7. The vaccine for Japanese encephalitis is:
   a. Live (mutant) vaccine
   b. Killed vaccine
   c. Live (attenuated) vaccine
   d. Live (recombinant) vaccine

8. In Bihar, the most affected children suffering from AES or encephalitis are:
   a. Gender
   b. Malnourished children
   c. Below age 5
   d. Culture specific

9. What are the symptoms of encephalitis or acute encephalitis syndrome, *except*?
   a. High fever
   b. Vomiting
   c. Confusion
   d. Pinkish skin color

10. Treatments given to encephalitis or AES patients are, *except*?
    a. Corticosteroids
    b. Mechanical ventilation
    c. Anticonvulsants
    d. Anthelmintic medicine

11. A patient presenting with a rapidly progressive course consisting of fever, focal abnormalities on neurologic examination, and evidence of increased intracranial pressure is MOST likely to have:
    a. Brain abscess
    b. Viral meningitis
    c. Intracranial hemorrhage
    d. Metabolic encephalopathy

12. Which of the following statements is/are true?
    a. Cranial osteomyelitis most frequently arises from the spread of bacteria through the bloodstream from an infection elsewhere in the body
    b. Subdural empyema is usually treated by administration of antibiotics without the need for surgical drainage
    c. Bacterial meningitis may lead to the development of hydrocephalus
    d. Bacterial brain abscesses are difficult to visualize by CT

13. What is a brain abscess?
    a. A pus-filled pocket inside the brain
    b. A sinus infection that causes postnasal drip
    c. An infection of the meninges
    d. A compound fracture where bone enters the brain

14. A patient with no prior head trauma is being treated for a brain abscess under your care. While she is in surgery to drain the

abscess, the parent wants to know what might have caused the condition. Which of the following would be the best reply?
a. Brain abscesses are caused by an infection that travels to the brain through the blood or other parts of the body
a. Brain abscesses are caused by uncontrolled cell division of glial cells
b. Brain abscesses are caused by the buildup of toxins in the blood, such as lead
c. Brain abscesses are caused by metabolic changes that happen during advanced liver disease

15. Early cerebritis can be developed in how many days?
    a. 1–4 days   b. 4–10 days
    c. 11–14 days   d. >14 days

16. Which of the following is causative organism for neurocysticercosis?
    a. *Taenia solium*   b. *Taenia sainata*
    c. *Taenia saginata*   d. *Taenia helex*

17. Which of the following health education is most suitable for a patient with neurocysticercosis?
    a. About diet
    b. About exercise
    c. About antiepileptic drug adherence
    d. About postoperative care

18. How is cysticercosis most commonly transmitted?
    a. Sexual contact
    b. Breathing in contaminated air
    c. Consuming contaminated water or food
    d. Coming in contact with an infected monkey

19. A person who is infected with cysticercosis may have cysts that grow throughout his or her body. What is the official term for these cysts?
    a. Granulomas   b. Tumors
    c. Calcification d. Benign cancer

20. Which of the following stage of neurocysticercosis shows maximum edema around the lesion on MRI?
    a. Vesicular   b. Colloid vesicular
    c. Granular nodular   d. Nodular calcified

ANSWERS

1. b	2. c	3. c	4. a
5. a	6. b	7. b	8. b
9. d	10. d	11. a	12. c
13. a	14. a	15. a	16. a
17. c	18. c	19. c	20. b

SUGGESTED READING

1. Ahmad R, Khan T, Ahmad B, Misra A, Balapure AK. Neurocysticercosis: a review on status in India, management, and current therapeutic interventions. Parasitol Res [Internet]. 2017 Jan 1 [cited 2021 Mar 30];116(1):21–33. Available from: http://www.cdc.gov/parasites/cysticercosis/biology.html
2. Archibald LK, Quisling RG. Central Nervous System Infections. In: Textbook of Neurointensive Care [Internet]. London: Springer London; 2013 [cited 2021 Feb 11]. p. 427–517. Available from: http://link.springer.com/10.1007/978-1-4471-5226-2_22
3. Bradshaw MJ, Venkatesan A. Herpes Simplex Virus-1 Encephalitis in Adults: Pathophysiology, Diagnosis, and Management. Neurotherapeutics [Internet]. 2016 Jul 22 [cited 2021 Mar 5];13(3):493–508. Available from: http://link.springer.com/10.1007/s13311-016-0433-7
4. Daroff RB. Bradley's neurology in clinical practice e-book. Elsevier Health Sciences; 2015. p. 644.
5. Dutta AK, Swaminathan S, Abitbol V, Kolhapure S, Sathyanarayanan S. A Comprehensive Review of Meningococcal Disease Burden in India. Infect Dis Ther [Internet]. 2020 Sep 23 [cited 2021 Jan 28];9(3):537–59. Available from: http://link.springer.com/10.1007/s40121-020-00323-4
6. Erdoğan E, Cansever T. Pyogenic brain abscess. Neurosurg Focus [Internet]. 2008 Jun 1 [cited 2021 Mar 19];24(6):E2. Available from: https://thejns.org/focus/view/journals/neurosurg-focus/24/6/article-pE2.xml
7. Mori I, Nishiyama Y, Yokochi T, Kimura Y. Olfactory transmission of neurotropic viruses. J Neurovirol [Internet]. 2005 Apr [cited 2021 Mar 5];11(2):129–37. Available from: https://pubmed.ncbi.nlm.nih.gov/16036791/
8. Muzumdar D, Jhawar S, Goel A. Brain abscess: An overview. Int J Surg. 2011;9(2):136-44.
9. Osenbach RK, Loftus CM. Diagnosis and management of brain abscess. Vol. 3, Neurosurgery clinics of North America. Elsevier; 1992. pp. 403-20.
10. Robertson FC, Lepard JR, Mekary RA, Davis MC, Yunusa I, Gormley WB, et al. Epidemiology of central nervous system infectious diseases: A meta-analysis and systematic review with implications for neurosurgeons worldwide. J Neurosurg [Internet]. 2019 Apr 1 [cited 2021 Mar 19];130(4):1107-26. Available from: https://pubmed.ncbi.nlm.nih.gov/29905514/
11. Roos KL. Meningitis, Fungal. In: Aminoff MJ, Daroff RBBT-E of the NS (Second E, eds. Oxford: Academic Press; 2014. pp. 1074-6. Available from: http://www.sciencedirect.com/science/article/pii/B9780123851574003584
12. Sejvar JJ. West Nile virus and "poliomyelitis." Neurology [Internet]. 2004 Jul 27 [cited 2021 Mar 5];63(2):206–7. Available from: https://pubmed.ncbi.nlm.nih.gov/15277609/
13. Sharma BS, Gupta SK, Khosla VK. Current concepts in the management of pyogenic brain abscess. Neurol India [Internet]. 2000 [cited 2021 Mar 19];48(2):105-11. Available from: https://pubmed.ncbi.nlm.nih.gov/10878771/
14. Shukla ND, Tiwari V, Valyi-Nagy T. Nectin-1-specific entry of herpes simplex virus 1 is sufficient for infection of the cornea and viral spread to the trigeminal ganglia. Mol Vis [Internet]. 2012 [cited 2021 Mar 5];18:2711. Available from: http://www.molvis.org/molvis/v18/a278
15. Stahl JP, Mailles A. Herpes simplex virus encephalitis update. Curr Opin Infect Dis [Internet]. 2019 Jun 1 [cited 2021 Mar 5];32(3):239-43. Available from: https://pubmed.ncbi.nlm.nih.gov/30921087/
16. Tsai J, Nagel MA, Gilden D. Skin rash in meningitis and meningoencephalitis. Neurology [Internet]. 2013 May 7 [cited 2021 Feb 11];80(19):1808-11. Available from:/pmc/articles/PMC3719428/
17. WHO Taeniasis Epidemiology [Internet]. WHO. World Health Organization; 2016 [cited 2021 Mar 30]. Available from: http://www.who.int/taeniasis/epidemiology/en/
18. Zunt JR, Kassebaum NJ, Blake N, Glennie L, Wright C, Nichols E, et al. Global, regional, and national burden of meningitis, 1990–2016: a systematic analysis for the Global Burden of Disease Study 2016. Lancet Neurol [Internet]. 2018 Dec 1 [cited 2021 Jan 28];17(12):1061-82. Available from: www.thelancet.com/neurology

CHAPTER 35

Nerve and Muscle Disorders

Priya Baby, Saraswathi Nashi

"Take up one idea. Make that one idea your life—think of it, dream of it, live on that idea. Let the brain, muscles, nerves, every part of your body, be full of that idea, and just leave every other idea alone. This is the way to success".
—**Swami Vivekananda**

LEARNING OBJECTIVES

After going through the chapter, the learner will be able to:
- Describe the etiopathogenesis of common nerve and muscle disorders (Guillain-Barre syndrome, myasthenia gravis, and muscular dystrophies).
- Discuss the various clinical manifestations of Guillain-Barre syndrome, myasthenia gravis, and Duchenne muscular dystrophy (DMD).
- Discuss the management of patients with Guillain-Barré syndrome, myasthenia gravis and DMD.
- Use the nursing process as a framework of care for patients with Guillain-Barre syndrome, myasthenia gravis, and DMD.

TERMS

- **Duchenne muscular dystrophy:** The most common form of muscular dystrophy which is characterized by progressive muscle weakness and follows an X-linked recessive pattern of inheritance.
- **Guillain-Barre syndrome:** An acute monophasic paralytic disease affecting the peripheral nerves and nerve roots.
- **Muscular dystrophy:** A heterogeneous group of neuromuscular disorders that are characterized by progressive muscle weakness caused due to degeneration of skeletal muscles.
- **Myasthenia crisis:** A life-threatening complication of myasthenia gravis that results in increased severity of the symptoms and results in respiratory failure.
- **Myasthenia Gravis:** A chronic autoimmune disorder of the neuromuscular junction characterized by weakness of skeletal muscles.

GUILLAIN-BARRÉ SYNDROME

INTRODUCTION

Guillain-Barré syndrome (GBS) is an acute monophasic paralytic radiculoneuropathy that progresses over a period of days to a maximum of 4 weeks. It is an immune-mediated disorder that affects the peripheral nervous system. It is a neurological emergency that affects about 100,000 people every year worldwide.

This condition was first described by Landry in 1859. The disease is named after two military Neurologists Guillain and Barré, who worked with paralyzed soldiers and identified unusual changes in their CSF, in 1916.

The reported incidence rate for GBS is 1–2 per 100,000 population. The incidence of GBS in tropical countries like India is higher when compared to the rest of the world. However, there are no population-based studies to do a statistical comparison. A seasonal increase in the prevalence of GBS is observed in India. This could be due to the increased incidence of gastroenteritis (which has a role in the etiopathogenesis of GBS) during summer. The disease is slightly more frequent in males than in females. The lifetime likelihood of any individual acquiring GBS is 1:1000.

ETIOLOGY AND PATHOGENESIS

GBS is a complex autoimmune disease of the peripheral nerves and nerve roots. Patients who develop GBS have a previous history of respiratory or gastrointestinal infection within the past 4 weeks. As many as two third of the adult patients with GBS have a history of such preceding infections. In Asian countries, *Campylobacter jejuni* is the pathogen predominantly causing preceding infections in GBS. Almost 25–50% of the adult patients have preceding *C. jejuni* infection causing GI symptoms prior to the onset of GBS. In Europe and Japan, respiratory tract infections caused by Cytomegalovirus (CMV) are linked to GBS. Epstein-Barr virus, influenza A virus, *Mycoplasma pneumoniae*, and *Haemophilus influenzae* are other pathogens that are linked to GBS.

The pathological basis for GBS is an aberrant autoimmune response that is induced by a preceding infection or other immune stimulation. The proposed theory for this response is of molecular mimicry. The close similarity between the microbial antigen and the nerve antigen results in an abnormal immune response directed toward the nerve antigens. The peripheral nerves and the spinal roots are attacked by the body's immune system causing unwanted autoreactivity. This is especially true in the case of infection with *C jejuni*. However, in all people who get infected with *C. jejuni*, the autoreactivity against the nerve antigens does not develop. There is a complex interplay between microbial and host factors that dictate if and how the immune response is shifted towards unwanted autoreactivity. Several of these factors which decide why autoreactivity develops in some people are not yet fully understood. Other than preceding infections, certain situations like surgery, immunization, and parturition are also seen as associated with GBS. The abnormal immune-mediated response is postulated as the cause of disease in all these conditions. Anti-ganglioside antibodies that react to self-ganglioside are identified as the pathological cause of autoreactivity. The autoantigenic gangliosides that are currently known are GD3, GM1, GM1b, GD1a, GalNAc-GD1a, GQ1b, GQ3, and GT1.

Newly emerging post-infectious forms of Guillain-Barré syndrome, such as those associated with arboviruses including Zika, were recently identified.

VARIANTS OF GUILLAIN-BARRÉ SYNDROME

GBS electrophysiologically is of two types, the demyelinating type, and the axonal type.

1. **Demyelinating type:** It is the one in which the immune attack is directed toward the myelin of the neuron. It is also commonly known as acute inflammatory demyelinating polyneuropathy (AIDP). Demyelination of the neurons due to lymphocytic and macrophagic infiltration is the most characteristic pathologic feature of the demyelinating type. In this type, there is a T cell-directed autoimmune attack against the proteins of the myelin sheath. This causes segmental demyelination. AIDP is the most prevalent form of GBS and accounts for 70–90% of the cases. Many times, GBS is synonymously used with AIDP, but AIDP is only one of the variants of GBS.

2. **Axonal type:** In this, the immune attack is directed at the axons rather than at the myelin. In the axonal type of GBS, the characteristic pathological changes include lengthening of the nodes of Ranvier and macrophagic attack at the nodal region. The axons are subsequently damaged by the macrophage activity. The two axonal types of GBS are acute motor axonal neuropathy (AMAN) and acute motor sensory axonal neuropathy (AMSAN). In AMAN, the motor nerves are affected, and in AMSAN, both motor and sensory nerves are affected. AMAN is characterized by acute or subacute onset of symmetric limb weakness and purely motor deficits, whereas AMSAN is characterized by both motor and sensory dysfunction.

Unlike AIDP, there is reduced lymphocytic infiltration in this type. Since the damage is mostly directed at the axons, delayed recovery is seen in axonal types. The pathological difference between the types of GBS is described in **Figure 35.1**.

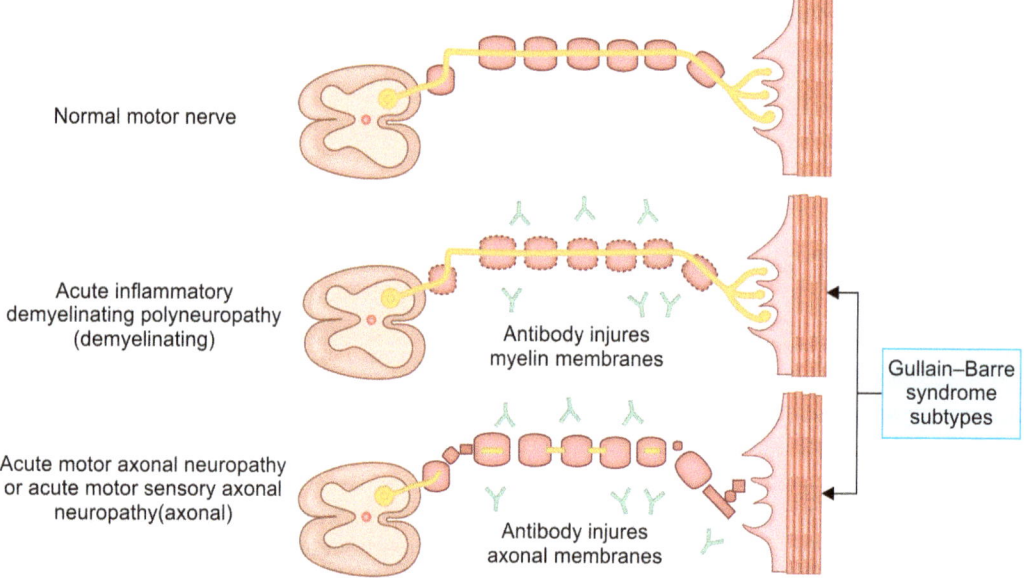

Fig. 35.1: Demyelination and axonal damage associated with subtypes of GBS.

TABLE 35.1: Differences between CIDP and AIDP.

CIDP	AIDP
Slowly progressive, usually more than 8 weeks	The course usually improves in 4 weeks or remains static
More frequency of relapses	Rarely relapses
Preceding infections are rare	Preceding infections are common
Respiratory failure uncommon	Respiratory failure common
Diffuse conduction slowing	Patchy conduction slowing
Responds to steroids	Usually does not respond to steroids

Miller-Fischer syndrome is another variant of GBS which is characterized by a triad of ophthalmoplegia, ataxia, and areflexia. It constitutes 5–10% of the GBS cases. Ataxia is primarily noted during gait and in the trunk, with lesser involvement of the limbs. Motor strength is characteristically spared. The usual course is one of gradual and complete recovery over weeks or months. In addition to the clinical features, they also have elevated CSF protein.

Chronic inflammatory demyelinating polyradiculoneuropathy (CIDP) is considered when the onset of the peak of weakness extends over more than 8 weeks. The differences between CIDP and AIDP are mentioned in **Table 35.1**.

CLINICAL FEATURES

GBS usually has an acute onset. The typical clinical manifestations begin as paresthesia of the distal limbs which progress into acute onset weakness of the limbs. The symptoms are relatively symmetric in pattern.

Flaccid paralysis: Acute onset weakness is the most characteristic feature of GBS. It usually manifests as rapidly evolving flaccid paralysis, typically affecting the lower extremities first and ascending upwards to involve the trunk and upper extremities. This usually evolves over a few days to weeks. Patients generally notice weakness in their legs, manifesting as "rubbery legs" or legs that tend to buckle. Even though the weakness is classically described as ascending, and usually starts in the distal lower extremities, it can also start more proximally in the legs or arms. Sometimes muscle weakness develops in the arms first (descending type) or in the arms and legs simultaneously. The weakness reaches its nadir (the peak of symptoms) in 2–4 weeks.

Dysautonomia is another common symptom of GBS, affecting about 70% of the patients. The manifestations of dysautonomia include tachycardia, hypotension/hypertension, cardiac arrhythmias, and urinary retention. Loss of vasomotor control is the cause of wide fluctuation in blood pressure causing hypo/hypertension. Patients may experience postural hypotension and facial flushing. Gastric dysmotility causing constipation, anhydrosis (no sweating) or diaphoresis (excessive sweating) may also occur. Dysautonomia is more frequent in patients with severe weakness and respiratory failure. The cold pressor test is a simple bedside test that can be used to check dysautonomia. In this, the patient's hand is dipped in ice-cold water for one minute. The variation in blood pressure and pulse is then checked. Patients having dysautonomia do not show much variation, whereas healthy subjects exhibit a rise in blood pressure.

Areflexia: The deep tendon reflexes of the affected limbs will be reduced or absent. But in some patients, during the initial period, the reflexes may seem intact.

Sensory disturbances: Can occur in some patients with GBS. This is more common in the demyelinating type of GBS. Patients may experience paresthesia in the fingers and toes which may then advance proximally. Loss of vibration, proprioception, and touch, distally may also be present. Pain (muscular or radicular) is a prominent symptom in 50% of patients. It is usually of deep aching or throbbing type especially felt in the weak muscles. Fatigue is a common sign which may persist for weeks to months.

Cranial nerve involvement: Can result in facial, ocular, or bulbar weakness. Frequently, the lower cranial nerves may be affected. This leads to bulbar weakness, causing oropharyngeal dysphagia, which includes difficulty in swallowing, drooling, and/or trouble maintaining an open airway. Respiratory difficulties can also occur due to bulbar involvement. One-third of the hospitalized GBS patients may need ventilator assistance due to the severe respiratory involvement.

Isolated cranial nerve involvement is usually seen in Miller-Fischer syndrome.

The clinical course of GBS is divided into three phases:
1. **Progressive phase:** This is the initial phase, which begins when the first definitive symptom develops and ends two to four weeks later, when no further deterioration is noted.
2. **The plateau phase:** This lasts several days to two weeks. The symptoms remain steady and no further deterioration happens in this phase.
3. **The recovery phase:** It coincides with remyelination and axonal process regrowth. This phase extends over four to six months. Patients with severe disease may take up to two years to recover, and recovery may not be complete.

GBS can cause life-threatening complications if the respiratory muscles are affected or if the autonomic nervous system is involved. About 5% of the patients diagnosed with GBS succumb to death. Many of the patients who recover from the acute phase are left with a disabling motor deficit and/or fatigue. The severity and duration of the disease are highly diverse in patients and can range from mild weakness, from which patients recover spontaneously, to patients becoming quadriplegic and ventilator-dependent without signs of recovery for several months or longer.

DIAGNOSTIC EVALUATION

The clinical presentation is the most useful ground on which a diagnosis of GBS is made. The common diagnostic features useful for the diagnosis of GBS are progressive weakness in limbs and areflexia. Usually, limb weakness is initially seen in the lower limbs alone. The additional symptoms which are helpful in GBS diagnosis are relative symmetry of weakness, presence of sensory or autonomic symptoms, pain, and cranial nerve involvement resulting in bilateral facial weakness.

The diagnosis may be confirmed by **cerebrospinal fluid (CSF) analysis and electrophysiological studies**. But both

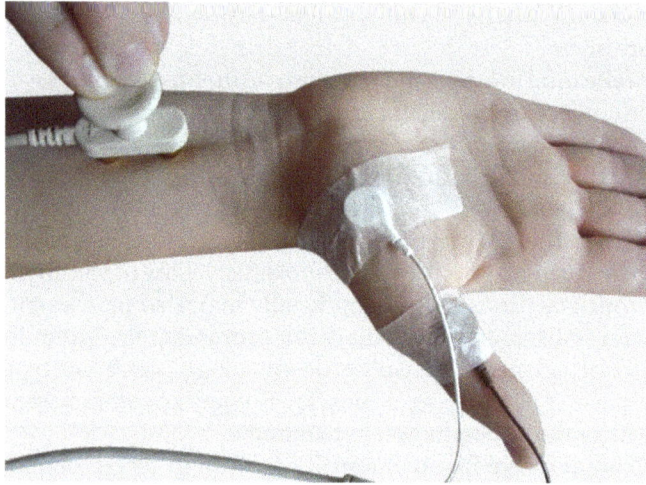

Fig. 35.2: Motor nerve conduction study showing electrical stimulus to median nerve and response recorded on abductor pollicis brevis (APB) muscle.

these investigations can yield normal findings in the early phase of GBS.

When GBS is suspected, electrophysiologic studies are essential to confirm the diagnosis and exclude its mimics. **Nerve conduction studies (NCS)** are the electrophysiologic studies done for GBS **(Fig. 35.2)**. These studies often demonstrate features of demyelination.

Motor NCS are performed by electrical stimulation of a peripheral nerve and recording from a muscle supplied by the nerve. After stimulation of a motor nerve, contraction of the appropriate muscle will occur. If electrodes are attached to the skin over the muscle, a Compound Muscle Action Potential (CMAP) can be recorded **(Figs. 35.3 and 35.4)**. The time between stimulation and response is measured and compared to the distance between the point of stimulation and the point of response to calculate the velocity. The time it takes for the electrical impulse to travel from the stimulation to the recording site is measured. This value is called the latency. The latencies and nerve conduction velocities get delayed due to demyelination. Other abnormal findings in NCS are temporal dispersion of waveforms, conduction block, prolonged or absent F waves, and prolonged or absent H-reflexes. All these findings are suggestive of demyelination.

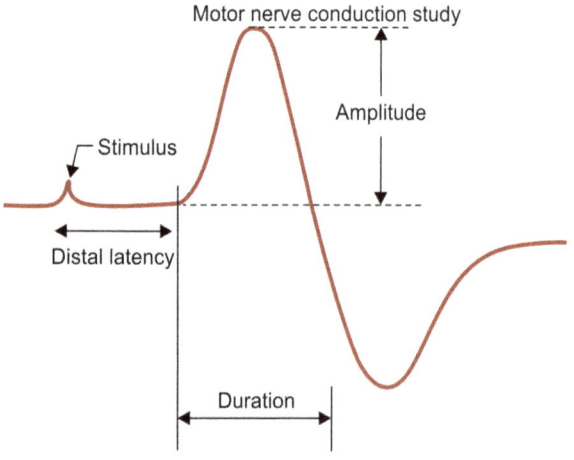

Fig. 35.3: Compound muscle action potential (CMAP).

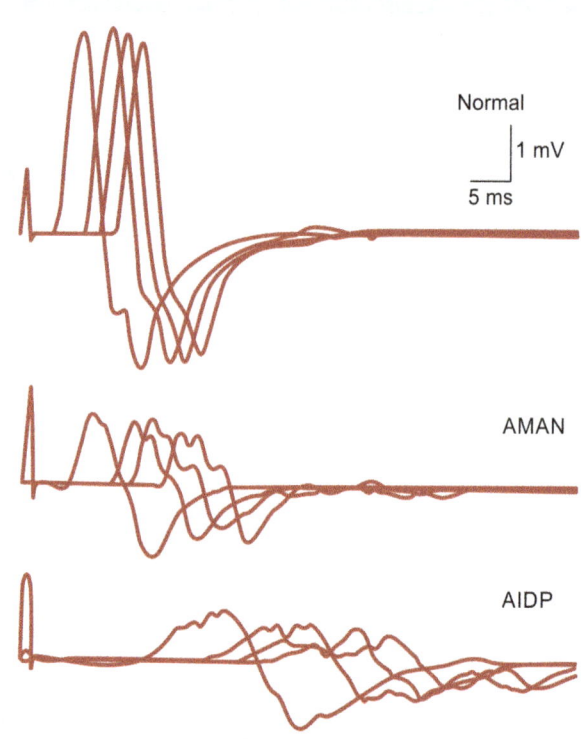

Fig. 35.4: Comparison of CMAP in a normal individual, AMAN and AIDP. *Note the reduction of amplitude with relatively preserved latencies in AMAN and the increase in latency with reduced amplitudes in AIDP.*

Different types of GBS are identified and categorized (such as acute inflammatory demyelinating polyneuropathy, acute motor axonal neuropathy, or acute motor and sensory axonal neuropathy) on the basis of the findings from the nerve conduction studies.

CSF analysis reveals an elevated CSF protein concentration and normal or mildly elevated white blood cell counts (<50 cells/mm^3). This is known as albuminocytologic dissociation. But in the initial phase of the illness, this finding cannot be seen in all the patients. By the peak of the disease, elevated CSF protein concentration occurs in more than 90% of the patients. The increase in CSF protein is thought to reflect the widespread inflammation of the nerve roots.

Albuminocytologic dissociation, findings of the nerve conduction studies, disease progression over days to four weeks, symmetry of symptoms, mild sensory abnormalities, cranial nerve involvement, autonomic dysfunction, and recovery that starts in two to four weeks are all supportive of a diagnosis of GBS.

Routine blood studies like complete blood count and blood chemistry are also done mainly to rule out other causes. Frequent evaluations of pulmonary function parameters should be performed at the bedside to monitor respiratory status and the need for ventilatory assistance.

Differential diagnosis: All diseases that attack the spinal cord, peripheral nerves, muscles, neuromuscular junctions, and cerebral vessels may result in weakness, like GBS, and need to be considered in the differential diagnosis. The differential of pure motor syndrome includes other diseases associated with quadriparesis/paralysis such as myasthenic crisis, idiopathic inflammatory myopathies and motor neuron disease. An increased lymphocyte count in CSF, usually points to other diseases like sarcoidosis, Lyme disease neuropathy, or recent HIV infection.

MANAGEMENT

GBS is a potentially life-threatening disease. It requires hospitalization and close monitoring. Immunological treatment and general supportive care are the major management strategies for GBS.

Intravenous immunoglobulin G (IVIG) therapy is an immunological therapy that has been shown to be effective in GBS. This treatment reduces both the severity of the disease and the residual deficits. IVIG is given in a dosage of 0.4 grams/kg body weight/day for a period of 5 days. Even though there are other regimes of IVIG therapy, this regime has fewer side effects and lesser treatment-related fluctuations. Adverse effects of IVIG include headache, nausea, chills, discomfort, muscle pains, and rarely acute renal failure, hyperviscosity syndromes which can lead to acute myocardial infarction, strokes, pulmonary embolism, and anaphylaxis (especially in patients with total IgA deficiency).

Plasma exchange therapy is an immunomodulatory therapy used in GBS. This is also known as plasmapheresis. In this therapy, the blood of the patient is removed and plasma is separated by an automated centrifuge. The plasma (200-250 mL plasma/kg body weight in five sessions) is separated and discarded so that the antibodies are removed from the blood along with the plasma. After separation of the plasma, the cells are returned to the patient along with replacement colloids. Five plasma exchange sessions (each exchange comprising 2-3 L of plasma according to body weight) over 2 weeks is the accepted, beneficial regimen. The plasma exchange therapy has to be started within the first 4 (preferably 2) weeks from the onset of symptoms in patients with GBS. Potential complications which could arise due to plasmapheresis include pneumothorax during insertion of central intravenous access, sepsis, hypotension, pulmonary embolism, hypocalcemia, coagulation abnormalities, and citrate toxicity.

There is no evidence to prove that combination of IVIG and plasma exchange is better than IVIG or plasma exchange alone. No evidence exists to show that a second course of IVIG is effective in patients with GBS who continue to deteriorate. One of the major disadvantages of IVIG is the high cost. New approaches to treatment using monoclonal antibodies are researched to study their possible use in GBS. Oral or IV steroids are not used in the treatment for GBS. Corticosteroids used as monotherapy is not found to significantly hasten recovery from GBS or affect long-term outcomes. However, in chronic inflammatory demyelinating polyneuropathy, corticosteroids are found to be extremely useful.

Pain management: Pain is highly prevalent and intense in patients with GBS. An adequate analgesic treatment is therefore of the utmost importance. Since the pain in GBS is neuropathic in origin, NSAIDS are not recommended. Drugs like gabapentin and, carbamazepine are useful for pain management. The analgesic effect of carbamazepine is attributed to blockage of the voltage-gated sodium channels that are essential for pain transmission. Pregabalin, which is an antiepileptic drug is also found useful for neuropathic pain in GBS. Pregabalin subtly reduces the synaptic release of several neurotransmitters and causes symptom control. Opioid analgesics are not used for pain management as they may aggravate the autonomic dysfunction and aggravate constipation and bladder distension.

Deep vein thrombosis (DVT) prophylaxis: Prophylaxis for DVT is essential as the disease is associated with immobility. Subcutaneous Heparin is administered to prevent thromboembolic events. Enoxaparin (40 mg daily) is commonly used for DVT prophylaxis.

One of the major aspects of management of GBS patients is the supportive care and monitoring of complications. Respiratory functions of the patients should be monitored closely and frequently. Timely transfer to ICU should be anticipated. Attention is needed for cardiac and hemodynamic monitoring so that emergencies arising from autonomic dysfunction can be identified early. Management of possible bladder and bowel dysfunction, early initiation of physiotherapy and rehabilitation, and psychosocial support are other aspects of the multidisciplinary management.

Prognosis

Majority of GBS patients recover within first few weeks from the onset of symptoms. Almost 85% of the patients return to their baseline functions within one year. About 5-10% might still have residual motor and sensory deficits. Relapse is usually uncommon, but can happen in 2-3% of the patients. Mortality in GBS is estimated at about 5%. The frequent causes of death in them include complications associated with respiratory compromise, aspiration pneumonia, sepsis, arrhythmias, and thromboembolic events.

NURSING MANAGEMENT

The role of a nurse in managing a GBS patient depends on:
- The point of the course of illness
- The severity of the symptoms
- The presence of respiratory distress
- The medical management the patient is receiving

If the patient is at the acute phase of the illness with acute onset of weakness, a proper history and physical examination is very essential to confirm the disease. History collection should identify any preceding infections in the past 2 to 4 weeks. Ask for any symptoms of respiratory or GI infections that the patient might have experienced in the recent past. Ask for a history of recent immunization, or surgical procedure.

Patients with GBS may stay in the hospital for several days to weeks. Hence a comprehensive supportive care is essential for them to make sure that they do not develop complications.

Monitoring Respiratory Status

Respiratory compromise can occur in GBS patients due to the weakness in respiratory muscles. Frequent monitoring is essential to pick up early signs of respiratory discomfort. In addition to the regular assessment of respiratory rate, rhythm, and depth, respiratory efficiency is checked by single breath count which is a simple bedside test. In this, the patient is asked to take a deep breath and hold it (maximal inspiration).

Holding their breath, the patient should count out loudly for as long as he or she can. The number at which the patient stops holding the breath is considered the value of a single breath count. Low single breath count indicates respiratory muscle involvement. Serial checking of the single breath count provides a quantitative picture of the drop or improvement in the respiratory ability of the individual. Ideally, serial pulmonary function tests can be done to identify any drop in vital capacity, mean inspiratory, or mean expiratory pressures. A drop in the vital capacity of less than 20 mL/kg or a single breath count as low as 15 can deem ventilator support. In such cases, patients should be shifted immediately to an ICU for ventilatory support.

Airway Protection

The weakness of pharyngeal and laryngeal muscles can lead to difficulty in clearing secretions and maintenance of patent airway. This can further increase the risk of aspiration and cause complications. Hence assessment for bulbar involvement and risk for aspiration has to be made for all patients. Modified feeds and NG tube feeding has to be considered in patients with dysphagia. Oropharyngeal suction may be required for patients who have difficulty clearing secretions. Nurses need to anticipate an exacerbation of respiratory symptoms and the need for intubation in patients. Sleep disturbances also occur in these patients owing to the respiratory muscle involvement. Monitor for sleep apnea and sleep behavioral problems in patients with respiratory involvement.

DVT Prophylaxis

As weakness and immobility occur due to demyelination, prevention of the complications of immobility is a prime responsibility of the nurse. The use of compression stockings helps to reduce venous stasis and thereby improve circulation. Fractionated or unfractionated heparin is also used to reduce the risk of venous thromboembolism.

Bowel and Bladder Management

Dysautonomia in GBS patients can cause reduced gut motility resulting in constipation. The immobility associated with the illness also promotes constipation. Hence abdomen should be auscultated to check for any reduction in bowel sounds. Bladder distension should be checked for, and catheterization may be initiated if necessary.

Autonomic Dysfunction

Serious and potentially fatal disturbances of autonomic function, including arrhythmias and extreme hypertension or hypotension, occur in approximately 20% of patients with GBS. Endotracheal suction and certain medications can actually precipitate these fatal disturbances. Patients with advanced generalized weakness and respiratory failure are more prone to fatal manifestations of autonomic dysfunction. Hence those patients should be on continuous ECG and vital monitoring. While checking the peripheral pulse, the nurse should palpate the pulse for an entire minute and any rhythm or rate abnormalities should be documented. Changes in position should be made cautiously to avoid falls due to orthostatic hypotension.

Physical Mobility

Physical therapy is considered as an integral part of supportive management in reducing the incidence of complications such as respiratory complications, deep vein thrombosis (DVT), pain management, and delayed mobilization. Mobility is compromised to varying degrees in patients with GBS. In patients who have no muscle power, passive exercises should be initiated. As the patient recovers from weakness, active exercises can be promoted. This ensures the prevention of several complications like venous thromboembolism and the development of contractures. A physical therapist can be involved in setting mobility goals and providing exercises for patients within their limits. In all these activities, active caregiver/family involvement is essential as it also acts as a bridge to the home care which the patient may need.

Treatment-related Aspects

Patients with GBS usually receive IVIG as a treatment. Although IVIG is relatively safe, adverse events occur in about 5% of patients. Hence nurses should monitor for common problems including infusion-related headache, myalgias, chills, and nausea. These can be managed by stopping the infusion temporarily and then resuming it at a slower rate. Symptomatic management using medications can also be helpful.

Patients who are undergoing plasma exchange therapy require special nursing attention as they are prone to several imbalances related to the therapy. They should be prepared well before initiating the treatment. The specific preparations include:

- ❖ Educate the patient about the purpose of the procedure.
- ❖ Obtain written informed consent for the therapy.
- ❖ Check the patient's body weight and the vital signs including blood pressure.
- ❖ Administer intravenous fluids as directed.
- ❖ Ensure adequate oral hydration.
- ❖ High protein diet, including egg whites, nuts, and dairy products should be encouraged.

The post-procedure care includes:

- ❖ Monitor the BP and vitals. Patients are prone to develop hypotension, after a plasma exchange session as it involves the removal of plasma.
- ❖ Administer IV fluids, including colloids like fresh frozen plasma and hydroxyethyl starch (HES) as advised.
- ❖ Check for signs of hypocalcemia, like perioral tingling, muscle cramps, Trousseaus sign, and Chvostek sign. Patients are prone to develop hypocalcemia due to the loss of calcium from blood due to the chelating action of anticoagulants (EDTA) used during the process of plasma exchange.
- ❖ Advise a calcium-rich diet and supplement calcium if necessary.
- ❖ Advise continuing a high protein diet. This will help to replace the proteins lost through plasma.

Psychosocial Aspects

The sensorimotor manifestations of GBS are usually so severe that it masks most of the psychological disturbances experienced by GBS patients. They may experience anxiety and depressive symptoms during illness. This can also be attributed to the prolonged course of illness. As the disease strikes acutely, hospitalization can burden the patient and family in a much unexpected way. Supportive care to the patient and the family is therefore a cardinal part of nursing care. Counseling the patient and family, listening to their concerns, and informing them about the course of the illness, its prognosis, and treatment options are necessary to ensure that they cope with the situation.

Even though the GBS patients are prone to several complications, meticulous nursing care helps to minimize the risk of mortality and eventually improves the outcomes. A hypothetical nursing care plan for a patient with GBS is summarized in **Table 35.2**.

TABLE 35.2: Hypothetical care plan for a patient with GBS.

Nursing diagnosis	Nursing interventions
Ineffective breathing pattern related to loss of respiratory functions	• Assess the respiratory ability of the patient by performing a single breath count • Assess the respiratory rate • Look for breathlessness while speaking • Use of accessory muscles of respiration to be observed • Periodically monitor the respiratory fatigue • Keep the head end elevated 30–45° • Assess oxygen saturation and arterial blood gas in case of dropping respiratory function • Anticipate airway intubation and ICU transfer • Suction secretions as appropriate, especially if the client is intubated or tracheostomy is done
Acute pain related to neuronal damage	• Assess the degree of pain • Administer neuropathic pain medications • Avoid opioids
Impaired physical mobility	• Assess the motor strength of the patient. • Encourage the patient to mobilize limbs as per the ability • Provide active ROM exercises in between rest periods • Provide change in position as tolerated • Use assistive devices to mobilize the patient • Assist in activities of daily living
Risk of injury (thromboembolism) related to immobility	• Encourage the patient to mobilize as tolerated • Apply compression stocking to promote venous return • Administer heparin injection as prescribed • Observe the calf muscles for any redness, warmth, or swelling and notify immediately
Risk of injury related to anticoagulant therapy	• Assess the injection site for local bruising and rotate the site to avoid tissue injury • Modify the environment to prevent falls and injuries • Do not leave the patient unattended anytime • Inform the patient to report any bleeding from gums, nose, or black tarry stools

Case Scenario

- Lakshman, a 42-year-old farmer noticed sudden the feeling of 'pins and needles' in his both legs. This was followed by difficulty in walking, and he felt that his legs were rubbery. The weakness increased and he became unable to walk. He also had pain in both lower limbs. He had a history of fever and diarrhea 2 weeks before which resolved spontaneously.
- His weakness was ascending and he was brought to the emergency when he started experiencing breathing difficulty. On examination, his deep tendon reflexes (DTR) was absent on both lower limbs. He had muscle strength of 0/5 in both his both lower limbs and 2/5 in the upper limbs. His pulse rate was 120 bpm and his BP was 170/90 mmHg. He also had an irregular heartbeat.
- Nerve conduction studies were performed and he was diagnosed to have acute inflammatory demyelinating polyneuropathy. Lumbar puncture was performed and CSF analysis revealed elevated protein levels.
- His condition worsened and he was intubated and shifted to ICU due to Type 2 respiratory failure. He was treated with plasma exchange therapy.
- Discuss the nursing care of Lakshman during his stay in the ICU.

SUMMARY

GBS is a typical post-infectious disorder, having a progressive, monophasic disease course. Molecular mimicry between microbial and nerve antigens is a major driving force behind the development of the disorder. Immunomodulatory therapies are the mainstay of medical management of this disorder. Diligent supportive care mainly focusing on the preservation of functions and prevention of complications can improve the outcome in these patients.

MYASTHENIA GRAVIS

INTRODUCTION

Myasthenia gravis (MG) is a chronic autoimmune disorder that affects the neuromuscular junction, which results in varying degrees of weakness of skeletal muscles. In MG, the autoimmune attack is directed to the acetylcholine receptors at the neuromuscular junction. This affects the impulse transmission from the nerves and the muscle contraction fails to get triggered, causing weakness. As it is a chronic disease which has no complete cure, appropriate disease management is essential to ensure a normal life for the patient.

EPIDEMIOLOGY

The exact prevalence of MG in the Indian population is not known, but globally the reported prevalence is 0.5–12.5 per 100,000. The annual incidence is 0.25–2 in one lakh population. Compared to the previous reports, there has been a clear trend toward an increase in the reported prevalence of myasthenia gravis.

MG affects all ages. However, gender and age are two factors that determine the incidence of MG. Females below 40 years of age are three times more vulnerable than their male counterparts. Peak incidence in females is between 20 and 30 years. In males above 50 years of age, the incidence of MG increases. MG can occur in childhood also. It comprises 10–15% of all MG cases.

PATHOPHYSIOLOGY

Myasthenia gravis is an autoimmune disease of the neuromuscular junction (NMJ). It is reported to coexist with other autoimmune diseases. It occurs due to the antibodies that attack components of the postsynaptic membrane and impair neuromuscular transmission. The normal NMJ transmits impulses using acetylcholine which acts as a neurotransmitter. It is synthesized in nerve terminals and stored in vesicles, which are then released into the synaptic cleft upon activation of the nerve. This gets attached to the Ach receptors (AChRs) on the post synaptic muscle membrane and triggers the action potential in the muscle. In MG, ACh is released normally, but its effect on the post-synaptic membrane is reduced.

Due to the autoimmune process in MG, circulating autoantibodies are formed against acetylcholine receptors (AChRs). Almost all the cases (>80%) are positive for these autoantibodies. This type of MG is known as seropositive MG. A less percentage of MG patients lack antibodies against AChRs; which is called seronegative MG.

However, in these patients, antibodies against other receptor proteins of the neuromuscular junction are reported. Antibody against muscle-specific tyrosine kinase (MuSK), localized to the postsynaptic membrane of the neuromuscular junction is reported in most seronegative MG patients.

There is an association between MG and thymus gland abnormalities. The Thymus gland is reported to be abnormal in 75% of the cases, with thymus hyperplasia in 65% and thymoma in 10% of the patients.

As the thymus is the primary lymphoid organ for immunological self-tolerance, thymic abnormalities result in an immune-mediated attack on AChRs in MG. Patients with thymomas usually have a severe form of illness with more circulating antibodies. There is also a correlation between the degree of follicular hyperplasia and the level of anti-AChRs antibodies. Neoplastic cells in thymoma express antigens similar to acetylcholine receptors and trigger the thymus gland to produce antibodies against them.

The post-synaptic muscle membrane in MG is distorted and simplified. The AChR concentration on the post synaptic muscle membrane is reduced and hence it becomes less sensitive to ACh. Loss of approximately 60% of AChRs is necessary to cause myasthenic weakness. The post-synaptic membrane loses structural integrity in terms of its normal folded shape due to the circulating antibodies **(Figs. 35.5A and B)**. This in turn reduces the number of available voltage-gated sodium channels available at the synapse for neurotransmission. Therefore, the threshold required to initiate a muscle action potential increases and neurotransmission fails.

CLINICAL MANIFESTATIONS

The hallmark symptoms of MG include fluctuating weakness of voluntary muscles that worsens after periods of activity and improves after periods of rest. The muscles involved include eye muscles, facial muscles, respiratory muscles, and limb muscles **(Table 35.3)**. The degree of muscle weakness involved in myasthenia gravis varies greatly among individuals. There is no abnormality reported in reflexes, sensation, cognition, and autonomic function.

TYPES OF MYASTHENIA GRAVIS

MG can be broadly classified into:
1. **Ocular myasthenia:** Only ocular symptoms might be present in approximately 15% of people with MG. Ocular symptoms are often the first symptoms to develop in MG. Later many of the patients may develop other generalized muscle weaknesses.
2. **Generalized myasthenia:** In this form of myasthenia, patients have generalized symptoms of muscles of the body along with ocular symptoms. Approximately 85% of people diagnosed with generalized MG have AChR autoantibodies present in their blood tests. Another 15% of the patients may not have these antibodies. Out of them, 50% of the patients might be positive for the antibodies against another major protein called muscle-specific kinase (MuSK) which is involved in neuromuscular impulse transmission.
3. **Seronegative myasthenia:** In this form of MG, autoantibodies (anti-AChR and anti-MuSK auto-antibodies) are not detectable in the blood. Approximately 10% of people with MG are considered seronegative.

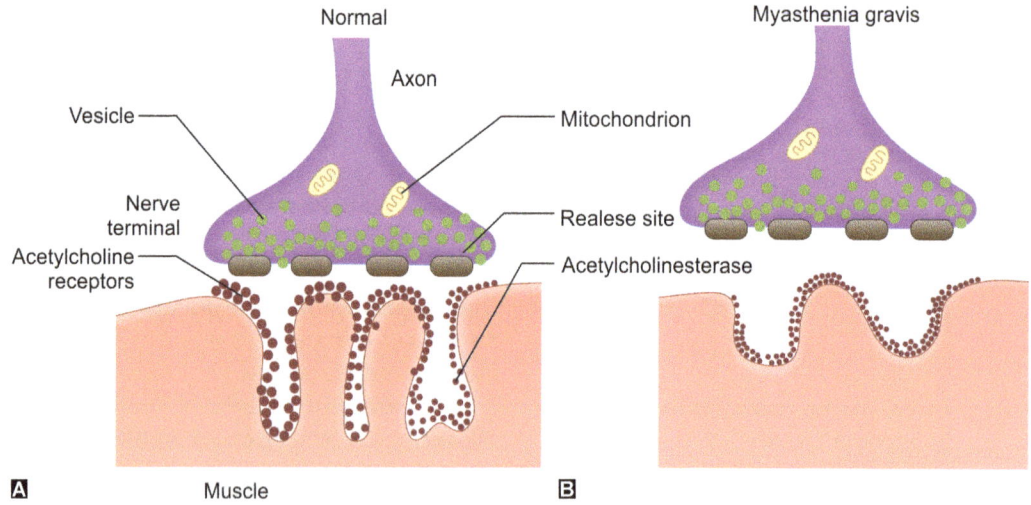

Figs. 35.5A and B:: (A) Normal neuromuscular junction; (B) Neuromuscular junction in MG.

TABLE 35.3: Clinical manifestations of myasthenia gravis.

Muscles involved	Clinical manifestations
Ocular muscles (Primarily due to levator palpebrae superioris complex and extraocular muscle are involved)	• Over 80% of the MG patients have ocular symptoms at initial presentation • These include ptosis or diplopia • Variable ptosis is usually observed in MG. It can be unilateral or bilateral and can be asymmetric if bilateral **(Figs. 35.6A and B)** • Diplopia can occur due to extraocular muscle involvement
Bulbar muscles (Muscles of the head and neck are involved)	• Over 15 % patients have bulbar muscle involvement as the initial sign • Difficulty in chewing, dysphagia, easy fatigability during chewing and frequent choking might be observed • Nasal twang of speech, hoarseness of voice, dysarthria might be present • Expressionless face
Respiratory muscles (Upper airway muscles and respiratory muscles can be involved)	• Dyspnea • Initially intercostal and accessory muscles are involved followed by diaphragm • Pronounced during myasthenic crisis
Limb muscles (Muscles of the extremities, usually proximal muscles more than distal muscles are involved)	• Upper extremity weakness is more common than lower extremity • It can be asymmetrical • Weakness increases with activity

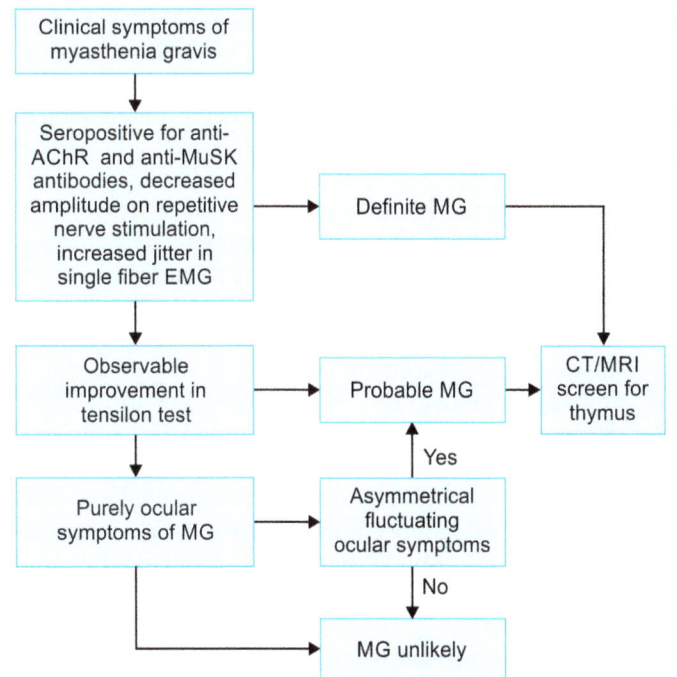

Flowchart 35.1: Diagnostic algorithm for patients with MG.

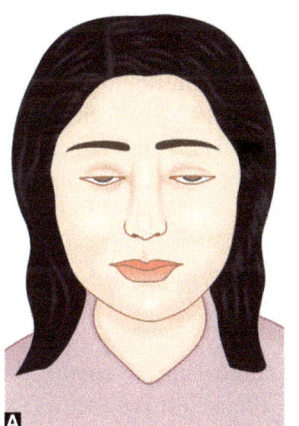 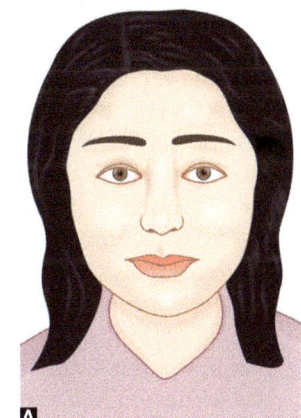

Figs. 35.6A and B: (A) Ptosis in MG; (B) Normal.

DIAGNOSTIC EVALUATION

The presence of characteristic manifestations of MG raises suspicion about the diagnosis. The most characteristic symptoms include diplopia, ptosis, dysarthria, muscle weakness of limbs with preserved deep tendon reflexes, weakness of trunk muscles, and respiratory symptoms. The weakness worsens with repeated use of the muscle. These features are typically directive towards myasthenia.

The most common tests used for diagnosis are the tensilon test, electrophysiological studies, serological tests, and imaging studies **(Flowchart 35.1)**.

❖ **Tensilon (edrophonium chloride) test:** Edrophonium chloride is a rapid onset, short-acting anticholinesterase drug. It prevents the degradation of acetylcholine at the NMJ. The test is performed by administering edrophonium intravenously and the patient is observed for objective improvement in muscle strength. At the beginning of the test 2 mg edrophonium is administered intravenously. The patient will receive subsequent doses of 2 mg edrophonium after each 60-second interval. Usually, after a 2–6 mg dose of edrophonium, the patient will show improvement. This is concluded as a positive result. In case of a positive result, the patients present with a dramatic improvement of ocular symptoms. They would be able to perform repeated actions with the same muscles without fatigue.

The test is contraindicated in patients with hypersensitivity to edrophonium and in patients with GI or urinary obstruction. Caution is advised when performing the test on asthmatic patients as it can precipitate bronchoconstriction and worsening of the condition. Heart rate and blood pressure are continuously monitored to assess for any adverse side effects including bradycardia, hypotension, or cardiac arrhythmias. Edrophonium can also cause increased salivation, sweating, and muscle fasciculations due to it cholinergic effects. Other side effects of edrophonium include increased salivation, sweating, nausea, stomach cramps, and muscle fasciculation. Atropine sulphate is administered in case of severe bradycardia.

❖ **Electrophysiological tests:** Diagnosis of MG is aided by two important electrophysiological studies; the repetitive nerve stimulation study and single fiber electromyography.

Repetitive nerve stimulation test: In this test, motor nerve fiber is repeatedly stimulated and the compound muscle action potential produced is recorded. With repeated stimulation, fewer muscle fibers respond in the case of MG. A 10% decrement between the first and the fifth evoked muscle action potential is diagnostic for MG.

The test is abnormal in approximately 50–75% of patients with MG.

Single-fiber electromyography (SFEMG): It is a type of selective electromyography (EMG), where the action potential is identified from individual muscle fibers. In SFEMG, when an action potential is elicited by nerve stimulation, it is recorded with an SFEMG electrode. The latency from the stimulus of the nerve to the response in the muscle fibre is the neuromuscular jitter. The jitter will increase in patients with MG as the transmission at the neuromuscular junction is reduced. Abnormal jitter in SFEMG is found in 95–99% of patients with MG. Proximal muscles are preferred for testing.

- **Serologic testing:** In this the antibodies to AChR or to MuSK is tested for the diagnosis of MG. Serological testing is highly specific for myasthenia gravis. Other autoimmune conditions usually co-exist in patients who suffer from MG. Hence other immune studies like antinuclear (ANA) antibodies, rheumatoid factor (RF), and baseline thyroid functions are recommended to be tested in MG patients.
- **Radio imaging studies:** CT of the chest is frequently used in MG patients to detect any thymus enlargement or thymoma.

MANAGEMENT

Myasthenia gravis is a treatable disease with most patients being able to live a healthy and active life with appropriate management. The main goals of management of patients with MG is to control the symptoms and allow patients to live life relatively normal. The management is dependent on the severity of the disease, age of the patient, and the pace of progression of the symptoms. As MG is heterogeneous the best treatment approach is decided based on the individual patient. Four basic types of therapies are available for the management of MG.

1. **Anticholinesterase drugs:** Anticholinesterase drugs are the first-line treatment for MG. They prevent the enzymatic degradation of acetylcholine and increase their availability at the neuromuscular junction. The drug of choice is pyridostigmine bromide (mestinon). It has a longer duration of action when compared to neostigmine. Oral pyridostigmine has a rapid onset of action within 15 to 30 minutes. The peak of action is reached in two hours and its effect lasts for about three to four hours. The dosing schedule of the drug is based on the individual patient's response to the therapy. It usually ranges from 60–90 mg every four to six hours. Anticholinesterase drugs increase the level of ACh not only in the post-synaptic muscle terminals but also in the autonomic nervous system causing various cholinergic symptoms in addition to nicotinic effects in the skeletal muscles. Cholinergic side effects include increased salivation and bronchial secretions, sweating, bradycardia, abdominal cramping, diarrhea, and nausea. These can be reduced using oral anticholinergic drugs like glycopyrrolate. Nicotinic side effects include muscle fasciculation and cramping.

   If the patient cannot be administered oral pyridostigmine due to swallowing difficulties, it is administered via the NG tube. In case the patient has acute bowel obstruction or other conditions which contraindicate enteral administration of pyridostigmine, neostigmine can be administered through the subcutaneous route. Neostigmine has a shorter half-life and hence requires frequent doses. It also has more marked cardio inhibitor side effects when compared to pyridostigmine.

2. **Long-term immunomodulating therapies:** Corticosteroids and other immunosuppressive agents are used in all patients who have not achieved remission with anticholinesterase drug therapy alone.

   Corticosteroids: When pyridostigmine is not adequately effective in managing MG, corticosteroids or other non-steroidal immunosuppressive agents can be used. However, once remission is achieved the dosage is tapered to the lowest possible dose. Continuing a low dose of corticosteroids for the long term can help to maintain the treatment goal. The preferred steroid used in MG is prednisolone. This is the preferred drug in pregnant ladies with MG as pyridostigmine may not be used in them due to the risk of inducing uterine contractions.

   Nonsteroidal immunosuppressive agents: The Nonsteroidal Immunosuppressive Agents used in MG are azathioprine, cyclosporine, mycophenolate mofetil, methotrexate, and tacrolimus. The first line of drugs in this group is Azathioprine. Even though cyclosporine is also preferred the drug interactions and adverse side effects associated with it make it a less preferred drug than azathioprine. These drugs are used along with steroids or alone when steroids are contraindicated. Rituximab is another drug for which the evidence of efficacy is building in MG management.

3. **Rapid immune-modulating therapies:** Therapeutic plasma exchange and intravenous immunoglobulin are used as rescue or bridge therapies in MG. Both of the therapies have a rapid onset of action and their effects are short-term. They are used in refractory MG to maintain remission in patients who are not well controlled with steroids or immune-modulatory drugs, in myasthenic crisis, and also in patients pre-thymectomy.

   Therapeutic plasma exchange/plasmapheresis: It removes AChR from the circulation thereby bringing clinical improvement. Even though the clinical improvement can be witnessed in a few days the effects last for only a few weeks. A typical course of treatment includes five plasma exchanges spanning over 7 to 14 days. The removed plasma is replaced with albumin and fresh frozen plasma transfusions. This is an established form of treatment in MG patients who are seriously ill.

4. **Intravenous immunoglobulin therapy (IVIG):** It is the pooled immunoglobulin that can quickly reverse life-threatening situations in MG. It can be used as a bridge to the slower-acting immune-modulating drugs and can achieve disease remission. The total dose of IVIG is 2 g/kg, usually over two to five days. IVIG may result in complications such as thrombosis or fluid overload and hence is used with caution in renal disease, congestive heart failure, and in older adults.

   Surgical management: Thymectomy is recommended for patients aged 18 to 50 years with stable, anti-AChR-positive MG, early in the disease course to improve clinical outcomes. This approach reduces the need for immunotherapy and decreases the number of exacerbations requiring hospitalization. However, it is not preferred in case of late-onset disease and in ocular myasthenia. The effect of thymectomy develops over many years.

Robotic-assisted thymectomy surgery (RATS), video-assisted thoracoscopic surgery (VATS), and open surgery are the various approaches used for thymectomy. RATS and VATS are minimally invasive and have clear advantages over open surgery in terms of shorter hospital stay and less intraoperative blood loss.

MYASTHENIA CRISIS

Certain life-threatening complications such as myasthenia crisis and cholinergic crisis can occur in myasthenia gravis.

Myasthenia Crisis

It is a life-threatening condition characterized by worsening of the symptoms usually presented as rapidly increasing muscle weakness, dysphagia, and respiratory failure. It is precipitated by concurrent infections, surgery, childbirth, or tapering of immunotherapeutic medications or by the use of certain drugs. It is estimated that 10–20% of MG patients experience myasthenic crisis. **Table 35.4** illustrates the drugs that should be used with caution in MG and can precipitate myasthenic crisis.

The clinical picture of a crisis should be promptly identified to allow early management. The patient requires close monitoring, usually in a critical care setting. Nurses have a pivotal role in identifying, monitoring, and managing MG patients in crisis. The care must be focused to support or assist in breathing, and maintaining gas exchange. ABG monitoring is mandatory to identify any development of respiratory failure. Keen observation of early signs of respiratory distress is needed and quick escalation to invasive ventilation might be needed to save the life of the patient. Nasogastric tube should be inserted early to administer medications as well as feeding. Nursing care should focus on the prevention of complications including aspiration, infections, pressure sores, etc. The primary management in MG patients in crisis involves IVIG and plasma exchange therapies.

TABLE 35.4: Drugs that can worsen myasthenia gravis.

Group of drugs	Examples
Anesthetic drugs	Neuromuscular blocking agents
Antibiotics	Aminoglycosides, e.g., neomycin
	Fluroquinolones, e.g., ciprofloxacin
	Macrolides, e.g., azithromycin
Beta blockers	Atenolol
Other drugs	Penicillamine
	Hydroxychloroquine
	Magnesium
	Botulinum toxin

Cholinergic Crisis

Cholinergic crisis is another emergency that is a potential side effect of excessive anticholinesterase medication. It is characterized by flaccid paralysis and respiratory failure. It is usually difficult to differentiate between worsening of myasthenia (myasthenic crisis) and cholinergic crisis as both involve worsening of weakness. However, the cholinergic crisis is rarer than myasthenic crisis and should not be assumed unless the dosage of anticholinesterase has been exceeded.

NURSING MANAGEMENT

Nursing management of the patient with myasthenia gravis is highly individualized and is often challenging. The nursing care depends on the course of the illness, the age of the patient, the type of pharmacological therapies used, the presence of adverse reactions to drugs and the psychosocial situation of the patient. Patients who are newly diagnosed need a detailed evaluation and teaching. A patient who is well managed on routine treatment does not require an extensive plan of care except for the maintenance of health and prevention of complications. An MG patient in crisis, pregnant or elderly MG patients, etc., are specific situations where nursing care is highly individualized and patient-specific.

Assessment of the Patient

A thorough understanding of the patient's concerns is necessary for the nurse to plan the care. Objective and subjective evaluation of the patient can provide information based on which objectives of care can be framed. It is important to remember that MG being a chronic disease, it not only has physical difficulties, but also affects the patient socially, emotionally, and financially. Occupation, education, and other productivity related matters should be taken into consideration for discussion. Family should be involved in the discussion and their concerns about the illness need to be understood. This comprehensive approach of evaluating the patient will help the nurse to plan nursing care based on a holistic approach.

The clinical history focuses on the symptoms experienced by the patient. The extent of weakness, diurnal changes in weakness, aggravating and relieving factors, etc need to be evaluated. Evaluate the daily routine of the patient and understand how the weakness associated with myasthenia is affecting the functionality of individual patients. This will help the nurse to prioritize the patient's needs. A thorough assessment of the physiological functions, nutrition, elimination pattern, and mobility needs to be performed. The current knowledge of the patient and family about the illness, willingness to make changes, family support, nature of the occupation, and socialization pattern also needs to be assessed.

A hypothetical nursing care plan for a patient with MG is summarized in **Table 35.5**.

Management of Specific Symptoms in MG

Fatigue: The fatigue experienced by patients with MG is different from the muscle fatigability which is a hallmark

TABLE 35.5: Nursing care plan for myasthenia gravis.

Nursing diagnoses	Interventions
Ineffective airway clearance related to copious oropharyngeal secretions	• Assess cough and gag reflex • Perform oral suction if required • Perform chest physiotherapy • Assess the need for intubation or tracheostomy • Position the patient in semi/high fowlers position • Consider drugs like glycopyrrolate to reduce oral secretions • Monitor respiratory rate, single breath count, and breath holding time. • Monitor ABG, and use bedside pulse oximetry for continuous evaluation • Administer oxygen if needed • Anticipate ventilator support if there is a steady decline in respiratory function
Impaired nutrition; less than body requirement related to impaired swallowing functions	• Monitor the intake and output • Measure the nutritional indices like anthropometric measures (mid-arm circumference and triceps skin fold thickness) • Weigh frequently to monitor changes • Encourage calorie-rich and potassium-rich diet • Assist the patient to find the best period for scheduling meal timing so that weakness does not impair with feeding. Usually, this corresponds to the period of maximal action of AChE inhibitors. • Provide small frequent meals as tolerated
Risk for aspiration related to poor swallowing	• Perform swallowing screen • Provide semisolid food in case of mild swallowing difficulty. Watch for nasal regurgitation. • Insert nasogastric tube in case of swallowing impairment
Activity intolerance related to muscle weakness	• Assess the ability to do activities and encourage the patient to maintain a fatigue log and chart activities that increase weakness • Ensure the patient receives adequate high-quality sleep • Assist in activities of daily living as needed. • Plan adequate rest periods before and after activities. Schedule a timetable based on the peak action time of drugs so that activities that need maximum energy (e.g., bathing) can be scheduled at such periods when weakness is the least.
Risk of infection related to use of immune-modulating therapies	• Avoid exposure to crowded places and people with active infections • Teach the patient to practice respiratory precautions such as wearing a mask when using public places, proper hand washing • Advise the patient to report early signs of fever, flu, etc., which might indicate an infection so that crisis can be prevented.
Impaired communication related to bulbar weakness and dysarthria	• Assess the ability of the patient to verbally communicate. • Foster the ability, display patience, acceptance and encouragement when verbally communicating • Allow the patient to use non-verbal cues • Use gestures, communication board, or written form of communication when appropriate • Ask closed-ended questions or questions that need brief reply • Watch for frustration and depression in not being able to communicate effectively. Display acceptance and patience.
Self-care deficit related to weakness	• Assist the patient's self-care activities if needed • Monitor dental hygiene as brushing can be affected due to poor hand strength and grip • Use mouth wash or an electronic brush for enhancing dental care • Accompany the patient to the bathroom and provide assistance in bathing as it may be needed
Knowledge deficit related to chronic disease and its management	• Assess the level of understanding about the illness and its possible management • Discuss in detail the pathology and the possible treatment options • Ensure that the patient understands the possible side effects of the drugs and ways of managing them • Teach the patient the required changes that they may need to make in life to adapt to the illness • Provide opportunities for the patient to meet other patients with the same illness and allow them to interact and learn from them • Provide written instructions about drugs, dosage, and dietary advice. Give written instructions about the red flags that the patient should be aware of and the course of action in case of such events

symptom of MG. It is a multifactorial symptom in MG and is experienced by around 80% of the MG patients during some stage of their illness. Primary fatigue occurs when there is muscle weakness. Another aspect of it is cognitive fatigue where they experience a 'brain fog'. Ensuring that the patient receives adequate sleep, nutrition and balanced rest and exercise can reduce the residual fatigue. However suitable exercise should be advised based on the stage of their illness.

Physical activity: MG patients tend to develop muscle stiffness and discomfort owing to the primary disease process. Reduced activities, corticosteroid therapy, and less efficient sleep will all contribute to gaining body weight. Hence appropriate physical activity is important to be ensured in them. Research has shown that MG patients are likely to become more sedentary even when asymptomatic. Once they initiate activities, they may quickly become breathless due to the conditioning rather than respiratory weakness. It is important to slowly de-condition this and initiate physical activities as they can tolerate it. Nurses should teach simple exercises that can increase balance and muscle strength.

Low mood and social withdrawal: As MG is a chronic illness, patients are likely to become depressed and anxious over time. The unpredictability associated with the disease, physical limitations, and variability in the course of treatment, corticosteroid therapy can all contribute to low mood. Nurses should be sensitive to pick up changes in the mood of the patient which can further affect their socialization, employment, and productivity. Psychological help should be given as needed. A vicious cycle of low mood and social withdrawal can worsen the patient significantly.

Respiratory difficulty: Impaired breathing is an important problem faced by MG patients. Nurses should teach the patients to do single breath count and breath holding time. In the single breath count test the patient is asked to take a deep breath and then start counting from one as far as they can without leaving the breath. The patient is instructed to do the counting in their normal speaking voice. To check the breath holding time the patient is advised to take a deep breath and check for the time that they can hold it. A stopwatch can be used for this. Depending on the respiratory ability the time may vary. However, both of these tests give an objective understanding of any worsening respiratory condition and can help the patient in self-monitoring.

Airway toileting, postural drainage and chest physiotherapy can help them to be relieved of the major problem of increased bronchial secretions. In patients who are on ventilator support, respiratory rehabilitation is needed to help them wean off the ventilator. This should be taken up by the nurses in conjunction with the critical care therapists. Even in the absence of respiratory muscle weakness, some MG patients may experience dysfunctional breathing and mild dyspnea. Teaching them relaxation techniques that help them relax intercostal and accessory muscles can help them regulate their breathing.

Dysphagia and aspiration: Determining the ability of the patient to perform safe swallowing is important to prevent complications associated with aspiration. Swallow evaluation by a trained speech and swallowing therapist is important. Alternate forms of feeding including nasogastric feeding or gastrostomy might be needed. Training related to swallowing

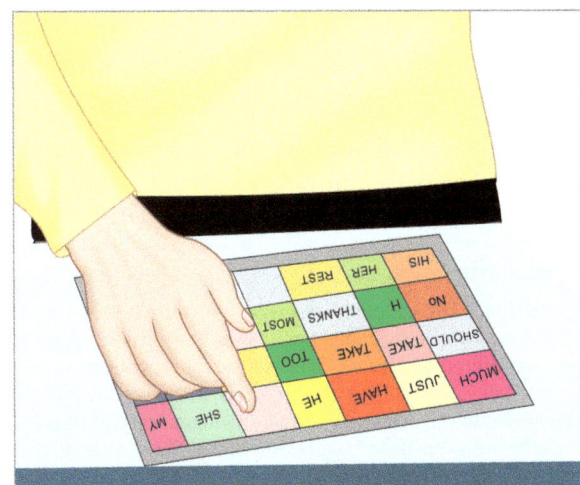

Fig. 35.7: Augmentative and alternative communication device for use in MG patients with speech difficulties.

can be given when the disabilities are less. Strengthening the muscles of mastication and oropharyngeal muscles can improve the abilities of the patient.

Speech and communication: MG patients who experience difficulty in speaking need an expert evaluation by a speech and language therapist. The patients may experience vocal fatigue. The marked nasal twang of speech is also possible due to imprecise articulation. The nurse should schedule speech therapy during peak medication hours which can avoid fatigue. The focus of speech therapy is to improve compensatory strategies and environmental modification which helps the patient communicate with maximal energy conservation. The use of augmentative and alternative communication (AAC) devices **(Fig. 35.7)** can be advised if needed. Voice rest and usage of short communication during a crisis need to be taught to the patient so that they effectively manage communication during the critical periods.

Managing side effects of drugs: The pharmacological management of MG entails adverse effects due to the long-term use of the medicines. The acetylcholinesterase inhibitors can cause abdominal cramps, bloating, diarrhea, urinary frequency, hypotension, bradycardia, sweating, salivation, lacrimation, and increased bronchial secretions. Most of these symptoms may reduce after the initial days. Propantheline is a drug that is administered to reduce the severity of these cholinergic symptoms. The importance of drug compliance should be taught to the patients. Sudden withdrawal of drugs can cause crisis and this should be emphasized on discharge. The side effects related to long-term steroid therapy should also be monitored in MG patients. These include gastric protection, prevention of osteoporosis, diabetes mellitus, and hypertension. Discharge advice for all patients on steroids should focus on potential excessive weight gain during steroid therapy, dietary changes, and exercise. The formation of cataracts, mood disturbances, sleep changes, and susceptibility to infections should also be notified to patients so that they will be able better cope with these changes and modify their lifestyle accordingly.

Pregnancy with MG: MG patients who are treated adequately can have a healthy pregnancy. As in other autoimmune conditions, the situation of the patient improves during pregnancy, but there is a risk of developing a crisis, during the postpartum period. It is safe to use pyridostigmine, corticosteroids, and azathioprine during pregnancy. Magnesium sulfate for the treatment of eclampsia should be avoided in MG. There are 10–15% chances of developing transient neonatal MG during the first three days of delivery in an infant due to the transplacental transfer of antibodies. Neonatal difficulty in breast feeding can occur because of this.

Case Scenario

- Ms Lakshmi a 26-year-old homemaker noticed occasional double vision and asymmetry of bilateral eyelids. She reported that she feels easily tired of chewing food and her family noticed a change in her quality of voice. She also reported having tiredness of upper extremities which worsened towards evening. She was unable to perform any household work by evening. She noticed that the symptoms were worsening. She consulted a physician and was referred to a neurologist.
- On physical examination, she had mild ptosis. She was subjected to a repetitive nerve stimulation test. On repetitive nerve stimulation, she had a >10% reduction in compound muscle action potential between the first and fifth stimulation. She was also positive for anti-AChR antibodies. She showed improvement in ptosis during the neostigmine test.
- She underwent a screening CT chest for detecting any thymus gland abnormality. It was found to be normal. She was started on pyridostigmine 60 mg 4th hourly and low-dose prednisolone. The treatment was effective and she noticed an improvement in her weakness. Later Lakshmi developed an acute exacerbation of her symptoms when she experienced upper respiratory tract infection. She was admitted to the ED. ABG revealed Type 2 respiratory failure. She was intubated and ventilated mechanically. She was treated with IVIG and large volume plasmapheresis. Prepare a nursing care plan for Lakshmi during the period of her acute hospitalization. Include discharge advice also for her.

SUMMARY

MG is a rare autoimmune disorder of the neuromuscular junction characterized by muscle weakness of skeletal muscles. The aim of management is prompt symptom control and induction of remission of the disease. Even though MG in itself is not life-threatening it can cause disabling symptoms and can lead to emergencies during exacerbation. Patients can have a good quality of life with multiple modalities of treatment like acetylcholinesterase inhibitors, immunomodulatory therapy, appropriate nursing care, and lifestyle modification. Optimizing the medical treatment and customizing the nursing care for an individual patient is a key aspect of MG care.

MUSCULAR DYSTROPHY

The term muscular dystrophy denotes disorders that are characterized by progressive muscle weakness caused due to degeneration of skeletal muscles. There are multiple types of muscular dystrophies, most of which have a genetic basis. A defect in the formation of a specific protein product is identified as the pathological basis of muscular dystrophy.

The most common muscular dystrophies and their characteristics are listed in **Table 35.6**. These disorders have a genetic basis and they have been mapped to over 29 different genetic loci.

DUCHENNE MUSCULAR DYSTROPHY

Duchenne muscular dystrophy (DMD) is the most common form of muscular dystrophy. It is a disabling disease, which is life-limiting and is characterized by progressive muscle weakness.

Etiology and Pathology

It is an X-linked recessive disorder where 50% of female offspring become carriers and 50% of male offspring develop the disease. The dystrophin gene has been found to be associated with dystrophy. The defective gene leads to the absence of dystrophin protein which is normally found on the muscle fibers. Lack of dystrophin causes instability of the muscle membrane causing muscle degeneration and fiber necrosis. Even though the damaged muscle fibers attempt to regenerate, the damage becomes marked as the disease progresses. Over the time, the necrotic muscle fibers get replaced by scarred fibrous tissue and fat. This looks like an apparent increase in the size of the muscle bulk, which is not true muscle tissue.

DMD is predominantly seen in males. The muscle wasting caused by the disorder makes the affected boys severely ill and disabled. The early symptoms include difficulty in climbing stairs and frequent falls. Usually, the symptoms begin early in childhood around 2–3 years of age. Waddling gait is another common abnormality identified early during the illness. One of the early manifestations is the difficulty in standing up from a sitting position. Hand pressure is applied

TABLE 35.6: Most common forms of muscular dystrophies.				
Sl. No.	Muscular dystrophy	Common presentation	Age at onset	Defective protein
1.	Duchenne muscular dystrophy (DMD)	Muscle weakness, wasting, scoliosis, dilated cardiomyopathy	Early childhood	Dystrophin
2.	Becker muscular dystrophy	Similar presentation as in DMD, slow progression and lesser severity when compared to DMD	Adolescence and adulthood	Dystrophin
3.	Fascio-scapulo-humeral muscular dystrophy	Weakness in the face, shoulder, and proximal upper extremities. Cardiac conduction abnormalities, hearing problems/retinal defects	Childhood/early adolescence	Not identified
4.	Congenital muscular dystrophies	Proximal limb muscle weakness. Seizures, cognitive and speech problems along with white matter changes. Joint contractures	At birth	Different proteins for each subtype
5.	Oculopharyngeal	Dysphagia, ptosis	From 4th decade of life	Poly-A-binding-protein 2

against the thigh when the child attempts to stand up. This 'climb up' is needed due to the weakness of the pelvic and proximal leg muscles. This is described as the Gower's sign which is a classic sign seen in DMD.

In advanced stages, the hands are used to obtain an upward thrust by placing them on the floor. Another feature of early DMD is the prone-crawl position where the child adopts a prone position before standing up. Physical examination may reveal hypertrophied calf muscles. The degenerated calf muscle tissue gets replaced by fat and fibrous tissue which appears like a (pseudo) hypertrophy of the calf muscle. Muscle degeneration and weakness progress and by 10–12 years of age, the child usually becomes wheelchair-bound and dependent. As the disease progresses, the involvement of respiratory muscles may warrant the need for mechanical ventilation. In the 2nd or 3rd decade of life, they usually succumb to respiratory or cardiac failure.

One-third of the affected children also present intellectual impairment and speech delay. Cardiomyopathy is a late manifestation.

Even though female carriers of the disorder do not present with symptoms, a small percentage (2.5–19%) of them can have some skeletal muscle weakness. They are also at risk for developing dilated cardiomyopathy.

Diagnosis and Genetic Screening

A suspected diagnosis of DMD is made based on the age of the child, gender, proximal muscle involvement, presence of hypertrophied calf, and Gowers sign. In children with suspected DMD, a prompt genetic diagnosis is warranted for accurate diagnosis.

The plasma creatine kinase, which is a marker of muscle damage, is very highly elevated in cases of DMD. Ongoing muscle damage can also cause other enzymes like alanine transaminase (ALT) and aspartate transaminase (AST) to be elevated. Electromyography and muscle biopsy are other investigations that can aid in diagnosis. A confirmatory diagnosis is made by identification of the genetic mutation.

Even though muscle biopsy can be helpful to understand the pathological changes in the muscles; it is not a mandatory test to diagnose DMD. Genetic tests can identify the causative mutation in the child which can then lead to a definitive diagnosis of DMD. Subsequently, genetic testing of the mother can be done to check if she is a carrier of the defective gene. If the mother is identified as a carrier, it has greater implications for the genetic screening of the maternal aunts and cousins. In mothers who are carriers, genetic counseling for subsequent pregnancies should be given as there is a 50% chance that she may have another son with DMD or a daughter who is a carrier.

Management

As DMD is a genetic disorder there is no curative treatment for the same. The multidisciplinary approach which focuses at the delayed progression of symptoms and rehabilitation ensures that the disease is well managed and the quality of life of the patient is improved. At various stages of the illness, the care is tailored so that the challenges of the disease are tackled adequately with the needs of a growing child.

The mainstay medical management of DMD includes corticosteroid therapy. The preferred drug is Deflazacort which is a derivative of prednisolone. It is used for the anti-inflammatory effects in the disease. Deflazacort has shown to reduce the mobility restriction and early use of wheel chair in children with DMD. However, long term use of corticosteroids is associated with several potential side effects including osteoporosis, immunosuppression and scoliosis. Newer drugs that target restoration of dystrophin production (e.g., ataluren) and those targeting to reduce the secondary effects of dystrophin deficiency (e.g., eteplirsen) are evaluated currently for use in DMD patients.

Nursing Management and Supportive Care

Owing to the progressive nature of the illness, and poor amenability to medical management, supportive care is the mainstay for DMD. Care focuses on all aspects of living and is mainly revolving around prevention of complications and palliation of symptoms. Nurses have a major role in ensuring that the child and family is supported from the diagnosis through the entire course of illness. Proper education about home management and assistance in setting goals for care can prove to be helpful for the families.

Physical therapy: As the hallmark symptom of DMD is loss of muscle function, physical therapy is of major importance. Scoliosis, contractures, and bone demineralization due to immobility and corticosteroid therapy are prevented and managed by physical therapy. Ambulation can be prolonged as much as possible in patients with optimum use of physical therapy. The use of orthoses should be promoted in patients who are ambulant. This can improve the stability and preserve the ambulatory capacity of the children. A well-planned schedule of light to moderate-intensity exercise with adequate rest periods in between can prove useful to reduce the ill effects of immobility. The home exercise practice should be easy to follow and manageable so that children remain adherent to it.

Nutrition and hydration: As the disease progresses, weakness of the oropharyngeal muscles set in resulting in dysphagia. In addition to this esophageal dysmotility and gastroesophageal reflux disease are also frequently found in patients with DMD. These conditions not only limit nutritional intake but also increase the risk of aspiration. Nasogastric tube feeding or percutaneous endoscopic gastrostomy feeding (PEG) needs to be initiated if the patient is at risk for aspiration. Pharmacological therapies to reduce gastric acid production, including proton pump inhibitors should be initiated in patients with GERD. Another frequent complaint observed in DMD patients is constipation and fecal impaction. Laxatives and enemas are needed in such situations.

The diet should be wholesome with adequate macro and micronutrients. Adequate calcium, vitamin D, and roughage should be included in the diet. Small frequent meals are advised in case of GERD. Due to immobility and reduced physical activity patients are at risk for being overweight and hence the advice to reduce processed food in the diet is imperative. Calorie intake should be individually tailored, based on the physical activity and energy demand.

Urinary symptoms: Urinary urgency, retention, and hesitancy are frequent urinary tract symptoms seen in males with DMD. Bladder dysfunction due to small size, hyperreflexive bladder, and lack of coordination of muscles result in these symptoms. Placing an indwelling urinary catheter may be warranted if there is urinary retention. Pharmacological management using oxybutynin can relieve lower urinary symptoms in most cases.

Monitoring the growth and development of children with DMD: The growth and development of a child with DMD happen hand in hand as the disease progresses. The course of illness and the steroid therapy can both impair the normal growth of children with DMD, affecting their bone health and delaying puberty. Hypogonadism might be seen in children and it should be discussed with an endocrinologist if puberty is delayed. Impaired cognition is usually seen in children with DMD. A psychological evaluation may prove useful to find the extent of impairment and educative support can be offered to patients and families on the basis of the evaluation. Co-occurrence of some psychological disturbances including ADHD, anxiety, and OCD might need a referral to a psychiatrist.

Involvement of family and care for parents: As DMD affects children, the disease has a great impact on the parents of the children. Multiple emotions including anxiety, isolation, and depression are often reported by the parents of these children. The maternal guilt of passing the disease to the child is a grave feeling that might require adequate counseling. Effective coping skills are taught to parents as the disease is long-standing. End-of-life caring for the child is a major area that parents might need support and assurance. Emotional well-being of the parents and families should be ensured throughout the course of illness as DMD affects multiple dimensions of family functioning. One of the major roles of a nurse who is involved in long-term care of DMD patients would be to allow patients and families to adapt to their disabilities. Healthy coping can allow patients and families to develop new perspectives towards the illness in spite of the progressive muscle weakness, loss of function and fatigue. Social interaction and support, fulfillment of individual needs, satisfaction with care, adequate recreational opportunities, and intimate relationships are few among several factors which can improve the quality of life of patients with DMD.

SUMMARY

Muscular dystrophy is a heterogeneous group of neuromuscular disorders which are inherited and marked by progressive weakness and muscle wasting. Even though the outcome depends on the type of dystrophy, most of them have poor outcome and are incurable. DMD is an X linked recessive disorder which is associated with marked weakness of the limb-girdle muscles which further progresses to involve other muscles of the body resulting in severe immobility, contractures, and respiratory difficulty. Even though there is no definitive or curative management, DMD is best managed using a multidimensional approach which is aimed at prolonging mobility, preserving muscle functions and improving the quality of life for patients and families. The long term and debilitating nature of the illness needs a comprehensive nursing approach to reduce the suffering for the patients and families.

GERIATRIC CONSIDERATIONS FOR NEUROMUSCULAR DISEASES

- ❖ Elderly patients with Guillain-Barre syndrome have more severe disease when compared to others. They are also found to have relatively poor prognosis at 3 months. They might require invasive mechanical ventilation and may remain dependent for care. Careful monitoring and prompt action are warranted in the elderly presenting with GBS.
- ❖ Late onset myasthenia gravis can occur in the elderly who may be above 60 years of age. The presence of other co-morbidities like hypertension, diabetes mellitus or hypothyroidism can worsen their functional capacity. They are also at risk for easy deterioration of respiratory functions. A quarter of such patients are found to require resuscitation in case of a crisis.
- ❖ The pharmacological management of MG in the elderly might be different when compared to young patients as steroids may have several adverse effects in them and may not be well tolerated. Azathioprine is more effective and well tolerated in the elderly when compared to steroids.
- ❖ Diagnostic delay can happen in the elderly presenting with neuromuscular symptoms. The presence of other comorbidities and several differentials including cerebrovascular disease or other somatic pathologies may result in diagnostic delay.

Case Scenario

- Kishan a 9-year-old boy was brought to the pediatrician by his parents who reported that he has frequent falls and experiences difficulty in climbing stairs. He was referred to a neurologist for further evaluation.
- On physical examination, Kishan denied any muscular pain and had a normal cranial nerve and sensory examination. Kishan was overweight and had calf hypertrophy bilaterally. He had difficulty in getting up from the sitting position and had a positive Gower's sign. He had normal intelligence for his age. The family history revealed consanguinity in the marriage of Kishan's parents. They also reported that his maternal uncle had a problem of weakness and died at a young age.
- With a suspected clinical diagnosis of muscular dystrophy serum creatine kinase and lactate dehydrogenase were performed and were found to be elevated. Genetic testing was done to positively confirm Duchenne muscular dystrophy.
- Kishan was initiated on low-dose steroids (Deflazacort). The diagnosis was difficult for the family and they had concerns about Kishan's future. Draw a multidisciplinary plan of care for Kishan

MULTIPLE CHOICE QUESTIONS

1. Tensilon test is performed on a patient who has complaints of double vision, ptosis, and muscle weakness. Which of the following observations is most likely for a diagnosis of myasthenia gravis?
   a. The patient develops worsening of muscle weakness
   b. The patient reports sudden tingling around the mouth with a deviation of face to a side
   c. The patient experiences improvement in muscle weakness
   d. The patient experiences tachycardia and drooling of saliva

2. Which of the following patients is most likely at risk for the myasthenic crisis?
   a. The patient with myasthenia gravis who has taken a double dose of pyridostigmine in the morning
   b. The patient with myasthenia Gravis who has undergone plasmapheresis recently

c. The patient with myasthenia gravis who had major abdominal surgery last week and has developed lower respiratory infection
d. The patient with myasthenia gravis who is compliant with drug therapy

3. While educating a myasthenia patient for planning home care, which of the following time is considered best for the patient to do exercise?
   a. Morning
   b. Evening
   c. Night
   d. After lunch

4. Your patient had a lumbar puncture just now. Which of the following positions should be given to the patient after the procedure?
   a. Sim's position
   b. Trendelenburg
   c. Supine
   d. Prone

5. While assessing a patient who is diagnosed to have Guillain-Barre syndrome, the presence of which of the following is considered an emergency?
   a. Patient complains of a crawling sensation on the lower limbs
   b. Patient has a muscle strength of 3/5
   c. Patient has weak cough reflex
   d. Patient has absent deep tendon reflex on the lower extremity

6. Which of the following assessment data is expected to be found for a GBS patient?
   a. Exaggerated startle reflex
   b. Ascending paralysis
   c. Cogwheel rigidity
   d. Hyperreflexia

7. A GBS patient is admitted in the ICU and is mechanically ventilated. Which of the following is the best strategy to communicate with the patient?
   a. Use a slate board for the patient to write
   b. Use yes or no questions and ask the patient to blink for no response
   c. Use call button at patients' reach
   d. Refer to a speech therapist for speech therapy

8. Which of the following interventions would a nurse expect for a patient admitted with weakness, tingling and numbness of lower extremities diagnosed to have Guillain-Barre syndrome?
   a. Insertion of the NG tube
   b. Mechanical ventilation
   c. IV methylprednisolone
   d. IV immunoglobulin therapy

9. The nurse is talking to the parents of a child who has been diagnosed with Duchenne muscular dystrophy. Which of the following should be mentioned to happen in the course of illness?
   a. Dry skin, gingival hyperplasia, and facial palsy
   b. Contractures, obesity, and pulmonary infections
   c. Tremors, urinary continence, and loss of hair
   d. Weakness of fingers, diarrhea, and loss of memory

10. The nurse is assessing a patient with suspected Duchenne muscular dystrophy. How can be a Gower's sign elicited?
    a. Asking the patient to walk in a straight line with one foot in front of the other
    b. Hop on one foot after other
    c. Hold the hand straight up for 3 minutes
    d. Asking the patient to stand up from a squatting position

ANSWERS

1. c 2. c 3. a 4. c
5. c 6. b 7. b 8. d
9. b 10. d

SUGGESTED READING

1. Mallik A, Weir AI, Nerve conduction studies: essentials and pitfalls in practice. Journal of neurology, neurosurgery and psychiatry. 76:2. available at http://dx.doi.org/10.1136/jnnp.2005.069138.
2. Beloor Suresh A, Asuncion RMD. Myasthenia Gravis. [Updated 2022 Sep 16]. In: StatPearls [Internet]. Treasure Island (FL): StatPearls Publishing; 2023.
3. Bogliun G, Beghi E. Italian GBS Registry Study Group. Incidence and clinical features of acute inflammatory polyradiculoneuropathy in Lombardy, Italy, 1996. Acta Neurol Scand. 2004;110:100-6.
4. Chiò A, Cocito D, Leone M, Giordana MT, Mora G, Mutani R. Guillain–Barré syndrome: A prospective, population based incidence and outcome survey. Neurology. 2003;60:1146-50.
5. Chopra JS, Lal V, Goyal MK. Tropical neuropathies In: Chopra JS, (Ed). Neurology in Tropics, 2nd edition. New Delhi: Reed Elsevier; 2016.
6. Duan D, Goemans N, Takeda S, et al. Duchenne muscular dystrophy. Nat Rev Dis Primers. 2021;7:13. https://doi.org/10.1038/s41572-021-00248-3.
7. Farrugia ME, Goodfellow JA. A Practical Approach to Managing Patients With Myasthenia Gravis-Opinions and a Review of the Literature. Front Neurol. 2020;11:604. doi: 10.3389/fneur.2020.00604. PMID: 32733360; PMCID: PMC7358547.
8. Fokke C, van den Berg B, Drenthen J, Walgaard C, van Doorn PA, Jacobs BC. Diagnosis of Guillain-Barré syndrome and validation of Brighton criteria. Brain. 2014;137:33-43.
9. Garg M. Respiratory Involvement in Guillain-Barre Syndrome: The Uncharted Road to Recovery. J Neurosci Rural Pract. 2017;8(3):325-326. doi: 10.4103/jnrp.jnrp_96_17R1. PMID: 28694605; PMCID: PMC5488546.
10. Hughes RA, van Doorn PA. Corticosteroids for Guillain-Barré syndrome. Cochrane Database Syst Rev. 2012;8:CD001446. doi: 10.1002/14651858.CD001446.pub4
11. Willison HJ, Jacobs BC, van Doorn PA. Guillain-Barré syndrome. Lancet. 2016;388:717-27.
12. Jacobs BC, Rothbarth PH, van der Meché FG, et al. The spectrum of antecedent infections in Guillain-Barré syndrome: a case-control study. Neurology. 1998;51:1110-5.
13. Kannan Kanikannan MA, Durga P, Venigalla NK, Kandadai RM, Jabeen SA Borgohain R Simple bedside predictors of mechanical ventilation in patients with Guillain-Barre syndrome. J Crit Care. 2014;29(2):219-23.
14. Lovering RM, Porter NC, Bloch RJ. The muscular dystrophies: from genes to therapies. Phys Ther. 2005;85(12):1372–88. PMID: 16305275; PMCID: PMC4496952.
15. Meena AK, Khadilkar SV, Murthy JM. Treatment guidelines for Guillain-Barre Syndrome. Ann Indian Acad Neurol. 2011;14(Suppl 1):S73-81. doi: 10.4103/0972-2327.83087. PMID: 21847334; PMCID: PMC3152164.
16. Moulin DE, Hagen N, Feasby TE, Amireh R, Hahn A. Pain in Guillain-Barré syndrome. Neurology. 1997;48:328-31.
17. Multidisciplinary care for Guillain-Barré syndrome. Cochrane Database Syst Rev. 2010;(10):CD008505.
18. Newswanger DL, Warren CR. Guillain-Barré syndrome. Am Fam Physician. 2004;69(10):2405-10.
19. Phillips WD, Vincent A. Pathogenesis of myasthenia gravis: update on disease types, models, and mechanisms. F1000Res. 2016;5:F1000 Faculty Rev-1513.

20. Plasma Exchange/Sandoglobulin Guillain-Barré Syndrome Trial Group. Randomised trial of plasma exchange, intravenous immunoglobulin, and combined treatments in Guillain-Barré syndrome. Lancet. 1997;349:225-30.
21. Raphaël JC, Chevret S, Hughes RA, Annane D. Plasma exchange for Guillain-Barré syndrome. Cochrane Database Syst Rev. 2012;7:CD001798.
22. Rolak LA. Neurology Secrets: Questions You Will Be Asked, 4th edition. Philadelphia, PA: Elsevier Mosby; 2005. p. 1045.
23. Roman GC. Tropical neurology. In: Bradely W, Marsden CD, Daroff RD (Eds), Neurological diseases, 2nd edition. London: Butterworth Heineman; 1995.
24. Samuels MA. Manual of Neurologic Therapeutics, 7th edition. Philadelphia, PA: Lippincott Williams & Wilkins; 2004. p. 2047.
25. Sanders DB, Wolfe GI, Benatar M, Evoli A, Gilhus NE, Illa I, et al. International consensus guidance for management of myasthenia gravis: Executive summary. Neurology. 2016;87(4):419-25.
26. Simatos Arsenault N, Vincent PO, Yu BH, Bastien R, Sweeney A. Influence of Exercise on Patients with Guillain-Barré Syndrome: A Systematic Review. Physiother Can. 2016;68(4):367-76.
27. Tan CY, Shahrizaila N, Yeoh KY, Goh KJ, Tan MP. Heart rate variability and baroreflex sensitivity abnormalities in Guillain-Barré syndrome: a pilot study. Clin Auton Res; 2018.
28. Tireli H, Yuksel G, Okay T, Tutkavul K. Role of thymus on prognosis of myasthenia gravis in Turkish population. North Clin Istanb. 2020;7(5):452-9. doi: 10.14744/nci.2020.51333. PMID: 33163880; PMCID: PMC7603859.
29. van den Berg B, Walgaard C, Drenthen J, Fokke C, Jacobs BC, van Doorn PA. Guillain-Barré syndrome: pathogenesis, diagnosis, treatment and prognosis. Nat Rev Neurol. 2014;10:469-82.
30. Wendell LC, Levine JM. Myasthenic crisis. Neurohospitalist. 2011;1(1):16-22. doi: 10.1177/1941875210382918. PMID: 23983833; PMCID: PMC3726100.
31. Willison HJ. The immunobiology of Guillain–Barré syndromes. J Peripher Nerv Syst. 2005;10:94-112.

CHAPTER 36

Movement Disorders

Priya Baby, Rohan R Mahale

"Don't imagine the worst… If you imagine the worst and it happens, you've lived it twice."
—The Ellen DeGeneres Show, 2012

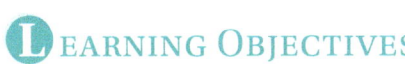

After going through the chapter, the learner will be able to:
- Describe the etiopathogenesis of common movement disorders.
- Differentiate between various types of movement disorders.
- Discuss the medical and surgical management of patients with various kinds of movement disorders.
- Use the nursing process as a framework of care for patients with movement disorders.
- Discuss the geriatric considerations for patients with movement disorders.

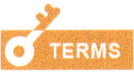

- **Chorea:** Involuntary movements that are abrupt, non-rhythmic, brief, and random flow of muscle contractions.
- **Dystonia:** Sustained or intermittent muscle contractions causing abnormal often repetitive movements or postures or both.
- **Movement disorders:** Neurological disorders in which the hallmark symptom is any abnormality related to movement.
- **Tremor:** Involuntary hyperkinetic movement disorder where there is rhythmic, oscillatory movements of one or more body parts, mostly the limbs.

INTRODUCTION

Movement disorders are a group of neurological disorders in which the hallmark symptom is any abnormality related to movement. A variety of diseases fall under this spectrum. They can be degenerative as in the case of Parkinson's disease, or can be induced by medications, inflammation, or trauma. There is often complex and variable clinical presentation in movement disorders. However, most often these are treated in ambulatory care settings.

CONCEPT AND DEFINITION

Movement disorders (MD) are a spectrum of neurological disorders in which there is excessive, uncontrolled, involuntary movement or paucity of movement. The symptoms of movement disorders are not attributable to weakness or spasticity or any other medical causes directly interfering with the musculoskeletal system.

EPIDEMIOLOGY

The prevalence of movement disorders increases with age, posing a growing challenge for older patients. Parkinson's disease is one of the most common debilitating movement disorders. Movement disorders constitute 3–8% of all neurological disorders prevalent in India. The crude prevalence rate of movement disorders in India varies from 31–45 per one lakh population in age above 60 years. These disorders are more frequent in rural India than in urban areas. Viral encephalitis is an important cause of acute onset of movement disorder in India, Japanese encephalitis being the most common (67.6%). However, there is significant under-recognition and under-treatment of these disorders by the general public.

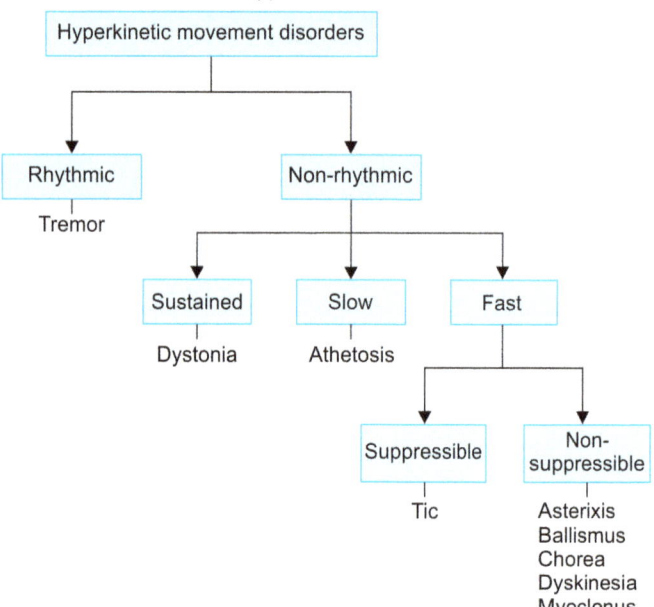

Flowchart 36.1: Hyperkinetic movement disorders.

Sydenham's chorea is a common problem encountered in developing countries, such as India. It was called St Vitus dance historically. It is named after Thomas Sydenham, an English physician who first described it. This chorea is seen as a neurological complication of acute rheumatic fever. In children, Sydenham's chorea is the most common cause of chorea. It affects females more than males. In acute rheumatic fever, the body produces antibodies against Group A beta hemolytic streptococcus. The cross-reaction of these antibodies in the neurons of basal ganglia describes the development of chorea. This can also be accompanied by some behavioral disturbances also. There are several causes for chorea, we discuss here Huntington's disease, an important cause of chorea.

Huntington's disease is an inherited, neurodegenerative disorder that is primarily characterized by choreic movements. Chorea, the typical feature of Huntington's disease was identified and described by George Huntington in 1872. Later after almost a century, when the disease was better understood; it was renamed Huntington's disease.

CLASSIFICATION

Movement disorders have been broadly subdivided into two types—hypokinetic and hyperkinetic MDs. Hyperkinetic movement disorders are characterized by excessive, involuntary movements which affect the normal flow of motor activity. These can be rhythmic or non-rhythmic. The classification of hyperkinetic movement disorders is depicted in **Flowchart 36.1**.

Hypokinetic movement disorders are characterized by the absence or slowness of movement. Parkinsonism is an important hypokinetic movement disorder.

As the spectrum of movement disorders is very varied, a few of the common disorders are discussed here. These include chorea, tremors dystonia, and a few others.

CHOREA

CONCEPT AND DEFINITION

Chorea can be defined as involuntary movements that are abrupt, non-rhythmic, brief, and random flow of muscle contractions. The word chorea is the Greek word for dance. The common causes of chorea are described in **Table 36.1**.

TABLE 36.1: Common causes of chorea.	
Genetic	• Huntington's disease • Wilson's disease • Benign familial chorea • Neuroacanthocytosis
Infectious	• Post-streptococcal infection (Sydenham's chorea)
Metabolic/hormonal	• Thyrotoxicosis • Hyper/hypoglycemia • Pregnancy-induced (chorea gravidarum)
Drug-induced	• Oral contraceptives • Estrogens • Antipsychotics • Antiepileptics

EPIDEMIOLOGY

In the Western population, the prevalence of Huntington's disease (HD) is estimated as 5–10 per 100,000. The mean age at onset of symptoms in HD is 30–50 years. In juvenile Huntington's disease, (10% of the cases) the symptoms start before 20 years of age. In late-onset HD, the symptoms may begin after 50 years of age. Huntington's disease occurs in all populations; however, its frequency is higher in people of European ancestry. In most Asian countries, the incidence is only one-tenth of that seen in European countries. There are only limited epidemiological data from countries, such as India about the incidence of Huntington's disease. However, the prevalence here is considered lesser than that seen in the west.

ETIOLOGY

Huntington's disease is a rare, genetically inherited disorder. It follows an autosomal dominant pattern of inheritance. All individuals with the affected gene develop the disease. It is caused by a defect in the Huntingtin gene **(Fig. 36.1)**. A CAG (Cytosine, adenine, guanine) trinucleotide repeats on the short arm of chromosome 4 is the typical genetic abnormality that results in the disease. If the repeat is more than 40, definite symptoms are seen. If the range of repeat

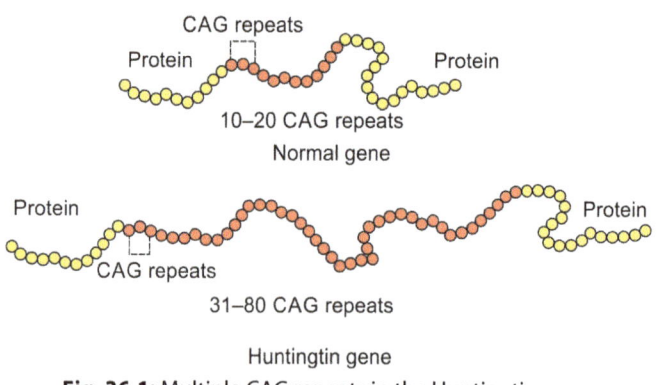

Fig. 36.1: Multiple CAG repeats in the Huntingtin gene.

is between 36 to 39 the disease may appear but has a very late onset. Thus, the disease onset is earlier when the CAG repeat is long.

PATHOPHYSIOLOGY

Several cellular functions get disrupted due to the aberrant behavior of the Huntingtin gene. The presence of the dysfunctional gene in the cells leads to neuronal destruction through various mechanisms, such as disruption of transcription and mitochondrial damage. Microscopic as well as macroscopic structural changes happen in the brain as the disease progresses.

CLINICAL MANIFESTATIONS

The classic clinical manifestation of Huntington's disease is the chorea. Other than chorea, patients may also experience several cognitive and emotional disturbances in the course of the illness. During the initial phase of the disease, abnormal movements often occur in the distal regions of the body including fingers and toes. The small movements of the facial muscles may not be initially noticeable by others or it may look, such as nervousness. The choreatic movements later involve other parts of the body. The facial movements may involve activities, such as lifting one eyebrow, turning the head to one side, and protruding the tongue. Another common choreatic movement involves the extension of the back muscles. An increase in muscle tone often marks one of the beginning signs of the illness. This often leads to abnormal postures, such as torticollis. Gait may become unsteady in most patients and is often described as 'drunk walking'. The progress in the motor symptoms eventually affects all activities of daily living. Patients experience frequent falls. Other motor manifestations of HD include dysphagia, dysarthria, hypokinesia, and rigidity.

At the very early stages of the illness itself, cognitive decline and psychiatric symptoms are frequently present. Patients experience difficulty in executing functions, and hence find even small tasks very difficult to perform. They have difficulty retaining attention and emotion recognition. Several neuropsychiatric symptoms, including apathy, anxiety, irritability, depression, obsessive-compulsive behavior, and psychosis are observed in Huntington's disease. These symptoms often precede motor symptoms. Psychosis and acoustic hallucinations usually appear in the later stages of the disease. Unintended weight loss, loss of appetite, increased sweating and sleep disturbances are the other constitutional symptoms experienced by the patients.

The disease has preclinical and clinical stages. The preclinical stage is the phase where symptoms of the disease have not appeared. This phase is further divided into at-risk stage and premanifest stage and the transition stage. In the clinical phase, the illness is manifested in various severities until it progresses to death. The clinical stage usually begins around the age of 45 years which then progress towards advanced illness and death. The median survival from the onset of motor symptoms is 18 years. The clinical stage has three phases. The stages of the illness are listed in **Table 36.2**.

TABLE 36.2: Staging of Huntington's disease and the manifestations.

Stage	Manifestations
Preclinical	
1. At risk	• Anxious about carriership of the gene (as it is not confirmed) • Care of affected parent
2. Premanifest	• Anxious and uncertain about the onset of symptoms as the carriership of the gene is confirmed
3. Transition phase	• Subtle cognitive, behavioral, and motor activity changes • Uncertainty is still present
Clinical	
1. Stage I	• The onset of motor or psychiatric symptoms • Chorea • Independent in ADL • The psychological burden on the patient as well as family • Death is rarely due to illness unless suicide
2. Stage II	• Motor manifestations become prominent • Dependence for activities • Death by euthanasia or suicide
3. Stage III	• Severe motor symptoms • Completely dependent for all ADLs • Death

Huntington's disease has a profound effect on the quality of life. The diagnosis of a parent and the subsequent caregiving process itself has a serious impact on the person. The functional capacity reduces as the disease progresses and later there is a need for totally dependent care. Pneumonia and suicide are the most common causes of death in these patients.

RELATED DIAGNOSTIC MODALITIES

The onset of symptoms in a person whose parent was diagnosed to have HD, points towards the diagnosis of HD. Confirmatory diagnosis is made by DNA testing which shows a CAG repeat of at least 36 in the Huntingtin gene. Imaging studies and blood investigations are not considered useful in diagnosis. These tests can help to rule out other conditions.

Chorea, being the most important presenting sign for HD, the other causes of chorea are ruled out for diagnosis.

Diagnosis of the disease in a fetus can be made before birth by DNA testing. Hence, prenatal diagnosis is also possible by obtaining cells from the fetus by chorionic villus sampling or amniocentesis. DNA testing can be carried out to identify the presence of a diseased gene. The decision regarding termination of pregnancy may be taken by the couple after the test if the fetus is identified to be carrying the gene. Historically, Huntington's gene was the first disease gene to be mapped.

MEDICAL MANAGEMENT

As the disease cannot be treated and halted from progression, the aim of management is basically to support the patient, control symptoms, and enhance the quality of life. The optimal management of HD is possible only by a multidisciplinary approach. Several health professionals including physicians, nurses, physical therapists, nutritionists, speech and language therapists, and occupational therapists need to be on the team. The aim of the management is to enhance the quality of life and anticipate the changing needs of the patient as the disease progresses. This is possible through various pharmacological and non-pharmacological interventions.

Pharmacological management of HD aims at the control of symptoms. The most classical sign of HD, chorea, is treated by typical and atypical neuroleptics. They exert an antichoreatic effect by dopamine receptor blocking. Tetrabenazine is a dopamine-depleting drug that is also used to treat chorea in Huntington's disease at a dosage of 50–75 mg per day. Olanzapine, risperidone, quetiapine, and sulpiride are other neuroleptic drugs that are used for HD patients.

Selective serotonin uptake inhibitors are used to treat depression. Neuroleptics can be useful in treating aggression and psychosis. Even though there is limited evidence, drugs, such as methylphenidate, atomoxetine, modafinil, amantadine, bromocriptine, and bupropion have been used to treat apathy. Emerging therapies that aim at lowering the levels of mutant genes and silencing them are on trial. These will be probably of hope for the patients in the near future.

Cognitive behavioral therapy is found to be useful in certain patients. Patients may be taught to employ coping strategies to deal with cognitive deficits. For example, a change of work setting or shifting oneself to a job that does not require multitasking may be needed. Even though several medical and non-medical treatment is available, these should be tailored for individual patients as there are wide differences among patients in their clinical course of the illness.

NURSING MANAGEMENT

The management and coordination of the multidisciplinary care of the patient and family is a major role of the nurse. The areas of the involvement of nurses in the management of HD patients involve, identifying the treatment and care goals, monitoring the effectiveness of the treatment and care regime, and reviewing the regime.

Huntington's disease impacts the life of not only the patient but also the families. The quality of life of the affected individual and the families worsen as the disease progresses. The initial stages of the illness entail several psychosocial, cognitive, and behavioral issues. Later these are dominated by motor symptoms and functional incapacity.

The inability to perform normal cognitive functions, such as planning, judgment, and decision-making affects the individual. They also may develop emotional disengagement and lack of impulse control, and multiple other areas of cognition including attention, language, learning, and memory are affected. This impacts their activities of daily living adversely. Hence, adequate changes have to be made in the environment and daily routines to incorporate changes according to the abilities of the individual.

The affected person experiences a loss of control, and autonomy as well as emotional and physical changes. They are aware of how the disease is overtaking them. As they notice themselves losing their abilities of independent living, it is a scary and emotional period for them. Hence, the care of HD patients is not just restricted to physical health but also sensitivity is needed in the emotional aspect of caring. The nursing care at each stage of the illness varies according to the deficits experienced by the patient. Multiple nursing interventions are important to help the person adapt to the changes which the disease brings to life. The most important aspects of care of a patient suffering from HD are mentioned in **Table 36.3**.

TABLE 36.3: Nursing care plan for Huntington's disease.

Nursing diagnosis	Nursing interventions
Risk for falls related to loss of balance	• Make environmental changes to prevent falls, such as using raised toilet seats, chairs with armrests, side rails, and padding on frequently bumped areas • Do not call the patient from behind as this increases the chance of a fall • Encourage the client to do transfers in the presence of others
Impaired cognitive function related to the disease process	• Demonstrate patience and understanding • Provide reassurance and encouragement • Teach the caregiver not to be offended by agitation and other disruptive and demanding behavior of the patients. Inform that these are primarily due to changes in the brain • Help the patient to make adequate modifications in daily routines and occupation, so that the cognitive abilities are less challenged
Impaired nutrition less than body requirement related to difficulty in feeding, and loss of sensation	• Watch for signs of aspiration, such as coughing, choking or frequent pneumonia, wet or gurgly voice • Minimize distractions during meals • Use modified utensils, such as double-handled cups, and cup with a cover on it, to help prevent spills • Special attention needs to be given while feeding hot beverages as heat sensitivity may be reduced
Self-care deficit related to loss of functional abilities	• Encourage tasks by prompting or giving cues • Change clothes often as people with HD tend to perspire profusely • Allow personal independence in doing activities, even if they are very minimal. This improves the sense of autonomy • Expect that the patients may experience the urge to urinate frequently as their thirst increases and the voiding becomes incomplete • Modify the teeth brushing using mouthwash or assist in brushing the teeth, if necessary, as choreatic movements make this part of daily activities very difficult • Encourage mouth care after each meal, as chances of pneumonia due to poor oral hygiene and regurgitation of food from the stomach, is very high in HD patients

Care during the late stages of illness mostly focuses on palliative care. The domains of care relevant for such patients include maintaining autonomy and dignity, fostering meaningful social interaction and communication, promoting comfort and safety, spirituality, enjoyment and entertainment, nutrition, and functional competence.

TREMOR

CONCEPT AND DEFINITION

Tremor is an involuntary hyperkinetic movement disorder where there are rhythmic, oscillatory movements of one or more body parts, mostly the limbs. Tremors can be broadly classified as rest tremors and action tremors. Rest tremor occurs when the affected limb is at rest and the muscles are relaxed. It usually disappears when the affected limb is moved. The typical Parkinson's disease tremor is an example of a rest tremor. Action tremor occurs when a person performs voluntary actions. It can be further classified into postural tremors, isometric tremors, and kinetic tremors. Postural tremor occurs when a person maintains a particular position against gravity, e.g., outstretching the hands against gravity. Isometric tremor occurs in situations when isometric muscle contraction occurs in a body part, e.g., pressing the hand or arm against a rigid resistance, or standing on feet. Kinetic tremors occur when a body part is moving, e.g., moving the hands to mouth while eating.

Tremors are commonly seen among middle-aged and older adults. Men and women have equal chances of having this disorder. The most important causes of tremors include neurodegenerative diseases, stroke, head injury, drugs and toxins, demyelinating disorders, systemic illnesses, metabolic disorders, etc.

The exact pathophysiology of tremors is not yet clearly understood. However, tremors are postulated to be generated by dysfunction of circuits within the brain which control the excitation and inhibition of movements. The two main circuits involved are the basal ganglia-cerebello-thalamic circuit (connecting the globus pallidus, ventrolateral thalamus, cerebellar nuclei, and motor cortex) and the dentate-olivary circuits (connecting the red nucleus, inferior olivary nucleus and dentate nucleus). The involvement of these circuits due to various lesions in the brain stem, extrapyramidal system, or cerebellum can cause tremors.

ESSENTIAL TREMOR (ET)

ET is a very common movement disorder. It classically affects the hands, head, and/or voice. Many patients with ET have a strong family history of the disease. Often most of the patients never seek medical attention as they have a very benign course. The tremor is usually symmetric and is characterized by postural or kinetic tremor which rarely can also be seen at rest during the later stage of the disease. It is seen that they improve with intake of alcohol. **Figure 36.2** illustrates the classic Archimedes spiral drawn by a normal person and an ET patient. Maximal tremor amplitude can be noted at an axis of 60°, which is characteristic of ET. Primidone, a deoxy barbiturate is the first line of management of essential tremors. Antiepileptics, such as topiramate, benzodiazepines,

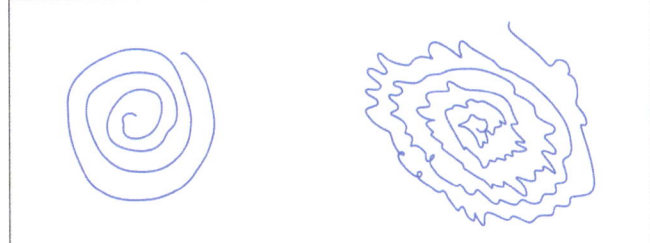

Fig. 36.2: Archimedean spiral showing the spiral drawn by a normal person and an ET patient.

and beta-blockers are also used for the treatment of ET. Botulinum toxin can also be used to reduce the severity of the tremors. However, this comes with significant weakness as a side effect which is often unacceptable. Deep brain stimulation (DBS) targeting the ventral intermediate (VIM) nucleus of the thalamus is a surgical option for essential tremor intractable to medical management. Paresthesia is an unwanted effect of the DBS on the VIM. One of the most recent treatment options for ET is magnetic resonance imaging (MRI)-guided focused ultrasound thalamotomy (FUT) which has shown promising results.

DRUG-INDUCED TREMORS

Drugs can induce tremors. Older people and patients with co-morbid renal or liver diseases are more prone to develop drug-induced tremors. Intake of several drugs (polypharmacy), with some having drug interactions with each other, also increases the risk of having drug-induced tremors. Nurses should be aware of the tremorogenic drugs which can cause or exacerbate the tremors. This will help in early recognition and prompt diagnosis so that unnecessary investigations can be avoided. Dopamine receptor blockers and neuroleptics are the most important group of drugs that can induce tremors. The common groups of drugs that can induce tremors are mentioned in **Table 36.4**. Drug-induced tremor can be rest tremor or action tremor depending on the drug. Alcohol is seen to reduce essential tremors; however,

TABLE 36.4: Drugs that can induce tremors.

Drug classification	Common drugs
Antiepileptic	Valproic acid, Gabapentin
Neuroleptics and dopamine depleters	Haloperidol, thioridazine, fluphenazine, chlorpromazine, cinnarizine
Antiemetics	Metoclopramide, promethazine, prochlorperazine
Bronchodilators	Salbutamol, salmeterol, theophylline, aminophylline
Antimicrobial	Co-trimoxazole, acyclovir, amphotericin
Antiarrhythmic	Amiodarone
Antidepressants and mood stabilizers	Imipramine, amitriptyline, lithium
Hormones	Levothyroxine, medroxyprogesterone, epinephrine, norepinephrine
Immunosuppressant	Tacrolimus, cyclosporine
Chemotherapeutic agents	Ifosfamide, thalidomide, cisplatin, tamoxifen

it can aggravate other forms of tremors. Cigarette smoking is also found to increase tremors.

PSYCHOGENIC TREMORS

Tremors are the most common manifestation of a psychogenic movement disorder. It is seen more in women and is most commonly observed in the hands and legs. Psychogenic tremors have an abrupt onset, are usually distractible, and may frequently switch between rest tremors and postural tremors. Other associated features of somatization may be observed in such cases. They usually have spontaneous remission.

SUPPORTIVE MANAGEMENT OF TREMORS

Other than medical or surgical management, several supportive management strategies can be used for reducing or eliminating tremors. These also help the patient to adapt oneself to the tremors. Physical therapy can be useful in improving muscle control and function. It strengthens coordination and balance. Splints and other adaptive equipments may be useful. Special plates, utensils, and other equipments for daily living can improve the ease of patients. Patients might be taught new ways of performing activities of daily living. Assessment of speech and swallowing by a Speech-language pathologist is necessary in case tremors have affected these functions. Patients can be taught to identify tremor-inducing substances which increase the intensity of tremors in them. Elimination or reduction of substances, such as caffeine can help improve tremors in some people. Some patients with tremors may find that alcohol reduced their symptoms. However, once the effect of alcohol wears off, the tremors may worsen.

DYSTONIA

Dystonia is characterized by abnormal and repetitive movements or postures or both. They occur due to sustained or intermittent muscle contractions. Dystonia can be classified as primary (including genetic forms and idiopathic) or secondary based on their etiologies. Secondary dystonia is mostly induced by drugs, such as neuroleptics, including haloperidol, risperidone, olanzapine, and antiemetics. These are called tardive dystonia. They appear after a few months of intake of neuroleptics. Other drugs that can induce dystonia include anticonvulsants and antidepressants. Other causes of secondary dystonia are post-encephalitis sequelae, cerebral palsy, hypoxic-ischemic encephalopathy, etc. Dystonia can involve only one body part termed as focal dystonia (e.g., blepharospasm), two contiguous body parts termed as segmental dystonia (e.g., neck and upper limb dystonia), two or more non-contiguous body parts termed as multifocal dystonia, and trunk with upper or lower limb termed as generalized dystonia.

The common forms and the associated manifestations of dystonias are given in **Table 36.5**.

The treatment of dystonia is based on the etiology. Intramuscular or intravenous anticholinergics (e.g.,

TABLE 36.5: Common forms of dystonias and the clinical manifestations.

Forms of dystonias	Clinical manifestations
Blepharospasm	Eyelid closure
Buccolingual crisis	Repetitive chewing, swallowing, facial asymmetry
Oculogyric crisis	Conjugate eye deviation
Larynx dystonia	Stridor
Torticollis	Cervical spasm
Opisthotonos	Trunk hyperextension

TABLE 36.6: Dystonia Severity Action Plan.

Grade	Severity
1.	Sits comfortably, regular periods of uninterrupted sleep
2.	Irritable, dystonic postures interferes with sitting; can only tolerate lying
3.	Not able to tolerate lying, sleep disturbed; no metabolic compensation with creatinine kinase <1,000 IU/L
4.	Not able to tolerate lying, sleep disturbed; pyrexia in absence of infection; evidence of metabolic decompensation with creatinine kinase >1,000 IU/L; myoglobinuria
5.	Features of grade 4 with full metabolic decompensation; respiratory, cardiovascular and renal compromise
6.	Trunk hyperextension

biperiden 5 mg IV, diphenhydramine 50 mg), or in milder cases, promethazine 50 mg IM are effective for acute dystonia. Baclofen, anticholinergics, and benzodiazepines, such as clonazepam is the first-line medications for patients with chronic dystonia. Botulinum neurotoxin (BoNT) injection into the dystonic muscles is the recommended treatment for drug-refractory cases of dystonia. If there is no improvement with medications, DBS of globus pallidus interna (GPi) and pallidotomy is the preferred surgical option for medication-refractory dystonia.

Status dystonicus (SD), or dystonic storm, is a medical emergency. It can occur due to aggravated symptoms of dystonia in which the patient may experience strong and painful muscle contractions involving the face and neck. This can affect respiratory function and can be life-threatening without prompt treatment. SD can be triggered by trauma, surgery, infection, fever, abrupt introduction, withdrawal, or change in medical treatment. Other complications, such as hyperpyrexia, dehydration, and rhabdomyolysis can be associated with it. SD is treated by inducing deep sedation using propofol and muscle relaxants. Nurses should use a clinical scoring system to monitor worsening dystonia and prevent status dystonicus. The Dystonia Severity Action Plan (DSAP) is a simple grading system that can be used by nurses for monitoring patients **(Table 36.6)**.

TOURETTE SYNDROME

Tourette syndrome (TS) is a disease of childhood characterized by multiple motor and vocal tics associated with multiple behavior and psychiatric comorbidities. The tics become most prominent when the child feels nervous or under stress. The medical management for tics includes typical and atypical neuroleptic drugs. Newer neuroleptics, such as olanzapine and risperidone are useful. Clonidine, which is an alpha blocker also has tic-suppressant effects and is used in children who have tics with attention deficit disorder. At times motor tics are so severe and multifocal that they are resistant to all forms of medical treatment and severely hamper the quality of life. Botulinum toxin can be used for focal, simple, and vocal tics; however, for complex tics, it is usually not desirable.

When both behavioral and medical therapy fail, patients with TS can be considered for deep brain stimulation (DBS). The targets that are being studied for DBS in TS include the centromedian para fascicular (Cm-Pf) nucleus and the ventralis oralis in the thalamus. The parents as well as teachers of the children with TS should be educated about the inability of the child to suppress the tics.

ATHETOSIS

Athetosis is a movement dysfunction manifested as a slow and continuous writhing movement of the hand or legs. It occurs due to pathology in the basal ganglia and is mostly seen as a symptom of organic lesions of the brain, such as anoxic encephalopathy or cerebral palsy.

NEURODEGENERATION WITH BRAIN IRON ACCUMULATION

Neurodegeneration with brain iron accumulation was earlier called Hallervorden-Spatz disease. It is a rare, autosomal recessive disorder that involves progressive extrapyramidal manifestations. The most common clinical presentation is progressive dystonia. Other manifestations include retrocollis (cervical dystonia in which the neck remains extended), oromandibular-facial dystonia, and chorea.

MYOCLONUS

Myoclonic movements are sudden, brief, involuntary muscle contractions that cause shock-like movements. Some myoclonus can be physiological. However, when pathological they can signify some underlying diseases, such as metabolic disorders—hyperammonemia, hypoglycemia, liver failure, renal failure, neurodegenerative diseases, such as prion diseases, and atypical parkinsonism.

TICS

Tics are a kind of movement disorder that is characterized by sudden jerky movements which are stereotypical in nature. Tics are predominantly seen in the face and neck. They can be divided into simple tics or complex tics. Examples of simple tics include repetitive eye blinking, nose wrinkling, shoulder shrugging, or throat clearing. Examples of complex tics include touching things, smelling objects, echopraxia, or jumping. Tics can be motor or phonic. Motor tics involve repetitive movements whereas phonic tics include repetitive sounds, sniffs, etc.

TARDIVE DYSKINESIA

Tardive dyskinesias are jerky and involuntary movements of the face and body. Half of all patients treated with some antipsychotic medications for mental illness develop this as a side effect of the therapy.

EMERGENCY IN MOVEMENT DISORDER

Even though most movement disorders are disabling they are usually not life-threatening. However, some of these can become an emergency in certain circumstances. This can include acute drug reactions which can result in acute dystonia or neuroleptic malignant syndrome. The neuroleptic malignant syndrome occurs due to an unexplained adverse reaction to antipsychotic therapy which is manifested as high fever, altered mental status, muscle rigidity, and other autonomic dysfunctions often posing a threat to life. Acute exacerbations of movement disorders, such as status dystonic, laryngeal dystonia, tic status, or lethal catatonia can also pose a threat to the life of the person.

BOTULINUM TOXIN IN MOVEMENT DISORDERS

Botulinum toxin is used widely for therapeutic use in movement disorders. Multiple movement disorders including blepharospasm, tics, and cervical and oromandibular dystonia can be treated using botulinum toxin. There are several subtypes of botulinum toxin. Out of these, types A and B are the ones that are used in movement disorders. The toxin is carefully injected into the target muscle. The selection of the muscle and site of injection is done with the assistance of electromyography and ultrasound. Botulinum toxin induces weakness in the muscle by inhibiting the release of acetylcholine at the neuromuscular junction. The therapeutic effect of botulinum lasts for around three months. When the site and dose of injection is carefully done, the procedure has mostly no side effects. Initially, the dosage is kept at the lowest possible and it is then increased based on the patient's response (**Fig. 36.3**).

SURGICAL MANAGEMENT OF MOVEMENT DISORDERS

The common surgical approaches for the treatment of movement disorders include deep brain stimulation (DBS) and neuroadaptive procedures. When pharmacological treatments have reached limits, the role of surgical interventions in these disorders is making a resurgence. When patients are appropriately selected for surgical management, these have compelling results in the treatment of movement disorders. DBS in movement disorders is targeted towards intracranial targets, such as subthalamic nucleus (STN) globus pallidus interna (GPi), and ventralis intermediate nucleus of the thalamus (VIM). Other than Parkinson's disease, a variety of movement disorders are recently considered for treatment by DBS. It is found to be useful for the treatment of essential tremors, primary dystonia, and Tourette's syndrome. Surgical management

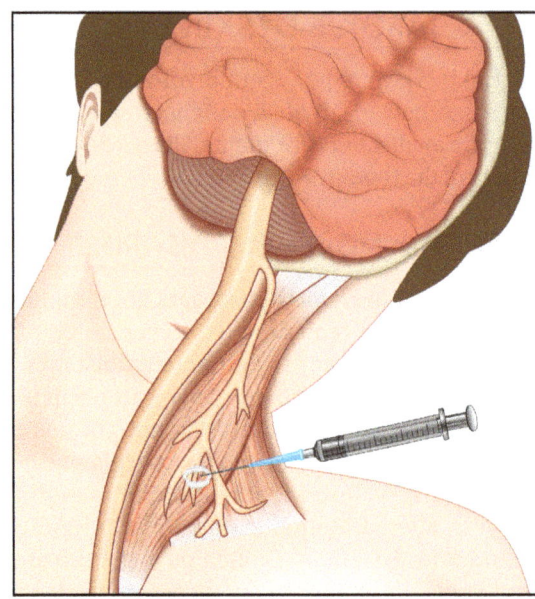

Fig. 36.3: Botulinum injection in cervical dystonia.

of movement disorders has gained importance and huge advancements are made in this field. This was possible with a clearer understanding of the neuroanatomical structures involved in movement disorders and the technological advancements in the field.

NURSING MANAGEMENT

Nursing management of movement disorders is basically supportive. When the major focus of medical treatment is on the maximal reduction of movement abnormalities, nurses should teach the patients and caregivers about the condition as well as address the psychosocial aspects of the disease. Focusing solely on the physical manifestations of the disorder is not enough for the holistic care of these patients. A study by Louis, et al., 2015 has shown that only 10% of patients with essential tremors were satisfied with their care.

The deficits associated with these disorders mostly interfere with the ability of the patients to perform ADLs. Several mental, social, and emotional needs of patients with movement disorders are usually overlooked. Most of the patients are uncomfortable in social situations due to their disorder and this causes embarrassment, social isolation, and anxiety.

Following are certain nursing interventions for patients with movement disorders:

- ❖ The most important aspect related to patient teaching is to discuss with the patient as well as their caregiver about the realistic goals of treatment of their disorders. Some of the disorders get controlled very well with pharmacological management, while others may show a progressive decline in response. For example, treatment options in dystonia are often not curative. Open discussion about the expected outcomes of treatment is necessary to prevent frustration and non-compliance to treatment.
- ❖ Assessment of the mental status of the patient is important to evaluate their overall response to treatment. Carefully evaluate for social anxiety and social avoidance behavior. A multidisciplinary approach involving mental health personnel may be needed to optimize the treatment of patients.
- ❖ Enhance self-care in patients to the optimum level. Modifications in the environment can support patients to carry out their activities of daily living with minimal support.
- ❖ Patients and their caregivers need support and education through the entire process of diagnosis and treatment. Research has shown that diagnosing dystonia can be delayed, with evidence concluding an average timeframe of 4–6 years in even the most common dystonia classifications (e.g., cervical dystonia).
- ❖ Monitoring the pharmacological treatment and carefully assessing side effects is necessary in movement disorders as the treatment is for a long term. As benzodiazepines are used frequently in treatment, the risk of dependency and abuse needs to be evaluated. These patients should also be educated about their increased risk of falls while on treatment. Adequate environmental alterations and safety precautions should be instituted.

Case Scenario

1. A 56-year-old man presented in the movement disorders clinic with a history of worsening symptoms from the past 5 years. His initial complaints included difficulty in walking, which progressively worsened as he developed choreic movements. He was working as a clerk in a private office and had to discontinue the job due to his motor symptoms. Family history was relevant with his father having similar symptoms. He passed away at the age of 70 years due to unrelated causes and was not investigated for Huntington's disease. Genetic testing confirmed Huntington's disease in the patient. He was started on tetrabenazine therapy 12.5 mg two times per day. The patient showed remarkable improvement in abnormal movements. Prepare a care plan for him anticipating the needs.
2. A 50-year-old school teacher consulted a physician with complaints of a general lack of coordination and shuffling gait. While collecting history, his spouse mentioned that he was appearing in a low mood lately and his colleagues and students have noticed a subtle decline in his memory and other mental abilities. No significant family history could be elicited. He was treated medically after confirming Huntington's disease with genetic testing. His symptoms gradually progressed and he developed choreic movements in the limbs. His cognitive abilities also declined over the next 5 years and he had to discontinue the job. His two sons were also screened for HD and both of them were found to be carrying the diseased gene. The family process got affected severely as the spouse became the only breadwinner of the family and had to perform the caregiver role continuously. The patient became partially dependent on daily activities as the disease further progressed. The sons were affected to witness the progressive decline in their father despite treatment. Supportive management of the patient with medicines, physical therapy, and nursing care continued. A multi-disciplinary approach towards the care of the family with psychosocial and spiritual care could ensure the well-being and coping among the family members. Draw a multidisciplinary action plan for him based on the needs.

SUMMARY

Movement disorders are neurological disorders that can present as excess of movement which is involuntary or paucity of voluntary movement. These disorders affect the fluency and quality of movement causing profound effects on the quality of life of the patients. The causes of movement disorders range from neurodegenerative or inflammatory to drug-induced and psychogenic. They are produced due to the incoordination in several interacting brain circuits. Movement disorders have a profound effect on health and quality of life of individuals. These disorders are managed by both medicines as well as with effective modification of individual living.

MULTIPLE CHOICE QUESTIONS

1. A nurse is caring for an elderly patient with essential tremors. Which of the following drugs should the nurse anticipate to increase the tremors in the patient?
   a. Acetaminophen
   b. Metoclopramide
   c. Phenytoin
   d. Aspirin

2. Which of the following is usually associated with dystonia?
   a. Difficulty in comprehending information
   b. Spasm of the neck muscles
   c. Bladder incontinence
   d. Low mood and poor judgment

3. Which of the following is the most common form of dystonia:
   a. Blepharospasm
   b. Truncal dystonia
   c. Cervical dystonia
   d. Laryngeal dystonia

4. A patient who has been treated with botulinum injection asks the nurse about the treatment. Which of the following responses by the nurse is appropriate?
   a. Botulinum is injected into the veins and can provide symptom relief for 2–3 years
   b. Botulinum injection is given into the muscle and can provide symptom relief for 1–2 years
   c. Botulinum injection is given into the vein and can provide symptom relief for few weeks to months
   d. Botulinum injection is given into the muscle and can provide symptom relief for few months

5. The nurse is caring for a patient who has been newly diagnosed with Huntingtons disease. While providing counseling to the family, the nurse understands that:
   a. The risk of the child inheriting the abnormal gene if one parent is affected, is 50%
   b. The children are at no risk of inheriting the disease unless both parents are affected
   c. Even if a child inherit the gene, he/she may not be affected by the illness
   d. If one child inherits the gene, other children will also be affected by the illness

6. Which of the following is the cause for brain tissue damage in patients with Huntington's disease?
   a. Hypoxic injury
   b. Electrolyte disturbances and metabolic derangement
   c. Congenital issues in brain development
   d. Abnormal protein

7. A nurse visits a patient with Huntington's disease who is cared at home by the family. Which of the following interventions will best ensure that contractures are prevented in the patient?
   a. The patient is provided a water bed with adequate cushioning
   b. The patient is repositioned every 2 hours in the bed
   c. The patient participates in range of motion exercise
   d. The patient has adequate modifications in the home environment to allow mobilization

8. The nurse is interacting with a newly diagnosed Huntington's disease patient. Which of the following responses from the patient should signal the need for more teaching?
   a. "I should seek help in case I feel suicidal"
   b. "I know that it is important for my children to get genetic screening for the disease"
   c. "I am sure that the medicines that I take can help me cure the disease"
   d. "My disease can get worsened over time, hence I need to keep my life plans accordingly"

9. Which of the following best describes status dystonicus?
   a. It is a type of dystonia that can be triggered by missing of treatment
   b. It is a exacerbated form of dystonia which is a medical emergency and requires immediate treatment including sedation
   c. Status dystonicus is an emergency which can be adequately controlled by providing large volumes of rapid IV fluids and antibiotics
   d. Status dystonicus can lead to extreme muscle flaccidity further progressing to respiratory compromise

10. Identify the movement disorder characterized by slow and continuous writhing movements of the hand or legs:
    a. Tardive dyskinesia
    b. Athetosis
    c. Neuroleptic malignant syndrome
    d. Tics

ANSWERS

1. b
2. b
3. c
4. d
5. a
6. d
7. c
8. c
9. b
10. b

SUGGESTED READING

1. Behari M, Srivastava A. Movement disorders: current understanding of pathophysiology and management. Astrocyte. 2018;5:55-62.
2. Booij SJ, Tibben A, Engberts DP, Marinus J, Roos RAC. Thinking about the end of life: a common issue for patients with Huntington's disease. J Neurol. 2014;261:2184-91.
3. Bridenbaugh SA, Kressig RW. Movement Disorders. In: Roller-Wirnsberger R, Singler K, Polidori M (Eds). Learning Geriatric Medicine. Practical Issues in Geriatrics. Springer, Cham. 2018. https://doi.org/10.1007/978-3-319-61997-2_20
4. Bruyn GW. Handbook of Clinical Neurology. In: Vinken PJ, Bruyn GW (Eds). Elsevier Amsterdam; Vol. 6. Huntington's Chorea: historical, clinical and laboratory synopsis. 1968; pp. 298-78.
5. Das SK, Ghosh B, Das G, Biswas A, Ray J. Movement disorders: Indian scenario: A clinic-genetic review. Neurol India. 2013;61:457-66.
6. Eddy CM, Parkinson EG, Rickards HE. Changes in mental state and behavior in Huntington's disease. Lancet Psychiatry. 2016;3:1076-86.
7. Hunington's disease collaborative research group. A novel gene containing a trinucleotide repeat that is expanded and unstable on Huntington's disease chromosomes. Cell. 1993;72:971–e 983. doi: 10.1016/0092-8674(93)90585-E
8. Klager J, Duckett A, Sandler S, Moskowitz C. Huntington's disease: a caring approach to the end of life. Care Manag J. 2008;9:75-81.
9. McColgan P, Tabrizi SJ. Huntington's disease: a clinical review Eur J Neurol. 2018;25(1):24-34. doi: 10.1111/ene.13413. Epub 2017 Sep 22.
10. Miao Xu, Zhi-Ying Wu Huntington Disease in Asia Chin Med J (Engl). 2015;128(13):1815-9.
11. Munhoz RP, Moscovich M, Araujo PD, Teive HA. Movement disorders emergencies: a review. Arq Neuropsiquiatr. 2012;70(6):453-61.
12. Ross CA, et al. Huntington disease: natural history, biomarkers and prospects for therapeutics. Nat. Rev. Neurol. 2014;10:204-16.
13. Tabrizi SJ, Scahill RI, Owen G, et al. Predictors of phenotypic progression and disease onset in re-manifest and early stage Huntington's disease in the TRACK-HD study analysis of 36–month observational data. Lancet Neurol. 2013;12:637-49.
14. van Duijn E, Kingma EM, van der Mast RC. Psychopathology in verified Huntington's disease gene carriers. J Neuropsychiatry Clin Neurosci. 2007;19:441-8.
15. Vuong K, Canning CG, Menant JC, Loy CT. Gait, balance, and falls in Huntington disease. Handb Clin Neurol. 2018;159:251-60.

CHAPTER 37

Cranial Nerve Disorders

Rakesh Sharma, Deepak Goel, Jitender Chaturvedi

"Safety is a sensual state. You cannot feel sensual unless you're feeling safe."

—Lebo Grand

LEARNING OBJECTIVES

After going through the chapter, the learner will be able to:
- Enumerate various cranial nerve disorders.
- Describe the epidemiology and etiopathogenesis of trigeminal neuralgia, Bell's palsy, Meniere's disease, and glossopharyngeal neuralgia.
- Recognize the clinical presentation of various cranial nerve disorders.
- Understand the diagnostic modalities of the cranial nerve disorders.
- Discuss the medical and nursing management of various cranial nerve disorders.
- Appreciate the collaborative care of various cranial nerve disorders.

TERMS

- **Bell's palsy:** Inflammation of seventh cranial nerve (facial nerve) resulting in weakness or paralysis of one side of face.
- **Bell's phenomenon:** It is also known as palpebral oculogyric reflex. In this a patient with orbicularis oculi muscle weakness tries to close eyes make upward and outward movement.
- **Endolymph:** It is also known as Scarpa fluid, clear fluid found in the inner ear of the membranous labyrinth.
- **Paroxysmal symptoms:** Sudden increase in intensity or reappearance of symptoms.
- **Tic douloureux:** It is painful twitch, disease of 5th cranial nerve, also known as trigeminal neuralgia.

INTRODUCTION

Some cranial nerves (CN) are susceptible to injury due to their location in the skull. These are the trigeminal nerve (CN-V), facial nerve (CN-VII), glossopharyngeal nerve (CN-IX), and vagus nerve (CN-X). In this chapter, four cranial nerve disorders are discussed: Trigeminal neuralgia, Bell palsy, Meniere's disease, and glossopharyngeal neuralgia.

TRIGEMINAL NEURALGIA

CONCEPT AND DEFINITION

Trigeminal neuralgia (TN) is defined as severe facial pain due to compression of the fifth cranial nerve (trigeminal nerve) or, more commonly, its maxillary or mandibular branches. It is also known as *tic douloureux*. Trigeminal neuralgia is the most devastating facial pain, ever known to mankind. Its presence may turn patients suicidal.

The prevalence of trigeminal neuralgia globally and in India is more common in females, and risk increases among age 40 years and older. Among three branches of 5th cranial nerve, the maxillary and mandibular branches are affected the most.

ETIOLOGY AND PATHOPHYSIOLOGY

There are no identified etiological factors for trigeminal neuralgia. The most common risk factors for trigeminal neuralgia are multiple sclerosis (MS), vascular compression, and hypertension, which causes symptoms among patients.

As per new classification, TN can be classified into three categories:
1. Classical
2. Secondary
3. Idiopathic.

CLINICAL MANIFESTATIONS

Trigeminal neuralgia is a unilateral, rarely bilateral, painful condition, where the pain is paroxysmal, sudden onset, and short-lived similar to an electric shock like sensation. It may be triggered by washing face, brushing teeth, smile, applying makeup, shaving, drinking, eating, a gust of cold wind, touch, or direct pressure over the nerve trunk.

The pain episode may be short-time, lasting for few seconds to a few hours or months, characterized by sharp, stabbing, shooting, like an electric shock. Once the pain episode start, the patient stop ("arresting") doing whatever activity they are performing.

Gradually, patients may lose weight, restrict activity of daily living, reduced quality of sleep, and quality of life with the fear of pain.

DIAGNOSTIC EVALUATION

Diagnostic criteria for trigeminal neuralgia defined by the International Headache Society, are:
1. Unilateral facial pain episodes for three or more times.
2. Pain originates in one of the branches of the trigeminal nerve with no radiation outside of the trigeminal nerve distribution.
3. Pain with three following characteristics, including paroxysmal pain attack for a second to two minutes, severe in intensity, and electric shock-like sensation with shooting, stabbing or sharp in nature.

As the reason of TN is usually unknown, other possible causes such as temporal arteritis, benign tumor of trigeminal nerve, multiple sclerosis, or other vascular abnormalities must be explored by complete blood count (CBC) analysis, surgical biopsy and, or imaging studies (X-ray, CT, and MRI) may help to make a confirmatory diagnosis.

MEDICAL MANAGEMENT

In TN, the first choice for treatment is carbamazepine. It is effective in almost 80% of the patients. It is started with 1,000 mg daily in divided doses and, most patients require maintenance doses of 200 mg daily, QID. An alternative to carbamazepine is oxcarbazepine given 300–1,200 mg daily.

If both the drugs are not tolerated and or not effective, lamotrigine 400 mg or phenytoin 300–400 mg daily are the other choices.

Baclofen with anticonvulsant may also be administered, with 5–10 mg TID, maximum up to 20 mg QID.

SURGICAL MANAGEMENT

If pharmacological management fails, surgical interventions need to be initiated.
- The most common is *microvascular decompression* to release pressure from the trigeminal nerve.
- *Gamma knife radiosurgery* is another therapy with lesser side effects.
- *Radiofrequency thermal rhizotomy* was used in the past. It helps in short-term relief from pain. It is a minimally invasive procedure; under fluoroscopy guidance, a radio-frequency needle is introduced via foramen ovale to heat the Gasserian ganglion.
- *Percutaneous balloon microcompression* is more suitable to relieve pain in the ophthalmic branch. In this procedure, selective nerve fibers are destroyed.

NURSING MANAGEMENT

Nursing management includes finding the triggering factors, frequency of spasms, and pain, monitoring effects of drug therapy, and providing emotional support and necessary information to the patient, such as warning for triggering factors and how to prevent them.

Nursing Assessment
- The nurse needs to collect a detailed history and perform a physical examination.
- A thorough examination of head, neck, eyes, ears, teeth, mouth, and the temporomandibular joint to find out other reasons of facial pain.
- The characteristics of pain should be assessed and documented, which will help evaluate therapy's effectiveness.

Nursing Diagnoses
1. Acute or chronic pain related to spasm or physiologic changes.
2. Knowledge deficit related to disease and triggers of spasm.
3. Self-care deficit related to fear of triggering pain.
4. Poor nutrition secondary to less than necessary intake related to fear of triggering spasm by chewing.
5. Ineffective individual coping related to severe pain, excessive threat to the self-alone.
6. Social isolation secondary to fear of triggering spasms with activity.
7. Anxiety related to prognosis of disease and changes in health.
8. Risk for injury to the eyes related to the risk factors like possible reduction in corneal sensation.

Nursing Interventions
- Assess the patients for triggering factors, educate them on methods of preventing triggers.
- Educate the patient about the drugs, doses, and importance of adherence.
- Teach and encourage communication methods without triggering pain.
- Educate ways to prevent or reducing pain by cleaning the face with cotton pads by normal room temperature water, keep the room temperature at normal range; only mouthwash after eating instead of brushing teeth; group the daily living activities.
- Encourage the patient to have a high nutritious diet, which should be comfortable to chew. The room temperature should be standard.

- Tell the patient to eat a small and frequent diet to avoid fatigue and pain.
- Advice for the use of nutritional supplements, if needed.
- Teach relaxation exercises such as breathing, meditation, and progressive muscle relaxation.
- Encourage to report of any side effects of drug therapy, such as dizziness, imbalance, and sedation, etc.
- Provide psychological support to the patients as well as to the family members in acute phase of disease.

Postoperative Care

- Assess neurological status with facial motor and sensory assessment.
- Assess eyes for dryness and redness. Administer artificial tear-forming drugs.
- Patients should be cautioned, avoid the use of the affected side to chew food.
- Observe for difficulty in eating and swallowing; if any, report to the surgeon immediately.

Case Scenario

- A female patient, 45 years of age, referred from primary health care center to a tertiary care center with the complaints of right facial pain.
- **Present health history:** The pain has been present for the past month. She states that it is a sharp shooting pain radiating over her right cheek. It is exacerbated by chewing, brushing her teeth. The pain interfere with her activities of daily living.
- The pain is 8/10 and continuous with intermittent increases to 9/10 when she is chewing. She has lost 5 kg of weight in the past month from not wanting to eat for fear of exacerbating the pain.
- There is no history of any hearing change, or change in taste.
- She is on acetaminophen with no improvement. Two weeks ago she was started on ibuprofen from nearby pharmacy.
- She has no other medical problems.
- Past history—no surgical history in the past; no history of any tooth extraction.
- Medication—she is currently taking ibuprofen 800 mg twice a day.
- There is no history of smoking or taking alcohol.
- **Family history:** There is no family history of headaches or other neurological problems.

Management
- Carbamazepine.
- Baclofen.
- Radiofrequency thermal rhizotomy, if symptoms are not relieved.

BELL'S PALSY

CONCEPT AND DEFINITION

Bell's palsy is an acute benign cranial polyneuropathy of facial nerve (CN-VII). It is facial paralysis or paresis of unknown cause. It is also known as facial paralysis, characterized by disruption of motor branch of CN-VII, mostly affecting one side of the face. Rarely, it may present as bilateral facial palsy.

The facial nerve controls the tear glands, the salivary glands, and muscles of middle ear. It is also responsible for taste sensations from the tongue.

INCIDENCE/PREVALENCE

Globally, the incidence rate is 15–20/1,00,000, and the lifetime risk of Bell's palsy is 1 in 60. The recurrence rate is 8–12%, and approximately 70% of patients recover completely without treatment. There are no specific gender, racial or age-related incidences. However, it occurs between 20–60 years of age but mostly in mid or late life with the onset at age of 40 years.

RISK FACTORS

Risk factors for Bell's palsy are diabetes, hypertension, obesity, pregnancy and pre-eclampsia. It occurs 3–4 times more frequently during pregnancy, usually at 35 weeks of gestation.

The exact etiology is unknown, but as per recent evidence, some of the viral infections such as herpes simplex virus (HSV), varicella-zoster virus, and Epstein-Barr virus may cause Bell's palsy.

PATHOPHYSIOLOGY

Due to unknown cause, infection or immune response results in the inflammation, edema, ischemia and finally demyelination of facial nerve. HSV was found in the endoneurial fluid suggests one of the most common cause. Similarly, varicella-zoster virus is associated with facial nerve paralysis and known to be the second most cause.

CLINICAL MANIFESTATIONS

- **Initial symptoms are:**
  - Herpetic vesicular lesions around the ear
  - Pain around the ear
  - Fever
  - Hearing deficit and tinnitus
- Maximum facial weakness begins by 48 hours of onset. Flaccidity of the affected side of the face, drooping of the mouth, along with drooling.
- Widened palpebral fissure.
- Flattening of the nasolabial fold.
- Inability to smile, frown, whistle and impaired chewing ability.
- Some of the patients may experience excessive tearing.
- Patient complaints of inability to close the eyelid, upward movement of eyeball while trying to close eye (Bell's phenomenon).
- Taste is lost unilaterally, on the side of the lesion
- **Presence of hyperacusis:** Hypersensitivity to particular sounds. Normal routine sounds will make uncomfortable to patient even sometimes painful.

COMPLICATIONS

- Psychological withdrawal, due to changes in the facial appearance.
- Malnutrition, dehydration, mucous membrane dryness and trauma.
- Corneal abrasions.
- Facial spasm and contractures.

DIAGNOSTIC EVALUATION

- A detailed history collection, pregnancy status (among women of reproductive age group), and neurological examination.

- There is no confirmative diagnostic test for Bell's palsy. The diagnosis and prognosis is made purely based upon the clinical manifestations of the patient.
- A complete blood count with ESR will suggest for presence of infection.
- MRI helps to show the edema and enhancement of the cranial nerve in unknown Bell's palsy.
- Electromyography (EMG) after 10 days of onset of symptoms suggest prognosis and recovery of the condition.
- It is also suggested to explore facial paralysis secondary to underlying conditions such as Guillain-Barre syndrome, tumor.

MEDICAL MANAGEMENT

- Primarily, patient is treated symptomatically and with an intention to prevent complications.
- Corticosteroid therapy, especially prednisone, 60–80 mg daily for the first 5 days followed by tapered doses for the next 5 days. It will help reducing inflammation, edema and pain.
- In addition to corticosteroid, valacyclovir may be marginally effective than prednisone alone in severe conditions. Embase, Web of Science, and the Cochrane Central Register of Controlled Trials were searched for studies published in all languages from 1984 to January 2009. Additional studies were identified from cited references. Selection criteria: Randomized controlled trials that compared steroids with the combination of steroids and antivirals for the treatment of Bell's palsy were included in this study. At least one month of follow-up and a primary end point of at least partial facial muscle recovery, as defined by a House-Brackmann grade of at least 2 (complete palsy is designated a grade of 6.
- Analgesics can be given to relieve pain.
- Other therapies include moist heat, facial massage, electrical stimulation of the nerve.

NURSING MANAGEMENT

Nursing Assessment

- Assess the motor and sensory responses of the facial nerve, specifically involving the face, eye, and tongue.
- Assess the ability of the patient to close the eyelids, lifting eyebrows, smiling, frowning, speaking clearly, drinking and eating.

Nursing Diagnoses

1. **Disturbed sensory perception:** Visual related to disturbed sensory function of facial nerve which eventually hamper closing and opening eyes, causes dryness.
2. Low self esteem related to alteration in structure and function for facial muscle secondary to Bell's palsy.
3. **Imbalanced nutrition:** Less than body requirement related to less intake of food due to weakness in facial and tongue muscles.
4. Anxiety related to the inadequate knowledge and prognosis of disease.

Nursing Interventions

The primary aims of nursing care will be to prevent eye injury, diet management and provide psychological support. In Bell's palsy, blink reflex is reduced or absent, and the patient can not close the eyelid frequently and completely. As the eye does not close, the chance of injury increases due to the entry of foreign particles or dust in the eye, or due to dryness of cornea, that may become ulcerated.

Eye Care

- Educate the patient to close eyelids manually before going to sleep.
- Lubricate eyes by administering artificial tears every 4–6 hours.
- Advice patients to use eye patches/shields.
- Instruct patients to wear sunglasses to prevent strain from sunlight; also, wrap-around sunglasses reduces evaporation from the eyes.

Face and Other Care at Home

- Due to weakness in the facial muscles, patient is unable to eat, drink and control saliva from the affected side. A small volume, frequent and soft diet is advised for patients.
- Encourage patients to be relaxed at mealtime, chew food slowly.
- To improve muscle strength, teach about moist heat application, facial exercise and massage, which can be performed at home.
- Some patients require electrostimulation therapy; this can be performed at outpatient basic.
- Emotional support is very important for the patient to cope with sudden bodily changes.

> **Case Scenario**
> - A female, 49 years old, complaining of left-sided facial weakness. She had difficulty closing her left eye and blinking, smiling. She had difficulty with closing left corner of the mouth.
> - Over few weeks, the weakness had progressed to involve the whole of the left side of her face.
> - There was no other limb weakness, and no hearing problems.
> - **Past history:** No such medical or surgical history evidenced.
> - **Family history:** There is no family history of any paralysis or other neurological problems.
> - **Medication:** Treated with prednisolone.
> - After six weeks she had made a near recovery, but not complete recovery.

MENIERE'S DISEASE

CONCEPT AND DEFINITION

Meniere's disease is also known as hydropic ear disease, a chronic disorder of the inner ear characterized by vertigo, tinnitus, hearing loss and aural fullness in the affected ear. Some of the patients may only have vertigo or hearing loss or tinnitus, but ultimately, they will have all the classical symptoms over the time.

Individuals may have isolated incidents of vertigo with/without hearing loss or tinnitus, but over time, the individual's condition will progress until the appearance of classic symptoms. It equally affects males and females, with commonly a unilateral (70–90%) presentation.

INCIDENCE/PREVALENCE

The prevalence of Meneire's disease is highest in Finland which is 513, and lowest in Japan 36 cases per 1,00,000 population. USA reports 190 cases per 1,00,000 population. The onset of symptoms is uncommon in children, but it starts in the 5th to 6th decade of life. In India, exact data regarding Meniere's disease are not available; as per a report, more than 50 lakh patients are diagnosed, and this number will increase due to exposure to air and noise pollution; and chemical toxicity.

ETIOLOGY AND PATHOPHYSIOLOGY

In Meniere's disease, there is an accumulation of endolymph in the endolymphatic space of the labyrinth (membranous labyrinth); this mechanism is known as endolymphatic hydrops.

The membranous labyrinth ruptures due to excessive accumulation of endolymph, and there is a mixing of high potassium endolymph with low-potassium perilymph.

CLINICAL MANIFESTATIONS

Vertigo: The attack of vertigo may be sudden or with little warning, lasting minutes to hours. Patient experiences feeling of pulled down to the ground ("drop attack"). Sometimes vertigo is accompanied by nausea and vomiting.
Aural fullness: Unpleasant sensation of fullness in the ear.
Tinnitus: Gradual raising tinnitus with a typical sound like "roar" or "like the ocean" characteristic.
Hearing loss: Decrease in hearing acuity.
Autonomic symptoms: Sweating, pallor, nausea, vomiting, tachycardia and headache.

DIAGNOSTIC EVALUATION

1. **Clinical history and physical examination:** A detailed history collection about family history, recent infection, allergic reaction, and neurological examination. Patient may show unidirectional nystagmus that may change during the attack. It is important to ask the history of frequency, duration, the severity of vertigo attack. Weber test may lateralize to the ear opposite the hearing loss.
2. Positive head-impulse test on the affected side.
3. **Caloric test:** Generally, confirm the vestibular asymmetry.
4. **Audiogram:** *Meniere's disease* patient will have pattern of sensorineural hearing loss on audiogram
5. **Dehydration test or glycerol dehydration test:**
   ➤ Osmotic diuretics are helped to inhibit the reabsorption of water and sodium and improve peripheral auditory and vestibular function.
   ➤ A baseline audiometric test is performed and followed by a solution of 20 g urea or glycerol (osmotic diuretics) mixed with unsweetened fruit juice (4 oz) being administered orally. Perform audiometric test after 3 hours (or as per physician's instructions) of ingestion solution.
   ➤ The patient is considered to be suffering from Meniere's disease if:
      • 10 dB or more improvement at two or more frequencies (250–2,000 Hz), or
      • 12% or more improvement in speech discrimination scores.
   ➤ *Side-effects of test*: Nausea, thirst, headache, emesis, diuresis, diarrhea, and dizziness.
6. **Electrocochleography (ECoG):** Finding may be normal or reduced vestibular results.

MEDICAL MANAGEMENT

Medical management of Meniere's disease is successful if treated with dietary modification and medications.

Pharmacological Management

During the acute phase of a vertigo attack, the vestibular suppressant and antiemetics to minimize vertigo, nausea, and vomiting are administered.
❖ **H1 and H3 antagonists:** These are used to increase cochlear blood circulation (e.g., citrizine).
❖ **Antiemetic:** Metoclopramide or prochlorperazine can be given for mild or moderate nausea/vomiting.
❖ **Corticosteroids:** During the acute phase, corticosteroids can be administered to relieve the symptoms (prednisolone 1 mg/kg body weight for one week with gradual dose tapering for 1–2 weeks).
❖ **Antihistamine:** For vertigo symptoms, e.g., meclizine, cyclizine
❖ **Sedative and hypnotics:** To control anxiety (e.g., benzodiazepines).
❖ **Diuretics:** To relieve the pressure osmotic diuretics (e.g., hydrochlorothiazide, triamterene) can be used. These are used during an acute attack.
❖ **Gentamycin:** Uncontrolled vertigo, gentamicin, intratympanic injection (40 mg/mL) may be given to destroy selective vestibular apparatus.

SURGICAL MANAGEMENT

If patients do not respond to pharmacological management, surgical interventions are next in the plan to treat Meniere's disease.
❖ **Endolymphatic sac decompression:** A shunt is introduced in the endolymphatic sac via a post-auricular incision to relieve symptoms.
❖ **Labyrinthectomy:** If a patient is experiencing hearing loss and severe vertigo attacks that interfere in the activity of daily living, labyrinthectomy can be performed.
❖ **Vestibular neurectomy or vestibular nerve section:** Sectioning the vestibular nerve is the last option in a patient who is not getting relief from any treatment. It has an excellent success rate to treat vertigo in patients with Meniere's disease.

NURSING MANAGEMENT

Nursing Assessment

- Assess the family history, history and episodes of whirling vertigo with duration.
- To assess balance, the nurse needs to perform Romberg test.
- **Audiometric examination:** This will find hearing loss in the affected ear. It includes a test to patients' ability check to tell the difference between words like "fit" and "sit."

Nursing Diagnoses

1. Self-care deficits related to labyrinth dysfunction and episodes of vertigo.
2. Anxiety related to threat of health status and disability effects of vertigo.
3. Risk for trauma related to impaired balance.
4. Feeding, bathing/hygiene, dressing/grooming, and toileting self-care deficits related to labyrinth dysfunction and episodes of vertigo.

Nursing Interventions

Meniere's disease patients are mainly treated as home-based therapy. They are hospitalized, in case the symptoms are aggravated and need surgical intervention. The primary aim of nursing care is to prevent injury secondary to falls after an acute attack of vertigo.

Care Regarding Safety

- Instruct the patient to identify the aura and keep themselves in a safe environment.
- Encourage to be in a lie-down position during vertigo attack, even with slight dizziness.
- If a patient is hospitalized, always keep the side rails up. Keep extra pillows on each side of the head.
- Educate about drug regimen; it will help to alleviate acute symptoms.
- Assist patient in ambulation whenever needed.
- Educate patients to avoid hazardous activities (e.g., driving, swimming, operating machinery) requiring continuous attention.

DIETARY MANAGEMENT

- Instruct the patient to limit foods that are high in salt and sugar.
- Encourage to have meals and snacks at a regular time and maintain a good hydration level.
- Educate about the use of fresh vegetables, fruits, and whole grains.
- Instruct to avoid canned, stored, or processed food. These foods consist of high salt and preservatives.
- Encourage to drink a good amount of water every day. Milk and low-sugar fruit juices can be used.
- Limit coffee, tea, soft drinks, alcohol. Alcohol can change the fluid volume concentration in the inner ear fluid and results in worsening the symptoms.
- Instruct to avoid the use of caffeine, as it acts as diuretic and may deteriorate the condition.
- Aspirin may cause tinnitus and dizziness, so avoid using aspirin.

Case Scenario

- A female patient, 42 years old with a past history of migraine since 2 years. She reported recurrent episodes of rotational vertigo (about 2 per month) lasting from a few minutes to 1–2 hours, often with a right ear fluctuating hearing loss.
- Migraine and vertigo never occurred together.
- She also reported the presence of tinnitus which increased before vertigo attacks.
- **Past history:** Patient reported the first attack of migraine at the age of years, which more typically occurred before menstruation, at a frequency of 1–2/month.
- **Family history:** Mother and one of three sisters have migraine history.

Radiodiagnosis: MRI demonstrated micro ischemic lesions.

Other tests:
- Audiometric test—low frequency sensorineural hearing loss.
- Acoustic evoked potentials were normal.
- Caloric tests demonstrated a right sided unilateral weakness

Management
- Cetirizine
- Prednisolone
- Meclizine
- Sedative and hypnotics—to control anxiety (e.g., benzodiazepines).
- Hydrochlorothiazide
- Gentamicin

GLOSSOPHARYNGEAL NEURALGIA

CONCEPT AND DEFINITION

Glossopharyngeal neuralgia is a ninth cranial nerve disorder, similar to pathophysiology of trigeminal neuralgia. It presents as an acute, unilateral paroxysmal pain in the base of the tongue at the tonsillar region and throat region. Pain may be localized or radiated in the ear or throat. It is also known as *Weisenberg syndrome*.

INCIDENCE/PREVALENCE

Glossopharyngeal neuralgia (GN) is a rare condition and account for 0.2–1.3% of all types of cranial neuralgias. It equally affects male and female, commonly present on the left side.

ETIOLOGY AND PATHOPHYSIOLOGY

Certain activities such as swallowing, coughing, laughing, or speaking act as triggering factors. Generally speaking, glossopharyngeal neuralgia occurs at the age of 40 years and older. There are no exact etiological factors, but the compression of vascular supply to the glossopharyngeal nerve may be one of the factors in the development of glossopharyngeal neuralgia. The secondary causes may be a malignancy or infection of the oropharyngeal area or any lesions at the cranial base.

CLINICAL MANIFESTATIONS

Pain: Intense pain, sudden onset, primarily unilateral, lasting few minutes to hours, localized or radiating from throat to the neck, triggered by swallowing, coughing, laughing, or speaking.

Cardiac symptoms: Bradycardia or asystole, hypotension, and fainting during an attack.

DIAGNOSTIC EVALUATION

- A detailed history of personal habits, recent infection, increased blood pressure, injury to the head and neck area.
- Patients are diagnosed based on the clinical features, neurological assessment (special attention to the glossopharyngeal nerve)
- MRI of the head and neck.

MANAGEMENT

Medical treatment of glossopharyngeal neuralgia is similar to trigeminal neuralgia. Along with general care, the first choice of drug is carbamazepine.

Surgical management: If medical therapy is unable to relieve the symptoms, surgical interventions include:
- Microvascular decompression to release vascular compression.
- Rhizotomy of ninth (glossopharyngeal) and tenth (vagus) nerve fibers.

NURSING MANAGEMENT

Nursing Assessment

- A detailed history of personal, family, past medical and surgical condition.
- Assess 9th cranial nerve assessment.
- Assess the characteristics of pain, and sign of cardiac symptoms.
- Assess nutritional status and coping mechanism.

Nursing Diagnoses

1. Acute pain related to damage to glossopharyngeal nerve.
2. **Imbalanced nutrition:** Less than body requirements related to pain during swallowing.
3. Ineffective individual coping related to severe pain and apprehension of death.
4. Anxiety related to prognosis of disease and changes in health

Nursing Interventions

The primary role of a nurse in the management of glossopharyngeal neuralgia is to prevent the injury (cardiac symptoms), symptomatic therapy, and teaching about home care.

Educate patients about the triggering factors which can induce pain; avoid blowing nose, eat slowly. The patient needs to maintain basic hygiene and maintain nutritional balance.

If a patient is undergoing a surgical procedure, the nursing care includes:

Preoperative Phase

- Education about the procedure to be done, possible mild to moderate cognitive deficit, psychological support, postoperative diet, rest, and exercise.

- **Preoperative:**
  - Explain about nothing by mouth (NBM) after midnight,
  - Part preparation, as per institutional policy.
  - Neurological assessment, vital assessment, prescribed drug administration.
  - Collect all the investigation reports and maintain all the records before shifting to the operating room.

Postoperative Phase

- Perform neurological assessment and vital recording,
- Positioning—the head of the bed elevated at 30 degrees, monitor for signs and symptoms of intracranial pressure (ICP)
- Administer drugs as per order
- Maintain intake—output chart
- Assess bowel sound and plan for ambulation.

GERIATRIC CONSIDERATIONS FOR CRANIAL NERVE DISORDERS

Numerous age-related changes occur in the nervous system, resulting gradual decline in sensory-motor functions. Due to old age, patients with cranial nerve disorders require additional care. The patient's diagnosis remains a great challenge due to similarity in symptoms, such as walking difficulties and falls, poor muscle power and control, etc.

These patients require special attention for care and preventive strategies for fall injury, malnutrition, pressure ulcers, and muscle contracture/rigidity. Most of them may become completely dependent, and the healthcare professionals must ensure daily personal hygiene, feeding, physical exercise, and drug administration as well as psychological support.

> **Case Scenario**
>
> - Mr X, 80 years old, with the complaint of intense and piercing pain for last 3 months, intermittent in nature, with a duration varying from a few seconds to a maximum of about two min, localized in the deep laterocervical site behind the right jaw angle and the base of the homolateral tongue.
> - Pain is aggravated by palpation at the root of the neck, by yawning or by coughing. Initially, pain was associated with solid food and then appeared with the swallowing of liquids. There is a loss of weight approximately 5–6 kg from the time the symptoms arose.
> - Pain arise suddenly without prior notice and to revert spontaneously.
> - On neurological examination a reduced sensitivity of the palatine veil, hoarseness and hyporeflexia of the pharyngeal reflex demonstrated.
> - Diagnostic studies—performed CT scans, CT angiogram of the supra-aortic vessels, and MRI of the cervical spine.
> - **Past history:** Tooth extraction of the third molars teeth without a clear diagnosis of the problem. Patient had a history of a hypertensive cardiopathy being treated with calcium channel blockers, diabetes being treated with metformin.
> - A careful neurological examination demonstrated a reduced sensitivity of the palatine veil, hoarseness and hyporeflexia of the pharyngeal reflex without distal neurological deficits.
>
> **Management:**
> - Carbamazepine.
> - Microvascular decompression to release vascular compression.

SUMMARY

In this chapter, cranial nerve disorders are discussed. Most of these conditions are treated on an outpatient department basis. When the condition are not managed medically then surgical interventions are considered. Nurses roles are more towards to teach about the symptomatic management and avoid aggravating factors. In surgical management nurses' roles are more in pre- and postoperative phases. While caring geriatric age group patients with cranial nerve disorders remember about the sensory and motor nerve changes. Nurses must assess comorbidities and their treatment while planning nursing care for old age patients.

MULTIPLE CHOICE QUESTIONS

1. A patient admitted in the ward with trigeminal neuralgia. On examination, the nurse found out that ophthalmic branch is also involved. Then what is the priority assessment to be done by the nurse?
   a. To check characteristics of pain
   b. To check previous history of medication and allergies
   c. To check corneal reflex
   d. Sensory assessment of hot and cold

2. In trigeminal neuralgia, trigger zones are least frequent in:
   a. Face
   b. Forehead
   c. Lips
   d. Tongue

3. Tic douloureux (trigeminal neuralgia) is associated with which of the following nerves:
   a. 7th nerve
   b. 3rd nerve
   c. 5th nerve
   a. 8th nerve

4. Analgesics are not effective in reducing the pain in:
   a. Chronic pulpitis
   a. Acute periodontitis
   b. Impacted molar
   c. Trigeminal neuralgia

5. The latest drug of the choice in the management in trigeminal neuralgia is:
   a. Valproic acid
   b. Carbamazepine
   c. Diphenhydantoin
   a. Eptoin

6. Trigeminal neuralgia is characterized by:
   a. Paralysis of one side of the face
   b. Uncontrollable twitching of muscles
   c. Sharp, excruciating pain of short duration
   d. Prolonged episodes of pain on one side of the face

7. A 31-year-old female patient arrives to emergency department. Her complaints are: sudden onset of left facial weakness that was noticed by her son. She denies fever, rash, or any other symptoms. On assessment, it was concluded that she has no other neurologic deficits other than what is shown. When asked to close her left eye, she cannot. Which of the following is the most possible diagnosis?
   a. Bell palsy
   b. Malingering
   c. Ramsay Hunt syndrome
   d. Brain tumor

8. In Bell's palsy, which cranial nerve is affected?
   a. Facial nerve
   a. Olfactory
   b. Optic
   c. Trigeminal

9. Temporary paralysis of seventh cranial nerve that causes paralysis only of the affected side of face is:
   a. Bell's palsy
   b. Trigeminal neuralgia
   c. Myelitis
   d. Multiple sclerosis

10. Cranial nerve which is responsible for taste sensation on the anterior 2/3rd of the tongue:
    a. Facial
    b. Trigeminal
    c. Glossopharyngeal
    d. Abducens

11. Meniere's disease is a disease of:
    a. Ear
    b. Nose
    c. Bone
    d. Heart

12. Ménière's disease has following clinical features, *except*:
    a. Fluctuating deafness
    b. Pulsatile tinnitus
    c. Sensorineural deafness
    d. Vertigo

13. In which of the following diseases condition, endolymphatic hydrops are present:
    a. Cholesteatoma
    b. Meniere's disease
    c. Otosclerosis
    d. Gradenigo's syndrome

14. Which of the following parts of the body plays a key role in balance?
    a. Labyrinth
    b. Pituitary
    c. External ear
    d. Hypothalamus

15. Meniere's disease is the disorder of:
    a. External ear
    b. Middle ear
    c. Inner ear
    d. Tympanic membrane

16. Which of the following clinical sign and symptoms present in a patient diagnosed with glossopharyngeal neuralgia?
    a. Bradycardia or asystole
    b. Paralysis of face
    c. Loss of smell
    d. Blurred vision

17. Weisenberg syndrome is also known as:
    a. Bell palsy
    b. Glossopharyngeal neuralgia
    c. Meniere's disease
    d. Trigeminal neuralgia

18. Cranial nerve affected in glossopharyngeal neuralgia is:
    a. VII
    b. VIII
    c. II
    d. IX

19. Which neurological disorder resembles glossopharyngeal neuralgia?
    a. Trigeminal neuralgia
    b. Cauda equina syndrome
    c. Gullian-Barre syndrome
    d. Bell's palsy

20. What is the surgical management of glossopharyngeal neuralgia?
    a. Microvascular decompression
    b. Macroscopic delusion
    c. Microgliosectomy
    d. Microastroctomy

ANSWERS

1. c	2. b	3. c	4. d
5. b	6. c	7. a	8. a
9. a	10. a	11. a	12. b
13. b	14. a	15. c	16. a
17. b	18. d	19. a	20. a

SUGGESTED READING

1. Alexander TH, Harris JP. Current Epidemiology of Meniere's Syndrome. Otolaryngol Clin North Am [Internet]. 2010 Oct [cited 2021 Apr 22];43(5):965-70. Available from: https://pubmed.ncbi.nlm.nih.gov/20713236/
2. Berg T, Bylund N, Marsk E, Jonsson L, Kanerva M, Hultcrantz M, et al. The effect of prednisolone on sequelae in Bell's palsy. Arch Otolaryngol—Head Neck Surg [Internet]. 2012 May 1 [cited 2021 Apr 17];138(5):445-9. Available from: https://jamanetwork.com/
3. Daroff RB. Bradley's neurology in clinical practice e-book; 2015. p. 1978.
4. De Toledo IP, Conti Réus J, Fernandes M, Porporatti AL, Peres MA, Takaschima A, et al. Prevalence of trigeminal neuralgia: A systematic review. J Am Dent Assoc [Internet]. 2016 Jul 1 [cited 2021 Apr 13];147(7):570-576.e2. Available from: https://pubmed.ncbi.nlm.nih.gov/27017183/

5. Duransoy YK, Mete M, Akçay E, Selçuki M. Differences in individual susceptibility affect the development of trigeminal neuralgia. Neural Regen Res [Internet]. 2013 May 15 [cited 2021 Apr 13];8(14):1337-42. Available from: /pmc/articles/PMC4107645/
6. Havia M, Kentala E, Pyykkö I. Prevalence of Menière's disease in general population of southern Finland. Otolaryngol—Head Neck Surg [Internet]. 2005 Nov [cited 2021 Apr 22];133(5):762-8. Available from: https://pubmed.ncbi.nlm.nih.gov/16274806/
7. Katheriya G, Chaurasia A, Khan N, Iqbal J. Prevalence of trigeminal neuralgia in Indian population visiting a higher dental care center in North India. Natl J Maxillofac Surg [Internet]. 2019 [cited 2021 Apr 13];10(2):199. Available from: http://www.njms.in/text.asp?2019/10/2/195/270728
8. Khajeh A, Fayyazi A, Soleimani G, Miri-Aliabad G, Shaykh Veisi S, Behrouz K. Comparison of the efficacy of combination therapy of prednisolone acyclovir with prednisolone alone in Bell's palsy. Iran J Child Neurol [Internet]. 2015 Feb 7 [cited 2021 Apr 17];9(2):17-20. Available from: /pmc/articles/PMC4515336/
9. Khan M, Nishi SE, Hassan SN, Islam MA, Gan SH. Trigeminal neuralgia, glossopharyngeal neuralgia, and myofascial pain dysfunction syndrome: An update. Pain Res Manag; 2017.
10. Linskey ME. Trigeminal Neuralgia: Diagnosis and Nonoperative Management. In: Youmans and Winn Neurological Surgery [Internet]. Elsevier Health Sciences; 2017. pp. 1397-1404.e2. Available from: http://www.clinicalkey.com.elibraryaiimsrishikesh.remotexs.in/#!/content/book/3-s2.0-B9780323287821001714
11. Longo DL, Jameson JL, Kaspe D. Harrison's Principles of Internal Medicine: 18th edition. MacGraw-Hill. 2012;2:3362.
12. Meniere's Disease In India: Audiologists Hearing the Call—Business Opportunities in India [Internet]. [cited 2021 Apr 22]. Available from: http://www.businessonlineindia.com/menieres-disease-in-india-audiologists-hearing-the-call/
13. Montano N, Conforti G, Di Bonaventura R, Meglio M, Fernandez E, Papacci F. Advances in diagnosis and treatment of trigeminal neuralgia. Ther Clin Risk Manag [Internet]. 2015 Feb 24 [cited 2021 Apr 16];11:289-99. Available from: /pmc/articles/PMC4348120/
14. Perez-Carpena P, Lopez-Escamez JA. Current Understanding and Clinical Management of Meniere's Disease: A Systematic Review. Semin Neurol [Internet]. 2020 Feb 1 [cited 2021 Apr 22];40(1):138-50. Available from: https://pubmed.ncbi.nlm.nih.gov/31887752/
15. Quant EC, Jeste SS, Muni RH, Cape AV, Bhussar MK, Peleg AY. The benefits of steroids versus steroids plus antivirals for treatment of Bell's palsy: A meta-analysis. BMJ [Internet]. 2009 Sep 19 [cited 2021 Apr 17];339(7722):685. Available from: https://pubmed.ncbi.nlm.nih.gov/19736282/
16. Shah RJ, Padalia D. Glossopharyngeal Neuralgia. Treasure Island (FL): StatPearls Publishing, Treasure Island (FL); 2021.
17. Shojaku H, Watanabe Y, Yagi T, Takahashi M, Takeda T, Ikezono T, et al. Changes in the characteristics of definite Meniere's disease over time in Japan: A long-term survey by the Peripheral Vestibular Disorder Research Committee of Japan, formerly the Meniere's Disease Research Committee of Japan. Acta Otolaryngol [Internet]. 2009 [cited 2021 Apr 22];129(2):155-60. Available from: https://pubmed.ncbi.nlm.nih.gov/18607900/
18. Spencer CR, Irving RM. Causes and management of facial nerve palsy. Br J Hosp Med [Internet]. 2016 Dec 1 [cited 2021 Apr 16];77(12):686-91. Available from: https://pubmed.ncbi.nlm.nih.gov/27937022/
19. The International Classification of Headache Disorders, 3rd edition (beta version). Cephalalgia [Internet]. 2013;14;33(9):629-808. Available from: https://doi.org/10.1177/0333102413485658
20. Yogesh G, Sharma R. CBS Nursing Drug Guide 2020-2021, 1st edition. CBS Publishers & Distributors Pvt. Ltd.; 2020.

CHAPTER 38

Neurodegenerative Diseases

Monaliza

"Learn how to develop a 'bulletproof' brain that will stay healthy for years and even decades".
—John Roberts

LEARNING OBJECTIVES

After going through the chapter, the learner will be able to:
- Enumerate various neurodegenerative diseases.
- Discuss the etiology, pathophysiology, clinical manifestations, and diagnostic tests of various neurodegenerative diseases.
- Understand the treatment modalities of various neurodegenerative diseases.
- Discuss the nursing interventions for various neurodegenerative diseases.
- Discuss the geriatric considerations of various neurodegenerative diseases.

TERMS

- **Akinesia:** Absence or difficulty in producing movements.
- **Amygdala:** It is an important part of the brain that helps in feeling emotions, detecting threats, and activation of appropriate behavior.
- **Amyloid beta protein (Aβ):** It is an amino acids peptide chain involved in Alzheimer's disease.
- **Ataxia:** Inability to synchronize walking movements. Loss of balance.
- **Atrophy:** The decrease in the volume of brain or muscle tissue.
- **Basal ganglia:** A group of subcortical nuclei that helps in motor control, motor learning, executive functions and behaviors, and emotions.
- **CAG repeat:** Repeating units of DNA present in all typical Huntington genes, which, when expanded to 36 or more units ("mutant") causes HD.
- **Cogwheel rigidity:** Stiffness in the muscles primarily of limbs, leading to movements in small increments accompanied by tremors.
- **Dysarthria:** Slurred or slow speech because of the weakening of the muscles involved in speech.
- **Dyskinesia:** Abnormal movements of the muscles of the face, arms, legs or trunk.
- **Dysphasia:** Difficulty in speaking.
- **Hippocampus:** Part of the limbic system which is primarily associated with memory.
- **Lhermitte's sign:** It is an electric shock-like transient sensation that travels down the spine, arm, legs, and sometimes the trunk. It occurs upon flexion and/or movement of the neck.
- **Lewy body:** Abnormal collections of protein developing within the nerve cells, causative of Parkinson's disease.
- **Neuritic plaques:** Extracellular amyloid beta (Aβ) deposits found in the brain.
- **Neurofibrillary tangles (NFTs):** Collections of hyperphosphorylated tau protein that are most commonly found in Alzheimer's disease.
- **Tau proteins:** Proteins that stabilize microtubules. In Alzheimer's and Parkinson's, tau proteins become defective and do not stabilize microtubules properly.

INTRODUCTION

Neurodegenerative diseases are a group of disorders affecting the brain (with or without spinal cord involvement) characterized by progressive impairment of brain function and loss of activities of daily living, behavioral alterations, and motor disturbances with relentless neuronal loss that is abnormal for the age. These are the leading cause of disability and public health concerns. The elderly population is increasing worldwide and accordingly the prevalence of various neurodegenerative disorders. Alzheimer's and Parkinson's illnesses are the most common of several neurodegenerative disorders. This chapter focuses on all facets of neurodegenerative illness, including the natural ageing process, and covers the related diagnostic techniques, treatment methods, and nursing management. It also discusses one of the demyelinating diseases (multiple sclerosis) in the end.

ALZHEIMER'S DISEASE

Alzheimer's disease is a progressive neurodegenerative disorder. It is the most common type of irreversible dementia manifested as a gradual loss of memory, intellect, rational thought, and social skills. Nearly 7 out of 10 people with dementia have Alzheimer's type. As per Shaheen E Lakhan, "Alzheimer's disease (AD) is a neurodegenerative disorder marked by cognitive and behavioral impairment that significantly interferes with social and occupational functioning. It is an incurable disease with a long preclinical period and progressive course."

EPIDEMIOLOGY

- ❖ Alzheimer's disease typically affects people of older age. With the increase in the proportion of elderly people worldwide, the number of patients with Alzheimer's disease is also expected to escalate.
- ❖ After the age of 65, the prevalence of Alzheimer's disease doubles every five years with <1% per year before age 65 to 6% per year after the age of 85 years.
- ❖ Women are slightly more likely than men to have Alzheimer's disease, particularly beyond the age of 85.

RISK FACTORS FOR ALZHEIMER'S DISEASE

Various risk factors of AD are:
- ❖ Advancing age
- ❖ Family history
- ❖ Head trauma
- ❖ Lack of mental stimulation "use it or lose it"
- ❖ Down's syndrome
- ❖ Environmental toxins: aluminum, mercury
- ❖ Oxidative stress due to accumulation of free radicals and/or low antioxidant levels
- ❖ Abnormal protein processing
- ❖ Neurotransmitter deficit
- ❖ Genetic polymorphism

CAUSES

The two main types of Alzheimer's disease is:
1. **Sporadic AD:** It is one of the most common types of AD. It usually occurs after age 65. Its cause is not fully understood.
2. **Familial AD:** It is also referred to as 'hereditary'. It is caused by a very rare genetic condition and results in dementia, usually in people in their 40s and 50s. This is known as younger onset dementia.

The causes of AD are not known. However, certain factors like neurochemical, environmental, and genetic and immunological are thought to be causing this disease.

- ❖ **Neurochemical factors:**
  - ➢ Acetylcholine
  - ➢ Somatostatin
  - ➢ Substance P
  - ➢ Norepinephrine
- ❖ **Environmental factors:**
  - ➢ Cigarette smoking
  - ➢ Certain infections
  - ➢ Metals, industrial, or other toxins
  - ➢ Use of cholesterol-lowering drugs (statin).
- ❖ **Genetic and immunological factors:** Oxidized LDL receptor 1 and Angiotensin 1-converting enzyme, are tied to the way the brain cells bind to Apolipoprotein 4 (APOE4) and reduce the buildup of harmful proteins, known as plaques, in the brain, respectively.

PATHOPHYSIOLOGY OF ALZHEIMER'S DISEASE

Neurons are the central/functional units and are the building blocks of the nervous system. These cells send electrical impulses and chemical signals to and from the brain. Signals pass along the connections between brain cells in the form of chemicals called neurotransmitters. In Alzheimer's disease, there is a destruction of these cells and neurotransmitters. Basically, there is an accumulation of abnormal neuritic plaques and neurofibrillary tangles. The beta-amyloid deposition and neurofibrillary tangles damage the synapses and neurons. According to the "amyloid cascade" hypothesis, it is the amyloid plaques that interfere with synaptic activity and initiate a series of downstream effects that cause increasing inter- and intraneuronal dysfunction and, ultimately, cell death. So, there is atrophy of the affected areas of the brain, basically starting at the mesial temporal lobe. This atrophy of the brain cells leads to disturbed memory, impaired thinking, impaired social skills, behavioral changes, and a person's ability to function normally **(Figs. 38.1A and B)**.

CLINICAL MANIFESTATIONS

Ten warning signs of Alzheimer's disease:
1. Difficulty performing familiar tasks
2. Memory loss
3. Language problem
4. Disorientation

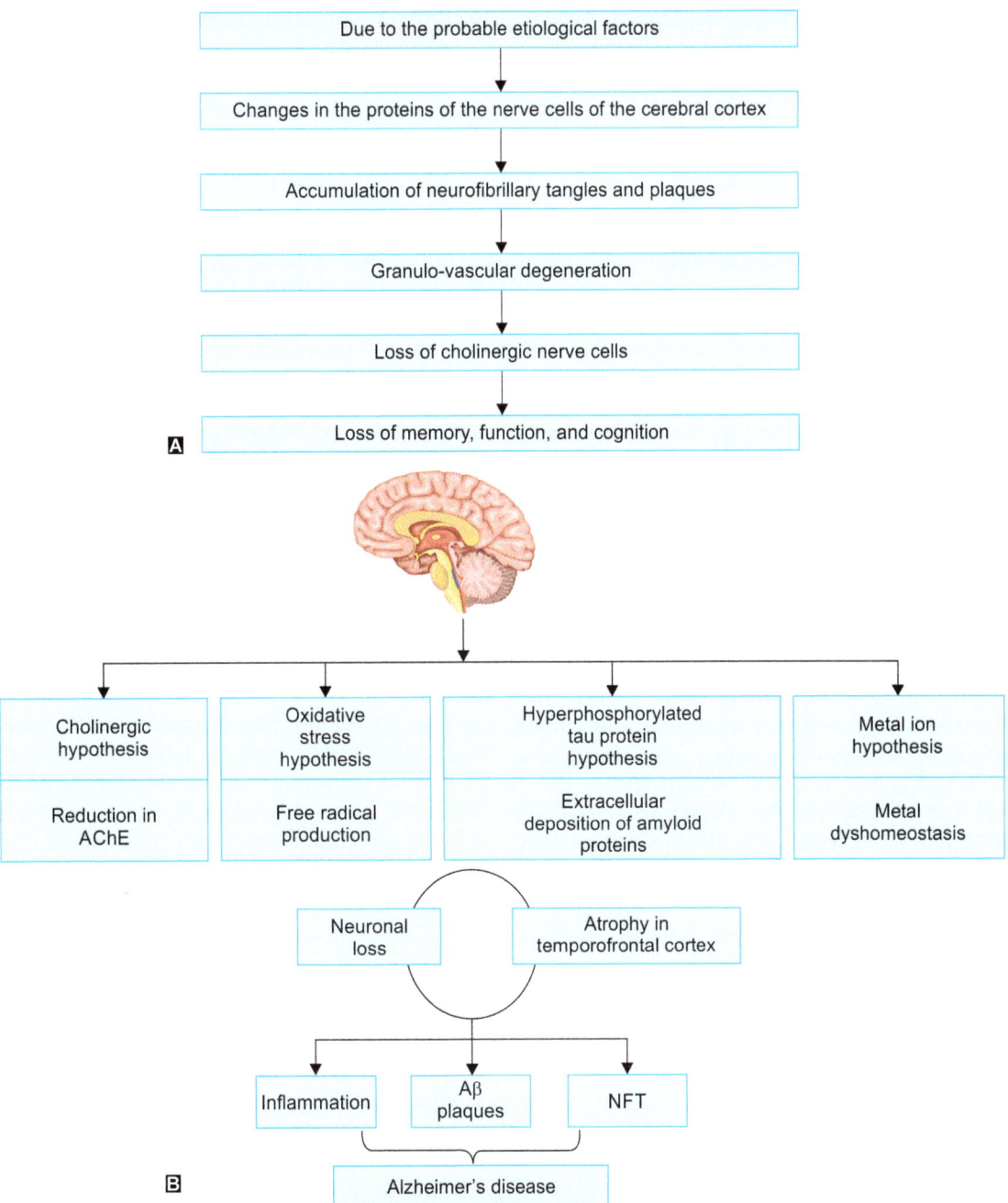

Figs. 38.1A and B: Pathophysiology of Alzheimer's disease.

5. Poor or decreased judgment
6. Impaired abstract thinking
7. Misplacing things
8. Changes in mood or behavior
9. Changes in personality
10. Loss of initiative

STAGES OF ALZHEIMER'S DISEASE

There are seven stages of AD:
- **Stage 1: Normal:** A normal mentally healthy individual.
- **Stage 2: Normal-aged forgetfulness:** Here a person over the age of 65 years experiences subjective complaints of cognitive and/or functional decline.
- **Stage 3: Mild cognitive impairment:** In this the capacity of an individual to perform certain functions, job performance, etc., gets compromised.
- **Stage 4: Mild Alzheimer's disease:** Here there is a decreased ability to manage instrumental activities of daily life, (e.g., ability to manage finances and prepare meals for guests, etc.). This can be very well assessed by using a scale called Instrumental Activities of Living by Lawton to assess which aspect of IADL is impaired.
- **Stage 5: Moderate Alzheimer's disease:** Here even a person's ability to choose proper clothing to wear as per weather is impaired.
- **Stage 6: Moderately severe Alzheimer's disease:** At this stage, even the ability of an individual to perform basic activities of daily life gets compromised.

- **Stages 7: Severe Alzheimer's disease:** There is a severe decline in cognitive functions and the patient become completely dependent on other for all his daily needs.

DIAGNOSTIC TESTS

Assessment

- Psychiatric assessment to determine if depression or any other mental health condition is causing or contributing to a person's symptoms.
- Mental status examination and neuropsychological assessment.

Laboratory Tests

1. **Brain scans:** CT, MRI, PET scan to rule out other possible causes for symptoms.
2. **CSF examination:** To measure the levels of proteins associated with Alzheimer's and related dementias.
3. Electroencephalogram (EEG).

MANAGEMENT

Medical Management

- **Acetylcholinesterase inhibitors:** These prevent the breakdown of acetylcholine, a chemical messenger important for learning and memory, e.g., Donepezil (Aricept), Rivastigmine (Exelon), Galantamine.
- **N-methyl d-aspartate receptor antagonist (NMDA):** Memantine-blocks the NMDA receptor and inhibit their overstimulation by glutamate (neurotransmitter)
- Antidepressants.
- Anxiolytics.
- Antipsychotics.
- Anticonvulsants

Psychosocial Intervention

- Behavioral approach
- Emotion-oriented approach
- Cognition-oriented approach
- Stimulation-oriented approach

NURSING MANAGEMENT

Caring for patients with AD is more than caring for conscious bedridden patients because here the patients are physically as well as mentally dependent on others. Apart from providing physical care, certain specific interventions for AD patients are:

- Provide a safe, orderly atmosphere at home to safeguard the patient from harm. Never leave the patient alone.
- Because of the patient's reduced cognitive capacities, establish an effective communication system with the patient and his family.
- Administer the prescribed medications. In case of swallowing problems, crush tablets or break open the capsules. It can then be mixed with semi-soft food and given to the patients.
- Establish a routine exercise schedule for the patients as per the capability of the patients. Encourage and motivate the patients to exercise as directed Allow rest times in between activities.
- Encourage and promote the patient to perform his activities of daily living to maintain independence. Assist the patient as necessary. Have patience and provide him with enough time to complete the tasks.
- Promote hydration and nourishment in moderation. Have a record of the patient's fluid and food intake to detect imbalances.
- Ensure the patient is aware of where the toilet is by taking him there at least every two hours.
- Inspect the patient's skin for evidence of trauma, such as bruises or skin breakdown.

> **Case Scenario**
>
> A 60-year-old female, working as a manager in a company, visited the OPD complaining of gradual cognitive decline, over the last three years. Because of her frequent forgetfulness, mistakes in calculations, and aggravation in recent memory impairments, she had to leave her job. She is having complaints of apraxia, apathy, disorientation to time and person, disturbed sleep waking up middle of the night, and self-talking. What are the confirmatory tests to be done in this case to diagnose AD and how will you manage such kind of patient?

DEMENTIA

Dementia affects the ability of thinking, memory, reasoning, personality, mood, and behavior. The decline in mental functions interferes with the activities of the daily life of an individual. About 50% of people aged 85 and older have dementia. As per Chertkow et al., "Dementia is typically defined as a clinical syndrome of cognitive decline that is sufficiently severe to interfere with social or occupational functioning."

CAUSES

Some of the causes of dementia or dementia-like symptoms can be reversed with treatment. They may include:

- **Infections and immune disorders:** Fever and other side effects of the body trying to fight off an illness can cause symptoms that resemble dementia.
- Dementia may also result from multiple sclerosis and other disorders where the immune system of the body attacks nerve cells.
- **Metabolic problems and endocrine abnormalities:** People with thyroid problems, low blood sugar, and too little or too much sodium or calcium, or problems absorbing vitamin B12 can develop dementia-like symptoms or other personality changes.
- **Nutritional deficiencies:** Not getting enough thiamine (vitamin B1), which is common in people with chronic alcoholism; and not getting enough vitamins B6 and B12 in the diet can cause dementia-like symptoms. Copper and vitamin E deficiencies also can cause symptoms of dementia.
- **Medication side effects:** Side effects of medications, a reaction to a medication, or an interaction of several medications can cause dementia-like symptoms.
- **Subdural hematomas:** Bleeding between the surface of the brain and the covering over the brain, which is common in the elderly after a fall, can cause symptoms like those of dementia.

TYPES OF DEMENTIAS

- **Alzheimer's disease:** This is the most common cause of dementia. Although not all causes of Alzheimer's disease are known, a small percentage are related to mutations of three genes, which can be passed down from parent to child. While several genes are probably involved in Alzheimer's disease, one important gene that increases risk is apolipoprotein E4 (APOE). Alzheimer's disease patients have plaques and tangles in their brains. Plaques are clumps of a protein called beta-amyloid, and tangles are fibrous tangles made up of tau protein. It is thought that these clumps damage healthy neurons and the fibers connecting them.
- **Vascular dementia:** This type of dementia is caused by damage to the vessels that supply blood to the brain. Blood vessel problems can cause strokes or affect the brain in other ways, such as by damaging the fibers in the white matter of the brain. The most common signs of vascular dementia include difficulties with problem-solving, slowed thinking, and loss of focus and organization. These tend to be more noticeable than memory loss.
- **Lewy body dementia:** Lewy bodies are abnormal balloon-like clumps of protein that have been found in the brains of people with Lewy body dementia, Alzheimer's disease, and Parkinson's disease. This is one of the more common types of progressive dementia. The patient experiences visual hallucinations, problems with focus and attention, uncoordinated or slow movement, tremors, and rigidity (parkinsonism).
- **Frontotemporal dementia:** In this, there is a breakdown of nerve cells and their connections in the frontal and temporal lobes of the brain. As these areas are associated with personality, behavior, and language, so behavior of an individual, personality, thinking, judgment, language, and movement, etc., are likely to get impaired in this type of dementia.
- **Mixed dementia:** Many types of dementia had a combination of several causes, such as Alzheimer's disease, vascular dementia, and Lewy body dementia.

CLINICAL MANIFESTATIONS

Generally, each individual patient exhibits the symptoms of dementia differently. It may depend upon various causes even as discussed earlier. As per the severity of the illness, the manifestations of dementia can be enumerated in three stages.

Early Stage

Usually, the symptoms of this stage are overlooked. These are gradual in onset. These are considered as part of ageing. Common symptoms may include:
- Forgetfulness
- Losing track of the time
- Becoming lost in familiar places.

Middle Stage

In this because of the progression of the disease, the symptoms become somewhat obvious. These may include:

- Becoming forgetful of recent events and people's names
- Becoming confused while at home
- Having increasing difficulty with communication
- Needing help with personal care
- Experiencing behavior changes, including wandering and repeated questioning.

Late Stage

Here the person is totally dependent on others. Memory disturbances are serious. The physical signs and symptoms become more obvious. These may include:
- Becoming unaware of the time and place
- Having difficulty recognizing relatives and friends
- Having an increasing need for self-care
- Having difficulty walking
- Experiencing behavior changes that may escalate and include aggression.

DIAGNOSTIC EVALUATION

- **History:** A thorough personal, medical, and family history needs to be taken. The specific questions include whether there is any family history of the disease, how and when symptoms began, changes in behavior and personality, and if the person is taking certain medications that might cause or worsen symptoms.
- **Psychiatric evaluation:** It is required to determine if depression or another mental health condition is causing or contributing to a person's symptoms.
- **Cognitive and neurological tests:** These tests include assessments of memory, problem-solving, language skills, and math skills, as well as balance, sensory response, and reflexes. These are done to evaluate thinking and physical functioning,
- **Brain scans:** These are done to identify changes in the brain's structure and function. The most common scans are CT, MRI, and PET.
- **Genetic tests:** These are done to know if there is any alteration in the genes.
- **Cerebrospinal fluid (CSF) tests:** CSF analysis is done to measure the levels of proteins or other substances in CSF that may be used to help diagnose Alzheimer's or other types of dementia.
- **Blood tests:** These are done to measure levels of beta-amyloid, a protein that accumulates abnormally in people with Alzheimer's.

MANAGEMENT

Most types of dementia cannot be cured, but symptomatic management can be done, which can help in improving the quality of life of the patients.

Medications

- **Cholinesterase inhibitors:** These medications-including donepezil (Aricept), rivastigmine (Exelon), and galantamine (Razadyne). These work by boosting levels of a chemical messenger involved in memory and judgment. Although primarily used to treat Alzheimer's disease, these medications might also be prescribed for other

dementias, including vascular dementia, Parkinson's disease dementia, and Lewy body dementia.
- Side effects can include nausea, vomiting, and diarrhea. Other possible side effects include slowed heart rate, fainting, and sleep disturbances.
- **Memantine:** Memantine (Namenda) works by regulating the activity of glutamate, a chemical messenger involved in brain functions, such as learning and memory. In some cases, memantine is prescribed with a cholinesterase inhibitor. A common side effect of memantine is dizziness.
- **Other medications:** Depending upon the other problems, the patients might be prescribed medications such as depression, sleep disturbances, hallucinations, parkinsonism, or agitation.

Therapies
- **Modifying the environment:** Reducing clutter and noise can make it easier for someone with dementia to focus and function. There could be a need to hide objects that can threaten safety, such as knives and car keys.
- **Simplifying tasks:** Break tasks into easier steps and focus on success, not failure. Structure and routine also help reduce confusion in people with dementia.

The nursing interventions are almost the same as has been discussed earlier in the management of Alzheimer's disease. Nurses can play a significant role in the prevention of dementia as well as in educating the public to maintain their physical and mental health. These are discussed as follows:

PREVENTION OF DEMENTIA

It is not sure, whether dementia can be prevented or not. However, there are steps that might be helpful to some extent. These steps otherwise also may help in the maintenance of the health of everyone.
- **Keep the mind active:** Certain mentally stimulating activities, such as reading, solving puzzles, playing word games, and memory training might delay the onset of dementia and decrease its effects.
- **Be physically active:** Spend At least one hour per day should be spent on some physical activity in any form like brisk walking, yoga, or any game.
- **Be socially active:** Social interaction with friends, family might delay the onset of dementia and reduce its symptoms.
- **Quit smoking:** Smoking might increase the risk of dementia. Quitting smoking will prevent the occurrence of other diseases and will improve overall health.
- **Consume adequate vitamins:** We should remember that all the vitamins are in our kitchens. So, avoid junk food and consume all the cereals, pulses, green leafy vegetables, etc. A diet such as the Mediterranean diet-rich in fruits, vegetables, whole grains, and omega-3 fatty acids, which are commonly found in certain fish and nuts, might promote health and lower the risk of developing dementia. This type of diet also improves cardiovascular health, which may help lower dementia risk.
- **Prevent cardiovascular risk factors:** Lose weight if overweight. Maintain physical and mental health. Eat a nutritious diet. Treat high blood pressure, high cholesterol, and diabetes. High blood pressure might lead to a higher risk of some types of dementia.
- Consult the doctors for treatment for depression or anxiety.
- **Maintain sleep hygiene:** Practice good sleep hygiene. Sleep for at least 6 to 8 hours. Snoring or other sleep-related problems should be discussed with the treating doctors.
- **Treat hearing problems:** People with hearing loss have a greater chance of developing cognitive decline. Early treatment of hearing loss, such as the use of hearing aids, might help decrease the risk.
- **Maintain mental health:** Focus on positive aspects of life. Be away from harmful substances. Practice all the above-said measures. These will help in maintaining mental health.

> **Case Scenario**
>
> A 63-year-old female with a 2-year history of repetitiveness memory loss, and loss of executive function with progressive decline in instrumental activities of daily living. She stopped driving a motor vehicle about 6 months back because of her memory problem. Past medical history revealed hypercholesterolemia and vitamin D deficiency. No surgical history was there. Mini-Mental State Examination (MMSE) scored 14/30 as well as poor visuospatial and executive skills. Neurological examination shows normal muscle tone and power, mild motor apraxia on performing commands for motor tasks with no suggestion of cerebellar dysfunction, and normal gait. A magnetic resonance imaging scan at age 58 revealed mild generalized cortical atrophy. After treatment with a cholinesterase inhibitor, her MMSE improved to 18/30 after 15 months. In the subsequent 4 years, she continued to decline in cognition and function, and then more dependence for her basic activities of daily living. Apart from this, she also developed muscle rigidity, motor apraxia, worsening perceptual, and language skills, and became totally dependent for all activities of daily living. Then she had respiratory distress for which was got hospitalized. CT brain imaging revealed marked generalized global cortical atrophy and marked hippocampal atrophy. She died at age 68 years of pneumonia after around 20 days of hospitalization. An autopsy was performed which showed numerous plaques and tangles with congophilic amyloid angiopathy.

DELIRIUM

Delirium is a serious change in intellectual abilities. It results in confused thinking and one loses awareness of his surroundings. The illness typically develops quickly in a matter of hours or days. Delirium can frequently be linked to one or more causes. A severe or persistent illness or an internal imbalance like low sodium are examples of some factors. Infection, surgery, certain medications, alcohol or drug use, or withdrawal are other potential causes of the illness. As per Kannayiram Alagiakrishnan, "delirium is defined as a transient, usually reversible, cause of mental dysfunction and manifests clinically with a wide range of neuropsychiatric abnormalities."

EPIDEMIOLOGY OF DELIRIUM

- In a systematic evaluation of 42 cohorts across 40 trials, delirium was diagnosed in 10–31% of newly admitted patients, while the incidence of delirium developing during hospitalization ranged from 3–29%.

- The prevalence of delirium among patients in intensive care units may exceed 80%.
- Though delirium can occur at any age, however, it is more prevalent in elderly patients and those who have altered mental status.
- Mortality rates in the patients who experience delirium during hospitalization range from 22–76%.

CAUSES

Delirium sometimes can be idiopathic. It always results from improper transmission and reception of brain impulses. Some potential factors include:
- Abuse or withdrawal from drugs or alcohol.
- Electrolyte imbalance such as hyponatremia or hypocalcemia.
- Stroke, heart attack, worsening lung or liver illness, a fall, any infection especially in elderly people.
- Serious, persistent illness that may result in mortality.
- Fever and a fresh infection, especially in youngsters.
- Exposure to a toxin, such as carbon monoxide, cyanide, or other poisons.
- Inadequate nourishment or excessive fluid loss.
- Insomnia or intense emotional distress.
- Pain.
- Surgery or any other medical treatment that requires being put the patient in a sleep-like state.
- Delirium may be brought on by certain specific medications when used alone or in combination. These medications as such may be used for certain conditions like pain, sleep issues, mood disorders like anxiety and depression, allergies, asthma, swelling, Parkinson's disease, and spasms or convulsions.

RISK FACTORS

The risk of delirium is increased by any illness that necessitates a hospital stay. Most of the time, this is true when a person is in critical care or recovering from surgery. Those who are older and those who reside in nursing homes are more likely to have delirium.

Some conditions that could increase the risk of delirium include:
- Previous delirium episodes
- Vision or hearing loss
- Multimorbidity
- Dementia, stroke, or Parkinson's disease

TYPES OF DELIRIUM

There are mainly three types of delirium:
1. **Hyperactive delirium:** It is simple to recognize. These individuals experience anxiety, quick mood swings, or delusions.
2. **Hypoactive delirium:** Individuals of this kind may be inactive. They frequently exhibit lethargy or sleepiness. They might come out as confused. They do not communicate with friends or family.
3. **Mixed delirium:** These patients exhibit the symptoms of both hypo and hyperactive delirium. Between being restless and being lethargic, the person may swiftly change states.

PATHOPHYSIOLOGY OF DELIRIUM

The pathophysiology of delirium has yet to be fully understood. Delirium can be considered a standard pathway resulting from multiple factors impairing brain function. In delirium, Inflammation, hypoxia, and oxidative stress increase brain exposure to toxins and create a hypo-cholinergic-hyperdopaminergic state. Inflammation increases blood-brain barrier permeability, making the brain susceptible to circulating deliriogenic medications, endogenous toxins, and proinflammatory cytokines that may cause delirium. Microaggregates of fibrin and neutrophils in the brain can cause episodes of decreased cerebral perfusion. These Transient hypoxic states lead to reduced synthesis of acetylcholine. Oxidative stress releases endogenous dopamine, which is responsible for the disturbances seen in delirium. In delirium, Melatonin deficiency is thought to result in sleep-wake cycle disruption and excess of norepinephrine and glutamate.

SYMPTOMS

The patients exhibit the symptoms of delirium usually over the course of a few hours or days. It depends upon the severity of the disease also. During daytime symptoms may or may not be there. However, the symptoms get worst at night because of darkness and things might appear unfamiliar. The primary symptom is reduced awareness of surroundings. This may result in:
- Being quickly distracted
- Having trouble concentrating
- Having trouble switching topics
- Becoming focused on an idea rather than responding to questions
- Having poor thinking skills.

This may appear as:
- Impaired memory, such as forgetting recent events
- Confusion of place or person
- Difficulties speaking or remembering words
- Rambling or incoherent speech
- Difficulty in understanding speech
- Difficulties with reading or writing

Behavior and emotional changes: These may include:
- Restless, anxious, aggression, anger
- Calling out, grumbling, or making other sounds
- Quiet and withdrawn, especially in older adults
- Slowing down or being sluggish
- Depression
- A short-tempered
- A sense of being elated
- Lack of interest and emotion
- Quick changes in mood
- Hallucination.
- Changes in sleeping patterns
- A change in the night-to-day sleep-wake cycle

DIAGNOSIS

The diagnosis of delirium is based on detailed personal and medical history; and mental status examination of the patients. Certain other factors such as side effects of medicines, etc., also need to be considered.

- **Medical history:** This involves asking questions about what has changed in the last few days. For example, Is there a new infection? Did the person put on some new medicine? Was there an injury or new pain? Did the person have taken alcohol or a legal or illegal drug?
- **Mental status examination:** It involves testing awareness, attention, and thinking. This may be done by talking with the person or it may be done with certain tests or screenings such as Mini Mental Status Examination. Information from family members or caregivers can be helpful.
- **Physical and neurological examination:** A physical examination is done to assess the signs and symptoms of any health problems or diseases. A neurological examination is carried out to check vision, balance, coordination, reflexes, etc. This can help determine if a stroke or another disease is causing delirium.
- **Other tests:** Blood, urine, and other tests are carried out to note any variation in the values. Brain-imaging tests may be done when a diagnosis cannot be made with other information.

MANAGEMENT

Identifying the causes or any triggering factor is the first step in treating delirium. This can include stopping a particular medication, managing an infection, or correcting any metabolic imbalance. The optimal environment for promoting physical and mental health is then created as the main goal of treatment.

Supportive Care

It aims to prevent any further complications in the patients.
- Avoid the use of physical restraints
- Protect the airway
- Provide fluids and nutrition
- Manage any kind of discomfort
- Address bowel and bladder problems
- Include family members or other familiar persons in the care.
- Periodically orient the patients to the environment.

Medications

Control the pain if it is causing delirium. Butyrophenone especially haloperidol is one of the high-potency antipsychotic drugs. It is the safest and one of the most effective antipsychotics for treating delirium. It also causes less sedation than phenothiazines and reduces the risk of exacerbating delirium. Rest, management of delirium depends upon its identified causes.

NURSING MANAGEMENT

Nursing Assessment

It should include:

Assessment of mental status: It must contain a description of the mental status of the patients. It also includes a thorough explanation of behavior, the flow of thought and speech defect, thought processes, sensorium and intellectual status, cognitive status, insight, and judgment.

Periodical Assessment

It is required to determine the fluctuation in the symptoms and also any other acute changes in mental status.

Nursing Diagnosis

1. Disturbed thought processes related to delusional thinking.
2. Chronic confusion related to cognitive impairment.
3. Impaired verbal communication related to cognitive impairment.
4. Risk for injury related to suicidal ideations, illusions, and hallucinations.
5. Impaired memory related to cognitive impairment.
6. Risk for other-directed violence related to suspiciousness of others.

Nursing Interventions

- **Assess the level of anxiety:** Evaluate the client's level of anxiety and any signs of rising anxiety. If the nurse can identify these signs, she or he may be able to intervene before violence breaks out.
- **Provide an appropriate environment:** Keep the environment of the room low-stimulus (low lighting, few people, minimal decor, low noise level). The patient may exhibit more anxiety in a high-stimulus environment.
- **Promote patient safety:** Remove all potentially dangerous objects from the patient's room. Because, in a disoriented, confused state, the patients may use objects to harm themselves or others.
- **Ask for assistance from others when needed:** The patient may get violent sometime. So, more staff may be required to execute a physical confrontation with the patients. Apart from taking care of the patients, the safety of the staff is equally important.
- **Stay calm and reassure the patient:** Maintain calm and quiet behavior with the patients. Do not attempt to frighten the patient unnecessarily, and provide continual reassurance and support.
- **Medicate or restrain the patient as prescribed:** When anxiety levels are particularly high, safeguard the client and others by using sedating drugs and gentle restraints as directed by a physician.
- **Observe the suicidal behavior of the patients:** Sit with the patient and observe the behavior regarding suicidal ideation. The safety of the patient is one of the top nursing priorities. Close observation may be necessary to prevent such kind of harm of the patients.

- **Teach relaxation exercises to the patients:** When the patient is in a normal state of mind, teach him certain relaxation exercises and motivate the patient to practice these exercises during the anxiety spells.

Also, teach the caregivers to recognize the behavior of their patients indicating anxiety and ways to intervene before violence occurs.

> **Case Scenario**
>
> An 80-year-old man was transferred to a medical ward after 20 days of admission in the ICU for Acute MI. The patient also developed a hospital-acquired infection in ICU itself due to which his ICU stay was prolonged. He is also a known case of DM type 2 and hypertension. Inside the ICU itself, he was also diagnosed with hypoactive delirium. Identify the causes of delirium in the patients. What investigations should be carried out to diagnose the problem? Discuss the nursing interventions to prevent such kind of episodes in the medical ward and also in his later life.

PARKINSON'S DISEASE

Parkinson's disease is a neurodegenerative disease that often manifests in later life and results in generalized slowness of movement (bradykinesia) and at least one additional symptom of resting tremor or rigidity. Other symptoms include loss of smell, mood swings, trouble sleeping, excessive salivation, constipation, and irregular, frequent limb movements while asleep. Lewy bodies and the degeneration of dopaminergic neurons in the substantia nigra are associated with the illness. In most cases, the cause is idiopathic. As per WHO "Parkinson's disease (PD) is a degenerative condition of the brain associated with motor symptoms (slow movement, tremor, rigidity, and imbalance) and other complications including cognitive impairment, mental health disorders, sleep disorders, and pain and sensory disturbances."

EPIDEMIOLOGY

- PD affects 1% of people over the age of 60. PD is more prevalent among ageing people, affecting 1–2 people per 1000 at any time.
- 5–10% of patients have a hereditary predisposition of the disease.
- Parkinson's disease affects more men than women, and incidence and prevalence rise with age.
- Only about 10% of cases have a genetic basis.

CAUSES

- PD has been linked to the use of herbicides, pesticides, and proximity to the industrial site.
- **Environmental factors:** Methyl-phenyl-tetrahydro-pyridine.
- Viral infections, such as encephalitis.
- In addition, some studies point out that the formation of free radicals and oxidation may potentiate the damage of thalamic nuclei.
- Family history plays a significant role in having PD. So, the gene plays a significant role in PD.
- The autopsy reveals that Lewy bodies are mainly composed of unusually high quantities of aggregated alpha-synuclein. It is assumed that altered alpha-synuclein function contributes to the etiology of PD.

PATHOPHYSIOLOGY

To classify, PD may be primary or idiopathic, secondary or acquired, hereditary parkinsonism or multiple system degeneration, or Parkinson's plus syndromes (They include dementia with Lewy bodies, corticobasal degeneration, multiple system atrophy, and progressive supranuclear palsy).

Parkinson's disease is characterized by the neuronal presence of alpha-synuclein in neuronal cell bodies called Lewy bodies and within neuronal cell processes called Lewy neurites. These changes cause the dopamine and acetylcholine imbalance in the substantia nigra of the brain. Dopaminergic neuronal cells in the substantia nigra are destroyed, resulting in a reduction of dopamine stores. Dopaminergic nigrostriatal pathway deterioration causes an Imbalance of Dopamine and acetylcholine neurotransmitters in the corpus striatum. This ultimately leads to the impairment of extrapyramidal pathways (controlling complex body movements) and leads to typical symptoms such as: (1) tremors, (2) rigidity, (3) bradykinesia, (4) postural changes **(Fig. 38.2)**.

STAGING OF PARKINSON'S DISEASE (HOEHN AND YAHR)

As per the symptoms, PD can be classified into five stages:
- **Stage 1:** Moderate symptoms on only one side (unilaterally), not debilitating, but friends notice.
- **Stage 2:** Bilateral symptoms like slight impairment, altered posture, and gait are all present.
- **Stage 3:** Substantial slowness and a relatively severe malfunction.
- **Stage 4:** Bradykinesia, rigidity, severe symptoms, and inability to live alone.
- **Stage 5:** Cachectic, unable to stand or move, completely invalidism, and in need of nursing care.

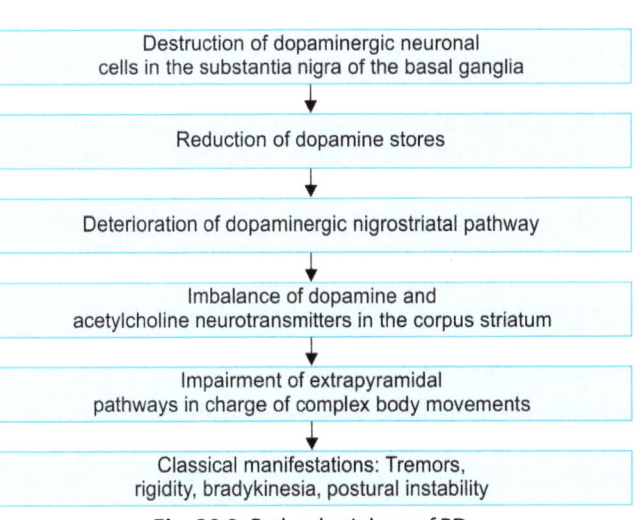

Fig. 38.2: Pathophysiology of PD.

DIAGNOSIS

Diagnosis is based on clinical features.
- **MRI:** It helps to rule out the secondary cause of the brain.
- **PET:** It is done to assess levodopa uptake and conversion to dopamine in the corpus striatum.
- **CT scans:** Do not show changes in the brain related to PD and is generally not helpful in diagnosis.

COMPLICATIONS

Various complications these patients are likely to develop include:
- Dementia
- Depression
- Psychosis
- Hallucinations
- Dysphagia
- Malnutrition
- Aspiration pneumonia
- Orthostatic hypotension

MANAGEMENT OF PARKINSON'S DISEASE

Anti-parkinsonism Medications

- **Levodopa:** It is the most efficient medication and the foundation of treatment for symptom control.
- **Sinemet:** It is made up of a combination of Levodopa and carbidopa. Levodopa enters the brain and is converted to dopamine; carbidopa boosts its potency and lessens levodopa's side effects, including nausea and vomiting.
- **Dopamine receptor agonists:** The drugs that activate or stimulate the dopamine receptors are known as dopamine receptor agonists, e.g., pramipexole, and ropinirole.
- **Ergot derivatives:** Bromocriptine or pergolide.
- **Non-ergot derivatives:** Ropinirole, pramipexole.
- **Monoamine oxidized inhibitors:** The medications Selegiline and Rasagiline, which stop the breakdown of dopamine and are generally used to treat motor fluctuation associated with levodopa treatment, are the most commonly used drugs.

Surgery

Surgery is the option only when there is no effectiveness of medicines.
- **Thalamotomy:** This surgical procedure creates an opening in the thalamus to improve overall brain function.
- **Deep brain stimulation:** A pulse generator sends high-frequency electrical impulses to the thalamus to regulate tremors by blocking the neural pathway. Parkinson's disease-related tremors and uncontrollable movements can be treated using deep brain stimulation. The neurostimulator (pacemaker device) is connected to the brain via surgically implanted electrodes.

Physiotherapy

In managing the patient, a combination of physiotherapeutic and pharmacological interventions is crucial. The patient's drugs and any potential side effects should be completely disclosed to the physical therapist. Peak dosage is when performance is supposed to be at its best, whereas the conclusion of the dose cycle is when performance starts to decline. Following interventions need to be carried out for the patients:
- Exercise training
- Strength training
- Balance training
- Correcting eating disorders.
- Practice verbal skills with breath control.

NURSING MANAGEMENT

Nursing Assessment

- Obtain a history of symptoms, including how they have affected their ability to work, move about, communicate, feed, and self-care.
- Evaluate cerebellar, cranial nerves, and motor function.
- Watch gait and performance of activities.
- Evaluate speech for clarity and space.
- Look for signs of depression.
- Evaluate family and social support.

Nursing Diagnoses

- Ineffective airway clearance related to tracheobronchial obstruction due to musculoskeletal changes.
- Improper nutrition less than body requirement related to bradykinesia, stiffness, and difficulty in swallowing, chewing, and eating.
- Impaired verbal communication related to low speech volume.
- Constipation related to inactivity and reduced motor function.
- Ineffective coping related to loss of independence and physical limitation.
- Risk for a fall-related injury because of impairment in motor functions.
- Impaired sleep pattern related to the disease condition.

Nursing Interventions

- Assess the neurological condition of the patient.
- Examine the ability to chew and swallow.
- Offer a soft diet high in calories, protein, and fiber with small, frequent feedings.
- Increase daily fluid intake to 2,000 mL.
- Encourage independence along with safety measures.
- Watch for constipation.
- Avoid rushing the patient with activities.
- Help with ambulation and provide assistive devices.
- Instruct the patient to wear low-heeled footwear.
- Instruct the patient to lift the feet when walking and avoid extended sitting.
- Offer a firm mattress, and position the patient prone, without a pillow, to encourage appropriate posture.
- Teach the patient how to hold the hands behind the back to keep the spine and neck erect and in proper posture.
- Advocate physical therapy and rehabilitation.
- Administer prescribed anticholinergic medications to treat rigidity and tremors and to inhibit the acetylcholine's effect.

- Administer antiparkinsonian medications to raise the level of dopamine in the central nervous system.
- Ask the patient to comply with the medication and other instructions to prevent complications.
- Advise the patient to avoid foods high in vitamin B6 because these foods interfere with the effects of antiparkinsonian medications.
- Tell the patient to avoid monoamine oxidase inhibitors because they trigger a hypertensive crisis.
- Educate the patients and their caregivers regarding the disease process.

GERIATRIC CONSIDERATIONS

The presenting signs and symptoms of PD may mimic advancing age. Sometimes it is difficult to tease apart these features. Many elderly individuals, experience the symptoms like slowness in performing their routine activities, stiffness of the body parts, curved posture, and also disturbance in gait. All these symptoms are there of PD also. So, it is important that the specific signs of PD are noted in elderly patients. Further investigations should be done to rule out the conditions at an early stage in order to prevent long-term complications in these patients.

Case Scenario

1. Mrs Goyal is a 64-year-old female. She is a retired housewife and now lives with her dog at home. Five years ago, Mrs. Goyal's husband passed away. She tripped over her dog and had a minor fall, landing on her right hand and inflicting wrist pain (about three months ago). She visited her doctor regarding her wrist but complained of recent balance issues and a slight hand tremor. She went to a neurologist and was identified as having a case of early-stage idiopathic Parkinson's Disease. She was referred to physiotherapy to perform a fall risk assessment, maintain her functional status, and address her worries regarding the condition. *Plan nursing interventions for the patient.*
2. A 59-year-old man presented with gait, increased stiffness and reduced range of motion (ROM), resting tremor, cogwheel rigidity, and coordination problems. The development of patient-centered goals included improving range of motion and coordination, enabling the patient to continue with his routine activities, and enhancing his ability to move more easily throughout his house. To achieve these aims, a 4-week training program was initiated that included both supervised training, a home exercise program, and an educational component. The patient shows improved balance and gait after completing this exercise program. He had improved confidence and was much less worried than during his initial assessment.

SUMMARY

Parkinson's disease (PD) is a chronic, degenerative disorder of the CNS that predominantly affects the motor system. In most cases, symptoms appear gradually, and as the disease progresses, non-motor symptoms increase in frequency. Tremor, rigidity, slow movement, and difficulty walking are the most prominent early signs. In addition to behavioral and cognitive problems, depression, anxiety, and apathy are common symptoms of PD. Although the exact cause of Parkinson's disease is unknown, it is believed that environmental and hereditary factors may contribute to it. Symptoms are generally employed to make a diagnosis in typical circumstances. Since Parkinson's disease has no known cure, the goal is to minimize the severity and impact of the symptoms.

AMYOTROPHIC LATERAL SCLEROSIS

INTRODUCTION

Amyotrophic lateral sclerosis (ALS) is also known as Lou Gehrig's illness. It is named for the famous New York Yankees baseball player who was the first diagnosed case. It is a progressive, degenerative disorder that involves both the upper and lower motor neurons. It damages the nerve cells in the brain and spinal cord, affecting the ability to control one's muscle movements. The initial symptoms of ALS are muscle twitching, slurred speech, and limb paralysis. Impaired muscles eventually cause speaking, moving, eating, or breathing difficulties. There is no cure for the disease condition.

Motor neurons die and deteriorate, stopping communication with the muscles, eventually leading to weakness, twitching (fasciculations), and atrophying (wasting away) of the muscles. The brain's capability to regulate voluntary motions eventually declines. As per Ryan G Brotman, Lou Gehrig's disease, ALS, is a neurological condition that affects the nerve cells, and motor neurons in the spinal cord and brain that regulate voluntary muscular contractions.

CAUSES

ALS affects motor neurons, which regulate voluntary muscle movements, including walking and speaking. As a result of ALS, the motor neurons slowly deteriorate and ultimately die. Motor neurons connect the brain, spinal cord, and muscles.

Damaged motor neuron leads to decrease communication with the muscles and inhibits muscles from contracting. In 5–10% of people, ALS is hereditary. The cause of the other cases is unknown.

RISK FACTORS

The following factors increase the risk of developing ALS:
- **Heredity:** Five to ten percent of those with ALS (familial ALS) inherit it from their parents.
- **Age:** It is most common in people between 40 and 60. The risk of ALS increases with age.
- **Sex:** Before age 65, males are slightly more likely to have ALS than women. After 70 years, both genders are at equal risk of ALS.
- **Genetics:** Studies have discovered several genetic similarities between people with non-inherited ALS and those with familial ALS. These genetic variants may increase a person's susceptibility to ALS.
- **Environmental factors:** The following environmental factors might trigger the disease:
  - *Smoking:* It is one of the main risk factors for ALS. Women appear to be at the most significant risk, especially after menopause.
  - *Environmental toxin exposure:* Certain evidence suggests that exposure to lead or other toxins at work or home might be linked to ALS. Numerous studies

have been conducted. However, no one substance or chemical has consistently been associated with ALS.
- *Military service:* Studies indicate that those in the armed forces are more likely to develop ALS. It is unclear what aspect of military service might manifest ALS. It might include exposure to certain metals or chemicals, traumatic injuries, viral infection, and intense exertion, etc.

PATHOPHYSIOLOGY

ALS is one of the most common progressive and devastating neurodegenerative diseases. The word "Amyotrophy" which is the atrophy of muscle fibers depicts the pathophysiology of the disease **(Fig. 38.3)**. The disease is characterized by Upper Motor Neurons (corticospinal motor neurons) and Lower Motor Neurons (bulbospinal motor neurons) degeneration and death, as well as reactive gliosis replacing dead neurons. Though the pathophysiology of the disease is quite complex and is multifactorial, certain mechanisms, which contribute to the neurodegeneration are abnormal mitochondria functioning, increased oxidative stress, increased free radicals, impaired axonal transport, sodium-potassium pump dysfunction, increased inflammatory mediators and increased secretion of toxins. A progressive UMN and LMN neurodegenerative disorder causing muscle weakness, disability, and eventual death.

CLINICAL MANIFESTATIONS

Early symptoms include:
- Twitching of the arm, shoulder, leg, or tongue muscle.
- Muscle jerks
- Muscle spasticity
- Weakness of arms, neck, leg, or diaphragm muscles
- Slurred speech
- Difficulty in swallowing
- Difficulty in chewing
- Muscle atrophy and weakness expand to other body areas as the condition gets worsen.

The person may develop other problems:
- Patients with ALS will gradually lose the capacity to independently get in or leave the bed and use their hands and arms.
- The inability to chew and swallow food (dysphagia)

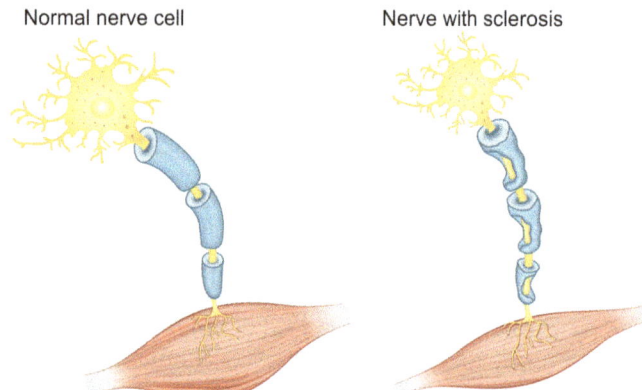

Fig. 38.3: Amyotrophic lateral sclerosis.

- Impairment of speech or word formation (dysarthria)
- Patients with ALS finally lose their ability to breathe on their own and have to rely on a ventilator.
- Maintaining steady weight.
- Malnourishment.
- Neuropathy and cramps in the muscles.
- With ALS, typically, people with anxiety and depression still retain the ability to reason, understand, recall, and are aware of their loss of function progressively.
- Experience problems with communication or decision-making.
- Over time, they acquire a type of dementia.

DIAGNOSTIC EVALUATION

- There is no single conclusive test for diagnosing ALS. It is required to evaluate with a thorough medical history and get a physical assessment. A neurologic examination is conducted to test reflexes, muscle strength, and other responses. Neurological examinations are routinely performed to check whether symptoms such as muscle weakness, muscle atrophy, and spasticity are worsening.
- Other diagnostic tests include:
  - *Electromyography (EMG):* This is a technique of recording the electrical activity of muscle fibers and is useful in diagnosing ALS. Fasciculations, Fibrillations, and positive sharp waves are also expected in EMG studies.
  - *Nerve conduction study (NCS):* It measures the electrical activity of the nerves and muscles by assessing the nerve's ability to transmit a signal along the nerve or to the muscle. In ALS, there may be normal or decreased compound muscle action potential (CMAP), prolongation of distal motor latency, and slowing of conduction velocity.
  - *Magnetic resonance imaging (MRI):* It creates fine-grained brain and spinal cord images using radio waves and magnetic fields and helps in the diagnosis of ALS.
  - *Muscle biopsy:* Under local anesthesia, a small muscle sample is taken and sent to the lab for analysis in case of suspicion of muscle involvement.

MANAGEMENT

Medications

- Riluzole (Rilutek, Exservan, Tiglutik kit). This medication can extend life by 3–6 months when taken orally. It may have side effects such as alterations in liver function, nausea, and dizziness.
- Edaravone (Radicava).
- Sodium phenylbutyrate taurursodiol (Relyvrio).

Other Therapeutic Modalities

- **Respiratory care:** As the respiratory muscles get weaken, the person eventually has more breathing difficulty. The doctor may do routine breathing tests and prescribe devices to help with nighttime breathing.
- **Physical therapy:** A physical therapist can address pain, walking, mobility, bracing, and equipment requirements

that support independence. Maintaining cardiovascular fitness, muscular strength, and range of motion for as long as possible can be accomplished by practicing low-impact exercises and workouts.
- **Regular exercise:** It will improve the sense of well-being. Stretching adequately can help prevent pain and can improve muscle performance.
- **Occupational therapy:** Despite hand and arm weakness, an occupational therapist can help determine ways to maintain independence. Adaptive equipment can make performing activities such as dressing, grooming, eating, and bathing easier.
- **Speech therapy:** A speech therapist can teach adaptive methods to improve speech comprehension. Speech therapists can help in exploring other ways of communication, such as an alphabet board or pen and paper.
- **Nutritional support:** Sometimes, a patient could require a feeding tube. The healthcare team with family and patient should ensure that the patient is eating foods that are easier to swallow and meeting nutritional needs.
- **Psychological and social support:** A team including a social worker, psychologists, social workers, and others can assist with money matters, insurance, obtaining the necessary equipment, and paying for devices and may offer emotional assistance.

Nursing Diagnoses

- Impaired mobility related to, weakness, spasticity, and muscle wasting.
- Impaired communication related to the impairment of the speaking muscles.
- High risk for aspiration related to the impairment of the swallowing muscles.
- Ineffective breathing pattern related to impaired muscles of breathing.
- Risk for injury related to falls and possible skin breakdown (pressure ulcers, abrasions), resulting from constant movement.
- Imbalanced nutrition, less than body requirements related to inadequate intake and dehydration due to swallowing or chewing disorders.
- Anxiety and impaired communication related to excessive grimacing and incomprehensible speech.
- Disturbed thought processes related to the disease condition
- Impaired social interaction related to the disease condition.

Nursing Interventions

- Offer and motivate the patients with intellectually stimulating activities because the patient typically experiences no cognitive deficits and retains mental abilities.
- Promote measures to improve body image.
- Encourage the patient and family to cope as they are dealing with the disease of poor prognosis and the grieving process.
- Provide referrals.
- Maximize functional abilities.
- Prevent complications of immobility.
- Encourage self-care.
- Maximize effective communication.
- Ensure adequate nutrition.
- Prevent respiratory complications.
- Promote measures to maintain an adequate airway.
- Promote measures to enhance gas exchange, such as oxygen therapy and ventilator assistance.
- Promote measures to prevent respiratory infection.
- Keep the skin meticulously clean.
- Prevent injury and potential skin breakdown.
- Pad the sides and head end of the bed.
- Secure the patient in a bed or chair with padding.
- Encourage ambulation with assistance to maintain muscle tone.

GERIATRIC CONSIDERATIONS

Neurodegenerative disease is more likely to be progressive in aged people, which may result in more significant disability. The risks and benefits should be carefully weighed before prescribing medication to recently diagnosed elderly patients. Clinical trial data are insufficient to predict how these medicines affect elderly patients. Symptomatic therapy may improve gait impairment, mood disruption, bladder and bowel dysfunction, neuropathic pain, and spasticity in elderly patients. Late onset appears to be more common and is likely to be under-recognized in elderly patients. In older patients, ALS should be considered a differential diagnosis. Potential reasons for older people being misdiagnosed with ALS include frequent presentations with symptoms such as dysphagia, frailty, or general weakness for other reasons. Pharmacotherapies, physical and occupational treatments are useful in this disease.

> **Case Scenario**
>
> A 28-year-old male presented to the neurology department with symptoms of a feeling of generalized weakness, cramps in muscles, and 5/10 pain in arms and legs. He was worried due to his recent falls. limiting the office work, and the limitation in performing certain day-to-day activities. During the initial assessment, he reported that he had stopped playing soccer as a result of increased cramping and weakness in his legs, he also has trouble in breathing while running in the field. His parents have noticed changes in his voice, he has noticed changes in his muscle mass. He was diagnosed with ALS and put on Riluzole medication.

HUNTINGTON'S DISEASE

Huntington's disease (HD) is a rare genetic condition in which there is a progressive destruction of brain nerve cells. The functional capacities of the patients are altered, which typically results in impairment of mobility, cognition, and behavior. As per Orlando De Jesus:

Huntington's disease (HD) is a "neurodegenerative autosomal dominant disorder, characterized by involuntary choreatic movements with cognitive and behavioral disturbances."

EPIDEMIOLOGY

- HD occurs in 2.7 per 100,000 inhabitants worldwide, and 10 per 100,000 in Europe, according to a new report of "Rare Disease Clinical Research".
- In some other populations, such as those of Japanese, Chinese, and African heritage, the illness seems to be less prevalent.

CAUSES

- Mutations in the HTT (Huntingtin) gene are the main leading cause of HD. Huntingtin is a protein that is made by the HTT gene. Its purpose is unknown, although brain neurons seem to depend on it in a significant way.
- The CAG trinucleotide repeat in the DNA is involved in the HTT mutation, which causes HD. Cytosine, adenine, and guanine, three DNA-building units that occur repeatedly in a row, make up this region. Within a gene, the CAG section is often repeated 10–35 times. People with Huntington's disease experience 36 to more than 120 repetitions of the CAG section.
- In people with 36–39 years, CAG repeats and those with 40 or more repeats have an equal chance of getting the disease.
- An increase in the size of the CAG segment results in the formation of an unusually lengthy variant of the huntingtin protein. Smaller, poisonous fragments of the elongated protein are broken down into smaller pieces that attach to one another and build up in neurons, interfering with their normal operations. HD is characterized by the impairment and eventual death of neurons in particular regions of the brain.

INHERITANCE

- The meaning of "heritage" has been widened. Since this illness is inherited in an autosomal dominant manner, only one copy of the mutated gene needs to exist in each cell for the disorder to manifest.
- The affected parent frequently passes on the mutated gene to their offspring.
- Rarely, a person with Huntington's disease has neither a parent with the condition.

PATHOPHYSIOLOGY OF HUNTINGTON'S DISEASE

Mutations in the HTT gene cause Huntington's disease. The HTT gene codes for protein huntingtin. It plays a vital role in brain nerve cells (neurons). The mutation in HTT, causes Huntington's disease. An increase in the size of the CAG segment causes the production of an abnormally long version of the huntingtin protein. Large protein is fragmented into smaller, toxic fragments that bind together and accumulate in neurons, interfering with their normal functions. The dysfunction and eventual death of neurons in specific brain areas lead to signs and symptoms of Huntington's disease.

CLINICAL FEATURES

Huntington's disease tends to develop in stages:

Early Stage Symptoms

- Difficulty making decisions
- Memory gaps
- Difficulty learning new things
- Loss of energy and fatigue
- Clumsiness
- Slow or abnormal eye movements
- Muscle problems (dystonia)
- Difficulty sleeping

Symptoms in the Middle Stage

Over time, symptoms start to disrupt the daily life of the patient more and more. The person might start dropping items or fall, for instance. Additionally, the person can have problems in swallowing or speaking. Maintaining an organization can be difficult. Changes in emotions may cause relationships to become disturbed. Common middle-stage symptoms include:

- Speech changes
- The decline in thinking abilities
- Uncontrolled twitching movements (chorea)
- Trouble walking
- Confusion
- Memory loss
- Personality changes
- Thoughts of death, dying, or suicide
- Weight loss
- Swallowing problems
- Breathing problems
- Weight loss
- Development of obsessive-compulsive disorder, bipolar disorder, or mania.

Symptoms in the Late Stages

At this point, the patients are usually dependent on others. The ability to move or communicate is not possible. There is a fair chance that the person will be aware of her nearby loved ones. The severity of Twitchy motions can change.

Juvenile Huntington's Disease Symptoms

Children and teenagers with Huntington's disease may have symptoms like:

- A sudden reduction in academic performance
- Stiff or uncomfortable walking
- Increased clumsiness
- Changes in speech
- Difficulty paying attention
- Behavioral issues
- Tremors

DIAGNOSIS

- **Preliminary:** A general physical examination, a study of the family medical history, and neurological and psychiatric tests are the main methods used to diagnose Huntington's disease.

- **Psychological testing:** The neurologist will interview the patient and do quick tests to evaluate the reflexes, muscle strength, and balance.
- **Sensory problems:** Include testing for hearing, vision, and tingling.
- **Psychiatric signs and symptoms:** Assessing for mental health and mood.
- **Neuropsychological testing:**
  - Spatial reasoning
  - Psychiatric evaluation
  - Memory
  - Reasoning
  - Mental agility
  - Language skills

  A psychiatrist may be asked to examine the person to look for:
  - Emotional state
  - Patterns of behaviors
  - Quality of judgment
  - Coping skills
  - Signs of disordered thinking
  - Evidence of substance abuse
- **Brain imaging and function tests:** In order to assess the anatomy or functionality of the brain, brain imaging tests are utilized. It is possible to use imaging methods that produce in-depth images of the brain, like MRI and CT scans. These images might show alterations in the brain which is affected by HD. Early in the disease's progression, these changes might not manifest.
- **Genetic testing and counselling:** If the symptoms substantially resemble Huntington's disease, a genetic test to screen for the unusual gene may be recommended by the doctor. The diagnosis can be verified by this test.
- The test will not yield information that may be utilized to create a treatment plan, but it may be helpful if there is no known family history of HD or if no other family member's diagnosis has been confirmed through genetic testing.
- The genetic counsellor will discuss the advantages and disadvantages of knowing test results before doing such a test.
- Predictive testing involves administering a genetic test to a person who has no symptoms but a family history of the disease.
- The stress of coping with a deadly illness may also be a problem.
- Federal regulations generally forbid discriminating against people who have genetic illnesses based on the results of genetic testing. Only after speaking with a genetic counsellor are these tests conducted.

MANAGEMENT

- The course of Huntington's disease cannot be altered by treatments. On the other hand, medication can help with some mobility and certain other symptoms.
- Medications will almost definitely change as the condition progresses, depending on the general objectives of treatment. Drugs that alleviate one set of symptoms could also have unintended side effects that make other symptoms worse. So, regular reviews and updates will be made to the treatment goals.

Treatments for Movement Disorders

- The following medicines are used to treat movement disorders—tetrabenazine and deutetrabenazine which have been authorized by the Food and Drug Administration to treat Huntington's disease-related chorea, which are uncontrollable jerking and writhing movements.
- Possible adverse effects include drowsiness, restlessness, and the chance of depression or other psychiatric problems worsening or developing.

  Antipsychotic medications, such as haloperidol and fluphenazine, can cause movement suppression.

  Other drugs, such as olanzapine (Zyprexa) and aripiprazole (Abilify), may have fewer adverse effects, but they still need to be used cautiously because they could exacerbate symptoms. Clonazepam, levetiracetam, and amantadine are a few additional drugs that could aid with chorea suppression.

Drugs to Treat Psychiatric Problems

Depending on the psychological problems and symptoms, different medications will be used to treat them. Following are some of the drugs:

- Drugs like citalopram, escitalopram, fluoxetine, and sertraline are examples of antidepressants.
- Antipsychotic medications like quetiapine and olanzapine can reduce agitation, irrational behavior, and other signs of psychosis or mood disorders. These medications, however, may result in various movement problems.
- Anticonvulsants such as carbamazepine (Tegretol, Carbatrol, Epitol, among others), lamotrigine (Lamictal), and divalproex (Depakote) are examples of mood-stabilizing medications that can help prevent the highs and lows connected with bipolar disorder.

Psychotherapy

A psychotherapist, such as a psychiatrist, psychologist, or clinical social worker, can aid in the treatment of behavioral issues, the development of coping mechanisms, the management as the disease advances, and the facilitation of family member communication.

Speech Therapy

The ability to regulate the mouth and throat muscles, which are crucial for speaking, eating, and swallowing, can be severely hampered by Huntington's disease.

A person can learn how to use communication aids like a board with drawings of common objects and activities from a speech therapist, who can also help the patient talk more clearly. Problems with the muscles needed for eating and swallowing can also be helped by speech therapists.

Physical Therapy

- Strength, flexibility, balance, and coordination can all be improved with the help of exercises. These exercises may help maintain the mobility of the patients for a longer period of time and reduce the risk of falling.
- It may be possible to minimize the severity of some movement issues by receiving instruction in good posture and using posture supports.

- The physical therapist can provide instructions on proper device use and posture when the use of a wheelchair or walker is necessary.
- Exercise regimens can also be changed to account for improved mobility.

Occupational Therapy
- Huntington's disease patients, their family members, and carers can learn how to use assistive technology to enhance their functional abilities from an occupational therapist.
- Assistive gadgets for tasks like bathing and dressing, as well as handrails in the home, are a few examples of such solutions.
- For those with weak fine motor skills, special utensils are used for eating and drinking.

Lifestyle and Home Remedies
- The patients, their families, and other in-home carers are all impacted by managing Huntington's disease. As the illness worsens, the patient's need for a primary carer will increase.
- There will be many problems to solve, and coping techniques will have to be adapted accordingly.

Eating and Nutrition
The following are some eating and nutrition factors:
- It is challenging to keep the weight of the patients in a healthy range. Having trouble eating, burning more calories as a result of physical activity, or undiscovered metabolic issues could all be the contributing factors.
- To receive enough nourishment, the individual might need to consume more than three meals a day and also take nutritional supplements.

NURSING MANAGEMENT

Nursing Diagnoses
- Risk for injury from falls resulting from constant movement.
- Imbalanced nutrition less than body requirements due to inadequate intake and dehydration resulting from swallowing or chewing disorders.
- Risk for aspiration related to swallowing difficulty.
- Anxiety and impaired communication from excessive grimacing and incoherent speech.
- Disturbed thought processes related to the disease condition.
- Impaired social interaction related to the disease condition.

Nursing Interventions
- Protect the patient from injury and possible skin breakdown.
- Pad the sides and head end of the bed, and keep the skin as clean as possible.
- Encourage ambulation with help to maintain muscle tone.
- Secure the patient in bed or a chair with padded protective devices.
- While feeding, keep the patient as upright as possible.
- While feeding, gently support the patient's head with one hand.
- The nurse must educate and support the patient and family as they adjust to the necessary lifestyle changes.
- Medication regimen actions and potential side effects must be taught, monitored, and adjusted to achieve the desired patient response.
- Regular moderate exercise can help to alleviate stiffness and tremors.
- The patient and family will require more care as the disease progresses.

Case Scenario
1. The patient is a right-handed 41-year-old male school teacher who has been identified as having Huntington's disease in its early stages. The treating doctor advised him that physiotherapy could be a suitable choice to assist him handle the various issues he has been experiencing at work, such as typing and writing with chalk. The patient complained that grading examinations were challenging since he was "having difficulty controlling his hands and fingers" as a result of uncontrollable, unintentional movements. He claimed that he used to rely on exercise as a stress reliever, but that he is now concerned about his ability to write safely since he finds it difficult to keep his fingers flexed on the handlebars of his bicycle. In spite of the fact that he can walk without the use of a gait aid and looks to be in fair physical condition when asked to sit down, he slumps heavily. The amount and quality of his sleep, he claims, haven't changed despite his increased exhaustion. Discuss the nursing interventions for this patient.
2. A 56-year-old man with undetected late-onset Huntington's disease displayed symptoms similar to those of Parkinson's disease, such as bradykinesia, or slowness of movement. He was identified appropriately when doctors discovered a family history of Huntington's disease and requested genetic testing. It is recommended that Huntington's disease be taken into consideration in older patients who display Parkinson's-like symptoms and have a family history of the condition given the diagnosis. In addition to the conventional symptoms including parkinsonism, ataxia, and dystonia, some patients may initially display abnormal movements. Discuss the treatment plan for this patient.

SUMMARY
A brain condition known as Huntington's disease (HD) runs in families and is inherited from one generation to the next. It is brought on by a mistake in the DNA instructions that create and keep our bodies functioning. The progression of the disease cannot currently be stopped, slowed down, or reversed by a cure or treatment. To address HD symptoms, there are several therapies and strategies available.

MULTIPLE SCLEROSIS

Multiple sclerosis is a chronic, progressive degenerative condition of central nervous system (CNS). This is characterized by damage of the myelin sheaths around the nerve fibers of brain and spinal cord, leading to generalized neurological impairment. There is disruption in the flow of information within and between the brain and body. As per Dawood Tafti multiple sclerosis "is an autoimmune disease of the central nervous system characterized by chronic inflammation, demyelination, gliosis, and neuronal loss."

EPIDEMIOLOGY

- Around 1 million persons in the US have MS (2019 study supported by the National MS Society).
- Previous estimates of clinically confirmed MS indicated a low prevalence of 1–3 per 100,000, except for the Parsee population, which reported a high frequency of approximately 20–25 per 100,000.
- Most MS cases are discovered in patients between 20 and 50, while it can also attack infants and elderly persons.
- Women are three times more likely to have MS than men. Possibly the hormones play a crucial role in determining MS vulnerability.
- It affects most ethnic groups, including Black Americans and Asians, and is also prevalent in white persons of northern European ancestry.
- African American women may be more susceptible to developing MS. The risk of developing MS differs among different populations.

ETIOLOGY

The exact cause of MS is unknown. Scientists believe that a group of factors may trigger MS. Research is continuing in the fields of immunology, epidemiology, genetics, and various infectious agents (such as viruses) to determine the cause of MS.

- **Immunologic factors:** In MS, a peculiar immune response results in brain damage and swelling. Several different cells are involved in this abnormal immunological response, immune cells, including T cells and B cells.
- **Environmental aspects:** According to studies, those who are relocated or migrated to a lower-risk area before age 15 and were born in a high-risk area for MS take on the risk of the new location. These findings imply that exposure to specific environmental agents may predispose an individual to MS later in life.
- **Vitamin D:** An increased risk of MS is linked with low vitamin D blood levels.
- **Smoking:** Various studies have reported that smoking increases the likelihood of getting MS, making the condition more severe and causing it to proceed more quickly.
- **Obesity:** According to several studies, obesity during childhood and adolescence especially in girls increases the likelihood of having multiple sclerosis (MS) in later life. Moreover, obesity may amplify MS activity and inflammation in those with the disease.
- **Vitamin B12 deficiency:** Vitamin B12 is used by the body to make myelin. The risk of neurological disorders like MS may increase if vitamin B12 is deficient in the body.
- **Genetic factors:** MS is not hereditary, and it cannot be passed from one generation to the next. But there is an inherited genetic risk for MS. The risk of acquiring MS is much less in identical twins than the other first-degree relatives (parents, siblings, and children) who already have the disease.
- **Infectious agents:** Measles, human herpes virus-6, canine distemper, Epstein-Barr virus (EBV), pneumonia and *Chlamydia* are a few viruses and bacteria being investigated to see their contribution to the onset of MS.
- **Unproven theories:** Numerous theories have been put up and investigated as potential causes of MS. However, many need more proof to be considered valid. These theories include the following:
  - Contact with domestic pet
  - Environmental allergies
  - Organic (chemical) solvents.
  - Exposure to heavy metals like mercury (including amalgam fillings for teeth), manganese, or lead.

PATHOPHYSIOLOGY

Multiple sclerosis is an inflammatory demyelinating disease of the central nervous system. The underlying cause of multiple sclerosis is unknown. Two critical processes constitute pathological processes in MS patients:

- Focal inflammation resulting in macroscopic plaques and injury to the blood-brain barrier (BBB).
- Neurodegeneration with microscopic injury involving different components of the CNS, including axons, neurons, and synapse.

Focal inflammation results in the formation of plaques. MS plaques predominantly center around small veins and venules and result in Myelin loss, edema, axonal injury, and also the disruption of the blood-brain barrier (BBB) **(Fig. 38.4)**

MS as defined by the 'International Advisory Committee on Clinical Trials of MS' in 1996 may take course as clinically isolated syndrome; relapsing-remitting MS; secondary progressive MS or primary progressive MS.

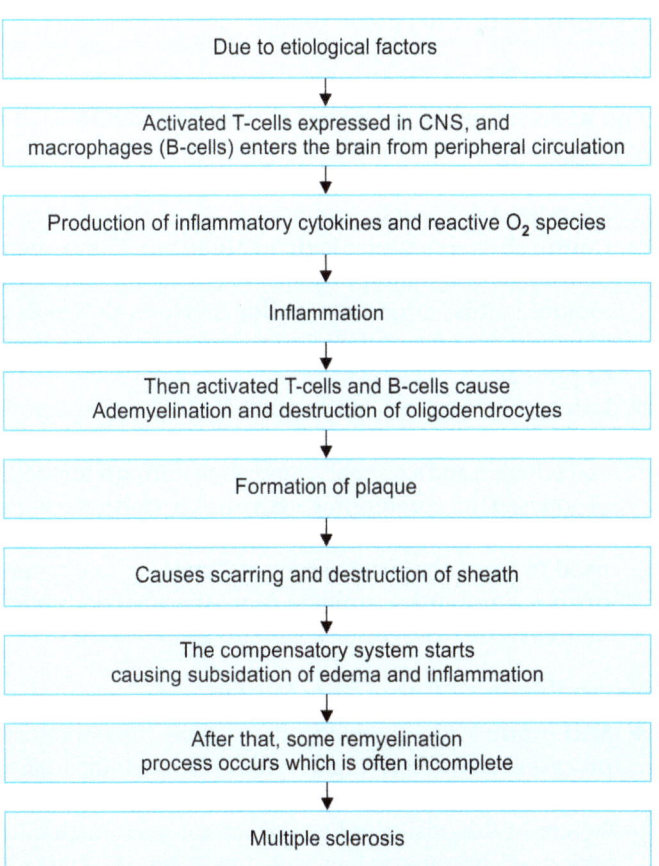

Fig. 38.4: Pathophysiology of MS.

- **Clinically isolated syndrome (CIS):** It is the first episode lasting for at least 24 hours of neurologic symptoms caused by inflammation and demyelination in the CNS. The symptoms may vary from person to person. However, the common symptoms include vision problems, vertigo, loss of sensation in the face, weakness in the arms and legs (one side of the body affected more than the other), loss of control of bodily movements, and bladder problems.
- **Relapsing-remitting MS (RRMS):** It is the most common course of the disease course. The defined attacks of new or increasing neurologic symptoms are followed by periods of partial or complete recovery, or remission. In remission, all the symptoms may disappear. Some of the symptoms may continue and become permanent. The disease does not look like progressing.
- **Secondary progressive MS (SPMS):** It course of the disease follows the initial relapsing-remitting course. Some of the patients with RRMS ultimately go into secondary progressive MS. In this, there is further worsening of the neurologic functions.
- **Primary progressive MS (PPMS):** During this course of the disease, the neurologic functions get further worsen leading to more disability with the accumulation of symptoms.

  Approximately 15% of people with MS are diagnosed with PPMS.

CLINICAL MANIFESTATIONS

Table 38.1 enumerates various manifestations of MS as per the area of dysfunction.

TABLE 38.1: Symptoms of MS.

Area of dysfunctions	Symptoms
Dysfunction of cranial nerves	• Blurred central vision, faded colors, blind spots (optic neuritis) • Diplopia • Facial weakness, numbness, pain • Dysphagia
Motor dysfunction	• Weakness paralysis • Spasticity • Abnormal gait • Fatigue
Sensory dysfunction	• Paresthesias • Lhermitte's sign • Decreased proprioception • Decreased temperature perception
Cerebellar dysfunction	• Dysarthria • Tremor • Incoordination • Ataxia • Vertigo
Bowel and bladder dysfunction	• Fecal urgency, constipation, incontinence urinary frequency, urgency, hesitancy, nocturia, retention, incontinence
Cognitive dysfunction	• Decreased short-term memory • Difficulty learning new information • Word-finding trouble • Short attention span • Decreased concentration • Mood alterations
Sexual dysfunction	• **Women:** Decreased libido, decreased orgasmic ability, decreased genital sensation • **Men:** Erectile, orgasmic, and ejaculatory dysfunction

DIAGNOSTIC CRITERIA

Assessment

The assessment of the patients with MS includes the following:
- **History:** Take a thorough history of past subjective episodes. Ask for all the symptoms.
- **Comprehensive neurologic evaluation:** A thorough neurologic evaluation includes checking the patient's mental status, motor, cerebellar, sensory, and reflex functions, and atypical clinical manifestations that may be present.
- **Exacerbation and remission clinical patterns:** A wide range of manifestations are present during an exacerbation and a normal examination during remission, as opposed to a chronic progressive pattern from the start. Numerous standardized assessment methods are used to track the progression of illness or to explain further a potential problem (e.g., the Kurtzke scale, neuropsychological testing, and urodynamic tests).

Neurodiagnostic/Laboratory Studies

- **MRI brain:** MRI can identify the chronic inflammatory process even without clinical symptoms and indications. It demonstrates the presence of plaques greater than 0.6 cm in the posterior fossa or lateral periventricular region, at least three to four white matter lesions, and one periventricular lesion and de-myelinization (the most sensitive test). Brain atrophy may also be seen.
- **MRI spine:** This test is extremely sensitive, particularly in the presence of FLAIR (fluid-attenuated inversion recovery).
- **Evoked potentials:** Visual-evoked slow, absent, or abnormal responses are seen in 85% of patients with definite MS and are the most useful. Brainstem auditory-evoked responses can identify pontine lesions in 67% of patients with MS. Sensory information can be detected by Sensory evoked responses.
- **Lumbar puncture:** CSF analysis is done if other tests are inconclusive. Electrophoresis of CSF reveals the presence of oligoclonal bands (OCB) and elevated IgG. Although OCB occurs in 90% of cases, additional causes should be ruled out (infections or other inflammatory conditions of the CNS).
- **EEG:** May show plaque and indicate a risk for seizure.
- **PET:** This shows the increased metabolism and the presence of plaque.

The 2017 Revisions to the McDonald Criteria

The primary requirement for the diagnosis of MS is evidence of widespread, time- and space-dependent impairment in the central nervous system. Demonstrating that damage occurred to different parts of the central nervous system [dissemination in space (DIS)] and at different times [dissemination in time (DIT)], setting apart MS from other neurological conditions.

The McDonald criteria use MRI evidence extensively and recommend that an MRI scan be performed on everyone for whom MS is suspected. People with few or no clinical symptoms may have lesions, indicating DIS. Another reliable MS indicator is the presence of oligoclonal bands in spinal fluid. It demonstrates that there has been previous disease activity and can be used as evidence of DIT.

MANAGEMENT

Although there is no cure for MS, however, to decrease the progression of the disease, lessen the severity of relapses, and easing the symptoms, drugs are available.

Anti-progression Medications

- These include the disease-modifying therapies (DMTs) available.
- These drugs function by altering the way the immune system works.

Treatment for MS Attack

- Corticosteroids such as oral prednisone and intravenous methylprednisolone are prescribed to reduce nerve inflammation.
- Possible side effects include insomnia, increased blood pressure, mood swings, and fluid retention.

Treatment to Modify Disease

- **Oral drugs:** Dimethyl fumarate, teriflunomide, fingolimod, siponimod.
- **Injectables:**
  - *Interferons:* These medications are the most often prescribed to treat MS. They function as immunomodulators. They are moderately efficient. They are injected subcutaneously and have the potential to reduce the frequency and severity of relapses.
  - *Glatiramer acetate:* It is an approved injectable for RRMS. It acts as an immunomodulator. It is also moderately efficient. It is given subcutaneously, 20 mg once a day.
  - *Ocrelizumab:* Unlike CD20, it is a monoclonal antibody. It is an approved therapy for RRMS and PPMS. It functions as an immunosuppressive drug. It has very high efficacy. It is administered 600 mg IV every 6 months.
  - *Ofatumumab:* It is a monoclonal antibody that works against CD20. It is used to treat RRMS. It acts as an immunosuppressive drug. It is highly efficient. It is administered 20 mg once a month subcutaneously.
  - *Natalizumab:* It works as an immunomodulator for treating RRMS. It works against α-4 integrin. It has high efficacy. It is administered 300 mg IV once a month.
  - *Alemtuzumab:* It acts as an anti-CD52 monoclonal antibody. It is used to treat RRMS. It is a nonselective immune suppressant drug. It has got high efficacy. It is administered 12 mg IV for five days continuously.
  - *Rituximab:* It acts as a monoclonal antibody against CD20. It is used to treat RRMS, SPMS, and PPMS. It is an immunosuppressive medication. It is a highly efficient drug. It is administered 1 g IV every six months.
  Other licensed Immunosuppressants that may be used to treat MS are azoran, mitoxantrone, methotrexate, and cyclophosphamide.

Surgical Management

Intrathecal baclofen is delivered by a surgically implantable pump to treat severe spasticity.

Adductor tenotomy and dorsal rhizotomy are two other surgical procedures for treating spasticity.

NURSING MANAGEMENT

Nursing Assessment

- Check gait, coordination, and motor strength.
- Assess the cranial nerves.
- Evaluate how well elimination works.
- Investigate coping, how it affects behavior and sexual function, and emotional adjustment.
- Analyze patient and family coping and support mechanisms.

Nursing Diagnoses

1. Impaired sensory perception related to loss of sensation, hyperesthesia, paresthesia, and diminished vibratory and position sensation.
2. Impaired physical mobility related to neuromuscular impairment, i.e., spasticity, motor weakness, useless hand syndrome, tremor, and weakness.
3. Alterations in visual perception related to optic nerve de-myelination or optic neuritis.
4. Chronic pain and discomfort related to dysesthetic pain, and radicular pain.
5. Impaired urinary elimination related to urinary urgency, urinary frequency, and urge incontinence resulting from detrusor hyperreflexia or detrusor-sphincter dyssynergia from spinal cord lesions.
6. Constipation related to immobility.
7. Sexual dysfunction related to diminished libido, erectile dysfunction (EDS), and deficient vaginal lubrication.
8. Activity intolerance related to fatigue.

Nursing Interventions

There could be overlapping of the nursing interventions in various nursing diagnoses enlisted above. So, the overall nursing interventions for various problems of patients with MS may include:

- Offer emotional and psychological support to the patient and his family, as well as give honest feedback to their questions.
- Stay by the patient's side during crisis periods. Encourage the patient by offering ways to cope with the illness.
- Provide assistance with physical therapy.
- Use massages and calming baths to relax patients and make them more comfortable.

- Ensure the water is not overly hot, which could temporarily exacerbate otherwise mild symptoms.
- Participate in active, resistive, and stretching activities to preserve muscle tone and joint mobility, reduce spasticity, enhance coordination, and boost morale.
- Exercises should be separated by rest periods because exhaustion and fatigue might exacerbate conditions.
- Encourage emotional stability.
- Assist the patient in establishing a daily routine to sustain optimal functioning.
- Tolerance level regulates activity level—promote regular rest periods to prevent fatigue.
- Have a bedpan or urinal close by because the urge to urinate is sudden.
- Evaluate the need for bowel and bladder training while the patient is in the hospital: Encourage regular urination and adequate fluid intake.
- Eventually, the patient may require urinary drainage via a condom catheter for men or a self-catheter.
- Practice all the infection control measures.

Patient Education

- Review the disease process, focusing on maximizing the patient's potential and avoiding exacerbations as much as possible.
- Explain to the patient any potential drug-related side effects and the medication regimen.
- Stress the value of avoiding infections, stress, and fatigue and maintaining independence by learning new ways to perform daily activities.
- Explain to the patient the significance of avoiding bacterial and viral infections.
- Stress the value of eating a healthy, nutritious, well-balanced diet with adequate fiber to prevent constipation.
- Encourage adequate fluid intake and frequent urination.
- Promote emotional stability.
- Help the patient develop a daily routine to maintain optimal functioning.
- Inform the patient that exacerbations are unpredictable and new physical and emotional lifestyle changes will be necessary.
- Inform the patient and his/her family about multiple sclerosis (MS)—highlight the importance of avoiding stress, fatigue, and infections.

Avoiding Exacerbation of MS

- Emphasize the value of maintaining independence by learning new skills to perform daily tasks.
- Inform the patient about the significance of preventing bacterial and viral infections.
- Reiterate the importance of exercise and inform the patient that walking can improve gait.
- Teach to walk with a broad base of support if motor dysfunction causes balance or coordination problems.
- Instruct the patient to keep an eye on his/her feet while walking if having trouble with position change.
- If in danger of falling, the patient might need a walker or a wheelchair.
- Stress the importance of taking rests, preferably lying down.
- Insist on the importance of eating a nutritious, well-balanced diet with adequate roughage to prevent constipation.
- Encourage adequate fluid intake and regular urination.
- Provide bowel and bladder training if needed.
- Teach the patient how to use suppositories to establish a regular bowel elimination pattern.
- Inform the patient that new physical and emotional lifestyle changes will be necessary because exacerbations are unpredicted.

Complementary and Alternative Therapies

The following therapies may help with different aspects of MS:
- Heat therapy, massage, and acupuncture for treating pain.
- Stress management to boost mood.
- Exercise to maintain strength and flexibility, reduce stiffness, and boost mood.
- A healthy diet with plenty of fresh fruits, vegetables, and fiber.
- Quitting or avoiding smoking.

Physical Therapy and Rehabilitation

Rehabilitation can improve a person's ability to perform effectively at home and at work. Typical programs include:
- **Physical therapy:** Aims to teach people how to maintain and restore their full range of motion and functional capacity.
- **Occupational therapy:** Work, self-care, and therapeutic play may aid in maintaining mental and physical health.
- **Speech and swallowing therapy:** A speech and language therapist will provide specialized training for those who require it.
- **Cognitive rehabilitation:** Helps people deal with specific issues with thinking and perception.
- **Vocational rehabilitation:** Supports a person whose life has been affected by MS in making career plans, learning employment skills, and obtaining a vocation.

Plasma Exchange

Plasma exchange involves:
- Taking blood from a person.
- Removing plasma.
- Replacing it with fresh plasma.
- Transfusing it back into the individual.

  This procedure eliminates antibodies in the blood that attack parts of the body, but it is uncertain whether it can benefit patients with MS.
- Plasma exchange is usually used in severe MS attacks.
- Scientists are studying stem cell therapy to regenerate various bodily cells and restore function to persons who have lost it due to a medical condition.
- According to researchers, stem cell treatment procedures will reverse MS damage and restore patients' functionality.

GERIATRIC CONSIDERATIONS

In older adults, MS is diagnosed less frequently. Potential mimics must be considered critically. A complete health history and physical examination, MRI, serum tests, and frequent cerebrospinal fluid tests are all important in diagnosing multiple sclerosis. Multiple sclerosis is more likely to be progressive in aged people, which may result in more significant disability. The risks and benefits should be carefully weighed before prescribing medication to recently diagnosed MS elderly patients. Clinical trial data are insufficient to predict how these medicines affect elderly patients. Symptomatic therapy may improve gait impairment, mood disruption, bladder and bowel dysfunction, neuropathic pain, and spasticity in elderly MS patients. Pharmacotherapies, physical and occupational treatments are useful in MS.

SUMMARY

Multiple sclerosis (MS) is a fatal neurological disorder. MS progression varies from person to person, making it challenging to forecast what will happen, but most patients do not experience significant disability. Newer medications offer great optimism for halting disease progression since they are safer and more effective than older ones. A person with MS can anticipate living the same number of years as someone without MS, provided they receive the proper treatment and follow a healthy lifestyle. It is important to have the support of others who understand what it is like to be diagnosed and live with MS.

Case Scenario

1. Ms Sita is a 35-years-old female who visited OPD for the evaluation of her long-term neurologic complaints. She reports noticing significant changes in neurologic functions for many years, particularly heat intolerance, resulting in a stumbling gait and a tendency to fall. Her vision also seemed to fluctuate over several years. She was under a lot of stress for the past two months and working very hard. She had the flu, and her neurologic condition deteriorated. She had difficulty holding objects in her hands, had significant tremors, and was extremely tired. She also had several missteps and experienced arthralgia on her right side. MRI scan revealed multifocal white matter disease—areas of increased T2 signal in both cerebral hemispheres. CSF analysis revealed the presence of oligoclonal bands. Visual evoked response testing showed abnormalities in optic nerve conduction. Write the management of the patient.
2. A 32-year-old Rita comes to an emergency with a 6-month history of unilateral visual impairment and facial numbness. Six months ago, she began to experience right-sided facial numbness and blurred vision that lasted several weeks. She said that three episodes have occurred in the last six months. There is no associated facial muscle weakness. The patient had right-sided impaired vision and right-sided numbness in her face when she woke up today. She said she has no muscle weakness, gait problems, fever, or urinary incontinence. What tests to are to be done to diagnose the condition? Discuss the management of the patient in detail.

SUMMARY

Degenerative disorders are frightening to the patient, since the patient experiences and recognize the changes brought on by the disease. The older patient may attribute early problems with memory, learning, concentration, calculation, judgment, restlessness, personality changes, or insomnia to normal ageing and may fail to seek medical assistance. Family members may also fail to acknowledge the seriousness of the symptoms until they become advanced. Denial is a protective mechanism that delays the inevitable diagnosis, which may be strongly suspected and generally unwelcome, especially if there is a family history or prevalence of degenerative disorders. With new scientific advances, increased public awareness, early diagnosis, and clinical management, patients with degenerative disorders can expect effective care in a variety of healthcare settings (e.g., ambulatory, home, acute, or long-term care). It is important to identify patients early for diagnosis and admission into the appropriate setting for health care management.

MULTIPLE CHOICE QUESTIONS

1. Alzheimer's disease is the most common form of which of these?
   a. Malnutrition   b. Dementia
   c. Fatigue   d. Psychosis
2. Physiologically, what happens to the brain as Alzheimer's disease progresses?
   a. Tissue swells   b. Fluid collects
   c. Many cells die   d. Brainstem atrophies
3. If you care for a relative with Alzheimer's disease, which of these measures will help stabilize the patient mentally?
   a. Move to a small apartment
   a. Correct "bad" behavior gently
   b. Establish a regular routine
   c. Repaint or buy new furniture
4. The word 'Dementia' comes from the Latin for what words?
   a. Without mind
   b. Partial mind
   c. Without soul
   d. Without hope
5. Dementia usually develops over __, while delirium occurs __.
   a. Years; suddenly   b. Suddenly; years
   c. Days; decades   d. Years; slowly
6. What is sundowning?
   a. When patients' symptoms become worse as night falls
   b. When patients' symptoms become better as nighttime approaches
   c. When patients' symptoms become worse in the morning
   d. When patients' symptoms persist without ceasing for two days or more
7. Parkinson disease is marked by a lack of which chemical in the brain?
   a. Dopamine   b. Serotonin
   c. GABA   d. Glutamate
8. The four primary signs of Parkinson's disease include:
   a. Ageusia, bradykinesia, dementia and rigidity
   b. Tremor, bradykinesia, rigidity and postural instability
   c. Tremor, bradykinesia, seborrhea, and constipation;
   d. Temor, bradykinesia, rigidity, and depression
9. What is often the first symptom of Parkinson disease?
   a. Vomiting   b. Blurred vision
   c. Headache   d. Shaking of a hand or foot.
10. What is the average age when Parkinson disease first appears?
    a. 30   b. 25
    c. 50   d. 60.
11. Bradykinesia, rigidity, severe symptoms, and inability to live alone is found in which stage of Parkinson's disease?
    a. Stage 1   b. Stage 2
    c. Stage 3   d. Stage 4
12. Which of the following is another name for amyotrophic lateral sclerosis (ALS)?
    a. Gaucher's disease b. Guillain-Barre syndrome
    c. Lou Gehrig's disease d. Graves' disease
13. Amyotrophic lateral sclerosis is also known as:
    a. Motor proton infection b. Auto neuron infection
    c. Auto proton infection   d. Motor neuron disease
14. Huntington disease is also known as:
    a. Huntington syndrome b. Huntington chorea
    c. Huntington neuritis d. Huntington reaction
15. HD mainly affects which body system?
    a. Lymphatic system   b. Nervous system
    c. Cardiovascular system d. Respiratory system

16. Early symptoms of HD include which of these?
    a. Mood swings
    b. Depression
    c. Irritability
    d. Hyperactivity
17. Which of the following symptoms do nearly all people with Multiple sclerosis experience during the course of their disease?
    a. Tremor
    b. Depression
    c. Fatigue
    d. Blurred vision
18. Inflammation and damage to which part of the body causes symptoms of multiple sclerosis?
    a. Muscles
    b. Myelin
    c. Lungs
    d. Bones
19. What usually prevents immune cells from entering the brain in healthy individuals?
    a. The immune-brain barrier
    b. Immune cells are never near the brain
    c. The skull
    d. The blood brain barrier
20. What is the most common type of MS?
    a. Secondary progressive MS (SPMS)
    b. Relapsing-remitting MS (RRMS)
    c. Primary progressive MS (PPMS)
    d. Primary relapsing MS (PRMS)

ANSWERS

1. b	2. d	3. c	4. a
5. a	6. a	7. a	8. b
9. d	10. d	11. d	12. c
13. d	14. b	15. b	16. c
17. c	18. b	19. d	20. b

SUGGESTED READING

1. Barker Ellen. Neuroscience Nursing "Spectrum of Care" 2nd edition. Published by Mosby.
2. Black JM, Hawks JH. Medical-Surgical Nursing, 8th edition. Elsevier, a division of Reed Elsevier India Private Limited. 2010. pp. 507-53.
3. Brunner LS, Suddarth DS. Textbook of Medical-Surgical Nursing, 5th edition. JB Lippincott Company.
4. Chugh SN. Textbook of Medical-Surgical Nursing, 1st edition. Avichal Publishing Company; 2013.
5. https://medlineplus.gov/genetics/condition/huntington-disease/#frequency
6. https://mstrust.org.uk/a-z/mcdonald-criteria#:~:text=The%20key%20requirement%20for%20a,of%20the%20central%20nervous%20system.
7. https://nms2cdn.azureedge.net/cmssite/nationalmssociety/media/msnational/professionals/diagnosing%20criteria/2018_dxcard_2018-01.png.
8. https://www.mayoclinic.org/diseases-conditions/huntingtons-disease/symptoms-causes/syc-20356117
9. https://www.medicalnewstoday.com/articles/37556#causes-and-risk-factors
10. https://www.medicalnewstoday.com/articles/37556#treatment calgaryguide.ucalgary.ca/multiple-sclerosis-ms/
11. https://www.nationalmssociety.org/What-is-MS/What-Causes-MS
12. https://www.ncbi.nlm.nih.gov/books/NBK556151/
13. https://www.ninds.nih.gov/health-information/disorders/amyotrophic-lateral-sclerosis-als
14. https://www.rnpedia.com/nursing-notes/medical-surgical-nursing-notes/amyotrophic-lateral-sclerosis-als-nursing-management/
15. https://www.rnpedia.com/nursing-notes/medical-surgical-nursing-notes/huntingtons-chorea-nursing-management/.
16. https://www.webmd.com/brain/hungtingtons-disease-causes-symptoms-treatment
17. Lewis SM, Heitkemper MM, Dirksen SR. Medical-Surgical Nursing, 6th edition. Section Editors.
18. Nair RN. Textbook of Medical and Surgical Nursing, 1st edition. Jaypee Brothers Medical Publishers (P) Ltd; 2009.

UNIT IV: Burns, Reconstructive and Cosmetic Surgery

OUTLINE

39. Burns, Reconstructive and Cosmetic Surgery
    Latika Rohilla, Vithal Malmande

CHAPTER 39

Burns, Reconstructive and Cosmetic Surgery

Latika Rohilla, Vithal Malmande

"I survived because the fire inside me burned brighter than the fire around me."
—A Burn Survivor

LEARNING OBJECTIVES

After going through the chapter, the learner will be able to:
- Enumerate and define various classification systems of the burn injury.
- Describe the pathophysiology and the associated clinical manifestations in terms of both systemic effects and local effects of a burn injury.
- Elaborate various aspects of management, such as diagnostic, medical, surgical and other non-pharmacological modalities.
- Identify the needs of a burn injury patient in all the three phases of burns, formulate the nursing diagnosis and enlist the nursing interventions for each one of them.
- Enumerate the potential complications along with the actions that are necessary to prevent them in a burn patient.
- Describe role of a nurse in various aspects of burn care, such as wound care, diet and nutrition, pain management, topical antimicrobial therapy, reconstructive and cosmetic surgery.

TERMS

- **Compartment syndrome in burns:** Reduced blood perfusion in underlying tissues due to either excessive fluid collection under the skin or by compression of the burnt tissue acting, such as a tourniquet, leading to necrosis in the closed space, often as a result of circumferential third degree burn or high voltage electric injury.
- **Contracture:** Shrinking of the skin tissues during the healing phase of a burn injury caused by collagen maturation.
- **Debridement:** An aseptic surgical process of removing the burnt and dead tissue from the wounds before dressing.
- **Donor site:** Part of the body from which the graft is taken mostly thighs or trunk.
- **Eschar:** A dark, dry and dead tissue that falls off or sheds from the surface of the skin after a deep burn wound.
- **Fasciotomy:** Surgical procedure of giving an incision in the muscle fascia to release pressure on the lower tissues and organs.
- **Split thickness skin graft (STSG):** A graft used to cover burn wounds (partial thickness), that contains the epidermis along with a portion of dermis. It does not have blood supply of its own and is dependent on the wound bed for graft in growth.
- **Total burn surface area (TBSA):** It is calculated by various methods, such as the rules of nines and the Lund and Browder method. It is used for estimating the fluid resuscitation needs.

INTRODUCTION

Burn injury, unlike other medical surgical conditions, has deep and long-lasting effect on psychology of the patient as patient tends to lose his/her very identity. However, various reconstructive and cosmetic surgeries have emerged today to ease the multiple problems of the burn patient during rehabilitation. This chapter highlights various aspects of burn injury and their management from immediate after injury to long term rehabilitation.

EPIDEMIOLOGY

World
- An estimated 180,000 deaths every year are caused by burns.

- Burn injuries (non-fatal) are among the leading causes of 'disability-adjusted life-years' (DALY) lost.
- Worldwide, over 10 million people are reported to have burn injuries each year.

India
- In India, over 1 million people are burnt every year.
- Burns are the second most common type of injury after road accidents.
- **Severity:** About 10% of burn injuries are life threatening. Over half of those who get hospitalized, do not survive. Nearly 2 lakh people get permanently disabled due to burns. They need many plastic surgeries and prolonged rehabilitation.
- **Age:** Most of the burn victims are in the age group of 15 to 40 years.
- **Gender:** There is a higher risk for mortality related to burns among females. The burn injuries are related to cooking related injuries (both LPG and kerosene stoves) because of which the loose clothing catch fire very easily.

CLASSIFICATION OF BURNS

Burns can be classified by the **mechanism of injury, depth, and extent of burn injury.** A brief description of all the three is given below:

1. **Mechanism of injury:** Burns are classified according to the causative agent and the related mechanism causing injury. A burn wound may be any one or a combination of the following:
   - *Thermal injury (dry heat):* Contact with hot object causes this type of burn. Fire flame injury is also categorized as thermal burns.
   - *Electrical injury:* It happens when a person is in contact with electric current for prolonged time. Electricity can affect internal tissues like muscles and the burn may appear on the skin. Electric burns are more injurious inside than they appear on the outside skin. Entry and exit point of the electric current are most severely injured.
   - *Scald injury (moist heat):* Contact with hot liquids, such as boiling water, hot beverages, oil or chemicals, such as acids to the skin can cause scald injury. Blisters are most common to appear after a scald burn.
   - *Chemical injury:* Any chemical erosion of the internal organs, such as eyes, oral or nasal cavity is termed as chemical injury.
   - *Cold injury (frost bite):* Frostbite is caused due to prolonged contact with freezing temperatures. It initially appears cold and red, followed by numbness and pale appearance.
   - *Ionizing radiations:* High-energy radiation used during radiotherapy for cancer patients.

2. **Depth of injury:** Burns are classified as first, second, third, and fourth degrees **(Table 39.1)**. The 'second' and 'third degree' wounds are also sometimes referred to as

Degree of burn	Tissue involved	Appearance of wound	Examples
First-degree (superficial) burns	Epidermis only	Red, painful, and dry appearance	Mild sunburn, quick contact with a hot object
Second-degree (partial thickness) burns **(Fig. 39.1A)**	Epidermis, part the dermis	Appears red, blistered, and swollen. They are painful	Hot liquids-water, oil, candle wax, etc., steam, friction burn
Third-degree (full thickness) burns	Complete loss of the epidermis and dermis, reaches the subcutaneous tissue	White or blackened and charred	Contact with hot object for long time, flame from a fire, electric, chemical burns
Fourth-degree burns **(Fig. 39.1B)**	Loss of all layers of the skin, underlying subcutaneous tissue and might involve muscle and bone	• Not painful • Exposed tissue appearance, which may be charred or black	Prolonged contact with fire, deep electric or chemical burns

TABLE 39.1: Classification of burns according to depth.

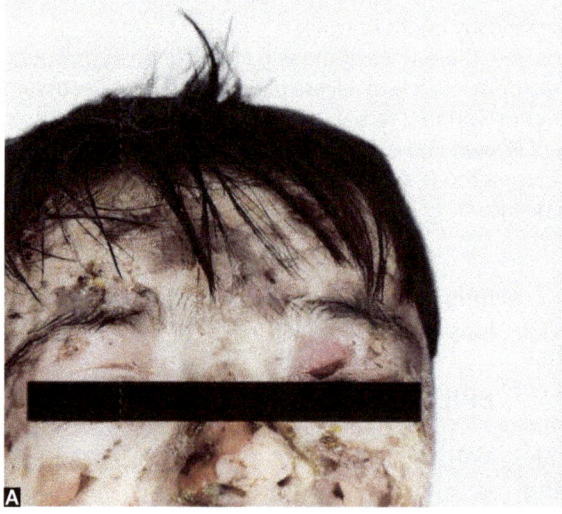
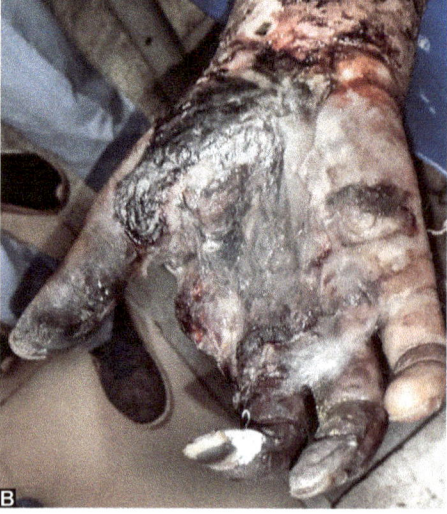

Figs. 39.1A and B: (A) Second degree (partial thickness burns); (B) Fourth degree burns.

'partial' and 'complete' thickness respectively according to the thickness of dermis involved.
3. **Extent of injury:** It involves classification of burns according to the total burn surface area (TBSA) of the body involved. It is very important to have accurate assessment of the TBSA as the fluid resuscitation is given according to TBSA and weight of the patient.

CALCULATING TOTAL BURN SURFACE AREA (TBSA)

It is important to calculate the total burn surface area to estimate the volume of fluid resuscitation. There are different methods to assess the TBSA.
- **Rule of nines:** It is the most commonly used method. The rule of nines is a quick and easy method of estimating the burn surface area in the emergency department. It divides the body into multiples of nine **(Fig. 39.2A)**.
- **Lund and Browder (L and B) method:** The L and B method is another method used for estimating TBSA among pediatric population. This takes different proportions of the body parts into account. So, with increasing age decreasing percent of body surface area for the head and increasing percent of body surface area for the legs, leads to a more accurate estimation **(Fig. 39.2B)**.

PATHOPHYSIOLOGY OF BURNS (FLOWCHART 39.1)

Burn injury affects the body in different ways, all adding up to an acute life-threatening emergency situation. Burn wounds have three zones. These are: (1) 'Coagulation zone', (2) 'Stasis zone', and (3) 'Hyperemic zone'.

- **Coagulation zone:** This is the zone of permanently destroyed tissues.
- **Stasis zone:** It is surrounding the coagulation zone, has damaged tissue with decreased perfusion, but it can still recover.
- **Hyperemic zone:** It is the tissue around the stasis zone that has minimal damage and can recover on its own.

The tissues in the zones of 'stasis' and 'hyperemia', are viable but can be damaged later due to perfusion loss, infection, or inflammation. This can lead to permanent damage to these tissues as well.
- The transfer of heat to the skin tissues leads to altered capillary permeability which causes the third space shift.
- Blisters are formed when plasma from damaged capillaries leaks into the interstitial space due to increased vascular permeability.
- The damaged epidermis then separates from the dermis below it. The high osmolarity of leaked fluid can cause water absorption from underlying tissue into the blister, leading to compartment syndrome. This causes a dual problem of reduced blood volume and increased interstitial pressure.
- Whereas the decreased blood volume leads to a hypovolemic shock that is systemic, compartment syndrome due to the increased pressure beneath the burn tissues especially in electric burns and circumferential deep wounds leads to progressive necrosis of the underlying tissues especially in legs and arms.
- **Skin barrier loss:** This leads to extensive loss of fluid by evaporation. This loss of fluid causes reduction in tissue perfusion and oxygenation. This hypovolemia results in hypoperfusion to all major body organs.

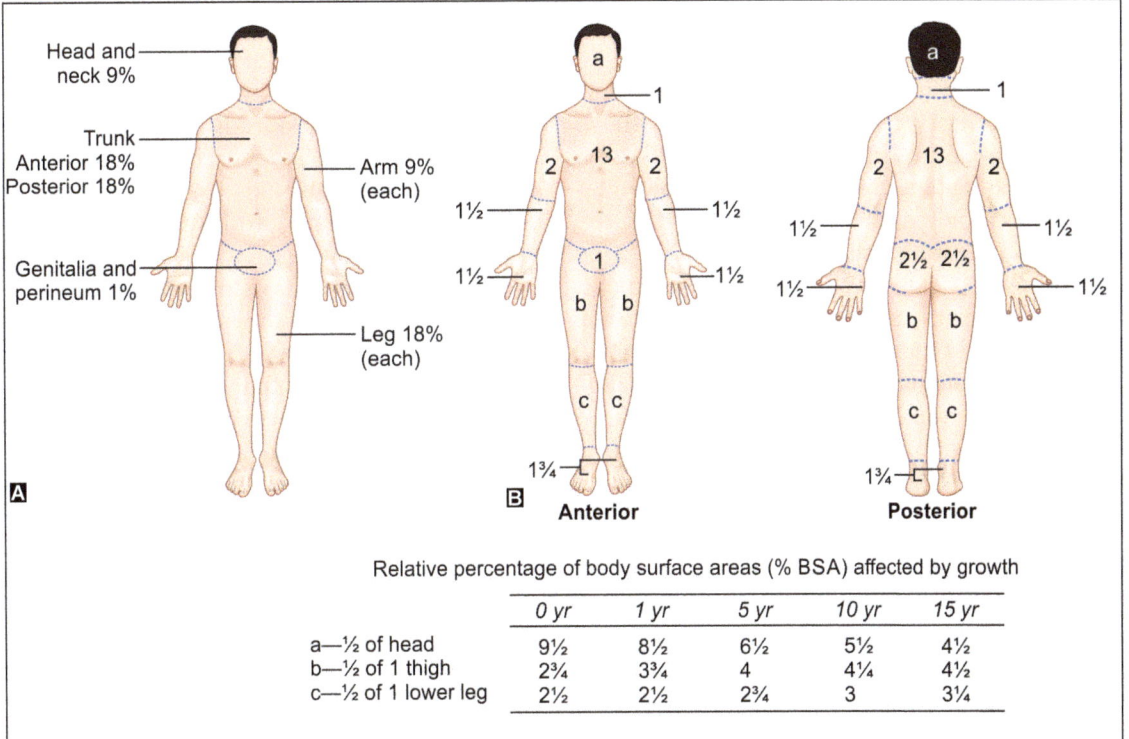

Figs. 39.2A and B: Estimating the total burn surface area (TBSA): (A) Rule of nine; (B) Lund-Browder diagram for estimating extent of burns.

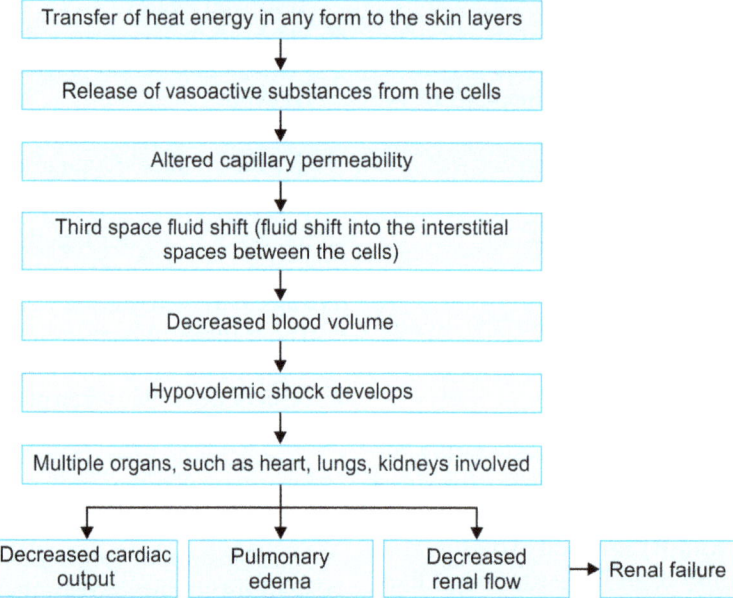

Flowchart 39.1: Pathophysiology of burns.

- **Multiorgan failure:** Tissues release many inflammatory substances after injury, which cause interstitial edema and multiple organ dysfunction. Multiorgan failure usually develops between the second and eighth week after injury and accounts for one-third of burn-related deaths. Increased age, increased TBSA burned, male sex, and the presence of inhalation injury all are associated with an increased chance of multiorgan failure after burn injury.
- **Systemic infections or sepsis:** Loss of the skin's immunity leads to an increase in susceptibility to infection. Systemic infection results from invasion of bacteria into the body through the burn wound. Immediately following injury, the burned area is sterile, but then bacteria quickly colonize the wound. Then, microorganisms rapidly gain access to the rest of the body through blood.
- **Cardiac effects:** Myocardial function may be depressed immediately after injury, but it improves within 48–72 hours. This is caused by circulating inflammatory agents and persisting hypovolemia. This is followed by a hyperdynamic cardiovascular response with an up-to-two-fold increase in cardiac output.
- **Metabolic changes:** Metabolic changes (e.g., 'metabolic acidosis', 'respiratory alkalosis', and 'electrolyte disturbances') are common. These include a rise in the intracellular concentrations of sodium and calcium and increase in the intravascular levels of potassium.

CLINICAL MANIFESTATIONS

The burn patient mostly reaches the emergency department in a state of shock due to pain and sudden hypovolemia.

Superficial to moderate partial thickness burns are painful, while deep burns involving full thickness are painless due to destroyed nerve endings. Fluid is not actually lost from the body, but it gets 'trapped in the interstitial spaces'. Consciousness is intact except in cases of hypoxia due to 'smoke inhalation', 'head trauma', or sedation. The specific signs and symptoms are:

1. **Immediate (within 24 hours):**
   - Pain and burning sensation over burn site
   - Reddening and blistering of the skin
   - Bleeding if skin is broken
   - Necrosis and skin is black in color
   - Lack of sensation (if nerve damage, as in deep wounds)
   - Anxiety
   - Tachycardia, tachypnea
   - Dizziness, particularly during change of position.
   - Fever (as an inflammatory response, not necessary a sign of infection)
   - Inhalation burns may also have breathlessness, stridor and cough
2. **Late manifestations (after 24 hours):**
   - Anasarca (generalized edema)
   - Decreased urine output
   - Bradycardia, bradypnea, hypotension, hypothermia
   - Shock (hypovolemic)
   - Increased thirst (polydipsia)
   - Nausea, vomiting
3. **Signs and symptoms of infection:**
   - Discoloration of the surrounding area around the burnt skin.
   - Purplish discoloration or swelling may also be seen.
   - Increase in thickness or depth of the burn (the burn extends deeper into the skin with infection)
   - Discharge (white to green color) or pus from the wound.
   - Fever

MANAGEMENT OF THE PATIENT

The burn patients have different needs and potential health issues that need to be managed accordingly. Therefore, the management of these patients is discussed under three

phases according to the time past the burn injury. These phases are:
1. The emergent phase (first 48–72 hours)
2. The acute or healing phase (after 72 hours to 15 days)
3. The rehabilitation phase of burn care (beyond 15 days)

The Emergent Phase (First 48–72 Hours)

This phase initiates with the start of the burn injury. It lasts till the fluid resuscitation is completed. It may be for the first 48 to 72 hours depending upon the severity of the burn injury. During this phase, priority of patient care involves maintaining an adequate airway, resuscitating the fluid and treating the patient for burn shock.

Medical Management

- ❖ **History taking**: As burns are a medicolegal emergency, history taking is very crucial step. The incidence should be reported in verbatim with details of the informer. History taking can give important clues to rule out homicidal cases. History taking is explained under the nursing management ahead.
- ❖ **Physical examination**: It includes assessment of the ABC (airway, breathing, and circulation) and the vital signs. Other parameters specific to the burn injury, such as the depth, degree and percentage of burn and inhalation injury are also assessed. Severity of burns is determined by:
  - ➤ *Is inhalation injury involved?* Inhalation injury requires prompt intubation and generally has a poor prognosis. Signs include: traces of carbon/soot on the face (around the mouth/nose), blisters on face and buccal cavity, or respiratory stridor.
  - ➤ *Depth:* Is it a first, second (partial thickness), third degree (full thickness) burn?
  - ➤ *Extent:* What is the TBSA?
  - ➤ *Age:* Is the patient from the more vulnerable age group? The very young (less than 10 years) and very old have a poor prognosis.
  - ➤ *Which area of the body has been burned?* The face, hands, feet, perineum, and circumferential burns need special attention.
  - ➤ *Any other injuries along with burns or any illness?* Medical history of the patient.
- ❖ **Laboratory investigations**: Later on investigations are performed to assess any complications, such as dehydration, infection, electrolyte imbalance, etc.
  The following blood samples are to be sent immediately at admission:
  - ➤ Arterial blood gas values
  - ➤ Electrolyte levels (sodium, potassium, chloride levels), blood glucose levels
  - ➤ Renal function test (blood urea nitrogen, uric acid, creatinine levels)
  - ➤ Liver function tests (ALT, AST)
  - ➤ Hematocrit (hemoglobin level, blood cell count)
  - ➤ Blood culture has to be sent for microorganism and sensitivity testing.
  - ➤ **'Serum lactate'**—helps detect acid-base imbalance.
  - ➤ Blood **'serum creatine-kinase'**—they are released in cases of injuries to internal organs, such as the kidneys or muscles. This can occur with electrical or deep third-degree burns.
  - ➤ **Blood type and cross-match**—Sever fluid loss or injury may require blood transfusion.

  Other investigatory tests include:
  - ➤ **Electrocardiogram (ECG):** To look for cardiac arrhythmias.
  - ➤ **Chest X-ray:** To detect atelectasis infections or pulmonary edema.
- ❖ **First aid for burns:**
  - ➤ This begins with the burn injury till the completion of fluid resuscitation (period of about the first 24 hours).
  - ➤ Maintaining an adequate airway and treating the patient for burn shock are nursing priorities during this time.
  - ➤ Stop the burning process and move the patient away from the site of injury.
  - ➤ In case of external wounds, wash the wound with tap water by continuous irrigation for 20 minutes. Prevent hypothermia too.
  - ➤ Maintain airway, breathing and circulation.
  - ➤ In case of fall from height accompanied with high voltage electric injury or fall from height, assess for any fractures or spinal injury. Shift the patient to the nearest medical facility as early as possible.
- ❖ **Burn care at hospital**

  Airway management:
  - ➤ Endotracheal intubation or tracheotomy for assisted ventilation may be required immediately to maintain adequate oxygenation.
  - ➤ Assess arterial blood gas values for respiratory or metabolic acidosis/alkalosis.
  - ➤ In case of circumferential burns on the chest wall and neck, escharotomy may be needed to relieve respiratory distress. Administration of humidified oxygen in case patient is not intubated.
  - ➤ Position the patient in high Fowler's position except in spinal cord injuries.
  - ➤ Encourage patient for coughing and deep breathing exercises, reposition every hour.
  - ➤ Provide chest physiotherapy and postural drainage.
  - ➤ Suction secretions when indicated.
  - ➤ Administration of bronchodilators may be necessary to relieve bronchospasm.

Carbon monoxide poisoning:
- ❖ Carbon monoxide has very high affinity for hemoglobin. It combines with hemoglobin in blood to form another chemical called carboxyhemoglobin.
- ❖ Carbon monoxide poisoning leads to a vasodilating effect.
- ❖ Early intubation and 100% oxygen administration may be needed.

Ensure proper circulation:

Signs of compromised circulation and impending shock are:
- ❖ Slow capillary refill (more than 5 seconds)
- ❖ Hypotension.
- ❖ Reduced urinary output.

Fluid management:
- In the initial hours after a major burn injury, loss of capillary permeability leads to intravascular fluid to flood into the extracellular space.
- In case of adults having more than 15% TBSA or a child having more than 10% TBSA, require immediately fluid resuscitation.
- Fluid replacement using solutions, such as crystalloids (usually 'Ringer's lactate') or colloids ('albumin'). The steps of fluid management are:
  - Insertion of at least one (and usually two) large bore catheter for administering Intra Venous fluids.
  - In case of large areas of burns vene-section or central line insertion may be necessary.
  - Calculating the TBSA involved.
  - Calculating the fluid needs according to one of the fluid resuscitation formulas **(Box 39.1)**:
    - Assessment of the adequacy of fluid replacement:
      - Urine output 30–50 mL/hour; 75–100 mL/hour for electrical burn patients (with evidence of hemoglobinuria or myoglobinuria).
      - Cardiopulmonary factors: BP (systolic >90 mm Hg), pulse rate <120 beats/minute.
    - After the first 24 hours, the amount of fluid infused is titrated according to the urine output.

Surgical management: Wound care
- Delayed until airway is patent and adequate fluid replacement is established.
- Cleaning and gentle debridement in a shower or at the patient's bed.
- Extensive surgical debridement is performed in an operating room.
- Releasing escharotomies or fasciotomies is done in the emergent phase, by burn physicians (plastic surgeons).
- Wound care is not only demanding on the patient but puts him at risk for heat loss, electrolyte depletion and cross contamination.
- Health care team members should ensure adequate infection control measures.
- Proper disinfection of the environment and the utilities is a must. Use of plastic liners prevents contamination of equipment.
- Face, eyes, fingers, perineum, hands, arms, ears and skin folds require particularly vigilant nursing care.
- Facial care is often performed by open method since dressings can be traumatizing to patients.
- Eye care for corneal burns and edema require antibiotic therapy. Artificial tears can be used to provide comfort. Assure patients that periorbital swelling is temporary.
- Hands and finger should be kept straight and elevated to prevent edema.
- Ears should be kept free of pressure as they have poor vasculature and are more prone to infection.
- Perineum should be kept clean and healthy and an indwelling catheter can prevent contamination of the wound.

Nutrition and dietary supplements
- Burn patients need high calories, high proteins diet to aid recovery. Egg white is most cost effective in our Indian scenario.
- Antioxidant rich fruits and vegetables.
- Reduce refined carbohydrates, white bread, and sugar.
- Caffeine, alcohol and tobacco are prohibited.
- 6–8 glasses water daily.
- A multivitamin to be given daily; containing the antioxidant vitamins A, C, E, the B-complex vitamins and trace minerals such as magnesium, calcium, zinc, and selenium.
- Vitamin C to promote new tissue growth. Vitamin E also promotes healing.
- L-glutamine supplement prevents movement of gut flora into blood capillaries and also supports immunity. These are contraindicated in hepatic encephalopathy, and severe liver disease with confusion.
- Probiotic supplement (which contains '*Lactobacillus acidophilus*'), 5–10 billion CFUs (colony forming units) in a day. Antibiotics upset the normal gut flora (bacteria). Probiotics are used to restore the balance, and also improve gastrointestinal and immune health.

Special Therapies

Pain Management
- Analgesics and sedatives should be started early and preferably using intravenous route.
- Morphine (opioid) is the first drug given for burn pain control, followed by hydromorphone and methadone.
- Anxiety and pain usually occur together in burn patients. The overall burn experience can cause severe anxiety, leading to exacerbation of pain. To mitigate the effect generally sedation with anxiolytic medications namely lorazepam and midazolam are often needed in addition to the usage of opioids.
- Using non-pharmacologic interventions are also effective in the burn pain management. These include relaxation and deep breathing exercises, yoga, cognitive behavioral therapy, guided imagery, hypnosis, therapeutic touch, humor, and music therapy **(Box 39.2)**.

BOX 39.1: Fluid resuscitation formulas.

"Parkland/Baxter Formula"
- **'Lactated Ringer's solution:** 4 mL × kg body weight × % TBSA burned
- **Day 1:** Half to be given in first 8 hours; half to be given over next 16 hours
- **Day 2:** Varies. Colloid is added.'

"Brooke Army Formula"
- **'Colloids:** 0.5 mL × kg body weight × % TBSA
- **Electrolytes (lactated Ringer's solution):** 1.5 mL × kg body weight × % TBSA
- **Glucose (5% in water):** 2,000 mL for insensible loss
- **Day 1:** Half to be given in first 8 hours; remaining over next 16 hours
- **Day 2:** Half of colloids; half of electrolytes; all of insensible fluid replacement.
- Second- and third-degree (partial- and full-thickness) burns exceeding 50% TBSA are calculated on the basis of 50% TBSA

> **BOX 39.2:** "Rohilla L, Agnihotri M, Kaur S, Sharma RK, Ghai S. Effect of music therapy on pain perception, anxiety, and opioid use during dressing change among patients with burns in India: A quasi-experimental, cross-over pilot study. Ostomy/wound Management. 2018;64(10):40-46. DOI: 10.25270/owm.2018.10.4046".
>
> **Introduction:** This study was conducted to assess the effectiveness of music for relief in pain as well as anxiety during change of burn dressing.
> **Methods:** Patients from a burn unit at a tertiary care hospital in North India, participated in this quasi-experimental and, cross-over study. aim was assessed using the NRS (numerical rating scale), and anxiety was assessed using the STAT (State Trait Anxiety Test).
> **Results:** Median pain and anxiety scores were significantly lower with music therapy during dressing changes.

Nursing Management during the Emergent Phase

Nursing Assessment

- **History taking should include:**
  - Age, height, weight and BMI of the patient.
  - Causative agent (electricity, fire flame, hot liquids, chemicals, gasoline, coal tar, radiation, etc.)
  - Duration or time of exposure to causative agent.
  - Circumstances around the injury (closed or open spacing, intentional or accidental, or burn to oneself, etc.
  - Initial treatment, first aid, emergency care (including fluids, intubation, etc.), or the care rendered in another health facility.
  - Preexisting medical problems and current medications.
  - Other injuries (e.g., associated fall, explosion, or assaults, etc.)
  - Evidence of inhalation injury (as explained in clinical manifestations above).
- Ongoing hemodynamic and respiratory assessment has to be performed every 6 hourly. This includes signs of infection, such as fever or foul-smelling discharge from wounds, etc.

Nursing Diagnoses

- Impaired gas (oxygen-carbon dioxide) exchange related to carbon monoxide or smoke inhalation, and/or obstruction of the upper airway.
- Risk for excess fluid volume related to fluid resuscitation.
- Ineffective thermoregulation related to reduced thermal regulation by the skin's barrier, hypothalamic response and/or infection.
- Risk for Infection related to altered immune response and lost skin barrier.

Nursing Interventions

Maintenance of adequate tissue oxygenation

- Assess respiratory status (breath sounds, respiratory rate, rhythm, and depth).
- Provide humidified oxygen.
- Observe for the following signs of inhalation injury:
  - Erythema or blistering near mouth and nose
  - Burnt or charred nostrils
  - Burns that involve face, neck/chest
  - Voice hoarseness
  - Soot/carbon in patient's sputum or respiratory secretions
- Monitor for signs of hypoxia (check arterial blood gas reports, pulse oximetry, etc.)
- Report signs of hypoxia, such as dyspnea, decreasing oxygen saturation, etc., immediately.
- Keep intubation and escharotomy tray ready.
- Monitor the mechanically ventilated (patients on ventilator) patients closely.

Facilitation of fluid balance

- Adjust fluid intake as tolerated.
- Maintain an hourly urine output of at least 50 mL. Maintain accurate intake and output charts.
- Check the patients' weight daily.
- Keep a check on the serum electrolytes and replace accordingly in intravenous fluids.
- Observe any signs of fluid overload and administer diuretics accordingly.

Promoting stable body temperature

- Do not expose wounds unnecessarily to minimize heat loss.
- Maintain warm temperature in environment.
- Use blowers/warmers, blankets, etc., to keep the patient warm.
- Keep top layer of dressing always dry to reduce evaporative heat loss.
- Use warm solutions for cleansing and dressing.

Avoiding infection (both local and systemic)

- Practice proper hand washing both before and after patient contact.
- Use barrier nursing (isolation, gown or plastic apron). Cover hair and wear masks.
- Use sterile gloves during dressing changes and all other nursing care activities involving contact with the patient.
- Provide tetanus prophylaxis.
- Change IV tubing and lines as per the hospital infection control protocol.
- Administer antibiotics, as prescribed.
- Assess wounds daily for local signs of infection. (swelling and redness, purulent discharge, discoloration, loss of grafts)
- Maintain personal hygiene of the patient (cleaning of unburned areas, mouth care, hair care, and care of IV and urinary catheter sites).
- Inspect the skin for pressure ulcers and skin breakdown.
- Report all signs of infections local or systemic immediately.

Potential Complications during Emergent Phase and their Management

- **Acute respiratory failure:**
  - Assess for respiratory distress, dyspnea, etc.
  - Monitor pulse oximetry for oxygen saturation and the arterial blood gas reports regularly (watch for decrease in PO_2 and increase in PCO_2).
  - X-ray examination of chest is needed to assess the status of lungs.
  - Assess for alteration in level of consciousness, confusion or delirium.

- **Distributive shock:**
  - Assess for decrease in urine output, blood pressure, or increase in pulse.
  - Check for peripheral or pulmonary edema due to third space fluid shifts.
  - Adjust fluid resuscitation accordingly.
- **Acute renal failure:**
  - Monitor urine output and renal function reports regularly.
  - Assess urine for hemoglobin or myoglobin loss.
  - Administer the fluids/diuretics if needed.
- **Compartment syndrome:** If the trunk or any extremity has circumferential burns, the nerves and blood vessels beneath the burn tissue get compressed due to the increase in interstitial fluid. This is called the compartment syndrome as the involved part gets 'compartmentalized' and separate from the whole body. The reduced or blocked blood and nerve supply can quickly progress the area to necrosis and non-viability. In case of delay in management, compartment syndrome can lead to loss of the extremity (amputation). For keeping a check on this, check the,
  - Peripheral pulses every two hours.
  - Warmth, loss of sensation, capillary refill time
  - Movement of extremities every two hours.

The Acute (Healing Phase)

Medical Management

After the first 48 hours, stage of shock resolves and physiological changes start appearing as follows:

- **Airway obstruction** is caused by upper airway edema. Intubation and mechanical ventilation is often needed. Frequent arterial blood gas analysis and continuous oxygen saturation monitoring using a pulse oximeter determines this need.
- **Risk of fluid overload** develops as the capillaries regain integrity and reversal of the third space shift occurs. Inadequate cardiac and renal function can cause congestive heart failure and pulmonary edema. Central venous or peripheral arterial catheters may be needed. (Monitor venous/arterial pressures, pulmonary artery pressures, and cardiac output).
- **Blood loss, anemia and hypoproteinemia** is treated by appropriate administration of blood components.
- **Infection progressing to septic shock** needs to be watched among those who have survived the first few days after a major burn.
- **Immunosuppression** is often seen after a major burn injury. It leads to a higher risk for sepsis. Infection from the burn site spreads quickly through the blood. Elevated body temperature due to septicemia can aggravate metabolic distress and increased oxygen needs of the tissues.

Infection Prevention

- When the burn wound is in the healing phase it needs to be protected from all sources of infection. However, after a severe burn, the gut becomes permeable and the gut flora is able to enter the systemic circulation. So, the source of infection can be either the environment or the patients' intestinal tract itself.
- Commonly, bacteria, such as '*Staphylococcus*,' '*Proteus*,' '*Pseudomonas*,' '*Escherichia coli*,' and '*Klebsiella*' and fungi, such as '*Candida albicans*' can be found in such cases.
- The infection can either be local at the wound site and second at the systemic circulation level.
- Infection slows the burn wound healing as it promotes excessive inflammation and tissue damages. Barrier nursing involves use of sterile cap, gown, gloves and mask at all times while caring for the burn patient.
- Blood and tissue specimens for culture are regularly taken to monitor for colonization of by any microbial organisms. Systemic antibiotics according to the sensitivity of the organism found in the tissue or blood culture report are administered.
- Not just the patient, but the whole burn unit requires frequent check on the microbial flora present there. Samples from surfaces and equipments are sent for bacterial colonization and systematic carbolization should be done daily, fogging of the entire unit should be done every 15 days. Careful attention should be paid to the antibiotic use among burn patients as inappropriate use can affect the microbial flora present in the burn unit significantly.

Antimicrobial Therapy

- Tetanus toxoid is given to the patients as early as possible.
- Systemic antibiotics are not recommended until there are evidences of systemic infections in blood cultures.
- Topical agents are used after the wound is cleansed.
- Topical therapy promotes healing of the wound. Criteria for choosing a topical agent are:
  - Effective for 'gram-negative organisms', '*Pseudomonas aeruginosa*', '*Staphylococcus aureus*', and fungi.
  - Not systemically toxic.
  - Cost-effective and acceptable to patient.
  - Should be easy to apply.
  - Commonly used topical agents include silver sulfadiazine (Silvadene), colloidal silver (megaheal), silver nitrate, etc.

Burn Wound Cleaning and Dressing Procedure

- Wound cleaning is usually performed every alternate day or daily as per the unit's protocol.
- Before the wound cleaning procedure, ensure adequate vital signs, nutrition and pain control as it is a challenging process for the patient.
- Tap water at room temperature is used for burn wound cleansing.
- Active participation of the patient is encouraged during the procedure.
- Unburned areas, including the hair are washed as well.
- During every dressing, the non-viable tissue over the wound is gently removed under aseptic conditions using forceps (mechanical debridement) or hydrogen peroxide (chemical debridement). Additionally, surgical debridement is performed in operation theatre if needed.
- After cleaning, the wound is gently patted with cotton towels/gauze dressing pads.

- A topical antimicrobial agent is then applied over the wounds.
- The wound is then covered with several layers of gauze and cotton pads and bandaged over.
- To allow for motion, a light dressing is used over joints.
- Circumferential dressings are applied distal to proximal.
- Fingers and toes are wrapped separately to prevent sticking together and promote adequate healing.
- Burns to the face are left open after cleaning and the topical agent is applied.

Burn Wound Grafting

Grafting is the surgical procedure whereby a necrosed burn tissue is removed and a healthy tissue substitute is placed over (or transplanted to) that wound area. If wounds are deep (full thickness) or extensive, grafting is done as spontaneous re-epithelialization is difficult. So, wound grafting is done to:
- Reduce infection risk.
- Reduce proteins, fluids, and electrolytes loss.
- Reduce burn surface area to minimize heat loss.
- Permit early functional ability and reduce risk of contractures.

Types of grafts

1. **Biological grafts:** The biological grafts include skin tissues either some recently deceased human or the amniotic membrane of the placenta (homograft), animal skin usually from pigs (xenografts) or the burn patients' skin itself from a non-burn area (autograft) **(Figs. 39.3A and B)**. Autografts can be either split thickness skin graft (STSG) which involves the dermis, and part of dermis or full thickness skin graft (FTSG) which involves the epidermis and whole of the dermis.

    The grafting procedure is always performed under strict sterile conditions in an operation theater. A tool called the 'Dermatome' which looks and functions like a vegetable peeler is used to raise a thin layer of skin from the patient's body which has not burnt. The burn wound is cleaned aggressively to remove all the debris and dead skin before putting the grafted skin. Then the graft is meshed and spread over the burn wound **(Figs. 39.3A and B)**.

2. **Biosynthetic and synthetic:** The biosynthetic and synthetic grafts have the properties of easy availability, sterility, and cost-efficient, e.g., **Biobrane** (nylon or silastic membrane that has collagen). It is semi-transparent, sterile and can be left intact for 3–4 weeks. It is used as an intermediate dressing until an autograft becomes available. Synthetic grafts are costly but very useful for patients who have higher TBSA leaving no possibility to raise an autograft. They are easy to apply. The grafting procedure can be done at the patients' bedside using local anesthesia as well. So, they are also suitable for the patients who are not hemodynamically stable to tolerate general anesthesia in operation theater.

3. **Dermal substitutes:**
    - *Artificial skin (Integra):* It is made up of two layers—epidermal, consisting of silastic, and dermal that is made up of animal collagen (usually cow or shark cartilage). It is used to cover the wound like a protective barrier, and it helps in re-growth of the skin.
    - *Alloderm:* It is a processed kind of dermis made from human cadaver skin. Alloderm grafts have a shelf life of about 2 years when stored in special refrigerators properly. They have very less scarring and post-grafting results are mostly acceptable. In India, allograft use is restricted to major cities and involve high cost.

Care of grafts

1. Blood, serum, or eschar between the wound area and graft, can cause graft loss.
2. Trauma during dressing changes, and infections are other reasons for graft loss.
3. Occlusive dressings are often used to immobilize the grafted area.
4. The grafts on torso or face can be immobilized using skin staples and left open.
5. The dressing after grafting is usually performed after 3–5 days.
6. If the graft gets displaced, apply sterile compresses (saline) to prevent drying.
7. Positioning and turning of the patient are done very carefully to avoid mishandling or pressure on the grafted area.

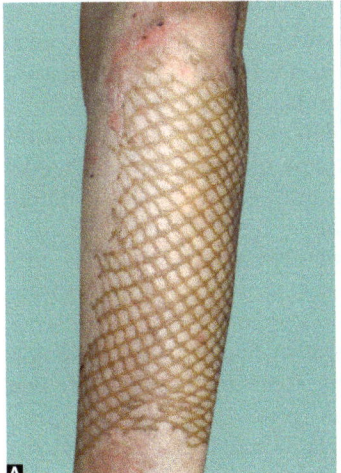 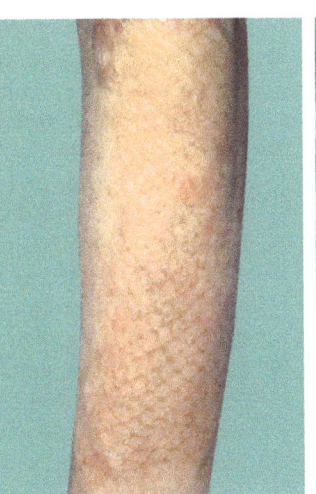 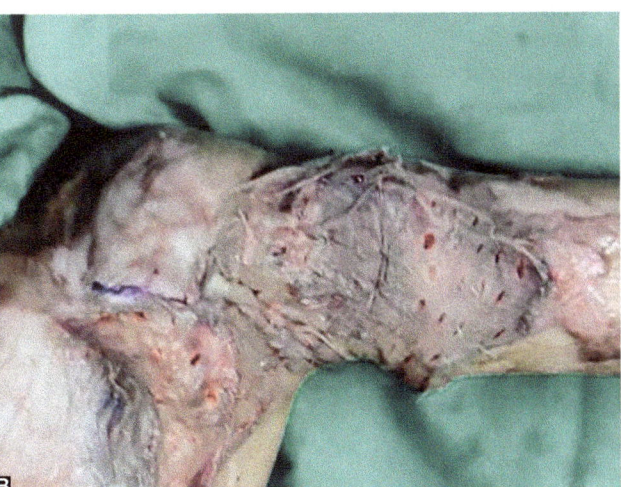

Figs. 39.3A and B: Split thickness skin graft: (A) An autograft application and after healing; (B) Intraoperative picture of applying a autograft.

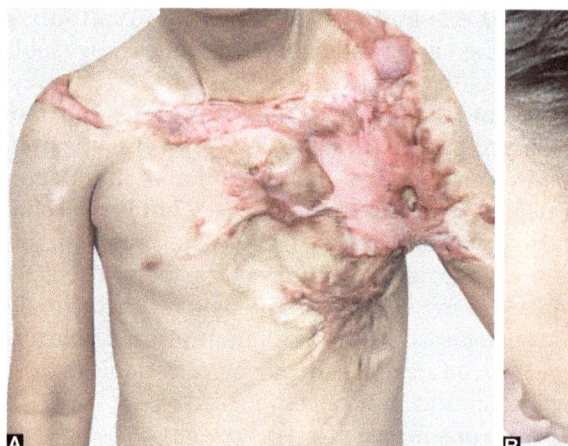 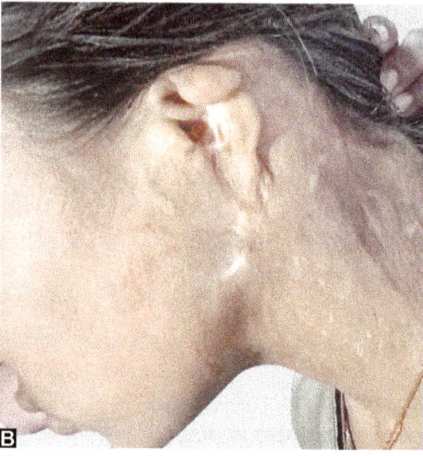 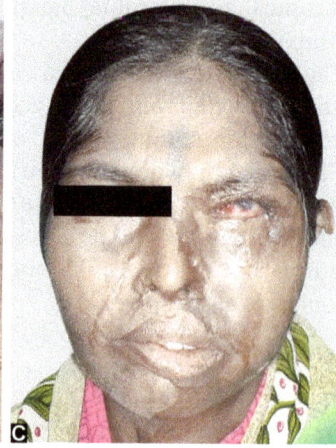

Figs. 39.4A to C: Disorders of burn wound healing: (A) Contractures; (B) Ear deformity; (C) Hypertrophic scarring and permanent mouth and eye deformity.

8. The extremity that has been grafted, should be kept elevated to minimize edema and improve venous return.
9. The patient is advised to begin exercise of the grafted area after 5–7 days of grafting.
10. Hypertrophic scarring, keloid formation and contractures are common disorders of burn wound healing that result from excessive abnormal healing. They are closely monitored for and prevented **(Figs. 39.4A to C)**.

Care of the donor site
- A moist gauze dressing is applied at the donor site immediately during the surgery. This is done to maintain some pressure on it to hault blood or fluid ooze from it. A thrombostatic agent, such as thrombin or adrenaline (epinephrine) is applied using a gauze dipped in it.
- The donor site may be dressed using a gauze with petrolatum, or biosynthetic dressing like 'Biobrane'.
- Donor sites should be kept clean, dry and pressure-free.

Nursing Management during the Acute (Healing) Phase (After 48 Hours to 15 Days)

Nursing Assessment
- Detailed respiratory assessment.
- Circulatory status assessment by checking blood pressure, heart rate.
- Strict intake-output monitoring.
- Round the clock temperature assessment for signs of infection.
- Pain assessment.

Nursing Goals
- Continuous assessment and maintenance of all body functions, such as the respiratory, circulatory and gastrointestinal function.
- Preventing infections, burn wound care (as explained previously)
- Analgesics for pain management.
- Nutritional support by means of oral intake, Ryle's tube feed or total parenteral nutrition.

Nursing Diagnosis
- Ineffective airway clearance related to inhalation injury and pulmonary edema
- Acute pain related to exposed nerves in burn wound.
- Impaired skin integrity related to burn injury and surgical interventions (donor sites).
- Imbalanced nutrition related to inability to increased metabolic needs and inability to intake orally.
- Impaired physical mobility related to peripheral edema and weakness.

Nursing Interventions

Maintain a patent airway and an adequate airway clearance:
- Maintain a patent airway at all times (Fowler's positioning, suctioning of secretions, and providing oxygen or artificial airway).
- Encourage patient to change positions, and practice deep breathing exercises.
- Incentive spirometry and coughing exercises are useful.

Reducing Pain
- Anticipatory analgesics are given round the clock. Regular pain assessment is done.
- Administer the analgesics before wound care and other procedures which can be painful.
- Oral analgesics should be given 30–45 minutes before the procedure.
- Reduce anxiety by explanations of all nursing procedures.
- Use relaxation techniques, guided imagery, meditation, etc., for pain and anxiety.

Protecting and Re-establishing the Integrity of the Skin
- Clean wounds and assist in dressing changes as per unit protocol. Use soap and water or any antimicrobial solution to wash the wounds. Dry them gently.
- After cleaning, the debridement procedure is performed. Gauze, scissors, or forceps may be used as needed. Debridement of the dead tissue is done for 20–30 minutes as tolerated by the patient.
- Apply topical bacteriostatic agents, such as silver sulfadiazine or colloidal silver as layer (1/8-inch (3-mm) thick).
- Using burn pads, gauze rolls, etc., layers of dressing are put over the wounds. Dressings are held in place using 6-inch rolled gauze.
- For grafted areas, caution is needed while removing dressings; observe for blood or pus discharge. Check the wounds daily and document the wound status as per protocol.

Maintaining Adequate Nutrition

- Oral fluids are initiated only after the bowel sounds have appeared back.
- Assess the patient's tolerance for fluids first. If tolerated well (no vomiting and or abdominal distention), intake is increased gradually. Progress to a normal diet or to Ryle's tube feeds.
- High proteins and high calories diet is given to these patients. Supplements for vitamin and mineral are given as a routine.
- If giving RT feeds, the volume of residual gastric secretions is checked. Parenteral nutrition may be indicated.
- The patient having anorexia is encouraged to increase food intake gradually.
- The patient's food preferences and pleasant surroundings can encourage food intake.

Promoting Physical Mobility

- Deep breathing exercises and frequent change of positioning are done. They help in preventing atelectasis/pneumonia, peripheral and pedal edema, pressure ulcers and contractures.
- Early sitting and early ambulation are good.
- When the lower extremities are involved in burns, elastic pressure bandages are applied to promote venous return and minimize swelling. Elevate lower limbs while patient is lying down.
- Practice both the passive and active ROM (range-of-motion) exercises daily.
- Use splints over the extremities for contracture control.
- Monitor the splinted areas frequently for any signs of distress (vascular insufficiency or nerve compression).

Rehabilitation Phase of Burn Care

This phase begins immediately after the injury and often continues for years. The main goals to be achieved in this phase are:

- Wound healing
- Restore maximum functional ability of the body in activities of daily living.
- Psychosocial support for enhancing self-image.
- Maintaining good fluid and nutritional status.
- Pre and post nursing care for reconstructive and aesthetic surgeries.

Nursing Management during the Rehabilitation Phase

Nursing Assessment

1. Patient's self-concept, current mental status.
2. Level of pain and physical discomfort.
3. Education and occupation status.
4. Cultural background.
5. Range of motion, functional ability for ambulation, eating, wound care, etc.

Nursing Diagnosis

- Activity intolerance related to pain, skin and joint contractures.
- Ineffective coping related to disturbed body image.
- Knowledge deficit related to post-discharge care at home.

Nursing Interventions

Promoting ability to perform the activities of daily living (ADLs):

- Encourage the patient to perform all ROM exercises with periods of rest in between.
- Prevent burn contractures by performing ROM exercises. Use pressure garments and splints to support during exercises.
- Position the patient such that adhesions and contractures are prevented.
- Provide pain management.
- Recreational therapy and spending time with loved ones can improve tolerance for physical activity.
- Help the patient achieve adequate sleep through medication and other environmental measures.
- Provide adequate sleep. Reassurance and administration of hypnotic drugs helps to promote sleep.
- Reduce metabolic stress by adequate relieving of pain helps in conserving energy for exercises.

Enhancing Coping Mechanisms

- Assess and respect the patient's current coping mechanisms.
- Listen to the patient. Explore alternate mechanisms with the patient.
- No false assurances should be given.
- Interpret patient behavior with the help of family members.
- Facilitate interaction with other burn survivors in the ward that may be admitted for reconstructive surgeries or during follow-ups.
- Appreciate the improvements made by the patient to improve self-esteem.
- Refer to psychologists, occupational therapists, medical social workers for assistance in enhancing emotional status as well as coping skills.

Preserving Positive Body Image and Self-concept

- Seek information on the patient's pre-burn self-image.
- Encourage the patient to express his concerns, when the patient is ready. Be honest, but positive when talking to the patient.
- Reinforce appropriate and effective coping shown by patient.
- Motivate the patient to talk with other burn survivors who are progressing satisfactorily.

Providing Discharge Teaching

- Stress on the need of regular ROM exercises because the contractures at joints are the most common sequel of burn injury which is easily preventable.
- Instruct the patient to wash the small areas to clean the open wounds and to apply topical agents. Emollients like coconut oil can be applied to the healed wounds to reduce scarring and keep wound soft and protected.
- Pain management and nutritional supplements continue for few months after discharge.
- Explain about when and where to come for follow-up. Also, explain what to expect during the follow-up visits.
- Teach them to recognize danger signs of infection like fever, swelling, discharge or pus in the wounds. Instruct them to report to physician immediately.

GERIATRIC CONSIDERATIONS

Burn injury during old age raises the risk of poor prognosis. It requires an extra attention by the nurse. The following points in each phase of management of burn injury need to be kept in mind.

1. **Emergency phase:**
   - Particular attention to pulmonary status, any other comorbidity or history of medications.
   - Cautious fluid resuscitation as risk of fluid overload in much more in the elderly patients. Acute renal failure can result.
   - Reduced immunological response make them more at risk for infections.
   - Close monitoring and prompt treatment of complications.
   - As skin is fragile, they are more prone to develop deep wounds.
2. **Acute phase:**
   - Aggressive pulmonary care by steam inhalation, breathing exercises and chest physiotherapy.
   - Early mobilization to prevent complications as well as pressure ulcers in case of prolonged hospitalization.
   - Along with fever, watch carefully for the other signs of infections locally at the wound area.
3. **Rehabilitation phase:**
   - Take into account previous limitations in physical activity that can be there like arthritis to plan range of motion activities.
   - Elderly patients may not be having many family members to provide emotional support during home care. Identify the person closest to the elderly and involve him in care.

CONCLUSION

A burn injury is a life-threatening injury. It always requires a timely intervention to manage the patient well. Fluid resuscitation forms the most important part of management at hospital. Barrier nursing is advocated in burn units as the patients are highly vulnerable to infections due to loss of protective skin accompanied by lowered immunity. Thus, the nurses working in the burn unit need to be very vigilant. Also, the burn pain is continuous and very severe. As a nurse, we should understand and able to interpret the pain level to provide relief to the patient accordingly.

Case Scenario

1. A woman carrying a pot of boiling water lost her balance and spilled the water on her right hand. How will you classify the burn? What will be the acute management for her?
2. A patient with 30% TBSA has just returned from the operation theater after "Debridement and grafting" surgery. What will be the special nursing considerations?
3. A female aged 25 years has reached the ER department with a history of stove blast? Is it a medicolegal case? If yes, what all should be noted and recorded immediately about the patients' condition?
4. A 55-year-old male patient with 90% TBSA including facial burns succumbed to the burn injuries and died. What are the special nursing considerations to be vigilant about?

SUMMARY

Any damage to the body's tissues which is most often caused by direct heat, chemicals, or electricity is called burn injury. There are four types of burns:
1. **First-degree burns:** Damage the outermost layer of skin, the epidermis.
2. **Second-degree burns:** Damage the epidermis and part of dermis.
3. **Third-degree burns:** Destroy both epidermis and dermis, reaches the subcutaneous tissue.
4. **Fourth degree burn** damages all layers of the skin, deeper tissues beneath, muscles and bones.

Burns can lead to blisters, lifelong scars, shock, or death. They can be a source of systemic infections. Treatment for burns depends on the cause, depth and TBSA involved. Antibiotic creams are used to prevent and treat infections of the burn wound. For major burns, treatment involves regular cleaning of the wound, replacing the skin with grafts, and making sure that the patient has adequate nutrition and fluids. Rehabilitation after the burn injury is as important as the acute phase management as the burns leave a devastating effect on the mind and body of a person. Emotional support is required in every phase of the burn management.

MULTIPLE CHOICE QUESTIONS

1. **This graft includes the epidermis and a part of the dermis. This graft is called:**
   a. Full thickness graft
   b. Dermal graft
   c. Epidermal graft
   d. Split thickness graft
2. **Burns are classified according to total burn surface area using which of the following formulas:**
   a. Lund and Browder formula
   b. Brooke Army formula
   c. Parkland formula
   d. Baxter formula
3. **According to Rule of Nines, a person with whole chest, abdomen and face burnt will have a TBSA of?**
   a. 10%
   b. 50%
   c. 45%
   d. 60%
4. **When providing care to a patient with massive full thickness electrical burn, the nurse should monitor the urine report for:**
   a. Potassium and urea
   b. Free iron and white blood cells
   c. Proteins and red blood cells
   d. Hemoglobin and myoglobin
5. **The .... layer of the skin regulates the body temperature:**
   a. Epidermis
   b. Endodermis
   c. Hyperdermis
   d. Muscle
6. **A 25-year-old male is received with burn on right leg. The burn area has small blisters, is pink, moist and shiny. The burn will be documented as:**
   a. 1st degree
   b. 2nd degree
   c. 3rd degree
   d. 4th degree
7. **Ramesh has been admitted with full-thickness burns involving the face and neck. It is priority to:**
   a. Prevent hypothermia
   b. Prevent hypotension
   c. Assess airway
   d. Prevent infection
8. **During the emergent phase of burn management, you would expect the following laboratory values:**
   a. Low sodium, low potassium, high glucose, low hematocrit
   b. High sodium, low potassium, low glucose, high hematocrit
   c. High sodium, high potassium, high glucose, low hematocrit
   d. Low sodium, high potassium, high glucose, high hematocrit

9. Best diet for a burn patient in acute phase shall include food that is?
   a. Low fiber, low calories, low protein
   b. High calorie, high protein and high carbohydrate
   c. High potassium, low carbohydrate, and low protein
   d. Low sodium, high protein, restrict fluids

10. A patient has deep burns on both arms and hands. It is nursing priority to:
    a. Elevate and extend the extremities
    b. Elevate and flex the extremities
    c. Keep extremities below heart level and extended
    d. Keep extremities level with the heart level and flexed.

11. A 7-year-old child has 3rd degree burns over 36% TBSA. What is the nursing priority during this initial phase management of this child?
    a. Fluid resuscitation   b. Grafting of wounds
    c. Thermoregulation   d. Pain management

12. A patient with sunburn is documented as:
    a. First degree
    b. Second degree partial thickness
    c. Third degree full thickness
    d. Fifth degree

13. Which burn will be painless to the patient?
    a. First degree   b. Second degree
    c. Third degree   d. Fourth degree

14. A child has experienced burns from the bathtub to both legs. The nurse knows that the percentage of the body according to rule of Nines?
    a. 15%   b. 30%
    c. 19%   d. 28%

15. The main cause of death in persons who initially survived major burns?
    a. Loss of skin barrier   b. Systemic infections
    c. Severe dehydration   d. B and C

16. What is the first aid for an electric burn?
    a. Put ice on the burnt area of contact.
    b. Cover the burn with sheet
    c. Ensure the person is not in contact with the electric source
    d. Putting water over the burn

17. If a patient has facial swelling and soot in the oral cavity, what management is a priority?
    a. Early intubation or tracheostomy
    b. 100% oxygen flow through nasal prongs
    c. Monitor respiratory status with pulse oximetry
    d. Admission to the burn unit

18. What is the most important step while sending a burn patient body to mortuary?
    a. Documentation of cause of death
    b. Removal of tubings
    c. Correct identification tagging at three places on the body.
    d. Plugging nostrils

19. Which type of graft is raised from the patient's own body?
    a. Allograft   b. Homograft
    c. Autograft   d. Xenograft

20. The physician removes the debris including the shedding tissue from over the burn wound using forceps prior to dressing. This procedure is called:
    a. Grafting   b. Wound dressing
    c. Cleaning   d. Debridement

ANSWERS

1. d	2. a	3. c	4. d
5. b	6. b	7. c	8. d
9. b	10. a	11. a	12. a
13. d	14. d	15. b	16. c
17. c	18. c	19. c	20. d

SUGGESTED READING

1. Hauser SL, Longo DL, Jameson JL, Kasper DL, Fauci AS, Braunwald E. Harrison's Principles of Internal Medicine.16th edition. USA: McGraw-Hill Companies; 2005. pp. 122-254.
2. Higashimori T, Kono T, Sakurai H, Nakazawa H, Groff W. Treatment of Mesh Skin Grafted Scars Using a Plasma Skin Regeneration System. Plastic Surgery International; 2010. pp. 1-4. doi:10.1155/2010/874348
3. Initial assessment and management of burn patients. In: Strauss S, Gillespie GL (eds). American Nurse Today. 2018;13(6):15-19.
4. Jong AEE, Middlekoop E, Faber AW, Loey NEE. Non pharmacological nursing interventions for procedural pain relief in adults with burns: A systematic review. Burns. 2007;33:811-27.
5. Nettina SM, Mills EJ, Lippincott Manual of Nursing Practice.10th Edition. Philadelphia: Lippincott Williams & Wilkins: 2013:1121-37.
6. Rohilla L, Agnihotri M, Kaur S, Sharma RK, Ghai S. Effect of music therapy on pain perception, anxiety, and opioid use during dressing change among patients with burns in India: A quasi-experimental, cross-over pilot study. Ostomy/wound Management. 2018;64(10):40-6. DOI: 10.25270/owm.2018.10.4046.
7. Smeltzer SC, Bare B. Brunner and Suddarth's Textbook of Medical-Surgical Nursing. 12th edition. Philadelphia: Lippincott Williams and Wilkins; 2010. pp. 1704-39.
8. Smolle C, Cambiaso-Daniel J, Forbes AA, Wurzer P, Hundeshagen G, Branski LK, et al. Recent trends in burn epidemiology worldwide: A systematic review. Burns. 2017; 43(2): 249-57. doi:10.1016/j.burns.2016.08.013.
9. Teague H, Swencki SA, Tang A. The Burned Patient: Assessment, Diagnosis, and Management in the ED. Trauma Reports; 2005. [Assessed on March 26, 2021]. Assessed from https://www.reliasmedia.com/articles/84953-the-burned-patient-assessment-diagnosis-and-management-in-the-ed

UNIT V

Oncological Disorders

OUTLINE

40. Cancer
Gurpreet Kaur, Latika Rohilla

41. Treatment Modalities of Cancer
Maninderdeep Kaur, Divya Dahiya, Pramod Kumar

42. Oncological Emergencies
Puneet Kaur, Sukhpal Kaur

43. Palliative Care
Sukhpal Kaur, Jyoti Kathwal

CHAPTER 40

Cancer

Gurpreet Kaur, Latika Rohilla

"When cancer happens, you don't put life on hold. You live now."
—**Fabi Powell, Caregiver**

LEARNING OBJECTIVES

After going through the chapter, the learner will be able to:
- Illustrate the epidemiology of cancer.
- Define the structure and characteristics of normal and cancer conditions.
- Elaborate the etiopathogenesis of cancer.
- Enumerate various factors of carcinoma.
- Discuss various diagnostic modalities for the diagnosis of cancer.
- Enlist the diagnostic procedures used to confirm the diagnosis of carcinoma.
- Discuss psychosocial aspects of cancer.

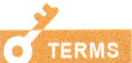

TERMS

- **Anaplasia:** Cells with a lack of normal cellular features in relation to cells of origin.
- **Benign:** A non-spreading carcinoma.
- **Chemotherapy:** Cancer treatment based upon chemo agents that may either kill or halt the growth of the cancer cells.
- **Dysplasia:** Unusual cell growth leading to cells with different features from the same type of tissue.
- **Hyperplasia:** Upsurge of the cell production in normal tissue or organ.
- **Mammogram:** It is an X-ray image of the breast.
- **Metaplasia:** Transformation of a particular type of cell into another type.
- **Metastasis:** Spreading of carcinoma from the place of origin to other body parts.
- **Neoplasia:** Uncontrolled cell growth in the absence of any physiologic demand.
- **Palliative care:** Comfort promotion and relief from pain to improve the quality of life.
- **PAP (Papanicolaou) test:** A test that collects cells from the cervix of the female to be further evaluated for cancer.
- **Staging:** Process to define the size of the tumor along with the extent of spread and metastasis.
- **Xerostomia:** Dryness of the mouth.

INTRODUCTION

Carcinoma or cancer is a disease condition in which cells of the body begin to multiply in an uncontrolled manner. This process can start almost anywhere in our body. Normally, the body cells multiply by cell division to form new cells. As the cells grow old, they die, and new cells replace them. Sometimes, this process is disturbed and abnormal cells grow and start multiplying. These cells then become a tumor, which is nothing but a lump of tissue. Tumors can be either cancerous or not cancerous (benign). Cancerous tumors can invade nearby tissues and can travel to other body parts to form new tumors.

CONCEPT AND DEFINITION

Cancer is a group of diseases that commence with the abnormal proliferation and growth of the cells. These cells can invade the surrounding cells and tissues, and further enter into the lymphatic and blood circulation. This process is known as metastasis when abnormal cancer cells enter the other bodily organs and impair their functioning.

EPIDEMIOLOGY OF CANCER

World

- Cancer is the most common cause of death worldwide, contributing to nearly 10 million deaths in 2020, and causing one in every 6th death.
- The overall incidence of cancer is higher among males in comparison to females and more in industrialized nations. The risk increases with age.
- According to the World Health Organization (WHO), the following sites were holding the given proportional figures:
  - Breast (2.26 million cases)
  - Lung (2.21 million cases)
  - Colon and rectum (1.93 million cases)
  - Prostate (1.41 million cases)
  - Skin (non-melanoma) (1.20 million cases)
  - Stomach (1.09 million cases)
- Cancer-related mortality in 2020 (WHO):
  - Lung (1.80 million deaths)
  - Colon and rectum (916 000 deaths)
  - Liver (830 000 deaths)
  - Stomach (769 000 deaths)
  - Breast (685 000 deaths).
- An estimated one-third of cancer-related mortality is attributed to tobacco and alcohol consumption along with higher body mass index, less consumption of fruits and vegetables, and a sedentary lifestyle.
- In the case of infection-induced cancers, human papilloma (HPV) viruses and hepatitis B and C accounted for approximately 30% of the cancer burden among the low and lower middle-income world countries.

India

- Estimated Indian figures for cancer cases and deaths were up to 1,157,294 and 784,821 respectively in the year 2018 (WHO, Cancer Country Profile 2020)
- In India, breast carcinoma is the leading cause contributing to cancer-related mortality (14%), followed by lip and oral cavity cancer (8.4%).

REVIEW OF STRUCTURE AND CHARACTERISTICS OF NORMAL AND CANCER CELL

A cell is the smallest unit of life that can live independently and further acts as the building block of all the living organisms and tissues of the body.

A normal cell consists of three parts, these are: (1) The cell membrane; (2) The nucleus; and (3) The cytoplasm. Within the cytoplasm lies intricate arrangements of fine fibers and hundreds or even thousands of minuscule but distinct structures called organelles. **Figures 40.1A and B** show the structure of a normal cell and a cancer cell.

Features of a Normal Cell

- Can control their growth and division using external signals, which means they divide only when required.
- As a part of normal development, they undergo programmed cell death (apoptosis). This helps to maintain tissue homeostasis.
- They intend to remain adhered to each other by selective adhesions, preventing their movement to the other body parts.
- While having the same genome they can differentiate into specialized cells with specific functions despite having different physical appearances.

Features of a Cancer Cell

Cancer causes specific changes in the genes of the cells. These changes disrupt the normal functioning mechanism of the cells, abruptly hampering normal cell functioning. This change specifically affects cell growth and division.

Various cells follow rapid proliferative patterns during their lifespan. These are:

- **Hyperplasia:** "Increase in the number of cells"
- **Metaplasia:** "Transformation of a particular type of cells into another type"
- **Dysplasia:** "Abnormal cell growth within a tissue with different features. It may indicate a stage prior to the development of cancer".
- **Anaplasia:** "Cells with lack of normal cellular features in relation to cells of origin"

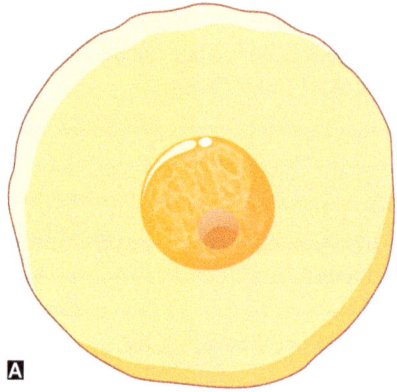

A

Normal cell (fine chromatin, single nucleus, single nucleolus, large cytoplasm)

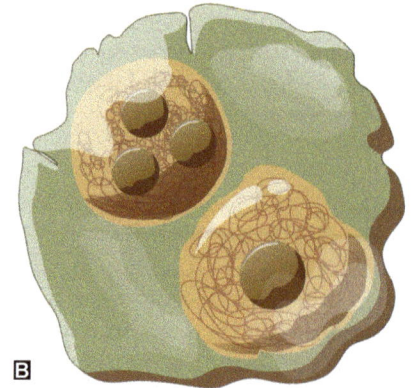

B

Cancer cell (coarse chromatin, multiple nuclei, single nucleoli, small cytoplasm)

Figs. 40.1A and B: Normal and cancer cell.

TABLE 40.1: Characteristics of malignant cells.	
	Characteristics of malignant Cells
Cellular features	Cells are atypical and often do not resemble the cells having origin from the same tissues
Growth patterns	Mostly grow in the periphery and send their processes, that infiltrate and destroy the neighboring tissues
Metastasis	Once cancer cells enter into the blood or lymphatic stream, easily spread out to the distant body parts
Tissue destruction	As a tumor increases in size, it leads to compromised blood flow to the area or may produce chemical substances leading to tissue damage, this uncontrolled squeal can lead to anemia, significant weight loss, and subsequently can lead to death also

- **Neoplasia:** "Uncontrolled cells growth in absence of any physiologic demand"

The cancerous cells are also known as 'malignant neoplasms'. The malignant transformation of the cell commences with a genetic mutation of the cell DNA. These cells start proliferating themselves abnormally, ignoring the growth-regulating mechanism and signals present in the surrounding cell environment. Cancer is not a single disease subset; but comprises of various definitive diseases, etiological causes, clinical presentations, and varied treatments and outcomes.

Characteristics of Malignant Cells

Table 40.1 explains the characteristics of the malignant cells. The features are described in terms of the cellular feature, growth patterns, metastasis, and tissue destruction.

ETIOPATHOGENESIS OF CANCER

Various agents and factors can cause cancer, including viruses, bacteria, and certain physiochemical agents. Besides this genetic predisposition, diet, and hormone supplements are also known to cause cancer.

- **Bacteria and viruses:** Viruses are considered to cause genetic changes in the genetic structure of the cells, thus causing cancer. For example, Epstein-Barr virus infection is closely associated with Burkitt's lymphoma, and a few types of non-Hodgkin's lymphoma and Hodgkin's disease. Human papilloma viruses 16,18,31,33 are known to cause cervix cancer. Similarly, human immunodeficiency virus has been associated with Kaposi's sarcoma. Helicobacter pylori can cause gastric malignancy secondary to the injury to the gastric cells.
- **Physical agents:** These may include exposure to sunlight or radiation, and tobacco consumption. These agents irritate the exposed cells, thus triggering the carcinogenesis process.
- **Chemical agents:** About 3/4th of different forms of cancer have been found to be associated with the environment. Tobacco products are known carcinogenic agents. Tobacco smoking is strongly associated with lung cancer. Chewing it can lead to buccal cavity cancer.
- **Genetic predisposition:** Genetic factors have been considered an important predisposing factor for cancer development. For example, *BRCA-1* and *BRCA-2* genes are associated with Ca breast.
- **Dietary factors:** Dietary intake of a high caloric diet, alcohol, smoked meat, and fat can predispose the individual to cancer risk. High fiber intake, and carotenoids (tomatoes, spinach, dark green- and yellow-colored vegetables) have been thought to reduce cancer risk.
- **Hormonal agents:** Either external administration or internal hormonal imbalance can promote tumor development. Diethylstilbestrol (DES) is known to cause vaginal carcinomas.
- **Immune system failure:** Immune suppression is known to trigger the development of certain types of cancer. Tumor-associated antigens are recognized by the macrophages and T-lymphocytes as foreign, and thus they trigger both cellular and immune responses. T-lymphocytes have cytotoxic properties also. Interferons (IFN) are produced in response to viral infections and possess antitumor properties as well. Similarly natural killer cells (NK), a sub-population of lymphocytes produces enzymes and lymphokines to kill cancer cells.

In cancer, the body fails to differentiate the abnormal malignant cells from 'normal', thus fail to trigger the immune cascade against the cancer cells. Besides this, tumor antigens can form complexes with antibodies, or tumor cells disguise themselves from immune defense mechanisms. Further, carcinogens, such as chemicals can further weaken the immune system, promoting tumor growth.

PATHOPHYSIOLOGY

The cancer pathophysiology has been explained in **Flowchart 40.1**. The basic cell division process that helps in the growth and proliferation of the body cells undergoes a genetic mutation that causes unprecedented growth or multiplication of the cells. These abnormally growing cells, gain access to blood or lymphatic circulation and are moved to other body parts leading to a spread also called metastasis.

Metastatic Pathways

Blood, and lymphatic channels are the key pathways via which cancer cells spread to other parts of the body.

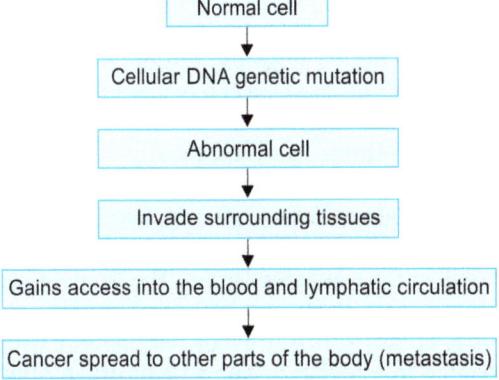

Flowchart 40.1: Pathophysiology of cancer.

Angiogenesis is another important process by which blood supply is ensured for the survival of the tumor cells.

- ❖ **Blood mechanism:** Cancer spread through this pathway directly depends upon the vascularity of the tumor. Malignant cells are capable of surviving in an environment that may lack blood supply and oxygen and attack from the body's own immune mechanism. These cells further adhere themselves to normal blood cells, such as platelets, and fibrin in order to escape the immune cascade. In order to gain entry into other cells, tumor cells secrete lysosome enzyme, which helps in its implantation into the normal cells.
- ❖ **Lymphatic mechanism:** Tumor arising from the enriched lymphatic supply areas are more likely to cause metastasis. For example, breast cancer. Because once tumor cells enter the lymphatic vessels, they are easily carried away with the lymphatic circulation to other parts of the body.
- ❖ **Angiogenesis:** In order to get nutrients and oxygen supply, cancer cells are capable of forming new capillaries from the area of their origin. This process is known as angiogenesis. Through this capillary network, cancer cells spread out to other distant sites.

STAGING OF CANCER

Staging is a process that describes how much cancer has spread across the body and which organs are involved. Staging helps to define the best available treatment options for the patient. For example, for small, localized tumors without spread, surgery or radiotherapy can be the best treatment options, and for blood cancers chemotherapy or immune therapy can be used. Staging can be done before the start of the treatment or during treatment.

Staging is cancer is done using the following different criteria:
- ❖ **Clinical staging:** It is done depending upon the physical examination, imaging results (CT or PET scan), biopsies or endoscopic results, and in blood cancer based upon the blood test and bone marrow aspirate results.
- ❖ **Pathological staging:** Here tumor or a piece of it is excised and sent for histopathological investigation. It helps to determine the pathological stage of the tumor. This gives a more precise view of the tumor which further helps the treating oncologists to determine the possibilities of other treatment options and to predict the prognosis also.
- ❖ **Recurrence or retreatment staging:** Restaging may also be done if cancer recurs or progresses. Here the new staging does not replace the original stage but is added to it.
- ❖ **TNM staging:** This is one of the most commonly used criteria for cancer staging. In this staging, cancer is described by three categories: tumor (T), node (N), and metastasis (M) in case cancer has spread to other parts of the body **(Table 40.2)**.
- ❖ **Ann Arbor system:** This is used as the landmark staging classification both for Hodgkin's and non-Hodgkin's disease. Hodgkin's disease staging classification meeting was held in 1971 at the US state of Michigan so the name of classification was agreed upon. The "staging," or extent of disease, for both HL and NHL, are similar:
    - ➤ *Stage I (early disease):* Single lymph node lymphoma located in a region or one area or organ outside the lymph node.

TABLE 40.2: TNM staging of cancer.

Tumor category	Staging
T (Primary tumor) Upon cancer detection, firstly its primary origin site is determined along with its spread across nearby areas	• **TX:** Means no information about the primary tumor/or not possible to measure • **T0:** No definite evidence of primary tumor • **Tis:** The tumor is not spread to the deeper layers and is confined to the site where it originated. Also termed as in situ or precancerous stage. • A numerical number following T (T1, T2, T3, T4) represents the extent of the tumor spread to other nearby parts of the body. The higher is the number more is the spread to the nearby organs
N (The lymph nodes) It describes the extent to which cancer has spread to the nearby lymph nodes	N letter accompanies a letter or a number: • **NX:** No symptoms of lymph node involvement or they cannot be assessed • **N0:** No evidence of nearby lymph node involvement • A numerical number following N (N1, N2, N3, N4) represents the size, location, and/or number of lymph nodes involved
M (Metastasis)	M letter represents the extent of tumor spread and it accompanies a letter or a number: • **M0:** This means cancer spread to distant organs has not been established • **M1:** Cancer has spread out to other distant parts of the body
Other notations	Many a times TNM staging is also done along with other notations by mentioning a lowercase alphabet preceding it. • "c": Represents clinical stage (e.g., cT3) • "p": Represents the pathological stage (e.g., cT3) For recurring/progressive cancers, the tumor category can also accompany another lower alphabet: • "y": Represents restaged cancers after treatment (e.g., ycT2 or ypT1) • "r": For restaged cancers after recurrence or progression (e.g., rcT2 or rpT1)

- ➤ *Stage II (locally advanced disease):* Lymphoma is located in two or more lymph node regions all located on the same side of the diaphragm or in one lymph node region and a nearby tissue or organ.
- ➤ *Stage III (advanced disease):* Two or more lymph node regions are involved, or one lymph node region and one organ, on opposite sides of the diaphragm.
- ➤ *Stage IV (disseminated disease or widespread disease):* Lymphoma is outside the lymph nodes and spleen and has spread to another area or organs such as the bone marrow, bone, or central nervous system.

Each stage is further subdivided into A and B categories depending upon the presence and absence of the following symptoms

- B category: B symptom—positive category:
  - Unexplained fever ≥38°C
  - Unexplained drenching night sweats
  - Loss of >10% body weight within the last 6 months
- A category: A is the one without B symptoms, such as fever (≥38°C), unexplained drenching night sweats, and loss of >10% body weight within the last 6 months.

Tumor Grading

It differentiates the cancer cells depending upon the degree of abnormality they look at during microscopy. Grading is further of two types:

1. **Low-grade cancers**—or well-differentiated cancer. They look nearly, such as normal cells and tend to grow slowly, often having a better prognosis.
2. **High-grade cancers**—or poorly differentiated cancers. They look more abnormal and are fast growing. And require additional and aggressive treatment in comparison to low-grade tumors.

Many a times other factors besides grading affect the line of cancer treatment. These could be:

- ❖ **Cell type:** Cancer can occur in a different types of cells in the same organ. And treatment is dependent upon the type of cells and thus can be a factor in staging. For example, cancers of the esophagus can either be squamous cell type or adenoma and the former is staged differently from esophageal carcinomas.
- ❖ **Location of the tumor:** The tumor's outlook or positioning is considered while staging. For example, cancer of the esophagus can develop in the upper, lower, or lower third of the esophagus.
- ❖ **Tumor marker levels:** The stage of cancer is affected by the blood level of the biomarkers or tumor markers. For example, in prostate cancer blood levels of prostate specific antigen (PSA) is considered while staging it.
- ❖ **Age of the patient:** Elderly are more likely to develop cancer.

DIAGNOSIS OF CANCER

Various test modalities are used for the diagnosis of cancer. The aim is to assess the presence and extent of the tumor; to assess tumor staging and grading. Various types of laboratories, imaging histopathology, and genetic tests are done for various types of cancers.

1. **Laboratory tests:** Following are the lab tests used for cancer diagnosis:
   - ➢ *Complete blood count (CBC):* This blood test helps to measure the various types of blood cells and is usually carried out to diagnose blood cancer.
   - ➢ *Blood proteins:* Various types of blood proteins are measured by electrophoresis. For example, M protein is used as an indicator for multiple myeloma.
   - ➢ *Tumor markers:* Investigation of the specific substances that are being produced by the tumor itself or by the body in response to the tumor. Various tumor markers are used to diagnose breast, colon, prostate (PSA), ovarian (CA 125), and lung cancer. For example, alpha-fetoprotein (AFP) is used in liver and germ cell cancer diagnosis.
   - ➢ *Blood test for studying the genetic material of the cancer cells:* These tests are performed to analyze the abnormal DNA structure of the cancer cells that are found in the blood.
2. **Imaging tests:** Various imaging tests performed to detect cancer are described in **Table 40.3**.
3. **Histopathology tests**: Tumor biopsies are done to remove small pieces of tumor to study under the microscope. The required tissues are removed through various procedures, such as endoscopy, incisional biopsy, fine needle aspiration, skin biopsy, etc.

ASSESSMENT OF PATIENTS WITH ONCOLOGICAL DISORDERS

Health assessment of patients with oncological disorders includes obtaining the patient's health history and performing

TABLE 40.3: Imaging-based diagnostic tests used for cancer diagnosis.

Imaging test	Explanation	Uses
Magnetic resonance imaging (MRI)	Radio-frequency and magnetic fields are used to form sectional images of body organs	Thoracic, abdominal, pelvic, and neurologic cancers
Computed tomography (CT scan)	Cross-sectional view of the successive layers of the body part under investigation is formed using a narrow beam of X-ray	Thoracic, abdominal, pelvic, and neurologic cancers
Fluoroscopy	Injected contrast agents are traced with the help of X-rays to find out tissue densities	Gastrointestinal, skin and lung cancers
Ultrasound	Deep body organ images are taken with the help of sound waves of high frequency, which are further converted electronically into images	Abdominal and pelvic cancers
Endoscopy	An endoscope is inserted into the body cavity for direct visualization. Tissue biopsies, fluid aspiration as well as therapeutic excision of small tumor can also be done during the procedure	Gastrointestinal and bronchial cancers
Positron emission tomography (PET) scan	Enhanced radio-isotope uptake by the desired organ or whole body is being assessed using computed cross-sectional images. Uptake is generally more in by the malignant tissues	Hodgkin's and non-Hodgkin's lymphoma, lung, colon, liver, breast, and gastric cancers
Radioimmunoconjugates	Radioisotopes labeled with monoclonal antibodies are injected into the body are further assessed for their aggregation at the tumor site, and are visualized with the help of scanners	Lymphomas, melanoma, breast, ovarian, colorectal, and head and neck tumors

physical assessment. This can be carried out in various settings including acute care, clinic, outpatient department, or home. Before the assessment of the patient rapport building is of utmost importance. Maintain eye-to-eye contact, listen carefully, and encourage honest communication.

- ❖ **Health history:** This should include the following components:
  - ➢ **Biographical data:** This includes the details about the patient's social profile, such as name, age, sex, marital status, occupation, and ethnicity. This can be done by interviewing the patient. Thus, rapport building before the interview is an essential step to have the trust of the patient.
  - ➢ **Chief complaints:** These complaints include the issues with which the client comes to the attention of the health care provider. For example, unexplained weight loss, and sudden fall in blood counts.
  - ➢ **Present health concern (or present illness):** It describes the road to the development of the patient's present illness. The history of the present health concern or illness is the single most important factor in helping the healthcare team to arrive at a diagnosis or determine the person's needs. It also helps in the selection of appropriate diagnostic tests for the patient. Present illness includes a recording of a series of episodes. For example, a patient with a chief complaint of episodes of post-coital vaginal bleeding for the last one month can prompt the examiner to go for a Pap smear for the patient to rule out cervical cancer. The details of the present illness are explained from the onset until the time of contact with the health care personnel. These facts are recorded in chronological order. It may also include the treatment the patient has sort before presenting with the present chief complaint. Warning signs and symptoms (pain, presence of a node, night sweating, change in bowel habits) are described in detail. The factors aggravating the current problem are also included.
  - ➢ **Past history:** After assessing the general health status, the interviewer may ask for the patient's previous health records. The medical history may include data regarding any allergies, immunization status, and the results of previous diagnostic tests, such as X-ray, mammogram, and Pap smear. It may also include information about personal health habits, diet and exercise. Physical inactivity and intake of a high salt diet have been proven predisposing factors for cancer development.
  - ➢ **Family history:** A family history of cancer is one of the predisposing risk factors for the cancer diagnosis. Genogram should be drawn to record the history of family members, including their age/sex and cause of death or, if living, their current health status. This helps to identify the disease that may have a genetic origin, such as Ca breast. The results of genetic testing or screening, if available, should be recorded.
  - ➢ **Review of systems:** This includes a detailed review of general health along with body system-specific symptoms. Assessment of body systems along with present and past symptoms helps in obtaining relevant data. Formal system-wise checklists can be used to obtain and record the information of the patient. Further, inspection, palpation, percussion, and auscultation should be used to assess the various body systems.
  - ➢ **Patient profile:** An extensive biographical information needs to be obtained for the patient. A person's ability to cope with the problem needs a critical analysis along with the chief complaints of the patient. A patient profile consists of the following content areas: Health-related past events:
    - Patient's education and occupation
    - Physical, spiritual, cultural, interpersonal environment
    - Habits
    - Any physical or mental disability
    - Self-concept
    - Sexual orientation
    - Risk or history for abuse
    - Stress and coping strategies, etc.
  - ➢ **Education and occupation:** Information pertaining to these factors helps to correlate the health status of an individual. For example, an apple grower may have excessive exposure to pesticides, which can be carcinogenic in nature, thus, exposing him to the development of hematological cancer.
  - ➢ **Environment:** It includes the type of housing, presence of hazards, and religious beliefs in relation to health and illness. Family relationships, customs, and value held also form the environment of the individual. The quality of relationships by the individual with the fellow beings also determines the interpersonal environment of the person. Health facilities availability also form an important part of the environment especially in cancer, as early diagnosis leads to more favorable outcomes.
  - ➢ **Lifestyle patterns:** Exercise has been a known factor in promoting healthy living. Inactivity causes a diminished quality of life among cancer survivors. According to WHO, mild-to-moderate physical activity for 30 min/day for 5 days a week helps to improve the overall quality of life of a person. Further sleep quality and duration, nutrition (24-hour diet recall, idiosyncrasies, restrictions); Caffeine (coffee, tea, cola, chocolate), the type and amount; Smoking (cigarette, pipe, cigar, marijuana)—the type amount per day, number of years, desire to quit; Alcohol-the type, amount, pattern over past years; drugs—the type, amount, route of administration should also be assessed, because these are the predisposing factors for the development of lung and GI cancers.
  - ➢ **Sexual habits:** Sexual habits need to be explored. For example, HIV is transmitted through sexual contact. And this predisposes a person to develop lymphomas.
- ❖ **Physical assessment:** This is done after the health history of the patient is completed. And it includes the system-wise assessment of the patients. The sequence of the physical assessment may vary according to the presenting complaints of the patients. For assessing a cancer patient, a detailed examination of all the systems is necessary. The four fundamental techniques used in the physical examination are inspection, palpation, percussion, and auscultation.
  1. *Inspection:* General observation of the patient on first contact provides an overall insight of the patient's health.

Among general observations that should be noted in the initial examination of the patient are posture and stature, body movements, nutrition, speech pattern, and vital signs. Cancer patients often suffer from fatigue and pallor. In case they have pain, then their general posture may be guarded. Facial grimace may be a sign of pain. The body parts should be inspected for the overgrowth, nodes, bleeding from the orifices, etc. Cancer patients usually have a loss of weight owing to poor nutrition or their body is not able to cope with the increased energy demands posed by cancer cells. So, they might appear thin and lean. Vital signs should be assessed. Due to cancer or accompanying infection, they may have fever, hypotension, and tachycardia. The fifth vital sign 'pain' should also be documented if present.

2. *Percussion:* This technique involves the application of physical force or tap against the body to produce a resonance. The technique of percussion translates the application of physical force into sound. The sound produced is related to the density of the organ. Through percussion, the level of fluid filled in the pleural cavity may be determined. These maneuvers are especially useful in assessing patients with gastrointestinal and thorax cancers.

3. *Auscultation:* This skill assesses the sounds created by the movement of the fluid in the body by using an instrument like a stethoscope. The frequency, intensity, and quality of the sounds are checked. This technique is very useful for the assessment of cancer patients. Being a non-invasive method, especially as cancer patients have a low resistance to infections, it helps as a diagnostic criterion. For example, murmur sounds of the heart can signify cardiotoxicities precipitated with chemotherapy. Similarly hyperactive, low, or absent bowel sounds can be present in GI cancer.

4. *Nutritional assessment:* Nutritional deficiencies are often observed among cancer patients during and after the treatment. Low dietary intake in patients with cancer secondary to anorexia, mucositis, diarrhea, and constipation is very common. Certain nutritional deficiencies can be easily assessed in cancer patients. 24-hour food recall helps to look into the intake of the patient. Patients with cancer can have physical signs indicative of nutritional deficiencies. For example, flaccid, lean, wasted muscles indicate unmet demands of the body owing to increased energy demand by the cancer cells. Similarly low skin turgor indicates dehydration. Further nausea and vomiting due to chemotherapy may also lead to lesser food intake and volume depletion. BMI is a ratio based on body weight and height. BMI below 20 is also an indicator of malnutrition, and those over 24 are at risk of obesity.

PREVENTION, SCREENING, EARLY DETECTION, WARNING SIGNS OF CANCER

Nurses and other healthcare team members are involved at every step starting from prevention to care and rehabilitation of cancer patients.

❖ **Primary prevention:** Nurses play an important role in prevention of cancer among the masses. This can involve imparting health education to the clients about the following preventive modalities to reduce the risk of developing cancer (adapted from American Cancer Society: "Taking control"):
  ➢ Avoid known carcinogens
  ➢ Adopting a healthy lifestyle (150 minutes per week moderate to high-intensity exercise program)
  ➢ Eating a healthy diet (more of fruits and vegetables, avoiding salty items such as pickles, red meat, etc.)
  ➢ Increase intake of vitamins A and C (Citrus fruits)
  ➢ Maintaining an adequate weight, reducing fat intake
  ➢ Stopping smoking cigarettes and cigars
  ➢ Reducing alcohol intake
  ➢ Wearing protective clothing in order to avoid sun exposure, thus reducing the risk of skin cancer.

  Further nurses can encourage the patients to participate in cancer awareness and prevention programs.

❖ **Secondary prevention:** Ongoing research across the globe is happening to understand the role of genetics in the carcinogenesis process. Inheritance of specific genetic mutations makes a person more susceptible to cancer. For e.g., *BRCA-1* and *BRCA-2* are associated with an increased risk of developing breast cancer. Thus, regular cancer screening among the person with increased risk can help to diagnose cancer at the earlier stages. **Table 40.4** shows the recommendations by the American Cancer Society (ACS) for the early detection of cancer among average-risk asymptomatic persons.

Public awareness of health promotion/warning signs of cancer can help to increase cancer awareness. Nurses are an integral part of these interventions, be it in health education planning and implementation, prevention, and screening programs.

The following health programs can be undertaken:
❖ Health education on the harmful effects of tobacco

TABLE 40.4: Screening recommendations for early detection of cancer.

Organ	Gender and age group	Evaluation and frequency
Colon/Rectum	Male/rectum ≥50 years	• Fecal testing for occult blood—yearly • Or colonoscopy—5 yearly • Or barium enema—every 5 yearly
Breast	Females 20–40 years	• Clinical breast examination—3 yearly • breast self-examination—every monthly • Mammogram—yearly
Prostate	≥50 years	• Prostate-specific antigen—yearly • Digital rectal examination—yearly
Cervix	Females ≥18 or sexually active females	• Papanicolaou (Pap) test—yearly

- **Vaccination:** In cancer of the cervix, human papillomavirus (HPV) vaccine has been proven to be effective against cervix cancer.
- Promotion of the importance of nutrition.
- Secondary prevention programs may include health education on breast and testicular self-examination, Papanicolaou (Pap) test, mammograms, digital rectal examination, etc.

WARNING SIGNS OF CANCER

A plethora of symptoms can appear with cancer. These symptoms can also accompany other health issues and are often difficult to distinguish. Depending upon the organ involved, cancer symptoms may include various symptoms as summarized in **Table 40.5**.

TABLE 40.5: Signs and symptoms of cancer/warning signs.	
Changes in breast	• Lump in the breast or armpit • Nipple changes or discharge • Breast skin is itchy, red, scaly, dimpled, or puckered
Urinary bladder changes	• Problem while urinating • Pain when urinating • Blood in the urine
Bleeding or bruising	From body cavity or part for no known reason
Bowel changes	• Blood in the stools • Changes in bowel habits
Cough	Cough or hoarseness that does not go away
Eating disorder	• Pain after eating (heartburn or indigestion that does not go away) • Dysphagia (trouble swallowing) • Abdominal pain • Nausea and vomiting • Change in appetite
Fatigue	Fatigue that is severe and lasting
Fever or night sweats	Patients with cancer usually complain of night sweat and fever
Changes in the oral cavity	• A white or red patch on the tongue or mouth • Bleeding, pain, or numbness in the mouth
Neurological problems	• Headaches • Seizures • Vision changes • Hearing changes • Drooping of the face
Skin changes	• A flesh-colored lump that bleeds or turns scaly • A new mole or a change in an existing mole • A sore that does not heal • Jaundice
Swelling or lumps	Swelling or lumps anywhere, such as in the neck, underarm, stomach, and groin
Changes in body weight	Weight gain or weight loss for no known reason

PSYCHOSOCIAL ASPECTS OF CANCER

- **Diagnosis:** The uncertainty of cancer prognosis is not easy to accept. A diagnosis of cancer threatens the feeling of security and balance in a person's life. Whereas some cancers are treatable, it is often believed that cancer represents pain, suffering, and death. A cancer diagnosis often also leads to complex behavior, giving a new meaning to life and death when the person's spiritual, and philosophical needs arise more than ever.
  - *Awareness about cancer:* A previous experience with cancer in the family or self encourages some to acquire medical help quickly. Sometimes, previous experiences may also lead to avoidance of seeking medical help. Sometimes, family members also support the acceptance of symptoms and keep delaying the visit to the doctor. Pain and generalized discomfort are often ignored to be minor symptoms. Lack of knowledge about other early signs of cancer in the general public also leads to delays in diagnosis.
  - *Knowing it is cancer:* It is always necessary to have the patient's trust in the physician. The family members often ask the doctor to avoid telling the patient that it is cancer fearing the patient's reaction that the shock of diagnosis will make him even sicker. But, the loss of trust in family and physician on knowing about it from another person worsens the management. Being open about the diagnosis and allowing the person autonomy in decision-making makes him or at least have some control of the situation. Remember, most persons accept the diagnosis over time.
  - *Patient's reaction to diagnosis:* The first response to the diagnosis of cancer is usually disbelief and anxiety. A cancer diagnosis is often associated with a surge of negative mood and distress for people. Most patients respond with denial which is often a protective mechanism from the impending threat. Intense emotions are a normal grief reaction and should be accepted. Most patients will accept the diagnosis after the initial denial phase is over. Answering all his questions and attending to all his concerns, providing him with all necessary treatment options, and allowing him to seek medical advice from another specialist as he feels, are some ways to ensure that the patient feels a sense of control. Intermittent episodes of intense emotions can still happen even after a long time of initial acceptance.
  - *Family reactions:* A family is equally vulnerable at the diagnosis of cancer as the patient is. It can be very stressful to see a loved one in a vulnerable situation. Some family members break down and give up and while others shield their emotions and take the role of caregiving. The financial burden of the treatment often adds to the misery. Being always "on duty" gives them physical and emotional burnout along with their innate fears of losing a loved one.
- **Response to cancer treatment:** After the diagnostic phase, once the treatment plan is finalized, the person as well as the family face different experiences that affect psychosocially.

Different treatment modalities have different psychosocial impacts. These include hospital stay, surgical interventions, in-situ intravenous access, chemotherapy, or other treatments. Despite of adequate level of education or awareness, a person may still feel unprepared to enter this unfamiliar world.

- ❖ **Response to terminal illness:** When aggressive, curative treatment does not show any improvement, the focus of the medical team moves to palliative care. This can often lead to various fears in a person or family members.
  - ➢ *Fear of death:* This is the most feared unknown entity for all persons. The patient often surrounds himself with questions like what will happen after his death, who will look after his family, about his future plans, etc.
  - ➢ *Fear of pain and suffering:* Cancer is often associated with unbearable pain by the patient and family members. They fear the pain of death and it makes them even more anxious and worried.
  - ➢ *Fear of abandonment:* As other treatment modalities fail, the cancer patient is shifted to palliative care. The end-of-life care often makes the patient feel abandoned by both family and the health care team.
  - ➢ *Loss of control:* When advancing cancer causes progressive weakness, fatigue, and confusion, patients have less opportunity to maintain control of the environment and what is happening to them.
  - ➢ *Loss of body image/self:* Deteriorating physique due to weakness and emaciation makes a person find it difficult to perform important personal care routines (e.g., bathing, grooming, shaving, etc.). The physical changes often are so marked that the person may not be recognizable.
- ❖ **Role of nurse in psychosocial care of a cancer patient:** All patients whether a new diagnosis, starting cancer treatment, and/or on continuing treatment, receive care by the oncology nurses. They must incorporate in their care an awareness of the tremendous psychosocial implications that the patient and family are going through. Nurses provide them the necessary knowledge and motivation to deal with side-effects and make decisions. Providing specific health education also enhances emotional support and helps in the development of a trusting nurse-patient relationship.

Points to remember while informing a cancer diagnosis:

- ❖ Provide privacy, time, and space to share information.
- ❖ Encourage the patient to bring one or more family members or friends to the meeting.
- ❖ Provide a written summary of the information given in the meeting.
- ❖ Monitor for signs of emotional distress and respond as per requirement.
- ❖ Give the information gradually as accepted by the person, rather than starting with the diagnosis. Listen to the patient's and family's concerns before beginning.
- ❖ Develop an alliance with the patient about the treatment plan.
- ❖ If the prognosis is very poor, avoid giving a definite time frame.
- ❖ Reinforce information given on subsequent visits.
- ❖ Provide necessary resources for follow-up support.

GERIATRIC CONSIDERATIONS

1. More than half of the patients undergoing cancer treatment are aged 65 years or above.
2. All side-effects of chemotherapy and radiation therapy are more intense in elderly.
3. They are also at increased risk for complications, such as septic shock, pneumonia and infection.
4. The elderly attribute various symptoms to old age and they must be motivated to report all symptoms immediately.

Case Scenario

1. Manorama is a 32-year-old female, recently diagnosed with Hodgkin's lymphoma, and is admitted to daycare for her first cycle of chemotherapy. How should the nurse at the daycare approach her? What are the special instructions to be given to Manorama?
2. Rajesh is a 72-year-old male who was diagnosed with prostate cancer 6 months back. Now, the last chest X-ray suggested multiple metastatic lesions in both lung fields. Rajesh has been explained the prognosis and referred for palliative care. Plan nursing care interventions for a patient requiring palliative care.

SUMMARY

Cancer or carcinoma is a broad category of diseases that involve abnormal growth and/or proliferation of body cells. Male gender, advancing age, genetic predisposition, and exposure to certain chemical agents or ionizing radiations are common risk factors. Cancer is diagnosed using certain specific tumor markers in blood investigations, the histological study of tissue biopsy as well as specific radio-diagnosis procedures, such as CT scan, MRI, and fluoroscopy. Treatment for cancer depends on the stage and grading of the carcinoma. Surgery, chemotherapy, and radiation therapy are the most commonly used therapies for the reduction or removal of carcinomas. Metastatic carcinomas are spread to more than one part of the body and severely restrict prognosis. Palliative care is the care given to a patient with end-stage carcinoma. This involves symptomatic relief and emotional support. It is important for nurses to be knowledgeable and skillful in addressing the fears of the patients and their families throughout the journey of treatment for cancer.

MULTIPLE CHOICE QUESTIONS

1. Cancer spread from one part to other is called metastasis. This usually spread through the:
   a. Blood and nervous system
   b. Blood and lymphatic system
   c. Nervous and lymphatic system
   d. Endocrine and lymphatic system
2. The development of new capillary system around a carcinoma is called:
   a. Capillarogenesis   b. Venogenesis
   c. Angiogenesis   d. Arteriogenesis
3. Prostate cancer is more common among men in which age group?
   a. 30–40 years   b. 20–30 years
   c. 50–60 years   d. Same risk at all ages
4. Which of the following is a vaccine preventable carcinoma?
   a. Cervix cancer   b. Lung cancer
   c. Prostate cancer   d. Breast cancer

5. The day care nurse just received the complete count report of Mr Ram, who is receiving his third cycle of radiotherapy involving the bone marrow today. Which of the following is a normal finding?
   a. Thrombocytopenia and leukopenia
   b. Elevated thrombocytes and reduced erythrocytes
   c. Elevated platelets
   d. Elevated red blood cells
6. Which is the most common cause of cancer-related mortality in the world?
   a. Lungs   b. Cervix
   c. Esophagus   d. Liver
7. Study of cancer tissues under microscope for diagnosis of cancer is known as:
   a. Histopathology   b. Biopsy
   c. Serology   d. Cytology
8. Pap smear is used to detect which cancer among females
   a. Breast cancer   b. Cervix cancer
   c. Thyroid cancer   d. Blood cancer
9. TNM staging system refers to:
   a. Tumor, node, metastasis   b. Type, node, metastasis
   c. Tumor, node and mode   d. Type, node and metastases
10. HPV vaccine is routinely recommended for which age group?
    a. 9–14 years   b. More than 60 years
    c. More than 45 years d. Less than 9 years
11. Colposcope is used to visualize:
    a. Uterus   b. Cervix
    c. Stomach   d. Oral cavity
12. PSA level is used as a tumor marker for which cancer?
    a. Prostrate   b. Cervical
    c. Breast   d. Lung

ANSWERS

1. b	2. c	3. c	4. a
5. a	6. a	7. a	8. b
9. a	10. a	11. b	12. a

SUGGESTED READING

1. Debela DT, Muzazu SG, Heraro KD, Ndalama MT, Mesele BW, Haile DC, et al. New approaches and procedures for cancer treatment: Current perspectives. SAGE Open Med. 2021;9:20503121211034366. doi: 10.1177/20503121211034366. PMID: 34408877; PMCID: PMC8366192
2. Dong ST, Costa DSJJ, Butow PN, Lovell MR, Agar M, Velikova G, et al. Symptom Clusters in Advanced Cancer Patients: An Empirical Comparison of Statistical Methods and the Impact on Quality of Life. J Pain Symptom Manage. 2016;51(1):88-98.
3. Ferrario L, Schettini F, Garagiola E, Cecchi A, Lugoboni L, Serra P, et al. Advanced Medical Devices for Preparation and Administration of Chemotherapeutic Agents: Results from a Multi-Dimensional Evaluation. Clinicoecon Outcomes Res. 2020;12:711-722. doi: 10.2147/CEOR.S267283. PMID: 33293839; PMCID: PMC7718866.
4. Kaur G, Prakash G, Malhotra P, Ghai S, Kaur S, Singh M, et al. Home-based Yoga Program for the Patients Suffering from Malignant Lymphoma during Chemotherapy: A Feasibility Study. Int J Yoga. 2018;11(3):249-54. doi: 10.4103/ijoy.IJOY_17_18. PMID: 30233121; PMCID: PMC6134742.
5. Kozachik SL, Bandeen-Roche K. Predictors of patterns of pain, fatigue and insomnia during the first year following a cancer diagnosis in the elderly. Cancer Nurs. 2008;31(5):334-44.
6. Mishra IS, Scherer RW, Snyder C, Geigle PT P, Gotay C. Are Exercise Programs Effective for Improving Health-related Quality of Life Among Cancer Survivors? A Systematic Review and Meta-Analysis. J Natl cancer Inst. 2018;41(6):E326-42.
7. Pituskin E. Cancer as a new chronic disease: Oncology nursing in the 21st Century. Can Oncol Nurs J. 2022;32(1):87-92. PMID: 35280062; PMCID: PMC8849169.
8. Pucci C, Martinelli C, Ciofani G. Innovative approaches for cancer treatment: current perspectives and new challenges. Ecancermedicalscience. 2019;13:961. doi: 10.3332/ecancer.2019.961. PMID: 31537986; PMCID: PMC6753017
9. Sitlinger A, Zafar SY. Health-Related Quality of Life: The Impact on Morbidity and Mortality. Surg Oncol Clin N Am. 2018;27(4):675-84.

CHAPTER 41

Treatment Modalities of Cancer

Maninderdeep Kaur, Divya Dahiya, Pramod Kumar

"Undergoing different treatment modalities of cancer may be quite challenging. Being positive can do wonders in life of a patient."
—Sukhpal

LEARNING OBJECTIVES

After going through the chapter, the learner will be able to:
- Describe the different treatment modalities of cancer.
- Identify the general principles of cancer surgery.
- Discuss the nursing management of the patients pre and postoperatively.
- Define the different types of stem cell transplantation.
- Describe the role of a nurse in various aspects of bone marrow and stem cell transplantation.
- Discuss the side effects of radiotherapy along with nursing interventions.
- Describe different types of chemotherapeutic drugs.
- Discuss the role of a nurse while administering immunotherapy.
- Describe hormone therapy along with examples.

TERMS

- **Adjuvant chemotherapy:** When chemotherapy is given after surgery.
- **Brachytherapy:** It is the type of radiation given internally to the body.
- **Lumpectomy:** Removal of the lump.
- **Mastectomy:** Surgical removal of the breast.
- **Mobilization:** A process of stimulating the stem cells out of the bone marrow space into the bloodstream so they are available for collection for future reinfusion.
- **Neo-adjuvant chemotherapy:** When chemotherapy is given before surgery.
- **Rehabilitation:** Strategies to improve a patient's mental or physical fitness prior to a treatment.
- **Teletherapy:** It is the type of radiation given externally to the body.

INTRODUCTION

Depending upon the stage and type of cancer, various treatment modalities are available worldwide **(Fig. 41.1)**. These modalities may be used alone or as a combination. The current chapter explains all these therapies.

SURGERY

Surgical oncology focuses on the surgical management of malignant neoplasm, including biopsy, staging, and surgical resection. The modality of surgical intervention is an important option in the treatment of cancer. The surgical procedure may be performed in order to prevent a cancer occurrence in the high-risk patient, to diagnose a primary or metastatic site of malignancy, to provide primary or secondary treatment of malignancy, to provide a route of administration of therapy, to rehabilitate by means of reconstructive intervention, or to offer palliative care through symptom management in advanced cancer.

The patients suffering from cancer usually undergo at least one surgical procedure at some point during the course of their disease. Nursing fulfils important roles in the care of these patients throughout the entire cancer experience. Nurses' involvement with the cancer patient may lead them to identify risk factors that prompt a preventive surgical procedure. They may play a significant role during the assessment and evaluation of symptoms,

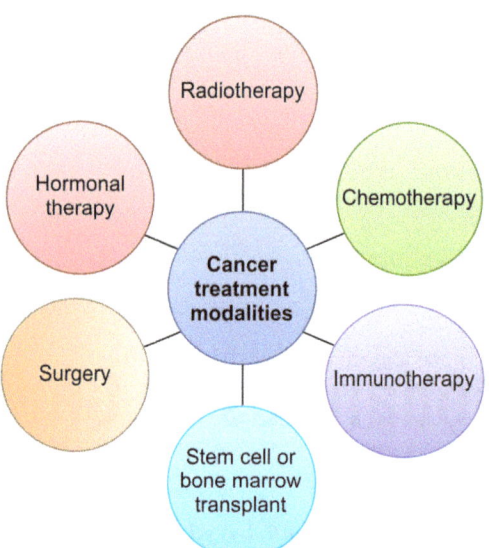

Fig. 41.1: Different treatment modalities for cancer patients.

testing, and diagnosis; and throughout the preoperative and postoperative care.

GENERAL PRINCIPLES OF CANCER SURGERY

Surgery is defined as treatment involving cutting or entering the body and removing or repairing body parts using tools or instruments. It may be employed in cancer care in a number of ways:

- ❖ To excise a tumor with curative intent (e.g., removal of a breast lump or bowel cancer)
- ❖ To remove a part of a tumor or metastases with palliative intent, which is often done to reduce symptoms (e.g., removal of a tumor that is causing spinal cord compression)
- ❖ To reduce the size of tumor to make it more amenable to other treatment (e.g., debulking surgery for a brain tumor)
- ❖ To diagnose cancer (surgical biopsy or excision of lymph nodes)
- ❖ To restore the form or function following the removal of a tumor (e.g., reconstructive breast surgery following mastectomy or formation of a stoma following bowel surgery).

TYPES OF SURGICAL THERAPIES FOR COMMON CANCERS

Surgery for Breast Cancer

It is a frequently occurring cancer among women worldwide. Surgery has been the mainstay option for the management of breast cancer for several decades. The two main surgical options for breast cancer are:
1. Mastectomy involving removing the entire breast.
2. Breast-conserving surgery involving removing just the cancerous area and a small amount of surrounding normal tissue.

Types of Mastectomy

- ❖ **Simple mastectomy:** In this procedure, the entire breast is removed without removing the axillary lymph nodes.

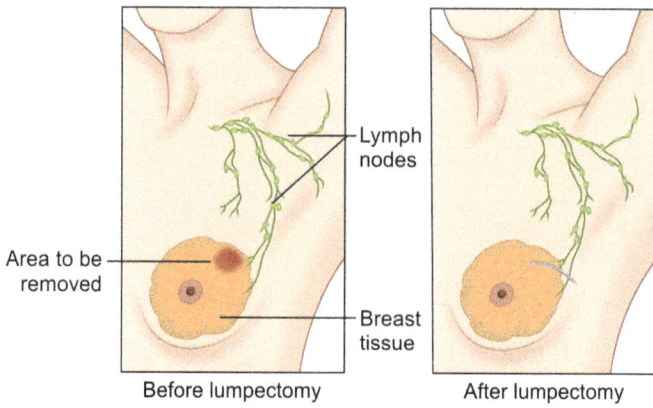

Fig. 41.2: Breast-conserving surgery.

- ❖ **Skin-sparing mastectomy:** In this, the nipple and areola are usually removed. But the rest of the skin over the breast is preserved.
- ❖ **Modified radical mastectomy:** It is the removal of the mammary gland, nipple, and areola, along with complete axillary lymph node dissection.
- ❖ **Breast-conserving surgery:** It is also known as lumpectomy, partial or segmental mastectomy, is the surgical procedure where a tumor as well as some surrounding normal tissue (clear margin) is removed but extensive maintenance of the breast tissue is done **(Fig. 41.2)**.

Surgery for Gynecologic Cancer

It involves the removal of the cervix, uterus, ovaries, and other pelvic organs depending upon the kind of disease and involvement of the organs. Various surgeries may include:

- ❖ **Debulking:** In this much of the cancerous tissue is removed. The remaining cancer is treated with chemotherapy and/or radiation.
- ❖ **Total hysterectomy:** It involves the removal of entire uterus and cervix.
- ❖ **Radical hysterectomy:** It involves the removal of the entire uterus, the tissue on both sides of the cervix, and the upper part of the vagina.
- ❖ **Salpingo-oophorectomy:** It involves the removal of the ovary and fallopian tubes. This type of surgery may be performed for ovarian and breast cancer.
- ❖ **Omentectomy:** It involves the removal of the omentum, an area of tissue rich in blood vessels covering the intestines and other organs in the abdomen.

Surgery for Head and Neck Cancer

- ❖ **Lobectomy:** In this surgery, one side or lobe of the thyroid that contains cancer is removed. A lobectomy is also called a partial thyroidectomy or hemi-thyroidectomy. This type of surgery is used to treat low-risk papillary thyroid cancer.
- ❖ **Total thyroidectomy:** To remove the entire thyroid gland. This surgery is usually performed in patients with follicular or papillary thyroid cancer.
- ❖ **Neck dissection:** It is carried out by having an incision in the neck. The three important structures in the neck closely involved in neck dissection are the internal jugular vein, the spinal accessory nerve, and the

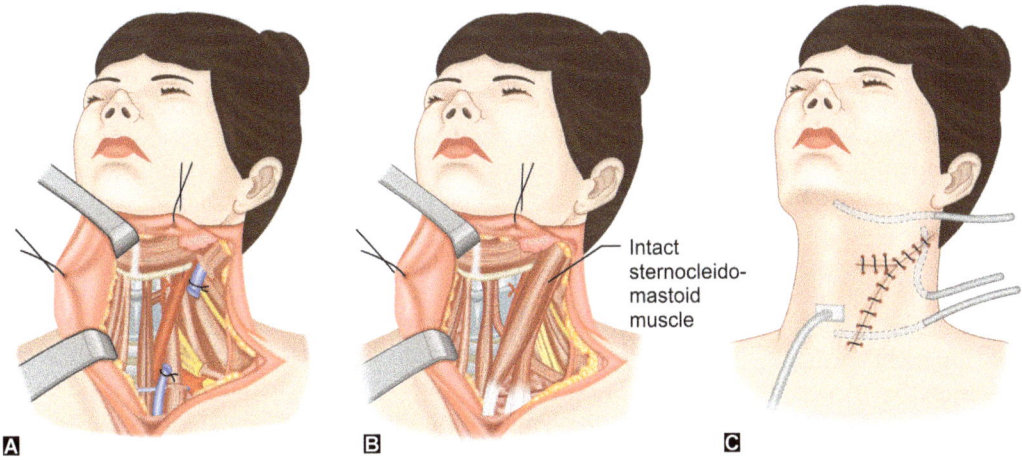

Figs. 41.3A to C: (A) Radical neck dissection; (B) Modified radical neck dissection; (C) Portable suction drainage.

sternocleidomastoid muscle. Neck dissection is classified by the zone from which the lymph nodes are removed. In radical neck dissection, all the nodes (zone I through V) and three structures are removed. If the nodes from zone I through V are removed and one of these three structures is preserved it is called a modified radical neck dissection. The surgery which does not involve all five zones, is called a selective neck dissection **(Figs. 41.3A to C)**.

Surgery for Gastrointestinal Cancer

- ❖ **Billroth surgery:** In this surgery partial resection of the stomach with anastomosis to the duodenum (Billroth I) or the jejunum (Billroth II) is done. It is performed in patients with stomach cancer.
- ❖ **Whipple surgery:** It is also called pancreatoduodenectomy. It is a surgical procedure to treat tumors of the pancreas, intestine, and the bile duct **(Fig. 41.4)**.

NURSING MANAGEMENT

Before Surgery

Pre- and postoperative nursing management of the patients is also discussed in detail along with each surgical condition in the respective chapters.

Information Giving and Informed Consent

After a treatment plan has been decided it is vital that information about the proposed surgery is given to the patients and their carer. This may include booklets, leaflets, or visual information. The information will allow the patient to prepare for the operation and be in a good position to give their informed consent for the operation.

The concept of informed consent is core to any procedure. The patient should be in receipt of all the information necessary to decide regarding the proposed treatment or choice of treatment. Consent has a particular importance

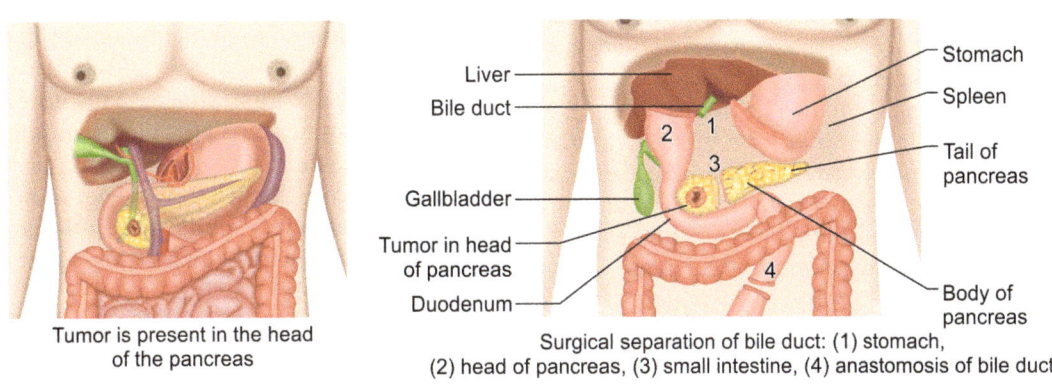

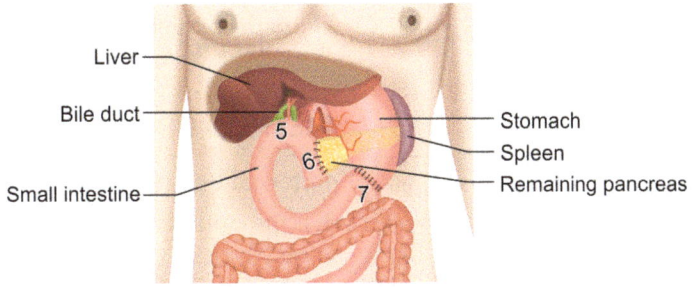

Fig. 41.4: Whipple surgery.

in cancer surgery as it may make temporary or permanent alterations to an individual's functional ability, appearance, and overall quality of life. When giving consent the patient should be able to make an assessment of whether the effects of any surgery are outweighed by the potential benefits. This is a crucial judgement in a situation where a surgical procedure might not be curative but offer prolongation of life or reduction in symptoms.

Rehabilitation and Enhanced Recovery Programs

Rehabilitation is the use of strategies to improve a patient's mental or physical fitness following the treatment. It should be carried out irrespective of any of the treatments such as surgery, radiotherapy, and chemotherapy. It generally involves:
- Physical activity
- Dietary support
- Psychological well-being

After Surgery

There are a number of key risks associated with cancer surgery. Most are common to all types of surgery.
- **Pain:** Preoperative pain assessment and education may reduce anxiety and pain after surgery. Postoperative pain should be managed with analgesics delivered by infusion, which ideally should be patient controlled in the first instance. Regular assessments of pain are vital in managing patient anxiety.
- **Hypovolemic shock/bleeding or disruption of clotting:** Anti-embolus aids should be used widely to help the patient get back to normal levels of mobility as quickly as possible. Observe wound sites and monitor all blood loss carefully.
- **Infection:** Maintain hygiene and a good hand-washing technique throughout the perioperative period and administer antibiotics. Thorough and regular observations are crucial as is frequent assessment of the wound sites for redness, swelling, smell, and exudates.
- **Nutrition:** Monitor weight and dietary input closely and refer the patient to the dietician for a full nutritional assessment. In case of prolonged recovery there may be a need for tube feeding or parenteral nutrition throughout the perioperative period, although this should be a last resort in patients with good gastrointestinal tract.
- **Psychological effects of surgery:** Many patients suffer from the psychological effects of cancer surgery. These may range from shorter side effects such as infection to a longer psychological trauma caused by a change in body image such as from the loss of a breast. These long-term changes can cause a loss of confidence and a range of psychological difficulties.

RADIOTHERAPY

Radiation therapy (RT) may play a key role in both the radical and palliative treatment pathways of many people living with cancer. Radiotherapy is not delivered in all hospitals and is only available within specialized cancer centers with a high level of demand. It is the use of high-energy ionizing radiation to treat diseases, usually cancer. Radiotherapy is a localized, targeted treatment that encompasses the treatment volume and an area of healthy tissue that is within the radiation beam or field of radiation. The treated volume is the tissue volume which is planned to receive at least a dose selected and specified by the radiation oncologist as being appropriate to achieve the purpose of the treatment. Radiotherapy requires achieving a balance between delivering an effective dose of radiation to the treatment volume and sparing or minimizing the dose received by healthy tissue and surrounding organs.

Radiotherapy is highly specialized. Each treatment is individually designed to account for the patient's unique anatomy, shape, and treatment site. A multidisciplinary team is responsible for the planning and delivery of a patient's radiotherapy. Core members of the team include oncologists, therapeutic radiographers, physicists, and nurses who provide expertise in treating and caring for patients with specific tumor sites.

Radiotherapy is delivered with a very high degree of accuracy often within 1 or 2 mm. This accuracy can be assured using a variety of verification techniques that may include indexed patient immobilization devices, patient set-up checks, and online imaging of the treatment area.

PRINCIPLES OF RADIATION THERAPY

Radiation kills cells primarily by damaging the DNA. Because the cells are mostly water, majority of the damage occurs when ionizing radiation interacts with cells' water to produce free radicals. These are highly reactive and cause breakage of DNA strands.

Fractionation, or dividing the total dose into equal daily fractions, takes advantage of the '4 Rs' of radiobiology. These are:
1. **Repair** is the ability of cells to recover from sublethal damage. Initially, both normal and tumor cells can recover but as the radiation dose accumulates the ability of the tumor cells to repair damage decreases.
2. **Redistribution** is based on the sensitivity of the cells to radiation at different phases of cell division. Dividing the radiation dose into smaller daily doses disrupts the cellular life cycle, causing a greater number of cells to enter into the more radiosensitive mitotic phase.
3. **Repopulation** refers to the regeneration of cells after radiation damage. Cellular repopulation that occurs between radiation fractions is greater in the normal tissue than in the tumor.
4. **Reoxygenation** is based on the fact that the presence of oxygen enhances the effect of ionizing radiation, particularly when X-rays or gamma rays are the sources. As the tumor shrinks the oxygen-deprived core is exposed to the oxygen-rich blood supply, increasing the tumor's sensitivity to radiation.

METHOD OF TREATMENT DELIVERY

External Beam Radiotherapy (EBRT)

It is the commonest treatment method in radiation therapy. It may be used alone or in combination with other cancer treatments. EBRT is delivered using a Linac (**Fig. 41.5**) which produces high-energy ionizing radiation. The radiation is electrically produced within the Linac and is directed toward the patient.

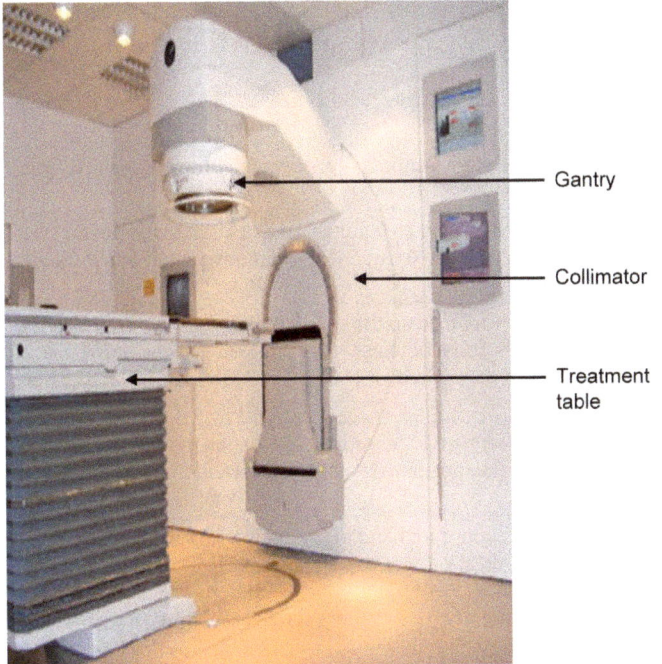

Fig. 41.5: Linac machine.

The patient will be positioned on a treatment couch, using the same immobilization equipment used during the CT planning scan. The radiographers will ensure that the patient is lying in the correct position for their treatment and perform quality checks to ensure that the setup is accurate. Once the radiographer is confident that the patient has been positioned correctly, they will inform the patient that they are leaving the room. The physician must leave the room to deliver the radiotherapy safely without exposing themselves to the radiation. From outside of the room, the radiographers can see and hear the patient at all times using a closed-circuit camera.

Once the treatment position has been verified, the radiographers will proceed to treatment delivery. During radiotherapy treatment, Linac will rotate around the patient to ensure delivery of an appropriate dose of radiation while minimizing the dose to any organ at risk. The patient will not be aware of the treatment except for hearing a louder buzzing noise from the machine. Radiotherapy treatment may only take a few minutes.

Following completion of each EBRT treatment which is called fraction, the patient is free to continue with their day-to-day life activities. Patients are not radioactive following the treatment and do not pose any risk to pregnant women and babies.

Internal Radiation Therapy or Brachytherapy

It is a procedure where a sealed radioactive source is placed close to, or inside a tumor to deliver a high dose of radiation to a small area. The radiation from these sources penetrates only to a few millimeters reducing the dose and toxicity to surrounding tissue.

Brachytherapy delivers a very precise treatment and can be completed in less overall time than other types of radiotherapy. It is commonly used to treat prostate, cervical, rectal, and breast cancers. Methods include interstitial implants or intracavitary implants. Interstitial implants may be in the form of needles, seeds, wires, or catheters. The radioactive source may be placed directly into the body cavity via an applicator.

Brachytherapy is administered by high dose rate (HDR) or low dose rate (LDR). In HDR one or more doses may be given over a few minutes and separated by at least 6 hours. LDR is administered continuously over several days after the patient is admitted to the hospital. Permanently sealed radioactive sources are left in the tissue indefinitely.

In gynecological cancers, applicators used to insert sources in the uterus and vagina and cervical cavity are the Fletcher Suit, interstitial implant with needles, and intracavity applicators. Sources used are cesium 137, cobalt 60, and iridium 192. The patient is placed on a low-fiber diet and receives diphenoxylate atropine to prevent bowel movement. Postoperative pain is managed by oral and intravenous medication.

In breast cancer surgically implanted catheters have been used in the past to deliver LDR and HDR radiation for partial breast irradiation. This method has been largely replaced by the mammosite radiation system, which entails placement of a balloon catheter in the lumpectomy cavity either at the time of surgery or a few weeks later with treatment delivered by HDR twice a day **(Figs. 41.6 and 41.7)**.

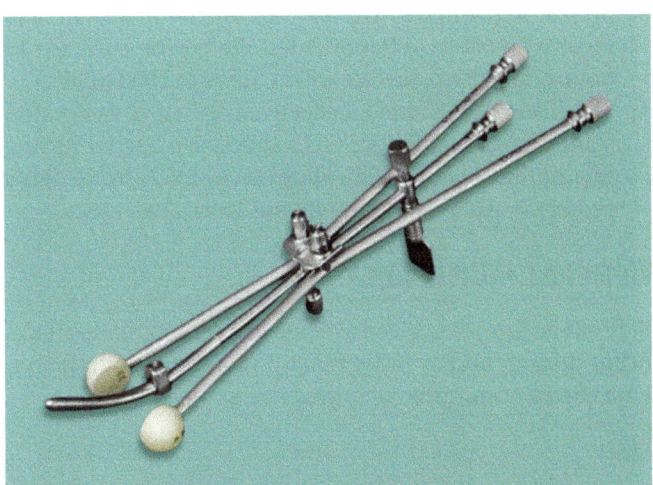

Fig. 41.6: Fletcher suit applicator.

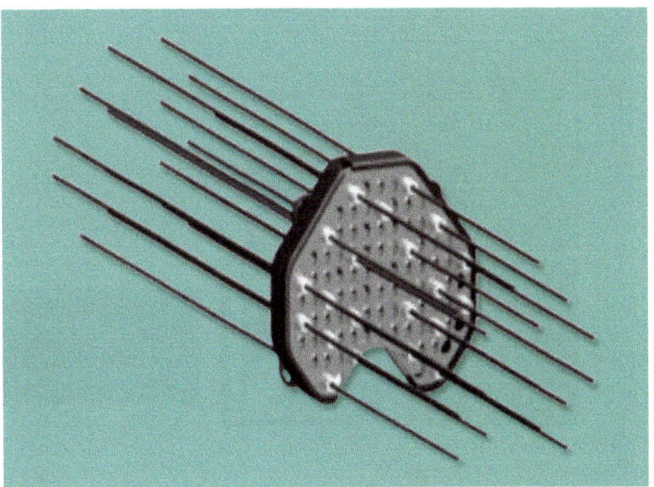

Fig. 41.7: Interstitial implant.

RADIATION SAFETY

With external beam radiation, there is minimal risk of exposure to radiation. Nursing care and radiation safety precautions required for implants are dependent on the type of radioactive isotope, the dose, and the method of administration. The nurse's knowledge of radiation biology can reduce anxiety and fear of exposure when caring for these patients.

Isolation precautions and film badges are necessary when caring for patients receiving radiation from sealed or unsealed sources. As Low As Reasonably Achievable (ALARA) is the acronym for a guideline used for radiation protection of staff involved in the care of patients receiving radiation. The techniques used to keep exposure ALARA are time, distance, and shielding **(Fig. 41.8)**. See **Table 41.1** for standard radiation safety precautions based on ALARA.

- ❖ **Distance:** Radiation is inversely proportional to the square of the distance from its source. Thus, increasing the distance from the source of radiation is a good protective measure. For example; if the dose rate is 100 mSv/h at 1 m, it will be 1 mSv/h at 10 m.
- ❖ **Time:** Radiation is directly proportional to the time spent near the source of radiation. Thus, as far as possible, less time should be spent near the source of radiation. For example, if the radiation dose rate is 100 mSv/h, and a person is staying in this field for one hour, she/he will receive a dose of 100 mSv, but if the person stays for 10 hours, the dose exposure will increase to 1000 mSv.
- ❖ **Shielding:** It is the most effective method of protection from external radiation. It is a protective barrier having appropriate features. Shielding can be made from highly protective materials like concrete, steel, lead, etc.

GENERAL SIDE EFFECTS

Side effects are categorized as acute or late. Acute side effects occur during therapy or within 2–3 months of completion. Late effects occur months to years later.

Skin

Ionizing radiation leads to various skin reactions by destroying the mitotic ability of stem cells within the rapidly proliferating, radiosensitive, basal layer of the epidermis. Depending upon treatment goals, a brisk skin reaction may be an anticipated outcome such as in the treatment of superficial skin cancers or chest wall. However, a radiation-induced skin reaction can greatly impact the quality of life and treatment outcomes of the patients.

TABLE 41.1: Comparison of radiation safety for sealed and unsealed radioactive sources.

Sealed sources	Unsealed sources
Private room	Private room
No minor or pregnant visitors allowed	No minor or pregnant visitors allowed
Adult visitors may spend 15 minutes per day at a distance of 10 feet	Adult visitors may spend 15 minutes per day at a distance of 10 feet
Staff and visitors are to keep the lead shield in the room between themselves and the patient	Staff and visitors are to keep the lead shield in the room between themselves and the patient
Radiation monitoring badges must be worn by nursing personnel	Radiation monitoring badges must be worn by nursing personnel
No special precautions for handling excreta, dishes, dressing, and bed linens	Body fluids are a source of radioactive contamination. Bed linens and gowns must be placed in separate plastic bags
Foley catheter for cervical implants	Must use the toilet if possible, flush the toilet 3 times
Regular utensils	Only use disposable utensils
The patient may be limited to bed rest depending on the location of the implant	The patient may walk in the room
Check for dislodgement of the source. If the source becomes dislodged it is handled with long forceps and placed in a lead container	—
When the implant is removed patient is no longer radioactive	The patient is checked by a radiation safety officer to determine for radioactivity and the patient is at a safe level for discharge

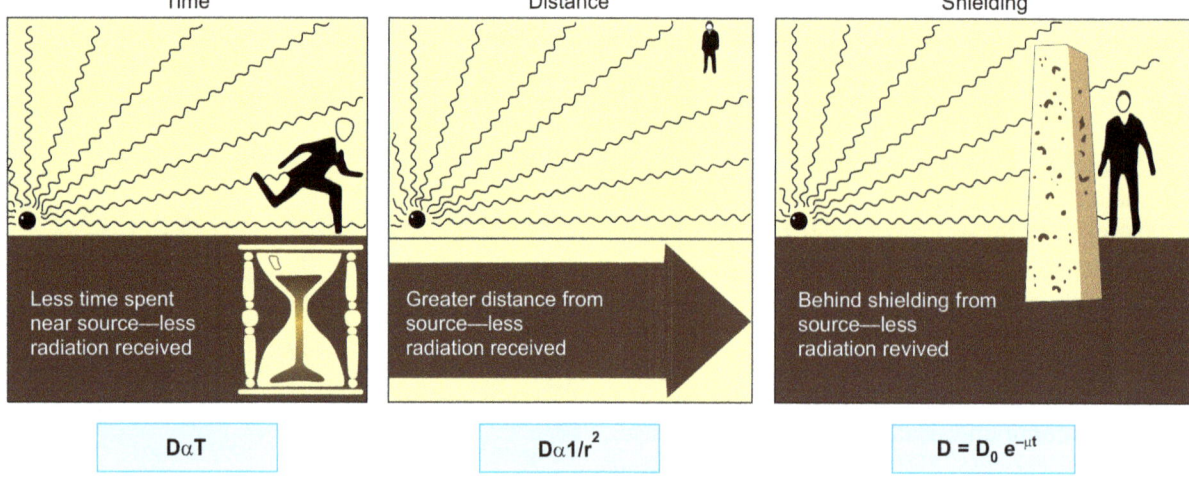

Fig. 41.8: Basic ways of controlling external radiation.

> **BOX 41.1:** Self-care instructions to minimize radiation skin reactions.
>
> - Wash the treated area gently with lukewarm water and mild soap and pat dry
> - Avoid applying any tape, rubbing, or scratching the marked site
> - Wear loose-fitting clothes having a soft texture
> - Make use of only an electric razor while shaving the treated area
> - Avoid sun exposure
> - Do not apply skin care products 4 hours prior to treatment

Factors that have an impact on the severity of radiodermatitis include the type of energy used, skin-to-source distance; sheet placed on the skin during treatment, and general skin condition. Skin reactions experienced during the course of radiation can range from erythema or hyperpigmentation to dry desquamation when basal layer stem cells become depleted; or moist desquamation when stem cells are eradicated from the basal layer. Skin changes may be seen within the first 2–4 weeks of treatment and usually peak in the 3–4 weeks. Although skin care protocols vary among institutions, an example of typical patient instructions is given in **Box 41.1**.

Fatigue

Fatigue because of cancer and its treatment modalities is one of the commonest side effects reported by patients. It occurs in about 90% of the patients undergoing treatment. During radiation therapy, fatigue gradually increases with the progression of treatment. It gets at its peak in the last week of treatment and slowly returns to pre-treatment level usually after around 3 months of the completion of the treatment. Patient education regarding these kinds of symptoms is very important in alleviating the fears that these could be manageable by adopting certain lifestyle modification techniques.

Bone Marrow Suppression

Patients receiving concurrent chemotherapy and radiation and total body radiation are at the greatest risk for bone marrow suppression. The patients and families are educated regarding possible decreased blood counts that could place them at risk for infection, bleeding, or fatigue. Growth factors or blood transfusions may be indicated when chemotherapy and radiation are combined. Patients and families are educated regarding the infection and bleeding precautions.

SITE-SPECIFIC SIDE EFFECTS

Breast Cancer

Patients undergoing radiotherapy may develop radiation skin reactions. They may experience the symptoms like pain, discomfort, irritation, itching, and burning at the site of the treatment throughout the course of treatment. These skin reactions may be classified as acute (hours or days) or late (months or years). The most common radiation skin reactions are summarized in **Table 41.2**.

Head and Neck

Radiotherapy to the head and neck causes a number of side effects. The most common side effects are shown in **Table 41.3**.

TABLE 41.2: Effects of radiotherapy treatment in women with breast cancer.

Telangiectasia	These dilated superficial blood vessels remain prominent at the irradiated skin area post-treatment. These may become permanent but may get reduced in severity over time
Cardiotoxicity	This may be the consequence primarily of left-sided radiotherapy. However, with the advances in radiotherapy planning and delivery, the incidence remains uncommon
Fibrosis	It is the thickening of the skin of the breast or chest wall after radiotherapy and may cause discomfort to the patients
Radiation pneumonitis	Radiation pneumonitis is the inflammation of the lungs caused by radiation
Secondary malignancy	There is a small chance that radiotherapy may lead to the development of secondary cancer at the site of treatment up to 20 years after the completion of radiotherapy

TABLE 41.3: Common side effects in patients receiving radiotherapy for head and neck cancers.

Side effects	Management
Changes in taste and smell	There is no specific management for this, but patients are made aware that it may happen. Patients are reviewed by an oncology dietitian for the management of dietary requirements throughout treatment
Xerostomia (dry mouth)	Occurs when there is not enough saliva or when saliva becomes very thick. From the start of treatment, patients are asked to use mouthwashes
Dysphagia	Inflammation in the mouth and throat leads to increased pain levels, making it difficult to swallow. Pain medication is given to patients as needed. Some patients also require the placement of feeding tubes to maintain their nutritional status
Mucositis	Patients are motivated to maintain good oral hygiene to decrease the risk of developing mouth ulcers. They are advised to use mouthwash such as saline solution and are asked to rinse their mouth regularly
Hoarse voice	Patients' voice may become hoarse as a direct result of the treatment. They are advised to rest their voice and may be referred to a speech therapist
Dyspepsia	This may occur if radiation fields extend quite inferiorly to include the upper part of the esophagus. Antacids and pain relief are prescribed to relieve symptoms
Breathing difficulty	Swelling inside the throat may occur due to inflammation causing breathing problems. Changes such as these could be deemed emergent and patients would be admitted for management

Thorax

Radiotherapy involving the thorax is used to treat many common cancers including breast and lung cancers. The side effects will of course depend on the area being treated (**Table 41.4**).

TABLE 41.4: Common side effects of radiotherapy involving the thorax.

Side effects	Treatment
Dysphagia	• Swallowing problems may be caused by irritation of the esophageal lining or if the tumor itself is blocking the esophagus • If it is radiation-induced analgesia, along with antacids, a soft diet may reduce the discomfort of the patient
Pneumonitis	• **Cough:** Acute radiation-induced cough may be treated with cough preparations such as simple linctus or codeine and should settle within a few weeks of completing the treatment
Chest infections	• Patients may become more susceptible to chest infections during treatment • Antibiotics may be prescribed
Lung fibrosis	• It is typically seen between 6 and 12 months after completion of the course of treatment • Most of the patients are asymptomatic, but some might have respiratory symptoms requiring symptomatic management

Abdomen

Abdominal sites encompass the gastric, liver, pancreas, and kidney **(Table 41.5)**.

TABLE 41.5: Common side effects of radiotherapy involving the abdomen.

Side effects	Treatment
Gastritis	• Radiation may cause inflammation of the stomach causing abdominal bloating or cramps, diarrhea, or a sense of urgency for bowel movements. Patients may be advised to avoid eating fiber-rich food such as bran, nuts, and wholegrain cereals or breads • Medication may be prescribed
Nausea and vomiting	It is generally less severe than nausea and vomiting caused by chemotherapy but it may last for a prolonged period in some patients. Side effects are clinically important and may be distressing. Treatment with antiemetics such as ondansetron is usually effective
Constipation	Medication is prescribed as required. The patient is motivated to take a high-fiber diet
Bone	Radiotherapy damages the bone in the area being treated. Patients are advised to take calcium-rich foods, to maintain the physical activity as far as possible

IMMUNOMODULATORS

Immunotherapy is a class of agents with immunomodulatory, antiangiogenic, or antineoplastic properties primarily targeting pathways related to multiple myeloma (e.g., thalidomide).

Cereblon is a human protein encoded by the CRBN gene. It has recently been identified as the primary target for this class of agents, as it is involved in the downregulation of interferon regulatory factor 4, tumor necrosis factor-alpha, and T cell immunomodulatory activity. Different types of drugs with their mechanism of action are depicted in **Table 41.6**.

MONOCLONAL ANTIBODIES

These are laboratory-made substances that mimic antibodies produced naturally by the human body as a part of the immune system response. They bind with proteins and antigens. Four types of monoclonal antibodies are shown in **Figure 41.9**.

1. **Murine:** Made from mice, for example, blinatumomab yttrium-90-ibritumomab
2. **Chimeric:** Part mouse and part human, for example, brentuximab, cetuximab, rituximab
3. **Humanized:** Small portions of mouse antibodies attached to human antibodies, for example, ado-trastuzumab, alemtuzumab, bevacizumab, pertuzumab, trastuzumab.

TABLE 41.6: Immunomodulators drugs.

Drug	Mechanism of action	Indications
Lenalidomide	Inhibits the proliferation and induces apoptosis of malignant hematopoietic cells; immunomodulatory effects include activation and increase in the number of T and NK cell	Multiple myeloma, myelodysplastic syndrome, mantle cell lymphoma
Pomalidomide	Inhibits the proliferation and induces apoptosis of malignant hematopoietic cells	Multiple myeloma
Thalidomide	Immunomodulatory, anti-inflammatory, and anti-angiogenic properties	Multiple myeloma

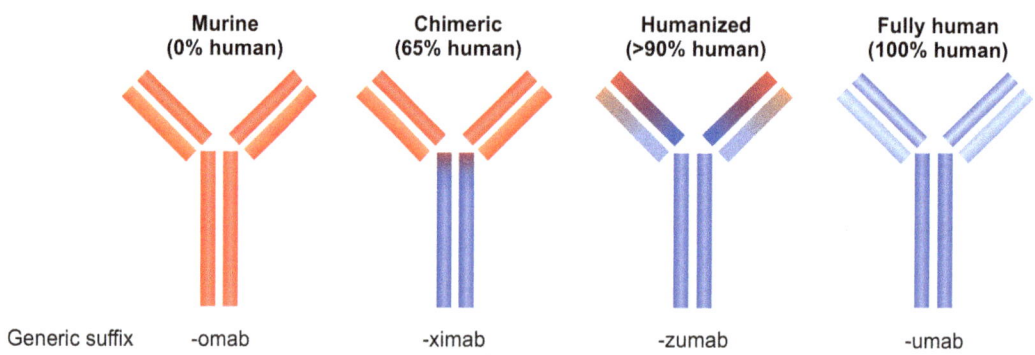

Fig. 41.9: Types of monoclonal antibodies.

4. **Human:** completely human antibodies, for example, daratumumab, denosumab, panitumumab.

MECHANISM OF ACTION

Monoclonal antibodies (mAbs) function in three manners:
- One is the mAbs ability to bind to cancer cells that contain tumor antigens. The antigens then prompt apoptosis.
- Another is the particular mAbs ability to bind to a receptor, blocking any antigens that would fuel cancer growth.
- Lastly, special antibodies can be conjugated to an element that is toxic to cancer cells (chemotherapy, radiotherapy, or other toxic). These antibodies can then be used to destroy tumor cells.

SIDE EFFECTS OF IMMUNOTHERAPY

The side effects of immunotherapy may be different from chemotherapy. They can cause inflammatory and autoimmune complications, which can affect any part of the body. Most frequently affected organs are the skin, colon, endocrine organs, liver, and lungs.

Examples of immune-related adverse events and some possible symptoms are depicted in **Figure 41.10**.

NURSING MANAGEMENT OF PATIENTS RECEIVING IMMUNOTHERAPY

- Educate the patients regarding the possible side effects of immunotherapy and the management of these adverse effects.
- They should also be made aware of various food items which can exacerbate gastrointestinal inflammation. They may need to follow certain dietary changes in case of immune-mediated colitis.
- Apart from patient education, the caregivers' queries regarding this treatment modality, financial implications, etc., should also be taken into consideration.
- They should be motivated to adhere to the long-term follow-up.
- Counsel the patients to avoid pregnancy during any of the therapeutic modalities. Educate them regarding reliable contraception methods such as intrauterine devices, oral contraceptive pills, etc.
- Encourage the patient to always carry a card showing the kind of treatment they are undergoing.

HORMONE THERAPY (ENDOCRINE THERAPY)

Hormones are natural substances or chemicals made by the organ and the glands of the endocrine system. These are carried around our bodies in the bloodstream and act as chemical messengers between various parts of the body.

Reproductive steroid hormones are involved in hormone-related cancers, namely breast and prostate cancer. Seventy percent of breast cancers are hormone positive. This means that their growth is driven by the hormones estrogen and/or progesterone. Prostate cancer growth is driven by androgen hormones mainly testosterone.

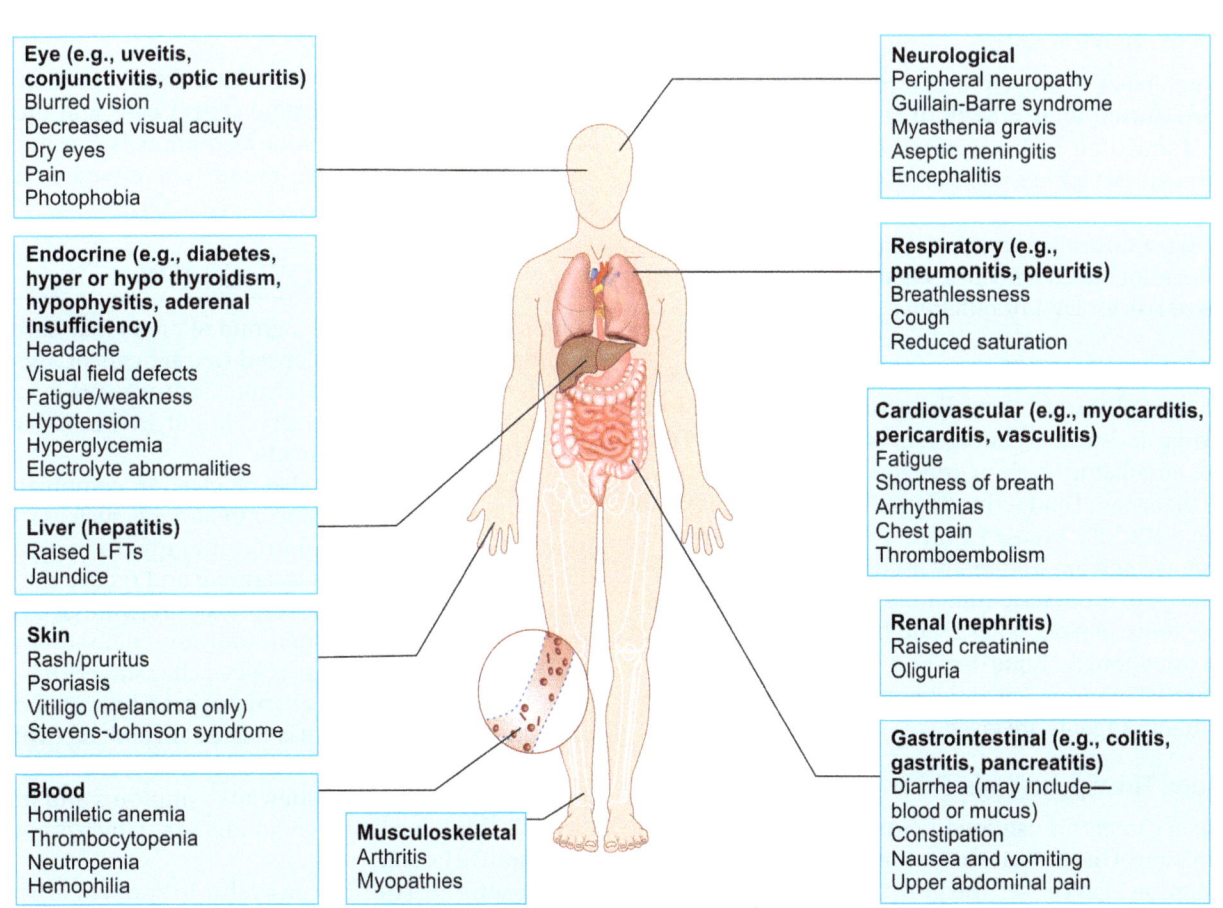

Fig. 41.10: Adverse effects of immunotherapy.

Reproductive steroid hormones are derived from cholesterol by a series of enzyme reactions within a cell. They are then bound to a protein in the bloodstream for transportation to the target cell. Here, the hormones cross the cell membrane and bind to the intracellular receptor, causing a change of shape that activates the receptor. The hormone and the receptor enter the nucleus of the cell together, where they bind to sections of DNA called hormone response elements. This stimulates or inhibits gene transcription causing protein synthesis and therefore the effects of the hormone.

HORMONE THERAPY TO TREAT BREAST CANCER

Approximately 70–80% of breast cancer are estrogen receptor positive (ER+) or estrogen receptor negative (ER-) and progesterone receptor positive (PR+) meaning they have estrogen receptor and/or progesterone receptors on their surface. Hormone receptor-positive tumors include estrogen receptor-positive (ER+) and/or progesterone receptor-positive (PR+) breast cancers.

Hormone therapy is used in patients with ER+ breast cancer in an attempt to block the effects of estrogen at its receptors or lower the amount of estrogen in the body to stop or slow down the growth of breast cancer. As hormone therapy is not effective in women with ER-breast cancer, it is only used in women with ER+ breast cancer.

TYPES OF HORMONE THERAPY FOR BREAST CANCER

Block Estrogen Receptors

Tamoxifen blocks estrogen receptors on breast cancer cells, thus preventing their growth. It is taken as a once-daily tablet. Tamoxifen is the endocrine therapy of choice in premenopausal women, used for ER+ breast cancer patients. While tamoxifen acts like an anti-estrogen in breast tissue, it acts like an estrogen in other tissues such as the uterus. Side effects include hot flushes, vaginal dryness, fatigue, and increased risk for DVT or pulmonary embolism.

Lower Estrogen Levels

Aromatase inhibitor blocks the aromatase enzyme from converting androgen to estrogen in adipose tissue and thus reduces circulating levels of estrogen. Aromatase inhibitors are the mainstay of endocrine treatment for postmenopausal women with ER+ breast cancer. Letrozole, anastrozole, and exemestane are frequently used aromatase inhibitors. Side effects of aromatase inhibitors include joint pain and stiffness, muscle pain, fatigue, and bone thinning that may lead to osteoporosis. Bone density is usually tested regularly in women taking aromatase inhibitors and appropriate bone-strengthening agents are given.

Hormone Therapy to Treat Prostate Cancer

Androgen namely testosterone is required for normal growth and function of the prostate in the male reproductive system. Testosterone also causes the growth and development of prostate cancer cells. Androgen exerts its effects by binding to prostate androgen receptors. Prostate cancer hormone therapy involves lowering androgen levels or blocking androgens from reaching prostate cancer cells to make prostate cancer shrinks or grow more slowly.

Types of Hormone Therapy for Prostate Cancer

Lower Testicular Androgen Production

Androgen deprivation therapy describes treatment to lower and ideally stop the testicles from making androgen namely testosterone. This is usually the first treatment men with prostate cancer receive.

GnRH (LHRH) Agonists are Injection or Implant

It daily stops or lowers the testicles from making androgen. This is usually the first treatment for prostate cancer. GnRH agonists are injections or implants administered to stop testicles from producing testosterone. When first given, GnRH agonists may cause a brief rise in testosterone before it falls to very low levels. Side effects include hot flushes, fatigue, shrinkage of testicles, and erectile dysfunction.

Lower Adrenal, Testicular, and Prostate Cancer Cell Androgen Production

Luteinizing hormone-releasing hormone (LHRH) agonists can stop the testicles from making androgen, but the adrenal and prostate cancer cells also make androgen hormones. Abiraterone blocks the cytochrome P45017α-hydroxylase/17, 20 lyase enzyme found in testicular, adrenal, and prostate cancer cells which are required to make testosterone hormone from cholesterol. Abiraterone, therefore, lowers testosterone production.

Androgen Receptor Blockers

Anti-androgen prevents testosterone from attaching to the androgen receptor on prostate cancer cells and therefore blocks the effect of testosterone on these cells. Enzalutamide and apalutamide are two recently licensed oral anti-androgens.

CHEMOTHERAPY

Chemotherapy comprises a group of drugs that have been developed, tested, and licensed to treat cancer. Cytotoxic literally means toxic to cells. Cytotoxic drugs work by causing cells to fail to complete the cell cycle and drive cells damaged by cytotoxic drugs to cell death.

Chemotherapy might also be given in combination or consecutively with other cancer treatments such as surgery, endocrine treatment, and radiotherapy, to increase the effectiveness of the cancer treatment and reduce the risk of cancer returning. Sometimes cytotoxic drugs are given before surgery, which is called 'neo-adjuvant chemotherapy' or NACT. When chemotherapy is given after surgery it is called 'adjuvant chemotherapy'. Sometimes it is administered at the same time as radiotherapy it is called concomitant treatment.

In patients who have metastatic disease, the intention of chemotherapy may be to alleviate symptoms and prolong survival. This is 'palliative chemotherapy' which is not given with curative intent.

The chemotherapy may be given via different routes including orally, intravenously, intramuscularly, subcutaneously, topically, intrathecally, and into body organs and cavities such as the bladder and peritoneum.

CYTOTOXIC DRUG CLASSIFICATION

Various types of chemotherapy drugs are grouped together taking into consideration that:
- Whether the drugs exert their effect at a specific phase of the cell cycle
- Pharmacological mechanism of action of the drug
- The chemical nature of the drug, for example when it contains platinum
- The source of the drug, for example, whether it is derived from plant or fungi

Cytotoxic drugs are commonly grouped as 'phase specific' or 'non-phase specific' defined by the effect of the drug during the cell cycle. Phase-specific cytotoxic drugs exert their mechanism of action in a specific phase of the cell cycle; e.g., methotrexate is classified as a synthesis (S phase) phase-specific drug, and vincristine is classified as a mitosis (M phase) phase-specific drug. These types of drugs tend to kill cells at lower doses compared to non-phase-specific drugs. The effect of cell cycle phase-specific drugs also plateaus at high doses. This is because only a certain proportion of cells in the tissue will be in that specific phase of the cell cycle at the time when the drug is administered so only those cells are killed. A higher dose of the drug would increase the severity of side effects but not the effectiveness of the drug. Nonphage-specific drugs such as cyclophosphamide, are equally toxic for quiescent cells that are in G0 as for the cell cycle between G1 and the mitosis phase.

CLASSES OF CYTOTOXIC DRUGS

Alkylating Agents
- Developed first of the anticancer agents.
- They are cell cycle nonspecific
- Cause breakage in DNA helix strand, thereby interfering with DNA replication and resulting in cell death.
- Dose-limiting toxicities include bone marrow suppression, GI toxicities, and organ-specific toxicities (renal and hepatic)
- **Example:** Busulfan, cyclophosphamide, cisplatin.

Antimetabolites
- Block the growth of DNA and RNA by interfering with enzymes
- Often divide into a folate analog, a purine analog, and a pyrimidine analog. Tumors with high growth rates or high parentage of cells in the S phase are the most susceptible to anti-metabolites.
- **Examples:** Capecitabine, cytrabine, 5-FU, gemcitabine, methotrexate.

Antitumor Antibiotics
- Interfere with DNA synthesis by binding with DNA at various points, preventing RNA synthesis.
- Myelosuppression, GI toxicities, and alopecia are common.
- Many are cardiotoxic or pulmonary toxic.
- **Examples:** Doxorubicin, bleomycin, epirubicin.

Nitrosoureas
- These have the capacity to cross the blood-brain barrier and are sometimes categorized with alkylating agents.
- Cause breakage in DNA helix strand, thereby interfering with DNA replication and resulting in cell death.
- **Examples:** Carmustine, lomustine, streptozocin.

Epipodophyllotoxins
- Antimicrotubular agents derived from the *Podophyllum pellatum* or mandre plant.
- Induce irreversible blockage of cells in the pre-mitotic phase of the cell cycle; interfere with topoisomerase II enzyme reaction.
- **Example:** Etoposide.

Taxanes
- Semisynthetic derivates of precursors from yew plants
- Stabilize microtubules, inhibiting cell division effectively in G and M phase
- **Examples:** Paclitaxel, docetaxel.

Vinca Alkaloids
- Derived from the *Vinca rosea* or periwinkle plant.
- Depolymerize microtubule and destroy mitotic spindles
- Drugs in these categories are vesicant.

NURSING INTERVENTIONS FOR THE GENERAL SIDE EFFECTS OF CHEMOTHERAPY

Nausea and Vomiting

Chemotherapy-induced nausea and vomiting may be experienced by up to 80% of patients with cancer. It is one of the most distressing side effects of cancer treatment. Oncology nurses must be knowledgeable and proactive when managing chemotherapy-induced nausea and vomiting (CINV).

The following interventions might be helpful:
- Encourage patients to eat small and frequent meals.
- Encourage the patient to eat a bland diet.
- Encourage patients to avoid fried food.
- Ensure the patients are eating enough protein and calories.
- Encourage the patients to avoid overeating.
- Instruct the patients to take anti-emetics as prescribed.
- The drugs should be reviewed if they are not effective to relieve nausea and vomiting.
- The patients should be reminded for taking anti-emetics before going for chemotherapy.

Bone Marrow Depression

Patients who are on chemotherapy and radiotherapy may develop bone marrow depression which leads to anemia, bleeding due to thrombocytopenia, and infection due to neutropenia.

Neutropenia

It is a significant reduction in the absolute neutrophil count (ANC) in the blood. They provide the first line of defense against infections. The severity of neutropenia is:

- **Mild:** ANC less than the lower limit of normal to 1500/mm³
- **Moderate:** ANC less than 1500/mm³ to 1000/mm³
- **Severe:** ANC less than 1000/mm³ to 500/mm³
- **Very severe:** ANC less than 500/mm³

Nursing Implications for Prevention of Infection

- **Hand hygiene:** Hand hygiene is the most simple and cost-effective measure to prevent the spread of infection. The patients and their caregivers should be sensitized regarding adherence to hand hygiene practices.
- **Diet:** Fresh fruits and vegetables should be restricted. Uncooked fruits and vegetables should be thoroughly washed.
- **Environment:** Protective and strict isolation helps in the prevention of infection among patients with cancer.
- **Plants and flowers:** Fresh or dried flowers could expose cancer patients to Aspergillus and Fusarium. So, these should not be kept in the patient's room.
- Treat the patient with granulocyte colony-stimulating factor (G-CSF).

Patient Education on Protective Measures for Neutropenic Precautions

Ask the patients to:
- Report fever, chills, and other signs and symptoms of infection immediately.
- Maintain personal hygiene.
- Wash hands frequently with soap and water or antiseptic hand rub.
- Bathe daily.
- Avoid activities that may affect skin integrity.
- Wear gloves when working in the garden.
- Perform regular oral care. Assess the oral cavity frequently to observe signs/symptoms of infection.
- Clean the perineal area from front to back after toileting.
- Avoid going to crowded places.
- Do not share food utensils.
- Eat the food properly washed and cooked.
- Avoid coming in contact with pets, farm animals, or animal excreta.
- Avoid going in the areas where construction material or debris has been placed or where fields have recently been ploughed.
- Avoid contact with persons who have been vaccinated within the past 30 days.

Thrombocytopenia Precautions

Platelet is an important blood cell that helps to stop bleeding by clamping and forming plugs in blood vessel injuries. The normal human platelet count ranges from 150,000–450,000 microliters of blood. Thrombocytopenia develops when the number of count falls under 150,000 microliters.

Various Signs and Symptoms of Thrombocytopenia

The deranged platelet count may affect each system of the body as enumerated below:

Cardiopulmonary
- Tachycardia, hypotension, orthopnea
- Dyspnea, tachypnoea, hemoptysis.

Head and Neck
- Petechiae at oral or nasal membranes
- Epistaxis
- Periorbital oedema, eye pain, blurred vision

Integumentary System
- Petechiae, bruising, pallor
- Bleeding from surgical devices or wound sites.

Neurologic
- Changes in mental status, confusion, and lethargy
- Widening pulse pressure, abnormal pupil size, diminished reflexes
- Headache

Gastrointestinal
- Abdominal pain
- rectal bleeding, tarry stools, hematemesis
- Enlarged liver

Nursing Implications for Thrombocytopenia

- Monitor the platelet count, PT, PTT, D-dimer, and fibrin level
- Test the stool, urine, and emesis for occult blood.
- Instruct the patients to avoid activities that may cause injury.
- Prevent the patients from falls.

Educate patients and families regarding various ways to maintain skin integrity by:
- Using a soft toothbrush
- Blowing nose gently
- Using an electric razor
- Using a water-soluble lubricant for sexual intercourse
- Avoiding any activity that may compromise skin or mucous membrane integrity
- Avoiding the use of tampons
- Using laxatives or stool softeners to avoid constipation
- Avoiding dental and other invasive procedures

Anemia

Many patients suffering from cancer and undergoing chemotherapy experience anemia. Severity may increase with comorbidities, concurrent radiation therapy, and insufficient nutritional intake.

Nursing Implications for Anemia

- Assess the nutritional intake for adequate content and quantity.
- Encourage frequent rest periods to conserve energy.
- Teach the importance of hydration.
- Provide supplemental oxygen in case of hypoxia.
- Give blood transfusions as advised by the physician.

Alopecia

- Explain to the patient that hair loss is temporary, and hair will regrow when the drug is stopped, though the texture of hair might be different.
- Use a mild, protein-based shampoo, and hair conditioner at least twice in a week.

- Minimize the use of an electric dyer.
- Avoid excessive brushing and combing of the air. Combing with a wide-tooth comb is preferred.
- Select a wig, cap, scarf, or turban before hair loss occurs.
- Keep head covered in summer to prevent sunburn and in winter to prevent heat loss.

Anorexia

- Perform nutritional assessment.
- Monitor the weight and compare it with the pre-treatment weight.
- Obtain the diet history from the patient.
- Refer to a dietician for early nutritional counselling.
- Encourage patients to eat small, frequent meals.
- Provide an attractive setting for meals.
- Use measures to control nausea and vomiting as discussed earlier.

Diarrhea

Some of the patients experience diarrhea during and after chemotherapy. Advise the patients:

- Avoid foods high in fiber, greasy or fried foods, lactose, legumes, caffeine, and alcohol. These may irritate the GI tract.
- Maintain fluid intake by drinking at least 8-10 large glasses/day of fluids in any form as per the liking of patients.
- Eat food at room temperature if not tolerated otherwise. Hot and cold foods aggravate diarrhea.
- Limit or avoids milk and other dairy products.

SAFE HANDLING OF CHEMOTHERAPEUTIC AGENTS

Clinical studies have indicated that many chemotherapeutics agents are carcinogenic, mutagenic, and teratogenic. Exposure to these agents can occur by inhalation, absorption, or digestion. Safe handling guidelines should be followed while preparing, administering, and disposing of these agents.

Drug Preparation

To ensure safe handling all chemotherapeutics drugs should be prepared according to the package insert in a class II Biologic Safety Cabinet (BSC). Venting to the outside where feasible is desirable. Personal protective equipment includes disposable latex gloves and a gown made of lint-free, low-permeability fabric with a closed front, long sleeves, and elastic cuffs. Eye protective splash goggles or a face shield must be worn when these drugs are prepared if a BSC is not used. Gloves should be changed between the preparation and administration of the drug and at least every 30 minutes during preparation and administration.

Drug Administration

Wear protective equipment. Explain to the patient that chemotherapeutic drugs are harmful to normal cells, so protective measures are used by healthcare personnel to minimize their exposure to these drugs. Healthcare professionals should administer these drugs in a safe, and unhurried manner. They should take measures during the administration of drugs to prevent any leakage by putting an absorbent pad under the tubing/IV cannula.

Disposal of Supplies and Unused Drugs

All unused supplies or drugs should be placed in a leak-proof, closable, puncture-proof, appropriately labelled container. Keep these containers in every area where drugs are prepared or administered so that waste materials need not be moved from one area to another. Dispose off containers filled with these agents as per the regulation of hazardous wastes or incinerate them at 1000°C.

BONE MARROW TRANSPLANTATION

Bone marrow transplant or hematopoietic stem cell transplant (HSCT) involves the administration of healthy bone marrow and hematopoietic stem cells in patients with dysfunctional or depleted bone marrow. Stem cells eventually proliferate into mature erythrocytes, leukocytes, and platelets.

Bone marrow transplantation involves the replacement of damaged or destroyed bone marrow with healthy bone marrow stem cells. Bone marrow is the soft, fatty tissue inside the bones. The bone marrow produces blood cells (RBCs, WBCs, and platelets). Stem cells are the immature cells in the bone marrow that give rise to various types of blood cells.

SOURCES OF BONE MARROW STEM CELLS (BOX 41.2)

BOX 41.2: Sources of hematopoietic stem cells.

- **Syngeneic:** From an identical twin
- **Allogenic:** From a sibling having HLA matching
- **Unrelated donor:** From a donor registry
- **Autologous:** From patients own marrow

TYPES OF HEMATOPOIETIC STEM CELL TRANSPLANTATION

Autologous Peripheral Blood Stem Cells

Although stem cells have been traditionally harvested from bone marrow cavities, functional hematopoietic stem cells are also found in circulating peripheral blood (PBSC). In this, the patient's own hematopoietic stem cells are removed before the high-dose chemotherapy and radiation therapy. After being removed, stem cells are stored (frozen) for later use. After chemotherapy or radiation is complete the harvested cells are thaws and returned to the patient. Steps of the procedure are shown in **Figure 41.11**.

The process of PBSC collection consists of two phases—mobilization and apheresis.

Mobilization

Peripheral blood in its steady state does not contain an adequate number of stem cells to allow for efficient collection. Bone marrow contains up to 100 times the number of stem cells found in the peripheral blood. To collect an adequate number of stem cells it is necessary to stimulate the production of PBSC through the process of mobilization. The most significant mobilization occurs when chemotherapy

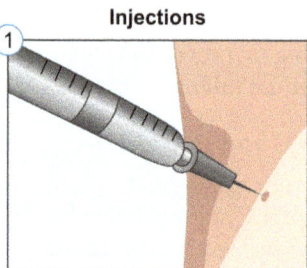
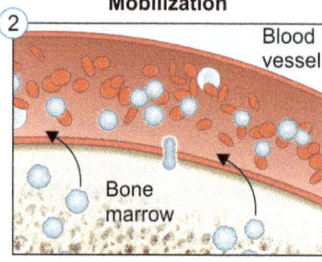
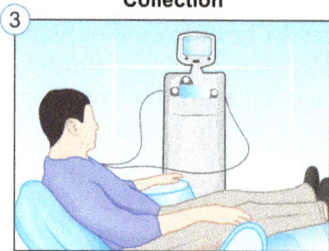
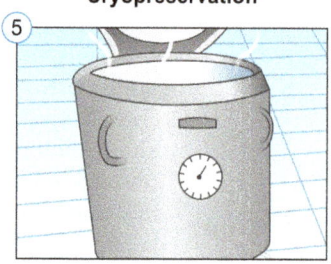
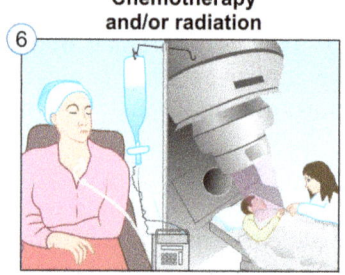
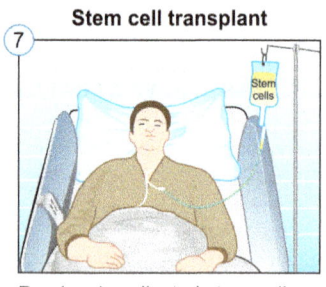
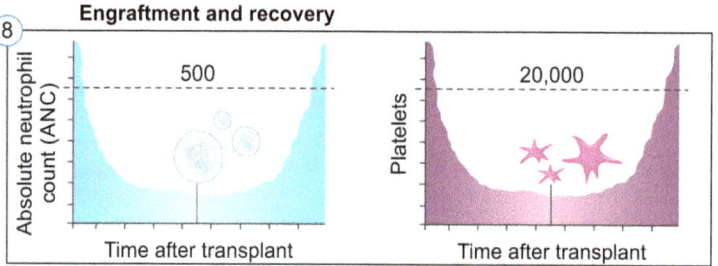

Fig. 41.11: Autologous bone marrow transplantation.

and growth factors are used together. In current clinical practice administration of chemotherapy combined with cytokines (granulocyte colony-stimulating factor G-CSF) is the preferred technique to mobilize autologous PBSC.

Apheresis

The PBSCs are collected by the process of apheresis using commercially available cell separators. The cell separators are programmed to collect either lymphocytes or low-density leukocytes. The remaining blood components are returned to the patient. Apheresis is performed for 1–3 days. Each session is 3–4 hours long but the duration is based on the rate of blood flow through the central venous catheter. After each collection, the stem cells are placed in a blood bag and cryopreserved using dimethyl sulphide (DMSO) as a cryoprotectant. The cells are kept frozen at –120°C.

Allogeneic Stem Cell Transplantation

In this type of stem cell transplantation, the donor of stem cells is another person having genetically similar blood cells to the patient. This person is often a sibling. For patients not having a compatible sibling, the donor can be a person who has been identified through a registry of possible donors. The donor's stem cells are collected in the same way as a patient's cells are collected in an autologous transplant. Once the patient has undergone conditioning, the donor's stem cells are infused into the patient **(Fig. 41.12)**.

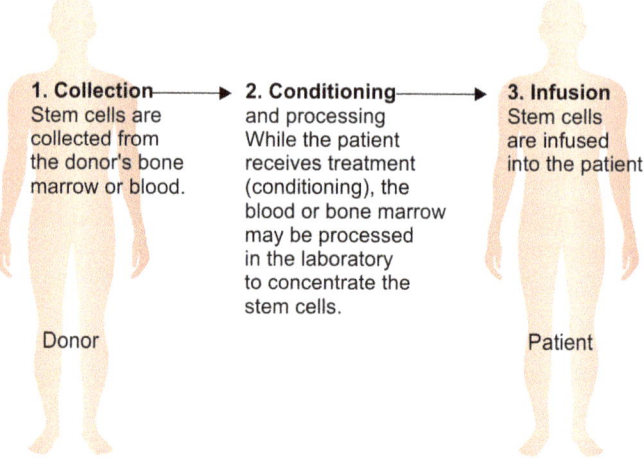

Fig. 41.12: Allogeneic bone marrow transplantation.

Allogeneic PBSC collection consists of two phases—mobilization and apheresis.

Mobilization
Mobilization of PBSC is necessary for the normal donor since there is not an adequate number available in the peripheral circulation in its steady state. With normal donors only the use of growth factor (G-CSF) is considered safe for mobilization.

Apheresis
Like the autologous PBSC, the allogeneic PBSC is collected by apheresis using standard cell separators. In normal donors, peripheral lines in the antecubital veins are commonly used for venous access.

PROCEDURE OF BONE MARROW TRANSPLANTATION

Donating Bone Marrow
Prior to donation, the donor is systematically examined. A thorough history is taken and a number of investigations are performed **(Box 41.3)**. A specialized marrow aspiration needle is used to aspirate the bone marrow **(Fig. 41.13)**. The donor marrow is obtained (harvested) by multiple aspirates from several sites on the iliac crests. The procedure is performed under general anesthesia, otherwise, it becomes very painful for the patients. The procedure lasts for about 45 minutes. In an adult 800–1,000 mL of bone marrow is aspirated and subsequently processed by a cell separator.

The separated red cells can be returned back to the donor. Transfusion of homologous blood is generally not required. Meanwhile, the white cells are processed into either a buffy coat or more commonly, mononuclear components. The preparation of mononuclear cells overcomes the problem of potential blood group (ABO) incompatibility and at the same time results in a small volume product that can be frozen in liquid nitrogen (cryopreserved).

Phases of HSCT: There are five phases of HSCT **(Fig. 41.14)**.

> **BOX 41.3:** Investigations performed before bone marrow donation.
> - Full blood count
> - Biochemistry profile
> - Virology
>   - CMV
>   - HSV
>   - HZV
>   - Hepatitis B
>   - HIV
> - Blood group
> - Chest X-ray
> - ECG

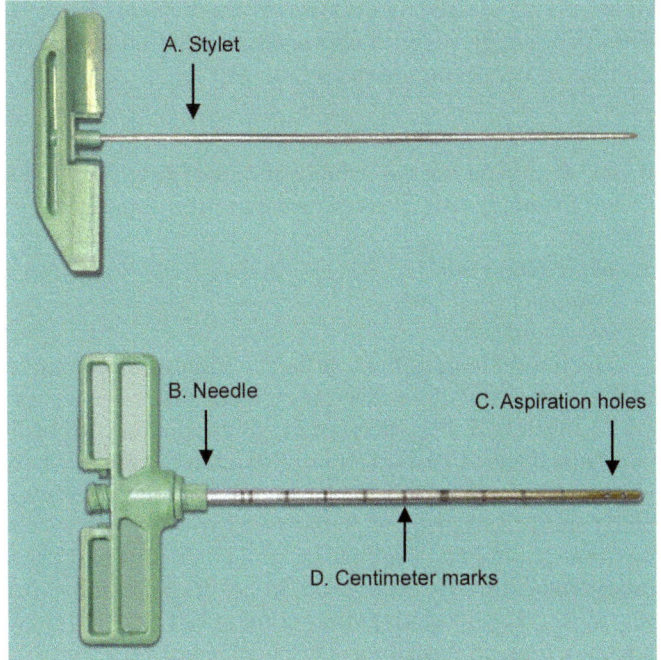

Fig. 41.13: Bone marrow aspiration needle.

Mobilization and Harvesting
Mobilization is the process to stimulate the bone marrow to produce more blood cells by giving granulocyte colony-stimulating factor (G-CSF) to the patient. In order to undergo a high dose of chemotherapy, first a predetermined minimum amount of hematopoietic stem cells needs to be collected. Previously, the removal of bone marrow from a patient's hip bones was the only available method. However, advances in technology now allow to collect stem cells from peripheral blood.

Conditioning Regimen
It involves the treatments used to prepare a patient for stem cell transplantation. It may include chemotherapy, monoclonal antibody therapy, and radiation to the entire body. It is done to help make room in the patient's bone marrow for new blood stem cells to grow, prevent the patient's body from rejecting the transplanted cells, and help kill any cancer cells that are in the body.

Reinfusion
It is a process in which stem cells are transplanted into the patient through intravenous (IV) infusion. For autologous transplants, the frozen stem cells are brought to the patient's room for transplant. The bag of cells is thawed in the normal saline bath drawn up in a large syringe and given through the rapid IV push via a central catheter. This process takes approximately 20–30 minutes. For allogeneic transplants,

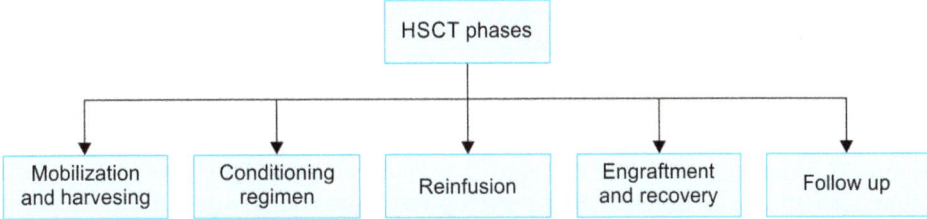

Fig. 41.14: Phases of HSCT.

stem cells are infused on the same day as they are collected. This procedure resembles an RBC transfusion and is transfused via a central venous catheter.

Engraftment and Recovery

It is a term used for the establishment of new stem cells within the bone marrow as evidenced by the appearance of (in order):
- White blood cells
- Platelets
- Red blood cells

The time of engraftment varies depending on the source of the stem cells. Bone marrow typically takes 2–3 weeks. PBSC may take 5 days (average 11–16 days), and cord cells take an average of 26 days. Transplanted stem cells begin to grow and reproduce healthy blood cells. For bone marrow or blood stem cell transplant, it may take two and three weeks for the engraftment to happen; for cord blood transplant, the process takes three to five weeks. Most of the patients have to stay in the hospital during this period to be protected from infection and monitored for side effects.

Follow-up

The patients are to be followed on a regular basis. They are monitored for signs of graft vs. host disease (GVHD) and also for complications related to chemotherapy or radiation, and cancer recurrence (relapse).

COMPLICATIONS OF HEMATOPOIETIC STEM CELL TRANSPLANTATION

Transplant recipients experience toxic complications associated with the procedure. Most complications result from the effects of the conditioning regimen. The major complications are infection, pneumonitis, veno-occlusive disease, GVHD, and graft failure.

Infection

Infection is the most common post-transplant complication. Alteration in the integrity of physical barriers and severe granulocytopenia from the pre-transplant regimen set up an environment for serious bacterial and fungal infections. One-half of all infection occurs in the first 4–6 weeks after transplant. Usually, the causative agents are from the patient's own microflora usually from GI and the integumentary system. During the first 6 weeks after the transplant, prevention of infection is crucial. Maintaining a protective environment, providing good hygiene, monitoring vital signs and head-to-toe assessment are essential.

Pulmonary Complications

During treatment, the patients are at risk for the development of pulmonary complications because their respiratory functions may become compromised. Pneumonia, inflammation of the airways, graft-versus-host disease, and bleeding are some of the things that singly or in combination may cause difficulty in breathing. The condition of the patient is closely monitored using pulse oximetry and chest X-rays. Antibiotics, fluid restriction, and oxygen therapy are administered as per requirement. If the condition worsens, the patient may need to be transferred to the intensive care unit for further management.

Veno-occlusive Disease (VOD)

VOD is the occlusion of the central veins of the liver resulting in venous congestion and stasis; this results in damage to the hepatic cells. The onset of VOD is usually within the first 3 weeks after transplantation but may occur later. VOD is usually diagnosed by its classic symptoms of weight gain, hepatomegaly, right upper quadrant pain, total serum bilirubin level more than normal, and ascites. Treatment is aimed at maintaining intravascular volume to minimize further liver damage and maintain renal perfusion.

Graft-versus-Host Disease (GVHD)

GVHD disease is a complication that can occur after allogeneic transplantation. It is the immune-mediated reaction of the newly grafted stem cells to the body of the recipient. Two types of GVHD have been identified: acute and chronic.

1. **Acute GVHD:** The risk factors related to the incidence of acute GVHD are advanced patient age, HLA mismatch, and donor-recipient gender mismatch. The skin, GI tract, and liver are the primary target organs of acute GVHD. Skin involvement is characterized by a maculopapular rash that can proceed to desquamating dermatitis. The GI involvement is characterized by nausea, vomiting, and diarrhea. Liver involvement is characterized by jaundice, elevated liver enzyme, and hepatomegaly. Because GVHD can be a life-threatening complication, means of preventing its occurrence are routinely administered. The most common medications used to prevent GVHD are cyclosporine, corticosteroid, tacrolimus, and methotrexate.
2. **Chronic GVHD:** The onset of chronic GVHD is arbitrarily defined as occurring 100 days after transplant; however, it can also occur at 70 days or years after transplant. It is characterized by scleroderma-like features and persistent immunodeficiency. It is a systemic multiorgan syndrome that resembles collagen vascular disease. Almost every organ of the body is affected but the basic effect is that of dermal thickening, fibrosis, and dryness. The standard treatment is prednisone and cyclosporine.

POST-BONE MARROW TRANSPLANT MANAGEMENT

It takes two to four weeks for the transplanted bone marrow to begin the process of hematopoiesis. During this time, the patient is at high risk for infection, bleeding, and other complications associated with bone marrow transplantation. Nurses play an important role in the prevention and management of these serious side effects.

Infection

Infection could be a significant contributing factor to morbidity and mortality in the BMT patient. So, infection prevention is extremely important during the immediate phase post-transplant. All the efforts should be directed toward the prevention of infection. The healthcare professionals should be vigilant to pick up the early signs and symptoms of infection. Vital signs should be checked and recorded hourly. Prompt interventions should be implemented at the first sign of an infectious process. The patient is kept in protective isolation in a laminar airflow room. It provides a sterile environment. The patient may also be placed in a reverse isolation room (some may be HEPA-filtered). All the protective precautions including thorough handwashing, wearing of mask, gown, and gloves should be meticulously followed by everyone whosoever is coming in contact with the patients. Since the skin is the first line of defense against infection, maintaining clean, intact skin and mucous membranes is an integral part of the care of a BMT patient. Sterile water and anti-bacterial soap are used to bathe the patients. The patient's linen should be properly sterilized. Anti-bacterial ointments should be applied to particular skin sites that tend to harbor microorganisms. The nurse must inspect the skin, mucous membranes, and central catheter site for pain, swelling, or redness every shift. As these patients are profoundly immunosuppressed, even normal GI tract flora and bacteria commonly found in food (particularly fresh fruits and vegetables) can be a source of infection. Therefore, the food is also sterilized before giving to the patients. Daily leukocyte count should be done. Only healthy immediate family members or significant friends are permitted to visit the patients.

Mucositis

Mucositis is one of the most frequent complications of the conditioning phase. It can lead to infection and bleeding in the oral cavity. Herpes simplex, *Candida*, or local infection may further deteriorate the condition of the patients. Meticulous mouth care should be provided. A thorough assessment of the mouth for ulcerations, redness, leukoplakia, bleeding, pain, etc., should be carried out at least once in each shift.

Thrombocytopenia

The patients following BMT are severely thrombocytopenic because of the disease itself and the conditioning regimen. The complications such as impaired skin and mucous membrane integrity, vomiting and diarrhea, infection, veno-occlusive disease, etc., can aggravate the patient's risk for bleeding. The nurses should be vigilant for the signs of bleeding—bruising, petechiae, hemoptysis, hematemesis, hematuria, melena, changes in vital signs or neurological status, irritability, and restlessness. Invasive procedures such as peripheral venipunctures, intramuscular injections, urinary catheterizations, and lumbar punctures should be avoided as far as possible. Rectal examinations, temperatures, and suppositories should also be avoided to prevent accidental tearing of the mucosa lining the rectum. These could cause bleeding and can become a source of infection for the patients. Certain exercises, such as bicycle riding or muscle strengthening, are restricted when the platelet count falls below 20,000. This is done to minimize the risk of bleeding into joints or muscles or intracranial bleeding due to increased blood pressure while exercising.

Veno-occlusive Disease

Veno-occlusive disease (VOD) is a form of liver disease. It occurs in around 20–30% of patients undergoing BMT one to three weeks after the conditioning chemotherapy. It is caused by the cytotoxic effects of the chemotherapy. Patients may experience various signs and symptoms like insidious weight gain, right upper quadrant pain, jaundice, hepatomegaly, ascites, elevated serum enzymes, and, in severe cases, hepatic encephalopathy. The nursing responsibilities for these patients include:

- ❖ Thorough assessment for signs and symptoms of VOD
- ❖ Maintaining a balanced fluid and electrolyte status
- ❖ Monitoring vital signs, and changes in neurological status
- ❖ Monitoring daily weight and abdominal girths
- ❖ Monitoring liver enzymes and hematology counts
- ❖ Administration of blood products and analgesic

Graft-versus-Host Disease

Graft-versus-host disease (GVHD) is a syndrome unique to BMT, especially allogeneic transplants. GVHD is a rejection process whereby the immunocompetent T lymphocytes of the transplanted marrow (graft) identify cells in the recipient (host) as foreign and attack them. The goals of nursing care of the patient with GVHD of the skin are to maintain intact skin and mucous membranes, maintain mobility, maintain patient comfort, and promote strategies to cope effectively with body image changes.

Other nursing interventions for the patient with GVHD are:

- ❖ Maintaining fluid and electrolyte balance
- ❖ Monitoring the amount, consistency, and characteristics of diarrhea
- ❖ Monitoring serum electrolytes and liver enzymes
- ❖ Monitoring vital signs, abdominal girths, and daily weights
- ❖ Administering anti-emetics and analgesics
- ❖ Providing emotional support to the patient and family.

GERIATRIC CONSIDERATIONS

For elderly persons, receiving any cancer therapy might be more difficult and complicated than the younger patients. This is because of the prevalence of existence of more comorbid illnesses in older persons. Their body will most likely react to treatment differently than a younger person's body, even when they are healthy. For instance, chemotherapy is more likely to cause severe adverse effects in older persons. So, before making any treatment decisions, the patients/caregivers should be informed about:

- ❖ The type of cancer, its stage, and its extent
- ❖ Various therapy options, together with the advantages and disadvantages of each
- ❖ Any additional medical issues that could complicate therapy or raise the possibility of negative effects
- ❖ How cancer treatment may impact lifestyle, mental health, and physical health.

> **Case Scenario**
>
> A 46-year-old patient was diagnosed with right breast cancer with FNAC and underwent total mastectomy with axillary lymph nodes dissection. Now, she is planned for external beam radiotherapy along with 6 cycles of taxane-based chemotherapy. After 10 fractions of radiotherapy and 3 cycles of chemotherapy, she complained about fever along with severe vomiting. Write the nursing management for this patient.

SUMMARY

Multiple treatment modalities are available for patients suffering from cancer. Surgery remains a cornerstone of cancer care and treatment and is increasingly employed alongside other types of treatment. Surgery may be used in a different oncology scenario with either curative or palliative intent. Radiotherapy is the treatment of cancer using radiation. The type of radiotherapy treatment to be chosen will depend on the type of cancer, cancer site, staging, and other contributing factors. The side effects are managed through a multidisciplinary approach. The dawn of immunotherapy is altering oncology care, as it has given hope and extended survival benefits to people with cancers that could not previously be treated effectively. There are a range of treatments that both target and use components of the immune system to treat cancer. Hormones are involved in the development of several cancers most commonly breast and prostate cancer. Hormone therapy may be most effectively used to achieve the best outcomes for our patients.

MULTIPLE CHOICE QUESTIONS

1. Which of the following is the most appropriate place to prepare the chemotherapeutic drugs?
    a. Patient's bedside
    b. Biological safety cabinet
    c. Nurses' duty room
    d. Inside the medicine cupboard
2. Salpingo-oophorectomy is:
    a. Removal of the ovary and fallopian tubes
    b. Removal of the uterus, ovary, and fallopian tubes
    c. Removal of the uterus and fallopian tubes
    d. Removal of ovary and uterus
3. ALARA is the acronym for a guideline used for radiation protection of staff involved in the care of patients receiving radiation.
    a. As low as reasonably achievable
    b. As long as radiation access
    c. As less as radioactivity access
    d. As low as reasonable access
4. Tamoxifen is used for:
    a. Breast cancer
    b. Prostate cancer
    c. Brain cancer
    d. Lung cancer
5. Very severe neutropenia occurs when:
    a. ANC <2000 mm^3
    b. ANC <1500 mm^3
    c. ANC <1000 mm^3
    d. ANC <500 mm^3
6. During radiation exposure:
    a. Radiation is directly proportional to the time
    b. Radiation is inversely proportional to the time
    c. Radiation is equal to the time
    d. Radiation is not dependent on time
7. The name of the surgery in which the nipple and areola are usually removed, but the rest of the skin over the breast is preserved is called:
    a. Modified radical mastectomy
    b. Skin-sparing mastectomy
    c. Breast-conserving surgery
    d. Simple mastectomy
8. In autologous bone marrow transplantation, bone marrow is taken from:
    a. Patient
    b. Parents
    c. Identical twin
    d. Siblings
9. Which of the following is NOT considered a radiation safety measure?
    a. Distance
    b. Time
    c. Shielding
    d. Environment
10. Which of the following category of chemotherapy is vesicant:
    a. Nitrosoureas
    b. Taxanes
    c. Vinca alkaloids
    d. Antimetabolites

ANSWERS

1. b	2. a	3. a	4. a
5. d	6. a	7. b	8. a
9. d	10. c		

SUGGESTED READING

1. Applebaum FR. The use of bone marrow and peripheral blood stem cell transplantation in the treatment of cancer. CA: Canc J Clin. 1996;46:142-64.
2. Bergkvist K, Larsen J, Johansson UB, Mattsson J, Svahn BM. Hospital care or home care after allogeneic hematopoietic stem cell transplantation—patients' experiences of care and support. Eur J Oncol Nurs. 2013;17(4):389-95.
3. Bevans M, Tierney DK, Bruch C, Burgunder M, Castro K, Ford R, et al. Hematopoietic stem cell transplantation nursing: a practice variation study. Oncol Nurs Forum. 2009;36(6):317-25.
4. Brown KA, Esper P, Kelleher LO, Neill B, Polovich M, White JM. Chemotherapy and biotherapy guidelines and recommendations for practice. Oncology Nursing Society; 2001.
5. Cassidy J. Chemotherapy administration: doses, infusions and choice of schedule. Ann Oncol. 1994;5(Suppl 4):25-9.
6. Crawford ED, Heidenreich A, Lawrentschuk N, Tombal B, Pompeo ACL, Mendoza-Valdes A, et al. Androgen-targeted therapy in men with prostate cancer: evolving practice and future considerations. Prostate Cancer Prostatic Dis. 2019;22(1):24-38.
7. Dodge-Palomba S. Providing compassionate care to pediatric patients undergoing enucleation of the eye. Insight. 2008;33:10-2.
8. Gilbert RW. Innovation in the surgical management of head and neck tumors. Hematol Oncol Clin North Am. 2008;22:1181-91.
9. Gyurkocza B, Sandmaier BM. Conditioning regimens for hematopoietic cell transplantation: one size does not fit all. Blood. 2014;124(3):344-53.
10. King RJB. Cancer biology. 3rd ed. London. Prentice Hall; 2006.
11. Lynch HT, Silva E, Wirtzfeld D, Hebbard P, Lynch J, Huntsman DG. Hereditary diffuse gastric cancer: prophylactic surgical oncology implications. Surg Clin North Am. 2008;88:759-78.
12. Mayer DK. Hazards of chemotherapy. Implementing safe handling practices. Cancer. 1992;70(4):988-92.
13. Mick J. Factors affecting the evolution of oncology nursing care. Clin J Oncol Nurs. 2008;12:307-13.
14. Milne JL, Spiers JA, Moore KN. Men's experience following laparoscopic radical prostatectomy: a qualitative descriptive study. Int J Nurs Stud. 2008;45:765-774.
15. Occupational Safety and Health Administration. Work practice guidelines for personnel dealing with cytotoxic (antineoplastic) drugs. Washington, DC: Office of Occupational Medicine; 1995.
16. Oseni T, Jatoi I. An overview of the role of prophylactic surgery in the management of individuals with a hereditary cancer predisposition. Surg Clin North Am. 2008;88:739-758.
17. Roe H, Lennan E. Role of nurses in the assessment and management of chemotherapy-related side effects in cancer patients. Nursing: Research and Reviews. 2014;4:103-15.
18. Scott EA. Surgery in America: From the Colonial Era to the Twentieth Century, Selected Writings. Philadelphia, PA: WB Saunders; 1965.
19. Shapiro GI, Harper JW. Anticancer drug targets: cell cycle and checkpoint control. J Clin Invest. 1999;104(12):1645-53.
20. Young LK, Mansfield B, Mandoza J. Nursing care of adult hematopoietic stem cell transplant patients and families in the intensive care unit: an evidence-based review. Crit Care Nurs Clin North Am. 2017;29(3):341-52.

CHAPTER 42

Oncological Emergencies

Puneet Kaur, Sukhpal Kaur

"Cancer is just a chapter in our lives and not the whole story".

—Allie Moreno

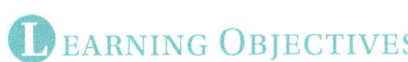

After going through the chapter, the learner will be able to:
- Understand various oncological emergencies.
- Identify assessment parameters of patients with oncological emergencies.
- Formulate strategies to prevent oncological emergencies.
- Describe medical and surgical management of oncological emergencies.
- Discuss the nursing interventions in various oncological emergencies.
- Discuss the geriatric considerations in oncological emergencies.

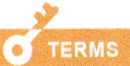

- **Curative treatment:** Therapies to destroy the cancer.
- **Cytotoxic:** Body cells killing drugs.
- **Ophthalmoplegia:** Paralysis of the muscles within or surrounding the eye.
- **Orthopnea:** Shortness of breath occurs when lying flat and is relieved by standing or sitting.
- **Pericardial effusion:** Buildup of fluid in space around the heart.
- **Plasmapheresis:** Process in which blood's liquid part, or plasma is separated from blood cells.
- **Extravasation:** It occurs when a vesicant drug leaks out of the vein into surrounding tissue.
- **Tachyphylaxis:** Acute, sudden decrease in response to a drug after its administration.

INTRODUCTION

Oncological emergencies are the acute health problems in patients suffering from cancer. These can be related to the disease itself like the compression of the vital organs by the aggressive tumor; or may be because of the side effects of treatment the patient is undergoing which may lead to metabolic and hormonal abnormalities. As these could be life-threatening, so, their immediate management is required. Many of these conditions develop gradually, however, many could be developed immediately requiring prompt interventions in order to save the life of the patients. It is very important that the nurses are aware of these emergencies in order to guide the patients during their management in the hospital so that the patients and their caregivers are empowered to recognize the manifestations at an early stage for their timely management.

In the current chapter, the common oncological emergencies are discussed system-wise for better clarity of the readers.

The common emergencies are depicted in **Figure 42.1**.

NEUROLOGIC EMERGENCIES

SPINAL CORD COMPRESSION (SCC)

SCC is a devastating complication of cancer affecting around 5% of terminal cancer patients. If it is not treated on time, it

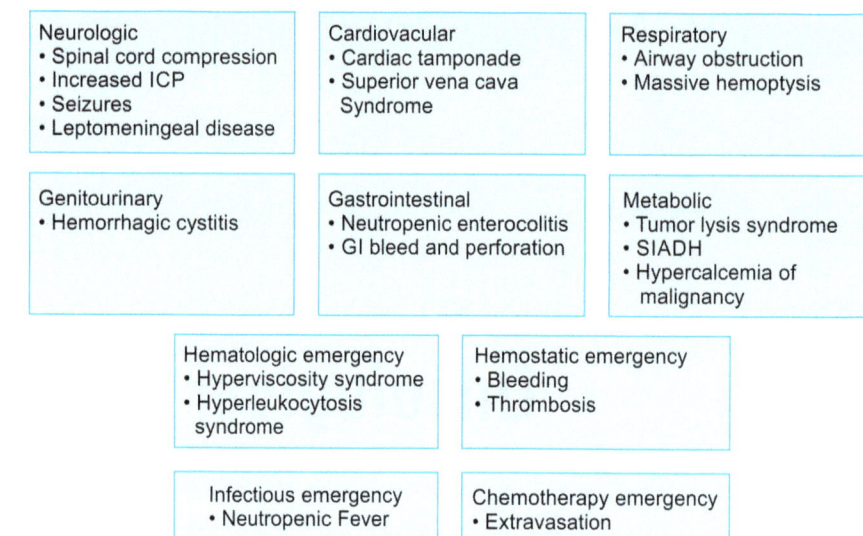

Fig. 42.1: Various oncological emergencies.

inevitably may lead to paralysis, loss of sensation, and loss of control of the anal sphincter. Around 15–20% of the patients having metastatic prostate, lung, or breast cancer develop SCC. Lymphoma, multiple myeloma, and kidney cancer are the other malignancies that frequently result in metastases to the spinal cord. In children, the tumors that spread to the spine most frequently are neuroblastoma, Ewing's sarcoma, osteogenic sarcoma, and rhabdomyosarcoma.

Since, the thoracic level of the spinal cord is the narrowest, in 60–70% of the individuals compression occurs there. It is followed by 30% in the lumbosacral area and 10% in the cervical spine. Dorsal kyphosis can further exacerbate the symptoms in the patients.

Signs and Symptoms

The degree and the site of cord involvement determine the neurologic impairment in the patients. Back pain is the commonest initial symptom occurring in around 90% of patients. Quadriplegia is caused by cervical compression; paraplegia is caused by thoracic compression; extensor plantar reflexes and bowel and bladder dysfunction are caused by upper lumbar involvement; and loss of bowel and bladder function and lower motor neuron weakening are caused by cauda equina involvement. Compression is most likely to affect the spinocerebellar pathways, posterior columns, and corticospinal tracts. With lateral compression, one may experience Brown-Squard syndrome. It is a "loss of vibratory and position senses on the side of compression and a contralateral loss of pain and temperature senses."

Diagnostic Methods

Apart from history taking, the following assessment and diagnostic tests are to be carried out:
- Tenderness at the level of compression
- Abnormal reflexes
- Sensory and motor abnormalities
- Other diagnostic tests include MRI, myelogram, spinal cord X-rays, bone scans, and CT scan. MRI is the gold standard for the diagnosis of SCC.

Medical Management

The goals of medical management include pain control, reducing complications, improving neurological functions, and maintaining the physical health and functional status of the patients. Once severe neuropathy develops, less than 10% of patients recover functional ability despite aggressive treatment. Immediate treatment includes the use of corticosteroids with dexamethasone as the drug of choice. The loading dose of dexamethasone is 10–100 mg followed by 4–24 mg four times daily. The dose can be adjusted as per the progression of symptoms. Steroids are then tapered off slowly during definitive therapy.

Radiation therapy: The recommended radiation range is two normal vertebrae above and below the boundary of the epidural tumor. Radiotherapy alone could help the patients in relieving the symptoms.

Surgery: In certain physiologically stable patients, who are in a position to tolerate surgery, anterior spinal decompression with stabilization may be performed.

Nursing Management

- Perform periodical neurofunction assessments to identify pre-existing and worsening deficits.
- Administer analgesia both by pharmacological and non-pharmacological methods
- Establish intermittent catheterization by demonstrating it to the patients or their caregivers.
- Initiate a bowel exercise program for those with bowel problems.
- Encourage the patients to perform range-of-motion exercises to maintain muscle tone.
- Encourage and support patients and families to cope with pain and changes in the functional capacity of the patients.

INCREASED INTRACRANIAL PRESSURE

Patients may experience elevated intracranial pressure due to the involvement of the brain parenchyma or obstruction of cerebrospinal fluid (CSF) flow through tumor tissue.

Signs and Symptoms

If the intracranial pressure exceeds 20 mm Hg, injury is likely and symptoms may occur. This is associated with loss of brain autoregulation and the development of ischemia or herniation.

The common presenting symptoms are headaches, nausea, vomiting, seizure, or focal neurological dysfunction. In the later stages involving imminent herniation, the patients present with the symptoms of Cushing triad exhibiting wide-pulse pressure, bradycardia, and rapid respiratory rate.

Management

- Dexamethasone is the drug of choice here also and the doses are similar to those used to relieve cord compression.
- Elevate the head end of the patient at 30° and keep it in the neutral position.
- Administer mannitol
- Correct hyperglycemia
- Maintain arterial PCO_2 between 35 and 45 mm Hg

For detailed management of the patients with increased ICP, kindly refer Chapter 29.

SEIZURES

Seizures may be the predominant symptom in 20–40% of patients with brain metastases. In addition, certain metabolic changes also can trigger seizures.

Management

Diazepam (5 mg) or lorazepam for prolonged seizures are used as part of proper acute seizure therapy. The patient must be protected from harm and the airways should be kept open. Patients should undergo a comprehensive diagnostic evaluation including imaging studies, cultures, drug levels (if indicated), and serum biochemistry.

In patients with extensive lesions, continuous anticonvulsants should be started with an initial dose of 15 mg/kg phenytoin and a maintenance dose of 300 mg/day.

LEPTOMENINGEAL DISEASE

Leukemias (5–15%), lymphomas (7–15%), and primary brain tumors (1–12%) are other solid tumors that can metastasize to the leptomeninges.

Leptomeningeal carcinomatosis occurs most frequently in advanced adenocarcinoma.

Clinical manifestations vary.

Signs and Symptoms

Patients may present with:
- Headache
- Changes in mental state
- Nausea/vomiting
- Localized weakness of the limb
- Seizures
- Pain distributed axially or radially
- Dermatome sensory loss
- Bladder and bowel dysfunction.
- Double vision, hearing loss, facial numbness, decreased vision, and ophthalmoplegia.

Diagnostic Tests

- **Lumbar puncture:** CSF cytology.
- Elevated protein, decreased glucose, and pleocytosis suggest leptomeningeal disease, but only CSF cytology is required for diagnosis.
- If leptomeningeal protuberances or nerve root clumps are present, imaging studies may also have to be carried out.

Management

A combination of surgery, radiation, and chemotherapy treatment better works for patients with leptomeningeal disease and improves the prognosis. Radiation therapy involves whole-brain irradiation for radiosensitive tumors. Patients may also be administered thiotepa (thioplex), cytarabine, or methotrexate with/without radiation therapy for less sensitive tumors, injected directly into the cerebrospinal fluid, either by lumbar puncture.

CARDIOVASCULAR EMERGENCIES

CARDIAC TAMPONADE

It is a medical emergency in which there is the accumulation of fluid in the pericardial sac, and the compression of the heart thereby leads to a decrease in cardiac output and the patient can go into shock. The most frequent cause of pericardial tamponade is malignant pericardial effusions. This illness should be recognized at the earliest because it can be very devastating despite having curable cancer and a favorable short-term outlook. Untreated patients have a median survival period of about 4 months, and 25% make it to their first year.

Primary pericardial tumors are usually uncommon causes of cardiac tamponade. Generally, it is because of metastatic tumors, such as lung and breast tumors, lymphomas, leukemia, and melanomas.

Signs and Symptoms

- Difficulty breathing and chest pain—sudden onset
- Cough
- Pyrexia
- Peripheral edema
- Hoarse voice
- Hiccups
- Nausea/vomiting

Diagnostic Evaluation

- Physical examination reveals hypotension, elevated jugular venous pressure, tachycardia, and narrow arterial pulse pressure.
- A chest X-ray shows a large "water-bottle heart" characteristic of slowly accumulating exudates.

Medical Management

Treatment is aimed at relieving acute symptoms and preventing recurrence. Temporary measures include IV infusion and oxygen administration.

For immediate relief of symptoms, pericardiocentesis is done. The aspirated fluid should be sent for chemical and cytological analysis. Methods to prevent fluid accumulation include systemic chemotherapy, catheter drainage, radiation therapy, or surgery. Chemotherapy injection into the pericardial space as a means of reducing the risk of recurrence of malignant pericardial effusions has been found beneficial for patients.

Appropriate systemic therapy should be started as per indication.

Surgical procedures include pericardiectomy, pleural pericardial window, or subxiphoid pericardiotomy.

Nursing Management

- Assess the consciousness level of the patients.
- Frequently check vital signs and oxygen saturation.
- Analyze the arterial blood gas and electrolyte values.
- Raise the head of the patient's bed as per the comfort of the patient.
- Lower the patient's physical activity to reduce oxygen needs; provide supplementary oxygen as needed.
- Ensure proper oral hygiene on a regular basis.
- Position every 2 hours and encourage the patient in deep breathing exercises to cough out secretions.
- Maintain patent IV line.
- Re-orient the patient to time, place, and person
- Provide supportive care and appropriate patient instruction as needed.

SUPERIOR VENA CAVA SYNDROME (SVCS)

In SVCS, there is obstruction of blood flow through the SVC. It can easily be compressed by tumors arising from lungs, mediastinal structure or lymph nodes. Malignant tumors are the most common cause of superior vena cava thrombosis (SVC) and superior vena cava syndrome (SVCS). Lung cancer leads to SVCS in 3–15% of patients. Lymphoma and tumors that have spread to the mediastinum are the other common causes of SVCS.

Signs and Symptoms

Clinical manifestations depend on the degree of SVC obstruction.
The common symptoms of SVCS include:
- Facial edema
- Difficulty in breathing
- Cough
- Orthopnea
- Edema of the neck and upper extremities.
- Dysphagia
- Headache
- Confusion

Diagnostic Evaluation

- Physical examination alone may be able to diagnose patients who have overt SVCS.
- The chest X-ray may show a mass on the right side of the chest and an enlarged mediastinum.
- Anatomical relationships between structures are defined by computed tomography (CT) and magnetic resonance imaging (MRI) scans, which also provide information on the intrinsic or extrinsic nature of collateral circulation and occlusion.
- The most conclusive diagnosis method is invasive contrast venography. It allows catheter access for thrombolytic treatment and precisely describes the etiology of blockage.

Management

Treatment depends on the severity of the symptoms and the type of malignancy. Patients rarely need urgent radiation therapy before they are diagnosed.

Depending on the tumor type, definitive treatment includes radiotherapy in high-dose fractions (300–400cGy) for the first 3 days, followed by low-dose fractionation (180–200 cGy).

The use of angioplasty, stents, and thrombolytic treatment are becoming more common. If delivered within 7 days of the onset of symptoms, thrombolytic therapy using streptokinase or urokinase may be beneficial.

Patients should continue taking anticoagulant medications, such as heparin or warfarin because they are more susceptible to developing new thromboses, including deep vein thrombosis. Low doses of warfarin can help lower the frequency of catheter-related thrombosis.

Nursing Management

- Identify patients at risk of developing SVCS.
- Monitor and report any clinical symptoms of SVCS.
- Elevate the head end side of the bed of the patients. Proper posture promotes breathing patterns. This helps promote well-being and reduce anxiety caused by dyspnea resulting from progressive edema.
- Provide supplemental oxygen.
- Monitor the intake output status of the patient and administer fluids watchfully to minimize edema.

RESPIRATORY EMERGENCIES

Cancer patients generally develop many respiratory complications. These may either be directly related to tumor growth and its invasion or indirectly to various treatment modalities.

MALIGNANT AIRWAY OBSTRUCTION

It can occur because of extrinsic compression from bronchial lesions or adjacent structures. Many patients with the cancer of tongue, thyroid, oropharynx, trachea, bronchi, and lungs may experience obstruction of the airways at some stage during the disease. Symptoms may be acute or subacute.

Signs and Symptoms

- Difficulty in breathing
- Wheezing
- Cough
- Heaviness in the neck
- Hemoptysis
- Dysphagia

Management

- Emergency treatment for impending obstruction includes intubation or tracheotomy.
- Provide supplemental oxygen and corticosteroids.

MASSIVE HEMOPTYSIS

Massive hemoptysis, the discharge of 400–600 mL of blood in 24 hours, is a rare occurrence. Massive hemoptysis is most frequently associated with bronchiectasis, pulmonary abscesses, aspergillosis, and bronchogenic cancer.

Diagnostic Evaluation

- Identifying the site of bleeding. A head and neck examination should be done to rule out extrapulmonary hemorrhagic foci.
- Bronchoscopy is the diagnostic procedure of choice.

Management

- Bed rest in a semi-upright position, humidified oxygen, sedation, blood and fluid replacement, platelet transfusions, and correction of abnormal coagulation parameters.
- Endobronchial tamponade can be used as a temporary measure until definitive treatment.
- Definitive treatment consists of surgical resection, neodymium-doped yttrium aluminium garnet (Nd:YAG) laser ablation, and bronchial artery catheterization and embolization.

GENITOURINARY EMERGENCIES

HEMORRHAGIC CYSTITIS

It can be caused by pelvic radiation, immune-interfering drugs (such as penicillin antibiotics), all invasive urothelial tumors. Despite prophylaxis with high-dose chemotherapy, the incidence of hemorrhagic cystitis can reach up to 40%, and mortality from uncontrolled bleeding is 2–4%. Bladder problems develop in 20% of patients who receive pelvic radiation.

Management

Once hemorrhagic cystitis develops, initial conservative therapy includes removal of blood clots, continuous bladder irrigation with saline or hydrocortisone, discontinuation of anticoagulant therapy, and control of the patient's predisposition to bleeding diathesis.

Second-line therapy includes cystoscopy and radiofrequency, intravesical formalin, intravesical prostaglandin (carboprost tromethamine], oral or parenteral conjugated estrogens, or intravesical administration of silver nitrate, phenol, or aluminum hydroxide. In resistant cases, urinary diversion, internal iliac artery ligation, embolization, or cystectomy may be required.

Preventive measures include aggressive fluid intake to promote frequent urination, continuous bladder irrigation, and administration of the uroprotectant Mesna (Mesnex). Mesna is a sulfhydryl compound that neutralizes acrolein without regenerating it, unlike N-acetylcysteine. It can be administered parenterally or orally.

GASTROINTESTINAL EMERGENCIES

NEUTROPENIC ENTEROCOLITIS

It is a severe inflammatory disorder of the intestine developing in neutropenic patients. It is characterized by stomach distension, right-side abdominal discomfort, watery diarrhea, and fever. Myelodysplastic syndromes, aplastic anemia, hematologic malignancies, and solid tumors are the conditions the syndrome is most frequently linked to. It can occur anywhere from 12% to 46% of the time. Mortality rates for these patients range from 50% to 100% and sepsis is typically the cause of death.

Bacterial invasion, direct damage to the intestinal mucosa, and bleeding into the intestinal wall with necrosis are the various risk factors for this complication. Nearly all patients who suffer from this disease have previously been treated with antibiotics, which has the unintended consequence of promoting fungal overgrowth and selection of aggressive microbes that can invade the intestinal wall.

Diagnostic Evaluation

- Plain X-ray abdomen shows a pattern of ileus with a dilated appendix
- CT scan—can reveal thickening of the bowel wall with pneumatosis.
- Endoscopies and invasive procedures, such as barium enema should be avoided as patients are at high risk of perforation.

Management

- Bowel rest, NPO
- Administer TPN
- Nasogastric suction

Surgery is indicated for perforation, bleeding, abscess formation, or failure of medical management. The necrotic bowel should be resected, and bowel diversion should be performed; primary anastomoses are unlikely to be successful in leukopenic patients.

GASTROINTESTINAL BLEEDING AND PERFORATION

Malignancy ranks third in importance among factors that induce gastrointestinal bleeding in cancer patients, after hemorrhagic gastritis and peptic ulcer disease. The most likely tumor to induce bleeding directly is a lymphoma. With lymphomas, perforation is a far less frequent consequence, happening in about 3–10% of cases.

Evaluation should be done carefully to rule out the cause of bleeding. Management is done as per the cause of bleeding.

METABOLIC EMERGENCIES

TUMOR LYSIS SYNDROME (TLS)

Rapidly destroying cancerous cells can produce intracellular ions and cellular breakdown products that might lead to potentially fatal metabolic disturbances. Burkitt's lymphoma, acute lymphocytic leukemia, and acute nonlymphocytic leukemia are among the tumors with a rapid proliferation index that exhibit tumor lysis syndrome. The condition typically appears after induction chemotherapy, although it can also occur spontaneously in individuals with a high tumor load, radiation therapy, corticosteroids, hormonal therapy (such as tamoxifen), biologic agents (such as interferon), or after treatment with hormonal agents, such as corticosteroids.

The syndrome exhibits hyperuricemia, hyperkalemia, hyperphosphatemia, and hypocalcemia metabolically. These can occur individually or in various combinations. If left unnoticed, calcium-phosphate complexes and uric acid can precipitate in the renal interstitium and renal tubules, respectively. Due to the impairment in renal function caused by these precipitates, metabolic acidosis may aggravate the condition.

Patients may be predisposed to tumor lysis syndrome due to high tumor burden, high serum lactate dehydrogenase (LDH), volume loss, acidic urine, and increased urinary urate excretion.

Signs and Symptoms
- Cardiac arrhythmias
- Seizure
- Fatigue
- Carpal spasms
- Neuromuscular hypersensitivity
- Signs of dehydration
- Impaired level of consciousness.
- Acidosis
- Nausea, and vomiting

Diagnosis
- Assess for the above-enlisted symptoms to clinically evaluate the patients.
- Lab findings showing two or more abnormal metabolic rates
- Assess the renal functions, cardiac abnormalities, seizures

Management
- To minimize morbidity and mortality from TLS, prevention, and prompt initiation of appropriate treatment are extremely important.
- Precautions, such as urine alkalinization, intensive fluid intake, and administration of allopurinol should be administered before initiating systemic therapy.
- Regularly monitor the electrolytes, blood urea nitrogen (BUN), creatinine, uric acid, phosphorus, and calcium levels.
- Fluid intake should exceed 3,000 mL/m² /day (200-300 mL/h).
- Sodium bicarbonate in an amount of 100 mEq/L can be added to intravenous fluids to alkalinize the urine.
- Allopurinol should be administered at a dose of 500 mg/m² on days 1 through 3, then reduced to 200 mg/m² throughout cytoreductive therapy. This regimen should be continued for at least 2-3 days after completing chemotherapy.
- Continuously monitor the patients for arrhythmias. Appropriate treatment with calcium and exchange resins should be initiated.
- Administer empirical antibiotic therapy for opportunistic infections.
- Hemodialysis may be required if conservative treatment fails. Hemodialysis is preferred over peritoneal dialysis because it removes uric acid and phosphorus more effectively.

Nursing Management
- Assessment of patients for signs and symptoms of electrolyte imbalances and teach them to report the same.
- Assess the urine output and the pH to confirm alkalization.

SYNDROME OF INAPPROPRIATE ANTIDIURETIC HORMONE SECRETION (SIADH)

SIADH is characterized by hyponatremia due to inappropriately concentrated urine. Around 1-2% of cancer patients develop SIADH. Small cell lung cancer is the most common cause. It accounts for 60% of all SIADH cases.

Signs and Symptoms
- Patients exhibit subtle mental and cognitive changes, such as memory loss, apathy, impaired abstract thinking, fatigue, anorexia, muscle aches, and headaches.
- Severe hyponatremia (serum sodium <115 mEq/L) or rapid-on-set hyponatremia is characterized by asterisks, altered mental status, confusion, lethargy, seizures, and ultimately coma.

Diagnostic Evaluation
- Physical examination may show papilledema, abnormal reflexes, and focal findings.
- Demonstration of normal thyroid and adrenal function and development of euvolemia is required prior to diagnosis of SIADH.
- Measure serum and urine electrolytes and osmolality, BUN, creatinine, serum cortisol and liver function test.
- In SIADH, urinary sodium concentrations are usually above 20 mmol/L.

Medical Management
- Fluid intake should be limited to <1000 mL/day, or <500 mL/day if the patient is unresponsive. Patients with refractory hyponatremia, or those who can be managed on an outpatient basis, can be treated with demeclocycline (decromycin) 600-1,200 mg daily in divided doses.
- Patients presenting with symptoms, such as coma and seizures can be treated with 3% hypertonic saline by slow infusion at a rate sufficient to raise serum sodium by 0.5-1.0 mEq/L/h
- Rapid correction (greater than 2 mEq/L/h) may be associated with central pontine myelination.
- Saline and intravenous furosemide may also be effective.

Nursing Management
- Maintain intake and output charts
- Assess the level of consciousness
- Monitor and record the vital signs accurately
- Monitor daily body weight
- Check urine-specific gravity.

- Also assess nausea, vomiting, loss of appetite, edema, fatigue.
- Monitor serum electrolyte levels, osmolality, blood urea nitrogen, creatinine, and urinary sodium levels.
- Minimize patient activity.
- Maintain proper oral hygiene. Maintaining environmental safety. Limit fluid intake as needed.
- Reorient the patient and provide guidance and encouragement as needed.

HYPERCALCEMIA OF MALIGNANCY

It is one of the most common metabolic events in cancer patients. Around 30% of cancer patients develop this complication during the course of their disease. The most common types of hypercalcemia-associated tumors are those of the breast, lung, kidney, and esophagus.

Malignant hypercalcemia occurs when the tumor develops systemic humoral factors that alter calcium metabolism in the bone, kidney, or intestine and at sites of tumor metastasis to the bone.

The disease is characterized by increased bone resorption, hypercalciuria, increased renal calcium absorption, increased renal cAMP, hypophosphatemia, and hyperphosphatemia.

SIGN AND SYMPTOMS

- Fatigue
- Lethargy
- Polyuria
- Constipation
- Coma
- Renal failure
- Cardiac arrhythmia

DIAGNOSTIC EVALUATION

- Laboratory results include elevated serum calcium (may exceed 14 mg/dL), low serum chloride, elevated or normal serum phosphate and bicarbonate, and elevated alkaline phosphatase.
- In contrast, only 25% of patients with primary hyperparathyroidism have serum calcium concentrations greater than 14 mg/dL. The chloride concentration is elevated above 112 mmol/L.
- ECG may show a shortened QT interval. Arrhythmias may also occur.

MANAGEMENT

- Treatment in the acute phase begins with aggressive hydration with saline. Initial treatment for hypercalcemia includes rapid IV hydration with an initial 1000-2000 mL bolus of normal saline accompanied by an infusion rate of 200-300 mL/h to reach 100-150 mL/h urine output. One needs to be cautious in case of heart failure.
- Cardiac monitoring should be performed in patients with severe hypercalcemia. Serum electrolytes should be carefully monitored and replaced as needed.
- Patients who cannot tolerate large exchanges can be treated with loop diuretics at doses of 20-100 mg every 1-2 hours with urine output at 300-500 mL/h. Thiazide diuretics can increase serum calcium levels and should be avoided. Vitamin supplements and parenchymal growth factors should also be avoided.

Gallium nitrate: It binds to bone and decreases the solubility of hydroxyapatite crystals in order to lower serum calcium levels. It has no effect on osteoclasts' ability to function. Gallium has a mean half-life of about 24 hours. Because it is poorly absorbed, the medication cannot be taken orally.

After the initial dose, the serum calcium level in the patient's blood gradually decreases until it reaches a minimum after 7-10 days. Nephrotoxicity, which manifests as an increase in BUN and creatinine, is one of the negative effects. Incidence estimates range from 8% to 15%. Reduced visual and auditory acuity, ocular neuritis, and pulmonary effusions and infiltrates are some other side effects of gallium. Gallium may be especially beneficial in treating hypercalcemia brought on by lymphoma since it directly inhibits the growth of the disease.

Plicamycin: It is an anti-cancer drug that lowers calcium by impairing osteoclast and bone resorption directly. Hemorrhage, thrombocytopenia, platelet deficiencies, renal insufficiency, hepatic damage, nausea, and vomiting are some of the toxic side effects that might happen after receiving repeated doses. Patients with impaired renal function should not use plicamycin,

Calcitonin: The medication of preference for quickly lowering a patient's serum calcium level is the calcitonin. It lowers calcium faster than bisphosphonates. It begins to reduce renal tubular calcium reabsorption within minutes. Additionally, calcitonin reduces calcium release from the skeleton and suppresses osteoclast activity.

Patients with organ failure can be given calcitonin safely, in contrast to other pharmacologic agents. The activity of calcitonin may be prolonged by the coadministration of glucocorticoids. Tachyphylaxis usually arises 72 hours after calcitonin is administered, and it restores serum calcium levels to baseline. Thus, in cases of life-threatening hypercalcemia, calcitonin is best administered as a temporary therapy until longer-acting medications can take action.

Bisphosphonates: Osteoclast activity is inhibited by synthetic pyrophosphate analogs known as bisphosphonates. The drugs that are used in clinical practice the most frequently are etidronate (Didronel) and pamidronate (Aredia).

Although etidronate can be given parenterally or orally, oral absorption is only moderate. Etidronate side effects include nephrotoxicity, metallic taste, bone demineralization after repeated high dosages, and accelerated phosphate absorption by the kidney with hyperphosphatemia. Patients with a blood creatinine level of more than 5 mg/dL should not be given etidronate.

Nursing Management

- Identification of the patients at risk and signs and symptoms for hypercalcemia.
- Educating patients and families about early detection and prevention to prevent any fatality.
- Encourage patients to have a daily intake of fluids 2-4 L unless contraindicated due to any cardiac and renal disease condition.

- Teach the use of dietary and pharmacologic interventions, such as stool softeners and laxatives for the management of constipation.
- Advice patient to maintain appropriate calcium levels and to get it checked often.
- Promote mobilization and teach the importance and prevention of demineralization and breakdown of bones.

HEMATOLOGIC EMERGENCIES

HYPERVISCOSITY SYNDROME (HVS)

It is characterized by a decrease in microvasculature circulation, decreased blood flow, and vascular congestion caused by markedly increased serum protein. Blood viscosity gets increased. Congestion occurs most commonly in peripheral, retinal, cerebral, and cardiac arteries. Multiple myeloma, polycythemia vera, Waldenstrom's macroglobulinemia, acute or chronic high cell count leukemia, dysproteinemia, and very rarely solid tumors are all associated with this disease. 85-90% of cases of Waldenstrom's macroglobulinemia are caused by this disease, and 5-10% by myeloma. Hyperviscosity syndrome may also be observed in light chain disorders with highly polymerized light chains.

Signs and Symptoms

The classic triad of HVC is:
- Skin bleeding
- Neurological deficits
- Vision Problems

Patients may also suffer from heart failure. Bleeding diathesis is usually manifested by epistaxis, ecchymosis, and mucosal bleeding. The hallmark of this syndrome is the tortuous, dilated, "sausage-like" retinal veins. Bleeding, exudate, and papilledema can occur as hyperviscosity syndrome progresses.

Diagnostic Evaluation

- Diagnosis is clinical and confirmed by measuring serum viscosity. The normal range for serum viscosity is 1.4–1.8 (compared to water). Most patients begin to develop symptoms when serum viscosity exceeds 4.0.
- Commonly observed laboratory findings include anemia and iron deficiency, increased red blood cell to blood volume, azotemia, rouleaux, elevated serum protein, and adrenal insufficiency.
- Look for thrombocytopenia, prolonged bleeding time, abnormal thrombus retraction, and abnormal platelet aggregation.

Management

- The main goal is reducing serum viscosity by the administration of IV fluid, plasmapheresis, or leukapheresis.
- Plasma pheresis is an emergency treatment for symptomatic Hyperviscosity. It is recommended to replace 3-4 L of plasma within 24 hours. Maintenance plasmapheresis of 1-2 L, 1-2 times a week may be required until definitive treatment is effective. Because it replaces immunoglobulins and clotting factors, it is usually replaced with fresh frozen plasma.
- Hypocalcemia associated with citrate anticoagulants may be observed. Plasmapheresis is more effective in IgM paraproteinemia because 80% of the protein is intravascular.

HYPERLEUKOCYTOSIS SYNDROME

It is most commonly seen in acute myeloid leukemia patients. It could be quite fatal because it is associated with respiratory failure, intracranial hemorrhage, and early death. Leukemia patients have significantly elevated white blood cell (WBC) counts, putting them at risk for end-organ damage due to leukemia infiltration and the impact of leukemic cells on the vasculature.

AML and CML in blast crisis with peripheral leukocyte counts >100,000/mL or rapidly increasing are the diseases that put patients at increased risk for leukostasis, Patients with lymphoblastic malignancies are less likely to develop symptomatic leukocytosis. There is no specific WBC number at which this condition is apparent.

Reduced deformability of leukemic blasts by microvasculature silting, local hypoxia due to blast cell oxygen consumption, the affinity of neoplastic cells for lung epithelium, and blast infiltration are some of the pathogenic pathways. When the hematocrit is reduced, Hyperviscosity usually does not occur.

Signs and Symptoms

The most frequently affected clinically are the pulmonary and nervous systems.
- Neurological symptoms—dizziness, blurred vision, tinnitus, ataxia, confusion, delirium, somnolence, papilledema, retinal vein dilation, retinal hemorrhage, coma, and intracranial hemorrhage.
- Pulmonary symptoms—fever, tachypnea, dyspnea, hypoxia, lung infiltrates, and respiratory failure.
- Hyper-leukocyte syndrome should be part of the differential diagnosis in all patients with minimal physical examination and chest radiographic findings related to respiratory failure.

Diagnostic Tests

- Oxygen consumption and leukocyte glycolysis in blood samples can artificially lower PO_2 and serum glucose, resulting in falsely elevated platelet counts.
- Pseudohyperkalemia may also be observed.
- Correlation with pulse oximetry should be established to assess the adequacy of oxygen replacement.

Management

- Administer oxygen, allopurinol, urine alkalinization, hydration, and immediate cytoreductive therapy.
- Initial treatment should include leukapheresis because cytotoxic chemotherapy can induce cytolysis and temporarily exacerbate symptoms.
- If leukapheresis is not available, hydroxyurea can be used at doses of 50-100 mg/kg/day (3-5 g/m^2) to induce rapid cytoreduction. The goal is to reduce the total white blood cell count by 20-60% in the first hours of treatment.

- Whole-brain irradiation at doses of 4-6 Gy is recommended for CNS lesions.
- Modifying the hemoglobin concentration above 10 g/dL is contraindicated as it may exacerbate symptoms.

HEMOSTATIC EMERGENCIES

BLEEDING

The hemostatic system can vary greatly depending on the disease and the kind of treatment. Various causes of bleeding in cancer patients:
- Disseminated intravascular coagulopathy
- Decreased clotting factors/abnormal clotting factors
- Primary fibrinolysis/fibrinolysis
- Platelet dysfunction
- Vascular defects
- Circulatory anticoagulants

Abnormal hemostasis test values are detected in 50% of patients with metastatic disease. Significant bleeding can occur in up to 10% of cancer patients.

Thrombocytopenia is the common cause of bleeding (50%). It is usually the result of chemotherapy or tumor involvement of the bone marrow, but can also be caused by coagulopathy, immune-mediated mechanisms, infection, or sequestration.

The use of prophylactic platelet infusion in such cases is controversial. However, because bleeding can be life-threatening, platelet infusions of 6-8 units every 1-2 days are recommended until the platelet count drops below 10,000–20,000/mm^3.

Multiple transfusion recipients frequently acquire alloantibodies to the class I HLA determinants on their platelets, which hastens the platelet clearance process. Alloimmunization ranges from 40% to 60% in leukemic patients and get close to 80–90% in aplastic anemia patients. Patients who develop this illness should have HLA-matched platelets from a single donor or a family member. Alloimmunization can be prevented by using leukocyte-depleted platelets, leukocyte filters, single donor platelets, and UV-irradiated platelets. These efforts help lessen the frequency of illnesses transmitted through blood transfusions, such as the cytomegalovirus (CMV), and febrile transfusion reactions.

Platelet pheresis can treat platelet dysfunction brought on by high platelet counts (more than 700,000/mm^3). The most frequent platelet functional abnormalities reported include poor platelet factor 3 release, insufficient alpha granules, and reduced aggregation to adenosine diphosphate (ADP) and epinephrine.

Numerous hematologic malignancies are also linked to acquired von Willebrand's disease. Treatment for the underlying malignancy usually helps the disease, and other therapeutic options include cryoprecipitate or desmopressin infusions.

Asparaginase (Elsper) therapy for acute leukemia has been shown to cause bleeding and thrombosis similar to those seen in disseminated intravascular coagulation (DIC). Bleeding can be managed by discontinuing asparagine therapy and administering cryoprecipitate and fresh frozen plasma.

Up to 50% of individuals with acute leukemia may experience DIC development, which can aggravate the disease. Procoagulant substances leading to DIC and fibrinolysis are found in myeloblasts, promyelocytes, monocytes, and lymphoblasts. Gastric, prostate, breast, and lung cancers are a few tumors that are frequently linked to DIC.

Clinical Manifestations of DIC
- Spontaneous bruising, petechiae, purpura,
- Gingival bleeding, bleeding from the sites of indwelling catheters.
- Fulminant DIC—bleeding in multiple sites simultaneously (pulmonary, CNS, gastrointestinal, or genitourinary sites).

Diagnostic Evaluation

Prolonged aPTT and thrombin time, decreased antithrombin III levels, increased fibrin degradation products, elevated D-dimer assay, and the presence of fragmented cells or schistocytes in the peripheral blood.

Management
- Patients with abnormal laboratory test findings but no clinical symptoms should receive antineoplastic treatment and antibiotics.
- Closely observe the patients. Induction chemotherapy with therapeutic dosages of 1,000 U/h heparin may reduce morbidity and death.
- Patients with heavy bleeding may benefit from the replacement of clotting factors and platelets. Cryoprecipitates and fresh frozen plasma are the best alternatives. Patients with fibrinogen levels <125 mg/dL should receive cryoprecipitate.

Nursing Management
- Maintain a consistent intake and output.
- Examine skin color and temperature.
- Assess the level of consciousness, headaches, vision problems, chest discomfort, reduced urine production, etc.
- Examine all body orifices, tube insertion sites, incisions, and bodily excretions for bleeding.
- Examine the findings of laboratory tests.
- Reduce physical activity to reduce risk of injury risks
- Prevent bleeding by applying pressure to all venipuncture sites and avoiding unnecessary invasive operations; use electric razors instead of straight-edged razors; avoid using tape on the skin; and encourage gentle and proper dental hygiene.
- Assist the patient in proper posture
- Reorient the patient, maintain a safe environment; and provide proper patient education and supportive measures.

THROMBOSIS

Deep venous thrombosis, arterial thrombosis, migratory thrombophlebitis, pulmonary embolism, and nonbacterial thrombotic endocarditis are some of the thromboembolic events that affect 5–10% of cancer patients. Infections are the leading cause of death in people with solid tumors, followed by thromboembolic events. The colon, gallbladder, gastric, lung (any cell type), myeloproliferative syndromes, ovary, pancreatic, and paraprotein diseases are a few cancers that are frequently linked to thrombotic events. Lung, pancreatic, and colon cancer patients can develop nonbacterial thrombotic endocarditis. The spleen is the organ most frequently infarcted, while the aortic valve is most frequently implicated.

Several pathways mediate hypercoagulability. Shortened aPTT and PT are symptoms of increased levels of clotting factors, including fibrinogen and factors I, V, VIII: C, IX, and XI. Increased levels of D-dimer and fibrin degradation products are symptoms of low-grade DIC. Acquired protein C, protein S, and antithrombin III deficiencies also show reductions in coagulation inhibitors.

Diagnostic Evaluation

- Physicians should closely monitor patients for thrombotic complications.
- Appropriate examinations include impedance plethysmography, phlebography, arteriography, ventilation/perfusion scans, etc.
- A complete coagulation profile should include PT, aPTT, platelet count, D-dimer, fibrin degradation products, fibrinogen, antithrombin III, protein S, and protein C.

Management

Medical management aims to treat the immediate event and lower the likelihood of recurrent episodes. For the underlying cancer, all patients should get antineoplastic therapy. Antiplatelet medications, such as dipyridamole or enteric-coated aspirin may be administered to asymptomatic patients.

Surgical procedures, such as embolectomy/vena cava interruption or thrombolytic therapy with streptokinase, urokinase, or plasminogen activators can be used to treat life-threatening thrombotic episodes. Heparin anticoagulation should then be used after treatment for the acute disease.

To treat severe thrombosis and reduce repeated occurrences, heparin and warfarin can be administered. To maintain an aPTT of 1.5–2.0 times control, heparin may be administered for 7–10 days. Starting oral warfarin on day 5 and continuing it for several days should follow the heparin therapy. Warfarin regimens that are less rigorous and have an international normalized ratio (INR) of 2.0 are nonetheless effective at preventing thromboembolism and carry a lower risk of bleeding.

EMERGENCIES CAUSED BY CHEMOTHERAPY

NEUTROPENIC FEVER

As a result of cancer treatment, particularly chemotherapy, neutropenic fever (NF) is one of the most well-known oncologic emergencies. Other risk factors include the rapid decline in absolute neutrophil count (ANC), and susceptibility to prior chemotherapy or immunosuppression.

Gram-positive cocci, such as *Staphylococcus aureus, Streptococcus pyogenes, Streptococcus pneumoniae, Streptococci viridans,* and *Enterococcus faecalis* and *faecium* are the most common causes of NF cases that have been confirmed by culture. *E Coli, Pseudomonas aeruginosa,* and *Klebsiella* species are some examples of gram-negative bacilli. The most prevalent fungal infection is *Candida ablicans*.

Presentation

The signs of neutropenic fever include a single oral temperature of 38.5°C or higher, a sustained temperature of 38°C or higher for an hour, and an ANC of less than 500 cells/mm^3 or a predicted drop of ANC to less than 500 cells/mm^3 in the upcoming 48 hours.

Diagnostic Evaluation

- Complete blood count (CBC)
- Renal and liver function test
- Urinalysis and analysis
- Chest X-ray
- *C. difficile* test and examining the stool cultures if the patient has diarrhea.

Management

Until they are afebrile for 48–72 hours and have ANC levels of at least 500 cells per mm^3 for 72 hours, patients with FN who are at high risk of complications should start receiving empiric antibiotics intravenously in the hospital environment.

Only sufficiently broad-spectrum medications, such as carbapenem, piperacillin-tazobactam, or fourth-generation cephalosporin cefepime, all of which have anti-pseudonomic action, are suitable for monotherapy.

Infections of the skin and soft tissues, pneumonia, or suspected device infections may benefit from the use of vancomycin rather than receiving it alone.

Patients with a persistent fever of unclear origin after 4–7 days of antibiotic therapy and those whose neutropenia is anticipated to remain longer than 7 days are advised to begin empirical antifungal therapy.

EXTRAVASATION OF CHEMOTHERAPY

Extravasation is the unintentional installation or leakage of cytotoxic drugs into the perivascular space during the infusion of these drugs. Three categories of cytotoxins—vesicants, irritants, and non-vesicant drugs—have been developed based on their subcutaneous toxicity.

Sign and Symptoms

The clinical presentation and intensity of the symptoms vary, and they may appear immediately or over the course of the next few days or weeks. Pain, induration, blistering, and discoloration are some of the initial signs. In severe cases, necrosis of the skin and underlying tissues may form, causing swelling, scarring, infection, a delay in treatment, functional disability, amputation, and, rarely, death. Erythema, swelling, and soreness are signs of irritating extravasation.

Management

The best strategy for dealing with an extravasation injury is prevention. Additionally, it is crucial to educate patients about dangers and symptoms. With the exception of vinca alkaloids and epipodophyllotoxins, it is advised to use ice (cooling), which produces vasoconstriction and lowers pain and the severity of local injury. Negative pressure wound healing and hyperbaric oxygen therapy are further methods. The use of nanoparticle medicines and liposomal chemotherapeutic agents results in less exposure to the surrounding tissue due to lower drug diffusion ability.

GERIATRIC CONSIDERATIONS

A substantial risk factor for many cancer is getting older. Age is an indirect risk factor for cancer since it increases exposure to carcinogenic substances and gives genetic alterations more time to accumulate, both of which could lead to the development of tumors. Geriatric patient treatment involves more difficulties as compared to young patients. Multisystem physiological changes develop as we grow old. Despite the fact that these changes are normal, they make older people less capable of handling stress on the body and more vulnerable to pharmacokinetic and pharmacodynamic interactions, which may result in toxicity. Thus, it is imperative that nurses caring for geriatric patients understand the unique challenges their patients may face to ensure that the care provided meets those needs.

Case Scenario

A 72-year-old female with newly diagnosed stage II diffuse large B cell lymphoma presents with fever to ER. She completed her first cycle of chemotherapy one week ago. She had chills this evening, with a fever of 100.4°F. There is no cough, urinary frequency, or urgency. No recent sick contact or recent travel history.

Physical examination: P-96, R-16, SaO_2-97%, no palpable LN, port site clean, non-tender, no erythema, resp—no rhonchi/rales, CVS—no murmurs, no organomegaly, no edema.

Possible diagnosis: Febrile neutropenia

Patients with cancer are subjected to infection prevention measures, with hand washing ranking as the most crucial non-pharmacological measure. Antimicrobials aimed at bacterial, viral, and fungal pathogen prevention are possible alternatives.

SUMMARY

A series of potentially fatal illnesses known as oncological emergencies develop as a direct or indirect effect of cancer or cancer treatment. Leukostasis, tumor lysis syndrome, superior vena cava, hypercalcemia, and neutropenic fever are just a few of these ailments. Patients with symptoms need to be evaluated quickly and receive specialized help as soon as possible. Always consider the therapeutic objectives in the management of the underlying oncologic illness (e.g., palliative care). Physicians must maintain a high level of suspicion in order to prevent and detect oncologic emergencies early, and they must properly inform patients about taking precautions and reporting symptoms.

MULTIPLE CHOICE QUESTIONS

1. Drug of choice in spinal cord compression is:
   a. Bleomycin
   b. Dexamethasone
   c. Heparin
   d. Sodium bicarbonate
2. "Water bottle heart" is a characteristic feature of which disorder?
   a. Tumor lysis syndrome
   b. Cardiac tamponade
   c. Neutropenic enterocolitis
   d. Hyperviscosity syndrome
3. A decrease in microvasculature circulation, decreased blood flow, and vascular congestion caused by markedly increased serum protein is suggestive of which of the following diagnosis?
   a. Pericardial tamponade
   b. Superior vena cava syndrome
   c. Congestive heart failure
   d. Hyperviscosity syndrome
4. Treatment of choice in hyperviscosity syndrome is:
   a. Blood transfusion
   b. Plasmapheresis
   c. Radiation therapy
   d. Chemotherapy
5. Hyponatremia as a complication is most commonly seen in:
   a. Tumor lysis syndrome
   b. SIADH
   c. DIC
   d. Cardiac tamponade
6. A 35-year-old woman with leukemia is admitted in the ward for chemotherapy. She complaints of generalized body weakness. Laboratory findings suggest pancytopenia, hyperkalemia (K 7.2), uric acid 15, and elevated LDH levels. What is the cause of this electrolyte imbalance?
   a. SIADH
   b. Hyperviscosity syndrome
   c. Tumor lysis syndrome
   d. Renal failure
7. A 72-year-old man with Ca lung was admitted as worsening of dyspnea. On examination, patient has distended neck veins, moon shaped face, exophthalmos, venous collaterals on his chest wall and murmurs. What is the most probable diagnosis?
   a. Congestive heart failure
   b. Superior vena cava syndrome
   c. Constrictive pericarditis
   d. Cardiac tamponade
8. Mesna is a drug of choice in which of the following disorder?
   a. Neutropenic enterocolitis
   b. Hemorrhagic cystitis
   c. Tumor lysis syndrome
   d. Hyperviscosity syndrome
9. Spinal cord compression occurs most commonly at which level?
   a. Lumbar
   b. Thoracic
   c. Cervical
   d. Sacral
10. A 42-year-old man admitted to ward with diagnosis of leukemia having fever 102°F, laboratory findings reveal leukocyte count of 800 with 27% polymorphonuclear cells. Which is the most appropriate treatment regimen?
    a. Cephalosporins
    b. Vancomycin, tazobactam and gentamycin
    c. Amikacin
    d. Doxycycline

ANSWERS

1. b	2. b	3. d	4. b
5. b	6. c	7. b	8. b
9. b	10. b		

SUGGESTED READING

1. Arrambide K, Toto RD. Tumor lysis syndrome. Semin Nephrol. 2018.13(5):27380.
2. Averbuch SD. New bisphosphonates in the treatment of bone metastases. Cancer. 2016.7(4):3443-52.
3. Baer MR. Management of unusual presentations of acute leukemia. Hematol Oncol Clin North Am. 2014;7(3):275-92.
4. Bates T. A review of local radiotherapy and cord compression. Int J Radiat Oncol Biol Phys. 2018;7(2):217-21.
5. Behl D, Hendrickson AW, Moynihan TJ. Oncological emergencies. Crit Care Clin. 2010;26:181-205, doi:10.1016/j.ccc.2009.09.004

6. Bick RL. Coagulation abnormalities in malignancy: A review. Sem in Thromb and Hemost. 2015;12(6):353-72.
7. Boogerd W, van der Sande JJ. Diagnosis and treatment of spinal cord compression in malignant disease. Cancer Treat Rev. 1993; 19:129-50.
8. Byrne TN. Spinal cord compression from epidural metastases. N Engl J Med. 2018; 27(6):614-9.
9. Campbell J, Mitchell CA. Acute leg ischemia as a manifestation of the hyperleukocytosis syndrome in acute myeloid leukemia. Am J Hematol. 2014;12(5):46-58.
10. Carter PW, Cohen HJ, Crawford J. Hyperviscosity syndrome in association with kappa light chain myeloma. Am J Med. 2013; 12(6):591-5.
11. Chamberlain MC. Current concepts in leptomeningeal metastasis. Curr Opin Oncol. 2018;15(5):533-9.
12. Choucair AK. Myelopathies in the cancer patient: Incidence, presentation, diagnosis, and management. Oncology. 2015;5(6).71-80.
13. Choucair AK. Myelopathies in the cancer patient: Incidence, presentation, diagnosis, and management. Oncology. 2021;5(7):25-37.
14. Colman RW, Rubin RN. Disseminated intravascular coagulation due to malignancy. Semin Oncol. 2015;7(3):172-86.
15. Dabrow MB, Wilkins JC. Management of hyperleukocytic syndrome, DIC, and thrombotic thrombocytopenic purpura. Postgrad Med. 2013;14(5):193-202.
16. DeVries CR, Freiha FS. Hemorrhagic cystitis. A review. J Urol. 2018;7(2):143-9.
17. Donahue LA, Frank IN. Intravesical formalin for hemorrhagic cystitis: Analysis of therapy. J Urol.14(6):809-12.
18. Dosik GM, Luna M, Valdivieso M, et al. Necrotizing colitis in patients with cancer. Am J Med. 2016;20(8):646-56.
19. Dunlau RW, Camp MA, Allon M, et al. Calcitriol in prolonged hypocalcemia due to the tumor lysis syndrome. Ann Intern Med. 2016;12(7):162-4.
20. Escalante CP. Causes and management of superior vena cava syndrome. Oncology. 1998;7(6):61-77.
21. Gartrell K, Rosenstrauch W: Hypoxemia in patients with hyperleukocytosis. True or spurious, and clinical implications. Leuk Res. 2014;12(4):915-9.
22. Geraci JM, Hansen RM, Kueck BD. Plasma cell leukemia and Hyperviscosity syndrome. South Med J. 2016;14(6):800-5.
23. Goenka P, Chait M, Hitti IF, et al. Acute leukostasis pulmonary distress syndrome. J Fam Pract. 2012;10(5):445-9.
24. Hall TG, Burns Schaiff RA. Update on the medical treatment of hypercalcemia of malignancy. Clin Pharm. 2011;9(3):117-25.
25. Helms SR, Carlson MD: Cardiovascular emergencies. Semin Oncol. 1989;16:463-70.
26. Heyman MR, Schiffer CA. Platelet transfusion therapy for the cancer patient. Semin Oncol. 2012;9(3):198-209.
27. Jafari A, Tavirani MR, Salimi M, Tavakkol R, Jafari Z. Oncological Emergencies from Pathophysiology and Diagnosis to Treatment: A Narrative Review. Social Work in Public Health. https://doi.org/10.1080/19371918.2020.1824844.
28. Kinirons MT. Newer agents for the treatment of malignant hypercalcemia. Am J Med Sci. 2012.8(4):403-6.
29. Klemencic S, Perkins J. Diagnosis and management of oncologic emergencies. Western Journal of Emergency Medicine. 2019;20(2):316-27.
30. Kreidieh FY, Moukadem HA, El Saghir NS. Overview, prevention and management of chemotherapy extravasation. World Journal of Clinical Oncology. 2016;7(1):87-95.
31. Kreisman H, Wolkove N. Pulmonary toxicity of antineoplastic therapy. In: Perry MC (Ed). The Chemotherapy Source Book. 2015; pp. 598-619.
32. Lascari AD. Improvement of leukemic hyperleukocytosis with only fluid and allopurinol therapy. Am J Dis Child. 2013;8(3):969-72.
33. Levine LA, Jarrard DF. Treatment of cyclophosphamide-induced hemorrhagic cystitis with intravesical carboprost tromethamine. J Urol. 2019;17(6):719-23.
34. Liu YK, Harty JI, Steinbock GS, et al. Treatment of radiation or cyclophosphamide-induced hemorrhagic cystitis using conjugated estrogen. J Urol. 2020;13(6):41-43.
35. Lyons MK, Meyer FB. Cerebrospinal fluid physiology and the management of increased intracranial pressure. Mayo Clin Proc. 1990;25(4):684-707.
36. Markman M. Common complications and emergencies associated with cancer and its therapy. Cleve Clin J Med. 2021;35(6):105-14.
37. Moses AM, Scheinman SJ. Ectopic secretion of neurohypophyseal peptides in patients with malignancy. Endocrinol Metab Clin North Am. 2009;21(13):489-506.
38. Nand S, Messmore H. Hemostasis in malignancy. Am J Hematol. 2014;15(7):45-55.
39. Nelson SC, Bruggers CS, Kurtzberg J, et al. Management of leukemic hyperleukocytosis with hydration, urinary alkalinization, and allopurinol. Are cranial irradiation and invasive cytoreduction necessary? Am J Pediat Hematol Oncol. 2018; 20(9):15:351-5.
40. Nussbaum SR. Pathophysiology and management of severe hypercalcemia. Endocrinol Metab Clin North Am. 2018;12(4):343-62.
41. Patterson WP, Caldwell CW, Doll DC. Hyperviscosity syndromes and coagulopathies. Semin Oncol. 2015;10(4):210-6.
42. Perrin RG. Metastatic tumors of the axial spine. Curr Opin Oncol. 2020;32(8):525-32.
43. Pestalozzi BC, Sotos GA, Choyke PL, et al. Typhlitis resulting from treatment with taxol and doxorubicin in patients with metastatic breast cancer. Cancer. 2014;12(4):1797-800.
44. Pierce ST. Paraendocrine syndromes. Curr Opin Oncol. 2014;9(3):639-45.
45. Pimentel L. Medical complications of oncologic disease. Emerg Med Clin North America. 2014;7(2)407-19.
46. Ringenberg QS, Doll DC. Acute nonlymphocytic leukemia. The first 48 hours. South Med J. 2014;12(7):83-93.
47. Rosol TJ, Capen CC. Mechanisms of cancer-induced hypercalcemia. Lab Invest. 2015;14(6):680-702.
48. Schiller JH, Jones JC. Paraneoplastic syndromes associated with lung cancer. Curr Opin Oncol. 1998;9(2):335-42.
49. Shepherd JD, Pringle LE, Barnett MJ, et al. Mesna versus hyperhydration for the prevention of cyclophosphamide-induced hemorrhagic cystitis in bone marrow transplantation. J Clin Oncol. 2018;12(4):2016-20.
50. Silverman P, Distelhorst CW. Metabolic emergencies in clinical oncology. Semin Oncol. 2016;14(7):504-15.
51. Soares FA, Landell GAM, Carduso MC. Pulmonary leukostasis without hyperleukocytosis: A clinicopathologic study of 16 cases. Am J Hematol. 2015;12(7):28-32.
52. Stellato TA, Shenk RR. Gastrointestinal emergencies in the oncology patient. Semin Oncol. 2015;1495):521-31.
53. Thomas CR, Dodhia N. Common emergencies in cancer medicine: Metabolic syndromes. J Natl Med Assoc. 2014;9(2):809-18.
54. Thomas CR, Edmondson EA. Common emergencies in cancer medicine: Cardiovascular and neurologic syndromes. J Natl Med Assoc. 2015;34(7)1001-17.
55. Vaitkus PT, Herrmann HC, LeWinter MM. Treatment of malignant pericardial effusion. JAMA. 1998;11(5):59-64.
56. Wade DS, Nava HR, Douglass HO. Neutropenic enterocolitis. Clinical diagnosis and treatment. Cancer. 2014;17(5):17-23.
57. Willson JKV, Masaryl TJ. Neurologic emergencies in the cancer patient. Semin Oncol. 2012;24(9):490-503.

CHAPTER 43

Palliative Care

Sukhpal Kaur, Jyoti Kathwal

"You matter to the last moment of your life, and we will do all we can, not only to help you die peacefully, but to live until you die."
—**Dame Cecily Saunders**

LEARNING OBJECTIVES

After going through the chapter, the learner will be able to:
- Define palliative care.
- Enumerate the principles of palliative care.
- Discuss the domains of palliative care.
- Describe the role of a multidisciplinary team in palliative care.
- Appreciate various models of palliative care.
- Understand various symptoms at the end of life and their management strategies.

TERMS

- **Hospice care:** It is a kind of care focusing on the quality of life, not prolonging life for patients whose life expectancy is not more than six months.
- **Hospice:** Providing home-like care.
- **Life limiting disease:** A disease condition which has no cure and the patient is dependent on medication for comfort and eventually dies due to the disease.
- **Palliative care:** It is comforting the life of an individual by providing them symptomatic relief.

INTRODUCTION

Death is an inevitable entity. Everyone has to die one day. But sudden death is very rare. In the past, people often use to die suddenly of diseases, infections, or accidents. Advances in medicine have transformed our society. Because of advancements in medications, technology, and more awareness among the public, people are living longer. With the increase in life expectancy, many health-related problems develop as we get older, such as cancer, various non-communicable diseases, communicable diseases, such as HIV/AIDS, etc. At the end of life, these may seriously impair the quality of life of an individual and burdened the family's economy, the society, and the healthcare system at large. People often had to spend many years living with serious and chronic illnesses. A significant number of people specifically residing in rural areas have poor access to health care and when available, the care may not be appropriate. To improve the care for people living with serious illnesses, and to ensure that they get the care as per their requirements, palliative care is required.

The current chapter acquaints the readers with the concept of palliative care and its related aspects, such as when to start palliative care, the domains and principles of palliative care, and management of the symptoms the patients requiring palliative care experience.

CONCEPT AND DEFINITION OF PALLIATIVE CARE

At the beginning of any illness, all the interventions aim at the curative aspects of the disease and prolong the life of the patients. But later once it is comprehended that these curative measures have become ineffective, the emphasis of care shifts to symptomatic management of the patients. This is what palliative care is. It is the active total care of

> **BOX 43.1:** Certain concepts of palliative care.
>
> - Palliative care is not only for cancer patients, but it is for all people living with any of serious illness.
> - Palliative care can be provided to the patients at any time during the course of a serious disease.
> - It is a multidisciplinary approach for the patients, their family members, and caregivers.
> - It is useful at any stage of a serious incurable disease.
> - The preventable physical, psychological, and social problems are identified at an early stage and are managed accordingly.
> - The sufferings of the patients are reduced to the minimum as far as possible to optimize their quality of life.
> - It can be provided in any setting (hospital, community, hospice, home).
> - It is a patient and family-centered approach to care.

patients whose disease is not or is no more responsive to the curative treatment. The concept of palliative care involves not adding years to life but adding life to years by providing "low tech and high touch" care to the patients. It is patient-centric and not disease-centered. The term "palliative care" has come from the word "palliate," which means, to make the effect of something less severe, intense, painful, harmful, or harsh. Thus, palliative care is provided to diminish the level of severity of the symptoms of a disease without curing the underlying cause with the main aim to improve the quality of life of the patients and their family and friends as well. WHO defined palliative care as, "an approach that improves the quality of life of patients and their families facing the problems associated with life-threatening illness, through the prevention and relief of suffering by means of early identification and impeccable assessment and treatment of pain and other problems, physical, psychosocial, and spiritual."

Palliative care offers a support system to the patient and family. It is not only for the end-stage cancer patients, but it is required for the elderly people, stroke, end-stage systemic diseases, neuromuscular disorders, HIV/AIDS, head injuries, spinal injuries, paraplegics, any mental and physical incapacitation, etc. Palliative care has gain more momentum since last two decades, though, it has been existing since the medieval era.

Certain concepts of palliative care are enumerated in **Box 43.1**.

BRIEF HISTORICAL ASPECTS OF PALLIATIVE CARE

Words, such as hospitality, hospice, hostel, and hospital all are derived from the Latin word "Hospes" which means guest. History reveals that the hospices were earlier managed by religious groups where the ill would come to get cured. Till the 19th century, there was no difference between the hospice and the hospital. King Asoka built eighteen institutions that were, such as hospice care units. Literature reveals the existence of such institutes in Buddhist, Islamic, and Christian traditions as well.

Dame Cicely Saunders was the founder of the hospice movement and improved palliative care. She took responsibility to improve palliative care when she lost her love to cancer and identified that quality of life is important in end-of-life care. She provided the concept of "total pain" which covered the physical, emotional, social, and spiritual aspects of distress.

India is evolving in palliative care. In 1975, Government of India started the National Cancer Control Programme. It was later modified in 1984 and included the pain relief services to be provided at PHC.

Palliative care was started in Gujarat in 1980 and provided pain clinic services under the Department of Anesthesia, followed by the formation of the Indian Association of Palliative Care (IAPC). The first hospice unit was established in 1986 under the guidance of Professor D'Souza named Shanti Avedna Ashram in Mumbai. Same time, many pain clinics were established in Kerala with the help of WHO. Since 1990, there has been a consistent increase in the palliative and hospice care units. In 1994, the IAPC was registered as Public Trust and society in Gujarat and in 1997 can support was founded which provided palliative care and home care support services in Northern India. Palliative care in India is still in the early developmental stage and need support from the medical and nursing field as well. About three percent of cancer patients gain access to pain relief services.

WHEN TO START PALLIATIVE CARE?

Figure 43.1 depicts the time of starting palliative care for the patients. At the bottom from left to right, it shows the time when an illness is diagnosed and the journey of the patient till death. From bottom to top, it depicts the different types of care, i.e., primarily initially curative care, which tries to cure disease or prolong life; and later primarily palliative care which tries to ease the suffering that comes along with serious illness. It also shows that palliative care can be started from the very beginning when the patients get diagnosed with an illness. It will be more of curative and less of palliative in the beginning and with the progression of disease and time, it becomes more of palliative and less of curative. Following the death of the patient, the family and other caregivers are counseled for bereavement support.

Palliative care often concentrates on symptom management in the early stages of sickness. It also begins to learn a patient's or family's beliefs so that those values may be used to guide the patient's present and future medical decisions. Palliative care increasingly becomes a more significant role when the illness enters its final stage and fewer and fewer therapies are effective in extending life

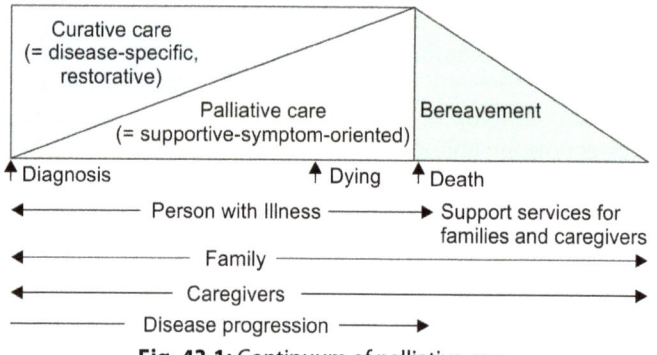

Fig. 43.1: Continuum of palliative care.

or treating the condition. This is significant since families frequently require more help as time goes on and a patient's symptoms worsen.

PALLIATIVE CARE TEAM

Palliative care is a holistic and interdisciplinary approach of providing care to patients and their caregivers. Palliative care teams often include doctors, nurses, social workers, psychologists, pharmacists, dieticians, etc., with the patient and the family at the central position **(Fig. 43.2)**. The palliative care team work in coordination with each other with the goal to help patients achieve the best possible quality of life. They perform multitasking. They develop a plan of care, manage pain and other symptoms, attend to the emotional, psychosocial, and spiritual aspects of dying and caregiving, teach the family how to provide care, advocate for the patient and family, and in the end provide bereavement care and counseling. Family members or carers play a key role in providing care and are central to the palliative care team. They are vulnerable to stress and social isolation and experience stress when providing care to their family member. They should be provided with information about the development of, such asly complications the patients may have and how they will impact their quality of life. So, they are counseled, and provided with practical aid, and training by the whole of the palliative care team.

PRINCIPLES OF PALLIATIVE CARE

The patients requiring palliative care are looked after keeping in mind the principles as that of a good clinical practice. A holistic approach considering the medical, nursing, alternative therapies, social, cultural, and spiritual aspects is taken into consideration. The palliative care approach has the following principles:

- ❖ **Patient and family are seen as one unit:** While planning care along with the patients, the needs of the family should also be taken into consideration. The family members, relatives, and friends are, such asly to have substantial emotional and physical distress, particularly if the patient is being managed at home. So, specific attention should be given to their needs, so that they are better able to cope and comply with the palliative care interventions. The success of palliative care may depend on the ability of the caregivers to cope.

  Apart from this, it is also important to understand that when patients, family, and other caregivers are involved in the care, it can lead to increased patient satisfaction, reduced stress, and increased empowerment among the caregivers.

- ❖ **Holistic and individualized care:** Every patient is a unique individual. In palliative care, each patient is managed as a 'whole' considering their physical, psychological, social, and spiritual needs. Patients with similar underlying diseases will have different physical, psychological, and social problems. So, because of the unique characteristics of each human being, the needs of each individual patient should be considered when planning care for them. All aspects of the suffering of patients and not just the medical, nursing, or social problems should be taken into consideration. A non-judgmental approach irrespective of caste, creed, ethnic background, or religious beliefs should be there while providing care to the patients. Cultural differences should be respected and the interventions should be planned in a culturally sensitive manner. Irrespective of the diagnosis, treatment, and life expectancy, the palliative care team must provide a respectful care to the patients. They should understand that the patients and their family members are going through the most difficult phase of their life.

- ❖ **Interdisciplinary approach:** Palliative care is a broad multi-disciplinary approach. The provision of comprehensive care to patients requires an interdisciplinary team who provide care to the patients as per their role as well as expertise. The whole of the palliative care team should be empathetic, and compassionate, and demonstrate a caring attitude towards the patients. Each team member should be able to see different aspects of the patients' suffering and provide appropriate care to them.

- ❖ **Palliative care can be initiated at any stage of illness:** Palliative care is not just for patients having terminal illnesses, but as soon as the disease condition is anticipated as incurable, it should be planned and implemented. It can be provided in conjunction with the ongoing interventions to treat an underlying disease. The overall plan of care should be established. It should be regularly reviewed as per the needs of the patients to prevent any physical and emotional crises that may occur with the progression of the disease. Some of the clinical problems can be predicted and prevented by implementing appropriate interventions, e.g., preventing bedsores in the bedridden patients.

- ❖ **Pain relief and comfort from other distressing symptoms:** The delivery of symptomatic and supportive care on a regular basis and providing comfort to the patients are important aspects of palliative care. The team should understand the cause of the distressing symptoms and their management. It shall be done based on the patient's condition and the feasibility of the intervention. The target is to provide relief without adding side effects or adding new problems to the patients. Pain management

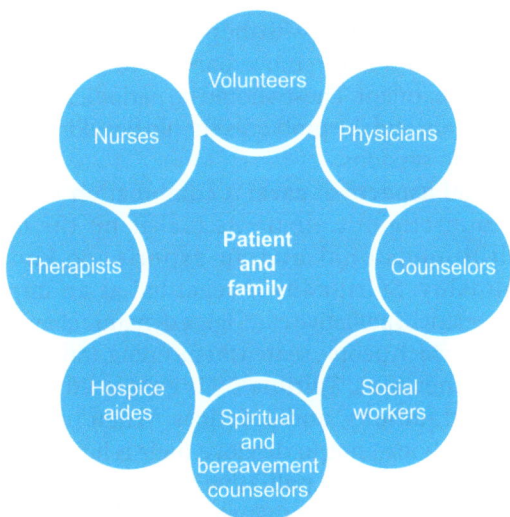

Fig. 43.2: Palliative care team.

should be done properly to enhance the comfort of the patients.

- ❖ **Affirm life and regards dying as a normal process:** Palliative care considers life and death as a normal and natural process. It neither hastens nor postpones death. All the efforts are directed towards the relief of suffering and enhancing the quality of life of the patients and not at the prolongation of life. All the treatment modalities should be appropriate to the stage of the disease and its prognosis. The active treatment known to be futile at the end of life should not be carried out further anymore in order to prevent unnecessary additional suffering which may be caused by that inappropriate active therapy.
- ❖ **Psychological and emotional aspects of care:** Palliative care goes beyond the physical aspects of providing care. The psychological and emotional issues which are very common in end-of-life care are also dealt with by the palliative care team. Their problems are listened to by the team. The support system and professional help are provided accordingly.
- ❖ **Respite care:** It involves having someone else to take care for the patient when their regular caretaker takes a brief break to relax and recuperate. This will give them some rest from their duties and may help prevent burnout. The palliative team may also help to provide such kind of support depending upon the availability of resources.
- ❖ **Bereavement support:** Bereavement is the grief of loved ones following the death of their patient. Following the death of a loved one, the focus of the team turns toward their family to provide support and counseling. So, palliative care apart from supporting the family to cope during the journey of illness of the patients, also helps them during their bereavement period through counseling.
- ❖ **Communication:** Communication in palliative care is extremely important amongst the team members as well as with the patients and their family members. The patient and the family members should be included in any of the discussions related to care. The consent of the patient and family is very imperative before starting any new treatment or in case of withdrawing anyone. They should be explained in simple understandable language without any medical jargon. Effective communication may support a family with decision-making.
- ❖ **Advance care planning:** It involves eliciting the end-of-life wishes, values, and preferences of the patients regarding their future treatments/last rites, etc. The patient may not be in a position to verbalize his/her wishes, so it is important to identify a family member who will be considered as a surrogate decision-maker and who is having some knowledge of the patient's wishes. Though many of these matters may be personal and of family affair, however, the palliative care team might help them to some extent. Planning all these in advance will help to prevent conflicts amongst the family members.

DOMAINS OF PALLIATIVE CARE

Various domains of palliative care are structure and processes of care; physical aspects of care; psychological aspects of care; social aspects of care; spiritual aspects of care; cultural aspects of care; care of imminently dying; and ethical and legal aspects of care. All these are further discussed as follows:

- ❖ **Structure/setting/processes of palliative care:** Principles and practices of palliative care can be incorporated into any of the settings including hospital, community, and home care settings. It should be ensured that we have the availability of a trained interdisciplinary team (IDT) in order to provide the best possible patient- and family-centered care. The emphasis on the involvement of patient and family, communication, care coordination, and continuity of treatment across healthcare facilities are the important requisites of palliative care.
- ❖ **Physical aspects of care:** The main emphasis of palliative care is symptomatic management. Pain, shortness of breath, exhaustion, nausea and vomiting, constipation, etc., are some of the most common symptoms these patients experience. Various management strategies include pharmacological, and non-pharmacological including behavioral, and complementary therapies. The ultimate goal is to preserve the functional status of the patients and improve their quality of life. The whole of the palliative care team works in collaboration with each other to achieve this aim.
- ❖ **Psychological aspects of care:** Along with physical health, there are a number of psychological issues these patients have to experience which are related to the disease itself, the kind of treatment the patient is undergoing, and the various-related symptoms. The interdisciplinary team addresses these psychological elements of care.
- ❖ **Social aspects of care:** The palliative care team addresses environmental and social elements that have an impact on patients and their families. Social determinants of health have a significant impact on the quality of care. The palliative care team collaborates with the patient and family to identify strengths and address their needs. There is a need to explore the social support system; financial constraints; and access to care, such as transportation and medicine, etc., available for the patients. Family meetings are an effective clinical strategy for concluding the process of thorough assessment and planning, recommendations, and cordial transfers to community/local service providers.

  Regular consultations with the patient and family can help identify issues and remove barriers to providing high-quality treatment. These should be periodically reviewed by the team and the problems should be addressed in the follow-up sessions.
- ❖ **Spiritual aspects of care:** A combination of religious and nonreligious elements makes up the diverse, multidimensional human experience known as spirituality. Spirituality is regarded as an important component of palliative care. It is a dynamic characteristic through which people search for meaning, transcendence, and connections. Spirituality is expressed via beliefs, values, traditions, and practices. When patients and families choose not to disclose their religious views or accept support, the palliative care team nonetheless provides care in a way that respects all spiritual beliefs and practices. Members of the care team must be aware of

their own spirituality. They should be provided assistance from a spiritual advisor, such as a priest, pastor, chaplain, rabbi, imam, or other religious figure.

- ❖ **Cultural aspects of care**: Cultural backgrounds have an impact on how patients and healthcare professionals see palliative and end-of-life care. Respect your family's traditions, attitudes, and viewpoints on matters of health, disease, and the duties of family carers. Include culturally appropriate tools and techniques in the treatment plan. By ensuring that language requirements are satisfied, communication obstacles may be eliminated. First, values, beliefs, and traditions are assessed and respected; second, care plans include culturally sensitive resources and strategies; third, grieving practices are respectfully acknowledged and culturally sensitive support is offered; and fourth, IDT members continuously increase awareness of their own biases and perceptions.
- ❖ **Care of imminently dying**: Make sure the patient's pain and other symptoms are managed appropriately. Avoid unnecessarily delaying death. Think about your spiritual and cultural requirements. Patients and their families are informed when there are warning signs or symptoms of approaching death. Help the family out by educating and supporting them. Help in making important decisions. Relieve potential burdens placed on cherished ones. Create a post-death care and follow-up strategy for grieving.
- ❖ **Ethical and legal aspects of care**: Discuss with the family members, the objectives of providing care to the patients. Choose the health proxies. Respect the decisions made by patients, legal proxies, or surrogate decision-makers. Uphold your limits as a professional. Prognosis communication is crucial for making informed decisions. The multidisciplinary team adheres to ethical standards while providing treatment for patients with life-threatening illnesses, including respecting patient wishes and surrogate decision-making.

MODELS OF PALLIATIVE CARE

Palliative care places the entire family as the center of care, not just the patient. Because a serious disease affects not only the patient but also the patient's family and carers, so, the palliative care team collaborates with the entire family. For instance, a major illness may necessitate additional assistance from the patient's spouse or children to care for their loved one or to manage their own emotions or social pressures. Being a carer for a loved one frequently results in psychological or emotional hardship and may require missing work or giving up a career. The pressure and stress of caring for a loved one's illness put carers at a larger risk of developing a serious disease themselves. They are sometimes called the 'silent patients.' So, it is better for them to be in close contact with their own healthcare providers.

In order to provide better direct medical care, palliative care also emphasizes knowing a patient's or family's values. These discussions must take place frequently over the course of the disease since values and hope frequently alter over time. Through these discussions, medical professionals can learn about a patient's or family's values and propose therapies that are in line with those beliefs. This occasionally prompts the writing of papers, such as living wills or the formulation of advanced treatment directives by a doctor, such as requests for different forms of life-sustaining care.

The models of palliative care basically talk about the kind of delivery of services to the patients requiring palliative care. The main models of care are hospital-based care (inpatient palliative care services); acute palliative care units (APCUs), outpatient palliative care clinics; community-based palliative care; telehealth; home-based palliative care; and hospice care. All these models complement one another in providing comprehensive supportive care to patients at the end of life. These models differ in their team structures, care processes, patient populations, location of care, etc. **Figure 43.3** depicts a picture of how these models intersect with each other.

Hospital-based Palliative Care

This model is one of the most established models of care and represents the backbone of palliative care. The inpatient model as the name suggests is used for patients who need hospitalization and palliative care services in the healthcare institution. The team of this model may vary across the hospitals but should constitute of physicians, nurses, psychologists, physiotherapists, dieticians, and social workers (SW). All these will have daily rounds of the patients individually or together. Their focus is on the symptomatic management of the patients in order to provide comfort and improve the quality of life of the patients. Because of the readily availability of services in the hospitals, there is better control of symptoms, less anxiety and depression in the patients as well as their caregivers, better family satisfaction and quality of life.

Acute Palliative Care Units (APCUs)

These are the dedicated units wherein the interdisciplinary palliative care teams provide comprehensive care taking into consideration the physical, emotional, and spiritual aspects of the suffering of the patients. These units are available only in the larger cancer hospitals because of the kind of resources and facilities required to run these units. Patients admitted in these units usually have very complex advanced cancer and severe and acute complications, such as intractable pain and refractory agitated delirium, etc. The patients might get benefitted from more intensive interdisciplinary management in APCU, e.g., rapid analgesic titration/rotation for intractable pain, and palliative sedation for refractory agitated delirium respectively. Palliative interventions are given simultaneously with other medical interventions.

Outpatient Palliative Care

This model is used for patients who are comparatively mobile and can travel and visit the OPD. The outpatient palliative care clinics represent the main setting to be approached by the patients. These require relatively fewer resources and can cater to many patients, as compared with the other models. Several variations of outpatient palliative care interventions are there. These include stand-alone clinics wherein only the palliative care multidisciplinary team takes care of the patients; embedded clinics wherein the palliative care team and the oncology team share the same

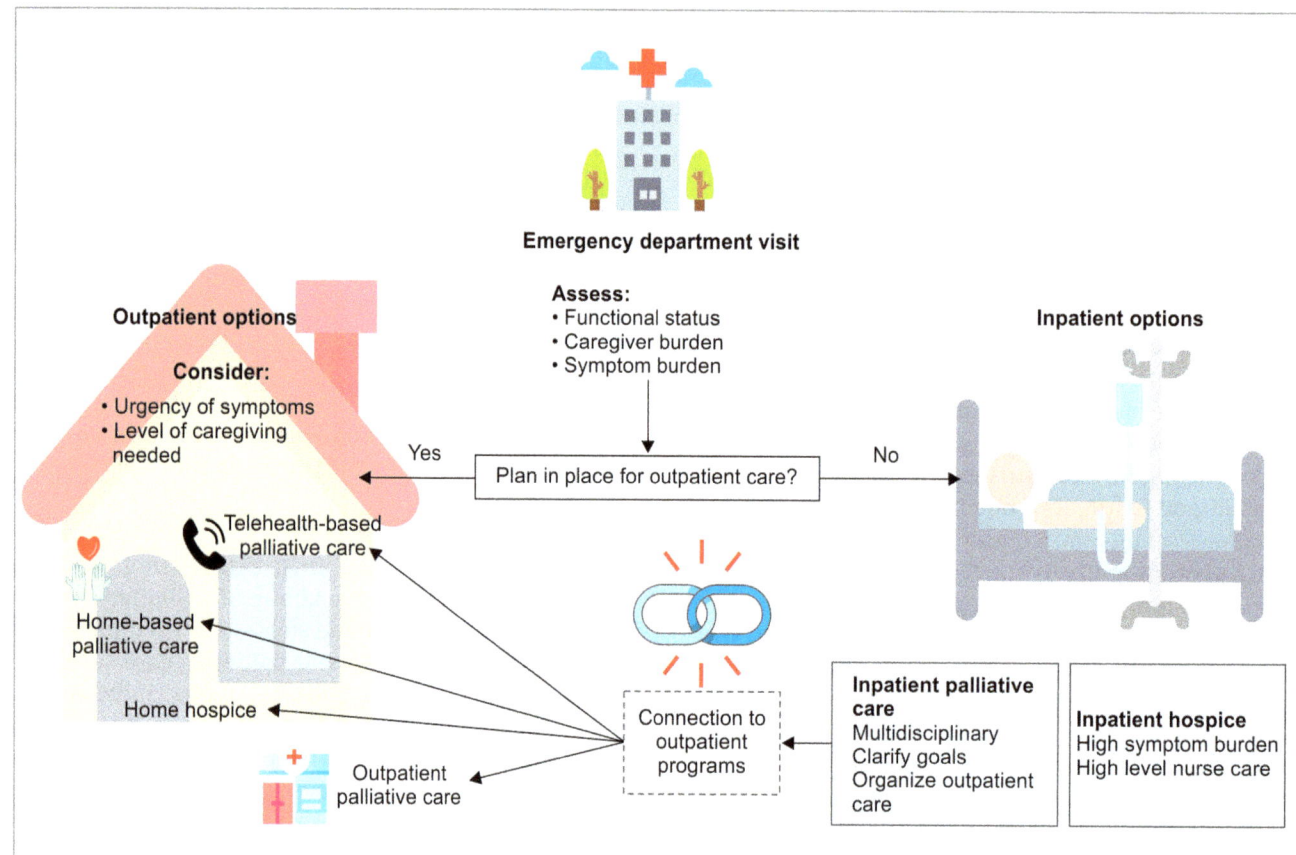

Fig. 43.3: Palliative care for emergency department patients living with advanced cancer.
(*Courtesy:* Grudzen CR et al.)

clinic space and see the same patients on the same day for the convenience of the patients; telehealth-based palliative care which involves making use of web-based interventions to connect to the patients and their caregivers. The outpatient palliative teams may include a physician, nurses, social workers, psychologists, and/or chaplains, etc. The benefits of outpatient palliative care include control of symptoms, satisfaction with care, decreased depression, improved quality of life, etc. However, the patients and their caregivers have to travel to OPDs involving the cost, leave from jobs, loss of daily wages, etc.

Community-based Palliative Care

This kind of model provides in-person visits, supplies, and telephone support for the patients at home or in community-based care facilities, such as nursing homes. The patients receiving such kinds of services are clinically stable though have a poor performance status, short expected survival, and have a desire to continue to care at ambulatory clinics. These are also attached to the hospice units to admit the patients as per requirement. The community-based palliative care programs provide physical, psychological, social, and spiritual support for the patients and respite and bereavement care for caregivers.

Kerala has progressed as a unique model in palliative care services through the community-based approach with 841 centers. It gives coverage of care to a large volume of patients solely through voluntary efforts. Kerala covers >12 million of India's population and is one of the largest networks in the world. The WHO considers the Kerala model of palliative care policy sustainable for developing countries with respect to the following domains—comprehensive high-quality care free of cost, economic self-sufficiency through voluntary community funds and resources, and active volunteering.

Telehealth-based Palliative Care

Telehealth interventions are particularly important for patients residing in rural areas where there is very poor access to healthcare services. Telehealth has been defined by the US Health Resources and Service Administration as "the use of electronic information and telecommunications technologies to support long-distance clinical health care, patient and professional health-related education, public health and health administration". The healthcare professionals provide education, counseling, and symptom monitoring in a cost-effective manner with the potential to improve adherence to the instructions. The prescription of medicines could be a major barrier for the nurses to independently providing telehealth services to the patients. This concept of remote monitoring of symptoms has taken extensive momentum, particularly during the covid pandemic. The patients really were benefitted from sitting in their homes with the health care professionals in the hospitals.

Home-based Palliative Care (HBPC)

Most of the patients want to stay home and spend their last days of life in their own homes. HBPC programs generally include nurses, social workers, physicians, chaplains, pharmacists, physical and occupational therapists, and health aides. The patients having a prognosis of more than

6 months, not qualifying for hospice admission, or those who wish to continue receiving life-prolonging therapies at home are enrolled in HBPC. These programs are designed in such a way that they provide comprehensive palliative care to patients in their homes to improve their quality of life. Unnecessary hospital visits are avoided. Apart from this, the travel costs and hospital admission charges are also avoided. The patients are provided care among their own family members. Though there are a number of benefits of this model, still standardization of practice guidelines is lacking.

The majority of people who have a terminal disease choose to care for their patients at home. The advantages of receiving palliative care at home include a sense of normalcy, freedom of choice, and comfort. It is also more affordable than receiving treatment in a hospital. Various aspects of care which may fall under the purview of family caregivers may include personal care (hygiene, feeding), domestic care (cleaning, meal preparation), auxiliary care (shopping, transportation), social care (informal counseling, emotional support, conversing), nursing care (administering medication, changing catheters), and planning care (establishing and coordinating support for the patient).

General practitioners, community nurses, and professional palliative care teams can provide high-quality palliative care to patients at home, with access to hospital facilities as needed. Family carers must devote a significant amount of time to providing care at home, and both their own needs and the needs of the patient must be taken into consideration.

Hospice Care

Patients with incurable cancer and a life expectancy of six months or less qualify for hospice. It provides comfort and quality of life for the individual who is dying. Comfort is the prime goal of hospice care. Most hospice care is provided through the home. Few residential hospices are also there. The family members provide routine day-to-day care to the patients. The hospice agency provides medications, equipment, and frequent visits by a palliative care team consisting of a nurse, social worker, chaplain, home health aide, and physician. As per the requirement of the patients, nurses visit the family once a week to as often as 3–4 times a week.

MANAGEMENT OF MAIN SYMPTOMS

Most patients requiring palliative care suffer from a variety of symptoms **(Box 43.2)**. These symptoms depend on the type of cancer, metastasis, kind of treatment, and associated comorbidities the patient is suffering from. Patients may experience multiple symptoms at a single point of time. Literature reveals that in advanced stages of cancer, 35–96% of the patients experience pain, 32–90% report fatigue, and 10–70% experience breathlessness. Pain, easy weariness, weakness, anorexia, lack of energy, dry mouth, constipation, early satiety, dyspnea, and weight loss are the commonest symptoms. Accurate assessment and diagnosis are paramount for effective management and better quality of life.

> **BOX 43.2:** Main symptoms at the end of life.
>
> - Pain
> - Dyspnea
> - Fatigue
> - **GI symptoms:**
>   – Nausea and vomiting
>   – Anorexia
>   – Constipation
> - Anxiety
> - Delirium

Principles of Symptom Management

❖ While treating, the patient should be considered as a whole. Along with the patients, their family members, and friends all are affected and their problems and needs should also be taken into consideration.
❖ Examine each symptom in detail by proper assessment. Take into account the probable reasons for each symptom. Think about how the symptom will affect the patient's quality of life.
❖ Communication with the patient and his caregivers is extremely important. Avoid medical jargon and explain in simple language. Patients' relatives should be informed of treatment alternatives included in the care plan.
❖ If the therapy is doable and not too burdensome, and is, such asly to reduce symptoms of the patients, it should be carried out. For example, going for palliative radiation for pain from metastatic bone disease.
❖ Non-pharmacological interventions, e.g., repositioning, complementary therapies, etc., can also assist in pain relief.
❖ Medications should be administered "as needed" (p.r.n.).
❖ The management regimen should be reviewed on a regular basis and modified accordingly.
❖ All the interventions should be planned in advance in to prevent delays in management.

PAIN

Pain is the frequently occurring symptom in patients with advanced cancer. It is the most important aspect of palliative care and inadequately treated pain is a global problem. Pain management is an essential component of palliative care. Its management at times can be difficult. The major cause of this may be the inadequacy in the assessment as pain is subjective, different misconceptions related to painkillers, and under-prescription of medications lead to sufferings among patients. Various other causes of pain are enumerated in **Table 43.1**.

Pain has been dealt in detail in Chapter 11 on pain in Vol-I. This chapter would focus on the management of pain in palliative care patients.

ASSESSMENT OF PAIN

Dame Cicely Saunders gave the term total pain where physical, psychological, and spiritual distress collectively affect the patient. Assessment of pain requires skill and a structured approach, active listening, and keen observation. Clinical expertise and good communication skills are the

TABLE 43.1: Causes of pain in cancer.

Disease-related	Treatment-related	Debility related	Comorbidities
Soft tissue infiltration	Surgery—postoperative scars or adhesions	Constipation	Low back pain
Visceral or bone nerve compression	Radiotherapy induced fibrosis	Pressure ulcers	Arthritis
Nerve infiltration	Chemotherapy-induced neuropathy	Bladder spasm	Angina
Muscle spasm		Stiff joints	Trauma
Raised intracranial pressure			

key to accurate assessment. Barriers to accurate assessment are physicians' underestimation of pain, patients' hesitance to report pain due to lack of knowledge, and changing attitudes of healthcare professionals which may lead to over or underestimation of pain.

PRINCIPLES OF PAIN ASSESSMENT

- Develop a trusting relationship
- Start the conversation with open-ended questions followed by the specific questions **(Table 43.2)**
- Allow the patient to speak the most in the conversation
- Look for clues related to pain, such as facial grimaces
- Avoid jumping to the conclusion

TABLE 43.2: Pain assessment questions.

Frequency	How frequently do you experience pain, intermittent/continuous? If intermittent how long does it occur and after how much duration does it occur again?
Impact on the activity of daily living	Does pain affect your routine life, such as sleep, work, or any other function?
Medications	What medicines you are taking for the pain? What route, and dose do you use, and how often do you have to repeat the medications? Do you experience any side effects from the medications you use?
Onset	Since how long you have been experiencing the pain?
Time	When was the first pain experienced?
Progression	What do you think, that the pain had become severe or reduced, how has it progressed with time?
Precipitating factors	Have you noticed any triggering factors for your pain? Anything which starts it or increases it.
Relieving factors	What do you do for relief from pain?
Quality	Can you explain the feeling of pain, is it a burning sensation or a pressing sensation, what is the pain, such as?
Site and radiation	Where do you feel pain. Do you think pain is fixed or it is moving or spreading towards any other area or body part?
Severity	How would you grade your pain in terms of severity?
Temporal/Relation to time or activity	How is your experience related to pain, is it more during the day or night? How is it with the body movement, increased or decreased?

The quality of pain can be assessed with the help of the pain scales. Self-reporting intensity pain scale, numeric pain scale, Wong Beker pain scale, Mc Gill questionnaire, and Brief Pain inventory are common tools used for pain assessment (Detail in Chapter 11 on pain in Vol-I).

PAIN MANAGEMENT

The aim of pain management is to prevent its recurrence, therefore always establish realistic goals. For example, if complete relief is not possible then management should aim to have sound sleep at night. Pain management can be targeted with:

- **By mouth method**—is simple yet effective as patients can take them home as well.
- **By clock method**—is suggested for continuous pain relief, for example, prescription of painkillers TDS or six hourly. It can be as and when required. This approach is helpful when there is a spike of pain intermittently, the aim is to reduce the suffering.
- **By ladder method:** Pain management is based on the WHO analgesic ladder where stronger analgesics are suggested for severe pain.
- **By Individual approach**—in this method, the prescription is individualized based on the comfort and medical condition of the patient.
- **Adjuvant approach**—is the use of additional drugs to enhance the effect of analgesics.

WHO Ladder

It is a flexible approach for managing cancer pain. It may be used to choose the best analgesics for the level of pain as per its severity. The analgesia should be given in a step-by-step fashion while moving up the ladder until the patient's pain is controlled.

In a similar way, the analgesics should be moved back down the ladder and end finally when the pain gets subside. At each level of the analgesic ladder, alternative analgesics, adjuvants, or non-pharmacological therapies should be taken into consideration. Regular assessment of pain should be done to identify the effectiveness of the therapy **(Fig. 43.4 and Table 43.3)**.

Nurses' Responsibility While Using the WHO Ladder

- Assess the level of pain on a regular basis.
- Morphine cause constipation, hence laxatives (Bisacodyl 10 mg HS) should be administered to the patient to prevent it.
- Nausea vomiting may occur with morphine and other strong opioid, so preventive measures shall be used, for initial three to five days.

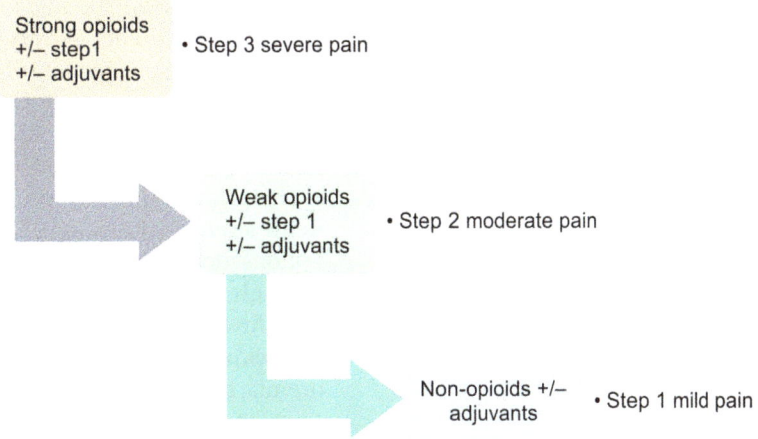

Fig. 43.4: WHO analgesic ladder.

TABLE 43.3: Medications used in WHO ladder.			
Non-opioids	*Weak opioids*	*Strong opioids*	*Adjuvants or coanalgesics*
PCM, Ibuprofen, diclofenac, aspirin	Tramadol, codeine, dihydrocodeine, hydrocodone, oxycodone	Morphine, fentanyl, methadone	Anti-emetics, antidepressants, muscle relaxants, antispasmodics

- Watch for warning signs, such as over-drowsiness, hallucinations, or confusion
  Potential side effects of opioid
- Nausea
- CNS depression/sedation
- Pruritis
- Constipation
- Delirium
- Endocrine dysfunction with long-term use

FATIGUE

It is a subjective term that incorporates the unpleasant feeling of being tired or exhausted, this may interfere with the activities of daily living. It is also referred to as Asthenia. Fatigue generally affects the patient negatively, and has contributing factors, such as anemia, malnutrition, endocrine dysfunction, and progressive disease condition. Asthenia (fatigue) limits activity and increases dependency and this leads to a sense of loss of control eventually making the quality-of-life poor.

The assessment of pain may be done by using various scales, such as the functional assessment of cancer therapy, QLQ-FA13, and Chalder Fatigue Scale Brief Fatigue Inventory.

MANAGEMENT

It involves pharmacological and non-pharmacological measures. Treat the contributing factors. Rest and activity cycles shall be maintained based on the strengths of the patient. Resistance training has an additional role in cancer, when patient experiences, cachexia. Music therapy, cognitive behavioral therapy, and expressive group therapy can be useful as non-pharmacological interventions.

Along with the non-pharmacological treatment, psychostimulant methylphenidate can be prescribed. IAPC has provided an algorithm for the management of fatigue.

DYSPNEA

Dyspnea is a subjective experience of breathing discomfort and restlessness. It can occur because of the primary cancer, because of metastasis, and the associated complications of the disease.

MANAGEMENT

Treatment is directed at the underlying cause. The most common reversible causes are bronchospasm, hypoxia, anemia, etc. Both non-pharmacological as well as pharmacological methods can be helpful. Under a non-pharmacological approach, reassurance to the patient and family can help. Adequate explanation of the situation and disease condition, clearing doubts about the artificial ventilation helps to reduce anxiety. Positioning in a propped-up position may reduce breathlessness. Anxiety and breathlessness make a vicious circle; therefore, anxiety shall be addressed first to bring relief in breathlessness. Reducing activity and working at a slow pace may help. Breathing retraining, such as deep breathing, pranayama, and abdominal breathing have shown positive results in the relief of breathlessness. Pursed lip breathing is significantly helpful in panic attacks. Distraction therapy works well in geriatric and pediatric patients. Relaxation methods, such as massage physiotherapy also have shown efficacy in relieving breathlessness.

The pharmacological approach starts with oxygen therapy based on the condition of the patient and the disease. Opioids are used for the management of refractory breathlessness.

However, the precise mechanism is not known. Opioids reduce respiratory rate and reduce the central perception of breathlessness. Nurses need to carefully monitor the respiratory status of patients.

NUTRITIONAL AND SUPPORTIVE CARE

Anorexia, oral candidiasis, and xerostomia affect the nutritional status of the patient significantly and these are mainly due to being immunocompromised status of the patient. Nurses need to be skilled in handling these problems effectively.

- **Oral candidiasis:** It is a whitish lesion on the oral mucosa and tongue. In the acute stage, it is easily removed but in the chronic or hyperplastic stage, it becomes non-removable. Treatment involves nystatin liquid two hourly, mycostatin lozenges, and clotrimax oral paint. In chronic state oral antifungals, such as ketoconazole, and fluconazole may be administered with intravenous amphotericin.

  Non-pharmacological management: Home remedies, such as garlic, honey coconut scrapings, etc., can be suggested for the acute stage. Beetle leaves with clove have an antiseptic effect and prove to be effective against oral thrush, however, literature may not support this remedy.

  Nystatin, ketoconazole, fluconazole, and other antifungal medications offer effective symptomatic relief.

- **Xerostomia:** It is also referred to as dry mouth that causes difficulty in speech and swallowing, and eventually leads to caries-producing bacterial growth. Mouth breathing, oral candidiasis, oxygen therapy, dehydration, anxiety, and drugs may be responsible for xerostomia. It can be managed by frequent sips of water, having slush (semi-frozen drinks), and artificial saliva. Cessation of smoking and tobacco chewing, sucking on ice chips, and chewing sugar-free gum or hard candies also may help. The application of desi ghee and butter also reduces the problem.

  Effervescent mouthwash tablets containing peppermint oil, clove oil, spearmint, menthol, and other ingredients are advised for therapy, which calls for rigorous oral hygiene every two hours. Hexidine exhibits antimicrobial action at 0.1%. Chewing gum, flavored candies, and pineapple chunks may be tried. Artificial saliva, a lot of fluid intake, and regular lip moisturization are also beneficial.

- **Stomatitis** is an inflammatory, and ulcerative condition of oral mucosa. It starts with an elevated white patch which is painful to touch and progresses to large painful lesions. Good oral hygiene, frequent sips of water, having slush (semi-frozen drinks), and artificial saliva is key for managing stomatitis. Tobacco, alcohol, and acidic food shall be avoided.

  Pharmacological management involves the local application of anesthetics, sucralfate, and silver nitrate.

  Homemade Sudarshan oral mix has proven to be the most effective. Sudharshan mix has one tablespoon of common salt, 5 mL Povidone-iodine solution, 3 mL hydrogen peroxide, one or two cloves, two mints units (polo two tablets) 200 mg, one tablet of metronidazole. All these ingredients are mixed and applied three to four times a day. The use of a soft brush helps to reduce the discomfort.

- **Halitosis:** Many cancer patients experience halitosis or the sensation of having bad breath. Smoking, eating foods, such as garlic, onions, or alcohol, or having a blockage in the stomach outlet are all potential causes. Treatment options include paying attention to oral hygiene, drinking enough water, treating oral candidiasis, and using mouthwashes.

- **Anorexia:** Fear of vomiting, unappealing food, dysphagia, uremia, radiation, chemotherapy, or psychogenic origins can all cause loss of appetite. The patient should be given psychological support and information regarding the, such asly cause of the anorexia. It should be advised to eat pleasant meals in small, frequent portions that are simple to digest. Try using appetite stimulants. Hyperalimentation may be administered in severe situations.

NAUSEA AND VOMITING

It is a potentially debilitating symptom near the end of life. It is majorly due to a variety of factors due to the treatment or its side effects. However, nurses need to understand the possible causes of nausea and vomiting. As mentioned earlier causes are multifactorial. Medications are prescribed as per need based not on a regular manner. Parenteral antiemetics may be necessary if there is substantial nausea and/or vomiting since the oral route may become momentarily ineffective.

CONSTIPATION

Palliative care patients may have constipation owing to a number of causes, including immobility, decreased intake of food and hydration, side effects of medication, intestinal pathology, and occasionally hypercalcemia. The diagnosis is often determined based on the history of decreased bowel movement frequency, the passage of tiny, firm stools, and the straining while passing stool. To aid with symptom improvement, take into account educating patients about the reasons for constipation, improving fluid intake, and making the proper dietary modifications.

GUIDELINES ON THE USE OF LAXATIVES IN CONSTIPATION

- Observe the cause of the constipation
- Always consider the preferences of the patient regarding the diet
- Provide the fiber-rich diet
- Suggest and try non-pharmacological interventions, before using any laxatives or medications
- Opioids generally cause constipation (side effect) and nurses need to assess this aspect before opting to inform the physician for laxative.
- Typically, a combination of a stool softener and a laxative stimulant is needed.
- Every two days, review laxatives and adjust the dosage as needed.

- If colic is evident, stay away from stimulant laxatives. Consider lowering the dosage of the softener if feces leak.
- Significant flatulence and bloating may be brought on by lactulose.
- Do not prescribe laxatives in the case of total bowel blockage without consulting a physician.
- Perform a rectal examination if it is safe and suitable to do so and adhere to local rectal measures if the bowels have not moved in three days.
- Abdominal exercises may be tried. The patients should be asked to contract and relax the abdominal muscles.

CACHEXIA

Cachexia is derived from a Greek word that means bad condition. It involves weight loss, lipolysis, loss of body protein leading to muscle wasting and visceral protein, nausea, and weakness.

STAGES OF CACHEXIA

- **Pre-cachexia:** In this, weight loss is <5% of body weight with metabolic changes and anorexia.
- **Cachexia:** Weight loss is >5% or BMI is <20 with a significant decrease in food intake and signs of inflammation is observed.
- **Refractory cachexia:** Has the involvement of cancer or any other disease, such as HIV/AIDS and is unresponsive to treatment. The prognosis is <3 months.

MANAGEMENT

Corticosteroids are prescribed, progestational agents are also prescribed and high-fat meal is given as these drugs are best absorbed with it. If the patient does not respond in two weeks, then megestrol acetate (progestational agent) is increased to 600–800 mg/day. Gastric emptying is increased with metoclopramide and domperidone.

Nutritional support is provided by Omega 3 fatty acids as they limit muscle proteolysis and inflammation. Exercise is also important as it is said "if you do not use, you lose", same is true for muscles, therefore active and passive exercises are performed. A rehabilitation program is designed for the patient depending on strength. Tube feeding or enteral feeding may be started to provide nutrition to palliative care patients.

GERIATRIC CONSIDERATIONS

Among geriatric patients, palliative care needs to be focused on comprehensive geriatric assessment as the geriatric syndrome influences the general health of elderly patients requiring palliative care. Comorbidities, age-related disabilities, such as impaired hearing or vision, diminished physiology, etc., contribute to increased health problems, which leads to atypical presentation of the disease. Apart from the physical issues, elderly patients requiring palliative care have psychological problems, such as dementia, depression, or impaired cognition and social problems, such as a financial burden, loneliness, or loss of a life partner. Neglect from the caregiver is a major contributor to the poor quality of life. All these can lead to polypharmacy, as they need to take medication as per their disease condition, but these medications may result in drug interaction and may sometime lead to adverse effects. Therefore, preventive interventions are extremely important for elderly patients especially in palliative care as the disease may have an atypical presentation.

Case Scenario

1. A 65-year-old female, suffering from Ca breast is having the symptoms of disabling pain due to side effects of chemotherapy, depression, functional decline, and social isolation. The family was also in distress. She had repeated ED visits and hospitalization for these symptoms. She was started with palliative care. There was expert pain management, 24/7 phone coverage, ongoing relationship with palliative care team, support from social worker, and other therapists. After some time, she could resume her work, her family role, and other religious activities. No hospitalization in the past 12 months.
2. Chris was a 15-year-old teenager when diagnosed with a medulloblastoma (a highly malignant brain tumor). He underwent surgery, chemotherapy, and radiotherapy. Two years later, he relapsed with metastases in his femur and thigh. With no further curative treatment options, radiotherapy was provided for symptom management. Chris was referred to palliative care and died 6 months later.

Identified Issues Were

- *Complex pain:* Main issue regarding rapid escalation of doses and changes from oral to intravenous along with adjuvant measures, such as radiotherapy.
- *Family issues:* Chris was the eldest son of the family and had a major role in family leadership and decision-making. This increasing loss required a great deal of support from the team.

Palliative Care Interventions that have been helpful

- Provided complex and timely analgesia, drug changes, and dose escalations at home and in the hospital.
- Maintained links with all other hospital teams and community services for optimal symptom and psychological support.
- Weekly home visits allowed the development of trust and intensive support-balancing Chris's right to know with traditional family roles and responsibilities as well as issues.
- Discussion with spirituality providers about how to support this family.
- Provided family-centered care which included liaison with clinicians to support siblings.
- Supported family goals for the end of life.
- Provided bereavement support

SUMMARY

A therapeutic strategy known as palliative care aims to improve the quality of life for patients who have serious or advanced diseases. It emphasizes communication between the treating physicians and the management of pain and other symptoms of the patients, assistance with patient decision-making regarding care, coordination of medical and other services, and support for carers. It is provided by a team with the main goal to provide appropriate symptomatic management and comfort for the patient's remaining life. A committed team consisting of a doctor, nurse, and support workers delivers palliative care. The use of artificial nutrition, treatment of malignant small intestinal obstruction, communication challenges, understanding patient preferences, advanced care planning, and bereavement support are crucial to palliative care. Palliative care facilities in India are short of its need. Advance directives are a crucial tool for facilitating this and are recognized as a key quality indicator in palliative care, which aims to alleviate suffering and support patients and their families in making medical decisions.

MULTIPLE CHOICE QUESTIONS

1. Who is the founder of hospice movement?
   a. Hippocrates
   b. Dame Cicely Saunders
   c. Thomson Edison
   d. Albert Einstein
2. Sudarshan mix is used for which of the following:
   a. Oral candidiasis
   b. Stomatitis
   c. Xerostomia
   d. Glossitis
3. In which year, the National Cancer Control Programme was started in India?
   a. 1970
   b. 1972
   c. 1975
   d. 1978
4. Which state was the first to start palliative care in India?
   a. Maharashtra
   b. Gujrat
   c. Karnataka
   d. Punjab
5. Name the first hospice in India?
   a. Shanti Aveda Ashram
   b. Shanti Niketan
   c. Sparsh hospice
   d. Jeevodaya hospice
6. In which year palliative care was started in India?
   a. 1975
   b. 1980
   c. 1986
   d. 1990
7. The word 'hospice' is derived from the Latin word "Hospes" which means:
   a. A guest
   b. A House
   c. A visitor

ANSWERS

1. b 2. b 3. c 4. b
5. a 6. b 7. a

SUGGESTED READING

1. Al Qadire M, Al Khalaileh M: Prevalence of symptoms and quality of life among Jordanian cancer patients. Clin Nurs Res. 2016;25: 174-91.
2. Alt-Epping B, Nejad RK, Jung K, Gross U, Nauck F. Symptoms of the oral cavity and their association with local microbiological and clinical findings—a prospective survey in palliative care. Support Care Cancer. 2012;20(3):531-7.
3. Arendorf TM, Walker DM. Oral candidal populations in health and disease. Br Dent J. 1979;147(10):267-72.
4. Baer WM, Hanson LC. Families' perception of the added value of hospice in the nursing home. J Am Geriatri Soc. 2000;48(8):879-82. doi: 10.1111/j.1532-5415.2000.tb06883.
5. Bausewein C, Currow D, Johnson M (Eds): Management of Chronic Breathlessness, in Palliative Care in Respiratory Disease. ERS Monograph. ERS, Sheffield, United Kingdom; 2016, pp. 153-71.
6. Bellior MN, Riou F. [Nursing staff, knowledge and attitudes concerning preventive oral hygiene in palliative care]. Article in French. Rech Soins Infirm. 2014;(117):75-84.
7. Bhatnagar M, Lagnese KR. Hospice Care. [Updated 2022 Mar 18]. In: StatPearls [Internet]. Treasure Island (FL): StatPearls Publishing; 2022. Available from: https://www.ncbi.nlm.nih.gov/books/NBK537296/
8. Bill O'Neill, Fallon M. ABC of palliative care: Principles of palliative care and pain control, Clinical Review. BMJ. 1997;315:801. doi: https://doi.org/10.1136/bmj.315.7111.80
9. Bruera E, Yennurajalingam S, Palmer JL, et al. Methylphenidate and/or a nursing telephone intervention for fatigue in patients with advanced cancer: A randomized, placebo-controlled, phase II trial. J Clin Oncol. 2013;31:2421-7.
10. Chalmers J, Johnson V, Tang JH, Titler MG. Evidence-based protocol: oral hygiene for functionally dependent and cognitively impaired older adults. J Gerontol Nurs. 2004;30(11):5-12.
11. Chen X, Clark JJ, Naorungroj S. Oral health in nursing home residents with different cognitive statuses. Gerodontology.
12. Chiu TY, Hu WY, Chen CY. Prevalence and severity of symptoms in terminal cancer patients: A study in Taiwan. Support Care Cancer. 2000;8:311-3.
13. Clark D. "From margins to the centre: a review of the history of palliative care in cancer". The Lancet. Oncology. 2007;8(5):430-8. doi:10.1016/S1470-2045(07)70138-9
14. Cooke C, Ahmedzai S, Mayberry J. Xerostomia—a review. Palliat Med. 1996;10(4):284-92.
15. Cramp F, Byron-Daniel J. Exercise for the management of cancer-related fatigue in adults. Cochrane Database Syst Rev. 20212;11:CD006145.
16. Dawes C. Physiological factors affecting salivary flow rate, oral sugar clearance, and the sensation of dry mouth in man. J Dent Res. 1987;66:648-3.
17. de Souza LJ, Lobo ZM. Symptom control problems in an Indian hospice. Ann Acad Med Singapore. 1994;23:287-91.
18. Good P, Afsharimani B, Movva R, et al. Therapeutic challenges in cancer pain management: A systematic review of methadone. J Pain Palliat Care Pharmacother. 2014;28:197-205.
19. Grudzen CR, Barker PC, Bischof JJ, et al. Palliative care models for patients living advanced cancer: a narrative review for the emergency department clinician. Emergency Cancer Care. 2022;1(10):1-10.
20. Higginson IJ, Costantini M. Dying with cancer, living well with advanced cancer. Eur J Cancer. 2008;44:1414-24.
21. Hui D, Bruera E. Models of Palliative Care Delivery for Patients With Cancer. J Clin Oncol. 2020;38:852-65. DOI https://doi.org/10.1200/JCO.18.02123
22. Kehl KA. Moving toward peace: An analysis of the concept of a good death. Am J Hosp Palliat Care. 2006;23:277-86.
23. Khosla D, Patel FD, Sharma SC. Palliative care in India: current progress and future needs. Indian J Palliat Care. 2012;18(3):149-54.
24. Lengacher CA, Reich RR, Paterson CL, et al. Examination of broad symptom improvement resulting from mindfulness-based stress reduction in breast cancer survivors: A randomized controlled trial. J Clin Oncol. 2016;34:2827-34.
25. Malik FA, Gysels M, Higginson IJ. Living with breathlessness: A survey of caregivers of breathless patients with lung cancer or heart failure. Palliat Med. 2013;27:647-56.
26. Miller SC, Mor V, Wu N, Gozalo P, Lapane K. Does receipt of hospice care in nursing homes improve the management of pain at the end of life? J Am Geriatr Soc. 2002;50(3):507-15. doi: 10.1046/j.1532-5415.2002.50118.
27. National Consensus Project for Quality Palliative Care. [Accessed October 10, 2022]; Clinical Practice Guidelines for Quality Palliative Care. 2013 https://www.hpna.org/multimedia/NCP_Clinical_Practice_Guidelines_3rd_Edition.pdf.
28. National Hospice and Palliative Care Organization; Hospice Care. http://www.nhpco.org/about/hospice-care. Updated 2016
29. Pappas PG, Kauffman CA, Andes D, et al. Clinical Practice Guidelines for the Management of Candidiasis: 2009 Update by the Infectious Diseases Society of America. Clin Infect Dis. 2009;48:503,535.
30. Parshall MB, Schwartzstein RM, Adams L, et al. An official American Thoracic Society statement: Update on the mechanisms, assessment, and management of dyspnea. Am J Respir Crit Care Med. 2012;185:435-52.
31. Peters MEWJ, Goedendorp MM, Verhagen SAHHVM, et al. A prospective analysis on fatigue and experienced burden in informal caregivers of cancer patients during cancer treatment in the palliative phase. Acta Oncol. 2015;54:500-6.
32. Plemons JM, Al-Hashimi I, Marek CL, American Dental Association Council on Scientific Affairs. Managing xerostomia and salivary gland hypofunction: executive summary of a report from the American Dental Association Council on Scientific Affairs. J Am Dent Assoc. 2014;145(8):867-73.

33. Poort H, Peters M, Bleijenberg G, et al. Psychosocial interventions for fatigue during cancer treatment with palliative intent. Cochrane Database Syst Rev. 2017;7:CD012030.
34. Portenoy RK, Thaler HT, Kornblith AB, et al. Symptom prevalence, characteristics and distress in a cancer population. Qual Life Res. 1994;3:183-9.
35. Rajagopal MR, Venkateswaran C. Palliative care in India: Successes and limitations. J Pain Palliat Care Pharmacotherapy. 2003;17: 121-8.
36. Ream E, Richardson A. Fatigue: A concept analysis. Int J Nurs Stud. 1996;33:519-29.
37. Ruddy KJ, Barton D, Loprinzi CL. Laying to rest psychostimulants for cancer-related fatigue. J Clin Oncol. 2014;32:1865-7.
38. Samaranayake LP, Lamey PJ. Oral candidosis: 1. Clinicopathological aspects. Dent Update. 1988;15(6):227-8, 230-1.
39. Solano JP, Gomes B, Higginson IJ. A comparison of symptom prevalence in far advanced cancer, AIDS, heart disease, chronic obstructive pulmonary disease and renal disease. J Pain Symptom Manage. 2006;31:58-69.
40. Stone P, Richards M, A'Hern R, et al. A study to investigate the prevalence, severity, and correlates of fatigue among patients with cancer in comparison with a control group of volunteers without cancer. Ann Oncol. 2000;11:561-7.
41. Stone PC. Methylphenidate in the management of cancer-related fatigue. J Clin Oncol. 2013;31:2372-3.
42. Sweeney MP, Bagg J. The mouth and palliative care. Am J Hosp Palliat Care. 2000;17(2):118-24. Dry Mouth. National Institute for Dental and Craniofacial Research Website. www.nidcr.nih.gov/oralhealth/Topics/DryMouth/DryMouth.htm. Published August 2014; accessed July 19, 2015.
43. Teno JM, Clarridge BR, Casey V, et al. Family perspectives on end-of-life care at the last place of care. JAMA. 2004;291:88-93.
44. Tomlinson D, Diorio C, Beyene J, et al. Effect of exercise on cancer-related fatigue: A meta-analysis. Am J Phys Med Rehabil. 2014;93:675-86.
45. Twycross RG. Introducing palliative care. Radcliffe Publishing; 2003.
46. Vivino FB, Al-Hashimi I, Khan Z, et al. Pilocarpine tablets for the treatment of dry mouth and dry eye symptoms in patients with Sjögren's syndrome: a randomized, placebo-controlled, fixed-dose, multicenter trial. P92-01 Study Group. Arch Intern Med. 1999;159(2):174-81.
47. What is telehealth? https:// www. hrsa. gov/ rural- health/ telehealth/ what is telehealth. Accessed 12 Mar 2022.
48. Wiseman M. The treatment of oral problems in the palliative patient. J Can Dent Assoc. 2006;72(5):453-8.
49. World Health Organization: Cancer pain relief: With a guide to opioid availability, 2nd edition http://www.who.int/iris/handle/10665/37896
50. World Health Organization; [Last accessed on 2012 Mar 02]. "WHO Definition of Palliative Care" Available from: http://www.who.int/cancer/palliative/definition/en.

UNIT VI

Emergency Nursing

OUTLINE

44. **Principles of Emergency Management**
 Santa De

45. **Disaster Management: Nursing Perspective**
 T Samuel Ravi Kumar

CHAPTER 44

Principles of Emergency Management

Santa De

"You treat a disease: You win, you lose. You treat a person, I guarantee you win—no matter the outcome."
—**Patch Adams**

LEARNING OBJECTIVES

After going through the chapter, the learner will be able to:
- Understand the role of an emergency nurse in identifying and managing various emergencies.
- Explain the principles of emergency nursing.
- Understand physical setup, staffing pattern, and equipments required in the emergency department.
- Discuss the triage system.
- Appreciate the qualities of nurses working in the emergency department.
- Recognize the common and emergent problems that require prompt medical and nursing attention.
- Interpret patient's conditions, develop an appropriate care plan, and monitor the patient's response towards it.
- Communicate sensitively with patients and their family members.
- Demonstrate professionalism in dealing with patients and co-workers.
- Discuss the medicolegal aspects of emergency care.
- Discuss geriatric considerations for the elderly in emergency nursing.

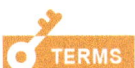

- **Carboxyhemoglobin:** It is formed in red blood cells upon contact with hemoglobin and carbon monoxide. Hence reduces the oxygen-carrying capacity of hemoglobin in the blood and results in hypoxemia.
- **Chilblain:** Cold injury developed from repeated exposure to cold and progressing to chronic vasculitis on the face, hands, anterior lower legs, and feet.
- **Corrosive chemicals:** Substance causing chemical action on living tissues at the site of contact leading to irreversible alteration.
- **Decompression sickness (Diver's disease):** It is a medical condition that occurs when the dissolved form of gases usually nitrogen emerges as bubbles from inside the body tissues upon a rapid decrease in barometric pressure.
- **Envenomation:** The process of poisonous secretions injected into the human body through a sting or bite of an animal.
- **Lyme disease:** A vector-borne multisystem disease in which an infected tick bites a human.
- **Polytrauma:** Multiple traumas occurring in severely injured patients. It describes the condition due to road traffic accidents, bullet injuries, falls from height, etc.
- **Primary survey:** It is done to identify life-threatening injuries and initiate appropriate resuscitation of trauma patients.
- **Rewarming:** It is the process of heating the body so that normal temperature is maintained. Rewarming should be started from the center of the body to the periphery.
- **Secondary survey:** It is done once the patient has been resuscitated and stabilized. A secondary survey is done to identify all potentially significant injuries. It is a systematic approach of identifying fractures or bleeding.
- **Triage:** It is a process of classifying the casualties into various categories to determine their health status and treat them as per their urgency.

INTRODUCTION

The term emergency is used for those patients or conditions who need prompt medical attention to prevent deterioration in their health status, long-term disability, and death. It is also needed for the stability of the patient's condition till the availability of services closest to the patients. The patients presenting to emergency are often physiologically unstable and their healthcare needs are often complex. The care provided to them is individualistic and focused on their unique needs.

Emergency nursing is one of the most challenging specialties in nursing. Emergency care is needed in a wide variety of settings. Emergency nurses are prepared to perform various tasks, from general nursing tasks to a range of complex nursing skills like managing a patient with life-saving resuscitation. They need to communicate effectively in order to provide competent care and should also demonstrate their skills working as an integral member of a large interdisciplinary care team. They work in a fast-paced often stressful environment that requires a unique skill to manage the situation. They need to remain calm yet exhibit confidence in the midst of uncertainty. The nurses should be compassionate yet confident in dealing with an emergency.

A lifelong commitment to learning is one of the important traits of emergency nurses. Emergency nurses must be prepared at all times to treat an extensive array of illnesses for patients ranging from neonates to geriatrics. To provide quality care to patients of all ages they need to have adequate knowledge of general and specific conditions and periodically update themselves in managing various crisis situations.

ROLE OF AN EMERGENCY NURSE

- ❖ **Care provider:** She/he provides direct care to the patients and their relatives. The role of an emergency nurse is to evaluate and monitor the patient regularly in order to prevent further complications in the patients.
- ❖ **Educator:** She/he is expected to provide up-to-date information to the patients and their relatives throughout their stay. They also provide education to the patient and their relatives based on their learning needs.
- ❖ **Manager:** The emergency nurses maintain the overall flow of the department. They coordinate the activities with the multidisciplinary team members in order to achieve the ultimate goal of providing emergency care.
- ❖ **Advocate:** It means preserving human dignity, and protecting the patients' rights. As patients' advocates, nurses help the patients navigate the complex healthcare system. These nurses work on behalf of patients to ensure quality care and maintain patient safety. For instance, if a patient does not agree with a treatment plan, a nurse will communicate with the treating doctor on behalf of the patient.

PRINCIPLES OF EMERGENCY MANAGEMENT

The principles of emergency management are quite broad and complex. These include some common rules or relationships that are preferably applied across all emergency management areas. The fundamental principles of emergency management include processes of preparation, mitigation, response, and recovery from an emergency. All these four processes basically deal with the disaster and are discussed in detail in Chapter 45 on the disaster.

Principles of emergency nursing also embrace three basic moralities, i.e., protecting any injury, preservation of life, and promotion of recovery.

- ❖ **Protecting any injury:** For a person working in an emergency, along with having the knowledge and skill that what should be done, it is important to know what not to be done. For example, moving an individual with a cervical injury can lead to spinal cord injury and later more complications for the patients.
- ❖ **Preservation of life:** Protecting the life of the patients is an extremely important principle of emergency care. All the efforts are carried out by the emergency team to preserve the life as per the condition (kindly see triaging in the following section of this chapter).
- ❖ **Promotion of recovery:** The process of recovery begins, immediately after the threat to the life of the patients has been subsided. All health promotion and restoration activities are to be carried out beyond the emergency period to fasten the recovery period of the patients.

Further principles of emergency nursing also involve early detection, early reporting, early response, care during transportation, and transporting to definite care **(Box 44.1)**.

- ❖ **Early detection:** Early recognition of critically ill patients is challenging. The nurses working in emergency need to ensure the safe and effective delivery of nursing care. They are responsible for the assessment, observation, monitoring, and charting of vital signs, planning, implementation, and evaluation of care.
- ❖ **Early reporting:** The physical status of a critically ill patient is unpredictable and may change at any time. They might need immediate decision-making at that point. Situation awareness (SA) is an important construct to have a positive patient outcome. This is the foundation of decision-making in order to determine the need for special treatment. Thus, these nurses should be able to perceive, interpret and project the patient's clinical cues so that the need for high-risk treatment can be assessed and decisions can be made at the earliest. Strategic decisions and overall care should be communicated to the patient's relatives.
- ❖ **Early response:** For prevention of further deterioration of the patient's status, recognition of early warning signs and immediate response to the situation is very significant to provide safe and effective care. In order to recognize an acute change in a patient's physiological status, a change in the level of consciousness and assessment of vital signs must first be done accurately. This is done to ensure patient safety and clinical stability. Early response helps the clinician to quickly intervene when alarming

---

BOX 44.1: Principles of emergency nursing.

- Early detection
- Early reporting
- Early response
- Care during transportation
- Transporting to definitive care

rapid changes occur. It is important to display high-value healthcare behavior during an emergency.

- **Care during transportation:** Transportation of critically ill patients can be intra-hospital transport or inter-hospital. Intra-hospital transport is the movement of a patient within the hospital premises, whereas inter-hospital transport is the patient's movement between two medical centers. The purpose of transportation is for diagnostic and therapeutic intervention. However, transportation may pose a potential risk of hypoxia, vascular access problems, organ or limb injury, etc.

   An established and organized transport can pave the way to patient safety. Pretransport coordination and communication by emergency nurses are very important. Shifting an unstable intubated patient should be accompanied by a nurse trained in emergency care and a physician trained in airway management and advanced cardiac life support. Accompanying medications, basic equipment, and emergency drugs should be checked before shifting the patient. The patient should be monitored continuously for ECG, pulse oximetry, blood pressure, pulse rate, and respiratory rate.

- **Transporting to definitive care:** Transporting the patient to definitive care means shifting the patient from one level to the next level of care. This is to ensure minimal interference and optimal continuity in care. A comprehensive and thorough handover to staff at the receiving unit is essential. It is necessary to ensure that all gear comes back with the caring team. Follow-up is important to report on the patient's progress after transfer.

ORGANIZATION OF EMERGENCY SERVICES

The emergency department is an integral part of a hospital. It is the front door of the hospital. It is the portal of entry for the highest volume of patients requiring emergent care. The function of the emergency department is to receive, stabilize and manage patients (adults and children) presenting with urgent medical and surgical conditions. Sometimes the patients report on their own in an emergency and sometimes they are shifted as the referred cases from other hospitals.

Location

- The emergency department should be situated on the ground floor and the entrance should be easily accessible to the ambulance.
- The unit should have separate entry and exit doors. The doors should be wide enough for the wheel chairs and stretchers to let freely in. The door should be swinging outward and not lockable from the inside. Immediately outside the main entrance, there should be the availability of enough wheel chairs and stretchers.
- The crash cart should be placed at a location where it is easily accessible.
- At the emergency unit there should be dedicated areas for triage and managing other emergency procedures like wound care and fracture handling. Articles to manage such procedures should always be kept ready. There should be an observation area. Other support areas include the nursing station and doctor's room. The hand washing area should be easily accessible to the health care staff.
- There should be a sufficient place to carry out patient care activity and patient circulation. A distance of 6 feet between beds is to be maintained at the observation ward in the emergency department. There should be an arrangement for the patients to provide privacy by drawing curtains.
- The emergency department should have scope for the management of mass casualty.
- There should be a facility for the storage of emergency medicine and consumables to manage mass casualty and sufficient space where mass casualty may be accommodated.
- Biomedical waste bins are to be placed as per biomedical waste (BMW) rules. A separate area should be identified to keep dirty linens and items. A distinct area for clean and a segregated area for dirty supplies should be there.
- There should be rapid access to all laboratory services to minimize the turnaround times for various investigations. Mechanical or pneumatic tube transport systems for specimen and electronic reporting of results are desirable.
- There should be a separate OT in the emergency department.
- There should be separate facilities for X-ray, ultrasonography, CT, etc.
- Emergency units using telemedicine facilities should have a dedicated, fully enclosed room with appropriate power and communications cabling provided.

Staffing Pattern in the Emergency Department

The staff requirement at the emergency department is unique. The emergency department is an essential part of any hospital as immediate care is provided in this department that saves lives of the patient in distress. The workload in the emergency department is unpredictable, so it is difficult to envisage an exact staffing pattern in the emergency department.

Usually, the Director of Emergency Medicine is the in-charge medical officer leading the team of emergency medicine doctors. A nurse manager (or in-charge nurse) leads a team of highly trained nurses. Care in any hospital emergency department is provided by highly trained professionals. The nursing interventions are carried out interdependently in consultation with or under the direction of a licensed physician.

An emergency nurse is a qualified registered nurse and specially trained to quickly triage the patient based on immediate observation, excellent assessment skills, and manage symptoms based on priority. She is an expert in assessing and identifying the healthcare problems in emergency and crisis situations. She also should support and attend to the families, and supervise allied health personnel. One should be flexible to the needs of the patient and respond immediately to the changes.

Other allied health professionals include radiographers, physiotherapists, and social workers. There are also administrative and support staff. The healthcare professionals in the emergency department work as a team to handle the situation and to provide quality care to the patients.

Equipments

The emergency department requires various equipments to aid in the provision of emergency care effectively. These can vary from basic stretchers to complex equipments being used in intensive care units and theaters. The emergency department of any hospital is arranged with a huge collection of complicated beeping and blinking equipment that serve an important purpose in saving the lives of the people.

The ability to use these equipments varies as per the qualification and competency of the healthcare professionals and the paramedics. Some of the important equipments required are:

- Ventilators, defibrillator, cardiac monitors, EKG machine.
- Central gas pipelines, plenty of IV fluids.
- Crash cart having all the emergency medicines
- IV lines and catheters of all size
- Nebulizers
- Dressing materials, plasters, dressing trolley
- Firefighting equipments
- Blood pressure and temperature monitoring equipments
- Stethoscope
- Generous number of orthopedic equipments
- Cervical collar
- **Jump-bag:** A large comprehensive bag with several pouches where bandages, syringes, pocket masks, ambu bag, drip sets, etc., are kept.
- **Bag and mask:** To manually give rescue breaths to a patient.
- Suction machines
- Suture tray containing equipment like a needle holder, forceps for holding the lacerated tissue, scissors, and small bowls for antiseptic solutions, etc.
- **Kendrick extrication device (Fig. 44.1):** This is a device used in the extrication (release) of victims of traffic collisions from motor vehicles. Typically, there are two head straps, three torso straps, and two legs straps which are used to adequately secure the device to the victim. The device uses a series of wooden or polymer bars in a nylon jacket, allowing the responders to immobilize the neck and upper spine and remove the victim from the vehicle or other confined space.

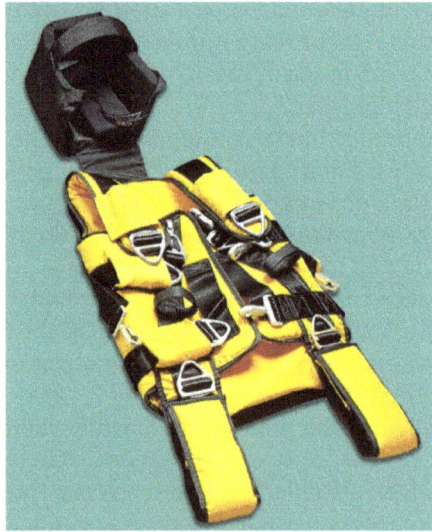

Fig. 44.1: Kendrick extrication device.

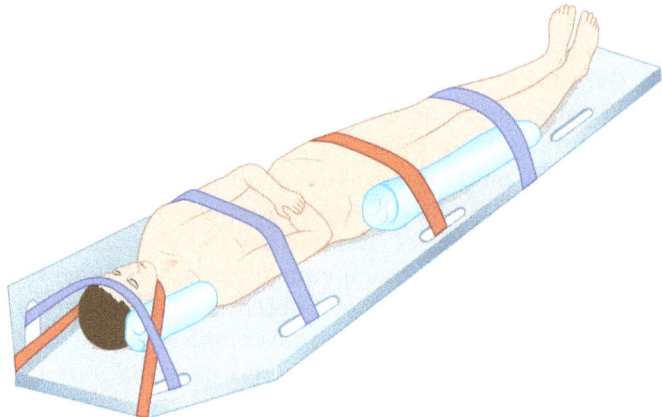

Fig. 44.2: Spine board.

- Spinal board to help reduce spinal cord injury (**Fig. 44.2**)
- Long backboard
- Incubator
- Infusion pumps
- Glucometer
- Slit lamp

It is important for the nurses to have audits of all the equipments frequently. The working of all these equipments should be checked in each shift.

COORDINATION AND INVOLVEMENT OF DIFFERENT DEPARTMENTS AND FACILITIES

The emergency department requires the effective participation of different professionals and specialists including physicians, nurses, paramedical staff, administrators and sometimes even members from outside the emergency department to work together. An interdisciplinary approach is integral to provide care in the emergency department. It is recognized that teamwork and effective communication in the emergency department is crucial to provide safe patient care. The role of every member of the team is linked with the common significant purpose of improving patient safety, minimizing clinical errors, and reduction in waiting time.

The emergency unit requires ready access to certain important related functional areas like the operation theater, radiography unit, pathology department, coronary care unit, blood bank, pharmacy, outpatient department, mortuary, etc. A designated area for medication is required for the storage of medications used within the emergency department. The entry should be secured with the self-closing door. There should be sufficient space for a refrigerator which is essential for the storage of heat-sensitive drugs.

MEDICOLEGAL ASPECTS OF EMERGENCY CARE

The purpose of medicolegal services in the emergency department is to collect medicolegal evidence and to provide meticulous care to the victims. Medicolegal issues are a major concern for the doctors and nurses practicing in the emergency care unit.

Medicolegal issues are situations where it is essential to inform the law authorities (police) to rule out whether any criminal incident or negligence has taken place behind this occurrence. Therefore, it is mandatory to inform any local police or law authorities, or law enforcers in some circumstances.

- ❖ **Privacy:** The nurses working at the emergency unit are accountable to the public for making nursing judgments and consequences for that. Nurses working in the emergency room are ethically and morally responsible to protect the privacy of their patients. Vigilance and sensitivity are very important to protect patients' privacy. Nurses and doctors caring for the patient must limit their conversation regarding the patient to those persons who need to know. They should discuss patient issues in suitable areas. Wrongful disclosure of individually identifiable information is a serious offense.
- ❖ **Autonomy:** As soon as the emergency duty team provides treatment to a person with multiple injuries or in a state of coma, the legal issues are involved with regard to informed consent. Autonomy is the capacity to think, decide and act freely and independently. It is important to ensure that there is an absence of controlling influences that determine the decision-making action by the treating team (team of doctors and nurses) in an emergency situation.
- ❖ **Consent:** Consent is acknowledgment and acceptance of medical treatment by the patient. Informed consent requires the capacity to consent. Informed consent occurs after full disclosure to the patient regarding the procedure. Obtaining patient consent is essential for any invasive procedure unless he/she is in a critical condition to take a decision or brought by strangers and the situation becomes lifesaving. Essential components of the consent include an explanation of the procedure, a discussion on potential risks and benefits of the procedure, any alternatives to the procedure, and confirmation that the patient understands the risks, benefits, and any alternatives and the fact should be documented. It should be ensured that the details of the treatment given are recorded stating the time of administration of the treatment, a note on the patient's condition, and response to treatment.
- ❖ **Documentation:** Documentation of care-related information is a very vital record in the emergency department. Because these emergencies are often due to accidents that eventually involve lawsuits. Without documentation, the communication related to nursing care is compromised.
  - ➢ **Emergency** department record forms should be well-planned, easy to read, and easy to fill out. It should be concise yet with essential details and framed in such an order that it is easy to complete. Adequate documentation may spell the difference between the success and failure of a lawsuit. Records of what was done in the emergency room should be as accurate as time and circumstances permit.
  - ➢ **Extreme** care is to be taken to make any entry in the accident register as it is a valid legal document in a court of law. The person from whom the history is taken is very clearly stated. The status of consciousness is important to mention as the court will decide the reliability of the statement on the basis of that. However, patient care, quality, and safety should always be the primary focus of ED providers.

ETHICS OF EMERGENCY NURSING

When a patient arrives in the emergency department, there is very little time to gather detailed information. Practically, a quick assessment is done and interventions are started based on protocols. The nurses working in the emergency room should have a high level of respect for all individuals and allow human dignity in care and communication. They demonstrate compassion and respect for every individual.

- ❖ **Individuality:** It denotes respect for the individual. The nurses should practice with compassion and respect for every individual. Human dignity and respect should be embedded in dealing with patients.
- ❖ Respect for the **autonomy** of the individual: Autonomy is the capacity to think, decide and act freely and independently. There is a need to ensure that there is an absence of controlling influences that determine their decision-making action.
- ❖ **Beneficence/non-maleficence:** The principle of beneficence is a moral obligation to act for the benefit of others in an emergency situation. Nurses' actions in the emergency room should promote good to others. Doing good means doing things that are best for the patient in an emergency situation. The principle of beneficence supports certain moral rules or obligations like protecting and defending the rights of others, removing conditions that are the potential to cause harm, helping persons with disabilities, rescuing persons in danger, etc.
- ❖ **Honesty:** Honest information regarding the patient's progress to be given to the patient's family members and relatives.

COMMON EMERGENCIES

Emergencies are conditions that appear unexpectedly. Such conditions may be life-threatening and might cause permanent damage or disability if not treated immediately.

POLYTRAUMA

Polytrauma and multiple trauma are terms describing the condition of a person who has been subjected to multiple traumatic injuries. This is a type of trauma where a person has sustained injuries in multiple areas of the body and caused a significant disability that may be life-threatening. It is a major cause of morbidity and mortality in both developed and underdeveloped countries. The younger generation, primarily males are the predominant victims of polytrauma. Types of traumas commonly occur in India are road traffic accidents, falls from heights, and assaults. Other causes of trauma are agriculture-related trauma, intentional self-harm, assault, fall of objects, natural calamities, disasters, terrorist attacks, etc.

The severity of the injury is determined by a number of systems involved, the severity of each injury alone and in combination. Immediately after the injury, the body reacts to the sudden hit with a systemic host-defense response that represents the physiological response to tissue injury, hypotension, hypoxemia, pain, and stress (antigenic load). In case of delay or absence in emergency intervention in the acute phase, there may be a failure in the host defense mechanism that may result in permanent disability or death. External evidences may be very mild or absent, but there may be internal injury.

TRIAGE

Triage is a process of rapidly determining the acuteness of a patient's health status. It is an advanced skill of classifying the casualties into various categories based on the severity of their health problems in order to treat them as per urgency. As the client arrives at the emergency department, she/he is triaged by an emergency nurse or an emergency doctor. The purpose is to determine the severity/acuteness of the condition in order to deliver

The most frequently used triage rating is:
- **Priority 1 (emergent/immediate care needed) (red color code):** Must be treated immediately to save the life of an individual. Casualty cannot wait for a space in the clinical area to be available.
- **Priority 2 (intermediate/urgent care needed) (yellow color):** Requires care within two to four hours. Can safely wait for a short period until a space in the clinical area is available.
- **Priority 3 (delayed care/non-urgent) (green color):** Requires treatment, but it can be delayed evaluation and possible treatment.
- **Priority 4 (dead) (black color):** It is confirmed that the patient is dead.

Patients who are critical, seriously affected, or having a threat to life are immediately taken to start appropriate intervention. Time-sensitive clinical decision-making and critical thinking ability are key competencies in triage. A well-developed interpersonal and communication skill is necessary.

- Prioritization of patients' needs is the most important activity by the ED nurse. The immediate attention includes recording vital parameters, taking note of medical history and personal information, pain assessment, weight recording, history of current events, history of allergy, neurological assessment, and screening for domestic violence.
- She is also responsible for monitoring waiting area patients, maintaining a safe environment, and liaison with patients' relatives. These data will help in the administration of suitable medication and treatment strategies. Recording of patient's condition, treatment, and medication, updating with electronic medical records as necessary.

Management

Kindly see Chapter 30 for the detailed management of traumatic conditions.

Primary Survey

Assess and Intervene

The patient is examined thoroughly and systematically to identify any potential threats. During the primary survey, the client is assessed for airway, breathing, circulation, disability, and exposure (ABCDE approach). ABCDE approach is universal for all in an emergency whether young or old and applied when critical injury is suspected. This approach is not recommended for patients in cardiac arrest.

- **Airway:**
  - Any patient with trauma at the face, head, or neck should be suspected of cervical spine injuries and immobilized using rigid cervical collars.
  - Check patency of the airway and assess breathing. Assess for the presence of a foreign body in the airway. Maintaining a patent airway should be the primary aim. Provide adequate ventilation. Open the airway using the jaw thrust maneuver avoiding hyperextension of the neck, and remove the foreign body if any. Airway maintenance should progress rapidly from the least (e.g., opening the airway using jaw thrust, suctioning, removal of foreign body) to the most invasive method (e.g., insertion of endotracheal intubation, ventilation) after ventilating the patient with 100% oxygen.
  - Look for any open chest wound and flail chest. If there is any penetrating object, leave it in position.
- **Breathing:**
  - Alteration in breathing is manifested as dyspnea, asymmetric chest wall movement (e.g. Flail chest), penetrating chest injuries, decreased or absent breath sound, cyanosis, etc.
  - The changes in breathing patterns may be due to asthma, allergic reaction, pulmonary embolism, pneumothorax, etc. The patient should be assessed for respiratory rate, oxygen saturation, use of accessory muscles, etc.
  - All patients brought to the emergency may need supplemental oxygen. It can be administered using high-flow oxygen (100%) via a nonrebreather mask. In extreme conditions, intubation may be required.
- **Circulation:**
  - The peripheral pulses may be absent due to the impact of injury or vasoconstriction. The palpable pulses may be felt by checking the central pulse (carotid, femoral pulses). Asses the rate and quality of the pulse.
  - Skin should be assessed for color, temperature, and moisture. Decreased perfusion may be manifested as pallor, sweating, and altered level of consciousness. Inspection of the skin gives clues to the problems of circulation.
  - An intravenous access should be obtained as soon as possible and saline or Ringer's lactate should be infused.
  - Blood samples may be drawn for blood grouping and cross-matching as a need for blood transfusion may arise at any time.
  - Pressure bandage to be applied at the obvious bleeding sites.
- **Disability:**
  - The degree of disability is determined by assessing the level of consciousness of the client.
  - AVPU method is applied for quick assessment of consciousness in emergency situations, where **A = Alertness, V = Verbal** responsiveness, **P** = response to **Painful stimuli, and U = Unresponsiveness.**

- Pupils to be assessed for size, shape, response to light, and equality.
- Blood glucose to be measured to assess the presence of hypoglycemia. Evidence of low blood glucose may be corrected immediately by oral or intravenous infusion of glucose.

❖ **Exposure:**
- Bearing in mind the dignity of the client, clothing is removed to allow a thorough physical examination and covering the patient using a blanket to prevent heat loss.
- A detailed physical examination is performed and the client is observed thoroughly for any sign of trauma, bleeding, skin rashes, etc.

Secondary Survey

This is a brief systematic process aimed to identify all injuries that are present in the patient's body.

- ❖ **Vital signs:** A full set of vital signs is recorded. This includes assessment for oxygen saturation, blood pressure, temperature, pulse rate heart rate. Depending on the patient's status of vital parameters it should be decided whether to proceed further with the secondary survey or not.
- ❖ **Family support:** Facilitating family presence gives them comfort as they can view themselves as the participation of the healthcare team in managing the emergency. One designated member of the healthcare team should explain the care rendered and be available to answer their question.
- ❖ **Give comfort measures:** Relief of pain can be initiated at the earliest by the nurses using both pharmacological (e.g., administration of analgesics or opioids as advised), and non-pharmacological measures (e.g., distractions). Some general measures that may be adopted are verbal reassurance, careful listening, and controlling environmental stimuli.
- ❖ **History:** Obtaining complete health history and history of the incident is important. Head-to-to assessment followed by diagnostic and laboratory testing is done.
- ❖ **Inspect:** Inspect the posterior surfaces. Trauma patients should be logrolled while inspecting the posterior side and looking for any abrasion, ecchymosis, and open wound. If there is a presence of an open wound, it needs to be cleaned. Cleansing is best achieved by high-pressure irrigation with normal saline. If there is a presence of hair around the wound, clipping is done. Consider the size and depth of the wound, and structures involved and then plan for suturing.

If the wound is due to a dog bite, suturing is not done because of the highly contaminated nature of the wound. Loose protective dressing should be applied before sending the patient out of the emergency department.

Taking care of patients with polytrauma is challenging. Patients with polytrauma are in life-threatening conditions. Caring for such a patient with multiple injuries requires a team approach. An organized polytrauma team consisting of a trauma leader, a trauma surgeon, an orthopedic surgeon, an anesthesiologist, two nurses, and any other subspecialist required by the trauma team leader. The leader in the trauma care team should be an experienced surgeon capable of managing all injury patterns. There should be a well-defined standard operating procedure to manage patients with polytrauma efficiently and effectively. The goal of management is to determine the extent of the injury and establish treatment based on priority as discussed previously.

Patients with polytrauma are taken care of as a case of spinal cord injury until it is confirmed. The initial survey should not take more than 3–5 minutes.

Any observation that suggests injury to vital organs and interfering with the vital physiologic function prompts a threat to life and needs the highest priority for immediate treatment. Simultaneously a thorough examination is carried out. Most missed injuries occur in unconscious patients. Therefore, all the clothes of the patients are removed or cut off and a rapid physical assessment is performed as soon as the patient is resuscitated. Patients' privacy and dignity are to be maintained during this process.

A powerful nursing observation is the key to preventing any complications and possible death. The advanced learning of the critical care nurse enriched with her experience and ability to make good assessments in critical situations are the key qualities in caring for polytraumatized patients.

Thus, the emergency nurse is the most important link in a multidisciplinary team that takes care of a patient with polytrauma. The nursing care of patients with polytrauma encompasses a wide range of interventions.

The nursing responsibility in managing patients with polytrauma includes: Assessment and monitoring the patient's vital parameters, ensuring and maintaining a patent airway, maintaining IV access, administration of prescribed medication, collecting samples for laboratory investigations, documentation of activities, and patient's response.

All these interventions have already been discussed in various other chapters and to avoid duplication are not being dealt here.

POISONING

Poisoning occurs when any substance interferes with normal body functions after being absorbed into the body. This may impair cellular metabolism, disrupt the structure, or disturb the normal functioning of the body. Poisons may be injurious to human health when introduced into the body by means of inhalation, ingestion, injection, or absorption through the skin. The danger of poisoning may range from short-term illness to brain damage, coma, and death. Short-term exposure to the poison is called acute poisoning whereas repeated long-term contact is called as chronic poisoning. Acute poisoning occurs when a single large dose or several small doses of harmful substance are taken over a short period of time, whereas chronic poisoning occurs when small doses of harmful substances are taken over a long period of time.

Poisonings can be accidental, occupational, recreational, or intentional. The severity of poisoning depends on the type, concentration, and route of exposure. They can cause effects when taken orally and swallowed, injected into the body, inhaled, or even rubbed on the skin. Commonly observed poisons are pesticides, organophosphates, carbon monoxide, heavy metals, and certain plants such as Datura, cannabis, opium, etc.

FOOD POISONING

Food poisoning calls for sudden illness that occurs after ingestion of contaminated food and drink. Often the food is contaminated with microorganisms or their products. Food poisoning is most often acute. In some cases, it can lead to complications like dehydration, electrolyte imbalance, etc.

Etiology

Most illnesses are due to eating undercooked food or contaminated food, improperly canned or preserved food, home preserved vegetable, and canned commercial products. Infection can also occur from the consumption of raw milk or unpasteurized milk or contaminated fruit juice. Drinking sewage-contaminated water or swimming in dirty water also gives rise to acute GI symptoms like food poisoning.

Food poisoning can be grouped as:
- Acute gastroenteritis due to bacterial infection, e.g., staphylococci, *Salmonella*, clostridial, etc.
- Neurologic symptoms from botulism, e.g., toxins from *Clostridium* botulism
- Poisonous chemicals, arsenic zinc, and potassium chlorate may contaminate foods.

Clinical Manifestations

Most signs and symptoms include nausea, vomiting, abdominal cramps, diarrhea, and in extreme cases some may have fever and chills. In the case of infection by botulism, symptoms may include constipation, distention, central nervous system symptoms like headache, dizziness, muscular incoordination, weakness, inability to talk or swallow, diplopia, breathing difficulties, paralysis, delirium, and coma.

Clinical manifestations of food poisoning caused by *E. coli* may vary from mild to severe bloody diarrhea. *E. coli* produces a powerful toxin and can cause severe illness. Diarrhea may start as watery but may progress to bloody diarrhea. There may be systemic complications that may be life-threatening like uremic syndrome and thrombocytopenic purpura that may lead to death.

Management

- The focus of intervention with food poisoning is to determine the source of poisoning, the type of food that caused the poisoning, and the prevention of the occurrence of infection. History to be obtained from the patient and family. If possible suspected food to be brought to the medical facility.
- The gastric content, vomitus, serum, and feces are collected for bacteriological examination.
- Since a large volume of fluid and electrolytes are lost due to severe vomiting and diarrhea, it is important to check the vital parameters, level of consciousness, monitoring of urinary output, muscular activity, and skin turgor for assessment of dehydration to evaluate whether the patient is progressing towards hypovolemic shock.
- Supportive care is needed to maintain intravascular volume through intravenous infusion to prevent dehydration and electrolyte imbalance.
- Measures to control nausea are important for the prevention of vomiting. In case of severe nausea injectable antiemetics as prescribed may be administered.
- Other therapies may include dialysis and plasmapheresis in case of hemolytic uremic syndrome and such cases are treated in ICU.
- Once nausea and vomiting subside, clear liquid is prescribed for 12–24 hours. The diet progressed to a low-residue bland diet.

INGESTED (SWALLOWED) POISONING

Swallowed poisons are substances that can cause tissue trauma to the GI tract. Contact with such agents causes tissue destruction. These may include drain cleaners, toilet cleaners, bleach, non-phosphate detergent, metal cleaners, rust removers, battery acid, etc.

If a corrosive substance is swallowed, there may be evidence of redness or burn in the mouth. There may be a presence of symptoms like:
- Weakness, dizziness, or fainting
- Decreased muscle coordination: Muscle spasms or seizures

Management of Ingested Poisoning

Measures are mainly concerned towards removing the toxin or decreasing the absorption. Efforts are taken to identify the nature of the substance, amount ingested, time since ingestion, vomiting, drooling, age, the weight of the patient, etc. An antidote is administered to diminish the effect of the toxin. In case of corrosive poisoning water or milk is given to drink to dilute the concentration of acid or alkaline substance. However, if there is evidence of edema, airway obstruction, or perforation of the esophagus, stomach, or intestine dilution is not attempted.

Blood samples are taken to determine the concentration of the drug or poison. ECG, vital signs, and neurologic status are monitored. Shock may occur due to cardio-depressant action of the substance.

Managing airway, ventilation, and oxygenation are most essential. An indwelling catheter is inserted to monitor kidney function. Monitoring the patient's vital parameters, fluid-electrolyte balance, and neurological status is very important. The prognosis largely depends on the successful management of respiration and circulation.

Prevention

Read the warnings and medical information on the labels of corrosive products before handling. In many cases, consumer education and proper use can prevent a serious medical emergency.

INHALED (CARBON MONOXIDE) POISONING

Carbon monoxide (CO) poisoning usually occurs by inhalation of a relatively high concentration of carbon monoxide gas.

The common sources of CO gas are incomplete combustion of organic compounds like vehicle exhaust, smoke from fires, and improperly maintained heating systems.

Etiology

Carbon monoxide poisoning may occur as a result of industrial poisoning, household poisoning, or attempted suicide. The sources of carbon monoxide (CO) poisoning are:

- **House fire:** The maximum concentration of CO in the air is around 5% in the immediate vicinity of a house fire.
- **Incomplete combustion of fuels,** e.g., charcoal, briquette, fuel gas, petroleum using a burner.
- **Heating or cooking equipment** with insufficient ventilation or improper maintenance.
- **Exhaust gas from vehicles** using internal combustion engines (the CO concentration in exhaust gas is less than a few percent).
- **Industrial accidents** such as those occurring at iron metalworks or chemical plants.

Symptoms

The toxic effect of carbon monoxide (CO) is due to its ability to bind with circulating hemoglobin and thus reduce the oxygen-carrying capacity of the blood. CO shows a high affinity for hemoglobin and other hemoproteins like myoglobin and cytochrome C oxidase. Hemoglobin absorbs carbon monoxide 200 times more readily than it absorbs oxygen. CO also binds to myoglobin in myocardium and skeletal muscle and about 15% of the total CO in the body is taken up by tissues. Carbon-monoxide-bound hemoglobin, called carboxy-hemoglobin does not transport oxygen. This may cause impairment of cardiac and neurological functions. A person with carbon monoxide poisoning may appear intoxicated with cerebral hypoxia, headache, palpitation, and muscular weakness that can progress toward coma.

Increased incidences of CO poisoning in the winter months of December to January in the northern part of India.

There may be radiological evidence of suspected CO poisoning. Diagnosis is made on the basis of history and response to supportive treatment. Some may have residual neurological damage as a result of hypoxic brain damage due to prolonged exposure to a toxic level of CO. Vascular permeability may be there due to prolonged tissue hypoxia that may cause accumulation of interstitial fluid with decreased circulating blood volume that may involve vital organs and may give rise to cerebral edema with neurological symptoms or unconsciousness; pulmonary edema with respiratory failure; cardiac symptoms like arrhythmia, decreased myocardial contractility, heart failure; renal failure, etc.

Management

The goal of management includes reversing cerebral and myocardial hypoxia. The treatment comprises immediate evacuation of the victim from exposure to fresh air. Open all doors and windows and loosen tight clothing. Carboxyhemoglobin level is analyzed on admission. Administration of high-flow or 100% oxygen by a nonrebreather reservoir oxygen mask or endotracheal tube is required for the elimination of carbon monoxide from blood as initial management.

Hyperbaric oxygen therapy can also be used as per availability. It is used to accelerate the elimination of CO and reverse the effects of inflammation and mitochondrial dysfunction induced by CO poisoning.

Management of the airway, intravenous access, and cardiac monitoring are required in the hospital as per the requirement of the patients.

CHEMICAL BURNS (SKIN CONTAMINATION)

A chemical burn occurs when the skin or mucous membrane comes in contact with irritants like alkali, acid, or any other corrosive chemicals or fumes produced by corrosive chemicals. Most of chemical burns are caused by the accidental misuse of a corrosive substance. The most commonly affected areas are the face, eyes, legs, and hands. The severity of a chemical burn is determined by the penetrating strength and concentration of the chemical, amount, and duration of exposure of skin to the chemical.

Chemical burns can occur at any place and are most commonly caused by exposure to acids or alkalis in the home, at school, workplace, where caustic and corrosive materials are handled. Chemical burns can affect anyone. However, the people who work in manufacturing facilities are at the highest risk. At home, children, and older adults with disability are at higher risk.

Some common products that can cause chemical burns are household cleaners such as bleach, ammonia, drain or toilet cleaners; skin, hair, and nail care products, and even teeth whitening kits; car batteries, etc.

SYMPTOMS

The symptoms of a chemical burn depend on the substance causing the chemical burn, the part of the body the substance came into contact with, the duration of exposure to the corrosive substance, and whether the substance was inhaled or ingested. Common manifestations of a chemical burn include:

- Redness, irritation, burning, or numbness at the site of contact
- Localized pain and edema at the surrounding tissue
- Discoloration of injured tissue
- Coughing, wheezing, and shortness of breath if the substance was inhaled or ingested
- Burning in eyes, blurry vision, or total loss of vision if the materials came into contact with the eyes.

MANAGEMENT

- Skin should be drenched immediately under running tap water.
- Asses responsiveness. If unresponsive, assess airway, breathing, and circulation before decontamination. If responsive monitor airway, breathing, and circulation.
- Watch patient with inhalation injury closely for signs of respiratory distress

- Brush dry chemicals from the skin before irrigation in case of lye and white phosphorus.
- Remove adherent clothing, shoes, watch, glasses, contact lenses, jewelry
- If burns of the eye, irrigate from inner to outer canthus with water
- Cover the burn area with a clean sheet
- Monitor pain, urine output
- Establish IV access with two large bore catheters if the burnt area is >15% TBSA
- Contact the poison control center for assistance
- Initiate medicolegal formalities

THERMAL EMERGENCIES

HEAT STROKE

This is the most serious heat-related condition. Heat stroke is a hyperthermic emergency condition when a client gets exposed to excessive heat.

Signs and Symptoms

The core temperature may be 105°F or 40.5°C or more. Often the client is comatose. Other symptoms may include hypotension, tachycardia, elevated body temperature, and hot flushed skin.

Treatment

- Intravenous infusion of normal saline to restore fluid volume.
- Institute cooling measures by removing the clothes and spraying tepid mist over the client's body while keeping him under the fan for adequate ventilation, giving cold therapy using ice packs on the scalp, neck, axilla, and groin.
- Frequently check oxygen saturation and body temperature.
- Gastric lavage with cold saline may be necessary to bring the core temperature down.
- Such measures should be continued until the temperature comes down to 101°F.
- Continuously monitor the client for muscle cramping and signs of neurological complications. Administration of calcium gluconate may be necessary in case of severe muscle cramps.

HEAT EXHAUSTION

Prolonged exposure to heat for hours or days leads to heat exhaustion. There is salt and water depletion due to prolonged exposure in an extremely hot environment.

Signs and Symptoms

It is a clinical syndrome characterized by fatigue, nausea, vomiting, extreme thirst, and a feeling of anxiety. There may be severe spasms in the muscles of the hands and legs, excessive perspiration leading to sodium depletion, dehydration due to excessive sweating, and heat exhaustion. The client may complain of light-headedness, headache, dizziness, nausea, and weakness. There may be mild hypotension and cold clammy skin.

Management

The patient should be placed in a cool area. Monitoring vital parameters is important in order to identify arrhythmias for the assessment of electrolyte imbalance.

FROSTBITE

Frostbite is damage to tissue and blood vessels as a result of prolonged exposure to cold. It is an extreme form of cold injury when ice crystals are formed and tissues freeze slowly. This occurs when tissues are frozen hard and are exposed suddenly to a temperature of –4°C or lower. At such a low temperature, damage to the tissues occurs due to a marked reduction in peripheral blood flow. The area may appear red and swollen. The commonly affected areas are fingers, toes, cheeks, ears, and nose.

Risk Factors

- **Age:** Elderly are more prone
- **Environmental temperature:** 35°C or less
- **Duration of exposure:** Prolonged exposure to cold
- **Pre-existing illness:** Diabetes, neuropathy, paraplegia, Raynaud's diseases
- **Use of alcohol or sedative drug:** Impaired judgement necessary to seek shelter
- **Smokers:** Vasoconstrictive effect due to nicotine.

Patients can have a combination of these injuries occurring in different body parts:

- **Frostnip** is a mild cold injury and completely reversible, seen on the face and hands. There may be pallor or numbness, tingling, or burning sensation. The patient may have a crunchy feeling.
- **Chilblain** is a more severe form of cold injury resulting from repeated exposure to cold progressing to chronic vasculitis on the face, hands, anterior lower legs, and feet. The skin has a violaceous color. There is pain and pruritis with cold exposure. Fingers and toes may become cyanotic.

Degrees of Frostbite

According to the severity, there are four degrees of frostbite.
- **Superficial frostbite:** It involves first and second degrees of frostbite.
  - *First-degree:* In first-degree frostbite, there is edema and redness in the affected part. If further freezing is arrested, this resolves fully. There may be cold sensitivity for a few weeks after recovery.
  - *Second-degree:* In second-degree frostbite, there is the involvement of partial thickness of skin and blister formation. These blisters may contain either clear or purple bloody fluid. A blackened crust (Eschar) may be formed from the dead tissues and dried secretion of the skin in 2–3 weeks that gets separated after 4 weeks. As a late consequence of this, the client may complain of paresthesia, tingling sensation, and reactive vasodilatation.
- **Deep frostbite:** This involves muscles, bones, and tendons. The third and fourth degrees of frost bites are included in this category.

- *Third degree:* The layers of tissue below the skin freeze. Skin appears lifeless and pale. There is bluish-gray discoloration that progresses till complete necrosis of the skin occurs and thereafter forms Eschar in 2 weeks causing damage even to the epiphyseal closure.
- *Fourth degree:* It involves the entire thickness of the skin, the structure below the skin, and varying depth of deeper tissues. The skin is hard and insensitive to touch. The affected area appeared mottled that gradually progress towards gangrene.

Management

- The affected areas need meticulous care as the injured tissues may be damaged easily.
- Clothing and jewelry may be removed as they may constrict and damage the extremity and decrease circulation.
- As soon as the client is removed from the cold environment, rewarming starts by keeping the affected limb immersed in lukewarm water for 20 minutes. The part should be handled gently. Blisters may be treated with utmost care keeping them intact. A sterile dressing is applied loosely. Daily dressing to be changed. The affected part should be kept elevated to control swelling. Heavy blankets and clothing should be avoided on the affected area because friction and weight may lead to the sloughing of damaged tissues.
- **An IV line to be started for the administration of medication:** Normal saline, injection of tetanus toxoid as prophylaxis, antibiotics for infection, and analgesics to relieve pain. Intravenous analgesia is administered to reduce pain associated with tissue thawing in severe frostbite and amputation in extreme cases.
- Monitor vital signs and urinary output. Assessment for systemic hypothermia is important.

HYPOTHERMIA

Hypothermia occurs when the core body temperature lowers 35°C (95°F). It occurs when heat produced by the body cannot compensate for the heat lost in the environment.

This may occur among individuals exposed to extremely cold weather for a long time or among victims of near drowning.

Etiology

- **Age:** Older adults are more prone to hypothermia due to decreased body fat, diminished energy reserve, and decreased sensory perceptions.
- **Medications:** Phenothiazines decrease the ability to shiver and hampers the body's innate ability to generate body heat.
- **Medical conditions:** People with concurrent illness, hypothyroidism, spinal cord injury.
- Environmental exposure to freezing temperature, cold wind, damp terrain in the presence of inadequate clothing, and physical exhaustion predisposes the individual to hypothermia.
- **Trauma victims:** These are at risk for hypothermia that results from treatment with cold fluid, and exposure during examination.

TABLE 44.1: Clinical features of hypothermia.

First stage	Cold and feeling of shivering as the body temperature falls
Second stage	- Shivering stops at 32° - Slurred speech - Impaired mobility - Respiration, circulation, and metabolism slow down - Drunken gait - Gradual loss of consciousness
Third stage	Death due to failure of function in vital centers

- Alcohol ingestion causes systemic vasodilation.
- Wet clothing increases evaporative heat loss 5 times more than normal.

Pathophysiology

Hypothermia leads to physiologic changes in all organ systems. In mild hypothermia, initially, peripheral vasoconstriction attempts to conserve body heat. As the body remains exposed to cold, there is increased heat loss. The body's only mechanism to produce heat is shivering and movement. There is progressive deterioration in CNS functioning leading to drowsiness, ataxia, pulmonary edema, impaired judgment, etc. With further exposure to cold, the body's self-worming mechanism becomes ineffective **(Table 44.1)**.

Management

Includes collaborative care. Management includes maintaining the CABs, rewarming the patient, and supportive care.

- **Monitoring:** Core body temperature is measured using a rectal thermometer. Monitoring of other parameters includes ECG monitoring, urine output, blood chemistry, blood urea, nitrogen, creatinine, ABG, chest X-ray, etc.
- **Rewarming:** Active internal rewarming is needed in case of moderate to severe hypothermia (28–32.2°C) and the patient should be monitored for ventricular fibrillation. Passive external rewarming by over-the-bed heaters to the extremities. Care must be taken to prevent burns due to the use of such devices as a patient may have altered sensation to feel the heat. Monitoring for arrhythmia and electrolyte imbalance is essential at this stage.
- **Supportive care:** Administration of worm IV fluids, to correct hypotension and maintain urine output, administration of sodium bicarbonate to correct metabolic acidosis, insertion of a urinary catheter to monitor kidney function test.

NEAR DROWNING

Drowning is the most common cause of unintentional injury death. Drowning is a condition where the person is underwater and survives for a limited period of time (at least 24 hours) without ventilation after submersion. The commonest consequence of drowning is hypoxemia.

The population at risk are children under 5 years of age and nearly 80% of people who die from drowning are male. Factors contributing to a higher rate of drowning among males include alcohol use, risk-taking behavior, and increased exposure to water (CDC 2019).

Factors associated with drowning are inability to swim, diving injuries, overestimation of swimming skills, hypothermia, extreme fatigue (exhaustion), and sudden illness (seizure, myocardial infarction, or hypoglycemia). Most downing events occur in natural water, lake, and swimming pools. Irrespective of the nature of the fluid aspirated, the ultimate result of drowning is pulmonary edema. The aspirated fluid washes out the alveolar surfactant and causes alveolar collapse, intrapulmonary shunting, decreased lung compliance, and hypoxemia. The nonfatal drowning process involves the onset of hypoxia, hypercapnia, bradycardia and dysrhythmias, and severe electrolyte imbalance.

MANAGEMENT

The aim of management is to maintain cerebral perfusion and adequate oxygenation.
- ❖ Begin assessment and intervention with ABCs. If there is the possibility of spinal cord injury the spinal cord should be immobilized.
- ❖ It is important to obtain a history of drowning events and consider the duration of submersion, temperature of water, nature of water, and associated injury. Observe for any effort of breathing; open the airway, look for manifestations of hypoxia, and obtain vital parameters.
- ❖ Monitoring ABG (to evaluate O_2, CO_2, HCO_3, and PH levels) to determine the type of ventilatory support is very important. The use of endotracheal intubation with PEEP improves oxygenation, prevents aspiration, and corrects ventilation-perfusion abnormalities for the patient who is not breathing spontaneously. Supplemental oxygen supply through a mask is needed for patients who are breathing spontaneously.
- ❖ Meanwhile client's wet clothing needs to be removed and wrapping with a warm blanket is done to initiate rewarming the patient. Determining the level of hypothermia is very important. ECG monitoring is done to assess dysrhythmia.
- ❖ Nasogastric intubation to decompress the stomach and catheterization by indwelling Foley catheter is done to measure urinary output.
- ❖ Close monitoring is continued with sequential recording of vital parameters, once the vital signs are stabilized, electrolyte imbalance and acid-base balance should be corrected. ABG analysis, serum electrolyte, chest X-ray, and assessment for increased ICP is very vital as the patient is at risk of developing ischemic cerebral injury. Close monitoring of neurologic status is essential.
- ❖ After a near drowning event the survivor is at risk of developing pulmonary edema, acute respiratory distress syndrome.

DECOMPRESSION SICKNESS (DCS)

It refers to the injuries caused by a rapid decrease in pressure surrounding the individual, i,e., air or water. This occurs most commonly among the individual engaged in scuba (Aqua-lung) or deep-sea diving. It also can occur during high-altitude or unpressurized air travel. Decompression sickness is also known as barotrauma or the bends. Proper decompression procedures during diving can help decrease the incidence of decompression sickness.

DCS can be classified as Type I and Type II.
- ❖ **Type I:** Skin, musculoskeletal and lymphatic system
- ❖ **Type II:** Symptoms that involve CNS

ETIOLOGY AND RISK FACTOR

Most decompression injuries are caused by changes in pressure. Most of the people at risk of decompression syndrome are those engaged in scuba diving in the deep sea. Air under high pressure is compressed. Each breath taken at depth contains more molecules than a breath taken at the surface. Oxygen is used continuously by the body, the extra oxygen molecules breathed under high pressure usually do not accumulate. However, the extra nitrogen molecule is accumulated in blood and tissue. Nitrogen bubbles may form in small blood vessels or in tissue themselves, tissue with high-fat content is likely to be affected as nitrogen dissolves rapidly in fat.

Individual factors contributing to increased risk for DCS include patent foramen ovale, dehydration, cold ambient (immediate surrounding) temperature, high body fat content, and alcoholism.

Type II DCS (neurological symptoms) are thought to occur from right to left shunting of venous bubbles.

The condition presents as dramatic and profound sudden onset injuries in patients engaged in tunnel work and compressed gas diving, including scuba. There is the occurrence of gas bubbles in extra pulmonic sites. There is also supersaturation of the tissue with dissolved gas and the subsequent evolution of gas bubbles. Gas embolism results from the direct transit of molecular gas from a pulmonary or intravascular origin into the arterial circulation causing occlusion of a distal locus **(Fig. 44.3)**.

SYMPTOMS

An individual exhibits the symptoms of **fatigue and pain in muscles and joints**. Other symptoms include numbness, tingling, arm or leg weakness, unsteadiness, vertigo (spinning), difficulty breathing, and chest pain which could be there in more severe cases.

PATHOPHYSIOLOGY

DCS is basically the formation of bubbles growth and elimination caused by a reduction in ambient pressure.

Sudden and too rapid a reduction in pressure (i.e., decompression) can cause the expansion of gases in the usual gas-containing cavities or organs in the body. This results in dysbarism (the formation of bubbles coming out of the solution). Tissue damage results from multiple mechanism including blockage of blood flow and vascular spasm.

Gas bubbles can cause endothelial damage that results in the activation of intrinsic clotting cascade with platelet activation. Inflammatory mediators are released and with increased endothelial permeability develop edema which leads to tissue ischemia. Other effects are due to the expansion of microscopic gas particles within the tissues of the body **(Fig. 44.4)**.

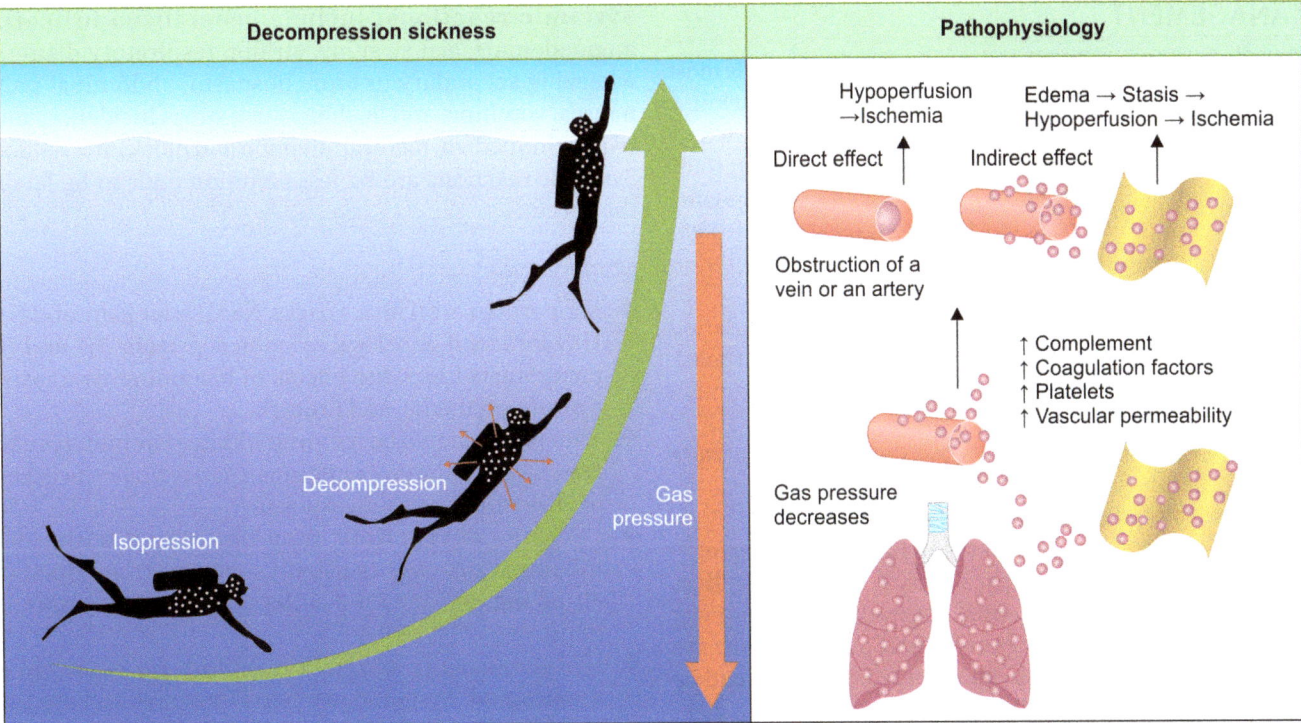

Fig. 44.3: Decompression sickness.

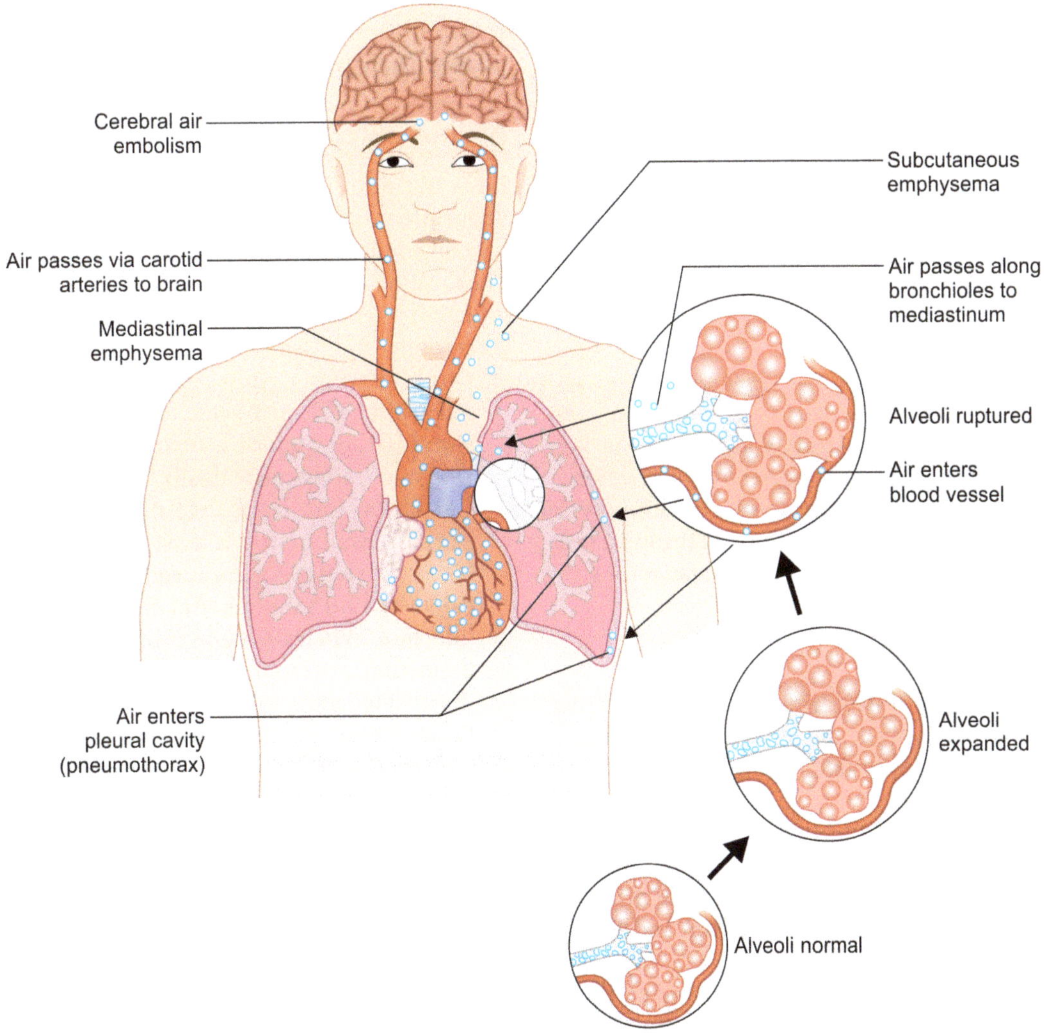

Fig. 44.4: Decompression sickness.

MANAGEMENT

Establishing a patent airway and adequate ventilation is most important. Immediate treatment for decompression sickness involves recompression therapy which is also known as hyperbaric oxygen therapy. Throughout the treatment, 100% oxygen is given. Treatment is directed towards increasing hydrostatic pressure, thus maximizing the gradient for gas reabsorption and dissolution and subsequently excretion via the lungs.

This is most effective and all patients should be started on high-flow oxygen at 15 L/min via a non-rebreather mask regardless of their oxygen saturation. There are three main effects of this recompression therapy:

1. Bubble crushing as per Boyle's law, the increased pressure decreases the volume of bubbles
2. Flushing out of nitrogen bubbles with oxygen
3. Healing the damaged tissues with hyperbaric oxygen

IV line started with Ringer's lactate or normal saline. Chest X-ray is taken to identify aspiration. Remove wet clothing and keep the patient warm. If possible, shift the patient to the hyperbaric chamber where treatment can be initiated at the earliest. In the case of air transport, the flight is kept at a low altitude. Nevertheless, if the patient is alert and awake and has no CNS deficit ground transportation may be done. Constant monitoring of the patient is done and changes are documented.

STINGS AND BITES

Stings occur when insects pierce the skin and one feels a sharp pain. Insects release saliva that may cause skin irritation. Sometimes part of the sting remains in the body of an affected person and is called a stinger. Stings may be managed with first aid but severe allergic reactions due to venom may be present. In these cases, there may be a danger to the life of the victim. Thus, immediate medical aid is required.

HYMENOPTERAN STINGS

Bee stings, hornet stings, ants, scorpions, and wasps, are usually painful rather than dangerous. Wasps, yellow jackets, and hornets are known to be more aggressive than others.

Some people are allergic and can develop severe anaphylactic reactions when toxins stimulate the mast cells. Multiple stings on the face and neck are also dangerous and can cause swelling and obstruction to the airway.

Clinical Manifestations

Clinical manifestation of bee and wasp stings include erythema, edema, and pain at the sting site. The onset of life-threatening, anaphylactic signs typically occurs within 10 minutes of the sting.

Most hymenopteran stings result in mild reactions in the form of a small area of local inflammation. Symptoms may include local edema, induration, increased warmth, and tenderness. These symptoms are self-limited and resolve within a few days.

Larger local reactions include induration and erythema around 10 cm, increased temperature locally, and lasting longer. They are more painful.

Systemic reactions: Include generalized urticaria, angioedema/facial swelling, stridor, respiratory distress/wheezing secondary to bronchospasm, abdominal pain, nausea, vomiting, and flushing. Such stings incidences may require immediate medical attention and quick intervention. Systemic reactions are far less common but can be fatal if they occur.

Management

- Supportive care with ice packs, NSAIDs for pain, and H1/H2 blockers if only local reaction is present. H1 and H2 antagonists block the effects of histamine-decreasing pruritis, erythema, and urticaria.
- The stinger should be removed within a few minutes after the sting by scraping rather than squeezing or tweezing to avoid further venom exposure.
- Large local reactions may be treated with anti-inflammatory agents usually a course of prednisone 40–60 mg per day for 3–5 days so that the symptoms improve.
- Life-threatening systemic reactions are managed at the hospital. Systemic reactions (anaphylaxis) are life-threatening and should be managed by maintaining ABC. Early intubation is recommended as the airway patency may be compromised within seconds to minutes.

An anaphylactic reaction may be managed by epinephrine, corticosteroids, and H1 and H2 antagonists. IV fluids should be started immediately. Such a situation is treated for managing anaphylactic shock.

ANIMAL AND HUMAN BITES

Bites are common reasons for visiting the emergency department. Biting incidents typically involve being bitten by a dog or cat and sometimes other domesticated animals. The location and type of the injury depends upon the animal inflicting the bite. Bite wounds can be puncturing wounds, lacerations, and tissue avulsion injuries.

- **Dog bites:** Most victims of dog bites usually know the dog. A dog bite can lead to scratches, deep open cuts, puncture wounds, crush injuries, and tearing away of a body part. Dog bites rarely cause death.
- **Cat bites:** Cats cause wounds mostly on the upper extremities or on the face with their teeth or claws. Cat bites cause deep punctured wounds involving joint capsules and tendons that can cause a greater risk of infection. When the hand is bitten, bacteria get into the tissue that is present in the skin folds and into the joint at the affected area.
- **Rodent bites:** Rat bites are commonest among rodents and often occur at night on the face or hands in children five years old or younger.
- **Human bites:** Children are the most common victims of human bites. They usually do this at the time of aggressive playing with one another. The skin may be punctured, or there may be a semi-circular or oval area of skin redness or bruising at the site of the bite. The usual sites of human bites are the face, upper extremities, or abdomen. Human bites may be at a high risk of infection from oral bacterial flora.

Appropriate information and physical examination are of prime importance in a client with a history of bites as early initiation of treatment and management will reduce the chance of infection. It is very important to collect and document information regarding the timeline since the bite has occurred, any signs of infection are very significant. Further information needed is how the bite has occurred, whether the animal was provoked, whether the animal has bitten someone else before, and the vaccination status of the animal.

A thorough medical history of the client is obtained including comorbidity and whether immunocompromised, vaccinated with tetanus prophylaxis or not. An aggressive wash with copious amounts of normal saline, or a virucidal povidone-iodine solution is essential. A very deep complicated wound may require surgical evaluation.

Pasteurella species, a gram-negative aerobic species is present in the oropharynx of most dogs and cats and can cause cellulitis in humans if not treated properly. This may lead to purulent discharge, fever, osteomyelitis, septic arthritis, and ultimately, septicemia with its consequences if left unchecked.

Management of Human and Animal Bites

Early medical management includes wound cleansing; prophylactic antibiotics to decrease the risk of infection; rabies postexposure treatment depending on the animal vaccination status; administration of tetanus vaccine if the person has not been adequately vaccinated.

This polymicrobial wound environment is composed of a broad mixture of aerobic and anaerobic organisms. Commonly involved aerobic species include *Neisseria*, *Corynebacterium*, and *Staphylococcus*. Anaerobes most frequently implicated in animal bite wounds include *Fusobacterium, Bacteroides, Prevotella, Propionibacterium, Peptostreptococcus,* and *Porphyromonas*.

Postexposure prophylaxis consists of local wound treatment with washouts and cleaning of the wound followed by tetanus prophylaxis, analgesics, and vaccination. Rabies prophylaxis is the most essential component to be considered in animal and human bites. An initial injection of rabies vaccine is administered to provide passive immunity and thereafter a series of injections are administered on 0, 3, 7, 14, and 28 days to provide active immunity.

Prophylactic antibiotics are administered for those at high risk of infection: Wounds over joints, punctured wounds, bites at the hand or foot, and wounds older than 6–12 hours.

SNAKEBITE

It is an acute life-threatening time-limiting medical emergency (National Health Mission). Snakebite envenoming is a life-threatening condition caused by toxins put in during the bite of a venomous snake. Envenoming is also caused by having venom sprayed into the eyes by certain species of snakes that have the ability to spit venom as a defense measure. A common problem in India especially in the tropical areas reason is heavy rainfall and humid climate. India accounts for 80% of global snakebite deaths.

There are about 236 species of snakes in India. Among them, 13 species are known to be venomous and 4 species are highly venomous. They are common Cobra, Russell's Vipers, saw-scaled vipers, and common kraits and are believed to be responsible for most of the snake bites in India. Common snakes seen in India (tropical area) are Rattle snakes, Vipers, Cobras, and common kraits. The envenomation effect depends on the type of snake. Venom from pit viper is hemolytic whereas coral snake venom is neurotoxic.

Local Reaction

One or two fang marks associated with pain, bruising, and edema within 36 hours of the bite.

Systemic Reaction

Nausea, vomiting, dizziness, tachycardia, muscle fasciculation, GI bleeding, and respiratory problems.

Management

Initial first aid management includes reassuring victims that death is not imminent and treatment is available.

Control anxiety as excitement will increase the heart rate and lead to the spread of venom. Make the victim lie keeping the bitten limb below the heart level and immobilize the limb using a splint. Shift the victim immediately to the nearest hospital where antivenom is available.

Parenteral fluids may be used to treat hypotension. Vascular access with a large bore intracath and administration of crystalloids to maintain blood pressure is essential in the emergency department.

Remove shoes, rings, watches, jewellery, and tight clothing from the bitten area. Tourniquets are not applied, no incision, no suction, and no washing with soap and water is recommended.

Airway breathing and circulation are the priority. ED team should be prepared to treat shock and provide CPR. In the emergency department, the initial evaluation is performed. The information includes when and where the bite occurred, the sequence of events, any medication given or not, signs of fang puncture, erythema, bite, and condition of nearby tissues.

Various investigations considered after a snake bite are 20 minutes blood clotting test of coagulation, Hb, platelet count, prothrombin time, D-dimer, fibrin degradation products (FDP), urine examination for proteinuria, RBC and hemoglobin, oxygen saturation, ABG, enzyme-linked immunosorbent assay (ELISA) to confirm the species of the snake. Course and prognosis depend on the part of the body in which the bite is, the kind and amount of venom injected, and the age and general health of the client. The client should be kept under observation for 24 hours and should not be left unattended.

Anti-snake venom is the mainstay treatment in India. The amount of antivenin required depends on the timing, type, and severity of envenomation.

TICK BITE

Ticks are blood-sucking parasitic insects that puncture the skin with a sharp beak. They are tiny crawling bugs in the spider family. Once the ticks are in contact with skin they migrate towards major skin folds (groin, armpit) where they implant themselves and do not begin to feed themselves until 12–24 hours.

Tick bites are common and are usually found in wooded areas. A tick bite can be the cause of local inflammation. Ticks transmit pathogens using saliva.

Ticks are vectors for numerous diseases like lyme disease, tick-borne meningoencephalitis, Q fever, Crimean–Congo hemorrhagic fever, tick-borne relapsing fever, tick-borne spotted fevers, babesiosis, ehrlichiosis, tularemia. In recent years, other tick-borne diseases, such as babesiosis, Ganjam virus (GANV), and Bhanja virus (BHAV) infections have also been reported in India.

Any tick found should be removed immediately and alive. Persons should be closely monitored after the removal of a tick for up to 30 days for signs and symptoms of tick-borne diseases. The number of ticks and tick-borne diseases should be regularly monitored in areas with a high risk of tick attacks.

LYME DISEASE

It is a multiorgan infection occurring in three different stages.
1. **The primary stage:** It is often characterized by erythema chronicum migrans (ECM), which is formed at the site of the tick bite. Lesions typically are found at the axilla, groin, or thigh areas and usually appear 2–20 days after the tick bite in 60–80% of cases. Untreated, ECM lesions are likely to remain for 3–4 weeks before resolving spontaneously and might recur in secondary stages.
2. **The secondary stage:** It is associated with the spreading of the spirochete within 4–10 weeks following the tick bite. This stage is characterized by multiple secondary annular (ring-shaped) red skin lesions (ECM), fever, adenopathy, neuropathies, cardiac abnormalities, and arthritic problems. These symptoms occur in up to 50% of infected patients. In this stage, approximately 15% of untreated patients develop neurologic symptoms like headache, neck stiffness, memory loss, poor motor coordination, joint pain (large joints), and cranial neuritis (usually unilateral or bilateral facial nerve palsy). In 8% of patients, there are cardiac manifestations such as myopericarditis or any type of atrioventricular (AV) block.
3. **The tertiary stage:** It can occur anytime from weeks to years after initial infection. It can be characterized by chronic arthritis, myalgia, myocarditis, and neuropathy. Symptoms can persist for a decade or more even after appropriate treatment.

Initially, the diagnosis is based on clinical features. Confirmation may be obtained via polymerase chain reaction (PCR) testing, polyvalent fluorescence immunoassay, or western immunoblot testing.

Management

Management consists of appropriate antibiotics. Treatment is mainly determined by clinical manifestations of the disease. In general, oral regimens are recommended for early localized disease. Most patients recover completely. In most cases, recovery is quicker and the sooner the treatment begins recovery is better. Treatment may be longer depending on the symptoms present.

The tick should be removed using tweezers or fine-pointed forceps. Grasp it as closely as possible to where it is attached to the skin and pull it gently upwards as a whole and not breaking it in parts. The risk of LB infection is not increased if the mouth parts are left behind. After removing the ticks, apply skin disinfectant to prevent infection.

Prevention

Prevention is an important part of management. Recommended measures for protection include wearing light-colored protective clothing with long sleeves, and long trousers tucked into socks or boots using tick repellents.

The best ways to avoid tick bites are to avoid tick-risk areas. One should also be informed about how to remove ticks and recognize early symptoms.

VIOLENCE, ABUSE, SEXUAL ASSAULT

Violence: Violence is a behavior that involves physical force with the intention of harming or killing someone. It is an aggressive behavior that is destructive in nature. Treating a person with cruelty or violence is called abuse. There are various forms of violence and abuse; domestic violence, physical abuse, emotional abuse, etc.

Sexual assault: It involves any sexual behavior that makes a person feel traumatized, uncomfortable, frightened, or threatened is termed sexual assault. It is a sexual activity to which a person does not consent. It can be verbal, visual, audio, or any other form which forces a person to participate in unwanted sexual contact or attention. It ranges from inappropriate touching to penetration or intercourse. Any forms of sexual contact are crimes.

Dealing with patients who have been subjected to sexual violence thus demands a broad range of skills. Essential skills needed are good communication skills, basic knowledge of the dynamics of sexual violence, information regarding legal issues related to sexual crimes, an understanding of relevant cultural and/or religious issues, empathy, and sensitivity.

Thus, a nurse working in the emergency unit has the opportunity to be trained as a sexual assault nurse examiner (SANE). This requires special training in forensic evidence collection, history taking, documentation, and ways to approach the patient and the family. Rape victims need an unusual degree of professional reassurance, acceptance, and understanding in regard to the therapeutic examination.

ASSESSMENT AND DIAGNOSTIC FINDINGS

The patient's reaction to rape is termed rape trauma syndrome. It is observed as an acute stress reaction and this is a life-threatening situation. Nurses dealing with such victims must be aware that the patient may go through several psychological reactions.

- ❖ **Phase of acute disorganization:** The victim may encounter shock, disbelief, fear, guilt, humiliation, anger, and other emotions. In some cases, the feelings may be hidden and the victim appears composed.
- ❖ **Phase of denial:** May be observed when the victim is unwilling to talk about the incident followed by a phase of intense anxiety and fear, hyper-alertness, sleep disturbances, and psychological reaction like loss of self-esteem.

❖ **Phase of reorganization:** The incident is put into perspective. Some may recover fully or some never fully recover and develop chronic stress disorder and phobias like post-traumatic stress disorder (PTSD).

MANAGEMENT OF PATIENTS WITH SEXUAL ASSAULT

The aim of management is directed towards reassurance and encouraging the victim to develop a sense of control over his/her own life. Privacy and sensitivity of the client to be respected. Patients should be dealt with, with the utmost care. The victim should not be left alone and assess the need for a support person.

Physical examination: An informed written consent needs to be obtained for physical examination. The victim should be undressed and draped properly. History of the incident obtained should be recorded in the victim's own words and thorough examination of head to toe for any injury should be done. Several laboratory specimens are collected during the physical examination. Each specimen is labeled with the victim's name, date and time of specimen collection, the body area from which the specimens are obtained, and the name of the person collecting the specimen. The specimens are then given to the designated laboratory and an itemized receipt is obtained.

The potential consequences of sexual assault should be dealt with, with the utmost care. Once the initial physical examination and management of associated physical injuries are treated and if the victim is a female of childbearing age antipregnancy measures need to be considered; a cleansing douche is given. Mouthwash and fresh clothing are offered. The client should not be left in isolation.

There may be physical, emotional, and psychological effects of the event on the victim. The person may experience pain, injury, nausea, vomiting, and headache. Victims may be impacted emotionally. The victim may experience shock, denial, irritability, anger, depression, social withdrawal, apathy, reduced ability to express emotions, nightmares, etc., There may be flashbacks of the event that may give rise to loss of self-esteem, the feeling of insecurity and lack of confidence, loss of trust in others, feeling of guilt, shame embarrassment, impaired memory and concentration, loss of appetite, suicidal ideation, substance abuse, and psychological disorders, etc. There may be hypervigilance, insomnia, self-mutilation, harming others panic attacks, etc.

It is important to counsel the family members along with the victim to help them prevent long-term psychological effects.

The victim needs to be encouraged to return to the previous level of functioning as early as possible.

PREVENTING SEXUAL ASSAULT

❖ At all times care should be taken to identify people and situations that may lead to sexual assault.
❖ Chances of being a victim can be lowered by training in self-defense and using common sense to choose people while being associated with them.
❖ Potentially dangerous situations while outside or at home can be avoided.
❖ One should be careful interacting with strangers and be sensible. It is advisable to avoid intimate or solo contact with unknown people. One should be vigilant in social events about food and drinks that are offered when that person is not in a protected environment.

GERIATRIC CONSIDERATIONS

Older adults have unique risks and their needs must be addressed carefully at the emergency department (ED). Older patients are at increased risk for a number of specific events. Often, they have impaired hearing and vision that limit their awareness regarding the place and poor adaptation to an unfamiliar environment. Many of them suffer from confusion, delirium, and poor balance that increase the risk of injuries in the typically designed healthcare facility. The geriatric-specific consideration should include adequate physical treatment space including material and space design. Assessment and evaluation of individual patients should include geriatric-specific protocol including comprehensive screening for ischemia and sepsis. Additional resources needed for managing older adults include decision support for medical care, complex pharmacy medication management, and social resources.

The physical parameters of a geriatric ED should focus on structural modifications that promote safety, comfort, mobility, memory cues, and sensorial perception. It should be an elderly-friendly setting. In fact, it will be better to have a separate emergency department for elderly patients. There should be proper lighting and enhanced signage. The method of transportation and need for transportation of older clients need to be reviewed for consideration for fall reduction. There should be availability of adequate staff to assist the older patients and low-risk transport methods within the treatment setting such as wheelchairs, carts, and gurneys (wheeled stretchers) should be readily available. Transportation of older adults can be minimized by the use of bedside radiography and portable laboratory assessment, which can avoid transfer injuries.

Case Scenario

1. Robin, a 45-year-old was brought to the emergency department in an unconscious state. He was found in an enclosed room with burning chula as the temperature outside was very cold. The duration of his exposure was unknown.

   On arrival in the emergency room, his heart rate was 126 beats per minute and his BP was 78/56 mm Hg. Initial ABG analysis revealed that pH = 7.32, PCO_2 = 33 mm Hg, PO_2 = 380 mm Hg, bicarbonate = 16 mEq/L, and a carboxyhemoglobin level of 24.0%. Sodium = 136 mEq/L, potassium 4.5 mEq/L, and calcium = 7.8 mg/dL. 12-lead ECG, chest X-ray, and CT brain were found to be normal.

   He was placed in a railed bed, in Fowler's position. Immediately he was administered 100% oxygen through a nonrebreather mask, and vital parameters were monitored frequently to assess the need for intubation. Hypotension was treated with IV fluids and parenteral norepinephrine. With initial management, his blood pressure recovered. His carboxyhemoglobin decreased to 1.3% after 5 hours of 100% oxygen administration. A repeated neurological assessment was done. He was warned of possible delayed neurological complications and advised follow-up of repeat medical and neurological examination in 2 weeks.

2. A 39-year-old construction worker, Chunilal, was brought to the emergency department in a hospital ambulance with a history of fall from a height of the 2nd floor at the site. Transportation from the accident site was delayed by 45 minutes. He has a penetrating chest wound by iron rods and a head injury. Assessment done en-route revealed that the patient was unconscious, rapid and feeble pulse and labored breath, and the wound site was stabilized and covered with a bulky dressing available at the site. He was log-rolled while transferring from trolly to bed anticipating a cervical fracture. Upon admission secondary assessment was performed, scalp wound was assessed, blood pressure 92/60 mm Hg, SPO_2 96%, cool and pale skin, bruise on face, bruise around the eyes and back, bleeding from the back side of the head. There was asymmetric chest movement and the airway was maintained with high-flow oxygen with a nonrebreather mask, IV line was accessed, and a blood sample was taken for baseline investigations. Indwelling urinary catheterization was done and 450 mL of urine was drained. Chest X-ray revealed a fracture at the 6th and 7th rib. Meanwhile, history was obtained from the eyewitness present at the site. The Glasgow coma scale was 8/15. He was reviewed by the emergency team and prepared for surgery as advised by the surgical team. Postoperative management was uneventful.

Critical thinking questions:
1. What other interventions are to be considered by the nurse?
2. Several family members of Chunilal including his wife are present in the emergency department. How will the nurse on duty approach the family members?
3. Based on the data presented write the nursing diagnosis.

SUMMARY

The emergency department is the first point of contact for critically sick patients requiring prompt management to save their lives and to avoid any long-term disability. It is a crossroad between in-patient and outpatient care. The emergency departments are managed by qualified healthcare professionals. Emergency nursing is an upcoming specialty in the field of nursing but is still at the infancy stage in India. There are numerous emergencies including trauma and medical emergencies which are managed by these professionals. While working in an emergency, apart from handling the emergencies very promptly and skilfully, they should ensure their own as well as the safety of others. A significant number of elderly people also attend the emergency department. With age, they become more susceptible to disease and disability. They have limited regenerative abilities and are more prone to multifaceted diseases and their complications than the younger adults. So, the emergency departments should be elderly friendly in order to prevent any further complications to this vulnerable group.

MULTIPLE CHOICE QUESTIONS

1. How much time should the medical responder spend on triaging each patient?
   a. Less than 1 minute
   b. Less than 2 minutes
   c. Less than 5 minutes
   d. Less than 10 seconds
2. A 33-years-old Mr Ratan was brought to the emergency department who suffered multiple injuries from a head-on collision car accident. Which of the following assessment should take the highest priority to take?
   a. Unequal pupil
   b. Irregular pulse rate
   c. Ecchymosis at the flank area
   d. Deviated trachea
3. The emergency medical service has transported a client with severe chest pain. As the client is being transferred to the emergency stretcher, the patient looked unresponsive, with cessation of breathing, and an unpalpable pulse. Which of the following task is appropriate to delegate to the nursing assistant?
   a. Assisting with the intubation
   b. Placing the defibrillator pads
   c. Doing chest compressions
   d. Initiating bag-valve-mask ventilation
4. Which of the following action to be carried out for a severe allergic reaction to an insect bite?
   a. Remove the sting
   b. Administer injection epinephrine
   c. Referring to immunologist
   d. Start IV line
5. What is the correct technical name of allergic reaction:
   a. Bronchospasm
   b. Urticaria
   c. Hypotension
   d. Anaphylaxis
6. On receiving a case of snakebite in the emergency unit which care is given to the client?
   a. Give the client an alcoholic drink
   b. Apply ice compression
   c. Start IV crystalloids using a thick bore needle
   d. Offer a cup of coffee
7. Decompression sickness is a diving-related disorder. Nitrogen dissolved in the blood and tissues by high pressure causes the formation of bubbles as pressure decreases. Which of the following tissues or organs is most likely to be affected?
   a. Brain and spinal cord
   b. GI tract
   c. Heart and lung
   d. Liver
8. While working in the emergency room you receive a patient with the complaints of midsternal chest pain and profuse sweating. Which of the following nursing action should get priority?
   a. Administer oxygen therapy via nasal cannula
   b. Put the patient on an ECG monitor
   c. Collect history
   d. Start an IV line
9. A client has been transferred to your emergency unit with complaints of severe chest pain. While transferring the client to the stretcher you noted that the patient is unresponsive, also there is a cessation of breathing and absence of a pulse. Which of the following task is most appropriate?
   a. Initiate bag mask valve ventilation
   b. Start CPR
   c. Assist for intubation
   d. Place defibrillator pads
10. In carbon monoxide (CO) poisoning carboxyhemoglobin level increases. Which of the following symptoms occur when carboxyhemoglobin level is 10–20%?
    a. Difficulty in concentrating
    b. Headache
    c. Loss of consciousness
    d. Impaired judgement cervical cord

ANSWERS

1. a	2. d	3. c	4. b
5. d	6. c	7. a	8. a
9. b	10. b		

SUGGESTED READING

1. Aggarwal A, Kaur S, Dhillon MS. Socio-demographic profile of road traffic accident victims admitted at emergency surgical OPD of a tertiary care hospital. Journal of Postgraduate Medicine, Education, and Research. 2012;46(1):15-8.
2. Bhagoria E, Kaur S, Singh A, et al. Making the Emergency OPD of a Tertiary Care Center Elderly Friendly Through Quality Assurance of Geriatric Syndrome Management Strategies. J Postgrad Med Edu Res. 2021;55(3):114-8.

3. Bhagoria E, Kaur S, Singh A, et al. The pattern of health problems amongst the elderly patients admitted in the emergency department of tertiary care hospital of North India. NMRJ. 2020;16(4):165-72. http://doi.org/10.33698/NRF0324
4. Black JM, Hawks JH. Black's Medical-Surgical Nursing: Clinical Management for Positive Outcomes, Vol II, 1st edition, Elsevier, chapter 57 & 64, page 1675.
5. Burton JH, Young J, Carol, Bernier CA. The Geriatric ED: Structure, Patient Care, and Considerations for the Emergency Department Geriatric Unit; International Journal of Gerontology. 2014;8:56-9.
6. Chemical burns: Causes, symptoms, treatment, prevention, care. Available from: https://www.webmd.com/first-aid/chemical-burns
7. Chintamani. Lewis's Medical Surgical Nursing Assessment and Management of clinical problems. Elsevier, chapter 30, section 8.
8. Cline DM, Ma O, Cydulka RK, Meckler GD, Handel DA, Thomas SH (Eds). Tintinalli's Emergency Medicine Manual, 7th edition. McGraw Hill; 2012. https://accessemergencymedicine.mhmedical.com/content.aspx?bookid=521&sectionid=41068918
9. Deshmukh CD, Pawar A. General Principles, Types, Diagnosis and Management of Poisoning; 2020. DOI: 10.36347/sajp.2020.v09i05.001
10. Emergency unit—guideline section—Indian Health facility guidelines. Available from https://india.healthfacilityguidelines.com/Guidelines/ViewPDF/HFG-India/part_b_emergency_unit,
11. Ertel WK, Kellam JF. General assessment and management of the polytrauma patient. DOI: 10.1055/b-0035-121623. https://musculoskeletalkey.com/1-4-general-assessment-and-management-of-the-polytrauma-patient/
12. Geriatric Emergency Department Guidelines. American College of Emergency Physicians. https://www.acep.org/globalassets/uploads/uploaded-files/acep/clinical-and-practice-anagement/resources/geriatrics/geri_ed_guidelines_final.pdf
13. Harding M, Kwong J, Roberts D, Hagler D, Reinisch C. Lewis's Medical-Surgical Nursing—Assessment and management of clinical problems, 11th edition. Elsevier, St. Louis, Missouri; 2020.
14. Harvard Health Publishing. Harvard medical school. Decompression sickness: what is it? https://www.health.harvard.edu/a_to_z/decompression-sickness-a-to-z
15. Hinkle JL, Cheever KH, Brunner and Siddharth's Textbook of Medical Surgical Nursing. SAE, 13th edition. New Delhi, Philadelphia, Baltimore, New York, Walter Kluwer. 2014;2:2128-9.
16. http://www.who.int/health-topics
17. https://www.ncbi.nlm.nih.gov/books/NBK518972/
18. https://www.pib.gov.in/PressReleasePage.aspx?PRID=1887097
19. https://www.who.int/news-room/fact-sheets/detail/road-traffic-injuries
20. Hurt JB, Maday KR. Management and treatment of animal bites. JAAPA. 2018;31(4):27-31. DOI: http://10.1097/01.JAA.0000531049.59137.cd PMID: 30973531.
21. Kaur J, Bhalla A, Gnanapandithan K, Kaur S. Does an Educational Program for Patient Bystanders Reduce the Incidence and Complications of Bedsores in the Medical Emergency? A Quasi Experimental Study. J Adv Res Nurs Sci. 2014;1(1):1-6.
22. Kaur M, Kaur S, Bhalla A. Knowledge regarding Cardiopulmonary Resuscitation among the Nursing Personnel Working in Emergency Department of a Tertiary Care Hospital. Journal of Nursing Science and Practice. 2012;2(2):37-41.
23. Kilner E, Sheppard LA. The role of teamwork and communication in the emergency department: a systematic review. Int Emerg Nurs. 2010;18(3):127-37. DOI: 10.1016/j.ienj.2009.05.006. Epub 2009 Jul 9. PMID: 20542238.
24. Kinoshita H, Türkan H, Vucinic S, Naqvi S, Bedair R, Rezaee R et al. Carbon monoxide poisoning. Toxicology report. 2020;7:169-73. https://doi.org/10.1016/j.toxrep.2020.01.005
25. Kumari MJ. Adult Health Nursing II, Medical Surgical Nursing. Jaypee Brother's Medical Publishers. Health Sciences Publishers, New Delhi; 2022.
26. Liu CC, Landeck L, Zheng M. Tick bite. Indian J Dermatol Venereol Leprol. 2014;80(3):269-70. DOI: http://10.4103/0378-6323.132265 PMID: 24823415.
27. Loewenherz JW. Pathophysiology and treatment of decompression sickness and gas embolism. J Fla Med Assoc. 1992;79(9):620-4. PMID: 1431793. https://pubmed.ncbi.nlm.nih.gov/1431793/
28. Lyme Borreliosis in Europe. Available from: https://www.euro.who.int/__data/assets/pdf_file/0008/246167/Fact-sheet-Lyme-borreliosis-Eng.pdf
29. Mahure D. Medicolegal issues in the emergency department. Available from: https://www.docplexus.com/posts/medicolegalissuesintheemergencydepartment
30. Manuel J, Raman M, Keith R. A tiny tick can cause a big health problem. Indian Journal of Ophthalmology. 2017;65(11):1228-32. DOI: 10.4103/ijo.IJO_411_17
31. Mohanan K, Kaur S, Das K, Bhalla A. Patient satisfaction regarding nursing care at emergency outpatient department in a tertiary care hospital. Journal of Mental Health and Human Behaviour. 2010;15(1):54-8.
32. Moon RE. Decompression sickness (Caison disease, the bends). Duke Univ Med Centre. Last review/revision Jun 2021 | Modified Sep 2022. Available from: https://www.msdmanuals.com/en-in/home/injuries-and-poisoning/diving-and-compressed-air-injuries/recompression-therapy
33. Negi T, Kandari LS, Arunachalam K. Update on prevalence and distribution pattern of tick-borne diseases among humans in India: a review. Parasitol Res. 2021;120(5):1523-39. DOI: http://10.1007/s00436-021-07114-x. Epub 2021 Apr 2. PMID: 33797610.
34. NursingAnswers.net. (November 2018). Emergency Triage and Rapid Assessment. Retrieved from https://nursinganswers.net/lectures/nursing/emergency-care/2-detailed.php?vref=1.
35. Nuttall PA. Tick saliva and its role in pathogen transmission. Received: 22 February 2019/Accepted: 9 April 2019 © The Author(s) 2019. https://doi.org/10.1007/s00508-019-1500-y
36. Payal P, Sonu G, Anil GK, Prachi V. Management of polytrauma patients in the emergency department: An experience of a tertiary care health institution of northern India. World J Emerg Med. 2013;4(1):15-9. DOI: 10.5847/wjem.j.issn.1920-8642.2013.01.003. PMID: 25215087; PMCID: PMC4129897.
37. Prasan H, Singh K. Management of Cold Injuries. Surgical Research Updates. 2013;1:20-5. DOI: 10.12970/2311-9888.2014.01.01.4
38. Rabies in India available from: https://www.who.int/india/health-topics/rabies
39. Sharma D, Kaur M, Chaudhary R, Kaur S, Agnihotri M, Bhalla A. Admission of Elderly in Emergency Units: Causes and Problems. Adv Practice Nurs. 2016;2(3). http://dx.doi.org/10.4172/apn.1000119.
40. Sharma S, Gupta R, Paul BS, Puri S, Garg S. Accidental carbon monoxide poisoning in our homes; Indian J Crit Care Med. 2009;13(3):169-70. DOI: 10.4103/0972-5229.58546.PMCID: PMC2823102.
41. Singh S, Singh G. Snake bite: Indian guidelines and protocols. Ch 94:424-6. Available from:https://www.sctimst.ac.in/Post-flood-Management/General-Health-Care/snake-insects/snake_bit_India.pdf
42. Sumbria T, Sharma A, Shina P, Kosey S, Devgan S. Introduction to Poisoning—A Systematic Review. International Journal of Pharmacy Teaching and Practices. 2015;6(4):2615-9.
43. Thim T, Krarup NH, Grove EL, Rohde CV, Løfgren B. Initial assessment and treatment with the Airway, Breathing, Circulation, Disability, Exposure (ABCDE) approach. Int J Gen Med. 2012;5:117-21. DOI: 10.2147/IJGM.S28478. Epub 2012 Jan 31. PMID: 22319249; PMCID: PMC3273374.
44. Thomas K. Medical surgical Nursing-Vol II, Emergency Management; 1st edition. Jaypee Brothers Medical Publishers, New Delhi. 2018;23:787-807.
45. Wm M, Kamrun J, David A. Cold Injury. Hand Clinics. 2009;25:481-96. http://dx.doi.org/10.1016/j.hcl.2009.06.004

CHAPTER 45

Disaster Management: Nursing Perspective

T Samuel Ravi Kumar

"We cannot stop natural disasters but we can arm ourselves with knowledge: so many lives wouldn't have to be lost if there was enough disaster preparedness."

—**Petra Nemcova**

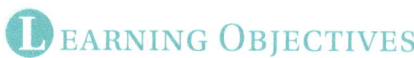 LEARNING OBJECTIVES

After going through the chapter, the learner will be able to:
- Define and classify disaster.
- Describe the disaster management cycle.
- Differentiate natural and manmade disaster.
- Describe the disaster management response both at the community and at the hospital level.
- Describe the role of nurses in disaster management.
- Identify a few areas of research in disaster management.

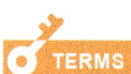 **TERMS**

- **Acceptable risk:** The level of potential losses that a society or community considers acceptable given existing social, economic, political, cultural, technical, and environmental conditions.
- **Capacity:** The combination of all the strengths, attributes, and resources available within a community, society, or organization that can be used to achieve agreed goals.
- **Critical facilities:** The primary physical structures, technical facilities, and systems that are socially, economically, or operationally essential to the functioning of a society or community, both in routine circumstances and in the extreme circumstances of an emergency.
- **Mitigation:** The lessening of the adverse impacts of disaster related hazards.
- **Multi-hazard early warning systems:** These address several hazards and/or impacts of similar or different types in contexts where hazardous events may occur alone, simultaneously, cascading, or cumulatively over time, and taking into account the potential interrelated effects.
- **Hazard:** It is a physical or human-made event that can potentially trigger a disaster. A process, phenomenon, or human activity that may cause loss of life, injury or other health impacts, property damage, social and economic disruption, or environmental degradation.
  - *Biological hazards* are of organic origin or conveyed by biological vectors, including pathogenic microorganisms, toxins, and bioactive substances.
  - *Environmental hazards* may include chemical, natural, and biological hazards.
  - *Geological or geophysical hazards* originate from internal earth processes.
  - *Hydrometeorological* factors are important contributors to some of these processes. Tsunamis are difficult to categorize: although they are triggered by undersea earthquakes and other geological events, they essentially become an oceanic process that is manifested as a coastal water-related hazard.
  - *Technological hazards* originate from technological or industrial conditions, dangerous procedures, infrastructure failures, or specific human activities.
- **Preparedness plan** establishes arrangements in advance to enable timely, effective, and appropriate responses to specific potential hazardous events or emerging disaster situations that might threaten society or the environment.

- **Prevention:** Measures taken to avert a disaster from occurring, if possible (to impede a hazard so that it does not have any harmful effects).
- **Risk:** It is the probability of an event happening and its impact.
- **Response:** Actions taken directly before, during, or immediately after a disaster in order to save lives, reduce health impacts, ensure public safety and meet the basic subsistence needs of the people affected.
- **Relief:** Measures that are taken for search and rescue of survivors, as well to meet the basic needs for shelter, water, food and health care.
- **Rehabilitation:** Actions taken in the aftermath of a disaster to:
  - Assist victims to repair their dwellings
  - Re-establish essential services
  - Revive key economic and social activities
- **Reconstruction:** Permanent measures to repair or replace damaged dwellings and infrastructure and to set the economy back on course.
- **Sustainable development:** Development that meets the needs of the present without compromising the ability of future generations to meet their own needs.
- **Vulnerability:** It is the susceptibility to harm of those at risk. It is also the conditions determined by physical, social, economic, and environmental factors or processes which increase the susceptibility of an individual, a community, assets, or systems to the impacts of hazards.

INTRODUCTION

Since the 2004 Tsunami, Disaster is a term that is well known by the public. The focus on Disaster Risk Reduction has increased at a larger scale. The ongoing pandemic has created much more awareness and impact on disaster management. The healthcare team, especially the nursing population has a crucial role in the prevention, mitigation, and management of disaster. Disasters can have both immediate and long-term impacts on individuals, communities, and even entire regions. They can lead to displacement, disruption of social and economic systems, and can cause physical and psychological trauma. Effective disaster management, which involves preparedness, response, recovery, and mitigation efforts, can help minimize the impact of disasters and facilitate a faster return to normalcy. The examples of some of the disaster include Atom Bombing of Hiroshima and Nagasaki, 1947; Bhopal Gas Tragedy 1988; Odisha cyclone 1999; Kargil War 1999; World trade center attack September 2001; Gujarat earthquake on 26th January 2001; Mumbai floods 2005; Mumbai attack 2008, etc.

The current chapter gives detailed content regarding disaster management including the personal experiences of the author for better understanding and application. All the references are from National and International Disaster Management Agencies which permit sharing of the content for the safe living and environment of the globe.

DISASTER

The term "DISASTER" owes its origin to the French word "Disastre", a combination of two words "Des" meaning "Bad" and "Aster" meaning "Star", thus the term Disaster refers to "Bad or Evil Star". A disaster is there when need gets exceeded than the availability of resources. It has been variedly defined. The World Health Organization (WHO) defines a disaster as "a sudden ecological phenomenon of sufficient magnitude to require external assistance". It is also defined as any event, typically occurring suddenly, that causes damage, ecological disruption, loss of human life, deterioration of health and health services, and which exceeds the capacity of the affected community on a scale sufficient to require outside assistance (Landsman, 2001). As per The International Federation of Red Cross and Red Crescent Societies (IFRC), "Disasters are serious disruptions to the functioning of a community that exceeds its capacity to cope using its own resources. Disasters can be caused by natural, man-made, and technological hazards, as well as various factors that influence the exposure and vulnerability of a community." According to UN Disaster Risk Reduction, disaster is "A serious disruption of the functioning of a community or a society at any scale due to hazardous events interacting with conditions of exposure, vulnerability, and capacity, leading to one or more of the following—human, material, economic and environmental losses and impacts." Alphabetically the word 'DISASTER' means

- ❖ **D**—Damage/Destruction
- ❖ **I**—Incidents
- ❖ **S**—Sufferings
- ❖ **A**—Administrative
- ❖ **S**—Sentiments
- ❖ **T**—Trauma/Tragedies
- ❖ **E**—Eruption of diseases
- ❖ **R**—Research program and its implementation

CHARACTERISTICS OF DISASTER

- ❖ **Predictability:** It means ascertaining the occurrence of a disaster. Sometimes it may be, and sometimes it may not be. Earthquakes have no pre-warning time whereas a cyclone warning system can prepare for forthcoming floods or cyclone related effects.
- ❖ **Controllability:** As in cyclone the people can be evacuated on time to reduce the effects.
- ❖ **Speed of onset:** Earthquakes, volcanoes, and mass casualty incidents, such as mass transit events have no predictable time factor.
- ❖ **Length of forewarning:** Timely warning can help in preparation for the disaster at the administrative as well as at an individual level.

- **Duration of impact:** The impact of an earthquake can have an impact for a long period of time requiring response, rehabilitation, and reconstruction.
- **Scope and intensity of impact:** Higher the impact, more will be the destruction.

CLASSIFICATION OF DISASTER

The disaster was earlier classified as natural and man made, whereas research has significantly changed the approach in classification as follows. Centre for Research on the Epidemiology of Disasters (CRED) and EM-DAT (Emergency Events Database) distinguishes between two generic categories for disasters—natural and technological. The natural disaster category is divided into 5 sub-groups, which in turn cover 15 disaster types and more than 30 sub-types. The technological disaster category is divided into 3 sub-groups which in turn cover 15 disaster types **(Table 45.1)**.

- **Natural disasters:** These are disasters caused by natural phenomena, such as earthquakes, hurricanes, floods, wildfires, landslides, and volcanic eruptions. Natural disasters are often unpredictable, and their impact can be devastating, resulting in loss of life, property, and infrastructure.
- **Technological disasters:** These are disasters caused by technological failures, such as nuclear accidents, chemical spills, and other man-made catastrophes. Technological disasters can have severe and long-lasting impacts on the environment and human health.
- **Human-made disasters:** These are disasters caused by human-made events, such as terrorist attacks, wars, and civil unrest. Human-made disasters can result in loss of life, property, and infrastructure and can have long-term social and economic consequences.
- **Health emergencies:** These are disasters caused by health emergencies, such as pandemics, epidemics, and outbreaks of infectious diseases. Health emergencies can have severe impacts on human health, and their control often requires significant resources and coordinated efforts.
- **Environmental disasters:** These are disasters caused by environmental factors, such as climate change, deforestation, and pollution. Environmental disasters can have long-lasting impacts on ecosystems, and their mitigation often requires significant changes in policies and human behavior.
  - *Hurricanes:* Hurricanes are severe tropical storms that can cause significant damage to infrastructure, property, and the environment. They are caused by warm ocean waters, high humidity, and low-pressure systems. The effects of hurricanes can include strong winds, heavy rainfall, storm surges, and flooding, which can lead to extensive property damage, loss of life, and disruptions to essential services.
  - *Tornadoes:* Tornadoes are violent windstorms that can cause significant damage to infrastructure and property. They are caused by the collision of warm and cold air masses, which creates rotating winds. The effects of tornadoes can include strong winds, hail, and flying debris, which can cause significant property damage, loss of life, and injuries.
  - *Earthquakes:* Earthquakes are sudden and violent shaking of the ground caused by tectonic plate movements. The effects of earthquakes can include building collapses, landslides, tsunamis, and disruptions to essential services. They can cause significant damage to infrastructure, property, and loss of life.

TABLE 45.1: Classification of disaster.

Disaster group	Disaster subgroup	Definition	Disaster main type
Natural	Geophysical	A hazard originating from solid earth. This term is used interchangeably with the term "geological hazard"	Earthquake, mass movement, volcanic activity
	Meteorological	A hazard caused by short-lived, micro- to meso-scale extreme weather and atmospheric conditions that last from minutes to days	Extreme temperature, fog, storm
	Hydrological	A hazard caused by the occurrence, movement, and distribution of surface and subsurface freshwater and saltwater	Flood, landslide, wave action
	Extraterrestrial	A hazard caused by asteroids, meteoroids, and comets as they pass near earth, enter the Earth's atmosphere, and/or strike the earth, and by changes in interplanetary conditions that affect the earth's magnetosphere, ionosphere, and thermosphere	Impact, space weather
Technological	Industrial accident	—	Chemical spill, collapse, explosion, fire, gas leak, poisoning, radiation
	Transport accident	—	Air, road, rail, water
	Miscellaneous accident	—	Collapse, explosion, fire

- *Volcanic eruptions:* Volcanic eruptions occur when molten rock, ash, and gas are expelled from a volcano. The effects of volcanic eruptions can include ash clouds, pyroclastic flows, lava flows, and landslides, which can cause significant damage to infrastructure, property, and the environment.
- *Floods:* Floods are caused by excessive rainfall, storm surges, or the overflow of bodies of water, such as rivers and lakes. The effects of floods can include property damage, infrastructure damage, loss of life, and disruptions to essential services, such as power and water supply.
- *Wildfires:* Wildfires are uncontrolled fires that can spread rapidly through forests, grasslands, and other vegetation. They are often caused by human activities, such as campfires, cigarettes, or deliberate arson, as well as by natural causes, such as lightning strikes. The effects of wildfires can include property damage, loss of life, and disruptions to essential services, such as power and water supply.

In summary, natural disasters can have severe impacts on infrastructure, property, the environment, and human life. Hurricanes, tornadoes, earthquakes, volcanic eruptions, floods, and wildfires are some examples of natural disasters, each with its own causes and effects. Effective disaster management, which involves preparedness, response, recovery, and mitigation efforts, is crucial in minimizing the impact of natural disasters and facilitating a faster return to normalcy.

❖ **Technological disasters:** Technological disasters are man-made incidents that can cause significant harm to the environment, infrastructure, and human life. Here are some examples of technological disasters:
  - *Nuclear accidents:* Nuclear accidents occur when nuclear reactors or weapons malfunction, resulting in radiation exposure. The effects of nuclear accidents can include radiation sickness, long-term health problems, environmental contamination, and forced evacuation of affected areas.
  - *Chemical spills:* Chemical spills can occur during transportation or storage of hazardous materials, such as oil, gas, or toxic chemicals. The effects of chemical spills can include environmental contamination, health problems, and property damage.
  - *Industrial accidents:* Industrial accidents can occur in factories, mines, or other industrial settings, resulting in explosions, fires, or chemical releases. The effects of industrial accidents can include property damage, environmental contamination, and loss of life.
  - *Cyber security breaches:* Cyber security breaches can occur when hackers gain access to sensitive information, such as personal data or financial information. The effects of cyber security breaches can include financial losses, identity theft, and damage to reputation.
  - *Transportation accidents:* Transportation accidents can occur during the transport of goods or people, such as plane crashes, train derailments, or shipwrecks. The effects of transportation accidents can include property damage, environmental contamination, and loss of life.
  - *Infrastructure failures:* Infrastructure failures can occur due to ageing or inadequate infrastructure, such as collapsing bridges, dams, or power grids. The effects of infrastructure failures can include property damage, power outages, and disruptions to essential services.

In summary, technological disasters are man-made incidents that can have severe impacts on infrastructure, property, the environment, and human life. Nuclear accidents, chemical spills, industrial accidents, cyber security breaches, transportation accidents, and infrastructure failures are some examples of technological disasters. Effective disaster management, which involves preparedness, response, recovery, and mitigation efforts, is crucial in minimizing the impact of technological disasters and facilitating a faster return to normalcy.

DISASTER PREPAREDNESS

Disaster preparedness is crucial in reducing the impact of disasters and saving lives. It involves taking proactive measures to minimize the impact of disasters through planning, early warning systems, and emergency response procedures. The following are some of the reasons why disaster preparedness is essential:

❖ **Saves lives:** Effective disaster preparedness can save lives by ensuring that emergency services, first responders, and evacuation procedures are in place and ready to act in the event of a disaster.

❖ **Minimizes damage:** Disaster preparedness measures can help minimize the impact of disasters on infrastructure, property, and the environment. For example, building codes and zoning regulations can help prevent buildings from collapsing during an earthquake, and flood control measures can prevent flood damage.

❖ **Reduces economic losses:** Disasters can have significant economic consequences, including the loss of jobs and the cost of rebuilding. Disaster preparedness measures can help minimize economic losses by ensuring that essential services remain operational during and after a disaster.

❖ **Increases community resilience:** Disaster preparedness can help build community resilience by ensuring that community members are informed and prepared for potential disasters. This can include educating community members about emergency procedures, providing emergency supplies, and conducting training exercises.

❖ **Provides early warning:** Early warning systems can provide advance notice of impending disasters, allowing people to evacuate or take other necessary precautions. This can be critical in minimizing the impact of disasters and saving lives.

❖ **Facilitates effective emergency response:** Disaster preparedness measures can help emergency responders and other first responders quickly and effectively respond to disasters. This can include ensuring that emergency equipment and supplies are available and that emergency services are coordinated.

In summary, disaster preparedness is essential in reducing the impact of disasters and saving lives. It involves planning, early warning systems, and emergency response procedures that can help minimize damage, reduce economic losses, increase community resilience, provide early warning, and facilitate effective emergency response.

DISASTER MANAGEMENT CYCLE

Earlier the focus of disaster management (DM) was on post relief and rehabilitation measures. However as per sec. 2(e) of DM Act 2005, disaster management is the coordination and integrated process of planning, coordinating and implementing measures which are necessary for prevention of danger or threat of any disaster; mitigation or reduction of risk of any disaster or its severity or its consequences; capacity building and preparedness to deal with any disaster; prompt response to any threatening disaster situation; assessing the severity or magnitude of effects of any disaster; evacuation, rescue and relief; and lastly rehabilitation and reconstruction.

Various principles of disaster management involve:
- DM is the responsibility of all spheres of government
- DM should use resources that exist for a day-to-day purpose.
- Organizations should function as an extension of their core business;
- Individuals are responsible for their own safety.
- DM planning should focus on large-scale events.
- DM planning should recognize the difference between incidents and disasters.
- DM planning must take account of the type of physical environment and the structure of the population.
- DM arrangements must recognize the involvement and potential role of non-government agencies.

The disaster cycle is a framework used to describe the various stages that a disaster typically goes through, from its initial occurrence to its eventual resolution. The cycle is generally divided into four main phases—preparedness, response, recovery, and mitigation. Disaster cycle has been given in various phases; the commonly used method is the four phases. It is important to note that the disaster cycle is not always linear, and different disasters may require different approaches to each phase. Additionally, each phase may occur concurrently or overlap with others. Some do 8 phases for a simpler manner to understand the role and response **(Figs. 45.1A and B)**.

1. **Preparedness:** It involves measures taken in anticipation of a disaster to ensure that appropriate and effective actions are taken in the aftermath. It includes risk assessments, planning, and training exercises to ensure that emergency responders and community members are ready to take action if a disaster strikes. It also involves preparation with respect to money, manpower and materials. It may also be based on the evaluation from the past experiences about disaster, location of disaster-prone areas, organization of communication, information and warning system, ensuring coordination and response mechanism, development of public education program, coordination with media, keeping stock of foods, drugs and other essential commodities. In fact, it is important to invest in preparedness and prevention of disaster in order to produce sustainable results, rather than spending money on relief after a disaster. Many disasters may be predictable, especially in their seasonality and the disaster-prone areas which are vulnerable. The community people should be involved in disaster preparedness for better outcome during disaster. International Day for Disaster Reduction is observed on 13th October every year. Special programs are organized in various universities and other public places regarding prevention and management of disaster.

2. **Response:** This phase begins when a disaster occurs and focuses on immediate actions to protect people and property. It includes mobilization of the necessary emergency services in order to save life, decreasing suffering, and limiting damage as far as possible. Response activities may include search and rescue efforts (SAR), medical care, and providing emergency shelter and supplies. It also involves actions taken immediately following the impact of a disaster when exceptional measures are required to meet the basic needs of the survivors.

3. **Recovery:** This phase involves the process of returning to normalcy after a disaster. So, it is the process undertaken by a disaster affected community to fully restore itself to pre-disaster level of functioning. Recovery efforts may include restoring essential services, such as water and electricity, repairing damaged infrastructure, and providing support to affected individuals and families. It also involves referring the people to mental health professionals, and helping the rehabilitation of the special group of people, such as elderly people, especially abled people, children and women.

4. **Mitigation:** This phase focuses on reducing the impact of future disasters by identifying and addressing underlying vulnerabilities. So, it involves the measures taken prior to the impact of a disaster to minimize its effects (sometimes referred to as structural and non-structural measures). Mitigation activities may include building stronger infrastructure, developing early warning systems, and educating communities on disaster preparedness. For example, improving structural qualities of schools, houses, and any other buildings in order to minimize the medical casualties.

EMERGENCY MANAGEMENT RESPONSE: 6 C's CONCEPT

The emergency response be it in community or at the hospital requires 6 C's Concept **(Fig. 45.2)**:

1. **Command:** The Incident Commander is crucial to control the Disaster Response.
2. **Contain:** As a team take measures to contain the event and not to let it affect more population, e.g., fire extinguish and evacuate.
3. **Control:** If on the field, i.e., at the disaster scene area than the control rests with the local administrative authorities, if within the hospital then it will be the hospital authority.
4. **Coordinate:** Human resources, logistics, operations have all to coordinate for the end results of the safety of the people.

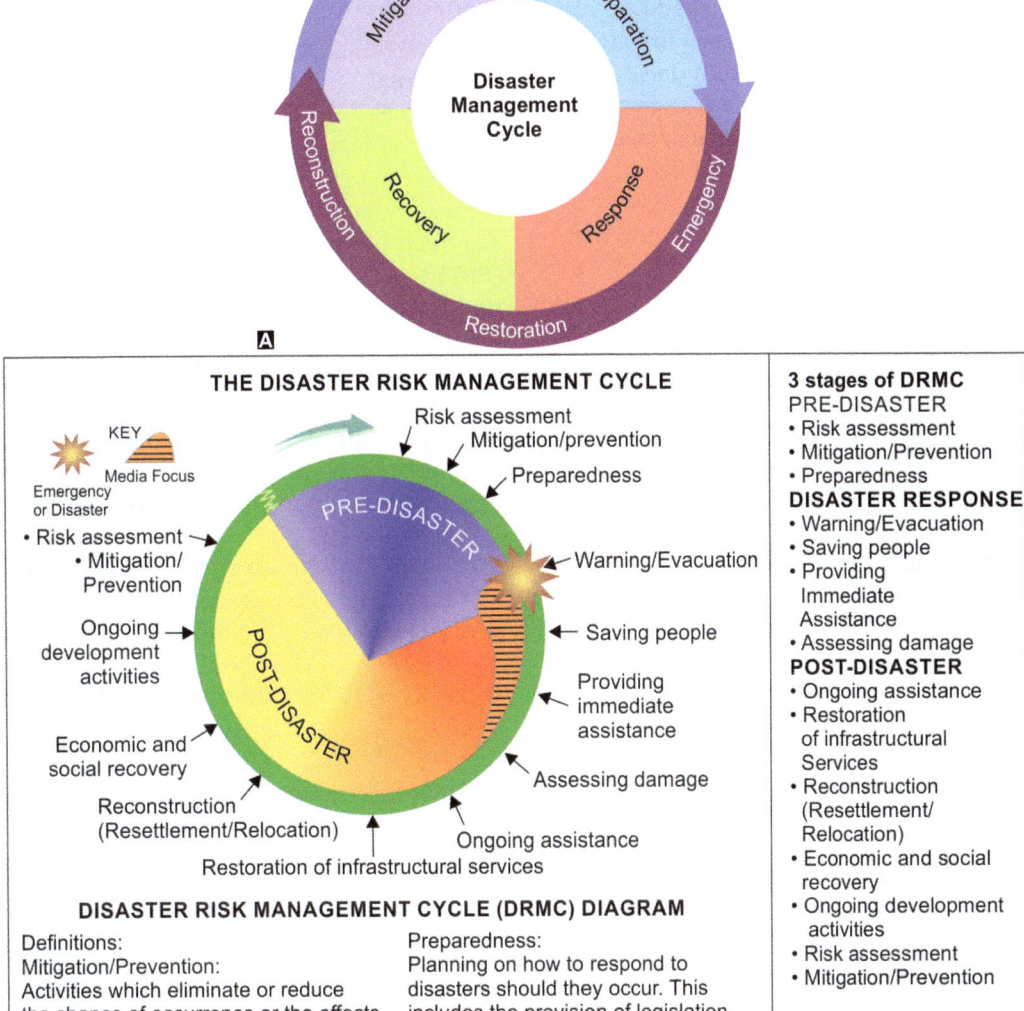

Figs. 45.1A and B: Disaster risk management cycle.

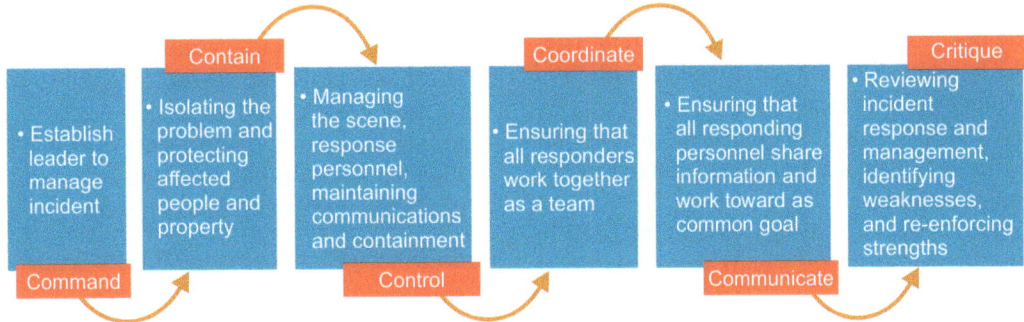

Fig. 45.2: Emergency management response: 6 C's Concept.

5. **Communicate:** Communication with the team and at all level dispersing only appropriate information.
6. **Critique:** After the response and safe evacuation of the people, appropriate medical care needs to be provided following a critique is mandatory. All the members involved in the rescue and care operations need to meet on the next day and collect open feedback as to what needs to be strengthened.

The above points briefly highlight the basics and foundation of disaster management for the benefit of practice by the healthcare team especially nurses.

ROLE OF NURSES IN DISASTER MANAGEMENT

Nursing affirmed as the Noble Profession by the society looks at its actives from the perspective of care encompassed by the scientific principles. Over a decade nursing has grown in reaching out to specialization, such as oncology, renal nursing, neuronursing, etc., one such area which has predominantly taken a global perspective is the trauma and disaster management. The pandemic revealed the role of nurse in disaster management in a powerful manner. The career options also have widened as trauma nurse, educator, trauma quality assurance within which is the sphere of mass casualty management and disaster management. The scope and practice of disaster nurse is so vast that it needs a book and not a chapter alone. The following text will briefly highlight the role of nurse in disaster management, both at community and at the hospital.

Disaster nursing refers to the specialized nursing practice that focuses on the care of individuals, families, and communities affected by natural or man-made disasters. It involves providing immediate and ongoing care, preventing further injury or illness, and responding to the physical and emotional needs of those affected by the disaster.

Disaster nursing requires specialized knowledge and skills in emergency care, triage, infection control, psychological support, and disaster management protocols. Disaster nurses work collaboratively with other healthcare professionals and first responders to ensure the best possible care for disaster victims.

The role of disaster nurses may include administering first aid, performing assessments and evaluations, assisting with evacuations, managing the flow of patients, coordinating care, and providing emotional support to both patients and their families.

Disaster nursing can occur in a variety of settings, including hospitals, clinics, shelters, and other emergency response locations. It plays a critical role in mitigating the impact of disasters on individuals and communities and can help to save lives and prevent further harm.

The role of a nurse in a disaster can vary depending on the type and severity of the disaster.

However, some general responsibilities of a nurse in a disaster include:

- **Emergency response:** Nurses are often called upon to be part of the first response team during disasters. They may be called to administer first aid, triage patients, and provide emergency care to those affected.
- **Evacuation:** Nurses may need to help evacuate patients from healthcare facilities or other areas affected by the disaster to safer locations.
- **Coordination:** Nurses play an essential role in coordinating the response efforts with other healthcare providers, emergency personnel, and community agencies.
- **Communication:** Nurses must communicate effectively with patients, families, and first responders during a disaster to provide accurate and timely information about the situation.
- **Psychological support:** Nurses can provide emotional support and counseling to traumatized patients and their families.

Overall, nurses are integral to the planning, response, and recovery efforts in the aftermath of a disaster. They bring their expertise, experience, and compassion to help those affected by the disaster to heal and rebuild their lives.

Role of the Nurse in Hospital Towards Disaster Management

Disaster management in hospital has two classifications:
1. External
2. Internal

External

A mass casualty or disaster event which has occurred externally in which the hospital Emergency Response Team (ERT) is activated to respond and provide medical care. In this, the emergency nurse plays a key role in coordinating, planning and providing resources (Human and material) and providing medical care at the site of Mass Casualty Event (MCE).

- Disaster pre-hospital care refers to the medical care and attention provided to injured or sick individuals by healthcare professionals during a disaster or emergency situation.
- The goal of disaster pre-hospital care is to provide immediate and essential medical assistance to prevent further damage to an individual's health and to increase their chances of survival.
- Disaster pre-hospital care includes providing basic first aid, stabilizing the injured or sick person, transporting patients to medical facilities, administering medications, and performing emergency medical procedures when necessary.
- Healthcare professionals involved in disaster pre-hospital care may include paramedics, emergency medical technicians, and nurses.
- Disaster pre-hospital care also involves effective communication and coordination between healthcare providers, emergency services, and other responders. This ensures a timely and efficient response in providing care and addressing patients' needs during a disaster.
- Disaster pre-hospital care is typically provided in a challenging and high-stress environment. Therefore, healthcare providers must be adequately trained, equipped, and prepared to respond to various disaster scenarios effectively.
- Preparedness and planning are essential components of disaster pre-hospital care to ensure effective and efficient medical support during a disaster.

Mass Casualty Management (MCM)—Sequence

A. TRIAGE— (Pre-hospital)
B. Extrication and evacuation
C. In hospital ER triage
D. Trauma level response
E. Resuscitation
F. Definitive care
G. Disposition–admission/operating room/discharge/death

The above sequence reveals that every phase of the MCM requires the active role of the nurse in the team. This also emphasizes the importance of disaster nursing training so as the disaster care will be of quality.

The master plan for mass casualty management will comprise of the following:

a. Alerting process	Fire and police
b. Scene assessment and response	Dr, Nurse, EMT
c. Field care	Dr, Nurse, EMT
d. First triage at the incident site	Emergency nurse
e. Care at advanced medical post	Dr, Emergency nurse
f. Communication in MCM	Police and Dr, In-charge
g. Incident command system	Dr, In-charge, police In-charge
h. Triage at receiving hospital	ER Nurse
i. Emergency and definitive care at hospital	Hospital emergency response plan

The master plan is self-explanatory to designate the role played by each member of the ERT especially the emergency nurse.

Figure 45.3 rescue chain is the schematic explanation of the pre-hospital field care:

1. The hospital emergency room receives the alert call
2. The ERT Commander along with pre designated team (Dr, ER Nurse, emergency medical technician) respond to the spot in ambulance
3. The search and rescue is carried out by the fire and rescue team, police and any other government designated team
4. Triage is performed by the emergency nurse and the patients are stabilized at the advanced medical post (AMP)
5. Victims are transported to the nearest hospital in appropriate ambulance.
6. Hospital activates its disaster response plan through the emergency department.

On a larger scale, the nurse also plays her role in different capacities depending upon the area of the service, such as nurse led disaster management program (Capacity for timely emergency service)

Internal

Internal disaster is an event which had occurred within the hospital requiring partial or full evacuation of the hospital to a surge capacity/alternate care site area.

Disaster hospital management: Refers to the process of ensuring efficient and effective management of healthcare facilities during a natural or man-made disaster. Hospitals are critical infrastructure during a disaster as they play a key role in providing medical care and treatment to the affected population. Effective disaster hospital management involves planning, preparedness, response, and recovery.

❖ **Planning:** This involves developing strategies, policies and protocols to address potential risks and hazards in hospital operations. Planning includes identifying potential disaster scenarios and developing plans to mitigate their impact. This also involves ensuring the availability of necessary resources, such as medical equipment, supplies, and staffing arrangements.

❖ **Preparedness:** This involves training of staff, testing and exercising the disaster response plan, and ensuring that all necessary resources are in place in case of an emergency.

❖ **Response:** This involves actual implementation of the disaster response plan during the emergency. Response activities include setting up triage areas, determining the level of patient care needed, identifying and responding to immediate threats, evacuation and transportation of patients, and communicating with emergency services.

❖ **Recovery:** This involves transition from the emergency phase to regular operations. This involves assessments, restoration of existing hospital services, ensuring ongoing patient care, and debriefing staff to improve future disaster readiness.

Proper disaster hospital management is essential for saving lives and ensuring the well-being of patients, staff and community during a disaster. It requires a multidisciplinary approach involving healthcare professionals, emergency services, government agencies, and the public at large.

Disaster preparedness: Nurses should be trained in disaster preparedness and have the necessary supplies and equipment to respond to any disaster effectively.

Nurse Led Disaster Management Program

Disaster and mass casualty management care rendered at:

1. **Sub-centers:** Immediate emergency care and refer
2. **Primary health centers:** Immediate emergency care and refer
3. **Community health centers:** Triage and emergency care
4. **District hospitals:** Triage, resuscitation and emergency care
5. Medical colleges and research institutions

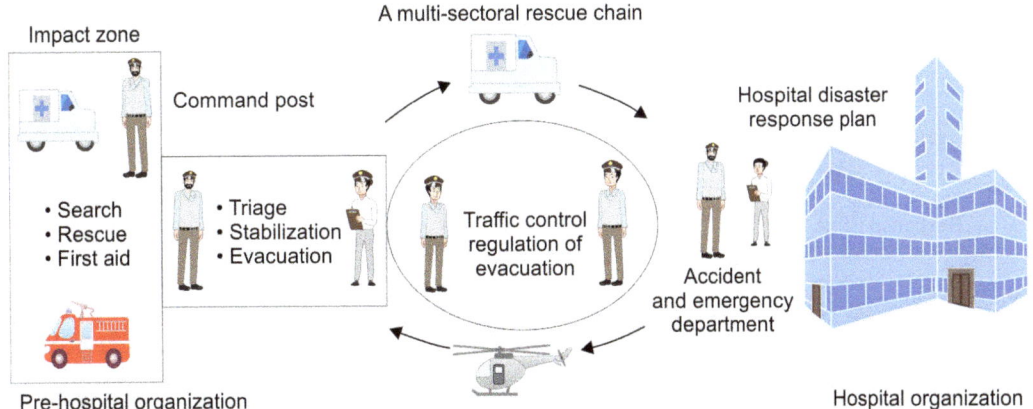

Fig. 45.3: Schematic explanation of the pre-hospital field care.

DISASTER MANAGEMENT

Government on the lead role (**Fig. 45.4**): The National Disaster Management Authority (NDMA) is a Government Agency of India responsible for handling natural or man-made disasters in the country. It was established in 2005 under the Disaster Management Act and functions under the Ministry of Home Affairs.

The key objectives of the NDMA are:
- To lay down policies and guidelines for disaster management in the country
- To promote a culture of prevention and preparedness for disasters
- To ensure timely and effective response to disasters
- To coordinate efforts of different stakeholders including government agencies, NGOs, and civil society organizations
- To create awareness among the masses about disaster prevention and management.

The NDMA works closely with state governments and district administrations to prepare for and respond to disasters. It also coordinates with international agencies in disaster response and management. The authority has developed a National Disaster Management Plan, which encompasses all aspects of disaster management, including prevention, preparedness, response, and recovery.

The National Disaster Response Force (NDRF) is a specialized disaster response agency of the Indian Government that was established in 2006. It is responsible for responding to natural disasters, such as earthquakes, cyclones, floods, landslides, and other such incidents.

The force is managed by the Ministry of Home Affairs and is composed of trained personnel from various government agencies, including the Indian Army, the Indian Air Force, and the Central Reserve Police Force.

The NDRF has a total of 12 battalions stationed in various parts of the country, each consisting of around 1,200 personnel. The force is equipped with the latest tools and technologies, such as satellite imagery, communication equipment, and specialized search and rescue equipment.

The NDRF is also responsible for conducting awareness programs and training workshops to enable communities to prepare for disasters and respond effectively in the event of a disaster.

The force has been involved in several major disaster response operations in the country, including the 2015 Nepal earthquake, Cyclone Fani in 2019, and the recent floods in the state of Assam in 2020.

Various nodal agencies for disaster management are shown in **Box 45.1**.

> **BOX 45.1:** Various nodal agencies for disaster management.
>
> - **Floods:** Ministry of Water Resources, CWC
> - **Cyclones:** Indian Meteorological Department
> - **Earthquakes:** Indian Meteorological Department
> - **Epidemics:** Ministry of Health and Family Welfare
> - **Avian Flu:** Ministry of Health, Ministry of Environment, Ministry of Agriculture and Animal Husbandry
> - **Chemical disasters:** Ministry of Environment and Forests
> - **Industrial disasters:** Ministry of Labour
> - **Rail accidents:** Ministry of Railways
> - **Air Accidents:** Ministry of Civil Aviation
> - **Fire:** Ministry of Home Affairs
> - **Nuclear Incidents:** Department of Atomic Energy
> - **Mine Disasters:** Department of Mines

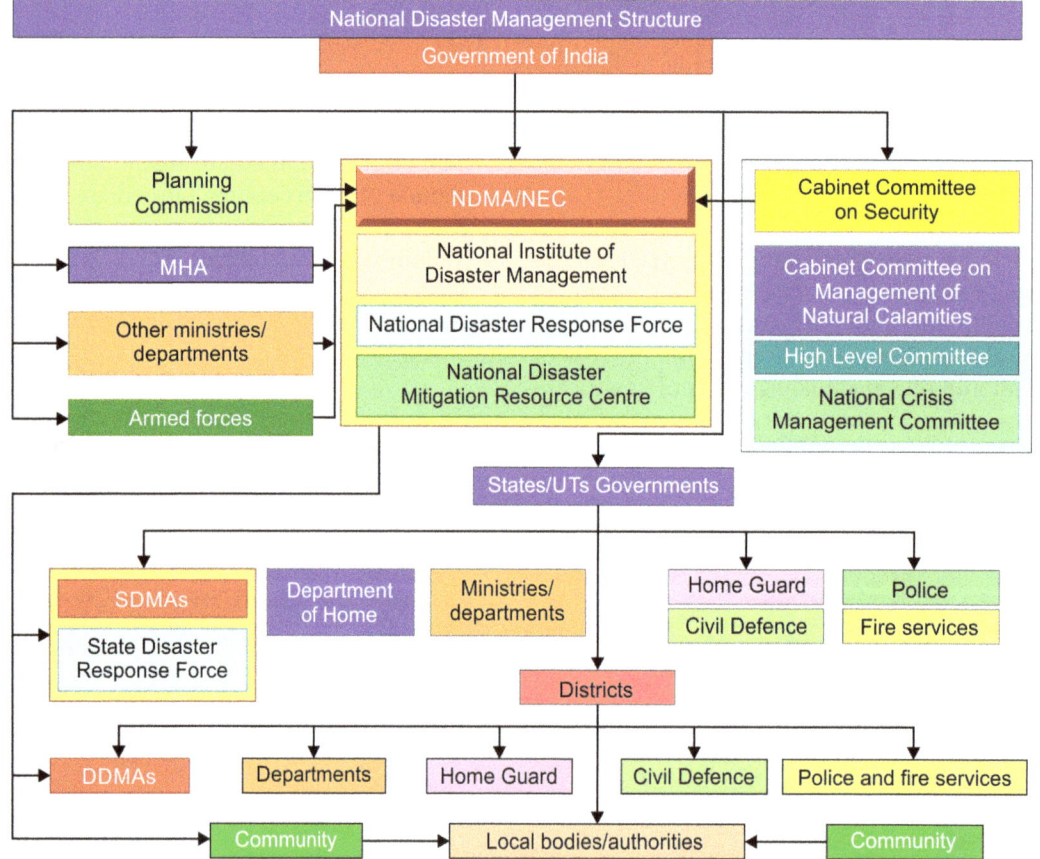

Fig. 45.4: Disaster management structure India.

Case Scenario

Case Study I
Scenario: Earthquake
Location: Nepal
Period of response: 07.05.2015–13.05.2015.
Team: CMC Emergency Response Team (CERT), Christian Medical College, Vellore, Tamil Nadu, India.
Introduction: India with a large landscape is vulnerable for multiple natural disasters. One such vulnerability is earthquake. An earthquake is a phenomenon that occurs without warning and involves violent shaking of the ground and everything over it. The earth's crust is divided into seven major plates, that are about 50 miles thick, which move slowly and continuously over the earth's interior and several minor plates. Earthquakes are tectonic in origin; that is the moving plates are responsible for the occurrence of violent shakes. The occurrence of an earthquake in a populated area may cause numerous casualties and injuries as well as extensive damage to property.
Background: The India tectonic plate is a minor tectonic plate that covers most of South Asia and a portion of the Indian Ocean. The Nepal earthquake of 2015 was a devastating natural disaster that occurred on April 25, 2015, with a magnitude of 7.8 Mw. It caused widespread damage and casualties in Nepal and neighboring countries.

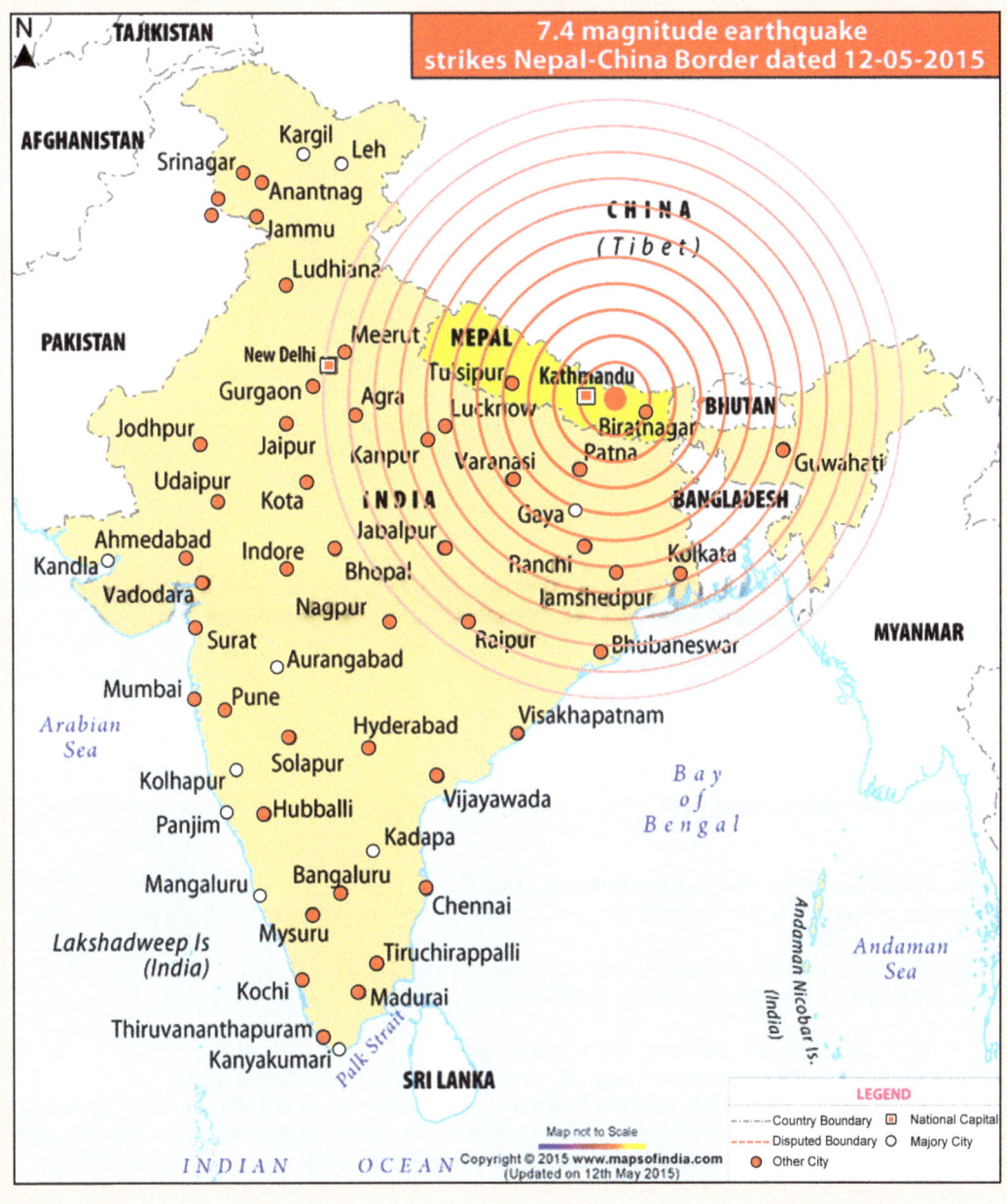

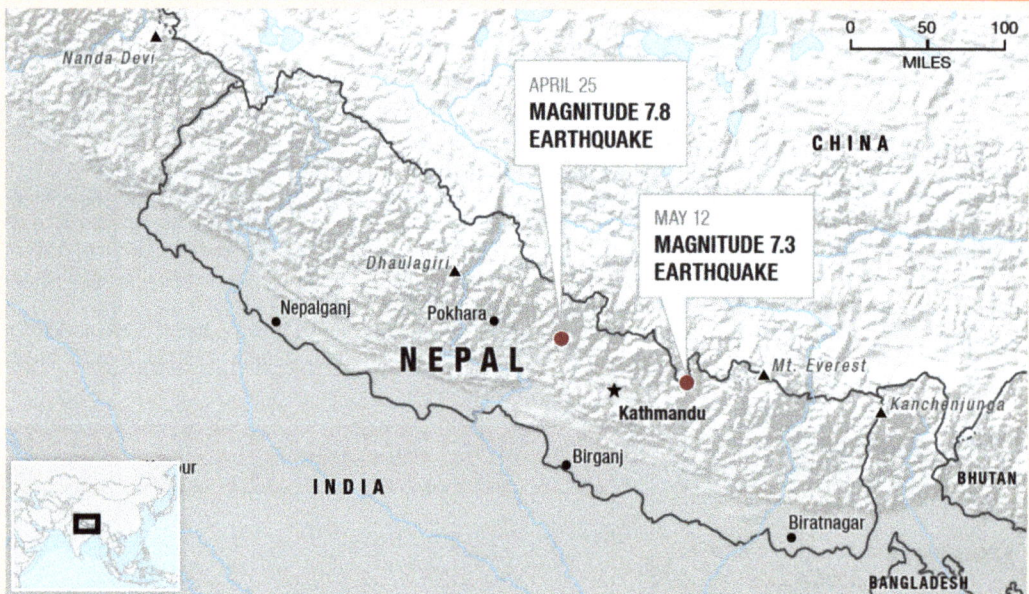

Salient findings:
- The earthquake killed about 9,000 people and injured more than 21,000 in Nepal and other countries.
- The earthquake triggered avalanches on Mount Everest and in the Langtang valley, killing dozens of climbers and villagers.
- The earthquake destroyed or damaged more than 600,000 structures in Kathmandu and other towns, including many historic and cultural sites.
- The earthquake was caused by the movement of the India tectonic plate under the Eurasian plate along the main Himalayan Thrust fault.
- The earthquake was followed by hundreds of aftershocks, including a major one on May 12 with a magnitude of 7.3 Mw.

Responding team for earthquake: In the wake of the Earthquake, CMC Vellore immediately convened the Emergency Response Team meeting for active response to meet the healthcare need of the affected population in Nepal.

About CMC: Christian Medical College, Vellore seeks to be a witness to the Healing Ministry of Christ, through excellence in education, service and research. As of 2015 during the period of 2015, CMC was 2500 bedded multispecialty tertiary level hospital. CMC has an active safety cell with an Emergency Response Team trained to respond to any emergencies and disasters.

Objectives:
1. To respond by providing appropriate health care to the affected victims as per FMT (Foreign Medical Team) guidelines by WHO.
2. To assess the situation at the affected area and report to CMC for future long-term plan in rehabilitation.

Plan of action:
A. Team preparation
B. Logistics
C. Transportation to Nepal
D. Coordination with local team at Nepal
E. Focus Healthcare needs
F. Primarily Team A and based on need Team B will join

A. **Team:**
   a. *Team coordinator:* Prof TS Ravi Kumar (Trauma nurse trained in disaster)
   b. Remaining members 2 nurses (Mr Arun and Muthu) and one Doctor (Dr Ramesh Karki) who is from Nepal serving in CMC
B. **Logistics:**
   – Medicines and stores items needed for health care, such as antibiotics, analgesics, POP, PPE, etc.
   – Total 11 boxes weighing 234 kg (Courtesy Jet Airways 180 kg of medicines were transported to Patna)
C. **Transportation:**
   – The team left on 07.05.2015 2345 hours from CMC with a word of prayer
   – Team reached Duncan Hospital Raxaul and coordinated with Medical Superintendent for further moves.
   – Volvo Company India had lent a Volvo of 50 seated bus for Nepal Disaster Relief through EHA. This was optimally used for transportation materials (Food, tent, mat, medicines, etc.) to Nepal as well as transferring affected people from the site to alternate camps.
D. **Base camp was established at Chitwan along Dhading district which is an affected area.**
   – *Base camp coordinator:* Mission Coordinator Nepal, who was playing a significant role. She and her team assisted the affected by providing the needed resources for daily need, tents for stay and helping them to re allot to newer living place. Area covered was Dhading, Gorkha and Pokhara District of Nepal.
   – This visit involved travel commencing 7 AM and returning back to the base by 12 midnight.
   – The team visited the disaster affected areas as mentioned above and communicated to the affected people through Dr Ramesh Karki.
   – It was shared by them that most of the sick had been airlifted to main districts hospitals by the government and the minimal injured are treated appropriately, the non-injured, but displaced are reluctant to come down from the hills as that is their livelihood.
   – We assisted in mobilizing and giving the non-medical relief materials to the people. We made contact with the district hospital and in person handed over the CMC Relief Medicines to the concerned authorities.

- Immediately they were dispatched and handed over to the concerned departments and camps. We visited a church which hosted as a clinic where they had two patients with probable spine and pelvic injuries. They were examined; as they were stable they were referred to the nearest district hospital.
- We conducted a health camp at Dhading. This involved assessment of their minimal injuries and normal check-up. The need as of now stood on reallotment of their houses and fulfilment of basic needs.
- *Health education:* Incidental health teachings were given by Dr Ramesh Karki to the affected people on hygiene, food habits, etc.
- A small training was offered to the mission volunteers to identify basic illness and referral to hospital. They were also guided to administer ORS wherever necessary for patients with diarrhea.
- A meeting was held with the mission field workers at Gorkha involving need assessment and future planning on rehabilitation.
- Medicines to the affected: A visit to the Dhading district hospital revealed that 90% of the patients were of trauma involving fractures and other vascular injuries. The district hospital is offering exemplary service to the victims and has good social services. We handed over the medicine to the appropriate authorities where upon it was immediately categorized and distributed to the respective areas concerned.
- We visited and met the patients who were mostly in post-traumatic stress. There was an increased need for Nepal speaking counseling as an on-going therapy.
- There was heavy rain in Pokhara during our visit. Team A planned to move further on.

On May 12, 2015 while traveling in the van, the team experienced the 7.4 Richter scale earthquakes in Kathmandu first hand. It was indeed frightening and was disturbing to see the building falling down and the uncertainty with which life moves on. Our prayers for Nepal as it stand to struggle with earthquake which was not far off for the rest of the country.

The Team A left Nepal and Team B took over in coordination with the local health authorities in providing the emergency healthcare services

Roadmap:
- Help construct safe accommodation for the health workers
- This health post has to be chosen depending on the population served.
- Most of these health posts are on top of the hill and this could be relocated midway making it easy for both those in the lower side of the hill (towards valley) and those on the top.
- Take up training of the health workers on disaster management, syllabus based. Could be modified for this region.
- Make plans to visit the hospitals run by these partners and see how we can improve the service provided by them. Add basic training component and help them adopt a needy village as their outreach centre.

https://en.wikipedia.org/wiki/April_2015_Nepal_earthquake

Case Study II
Scenario: Cyclone and floods
Location: Tamil Nadu
Period of Response: 8/11/2015–14/12/2015.
Team: CMC Emergency Response Team (CERT), Christian Medical College, Vellore.

Introduction: The Chennai metropolitan region (CMA), with an area of 1,189 sq km and a population of 8,653,521, is the fourth-largest populated city in India. In November and December of 2015, Chennai received unprecedented levels of rainfall leading to the overflow of the arterial Adyar River, which in turn led to floods in the city. Multiple low-lying areas in the city were inundated for days together; massive rescue and evacuation efforts had to be undertaken in areas where houses were getting submerged. The city was no stranger to flooding. In 2007, a Drescher et al. study on risk perception consisting of analysis of flood risk exposure and the development of flood risk maps showed that flooding is a regular occurrence.

Background: The 2015 South India floods resulted from heavy rainfall generated by the annual Northeast monsoon in November–December 2015. The unprecedented Monsoon rainfall affected and paralyzed the whole city and suburbs including hospitals and healthcare services. The affected people are as cited in **Figure 45.5**.

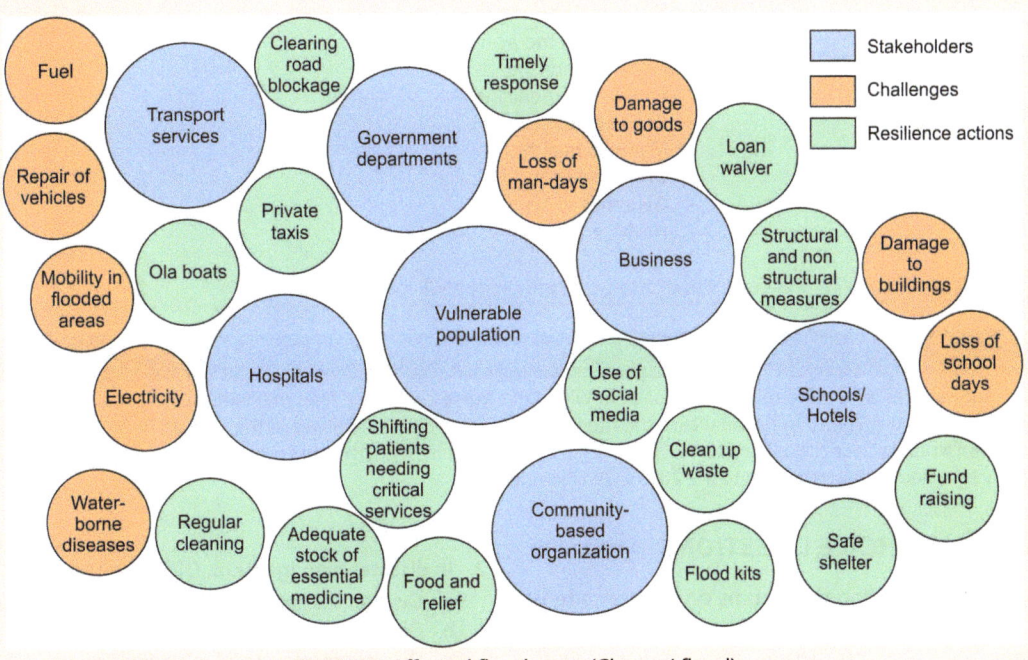

Fig. 45.5: Affected flood areas (Chennai flood).

Responding team for monsoon flood: In the wake of the flood, CMC Vellore immediately convened the emergency response team meeting for active response to meet the healthcare need of the affected population in Tamil Nadu.

Objectives:
1. To respond by providing appropriate health care to the affected victims as per guidelines by WHO.
2. To assess the situation at the affected area and report to CMC for future long-term plan in rehabilitation.

Plan of action:
A. Team preparation
B. Logistics
C. Transportation to flood affected areas
D. Coordination with local team at various flood affected areas
E. Focus: Healthcare needs
F. Primarily Team A and based on need Team B will join

A. **Team:**
  – *A-team coordinator:* Prof TS Ravi Kumar (Trauma nurse trained in disaster)
  – Every day new teams responding in different directions, team comprised of Drs, nurses, pharmacist, technicians and volunteers

B. **Logistics:** Every day medicine and relief materials were moved to the affected zones

C. **Transportation:** Every day a mini van will transport the team to a base at the affected area and establish a mobile clinic there

D. The daily team will coordinate with local healthcare services and render the needed clinic and services.

The overall report is provided as follows:

Disaster Response Report of the Chennai Flood December 2015

1.	Type of disaster	Brief report and documentation Monsoon flood	Chennai Kanchipuram Thiruvallur Cuddalore
2.	Teams network	• CSI Hospital, Kanchipuram • AG Church, Cuddalore • RC Church, Vadalur • Lions Club, Vellore • Ashok Leyland, Chennai • Tata Groups	
3.	Total number of days	10 (Mostly daily trips, 2 occasion it was for 2 days each)	
4.	Number of camps	27	
5.	Total number of people	6130 (Adult and children)	
6.	Distance covered	2750 km	
7.	Team members (Field work)	65 (Multi-disciplinary)	

8.	Type of relief activities	1. Relief materials
		2. Food, water, fruits and biscuits
		3. Healthcare camps:
		  – Community medicine,
		  – General medicine,
		  – Emergency medicine,
		  – Child health,
		  – Maternal health,
		  – Orthopedics and
		  – Geriatrics
		  – Health education	

https://www.mei.edu/publications/2015-chennai-flood-case-developing-city-resilience-strategies

SUMMARY

Disaster management requires a multidisciplinary approach in which the nurse can take a lead role with experience and training to enhance a qualitative disaster care. From triage to in-hospital care the nurse can aggressively be involved in the care. In India, every nursing program as approved by the Indian Nursing Council has Disaster Nursing within the curriculum. Thus, the nurses of India are well prepared for disaster nursing which was evidently revealed in their response to the 2019 COVID Pandemic.

MULTIPLE CHOICE QUESTIONS

1. Prioritizing and color coding the victims on disaster site is termed as:
   a. Mitigation
   b. Triage
   c. Resilience
   d. Prevention

2. In disaster management, DRR means:
   a. Disaster resilience and rehabilitation
   b. Disaster response and recovery
   c. Disaster recovery and rehabilitation
   d. Disaster risk reduction

3. The elements of disaster cycle involves:
   a. Prevention
   b. Mitigation
   c. Response
   d. All of the above
4. Man made disaster:
   a. Earthquake
   b. Cyclone
   c. Bomb blast
   d. Flood
5. A physical event that can trigger a disaster is termed as:
   a. Hazard
   b. Mitigation
   c. Prevention
   d. Capacity
6. An exercise in which people simulate the circumstances of a disaster so that they have an opportunity to practice their responses is termed as:
   a. Class
   b. Rescue
   c. Drill
   d. Triage
7. In disaster triage, the color code for severely injured is:
   a. Red
   b. Yellow
   c. Green
   d. Black
8. MCM refers to:
   a. Medical casualty management
   b. Mass casualty management
   c. Mild casualty management
   d. Moderate casualty management
9. An action that reduces or eliminates long-term risk to people and property from natural hazards and their effects is termed as:
   a. Mitigation
   b. Preparation
   c. Recovery
   d. Response
10. The number one concern in disaster response is:
    a. Speed
    b. Communication
    c. Documentation
    d. Safety

ANSWERS

1. b	2. d	3. d	4. c
5. a	6. c	7. a	8. b
9. a	10. d		

SUGGESTED READING

1. American Red Cross. https://www.redcross.org/
2. Centers for Disease Control and Prevention (CDC). https://www.cdc.gov/
3. Emergency Management Institute (EMI). https://training.fema.gov/emi.aspx
4. Federal Emergency Management Agency (FEMA). https://www.fema.gov/
5. http://unisdr.org/files/7817_UNISDRTerminologyEnglish.pdf
6. http://www.emdat.be/
7. http://www.oxforddictionaries.com/definition/english/disaster Ministry of Home Affairs, Govt. of India, Disaster Management in India
8. http://www.unisdr.org/we/inform/terminology 9
9. https://disaster-management.piarc.org/en/
10. https://ndma.gov.in/Resources/Reports-Studies
11. https://nidm.gov.in/PDF/pubs/NDMA/18.pdf Hospital Safety
12. https://steadypoint.wordpress.com/2016/07/13/chapter-1-2-introduction-to-disaster-management/
13. https://www.ifrc.org/en/what-we-do/disaster-management/about-disaster-management/
14. International Federation of Red Cross and Red Crescent Societies (IFRC). https://www.ifrc.org/en/
15. Module 4 - Capacity Building in Asia using Information Technology Applications (CASITA)—Asian Disaster Preparedness Center (ADPC),Bangkok .
16. National Emergency Management Association (NEMA). https://www.nemaweb.org/
17. National Institute of Standards and Technology (NIST) Disaster Resilience Program. https://www.nist.gov/topics/disaster-resilience-program
18. National Weather Service (NWS). https://www.weather.gov/
19. United Nations Office for Disaster Risk Reduction (UNDRR). https://www.undrr.org/
20. World Health Organization (WHO). https://www.who.int/
21. "Establishing a Mass Casualty Management System" French Ministry of Cooperation and Cultural Affairs and the Overseas Development Administration of the United Kingdom.

UNIT VII

Geriatric Nursing

OUTLINE

46. **Ageing: Demography, Classification, Myths and Realities, and Theories**
    Sukhpal Kaur, Manjeet Singh

47. **Age-related Body System Changes and Common Health Problems in Elderly**
    Manjeet Singh, Alisha Talwar, Sukhpal Kaur

48. **Elderly Abuse, Legal and Ethical Issues of the Elderly**
    Nitasha Sharma, Sunita Sharma

49. **Provisions and Programs for Elderly**
    Ruchi Saini, Nitasha Sharma, Sukhpal Kaur

50. **Care of Elders**
    Sukhpal Kaur, Alisha Talwar

CHAPTER 46

Ageing: Demography, Classification, Myths and Realities, and Theories

Sukhpal Kaur, Manjeet Singh

"Age is just a number. It carries no weight. The real weight is in impacts. The truth is that you can do it at any age. Get up and be willing to leave a mark."

—Israelmore Ayivor

Learning Objectives

After going through the chapter, the learner will be able to:
- Discuss the demographic transition of ageing.
- Understand the classification of ageing.
- Deliberate various myths and realities of ageing.
- Enumerate various theories of ageing.
- Discuss various theories of ageing.
- Compare the biological, social, and psychological theories of ageing.

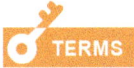

TERMS

- **Antioxidants:** These are the natural substances help/prevent/delay some types of cell damage.
- **Chronological:** It is listing, describing, or discussing the events as happened as per the timeline.
- **Disengagement:** It is the process of losing interest in involvement in any activity, situation, or group.
- **Errors:** It is the deviation from precision.
- **Free radical:** It is an unstable molecule containing an unpaired electron generated at the time of normal cell metabolism.
- **Immunity:** The ability of the body to prevent the invasion by the disease causing organisms.
- **Immunosenescence:** Immune dysfunction related to ageing predisposing elderly to infections, immune mediated diseases and cancer.

INTRODUCTION

Ageing is a natural phenomenon and is the buildup of changes in an organism over a time period. The ageing population has emerged as a major demographic trend worldwide and time is not far from when we will have more of elderly people as compared to children. It is the result of declining fertility and mortality rates, improved healthcare facilities, and advances in medical technology. The continuous increase in life expectancy is the consequence of all these developments. However, this increase in longevity is associated with several physical, physiological, psychological, and social issues. Several societal and economic implications are associated with the rapid increase in the elderly population. With increasing age, apart from developing health-related issues, there is a loss of employment and income among the elderly, loss of physical strength and stamina, and increasing dependency on others to handle their old age-related issues and requirements. All these affect their self-esteem and their well-being further. Even they are more prone to various kinds of crimes such as murder, theft, cheating, etc. All these pose major challenges for the elderly people who in fact are the valuable resources for our society.

The current chapter gives us an overview of the demographic transition of the elderly population; the classification of ageing; myths, and realities of the elderly, and theories of ageing.

DEMOGRAPHIC TRANSITION

Worldwide there is an exponential increase in the proportion of the elderly in the general population both in absolute and relative terms. This demographic transition is an inevitable reality and owes to the decrease in fertility rates because of better access to contraceptives, late marriage, decreasing infant mortality rate, etc. Life expectancy has increased because of advancements in medical science and technology, better health facilities, awareness of the public regarding health, economic well-being, access to better nutrition, etc. With the rapid progression in medical science, it is comparatively easy to prevent and control various diseases, earlier which were the reasons for high mortality.

Life expectancy is the number of years a person born today is expected to live, on an average, after attaining that particular age. There is a dramatic increase in life expectancy at the age of 60. It was 12 years in 1950 and increased to 18 years in 2015. Further, by 2050, it is projected to rise to more than 21 years. The global life expectancy at birth was 72.8 years in 2019 and it is projected to be around 77.2 years by 2050. Females are in an advantageous position in life expectancy and outnumber men at older ages even. It has also been reported that the global life expectancy at birth fell to 71.0 years in 2021, down from 72.8 in 2019, because of the impact of the COVID-19 pandemic. (World Population Prospects 2022, United Nations New York, 2022, Department of Economic and Social Affairs Population Division).

The two most populous countries of the world are China and India, having more than 1 billion population. About 18% of the total world's population is constituted by both these countries individually. India has overtaken China as the world's most populous country **(Fig. 46.1)**.

Now talking about the elderly population, worldwide the proportion of persons aged 65 or over is projected to increase between 2022 and 2050. It is expected that by 2030, in 34 nations, 20% of the population will be more than 65 years. In 1980, there were 258 million people above 65 years, and the number increased three times in 2022 with 771 million people aged 65 years or over. This population is likely to reach 994 million by 2030 and 1.6 billion by 2050. So, it is projected to rise from 10% in 2022, 12% by 2030 to 16% in 2050. Further, it is also expected that by 2050, the number of persons aged 65 years or over is projected to be more than twice the number of children under age 5 and about the same as the number of children under age 12. Regarding gender-wise distribution, globally, in 2022, women aged 65 or older outnumbered men by 55.7%, but, they are expected to decline slightly to 54.5% by 2050. Europe and Northern America had the largest proportion of the older population in 2022, with about 19% aged 65 or over, followed by Australia

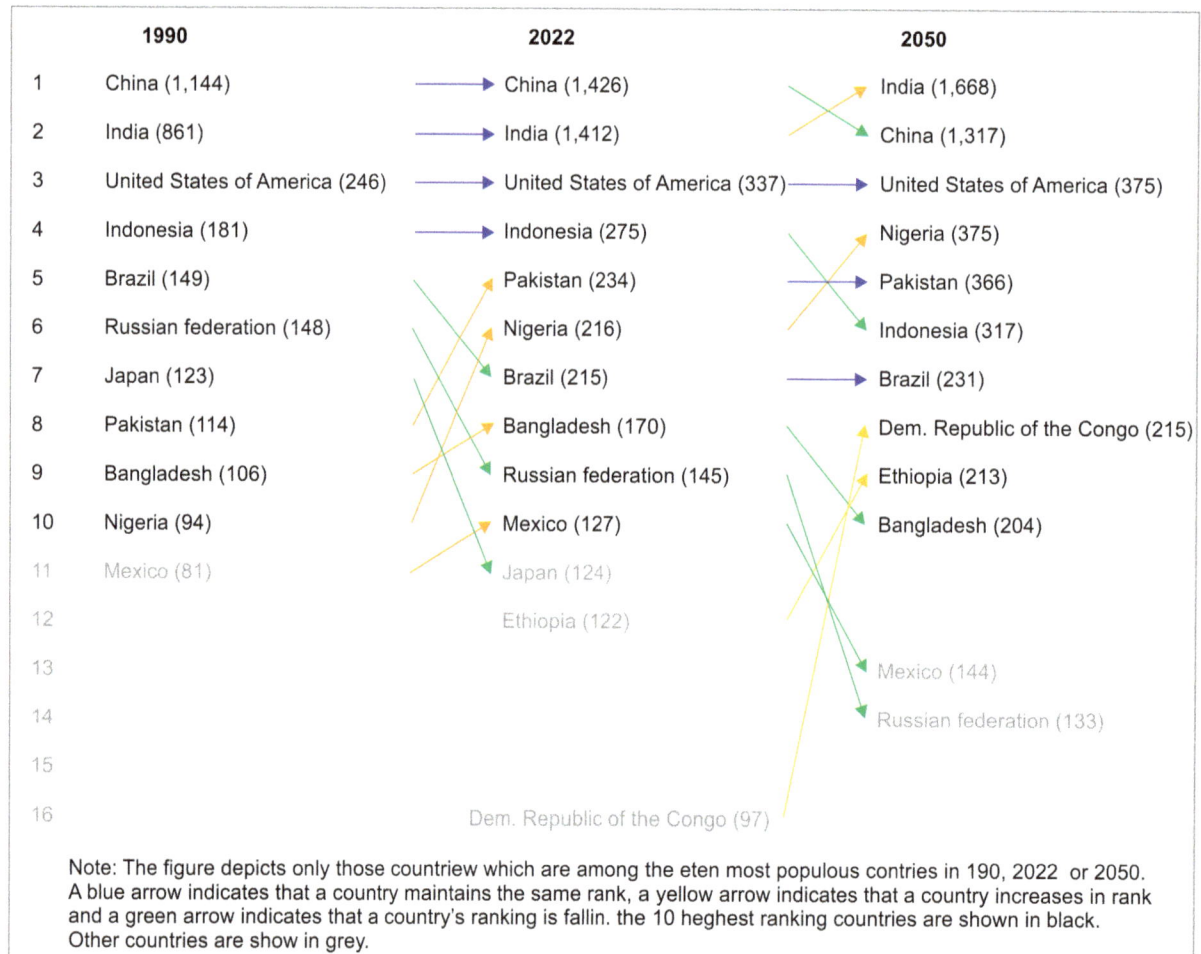

Fig. 46.1: Rankings of the world's ten most populous countries, 1990 and 2022, and medium scenario, 2050 (numbers in parentheses refer to total population in millions).

(*Source:* "World Population Prospects 2022, United Nations New York, 2022")

and New Zealand (16.6%). Both regions are continuing to age further. It has been projected that by 2050 one in every four persons in Europe and Northern America could be aged 65 years or over. (World Population Prospects 2022). By 2030, 1 in 6 people in the world will be aged 60 years or over. The number of persons aged 80 years or older is expected to triple between 2020 and 2050 to reach 426 million. (https://www.who.int/news-room/fact-sheets/detail/ageing-and-health).

In India, the elderly (60 and above) are anticipated to upsurge from 20 million in 1951, 71 million in 2001, 144 million in 2011, to 179 million in 2031, and further to 301 million in 2051. In 1961, the elderly constituted 5.6% of the total population. According to Census 2011, this number was 8.6% of the total population. It further increased to 10.1% in 2021 and is expected to increase to 13.1% in 2031.

As per gender-wise distribution, the number of elderly females is more as compared to elderly males. In 2021, there were 71 million females with 67 million males. In 2031 it is projected to have 93 million males and 101 million females **(Fig. 46.2)**. The dependency ratio of females is also more as compared to males **(Fig. 46.3)**. A similar trend is there in the rural as well as in urban areas. In rural areas, the elderly

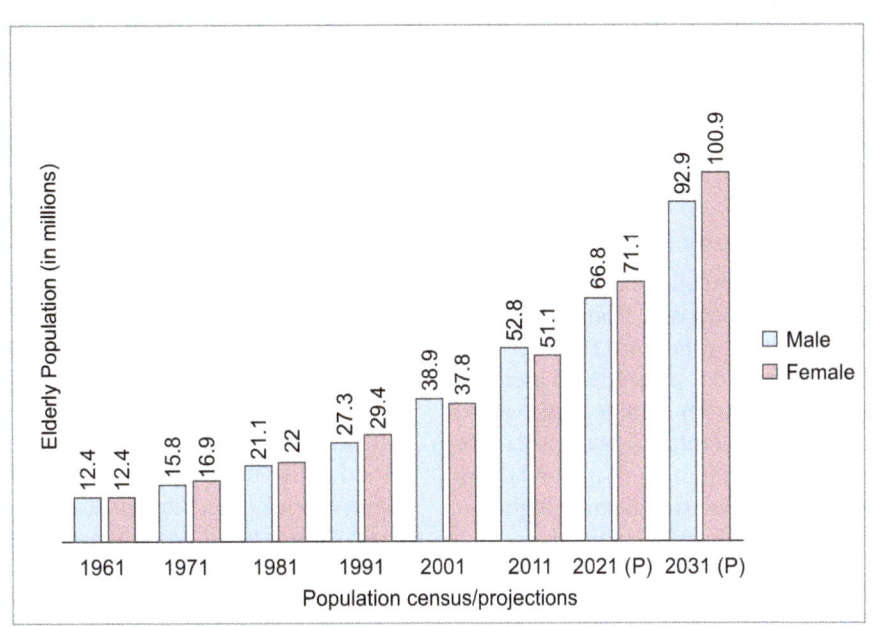

Fig. 46.2: Sex-wise distribution of the elderly population (aged 60 years and above) in India.
(*Source:* Govt of India 2021).

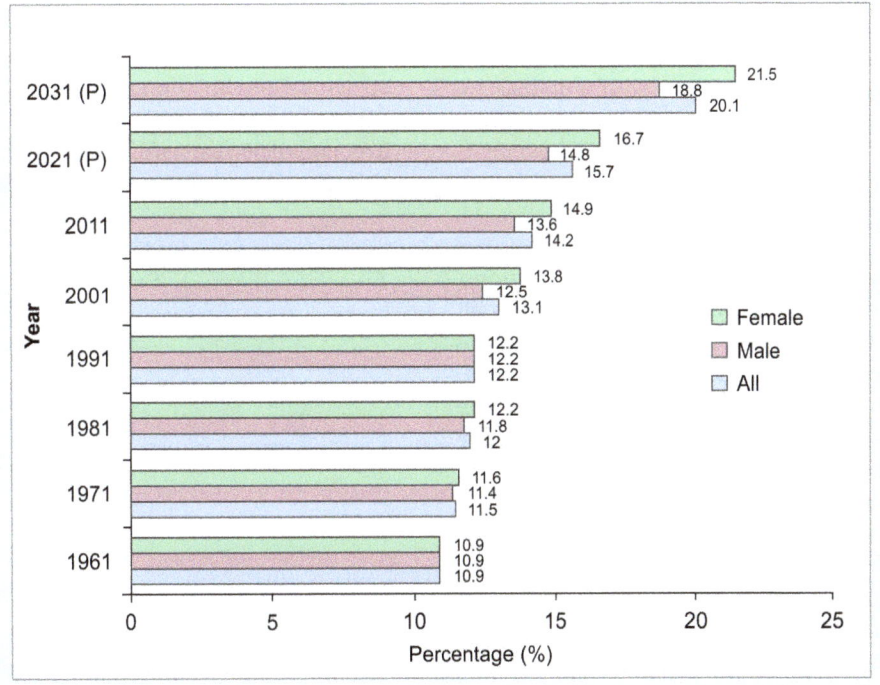

Fig. 46.3: Old age dependency ratio in India by sex.
(*Source:* Govt of India 2021).

population has increased from 5.8% in 1961 to 8.8% in 2011, whereas in urban areas, this number has increased from 4.7–8.1% during 1961 to 2011.

State-wise Data

As per the Report of the "Technical Group on Population Projections for India and States 2011–2036", the state-wise data on the elderly population of 21 major states reveal that in 2021, Kerala has outnumbered the elderly population (16.5%). It is followed by Tamil Nadu (13.6%), Himachal Pradesh (13.1%), Punjab (12.6%), and Andhra Pradesh (12.4%). However, the least proportion of elderly was in the State of Bihar (7.7%). It was followed by Uttar Pradesh (8.1%) and Assam (8.2%). The projection of the states regarding elderly population is going to be the same a decade from now, with Kerala (20.9%) followed by Tamil Nadu (18.2%), Himachal Pradesh (17.1%), Andhra Pradesh (16.4%) and Punjab (16.2%).

The Economic Status of the Elderly Population

With the increase in age, a significant increase in the old-age dependency ratio has also been observed. There is a steady increase in the old age dependency ratio from 10.9% in 1961 to 14.2% in 2011, 15.7% in 2021, and is projected to increase to 20.1% in 2031. The overall old-age dependency ratio varied from 10.4% in Delhi to 19.6% in Kerala (Census, 2021). In 2031, it could vary from 15.6% in Bihar to 34.3% in Kerala. The female old-age dependency ratio was significantly higher in Kerala, Tamil Nadu, Himachal Pradesh, and Punjab.

Literacy Level

Only 28% of female elderly were literate as against 59% of males as per Population Census 2011. The literacy levels among elderly males and females have improved over time in both rural and urban areas, though the urban areas are significantly better than the rural areas. The average number of years in formal education among persons aged 60+ is the highest in Chandigarh (12.7 years) followed by Delhi (10.7 years) and is the lowest in Sikkim (6.2 years), followed by Mizoram (6.3 years) and Daman & Diu (6.5 years). (Elderly in India, 2021)

CLASSIFICATION OF AGEING

Ageing is a part of the life cycle. It is a natural, continuous, irreversible, universal process, starting from conception till the death of an individual. However, the age at which there is a decline in the productive contribution of an individual, and has to be economically dependent, can probably be the onset of the old age stage of life. National Elderly Policy defines people of the 60+ age group as elderly. Each nation, government, and nongovernment organization has different ways of classifying age. In India, senior citizenship is also considered as per the age of superannuation for a person working in public places (Govt places). It varies from 58 to 65 years. In private and corporate places there is no limitation of the age of working. A person can work till his health permits him to work.

The population aged 65 and older is often categorized into three categories: young-old (65–74), middle-old (75–84), and oldest-old (≥85). In the last few years, medical science has identified a new group within the senior citizen category: the super-agers for people in their 70s and 80s having the mental or physical capability of their decades-younger counterparts.

Phases of Ageing

The categorization of old age is quite broad and complex. Some people consider ageing to simply be a state of mind, and others go by how the mind and body naturally change over time. Theoretically speaking, various phases of ageing can be categorized as chronological, biological, psychological, and social. However, all these phases are interdependent, and interrelated, and cannot be separated from each other **(Fig. 46.4)**.

❖ **Chronological age:** This is the most straightforward definition of ageing. It is the age of an individual in years, months, and days after birth means how old a person is. It is a matter of fact that the chronological age of an individual does not correlate perfectly with the biological/functional age. This means that two persons may be of the same chronological age, but may differ in their mental and physical capacities.

❖ **Biological ageing:** It is also known as the physiological age or functional age. It is defined by a person's "present position with respect to his potential life span". It is measured by the "assessment of functional capacities of vital or life-limiting organ systems". It refers to how old a person looks like. Biological ageing denotes to the various ways the human body naturally changes over time. For example, with age, there are changes in digestion affecting the nutritional status; our joints affecting movement and daily functioning; the immune system making it difficult to fight infections; and changes in vital organs, hearing, vision, oral health, etc. So, biological ageing depends upon the condition of a person's organs and body system. An individual's biological functioning and physical appearance may differ from other persons of the same chronological age. It is used for expressing structural and functional losses. It is an index of one's level of competence in carrying out specific tasks. For example, a worker of 60 years of age performs adequately on the job as a 20-year-old. Biological age is influenced by various

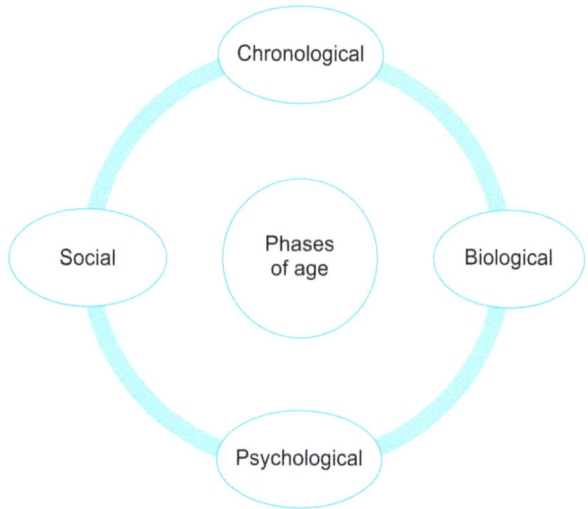

Fig. 46.4: Phases of age.

factors. Though genetics plays a significant role, other factors such as diet and nutrition also affect the biological age of an individual. A person can age well biologically by regular exercising, maintaining body weight, managing stress, being proactive about recommended health screenings, and eating fresh fruits and vegetables, etc.

- **Psychological ageing:** It is an individual's adaptive capacities means his/her ability to adapt to the changing environment. Psychological age is defined as the "behavioral capacities of individuals to adapt to changing demands", including the uses of "memory, learning, intelligence, skills, feelings, motivations, and emotion for exercising behavioral control or self-regulation". With age, there is a decrease in perception, cognitive abilities, and problem-solving abilities. Individuals adapt to their environment by drawing on various psychological characteristics. These may be with regard to intelligence, emotional control, motivational strengths, coping styles, etc. how an individual adapts to or reacts to that particular environment.

  Certain important points that can help the elderly to improve their psychological ageing include having healthy emotional outlets by talking with their friends/family members, getting good support from their dear ones for all of their day-to-day needs; maintaining nutritional status by eating healthy foods; and early identification of any of the mental or physical disorders, etc. The biological aspects of ageing could also affect older people psychologically. For instance, if there are untreated health-related issues, and no one is there to take care, it may affect the behavior of the elderly.

- **Social ageing/sociological age:** Social habits and behaviors change over the period of time. Each society has its own expectations about roles to play and goals to attain from the individuals in each phase of life-like from the young, middle, and older adults. From elderly people, social ageing is the society's expectations of how people should act as they grow older. It is also the social roles and expectations people hold for themselves as well as those who impose on them. The social age is defined by the person's "roles and habits with respect to other members of the society of which he is a part. An individual may be older or younger depending on the extent to which he shows the age-graded behavior expected of him by his particular society or culture" (Birren and Cunningham). Ageing can present unique challenges for older adults. As per their capabilities, the elderly should be involved in various household chores.

  Certain points that may help elderly people to age well socially include "maintaining healthy relationships with friends and family members, exploring new ways to engage socially as per the change in life circumstances, and getting assistance for the physical limitations that could be affecting social interactions".

MYTHS ABOUT AGEING

Many people think negatively about getting older. They are of the opinion that old age is going to affect them adversely in all facets of their life. Definitely, it may be to some extent. Certainly, with age, there is some transition in our body and mind, but it does not mean that our quality and value of life get completely impaired as we grow older. It is important to understand the positive aspects of ageing as well. It has been reported that we age well when we have a positive attitude towards it, we have a sense of independence, we adopt a healthy lifestyle, there is a purpose in life, and we are active socially, etc. We all need to remember that age is just a number. So, we need to forget our age in order to lead a positive and fruitful life. Each moment of life that passes away will not come again. So, live that moment to the best. In fact, these are the golden years of life.

Following are certain myths related to ageing and the realities behind each.

Myth 1: *Loneliness is normal and is expected in older people.*
As people age, some may find themselves feeling lonely. Certain factors like the changed family system of the nuclear family, the children going out for their professional carrier, and on top of that, in old age, there could be the loss of a life partner, it is true that older people have the feeling of Empty Nests. But many of the older people can volunteer themselves in various social activities, involve in various household chores like gardening, care for grandchildren, and spend quality time with friends of their own age, etc. Even they can devote more to their relationships with their relatives or friends, which they were not able to do when they were in their jobs and working full-time and even were busy raising their kids. Many wish to remarry with their new eligible partners. All of these can prevent loneliness in them.

Myth 2: *My genes will determine my longevity.*
It is true to some extent that the longevity, family history of certain disorders, etc., will mirror that of the blood relations (parents, grandparents, siblings, or other blood relations). But we can remain healthy if we have a healthy lifestyle with respect to diet, sleep hygiene, regular exercise, avoiding alcohol/smoking/stress, etc. So, if we adopt healthy habits and stick to them throughout our life, we will improve our chances of living longer.

Myth 3: *Getting old is a synonym for weak/frail/feeble/sick individual, etc.*
With age, there are certain physiological changes that happen for sure. But this is also a fact that if we stay active with age, we can remain fit throughout the tenure of our life. It is all about the lifelong maintenance of our health. In fact, healthy lifestyle habits should start from childhood itself, so that a person develops those habits forever to be continued throughout life. Osteoporosis may affect both men and women. But it can be preventable and treatable. Exercising will also maintain a healthy weight in elderly people.

Myth 4: *Depression is normal and is expected in older adults.*
These are the mood disorders that can happen at any age. Very effective treatments are available for all these disorders. Depression, anxiety, sadness, etc., are not as such a normal part of ageing. Even if these are there, most of the elderly have less obvious symptoms and are less likely to discuss such kind of feelings. By this age, they become too contended and patient. It has been reported that elderly people are less likely to experience depression than young adults. They usually have long-lasting relationships with their friends

and family. They have a plethora of lifetime memories to share with their loved ones to give them happiness.

Myth 5: *Older people need less sleep.*
It is a common misconception that there is a decline in sleeping hours in older persons. However, this is not a fact. They all need the same about 7–9 hours of sleep as all adults. Getting enough sleep, and maintaining sleep hygiene also helps reduce the risk of falls in the elderly. It has been seen that if they have the habit of getting up early in the morning during the earlier/adult years of life, they continue with the same routine in this new inning of their life period. In fact, such kinds of habits keep them fit and healthy both physically and mentally.

Myth 6: *Older adults end with their cognitive development and can't learn new things.*
Many people are of the opinion that elderly people cannot learn new things. It is true that there could be some changes in their thinking and cognition, but still, they have the ability to learn. It has been reported that cognitive development continues throughout life. Trying and learning new skills may even improve their cognitive abilities. Pursuing new interests, and learning new skills, that stimulate the brain can help to improve their cognitive ability and memory. They should consider taking up a new hobby, learning a new language, gardening, cooking, photography, brain games, or even mindful meditation to stimulate their brain and bring joy to their daily routine.

Myth 7: *Older people definitely have some memory disorders or dementia or Alzheimer's disease.*
Many people worry about having memory loss or certain disorders like Alzheimer's disease and dementia with age. Some forgetfulness is not uncommon as we age. It is normal. However, dementia is not a normal part of ageing. Although its risk increases with age, it is not certain that all older individuals are going to get it. Many people live long without the significant declines in thinking and behavior that characterize dementia. The causes of dementia may be different, some of which may be treatable or reversible and accordingly management can be done.

Regarding Alzheimer's disease, if there is a family history of the disease, there could be more risk of having this disease. Environmental and lifestyle factors, such as exercise, diet, exposure to pollutants, and smoking also may affect a person's risk for Alzheimer's. While one cannot control the genes one inherits from their parents but can take steps to stay healthy, such as getting regular exercise, controlling high blood pressure, and not smoking, etc.

Myth 8: *Older adults should not exercise, because of more prone to injury.*
Because of more prevalence of osteoporosis in elderly people, there could be some fear of injury while exercising. Some of the elderly people, because of the inactivity, land up into some problems. Engaging in some form of exercise and being active, could be very beneficial for elderly people to maintain physical and mental health. These can help in the prevention of obesity, diabetes, hypertension, and many other non-communicable diseases. These will improve bone health and balance. Having strong bones and muscles, good balance, and overall good health will prevent falls in the elderly which is extremely important because sometimes it can be very devastating. Moreover, moving out of the home for a walk, or exercise can also increase social interaction with others.

Myth 9: *Older people will have to give up driving.*
There could be some constraints like diminished vision, hearing problems, slow speed of driving, etc., but age is not the criterion to give up driving. Even age is not the criterion to learn driving. Many people have been seen learning to drive after superannuation. This enhances their confidence to be self-dependence.

THEORIES OF AGEING

Ageing is a universal, ongoing, time-related alteration of the physiological functions of the body. It is not reducible to any single cause but is a multifactorial process involving the sequence of events happening from conception to the death of an individual. It is defined as "the progressive accumulation of damage over time, leading to disturbed function on the cellular, tissue, and organ level and eventually to disease and death". It is a multifactorial process where genetic, endogenous, and environmental factors play a role.

There are more than three hundred theories of ageing explaining and exploring various dimensions of ageing. But it has been seen that a single theory does not explain all the aspects of ageing. Rather, many theories may be combined to explain various dimensions of this complex phenomenon of ageing. In the current chapters, the important theories of ageing are discussed under three main headings, i.e., Biological; Social; and Psychological **(Flowchart 46.1)**.

I. Biological Theories

These theories talk about the basic questions regarding the physiologic processes happening in all living organisms over a period as they age. Various biological theories are discussed as follows:

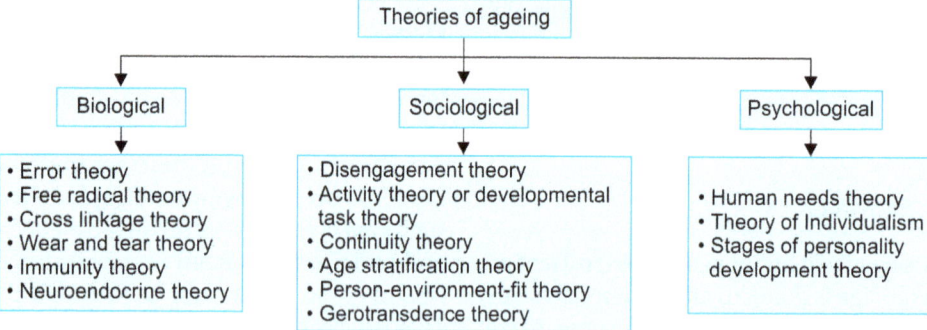

Flowchart 46.1: Theories of ageing.

- **Errors theory:** This theory was proposed by Dr Leslie Orgel in 1963. Orgel suggested that "an error in the machinery for making protein could be catastrophic." So, in this context, this is also known as Error Catastrophe Theory. This theory is based on the idea that the production of proteins and the reproduction of DNA sometimes are not carried out with accuracy. Errors can occur in the transcription of the synthesis of DNA with respect to not copying the original one. So, it is likely that the next transcription would again contain an error. The body's DNA is so vital that the natural repair processes kick in when an error is made. However, each time, perfect repairs on these molecules may not be possible. The accumulation of these flawed molecules can cause diseases and other age-related changes. With the continued effect through several generations of proteins, the end product may not even resemble the original cell and its functional ability would be decreased **(Fig. 46.5)**. This ultimately leads to either the ageing or the actual death of a cell.

- **Free radical theory:** This theory was proposed initially by Denham Harman, an American scientist in the 1950s. This is one of the most popular theories of ageing. This theory suggests that ageing is the cumulative result of oxidative damage to the cells and tissues of the body caused by free radicals produced primarily as a result of aerobic metabolism. When these byproducts accumulate, they damage the cell membrane, which decreases its efficiency. Free radicals are atoms or molecules that have at least one unpaired electron and are therefore highly unstable and highly reactive. In order to gain their stability, they take electrons from other atoms **(Fig. 46.6)**. If this continues to happen, it begins a process called oxidative stress. This oxidative stress can damage the body's cells, leading to a range of diseases and causing symptoms of ageing. **Free radicals** and other reactive oxygen species (ROS) are produced during normal cell metabolism in the human body as well as exposure to exogenous sources such as tobacco smoke, pesticides, radiation, excessive alcohol, air pollution, industrial chemicals, excessive fried foods, etc. Free radicals break cells down over time **(Fig. 46.7)**. As the body ages, it loses its ability to fight the effects of free radicals. The result is more free radicals, more oxidative stress, and more damage to cells, which lead to degenerative processes, as well as "normal" ageing. So, free radicals are linked to ageing and a host of diseases. They are responsible for damage associated with ageing. The body produces antioxidants that scavenge the free radicals. Antioxidants are important to fight all the free radicals. Antioxidants are also known as "free radical scavengers." With ageing the antioxidant systems are unable to counterbalance all the free radicals continuously generated during the life of the cell. Antioxidants are chemicals that interact with and neutralize free radicals, thus preventing them from causing damage.

- **Cross linkage theory:** This theory was first proposed in 1942 by Johan Bjorksten. This theory is also known as connective tissue theory. With age, it has been theorized that some proteins in the body become cross-linked, entangled, and trapped inappropriately leading to irreversible protein structural changes and thereby altered protein functioning. Normal activities of the body get impaired and the waste products start accumulating in the cells. The cross-linking hypothesis is based on the observation that with age, our proteins, DNA, and other structural molecules develop inappropriate attachments or cross-links to one another. These unnecessary links or bonds decrease the mobility or elasticity of proteins and other molecules. Elastin dries up and crack with age. For example, the changes associated with ageing skin. The skin of a baby is very soft and pliable, whereas the ageing skin losses much of its suppleness and elasticity. The theorist applied this theory to ageing diseases such as sclerosis, a declining immune system, and the loss of elasticity in the skin.

- **Wear-and-tear theory:** Dr August Weismann, a German biologist, introduced this theory in 1882. It hypothesizes that ageing is the result of use. This theory equates man

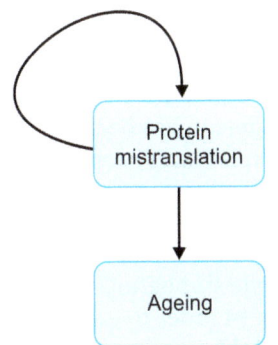

Fig. 46.5: Error theory of ageing.

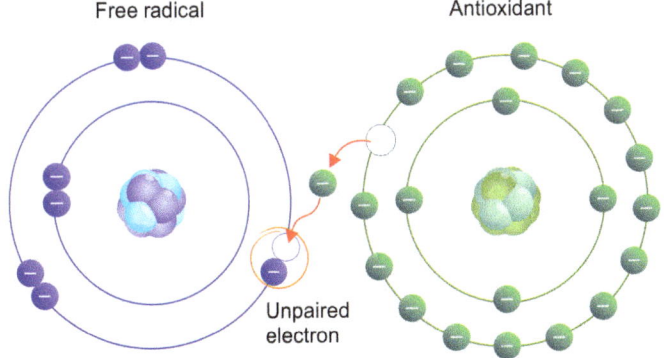

Fig. 46.6: Free radicals.

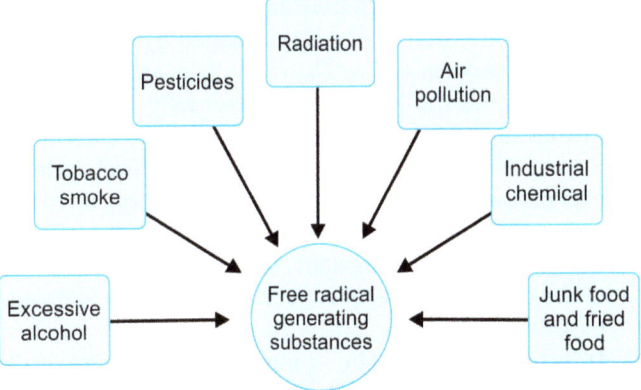

Fig. 46.7: Free radical generating substances.

with machine. Just as a machine gets worn out with use, similarly the body cells get damaged by overuse and abuse. The worn-out will be more if we are more prone to toxins internally as well as externally. The theorist further suggested that wear and tear are not confined to the organs; it also takes place at the cellular level. All living organisms have a limited amount of energy available to them. It ultimately gets worn out when the allotted energy ends and eventually, there will be death of the entire organism when it is not possible for the worn-out tissue to recover.

- ❖ **Immunity theory:** The immune system is one of the important systems of our body. It is composed of different organs, cells, tissues, and proteins that work together to protect our body. It has a vital role to protects our body from harmful substances, and germs (bacteria, viruses, fungi, and toxins), by differentiating self from non-self. The function of the immune system peaks at around puberty and thereafter gradually starts declining with the advancement in age. However, it undergoes dramatic ageing-related changes after around the sixth decade of our life. Thereafter, the ability of the immune system to protect against infections and other diseases gets impaired. This age-related decrease in functions of the body is immunosenescence.

  The T and B cells, both are vital components of the immune system. Both these cells protect our body from the attack of the organisms, though one may provide more protection in certain situations. T cells are responsible for cell-mediated immunity and help protect the body from infection and cancer by destroying the infected and the cancerous cells. B cells also called B lymphocytes create a type of protein called antibody. These antibodies are responsible for humoral immunity. As a result of ageing, the changes occur most specifically with the T lymphocytes. This change makes an individual more vulnerable to disease. Changes also occur in the functioning capabilities of B-lymphocytes. So, with age, there is a decrease in the body's defense against foreign organisms, thus, there is an increased incidence of various infectious as well as other diseases.

- ❖ **Neuroendocrine theory:** This theory was described in the year 1954 by Dr Vladimir Dilman, a Russian scientist. This theory of ageing states that "The effectiveness of the body's homeostatic adjustments declines with ageing leading to the failure of adaptive mechanisms, ageing, and death." The neuroendocrine system releases hormones in the general circulation. They travel throughout the body to act on body tissues wherever their receptors are located. Hypothalamus is a small but very important part of the brain. It acts as a coordinating center and also maintains the body's internal balance. It instructs the other organs and glands to release their hormones. It also responds to the body's hormone levels as a guide to the overall hormonal activity. But as we grow old the hypothalamus loses its functions of regulation. So, the hormones which are very important for repairing and regulating bodily functions, their secretions are reduced which leads to a decline in the body's ability to repair and regulate itself as well.

II. Sociological Theories

Sociologic theories focus on the changing roles and relationships wherein people are engaged in their later life. These also relate to various social adaptations in the lives of older adults. This can also be viewed within the context of the societal values in which they were developed.

Various sociological theories are elaborated as follows:

- ❖ **Disengagement theory:** Cumming and Henry introduced this theory in 1961. This theory suggests that with ageing, many of the relationships between a person and other members of society are detached as well as for many there is an alteration in the quality of relationships. New types of relationships are developed with the society. The withdrawal of the relationship may be partial or total. But it is also true that a large number of older people do not withdraw from society. So, this theory is controversial in this context and is not much supported.

- ❖ **Activity theory or developmental task theory:** As per this theory, involvement in various social activities is very important to maintain personal life satisfaction and a positive self-concept. By remaining active, adopting new roles, and showing their involvement as per their physical and intellectual capability, they stay young and do not withdraw from society. This theory is based on the assumptions that it is better to be active throughout our life instead of becoming inactive; it is extremely important to be happy than unhappy. It is also said that an older individual is the best judge of his or her own success in achieving these two assumptions. Practicing all these can help an older person remain active, thereby achieving a sense of life satisfaction.

- ❖ **Continuity theory:** Old age should not be regarded as a terminal part of the life cycle. It cannot be separated from the rest of life. It should be considered an integral component of the entire life cycle. This theory proposes that this new inning of life (entering old age) is a continuation of the earlier part of the elderly people. It also emphasizes that continuation through the remainder part of life is how a person has been throughout his previous life. It recommends that as people age, they try to maintain or continue previous habits, preferences, commitments, values, beliefs, and all the factors that have contributed to their personalities. So, it is better that all individuals follow a healthy lifestyle throughout their life before entering into this inning in order to enjoy a better quality of life throughout their life.

- ❖ **Age stratification theory:** This theory was started in the 1970s. The key societal issue being addressed in this theory is the concept of interdependence between the ageing person and society at large. This theory is only one example of a theory addressing societal values. This theory views an elderly person as an individual and an important part of society. The theory attempts to explain the interdependence between older adults and society and how they are constantly influencing each other in a variety of ways. Riley (1985) identifies the five major concepts of this theory: "(1) each individual progresses through society in groups of cohorts that are collectively ageing socially, biologically, and psychologically; (2) new cohorts are continually being born, and each of them experiences their own unique sense of history; (3) society itself can be divided into various strata according to the parameters of age and roles; (4) not only are people and roles within every stratum continuously changing, but so is society at large; and (5) the interaction between individual ageing people and the entire society is not stagnant but remains dynamic."

- ❖ **Person-environment-fit theory:** This theory was proposed by Lawton (1982). It examines the concept of interrelationships among the competencies of a group of persons, older adults, and their society or environment. Everyone, including older persons, has certain personal competencies that help mold and shape them throughout life. Lawton identified these personal competencies as including ego strength; level of motor skills, individual biologic health, and cognitive and sensory-perceptual capacities. Ego strength is the ability of an individual to manage the demands of the id, the superego, and reality. All of these help a person deal with the environment in which he/she lives. As a person ages, there may be changes or even decrease in some of these personal competencies. These changes influence the individual's ability to interrelate with the environment. If a person develops one or more chronic diseases, such as rheumatoid arthritis or cardiovascular disease, then competencies may be impaired and the level of interrelatedness may be limited. The theory further proposes that, as a person ages, the environment becomes more threatening and one may feel incompetent dealing with it.
- ❖ **Gerotransdence theory:** This theory was proposed by Lars Tornstam in 1989. This is also named a developmental theory of positive ageing. It is composed of two words: Gero which means 'old' and transcendence refers to 'rising above'. Thus, this theory focuses on two phenomena: the old person and the ageing process itself. The theory describes both the experience of growing old and the characteristics of a normal and positive old age. It explains ageing from a psychosocial perspective. It is regarded as the final stage of life in a natural progression toward maturation and wisdom and also describes the development of an individual regarding new understandings of the self and relationships with others. This theory also emphasizes that with age an individual might experience a decreased interest in material things and a greater need for meditation. According to Tornstam (1997), "It is a shift in meta-perspective from a materialistic and rational view of the world to a more cosmic and transcendent one, normally followed by an increase in life satisfaction". Individuals have less fear of death and a new understanding of life and death.

III. Psychological Theories

The psychological theories of ageing involve the psychological changes that are the result of ageing, just like the physiological changes are related to biological theories of ageing. Distinguishing psychological theories from other theories of ageing such as social, biological, and psychosocial is very difficult. Theoretically, the differentiation might be done, however, practically, it might not be possible because of the overlapping of many concepts of ageing. Further, to make it clear, just like an individual's "psyche" cannot be analyzed in isolation, one should not make assumptions about individuals without taking into account their immediate social, cultural, and historical context. Also, psychological theories are controlled and influenced by biology and sociology.

Various psychological theories are discussed as follows:

- ❖ **Human needs theory of ageing:** This theory was proposed by Maslow, a psychologist (1954). In this theory, Maslow has inferred that human behavior is motivated by their five needs with age. These are "physiological, safety and security, love and belongingness, self-esteem, and actualization" having different orders of priority **(Fig. 46.8)**. All these five human needs are shown as a pyramid with the most basic needs at the base which are related to physiologic needs and is required for the basic survival of a person. Of utmost importance is the need for food which is required to survive. Because until this need is not met, the other needs become meaningless. After fulfilling this need, the next apprehension is about safety and security which is also important at least to some extent, before going to the next needs of love, acceptance, and a feeling of belonging, self-esteem, and actualization which are there in the pyramid as we go up. Maslow asserted that failure to grow leads to feelings of failure, depression, and the perception that life is meaningless.

  Further, it has been emphasized by the author that when an individual achieves the fulfillment of their basic needs, they attempt to the next level. This process is continued till the highest order of needs is grasped. The self-actualized person displays high levels of "perception of reality; acceptance of self, others, and nature; spontaneity; problem-solving ability; self-direction; detachment and the desire for privacy; the freshness of peak experiences; identification with other human beings; satisfying and changing relationships with other people; a democratic character structure; creativity; and a sense of values". It has also been said that only about 1% of the population is the ideal self-actualized person.

- ❖ **Theory of individualism:** This theory was proposed by Carl Jung who was a Swiss psychologist in 1960. Jung defined individuation, the therapeutic goal of analytical psychology belonging to the second half of life, as the process by which a person becomes a psychological individual, a separate indivisible unity or whole, recognizing his innermost uniqueness. Jung proposed a theory of personality development throughout all the phases of life (childhood, youth, young adulthood, middle age, and old age). According to this theory, a person's personality could be either extroverted or introverted. A balance between these two is important to maintain mental health. As the person ages chronologically, the personality often begins to change from being outwardly focused, and concerned about establishing oneself in society, to becoming more inward, as the individual begins to search for answers from within. Successful ageing, when viewed from Jung's theory, is when a person

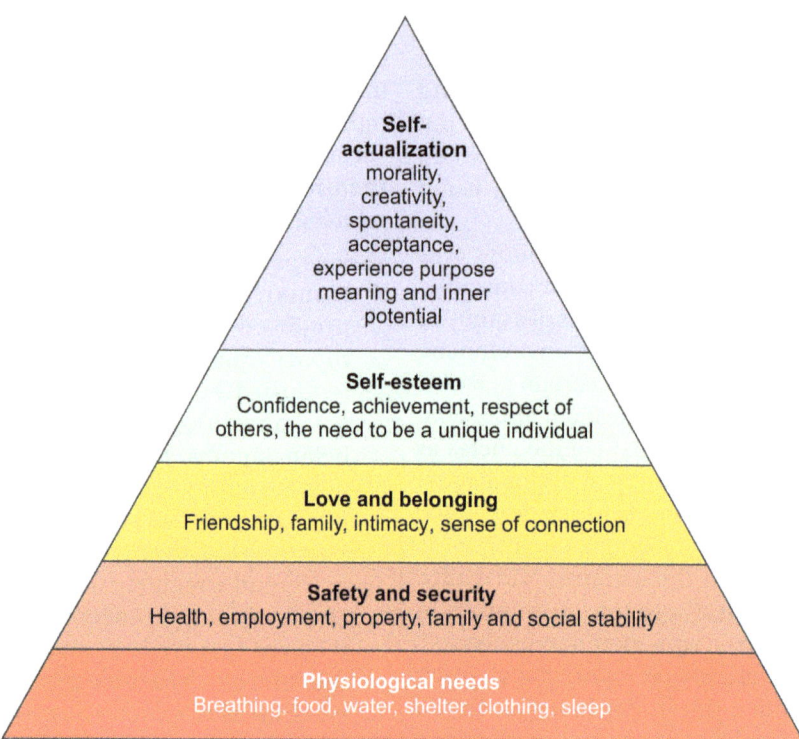

Fig. 46.8: Maslow's hierarchy of needs.

looks inward and values oneself for more than just current physical limitations or losses. The individual accepts past accomplishments and limitations.

As individuals age, they begin to reflect on their beliefs and life accomplishments. According to Jung, one age successfully when he/she accepts the past, adapts to physical decline, and cope with the loss of significant others. Introspection is a part of healthy ageing.

Applying Jung's theory to individuals as they progress through life, it is at the onset of middle age that the person begins to question values, beliefs, and possible dreams left undone. The phrase "midlife crisis" became popular based on this theory and refers to a period of emotional, and sometimes behavioral, the turmoil that heralds the onset of middle age. This period may last for several years, with the exact time and duration varies from person to person. During this period, the individual often searches for answers about reaching goals-questioning whether a part of their personality or "true self" has been neglected and whether time is running out for the completion of these quests.

❖ **Stages of personality development theory:** The theory was proposed by Erik Erikson in 1963. It specifically focuses on one's personality development. This theory states that personality develops in eight distinct stages from birth to death **(Fig. 46.9)**. Each stage is associated with a life task at which one may succeed or fail. The last stage, ego integrity vs. despair, begins at age 65 and continues until death. In this stage, older adults search for the meaning of their lives and evaluate the accomplishments of their lives. From this period of introspection, feelings of satisfaction lead to integrity, while dissatisfaction creates a sense of despair (Erikson, 1963). Older adults specifically face additional

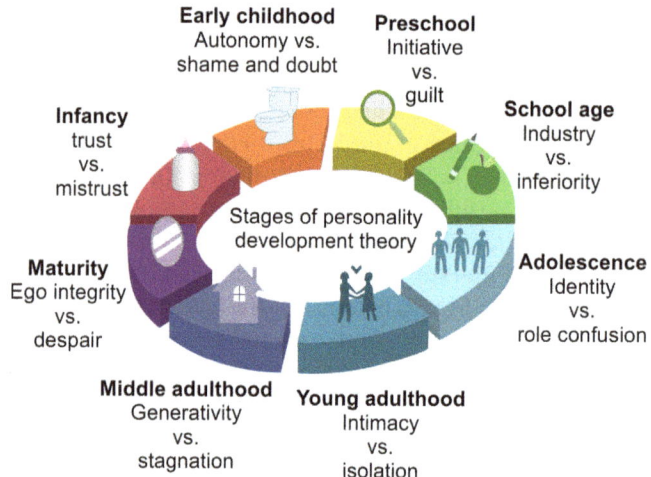

Fig. 46.9: Erikson' stages of personality development.

challenges or life tasks including physical and mental decline, accepting the care of others, and detaching from life. Theorists of the stages of personality development define "integrity vs. despair" to include three more challenges: creating a meaningful life after retirement, dealing with an empty nest as children move away, and contemplating the inevitability of death. The stages of personality development theory are widely employed in the behavioral sciences. In nursing, this model is used as a framework to examine the challenges faced by different age groups. Research has found that older adults who expressed elevated levels of energy and meaning in life described a sense of connectedness, self-worth, love, and respect that was absent among participants who felt unfulfilled.

Case Scenario

A 70-year-old female expressed that she wanted to be involved with a community program for females in her village. But the family members restricted her to participate in any of the outdoor activities because they consider her weak and vulnerable to injury while going out to participate in such activities. They are of the opinion that older adults should be limiting their social participation. However, it is important to understand that such types of restrictions may lead to loneliness and social disengagement in the elderly. So, there is an urgent need to tackle loneliness in old age. The value of social participation, with emphasis on community-based activities and interpersonal interactions, is imperative.

SUMMARY

Life at any age can be gratifying and rewarding. However, many of us resist the thought of growing older. However, numerous welcome this phase of old age very gracefully. It is important to understand that wisdom comes with age, which gives us the ability to make smart choices to make our mind and body healthy. The elderly population in India is increasing at a fast pace. Growing older is synonymous with going nearer towards many unwanted realities. Ageing is a gradual but inevitable process of life. It involves the degeneration of the structure and function of organisms. With advancing age, elderly people may have to face many biopsychosociological challenges which may not be much evident in the beginning but later begins to be more pronounced. These may differ from person to person. There are many myths about ageing, but the reality is that if you are physically, socially, and psychologically healthy, you will be fit to fight any of the untoward incidence related to ageing. There are a number of theories of ageing. Many ageing theories need to be combined to explain various dimensions of ageing because a single theory does not explain all the aspects of ageing.

MULTIPLE CHOICE QUESTIONS

1. What is the expected percentage of elderly Worldwide by 2030?
   a. 6%
   b. 8%
   c. 10%
   d. 12%
2. What is the expected percentage of elderly in India by 2031?
   a. 7%
   b. 9%
   c. 11%
   d. 13%
3. In India which state outnumbered with regard to the elderly population in 2021?
   a. Kerala
   b. Tamil Nadu
   c. Himachal Pradesh
   d. Punjab
4. Who proposed the error theory of ageing?
   a. Dr Leslie Orgel
   b. Dr Denham Harman
   c. Dr Johan Bjorksten
   d. Dr August Weismann
5. Which of the following ageing theories suggests that ageing is the cumulative result of oxidative damage to the cells and tissues of the body?
   a. Error theory
   b. Free radical theory
   c. Cross linkage theory
   d. Immunity theory
6. Which of the following ageing theory is also known as connective tissue theory?
   a. Cross linkage theory
   b. Wear-and-tear theory
   c. Neuroendocrine theory
   d. Free radical theory
7. Which of the following ageing theory equates man with the machine?
   a. Disengagement theory
   b. Wear-and-tear theory
   c. Error theory
   d. Continuity theory
8. Which of the following ageing theories is also named as developmental theory of positive ageing?
   a. Person-environment-fit theory
   b. Gerotransdence theory
   c. Age stratification theory
   d. Continuity theory
9. The human needs theory of ageing is categorized under which of the following domains of theories?
   a. Biological theories
   b. Social theories
   c. Psychological theories
   d. Moral theories
10. Who proposed the theory of individualism?
    a. Dr Abraham Harold Maslow
    b. Dr Carl Jung
    c. Dr Erik Erikson
    d. Dr Lars Torstam

ANSWERS

1. d	2. d	3. a	4. a
5. b	6. a	7. b	8. b
9. c	10. b		

SUGGESTED READING

1. Birren JE, Cunningham WR. Research on the psychology of aging: Principles, concepts and theory. In: JE Birren and KW Schaie (Eds). Handbook of Aging and Psychology (pp. 3–34). Van Nostrand Reinhold; 1985.
2. Elderly in India 2021. Government of India, Ministry of Statistics and Programme Implementation, National Statistics Office, Social Statistics Division, www.mospi.gov.in
3. http://www.transgenerational.org/aging/demographics.htm#ixzz197ovW51L, retrieved on 25th Dec 2010
4. https://www.un.org/en/desa/india-overtake-china-world-most-populous-country-april-2023-united-nations-projects
5. Kaur S, Singh AJ, Kumari S, Bhalla A. Assessment of functional status and daily life problems faced by elderly in a North Indian city. Psychogeriatrics. 2019. doi:10.1111/psyg.12406.
6. Rajan SI, Sarma PS, Mishra US. Demography of Indian aging, 2001-2051. J Aging Soc Policy. 2003;15(2-3):11-30. doi: 10.1300/J031v15n02_02.
7. Rudnicka E, Napierała P, Podfigurna A, Męczekalski B, Smolarczyka R, Grymowicz M. The World Health Organization (WHO) approach to healthy ageing. Maturitas. 2020;139:6-11.
8. Sharma S, Thakur M, Kaur S. Assessment of dependency level in the performance of activities of daily living amongst elderly in a suburban population of India. International Journal of Nursing Education. 2012;4(1):94-6.
9. Vina J, Borras C, Miquel J. Critical review-Theories of ageing. IUBMB Life. 2007;59 (4-5):249-54.

Age-related Body System Changes and Common Health Problems in Elderly

Manjeet Singh, Alisha Talwar, Sukhpal Kaur

"Do not be afraid of ageing. It is inevitable. Adopting a healthy lifestyle will facilitate ageing gracefully".
—**Sukhpal**

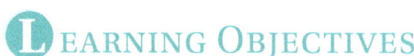 Learning Objectives

After going through the chapter, the learner will be able to:
- Understand the age-related body system changes.
- Enumerate the common age-related health problems.
- Discuss system-wise problems in the elderly.

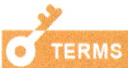 **TERMS**

- **Cognitive changes:** Changes in thinking, remembering things, etc., with age.
- **Emotional well-being:** Emotional experiences influenced by various life events and social relationships.
- **Physical changes:** Changes in the skin, hair, muscle mass, bone density, and sensory perception, etc., with age.
- **Senescent bone loss:** Bone loss with ageing.

INTRODUCTION

Ageing is a universal and irreversible process that all living beings go through. It involves changes in the body and mind over time, leading to a gradual decline in various physiological functions which is associated with several health conditions like hypertension, cardiovascular disease, osteoporosis, diabetes, cancer, and dementia apart from many other diseases. Multiple morbidities are quite common in this age which further multiply the complexity of health problems compromising the quality of life of an individual in old age. While ageing is a normal part of life, its pace and impact can vary from person to person. Factors such as genetics, lifestyle, and environment can influence the ageing process.

The current chapter elaborates on the age-related body system changes, subsequent to which, various related disorders are summarized. For a detailed description of each disorder, kindly refer to the related chapter also.

CARDIOVASCULAR SYSTEM

Myocardial muscle cells gradually decrease in number while cell volume increases, leading to a reduction in fat cells and fibrous tissues. Consequently, the heart becomes flabbier and less robust. The heart valves experience thickening, lose their elasticity, and may undergo calcification. This process could result in a decline in the discharge of the SA node and disturbances in the atrioventricular (AV) system **(Fig. 47.1)**.

Cardiac impulse generation and conductivity may remain normal, but the duration of contraction and relaxation is prolonged. However, due to ischemic changes or otherwise, SA node and other conducting tissues may also become dysfunctional requiring artificial impulse generation. Cardiovascular reflexes are blunted especially heart rate in response to hypotension or orthostasis. These reflexes are because of decreased β-adrenergic responsiveness.

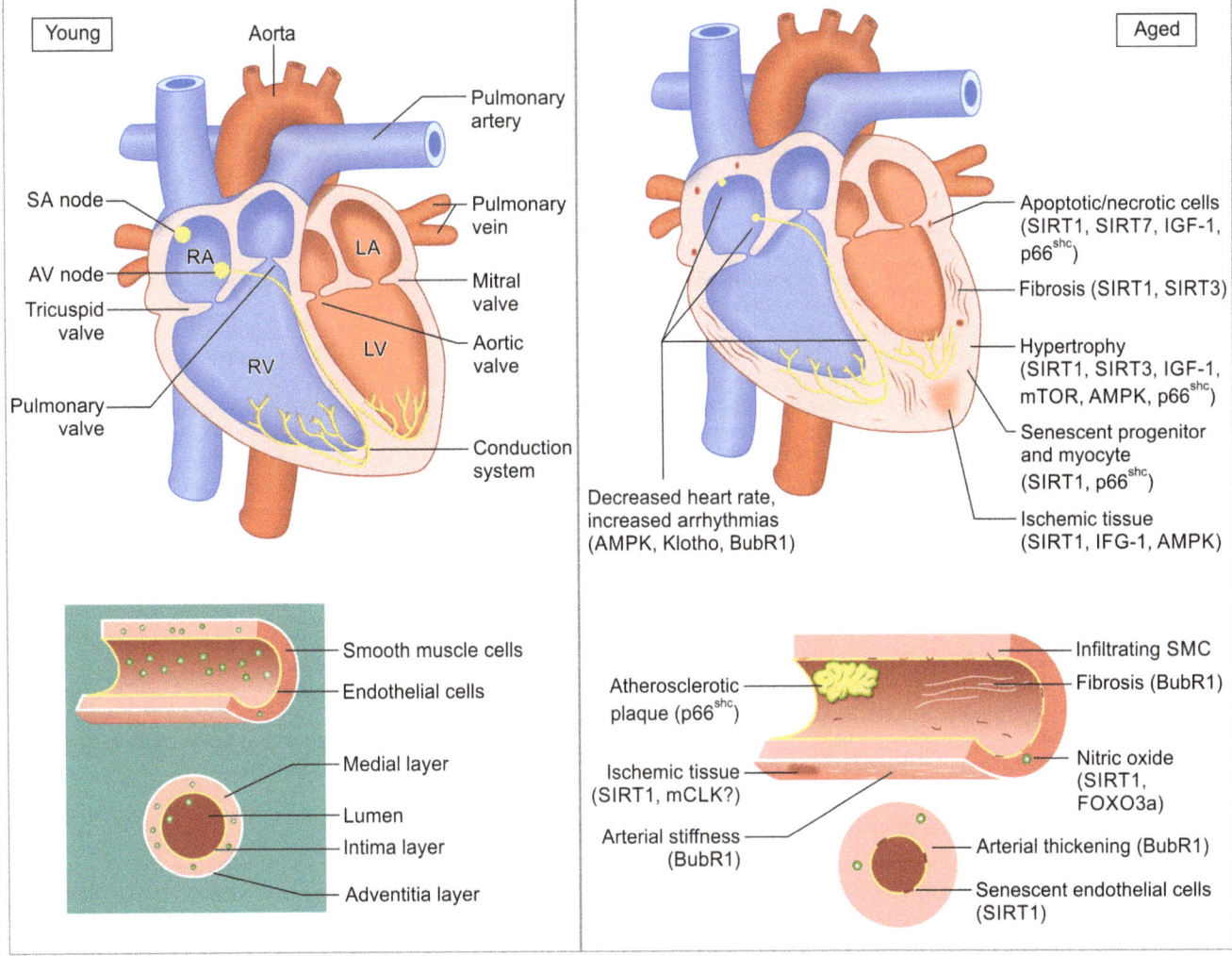

Fig. 47.1: Age-related changes in the cardiovascular system.

The other cardiovascular age-related changes are:
- ❖ **Structural changes:**
  - ➢ *Cardiac muscle:* The heart muscles may thicken or become stiffer over time, which can affect the heart's ability to pump blood efficiently.
  - ➢ *Heart size:* The heart may slightly increase in size with age, particularly the left ventricle.
- ❖ **Changes in heart rate and rhythm:**
  - ➢ *Resting heart rate:* Resting heart rate may slightly decrease with age.
  - ➢ *Arrhythmias:* Older adults may be more prone to develop irregular heart rhythms (arrhythmias).
- ❖ **Cardiac output:** The heart's ability to pump blood may decrease with age.
- ❖ **Blood pressure:** Blood pressure tends to increase with age, and hypertension is more common in older adults.
- ❖ **Exercise tolerance:** Older adults may experience a decline in exercise tolerance due to reduced cardiac reserve.
- ❖ **Baroreceptor sensitivity:** Baroreceptors, which help regulate blood pressure, may become less sensitive with age, affecting blood pressure regulation.

These age-related changes in the cardiovascular system can contribute to an increased risk of cardiovascular diseases and conditions, such as hypertension, atherosclerosis, heart failure, and arrhythmias **(Table 47.1)**. It is important for older adults to be proactive in maintaining heart health through lifestyle modifications, regular exercise, a heart-healthy diet, manageing blood pressure and cholesterol levels, avoiding smoking, and seeking appropriate medical care. Regular check-ups with healthcare professionals can help monitor and address any potential cardiovascular issues as individuals age.

RESPIRATORY SYSTEM

In the larger airways and bronchi, a decline in the number of glandular epithelial cells results in reduced production of protective mucus, increasing the susceptibility to infections. In the smaller airways and air spaces, the loss of supportive elastin and collagen causes the widening of alveolar ducts and air spaces, leading to senile emphysema. Although the alveoli become larger, their overall count decreases, resulting in a diminished alveolar surface area and less efficient gas exchange. Age-related alterations in muscle structure led to weakened respiratory muscles, contributing to reduced strength.

The thoracic cage undergoes stiffening and rigidity due to the ossification of costal cartilages and the development of spinal kyphosis, which further impedes proper ventilation. The body's respiratory responses to both low oxygen levels

TABLE 47.1: Age-related cardiovascular conditions.

Disorders	Management
Hypertension	
<ul><li>Most common health problem in old age and it is more prevalent in older adults compared to younger age groups. As individuals age, the risk of developing hypertension increases due to various factors, including changes in blood vessel elasticity and hormonal influences.</li><li>Undiagnosed and under-treatment are common.</li><li>Among the elderly population, there is a tendency for systolic blood pressure to rise more prominently compared to diastolic blood pressure. This phenomenon is referred to as isolated systolic hypertension and is prevalent among older individuals. Systolic blood pressure holds a higher degree of predictability for vascular events such as stroke, ischemic heart disease, congestive heart failure, renal failure, and mortality, surpassing the predictability of diastolic blood pressure.</li><li>HTN accelerates cognitive decline in the elderly which also hampers the management of other comorbid conditions. Hypertension is a significant risk factor for cardiovascular diseases such as heart attack, stroke, heart failure, and peripheral artery disease. The risk of these conditions further increases in the presence of other cardiovascular risk factors, such as high cholesterol, diabetes, and smoking.</li><li>Some older adults may experience "white coat hypertension," where their blood pressure readings are elevated when taken in a medical setting due to anxiety or stress. Regular blood pressure monitoring at home or over 24 hours may help differentiate between true hypertension and white-coat hypertension.</li></ul>	<ul><li>The appropriate management produces major benefits for the elderly and reduces the adverse consequences.</li><li>Managing hypertension in the elderly requires a comprehensive and individualized approach to promote cardiovascular health and overall well-being.</li><li>Lifestyle modification with salt restriction, weight control, lipid control and exercise are inseparable and the most important components of management.</li><li>The main goal is to achieve a blood pressure of <140/90 mm Hg.</li><li>Common drugs used for the management are: diuretics, calcium channel blockers (nifedipine, amlodipine, and clinidipine, etc.), ACEIs (angiotensin converting enzyme inhibitors like enalapril, lisinopril, ramipril, etc.)/ARBs (angiotensin receptor blockers e.g., losartan, telmisartan, olmesartan etc.), need-based β-blockers (bisoprolol, metoprolol, carvedilol, etc.), α-blockers and vasodilators, etc.</li><li>Common side effects of antihypertensive include:<ul><li>Pedal edema (calcium channel blockers)</li><li>Bradycardia, aggravation of asthma, and peripheral vascular disease (β-blockers)</li><li>Cough (ACEI)</li><li>Orthostatic fall of blood pressure (drugs like α-blockers, high dose diuretics and peripheral adrenergic blockers).</li><li>Centrally acting drugs like clonidine need caution regarding cognitive impairment.</li><li>α-blockers in addition have added advantages for prostatic hyperplasia, so common to elder males.</li></ul></li></ul>
Ischemic heart disease	
Ischemic heart disease, also known as coronary artery disease (CAD), is a common cardiovascular condition that affects many elderly individuals. It occurs when there is reduced blood flow to the heart muscle due to atherosclerosis, a build-up of plaque in the coronary arteries. As people age, the risk of developing ischemic heart disease increases due to various factors such as the cumulative effects of unhealthy lifestyle choices, genetics, and the natural ageing process. Symptoms of ischemic heart disease in the elderly:<ul><li>Chest pain or discomfort (angina) that may radiate to the arm, jaw, or back.</li><li>Shortness of breath.</li><li>Fatigue or weakness.</li><li>Dizziness or fainting.</li><li>Nausea.</li></ul>	Management of ischemic heart disease in the elderly:<ul><li>**Lifestyle modifications:** Encouraging elderly patients to adopt a healthy lifestyle is crucial. This includes quitting smoking, following a heart-healthy diet (low in saturated fats, cholesterol, and salt), maintaining a healthy weight, engaging in regular physical activity appropriate for their condition, and managing stress.</li><li>**Medications:** Several medications are commonly prescribed to elderly individuals with ischemic heart disease to manage their symptoms and reduce the risk of complications. These may include:<ul><li>Aspirin or other antiplatelet agents to reduce the risk of blood clots.</li><li>Beta-blockers to slow the heart rate and reduce its workload.</li><li>Statins to lower cholesterol levels.</li><li>Angiotensin-converting enzyme (ACE) inhibitors or angiotensin receptor blockers (ARBs) to control blood pressure and protect the heart.</li></ul></li><li>**Cardiac rehabilitation:** For elderly patients who have experienced a heart attack or undergone heart-related procedures, cardiac rehabilitation programs can be beneficial. These programs provide supervised exercise, education on heart-healthy living, and emotional support.</li><li>**Interventional procedures:** In some cases, elderly patients with severe coronary artery disease may benefit from procedures such as angioplasty and stent placement to open blocked arteries and restore blood flow. For some individuals, coronary artery bypass grafting (CABG) may be recommended.</li></ul>
Heart failure (HF)	
<ul><li>The incidence of heart failure grows exponentially with age. It affects about 2% of the adult population. However, above 65 years of age, the prevalence may be as high as 6–10%.</li><li>Due to the frequent use of diuretics for dependent edema in the elderly, HF may be underdiagnosed.</li><li>The relative incidence of HF though is less in women but because of longer life expectancy, they constitute at least half of the HF patients.</li></ul>	<ul><li>The management of heart failure in the elderly focuses on enhancing the outcomes associated with heart failure rather than solely addressing the underlying primary condition.</li><li>The prognosis needs to be discussed with the family with all the certainties of poor outcomes in spite of the best efforts.</li><li>With apparently comfortable results initially, HF eventually follows a downhill and progressive course which is quite a frustrating experience for the patient, the family as well as the treating physician.</li></ul>

Contd...

Contd...

Disorders	Management
<ul><li>Hypertension, coronary artery disease, diabetes mellitus, and valvular heart disease are the well-recognized causes of cardiac failure in old age.</li><li>Anemia, is a frequent association but is often ignored as the precipitating cause of HF.</li><li>The common symptoms of exertional dyspnea may be absent due to lack of physical efforts, especially in bedridden patients, and symptoms may be nonspecific in the form of fatigue, weakness, and tiredness.</li><li>On the other hand, fluid overload may be there in the absence of cardiac failure due to prolonged immobility, malnutrition, hypoproteinemia and venous insufficiency, etc.</li><li>HF carries a poor prognosis with a mortality of around 30–40% during the first year after the diagnosis and 60–70% within 5 years.</li></ul>	<ul><li>Renal functions and electrolytes need frequent monitoring.</li><li>Diuretics, which constitute an important constituent of the armamentarium to manage HF may not be well tolerated by the elderly.</li><li>ACEI/ARBs/Neprilysin inhibitors have a very useful role in HF and have survival benefits.</li><li>β-blockers, thought earlier to be contraindicated in HF have now proved to be the most important drugs in the fight against HF. Electrolyte imbalance in the form of hypo and hyperkalemia, hyponatremia, hypercalcemia as well as uremia and hyperglycemia are not uncommon.</li><li>Patients may have incontinence or retention of urine, postural and supine hypotension, hearing impairment and osteoporosis, etc. as a consequence of diuretic usage which needs observation and monitoring.</li></ul>
Syncope	
<ul><li>Syncope or fainting is not uncommon in old age. In fact, it may be an important initiating event ending in morbidity in a large number of elderly.</li><li>Syncope refers to a momentary loss of consciousness accompanied by a lack of control over one's posture, often leading to a fall. This condition is followed by a complete recovery without the need for medical intervention. Syncope occurs due to a brief interruption of cerebral function, caused by a sudden and temporary decrease in blood flow to the brain regions responsible for consciousness.</li><li>The onset of syncope can occur suddenly or be preceded by certain symptoms, which are referred to as presyncope. These symptoms include sweating, nausea, dizziness, light-headedness, a sensation of warmth, blurred vision, or momentary blackout.</li><li>It is important to differentiate syncope from seizures. Neurocardiogenic syncope can be precipitated by situations like hot or crowded environment, alcohol, extreme fatigue, severe pain, hunger, prolonged standing, and emotional or stressful situations. An episode may be prolonged by presyncope lasting seconds to minutes and may rarely occur in a supine position also.</li><li>Situational syncope can occur with cough especially prolonged coughing in patients of chronic obstructive airways disease (COAD), during or after micturition, especially in patients with BPH or other obstructive urinary disorders, and while straining in constipation. These activities are associated with Valsalva-like maneuvers resulting in decreased venous return to the heart. Due to increased intrathoracic and intracerebral pressure cerebral perfusion is decreased.</li><li>Cardiac syncope results from decreased cardiac output. The most common cause is arrhythmias (supraventricular and ventricular arrhythmias).</li><li>Other cardiac causes of syncope include myocardial infarction, aortic stenosis, cardiogenic shock, hypertrophic obstructive cardiomyopathy and other obstructive lesions, sick sinus syndrome, and AV blocks, and severe pulmonary hypertension.</li><li>Other important causes of syncope include carotid sinus syndrome, orthostatic hypotension, epilepsy, and transient ischemic attacks (TIAs). One also needs to differentiate syncope from accidental falls, seizures, dizziness, and vertigo. Syncope occurs due to reduced cerebral blood flow or vascular tone, or cerebrovascular accident (CVA). Anemia may be an important though often ignored co-morbidity. More than one cause will usually coexist in the elderly. Age-related changes in cerebral autoregulation, baroreflex sensitivity, and volume regulation make the elderly particularly vulnerable to syncope. Multiple age-related diseases, medication affecting blood circulation, altered control of gait and stance and cognitive dysfunction predispose as well as influence the outcome of syncope in the elderly.</li></ul>	<ul><li>It is generally assumed that syncope is the marker of underlying cardiovascular disease. However, syncope can manifest as a diverse range of conditions, varying from benign to potentially life-threatening. Despite thorough evaluations, the underlying cause of syncope remains unidentified in up to half of the cases. The manifestations and management of cardiovascular causes of syncope have been well characterized.</li><li>If the underlying cause of cerebral ischemia is corrected, the pre-syncope symptoms may resolve or otherwise they may persist for variable duration culminating into syncope.</li><li>These episodes usually occur in upright position and as soon as the causative factor is corrected or the person is made to lie in supine position (assisted or spontaneously as a result of fall), the patients start improving.</li><li>Circumstances and situations leading to neurocardiogenic syncope needs to be identified, evaluated, and corrected.</li><li>Treatment of situational syncope also involves managing the underlying cause.</li><li>The treatment of cardiac syncope may involve antiarrhythmic drugs, management of ischemia, anemia and pacemaker where required.</li><li>Syncope and falls hold significant significance in old age due to their potential to cause severe injuries, including fractures and intracranial bleeding. These injuries can lead to hospitalization, reduced mobility, and subsequent related complications. Furthermore, they can result in a loss of confidence and a decrease in independence among older individuals.</li><li>Prevention of fall in elderly is a subject in itself and all efforts, management strategies and underlying disease correction needs to be carefully planned to prevent falls in them.</li></ul>

Contd...

Contd...

Disorders	Management
Other conditions	
• These include peripheral vascular diseases (PVD), heart blocks, atrial fibrillation and other arrhythmias, pulmonary and cerebral thromboembolism, and aortic stenosis. PVD is the equivalent of IHD, and the general management is on the same lines. • Heart blocks may be a consequence of various cardiac diseases including IHD, Cardiomyopathy, or drug effect. • Atrial fibrillation may also be a result of various cardiac ailments affecting atria.	• Peripheral vascular disease needs to be managed on the pattern of cardiovascular disease with antiplatelets (aspirin, clopidogrel, ticaglor), statins (atorvastatin, rosuvastatin, etc.), and revascularization where possible. • Heart blocks are managed on the same pattern as in younger adults and may need pacemaker insertion. • Valvular diseases and other structural diseases, relatively asymptomatic, may become symptomatic as age advances and will need intervention. • Treatment of the basic diseases as well as control of heart rate is the aim while treating atrial fibrillation.

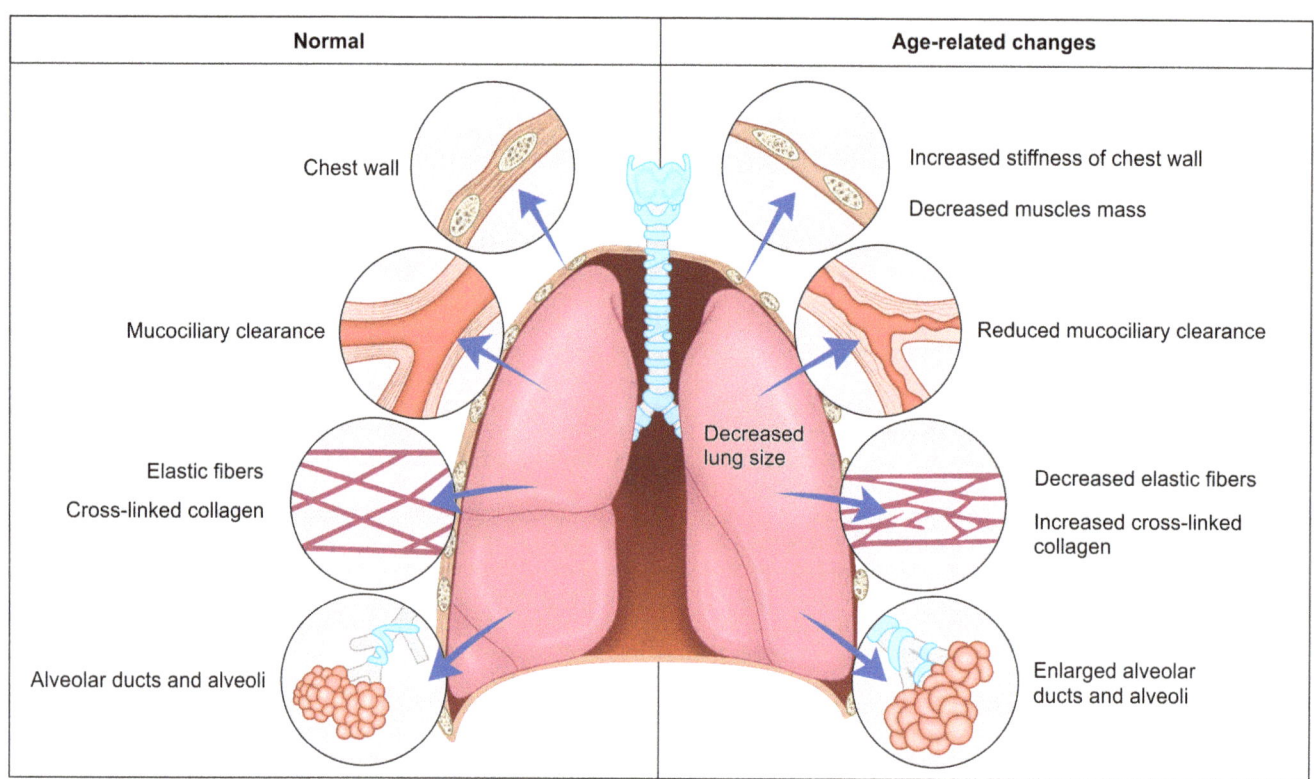

Fig. 47.2: Age-related changes in the respiratory system.

(hypoxia) and high carbon dioxide levels (hypercarbia) are dulled with advancing age. Additionally, the central control of breathing becomes impaired over time. A diminished cough reflex and impaired ciliary action create an environment conducive to bacterial colonization in the respiratory tract. These changes are exacerbated by factors such as smoking or exposure to air pollution, compounding their impact.

It is essential to note that while these age-related changes are common, not all older adults will experience the same respiratory changes, and many individuals maintain good respiratory health as they age **(Fig. 47.2)**. Maintaining a healthy lifestyle during youth and middle age goes a long way in the prevention of age-related organ dysfunction and maintaining performance levels. Yoga, breathing exercise, and avoiding active and passive smoking are very important in the maintenance of respiratory health. Engaging in regular physical activity, avoiding exposure to respiratory irritants (e.g., smoking and pollution), getting vaccinated against respiratory infections, and maintaining overall health through a healthy lifestyle can help support respiratory function and promote lung health in the elderly. Prevention of air pollution has an overall impact on the respiratory and overall health of humanity, the elderly in particular. Regular check-ups with healthcare professionals can help monitor respiratory health and address any specific concerns or conditions as individuals age.

Various age-related respiratory conditions are shown in **Table 47.2**.

GASTROINTESTINAL SYSTEM

The movement of food through the gastrointestinal (GI) tract slows down with age, which can lead to constipation and a higher risk of bowel obstruction. The production of stomach acid and digestive enzymes continues to decline in older adults, affecting digestion and nutrient absorption **(Fig. 47.3)**.

With age, the oral mucosal membrane also atrophies. Teeth are lost due to periodontal diseases and resorption of the mandible. The muscles of mastication become weak. The number of taste buds decreases causing diminished taste and smell sensations that can affect appetite and food intake in

TABLE 47.2: Age-related respiratory conditions.

Disorders	Management
Pneumonia	
<ul><li>Susceptibility to pneumonia in old age is increased due to poor cough reflex, reduced ciliary action, and immune system changes. 50% of old-age deaths are due to pneumonia.</li><li>After myocardial infarction and stroke, pneumonia is the third most common cause of hospitalization in the elderly.</li><li>Pneumonia is invariably a terminal event in old patients with cerebrovascular accidents, degenerative neuromuscular diseases, dementia, congestive cardiac failure, and malignancies. Nearly 1/3rd of elderly patients admitted with pneumonia die despite all advancements in treatment with antibiotics and intensive care. Pneumonia may be acquired at home or in a hospital while admitted for an unrelated illness. The place of infection decides the type of organism. *Streptococcus pneumoniae* and *Haemophilus influenzae* are common community-acquired organisms whereas gram-negative bacilli and *Staphylococcus aureus* are frequent hospital-acquired bacteria. The organisms responsible for hospital-acquired infections have higher virulence and multiple antibiotic resistance.</li><li>Pneumonia tends to present differently in the elderly compared to younger individuals, both in terms of its clinical symptoms and eventual outcomes. Classical signs of inflammation such as fever, rapid heart rate (tachycardia), and elevated white blood cell count (leukocytosis) may not always be evident in older patients. Many elderly patients already have some form of underlying health issue, with chronic obstructive airways disease (COAD) being the most common.</li><li>These distinctions become particularly important for individuals who live alone, as the disease can progress silently without the patient seeking medical attention. Moreover, in older adults, the progression and resolution of pneumonia tend to be slower, leading to extended hospital stays. The absence of fever, low blood pressure (hypotension), inadequate oxygen levels (hypoxia), and urinary incontinence are indicators of a poorer prognosis.</li><li>Respiratory infections, including pneumonia, carry a significantly higher mortality rate in the elderly compared to younger patients. This underscores the importance of careful monitoring, early medical intervention, and tailored management strategies for pneumonia in the elderly population.</li></ul>	<ul><li>Diagnosis of pneumonia is clinical, confirmed by X-ray. With the more frequent availability, CT scan adds to the diagnostic understanding of the underlying pathology and comorbidities. Bacteriological confirmation is usually difficult to achieve in most patients. As symptoms and X-ray features are nonspecific, treatment is aimed to empirically cover the common pathogens with beta-lactams and macrolides for ambulatory patients and parenteral antibiotics for hospitalized patients.</li><li>The presence of coexisting illnesses and complications of pneumonia generally influence the duration of antibiotic therapy. However, most of the organisms will require one to two weeks of treatment with initial three to six days of parenteral therapy. The presence of risk factors is an indication for hospitalization, e.g., age more than 65 years, COAD, diabetes, chronic renal failure, heart failure, dementia, liver diseases, tachypnea, hypotension, high fever, altered sensorium, leukopenia, hypoxia, uremia, etc., as these risk factors increase the mortality.</li></ul>
Tuberculosis	
<ul><li>Infection with *Mycobacterium tuberculosis* is widespread, although the prevalence of the disease varies among different populations due to socioeconomic factors. In the elderly, the prevalence of tuberculosis tends to be higher compared to younger individuals, primarily due to reactivation or reinfection as a result of declining immunity.</li><li>Unlike younger patients, elderly individuals with tuberculosis often do not display typical symptoms such as fever, night sweats, hemoptysis (coughing up blood), and persistent cough. Instead, they may present with nonspecific symptoms, and weight loss is a prominent feature. In contrast to the classic upper lobe lesions typically seen in younger patients, elderly patients often exhibit widespread and patchy infiltrates, as well as a form of tuberculosis known as miliary tuberculosis.</li><li>Tuberculin skin test is commonly used for diagnosing tuberculosis, may yield negative results in some elderly individuals. This further underscores the atypical nature of tuberculosis presentation in the ageing population.</li></ul>	<ul><li>Treatment is similar to that in younger subjects. Short-course chemotherapy preferably directly observed (DOTS) now available in all healthcare institutions in India is the preferred form of treatment with isoniazid: 5 mg/kg/day (4–6 mg), ethambutol: 15 mg/kg/day (12–18 mg), pyrazinamide: 25 mg/kg/day (20–30 mg) and rifampicin: 10 mg/kg/day (8–12 mg). It is advisable to avoid streptomycin in the elderly in view of ototoxicity. Though adverse effects are frequent in old age, the risk of hepatoxicity is similar for younger ones. However, in view of the emergence of multidrug-resistant and extended drug-resistant tuberculosis increasing in prevalence, drug treatment is now more and more based on culture sensitivity reports. Also, treatment regimens have been defined for drug-sensitive and drug-resistant cases.</li><li>Government of India under the National TB Elimination Programme has simplified the investigations and management along with the financial support to the patient.</li></ul>
Bronchial asthma	
<ul><li>Bronchial asthma and chronic obstructive pulmonary disease (COPD) can be easily mistaken for each other, especially among the elderly population, even though they are distinct conditions. While asthma often originates in early life for most elderly patients, it remains a separate condition from COPD.</li></ul>	Acute asthma should be managed with oxygen inhalation and nebulization with short-acting β_2 agonists like salbutamol with or without short-acting anticholinergics like ipratropium. A short course of steroids acts as a lifesaving rescue management for acute severe asthma. Xanthine derivatives like theophylline may be useful as an add-on therapy in few patients. Patients who do not respond, with rising CO_2 levels and impending exhaustion may need mechanical ventilation.

Contd...

Contd...

Disorders	Management
• In older individuals, asthma may manifest as intermittent symptoms like coughing, wheezing, and breathlessness. These characteristics can be misleading and may be wrongly attributed to COPD or left ventricular heart failure, which are more prevalent in old age. It is not uncommon for these conditions to coexist in elderly patients, adding to the complexity of diagnosis and management. • Management of acute or chronic phases of asthma is same for old patients as for youngsters. Complications and mortality may be higher with advancing age. Peak flow monitoring helps in the proper management of these patients.	Symptomatically, chronic bronchial asthma is usually managed with inhaled short-acting β_2 agonists with or without short-acting anticholinergics as and when required for reliever purposes, whereas long-acting β_2 agonists (salmeterol/formoterol) with or without long-acting anticholinergics (tiotropium) are used for long-term maintenance therapy. However, the mainstay of long-term asthma preventive treatment is the use of inhaled steroids (beclomethasone/budesonide/ciclesonide, etc.) to keep inflammation under control. For elderly patients, who have coordination problems with MDI or are not comfortable with the use of a spacer, dry powder inhalers (DPI) and now breath-actuated devices are better options. Chronic severe asthma for good control may sometime require oral steroids for variable periods of time. Antileukotriene montelukast is also a good add-on treatment for chronic severe asthma.
Chronic obstructive pulmonary/airway disease (COPD/COAD)	
• COPD or COAD is a slowly progressive inflammatory airway obstruction that does not change markedly over many months sometimes years. Smoking is the most common cause of COPD. After many years of smoking, there is an asymptomatic phase of decline in respiratory function which gets manifest by the age of 50–60 years. Nearly one-third of elderly subjects may have COPD, though half of them are not diagnosed or are untreated. It starts with a smoker's cough which goes on to become chronic bronchitis and with a fall in forced expiratory volume (FEV) below 60% breathlessness sets in. Symptoms of hypoxia include fatigue, malaise, weight loss, and sleep disturbances. Signs include hyperinflated chest, wheezing, polycythemia, cyanosis, and eventually edema and raised jugular venous pressure (JVP) as a manifestation of right heart failure. Clinical features and an X-ray chest are diagnostic; however, spirometry confirms the obstructive defect. • Acute exacerbations of COPD are the most common cause of hospitalizations among these patients. Upper or lower respiratory tract infections are the usual triggers of acute exacerbations causing hypoxia and sometimes death.	Treatment of COPD involves relief of airway obstruction by: • Inhaled β-2 agonists (salbutamol for immediate relief as a short-acting drug and salmeterol/formoterol for long-term maintenance being long-acting). • Inhaled anticholinergic bronchodilators (ipratropium for immediate relief as a short-acting drug and tiotropium for long-term maintenance being long-acting. • Inhaled steroids in the form of beclomethasone/budesonide/ciclesonide, etc. Oral drugs from the above categories are better avoided, however, short-term oral steroids are helpful as rescue therapy during exacerbations. Sustained release of theophylline as an add-on at bedtime helps in preventing nocturnal symptoms. As COPD patients frequently develop exacerbations, they require antibiotics during the episodes of increased cough/purulence or increased quantity of expectoration. Vaccination against influenza and pneumonia will avoid exacerbations and thereby reduce morbidity and mortality. Long-term domiciliary oxygen administration is recommended in patients with persistent hypoxia (PaO_2 <55). Pulmonary rehabilitation improves exercise tolerance and includes: • Aerobic exercises and exercise training • Resistive respiratory muscle exercises • Maintaining physical activity
Lung cancer	
• Lung cancer holds the distinction of being the most prevalent cancer among elderly men worldwide. Furthermore, its prevalence is on the rise among women as well. Notably, a substantial 95% of these cases are directly linked to cigarette smoking. • Clinical presentations of lung cancer commonly encompass symptoms such as persistent cough, hemoptysis (coughing up blood), chest pain, and weight loss. • It's important to note that a significant portion of older patients tend to present in advanced stages of the disease. The process of diagnosing lung cancer involves obtaining tissue samples for accurate identification, and the assessment of operability hinges on both anatomical and functional considerations.	• Diagnostic evaluation and staging protocols for lung cancer remain consistent across different age groups, including the elderly. The distribution of lung cancer subtypes is notable, with squamous cell carcinoma accounting for 50–70% of cases, followed by small cell carcinoma at approximately 25%. • While surgical resection is the preferred treatment, many patients, including a significant number of elderly individuals, may necessitate radiotherapy. Chemotherapy is typically reserved for cases of small cell carcinoma and is often associated with poor tolerance. • In addition to medical interventions, essential components of treatment encompass dietary management, teaching relaxation techniques, and providing psychological support. These aspects contribute to a comprehensive approach in managing lung cancer in the elderly and other age groups alike.

the elderly. Salivary secretions are reduced. The swallowing mechanism is affected by weakened oropharyngeal muscles and disturbed coordination between the oropharyngeal muscles and the upper esophageal sphincter. As a result, elderly people are susceptible to dysphagia and aspiration.

The muscles in the GI tract can get weaken further with age, potentially leading to conditions like gastroparesis (delayed stomach emptying) and fecal incontinence. The risk of gastrointestinal disorders, such as gastroesophageal reflux disease (GERD), peptic ulcers, and inflammatory bowel disease (IBD), is higher in the elderly **(Table 47.3)**.

Age-related changes in gut bacteria composition may impact digestion, metabolism, and immune function. Gastric emptying of liquids is delayed. Gastric acid secretion may increase or decrease depending upon infection with *Helicobacter pylori* or the use of drugs. Absorption of

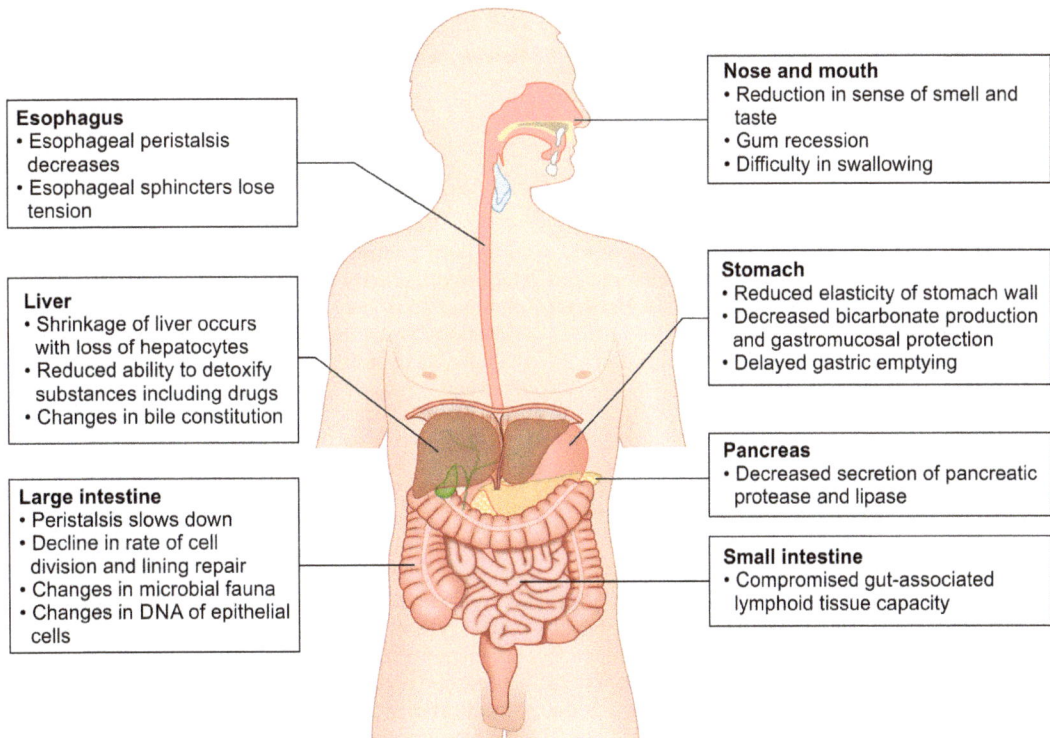

Fig. 47.3: Age-related changes in GI system.

TABLE 47.3: Age-related GI conditions.

Disorders	Management
Hiatal hernia and gastroesophageal reflux	
These are the most common problems of the upper GI tract in old age. Their prevalence increases after the age of 50 and may be present in as many as two-thirds of the people over 60 years, being more common in women. Symptoms include heartburn, dysphagia, pain in the region of the lower sternum, belching, reflux of food, and vomiting. Overeating, excess of tea/coffee/alcohol/obesity/stress, etc., could be triggering/aggravating factors. Their identification helps in the non-pharmacological management of the disease.	Interventions to correct the symptoms include-weight loss in obese patients, small frequent meals, and a bland but nutritious diet. One should avoid alcohol, tea, coffee, cold drinks, spices, and fried foods. The amount of fat in the diet should be minimized. Sleeping in a semi-upright position gives relief to the symptoms. Early dinner and elevation of the head end of the bed do help in a meaningful manner. Prokinetics, proton pump inhibitors and H_2-blockers in a rational manner do give significant relief. Antacids and skimmed milk also help with symptomatic relief.
NSAID gastropathy and peptic ulcer	
Nonsteroidal anti-inflammatory drugs (NSAIDs) are frequently prescribed to older patients for pain and inflammation caused by various ailments. Acute toxicity is dose-dependent and 100% of NSAID users develop gastropathy during the first one or two weeks of treatment. A small but significant proportion of chronic NSAID users develop serious toxicity, including ulcer disease. Manifestations may vary from non-ulcer dyspepsia to severe and life-threatening hemorrhage.	Simultaneous use of proton pump inhibitors (omeprazole/pantoprazole/rabeprazole, etc.) can prevent NSAID use toxicity. Peptic ulcers induced by NSAIDs, and *H. pylori* tend to be very virulent in old age. Presentation of ulcer disease is usually acute, often with bleed or perforation, though gastric ulcers may remain subtle. Anemia due to chronic blood loss, fatigue, or weight loss may be the only complaint in some patients. The risk of complications from peptic ulcer disease is very high in old age, though the response to drugs is good. Older patients should not be denied surgery for complications.
Nonulcer dyspepsia (NUD)	
Dyspeptic symptoms without any endoscopic evidence of ulcer are a frequent complaint in old age. Although psychogenic factors, gastrointestinal dysmotility, *H. pylori,* etc., have been frequently considered to be causative, the exact cause of NUD largely remains unknown in a given subject.	These patients usually respond well to peptic ulcer therapy. Gastric cancer may mimic peptic ulcer or NUD in the early stages and must be excluded if the older patients show atypical manifestations.
Cancer of GIT	
The incidence of GI cancers increases with age. Cancer of the rectum is more common in men, whereas colon cancer is more prevalent in women. Symptoms include a change in bowel habits, i.e., new onset diarrhea or constipation, decrease in size of stool, blood in stool, loss of appetite, wasting, weight loss, weakness, and dull pain radiating to the back. Colorectal cancers carry a high rate of morbidity and mortality. Digital rectal examination and checking stool for occult blood should be part of routine health checks for older people.	Oral screening for sores and other signs of cancer should be done, especially among persons who are at high risk from smoking, tobacco chewing, drinking alcohol, or especially hot beverages regularly. Similarly, elderly patients with GI bleed, dysphagia, and altered bowel habits must be screened early to detect cancers at curable stage.

Contd...

Contd...

Disorders	Management
The incidence of oral cavity, esophagus, and stomach malignancies also increases with age. Probably dietary factors and tobacco chewing, etc., do contribute. The incidence of these cancers is high in certain ethnic groups.	
Constipation	
Older people complain of constipation quite often and do have more constipation than youngsters. The most probable contributory factors appear to be diet deficiency in fibers and poor fluid intake. However, other contributory factors could be: • Drugs: Diuretics, anticholinergics, opiates, antidepressants, etc. • Mental health problems: Depression and dementia, etc. • Laxative abuse • Inadequate fluid consumption • Inadequate fibers (fruits and vegetables) in the diet • Chronic debilitating diseases and functional disability • Lack of physical exercise	Long-term complications of constipation include fecal impaction, megacolon, urinary infection, incontinence, and a confusional state. Impacted stool may be required to be removed manually which is unpleasant, embarrassing, and may cause rectal trauma and bleeding. The right blend of lifestyle changes and laxatives can relieve constipation in old age.
Hepatobiliary disease	
Hepatobiliary diseases are conditions that affect the liver, gallbladder, and bile ducts. These diseases can have a significant impact on the health and well-being of elderly individuals. As people age, their liver function and bile production may decline, making them more susceptible to hepatobiliary disorders. Some common hepatobiliary diseases in the elderly include: • **Nonalcoholic fatty liver disease (NAFLD) and nonalcoholic steatohepatitis (NASH):** These conditions involve the accumulation of fat in the liver (NAFLD) and inflammation with potential liver damage (NASH) in individuals who do not consume significant amounts of alcohol. Risk factors for these conditions include obesity, insulin resistance, and metabolic syndrome.	Management of hepatobiliary diseases in the elderly • **Lifestyle modifications:** Encouraging a healthy diet, weight management, and exercise can be beneficial for managing various hepatobiliary conditions. • **Medications:** Specific medications may be prescribed to manage liver disease or complications such as antiviral medications for viral hepatitis or ursodeoxycholic acid for certain bile duct disorders.
• **Alcoholic liver disease:** Chronic alcohol consumption can lead to liver damage, including fatty liver, alcoholic hepatitis, and cirrhosis. Older adults may be more vulnerable to the effects of alcohol on the liver due to age-related changes in metabolism and liver function. • **Viral hepatitis:** Hepatitis B and C are viral infections that can cause inflammation of the liver and lead to chronic liver disease. These infections can be acquired earlier in life and persist into old age, or they may be acquired later in life due to healthcare exposures or other risk factors. • **Biliary tract diseases:** Conditions that affect the bile ducts and gallbladder, such as gallstones, cholecystitis (inflammation of the gallbladder), and bile duct obstruction, can occur in the elderly population. • **Liver cirrhosis:** Cirrhosis is a late stage of scarring (fibrosis) of the liver caused by many forms of liver diseases and conditions. It can result from chronic hepatitis, alcoholism, or other causes. Liver cirrhosis can lead to liver failure and other complications. • **Liver cancer:** Elderly individuals may be at a higher risk of developing primary liver cancer (hepatocellular carcinoma) due to a long history of chronic liver disease, viral hepatitis, or other risk factors.	• **Avoidance of alcohol and hepatotoxic medications:** For individuals with liver diseases, including alcoholic liver disease, it is crucial to avoid alcohol and medications that can harm the liver. • **Screening and vaccination:** Regular screening for viral hepatitis and appropriate vaccination for hepatitis A and B can help prevent or manage these infections. • **Treatment of complications:** Complications of hepatobiliary diseases, such as portal hypertension, hepatic encephalopathy, or ascites, may require specific management and interventions. • **Transplantation:** In severe cases of liver failure or end-stage liver disease, liver transplantation may be considered for eligible elderly patients. It is essential for elderly individuals with hepatobiliary diseases to work closely with their healthcare providers to develop a comprehensive treatment plan tailored to their specific health needs and considerations related to their age. Regular follow-up, monitoring, and adherence to medical recommendations are vital for managing these conditions effectively.

multiple nutrients in the small intestine is reduced leading to malabsorption, but steatorrhea is unusual as pancreatic functions remain normal. Though the large intestine function remains normal, decreased tone of abdominal muscles may affect peristalsis and evacuation may not be complete. Liver volume, blood flow, and perfusion decline with age. As a result, the ability to metabolize and detoxify toxins, hormones, and drugs is significantly impaired.

Managing the GI health of elderly individuals requires extra attention and care. Some strategies to support their GI system include:
❖ Encouraging a well-balanced diet rich in fiber, fruits, and vegetables to prevent constipation.
❖ Promoting regular physical activity to maintain muscle tone and stimulate bowel movements.
❖ Ensuring adequate hydration to prevent dehydration and maintain proper digestion.
❖ Regular medical check-ups to monitor GI health and detect any issues early.
❖ Adjusting medications and dosages, if needed, considering potential changes in drug metabolism.

URINARY SYSTEM

One of the most significant age-related changes is a decline in kidney function, known as an age-related decline in glomerular filtration rate (GFR). GFR is a measure of how well the kidneys filter waste and toxins from the blood. As GFR decreases, the kidneys may not efficiently remove waste products, leading to a buildup of waste in the bloodstream.

The bladder's capacity to hold urine may decrease with age, leading to more frequent urination and potentially an increased risk of urinary incontinence. The muscles of the bladder may weaken over time, leading to difficulties in fully emptying the bladder and contributing to urinary retention **(Fig. 47.4)**.

Age-related changes in the urinary system, coupled with weakened pelvic floor muscles, may lead to urinary incontinence, which is the involuntary leakage of urine. Reduced bladder emptying and weakened immune responses in older adults increase the risk of urinary tract infections (UTIs) **(Table 47.4)**.

Ageing kidneys may have difficulties regulating fluid and electrolyte balance, which can lead to dehydration or imbalances in sodium, potassium, and other electrolytes. The ageing kidney's reduced ability to filter drugs from the bloodstream can lead to drug accumulation and potentially adverse drug reactions. The kidneys' ability to adapt to stress or injury, known as renal reserve, decreases with age, making elderly individuals more vulnerable to kidney damage in the face of acute illnesses or dehydration.

To support the excretory system and promote kidney health in the elderly, the following measures are essential:
- ❖ Staying adequately hydrated to support kidney function and prevent urinary tract infections.
- ❖ Maintaining a healthy diet that is low in sodium and includes foods that support kidney health, such as fruits, vegetables, and whole grains.

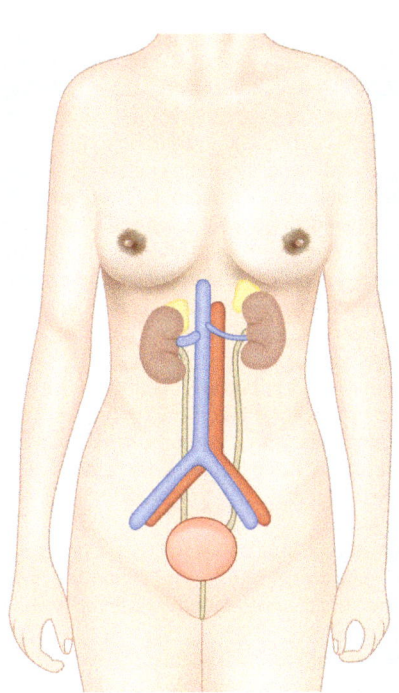

Fig. 47.4: Age-related changes in the urinary system.

TABLE 47.4: Age-related urinary system conditions.	
Disorders	**Management**
Urinary tract infection	
• Significant bacteriuria or the presence of >10 microorganisms per mL of urine with or without symptoms is considered a urinary tract infection (UTI). • The prevalence of bacteriuria increases with age though it is more common in women. Asymptomatic bacteriuria can be detected in 30% of elderly females and 10% of elderly males above the age of 65 years. • The prevalence of asymptomatic bacteriuria is much higher in chronically ill patients and can be detected in up to 20% of males and 60% of females. • Asymptomatic bacteriuria does not require therapy and is not significantly associated with serious renal disease. Antibiotic therapy of asymptomatic bacteriuria only results in temporary clearance of infection. • Symptomatic urinary tract infection in elderly patients is nearly always secondary to the introduction of the organism to the urinary tract by catheterization or any other instrumentation.	In patients living in community settings, *E. coli* is the most common isolated organism in 85% of cases. In the institutionalized elderly, the profile changes to *Proteus, Klebsiella,* and *Pseudomonas*. Symptomatic UTI always needs to be treated. Five to seven days course of therapy with amoxicillin, cotrimoxazole, norfloxacin, or ciprofloxacin is effective. In the presence of shock and septicemia, parenteral antibiotic therapy with ciprofloxacin, cephalosporin, or aminoglycosides and hospitalization are required. Management of UTI in a catheterized patient becomes a challenging task at times.

Contd...

Contd...

Disorders	Management

• Factors that encourage the growth and persistence of the infection in the urinary tract are:
   – Structural abnormalities in the urinary tract (prostatic hypertrophy, uterine prolapse, strictures, stones, and neurogenic bladder)
   – Renal scars associated with vesicoureteric reflux
   – Vascular insufficiency
   – Declining immunity	

Benign prostatic hypertrophy (BPH)	
It is an extremely common problem of advancing age. Enlargement of the periurethral portion of the prostate leads to the obstruction of urinary flow. The symptom complex associated with BPH begins with features of prostatic hyperplasia and ends up with urinary obstruction. Diagnosis is usually made by rectal digital examination and ultrasound of the bladder and prostate. Urodynamic studies sometimes may be helpful in therapeutic decision-making.	A few decades back, surgery, initially abdominal and later transurethral was the only mode of therapy for BPH. However, in recent years medical management with long-acting α-1 adrenergic antagonists like terazosin, doxazosin, tamsulosin, alfuzosin, and 5-α reductase inhibitors like finasteride, dutasteride, etc., have been used with excellent results.
Urinary incontinence (UI)	

• It is a major problem for elders, afflicting up to 30% of community-dwelling elders and 50% of nursing home residents. Up to 80 years of age, UI affects women twice as commonly as men, whereas after 80 years, both sexes are affected equally. In addition to the great impact of UI on patients' well-being, including embarrassment, social isolation, and depression, UI is also a risk factor for nursing home placement. While certainly not an essential component of ageing, advanced age, functional impairment, dementia, obesity, smoking, affective disorders, constipation, COPD, heart failure, and a history of pelvic surgery, etc., are associated with UI in various combinations.
• UI can be classified as either acute or chronic.
• Acute or sudden incontinence can be due to urinary tract infection, vaginal infections, fecal impaction, medication use (diuretics, α-adrenergic agonists or antagonists, anticholinergics like psychotropics, antidepressants, and anti-parkinsonians, etc.) confusion, and systemic sepsis. Acute incontinence resolves as soon as the underlying cause is treated.
• Chronic incontinence can be:
   – **Stress incontinence:** Loss of urine during coughing, sneezing, laughing, or any other activity that increases abdominal pressure.
   – **Urge incontinence:** Loss of urine associated with an abrupt and strong desire to void.
   – **Overflow incontinence:** Loss of urine associated with over-distension of the bladder.
	• Management of incontinence depends on the type of incontinence. Drugs and surgery are sometimes needed; however, most symptoms can be minimized by behavioral techniques and adaption to the environment.
	• Stress incontinence is usually managed by improving the strength of pelvic musculature. Urge incontinence is managed by anti-cholinergic drugs and pelvic muscle exercise. Overflow incontinence is associated with a full bladder and requires intervention for the primary disease. In the presence of an irreversible condition such as neurogenic bladder, catheterization may be required.
	• In addition, the patient needs to be educated about several behavioral interventions, such as:
	   – Bladder training by regular voiding at 2-hour intervals even if there is no urge.
	   – Limiting fluid intake to daytime.
	   – Using some type of protection because leakage and accidents are common.
	   – Wearing loose clothing so that changing clothes is easier.
	   – Avoiding strenuous exercises.
	   – Limiting the use of dietary irritants like caffeine and carbonated drinks.
	   – Practicing relaxation techniques.
	   – Maintaining good skin care and good hygiene.
	   – Monitoring for urinary tract infection.

❖ Managing chronic conditions, such as diabetes and hypertension, that can affect kidney function.
❖ Regular monitoring of kidney function through medical check-ups and blood tests.
❖ Avoiding excessive use of medications that can be harmful to the kidneys, if possible.
❖ Engaging in regular physical activity to promote overall health and circulation.

MUSCULOSKELETAL SYSTEM

With advancing age, there is a gradual loss of muscle mass (sarcopenia) and a decrease in muscle strength (dynapenia). This can lead to reduced physical performance and increased frailty. Bone mineral density tends to decline with age, resulting in an increased risk of osteoporosis and fractures. The cartilage within joints may wear down over time, leading to osteoarthritis, a degenerative joint disease that causes pain, stiffness, and limited range of motion. Ligaments and tendons may become less flexible and more prone to injury or tears in elderly individuals **(Figs. 47.5, 47.6 and Table 47.5)**.

Ageing can affect posture and balance, making older adults more susceptible to falls and fractures. Older adults may experience changes in their gait patterns, leading to alterations in walking and mobility.

To maintain musculoskeletal health in elderly individuals, it is essential to adopt a healthy lifestyle that includes regular exercise, a balanced diet with adequate protein and calcium intake, and fall prevention strategies.

ENDOCRINE SYSTEM

Some of the age-related changes in the endocrine system in elderly individuals include **(Fig. 47.7)**:
❖ **Hormone production:** With age, certain endocrine glands may produce hormones at a reduced rate. For example, the pituitary gland may produce less growth hormone, and the adrenal glands may produce less cortisol.
❖ **Thyroid function:** The thyroid gland's activity may decrease with age, leading to a condition known as hypothyroidism, which can cause fatigue, weight gain, and other symptoms.

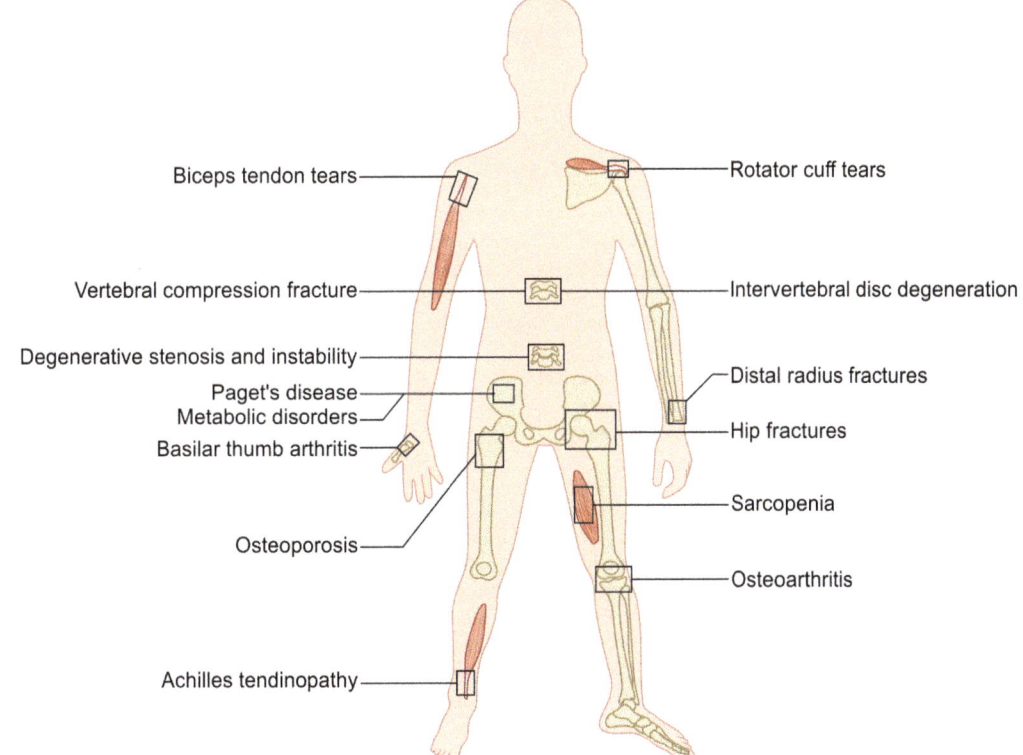

Fig. 47.5: Age-related changes in musculoskeletal system.

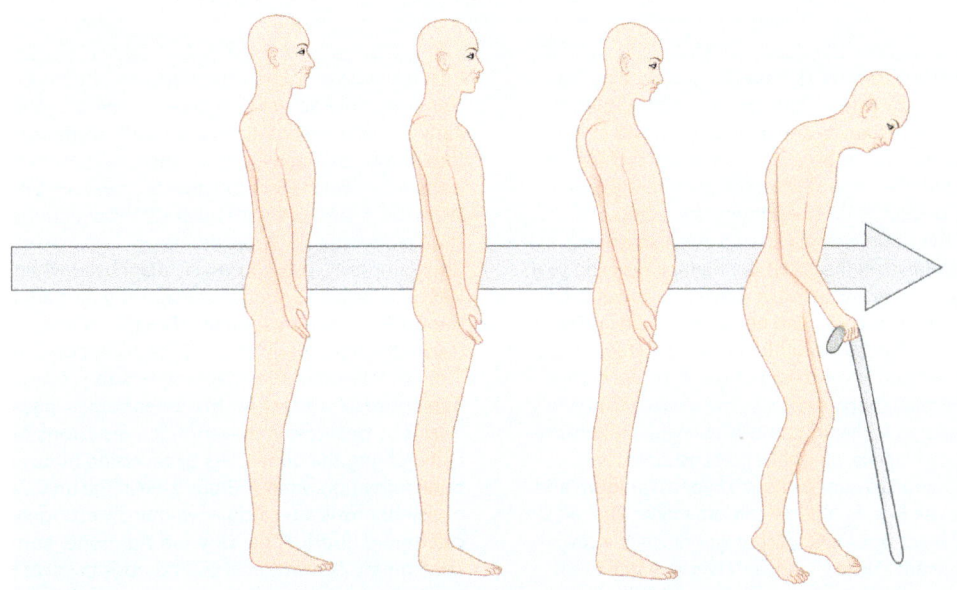

Fig. 47.6: Age-related postural changes.

- ❖ **Menopause and andropause**: In women, menopause occurs as the ovaries stop producing estrogen and progesterone, leading to various physical and hormonal changes. Similarly, in men, there is a gradual decline in testosterone production, known as andropause.
- ❖ **Insulin sensitivity**: Insulin sensitivity may decrease with age, contributing to a higher risk of insulin resistance and type 2 diabetes.
- ❖ **Growth hormone deficiency**: Some elderly individuals may experience a deficiency in growth hormone, leading to reduced muscle mass, increased body fat, and decreased bone density.
- ❖ **Cortisol regulation**: The body's ability to regulate cortisol, a stress hormone, may change with age, affecting the response to stress and the sleep-wake cycle.
- ❖ **Parathyroid function**: The parathyroid glands may experience alterations in hormone secretion, leading to changes in calcium metabolism and potential bone loss.
- ❖ **Reproductive hormones**: In both men and women, there is a decline in reproductive hormones, leading to reduced fertility and changes in sexual function.
- ❖ **Melatonin production**: Melatonin, a hormone involved in regulating sleep-wake cycles, may be produced in lower amounts in older adults, potentially affecting sleep patterns.

TABLE 47.5: Age-related musculoskeletal system conditions.

Disorders	Management
Osteoarthritis (OA)	
OA is a degenerative disease of the joints. OA of the knees is the most important cause of pain in the elderly. There is loss of cartilage and change in the composition of cartilage leading to failure of normal response to stress. As a result, the cartilage breaks down and the bone is exposed. Thus, a clinical syndrome of pain and disability is established. OA is usually a result of excessive and inappropriate stress, or it follows joint disease secondary to trauma, infection, inflammation, or metabolic disease. In a significant number of patients, no cause can be demonstrated. It usually involves weight-bearing joints and includes knees, hips, lower spine, cervical spine, and fingers. The onset is usually gradual. Radiological changes include loss of joint space, marginal osteophytes, subchondral sclerosis, and loss of alignments and these changes are usually diagnostic.	Being a degenerative disease, the treatment of OA is limited to symptomatic relief with analgesics and physiotherapy. Calcium helps in taking care of OA. Drugs like glucosamine, collagen peptides, chondroitin sulfate, diacerein, etc., may be useful in early OA. Intra-articular hyaluronic acid, steroids, and other medicines do help in selected cases. Replacement of hip and knee is very useful.
Rheumatoid arthritis (RA)	
• RA is usually insidious in onset with inflammatory synovitis. Symptoms include pain, swelling, tenderness, and stiffness which are maximum during morning hours or after rest. Hands, wrists, elbows, hips, knees, and feet are frequently involved joints. The involvement of the joints is usually bilaterally symmetrical. Malaise and fatigue are common systemic symptoms. • Diagnosis is usually clinically supported by radiological abnormalities and the presence of rheumatoid factors in serum. • The course of the disease is progressive with remissions and relapses. Early diagnosis, prompt treatment, and appropriate control of symptoms and disease activity are very important in the prevention of chronic complications.	Treatment involves analgesia with NSAIDs, disease-modifying drugs (methotrexate, hydroxychloroquine, sulfasalazine, corticosteroids, leflunomide, etc.), rehabilitation, and corrective surgery if required. RA in older patients can have specific problems like immobility, the effect of comorbid conditions, and the risk of adverse effects from NSAIDs and other drugs. The target of treatment is disease remission or low disease activity. Where, the above drugs fail to achieve the target, newer biological have got a good role to play. These drugs include TNF-alpha inhibitors (infliximab, etanercept, adalimumab, golimumab, certolizumab), IL-1 inhibitors (anakinra), IL-6 inhibitors (tocilizumab), CD20 inhibitors (rituximab) and cytotoxic T-lymphocyte associated antigen (CLTA)-4 inhibitor abatacept.
Osteoporosis	
• Osteoporosis is a systemic skeletal disease characterized by low bone mass and microarchitectural deterioration of the skeleton, leading to increased bone fragility and increased risk of fracture. Osteoporosis is now recognized as a common health problem in old age. It is estimated that about 40% of the postmenopausal women in India are osteoporotic. The primary risk factors are increasing age, heredity, and estrogen status. Because women accumulate less skeletal mass than men during their growing years (particularly during puberty), resulting in smaller, narrower, more fragile bones with thinner cortices, and because women undergo menopausal bone loss, women are at higher risk for osteoporosis and osteopenia. Other factors which can cause osteoporosis are premature and surgical menopause, heavy tobacco and caffeine use, alcoholism, inadequate dietary calcium, and vitamin D intake, small build, sedentary lifestyle, drugs like corticosteroids and antiepileptics, and comorbid conditions like hyperthyroidism and diabetes, etc. These risk factors, like low calcium intake, vitamin D deficiency, physical inactivity, being part of ignorance or a casual lifestyle approach are amenable to early intervention that helps attain peak bone mass and better musculoskeletal health. • Purely menopausal bone loss increases the risk of vertebral and Colles' fractures disproportionately. Similarly, senescent bone loss increases the risk of vertebral and hip fractures. In general, the elderly typically develops fractures in the spine or proximal long bones (e.g., hip fractures) secondary to minimal forces; this contrasts with younger adults, who often develop fractures in the middle of bones secondary to maximal forces. • Osteoporosis is usually silent until an osteoporotic fracture occurs. The most common fractures to occur are those of the wrist, the hip, and the vertebra. Hip fractures are the more severe and are associated with significant morbidity and mortality. A significant collapse of one vertebral body usually leads to severe pain. In addition to pain, numerous such fractures result in loss of height and often significant kyphosis resulting in cardiopulmonary embarrassment and severely reduced exercise tolerance, and marked physical disability.	• Earlier, the diagnosis of osteoporosis was used to be made with the occurrence of fracture. The current trend is to make the diagnosis early to make interventions work. Early diagnosis can be made by measuring bone density. Dual-energy-X-ray-absorptiometry (DEXA) is the most reliable investigation for measuring bone density. Women 50 years of age or older with four or more risk factors should undergo bone densitometry. • Conventionally, osteoporosis is diagnosed when bone density is at least 2.5 standard deviations below the young adult mean; when bone density is between 1 standard deviation and 2.5 standard deviations below the young adult mean, the condition is termed osteopenia. The primary goal of management is to prevent the occurrence of osteoporosis, and when the osteoporosis has already set in, the goal is to treat it and prevent fractures. Drugs for osteoporosis aim at increasing the bone mass by reversing bone loss and stimulating bone formation. Various drugs used in the treatment and prevention of osteoporosis are calcium, vitamin D, estrogen, bisphosphonates, calcitonin, fluoride, parathyroid hormone, and anabolic steroids. The primary prevention of osteoporosis involves taking a diet rich in calcium and vitamin D, avoiding tobacco, alcohol, and excess tea and coffee, brisk physical exercise, and hormonal replacement therapy for postmenopausal women. • Hip fracture which occurs from falls is a serious threat to the health of older people and can lead to major disability and often death. Since most musculoskeletal disorders are irreversible, interventions for adaptation to the environment are required so that the activities of daily living are minimally affected. It is very important to anticipate the needs of old people with these conditions. Adaptation in clothing, modifications in the home environment in providing fixed supports to avoid falls, periodic rest, avoidance of excessive exercise, and weight loss for overweight and obese are some of the recommendations which can be useful in elderly patients with musculoskeletal disorders in the prevention of falls and fractures. The need for a safe environment cannot be overemphasized. In elderly people, all the possible strategies are required to be adopted for the prevention of falls.

Contd...

Contd...

Disorders	Management
Fracture	
Fractures are relatively common in elderly individuals due to age-related changes in bone density and increased risk of falls. Some of the most common fractures seen in the elderly population include: • **Hip fractures:** These are among the most serious fractures in the elderly and often occur as a result of falls. They can significantly impact mobility and independence. • **Wrist fractures:** Fractures of the distal radius (the larger of the two bones in the forearm) are common in older individuals, especially in postmenopausal women with osteoporosis. • **Spine fractures (vertebral compression fractures):** These are often associated with osteoporosis and can lead to loss of height, chronic pain, and changes in posture. • **Ankle fractures:** Fractures of the ankle joint are common in elderly individuals, especially after falls or twisting injuries. • **Shoulder fractures:** Fractures of the proximal humerus can occur due to falls or trauma. • **Pelvic fractures:** Fractures of the pelvis can be serious and are often due to high-energy traumas, such as motor vehicle accidents or falls from a significant height. • **Rib fractures:** Elderly individuals may experience rib fractures, especially after falls or chest injuries, and these can be painful and limit breathing. • **Forearm fractures:** Fractures of the ulna or radius bones in the forearm can occur due to falls or direct trauma.	It is important to note that osteoporosis, a condition characterized by low bone density and increased susceptibility to fractures, is a significant risk factor for fractures in the elderly. Preventive measures such as regular exercise, a balanced diet with adequate calcium and vitamin D, and fall prevention strategies can help reduce the risk of fractures in this population. For the people at risk of fractures, it is essential to seek medical advice and take appropriate precautions.

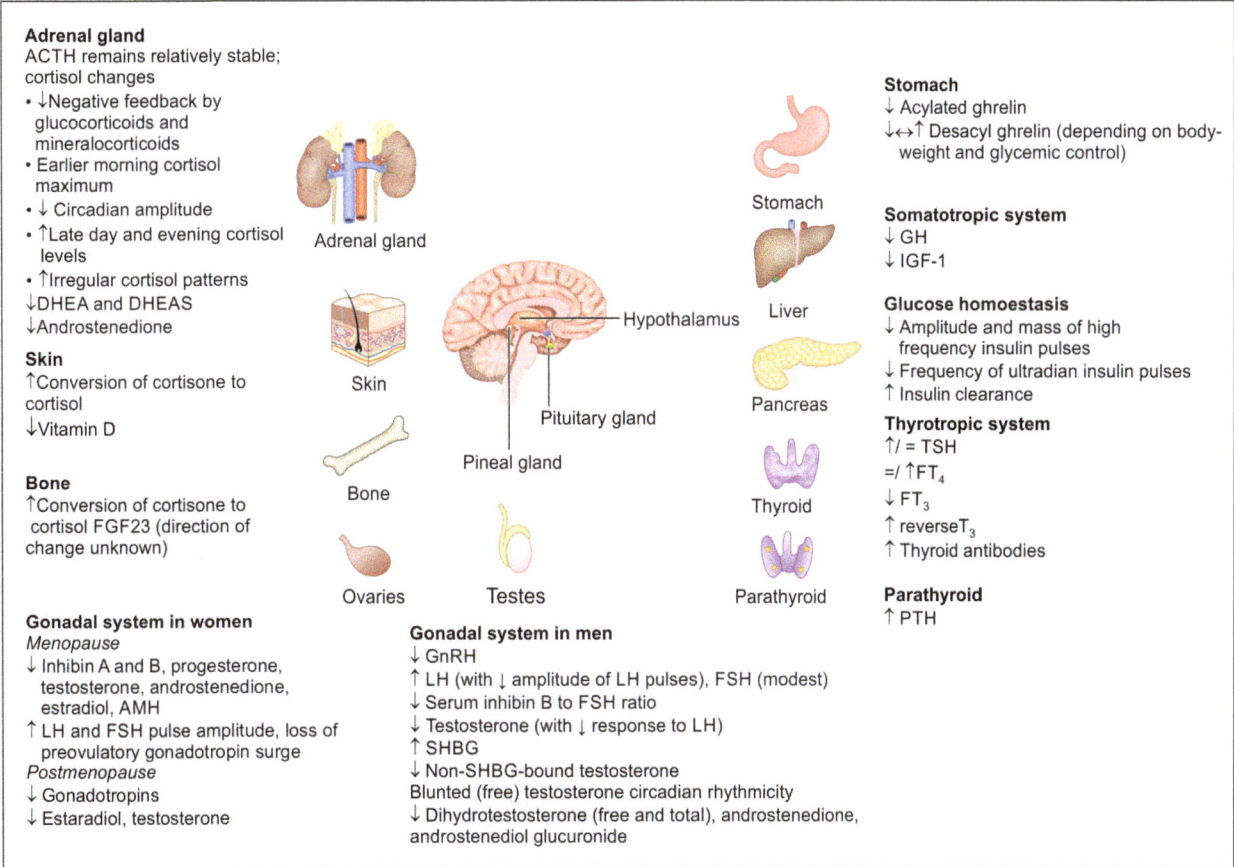

Fig. 47.7: Age-related changes in the endocrine system.

❖ **Ovarian and testicular changes**: In women, the ovaries may shrink and produce fewer eggs with age, while in men, testicular size may decrease, leading to reduced sperm production.

Various age-related endocrine disorders are depicted in **Table 47.6**.

REPRODUCTIVE SYSTEM

Age-related changes differ between males and females and can have significant effects on reproductive function and overall health.

TABLE 47.6: Age-related endocrine system conditions.

Disorders	Management
Diabetes mellitus	
• After hypertension, diabetes mellitus (DM) is probably the second most common condition whose prevalence increases with age. The estimated prevalence of DM is about 15–20% in those >65 years. While hypertension accelerates cognitive decline, DM contributes to accelerating functional decline. Diabetes is also associated with greater risk and severity of urinary incontinence and falls in older women. Also, DM and stroke are the conditions most consistently associated with a diminished capacity for functional recovery in the aged. • It is a common health problem in old age as more than 50% of all diabetics are over the age of 60 years. However, only 50% of elderly diabetics are diagnosed and only a small minority can achieve good glycemic control making them vulnerable to chronic complications like nephropathy, retinopathy, and neuropathy. Many of these diabetics have non-insulin-dependent diabetes, though insulin-dependent diabetics are also now living to ripe old age due to better management. Older diabetics with vascular and neurological complications of diabetes burden the hospital services two to three times more than the general non-diabetic population. Most long-term complications of diabetes such as hypertension, diabetic foot disease, and diabetic neuropathy are diseases of advancing age. Diabetes increases the risk of mortality and is associated with reduced life expectancy. Diabetes is also associated with a higher risk of dementia.	The aims of managing diabetes in the elderly are: • To relieve symptoms of hyperglycemia, prevent undesirable weight loss or weight gain and avoid hypoglycemia and other adverse drug reactions. • To assess the impact of coexisting hypertension and ischemic heart disease. • To screen for and prevent complications of diabetes. • To minimize disability, and maintain well-being and quality of life. Various problems faced during the management of diabetes are: • Irregular oral intake due to confusion, poor appetite, and concurrent illness, etc. • Recurrent infections like urinary tract, lower respiratory tract, and skin infections, etc. • Leg ulcers and bedsores. • Increased vulnerability to hypoglycemia. • Concurrent systemic diseases like cardiac and renal failure. • Difficulty in communication. • Lack of infrastructure (experienced health professionals and monitoring facilities). • Isolation and all its consequences. Control of blood sugar can be achieved by: • Adequate diet (calories and composition) • Physical exercise • Appropriate prescription drugs (OHAs and insulin, etc.) Insulin is sometimes required in type 2 diabetes for proper control of diabetes despite oral drugs in the presence of infection, ketosis, and hyperosmolar state and during surgery, and sometimes in the presence of neuropathy. It is very important to educate the patient regarding the need to follow a planned diet, insulin injections, symptoms of hypoglycemia, care of feet, regular eye check-ups, and blood pressure monitoring.
Hypothyroidism	
• Hypothyroidism is a clinical state which results from the decreased production of thyroid hormones. The most common cause is primary dysfunction of the thyroid gland and infrequently secondary to pituitary or hypothalamic failure to secrete TSH and TRH respectively. Prevalence of hypothyroidism increases with advancing age. • Hypothyroidism is a common problem with a strong predilection for female sex. More common underlying causes of primary hypothyroidism in old age are immune-mediated thyroid destruction, burnt-out Grave's disease, radioablation, and surgical removal of the thyroid gland. Hypothyroidism in old age presents insidiously developing over many years. As a result, patients and family members are rarely aware of the disease, and all the alterations are wrongly attributed to the ageing process. Clinical features of hypothyroidism are detected in only 10% of the laboratory-confirmed cases. Neuropsychiatric manifestations are most frequent which may include cognitive impairment, depression, and delirium. Stressful conditions can precipitate an acute decline in mental status presenting as coma. • Obesity, deafness, coarse skin, cold intolerance, hoarse and slurred voice, fatigue, arthralgia, entrapment neuropathy, and a low cardiac output state with bradycardia are other common features of hypothyroidism in old age.	Definitive diagnosis requires the demonstration of high TSH with low T3 and T4 concentrations. Regular monitoring and thyroid hormone replacement can solve the issue. While starting thyroid replacement therapy in the elderly, it is advisable to start initially with a lower dose for days and then increase the dose as starting with a high dose can precipitate tachyarrhythmias.
Hyperthyroidism	
Overproduction of thyroid hormones leads to the clinical condition of hyperthyroidism. This disease is common in old age and 20% of all thyrotoxicosis patients are aged 60 years or more. In contrast to younger patients, hyperthyroidism in old age is more likely to be due to multinodular toxic goiter than Graves' disease. Other causes include toxic adenoma, thyroid supplementation, and ingestion of iodine or iodine-containing substances. The clinical presentation of thyrotoxicosis in old age is rarely classic and includes a progressive functional decline, anorexia, weight loss, fatigue, cardiac arrhythmias, and cardiac failure. A syndrome termed "apathetic hyperthyroidism" comprising weakness, lethargy, listlessness, depression, and chronic wasting may be the presenting feature. Classical features of hyperactivity, irritability, and restlessness common in younger age groups may be absent. Subclinical hyperthyroidism in older patients may present itself as refractory atrial fibrillation.	• The diagnosis of thyrotoxicosis requires the demonstration of high circulating T3 and T4 with low TSH values in the blood. A thyroid scan is essential to delineate thyroid anatomy and planning of treatment. • The management of thyrotoxicosis in old age requires early control of cardiovascular manifestations by β-adrenergic blockers (propranolol, atenolol) and control of toxic symptoms by antithyroid drugs (carbimazole or propylthiouracil). Thyroid ablation by radioactive iodine is a good option in older patients, which provides one-time treatment without resorting to surgery.

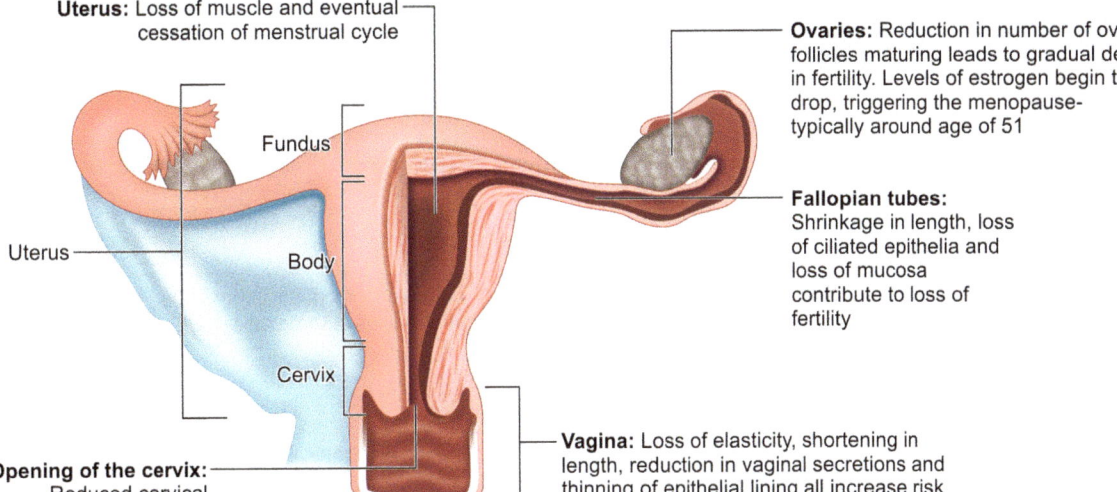

Fig. 47.8: Age-related changes in the female reproductive system.

In females (Fig. 47.8):
- **Menopause:** Menopause is a natural part of the ageing process for females and typically occurs between the ages of 45 and 55. During menopause, a woman's ovaries stop producing eggs, and hormone levels (estrogen and progesterone) decline, leading to the end of menstruation. Menopause can also be accompanied by symptoms such as hot flashes, mood swings, and vaginal dryness.
- **Vaginal changes:** As estrogen levels decline, the vaginal walls may become thinner and less elastic, leading to vaginal dryness and an increased risk of urinary tract infections.
- **Changes in breasts:** Breasts may lose some of their firmness and fatty tissue as women age. Menopause can also increase the risk of breast-related conditions like breast cancer.
- **Bone health:** After menopause, women are at an increased risk of osteoporosis, a condition where bones become weaker and more prone to fractures.

In males (Fig. 47.9):
- **Andropause:** Also known as "male menopause," it is a gradual decline in testosterone levels in older men. This decline usually begins around the age of 40 or 50 and continues at a slower rate compared to women's menopause. The effects of andropause can vary but may include decreased libido, reduced muscle mass, fatigue, and mood changes.
- **Prostate changes:** The prostate gland may enlarge with age, a condition known as benign prostatic hyperplasia (BPH). BPH can cause urinary symptoms like frequent urination, weak urine stream, or difficulty emptying the bladder.
- **Erectile dysfunction:** Ageing can lead to changes in blood flow and nerve function, contributing to erectile dysfunction (ED) in some men.
- **Sperm quality:** While men can continue to produce sperm throughout their lives, the quality of sperm may decline with age, potentially leading to reduced fertility in some cases.

General changes:
- **Fertility decline:** Both men and women experience a natural decline in fertility with age. The chances of

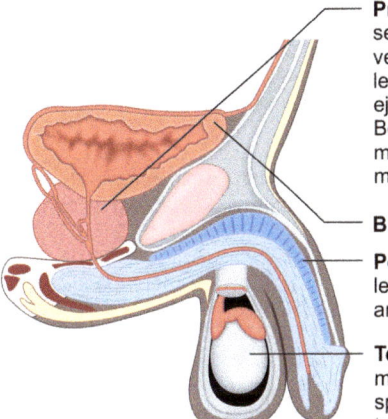

Fig. 47.9: Age-related changes in the male reproductive system.

conceiving decrease, and the risk of age-related birth defects and complications during pregnancy increases.
- **Hormonal changes:** Both males and females experience changes in hormone levels as they age, which can impact overall health and well-being.

The age-related reproductive system disorders are shown in **Table 47.7**.

NEUROLOGICAL SYSTEM

Cerebral blood flow may decrease with age, leading to reduced oxygen and nutrient supply to brain cells. There may be alterations in the production and function of neurotransmitters, affecting communication between nerve cells. Nerve conduction velocity may slow down, leading to a decline in reflexes and reaction times **(Figs. 47.10A to D)**.

Ageing can lead to alterations in sleep patterns, with older adults experiencing more fragmented sleep and reduced rapid eye movement (REM) sleep. It also affects motor coordination, balance, and fine motor skills.

Neuroplasticity, the brain's ability to reorganize and adapt to new experiences, may decline with age.

Various age-related neurological conditions are shown in **Table 47.8**.

TABLE 47.7: Age-related reproductive system conditions.

Disorders	Management
Erectile dysfunction (ED)	
It is a prevalent disorder in ageing males. It is characterized by the inability to achieve or maintain an erection sufficient for sexual activity. ED can be caused by various factors, including reduced blood flow to the penis, hormonal imbalances, and psychological factors.	Treatment options include medications (e.g., sildenafil, tadalafil), lifestyle changes, counseling, and vacuum erection devices
Benign prostatic hyperplasia (BPH)	
It is a noncancerous enlargement of the prostate gland that commonly occurs in ageing men. It can lead to urinary symptoms such as frequent urination, difficulty starting and stopping urination, and a weak urine stream.	Treatment options include medications (alpha-blockers, 5-alpha-reductase inhibitors) or, in some cases, surgery to relieve obstruction.
Vaginal atrophy	
It is a condition that affects postmenopausal women. It is characterized by the thinning, drying, and inflammation of the vaginal walls due to decreased estrogen levels. Symptoms may include vaginal dryness, itching, discomfort during intercourse, and an increased risk of urinary tract infections.	It can be managed with topical estrogen creams, vaginal moisturizers, and lubricants.
Pelvic organ prolapse	
It is a condition in which the pelvic organs (such as the bladder, uterus, or rectum) descend into the vaginal canal due to weakened pelvic support. It is more common in postmenopausal women.	Managed with pelvic floor exercises, pessaries (devices inserted into the vagina to support the organs), and surgical repair.
Testosterone deficiency	
Some older men may experience a decline in testosterone levels, leading to symptoms like decreased libido, fatigue, and reduced muscle mass.	Testosterone replacement therapy may be considered in certain cases, but it should be carefully managed due to potential risks.
Gynecological cancers	
The risk of gynecological cancers, such as ovarian, uterine, and cervical cancer, increases with age in women.	Regular screenings and early detection are crucial for successful management and treatment.
Malignancy of prostate	
Cancer of the prostate is a common malignancy of old age that can be detected early by screening and managed satisfactorily. Clinical manifestations are either silent or similar to benign hypertrophy in the early stages. In late stages when skeletal metastasis is frequent, it becomes one of the most painful conditions. Unfortunately, a majority of patients with cancer of prostate present with metastatic disease.	Management includes radical surgery in the early stages and in younger patients. Other options include hormonal manipulations and include: 1. LHRH agonists like goserelin, triptorelin, histrelin, leuprolide (all injectables) 2. LHRH agonist: Degareflix 3. Antiandrogens: Bialutamide, flutamide, nulotamide (all oral) 4. Receptor signalling pathway inhibitor: Enzalutamide (oral) 5. Pregnaolone analogue: Arberaterone (oral) 6. Targeted therapy (PARP inhibitors): Olaparib, rucaparib, tolazoparib. 7. Chemotherapy 8. Bilateral orchidectomy 9. Radiotherapy Various treatment modalities are decided based on the stage of the disease and the life expectancy of the patient. Early detection with digital examination and an assay of a specific marker PSA (prostate-specific antigen) has currently emerged as a useful strategy for secondary prevention.

SENSE ORGANS

- ❖ **Vision (Fig. 47.11):**
  - ➢ *Presbyopia:* The lens of the eye becomes less flexible, leading to difficulty focusing on close objects, such as when reading.
  - ➢ *Reduced visual acuity:* Ageing can lead to a decline in visual acuity, making it harder to see fine details or read small print.
  - ➢ *Increased sensitivity to glare:* Older adults may become more sensitive to glare from bright lights or sunlight.
  - ➢ *Reduced depth perception:* Depth perception may decline, affecting tasks that require judging distances accurately.
  - ➢ *Increased risk of eye conditions:* The risk of age-related eye conditions, such as cataracts, macular degeneration, and glaucoma, rises with age.
- ❖ **Hearing (Fig. 47.12):**
  - ➢ *Presbycusis:* Age-related hearing loss, known as presbycusis, affects the ability to hear high-pitched sounds and understand speech in noisy environments.
  - ➢ *Reduced auditory discrimination:* Older adults may have difficulty distinguishing between similar sounds or understanding speech with background noise.
- ❖ **Taste and smell:**
  - ➢ **Reduced taste sensitivity:** The ability to taste certain flavors may decline with age, leading to a decreased perception of sweet, salty, sour, and bitter tastes.

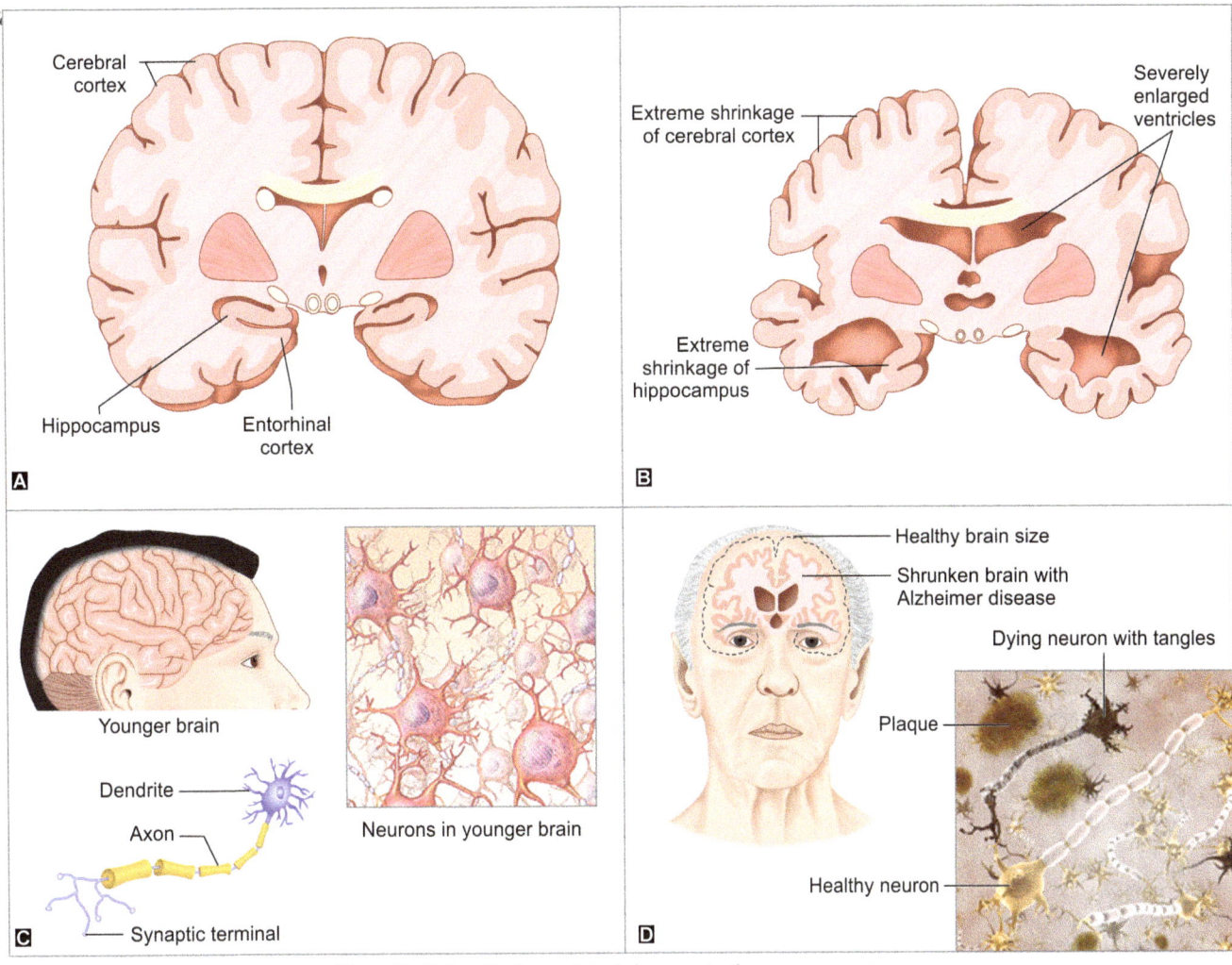

Figs. 47.10A to D: Age-related changes in the nervous system.

TABLE 47.8: Age-related neurological conditions.	
Disorders	*Management*
Alzheimer's disease	
Alzheimer's disease is a progressive and irreversible neurological disorder that primarily affects the elderly population, especially those aged 65 and older. It is the most common cause of dementia, accounting for approximately 60–80% of all dementia cases. The disease gradually damages and destroys brain cells, leading to a decline in memory, thinking, and cognitive abilities. As the condition progresses, it interferes with an individual's ability to carry out daily activities and eventually affects their overall quality of life. Key features of Alzheimer's disease in the elderly include: • **Memory loss:** One of the earliest and most prominent symptoms of Alzheimer's is the loss of short-term memory. People with Alzheimer's may forget recent conversations, events, or appointments. As the disease progresses, long-term memory may also become affected. • **Cognitive decline:** Alzheimer's leads to difficulties in thinking and problem-solving. Individuals may struggle with tasks that used to be routine, such as managing finances or following directions. • **Language problems:** Communication becomes challenging, and individuals may have trouble finding the right words or understanding written or spoken language. • **Disorientation:** People with Alzheimer's often become disoriented to time and space. They may get lost in familiar places or forget the date or season. • **Behavioral changes:** Alzheimer's can cause changes in mood and behavior. Individuals may become anxious, agitated, or withdrawn.	There is currently no cure for Alzheimer's disease, but various treatment approaches and interventions can help manage symptoms and improve the individual's quality of life. It includes: • **Medications:** There are medications available that can temporarily improve memory and cognitive function or manage behavioral symptoms. • **Cognitive stimulation:** Engaging in mentally stimulating activities may help slow cognitive decline. • **Supportive care:** Creating a safe and supportive environment for the individual can reduce stress and agitation. • **Healthy lifestyle:** Encouraging a balanced diet, regular exercise, and social engagement may help support brain health.

Contd...

Contd...

Disorders	Management
• **Inability to recognize loved ones:** As the disease progresses, individuals may no longer recognize family members and close friends. • **Difficulty with self-care:** Alzheimer's disease can impair the ability to perform everyday activities, such as dressing, bathing, and eating.	
Parkinson's disease	

Parkinson's disease is a neurodegenerative disorder that primarily affects the elderly population, although it can occur in younger individuals as well. It is the second most common neurodegenerative disorder after Alzheimer's disease. Parkinson's disease is characterized by the progressive degeneration of dopamine-producing neurons in a region of the brain called the substantia nigra. The loss of dopamine leads to motor symptoms and various non-motor symptoms.
Features of Parkinson's disease in the elderly include:
• **Motor symptoms:** The cardinal motor symptoms of Parkinson's disease include:
  – *Tremors:* Typically, resting tremors that affect hands, fingers, or other parts of the body.
  – *Bradykinesia:* Slowed movements and difficulty initiating movements.
  – *Muscle rigidity:* Stiffness and resistance to passive movement of limbs.
  – *Postural instability:* Impaired balance and increased risk of falls.
• **Nonmotor symptoms:** Parkinson's disease can also cause a range of nonmotor symptoms, which may include:
  – *Cognitive changes:* Problems with memory, attention, and executive function.
  – *Mood disorders:* Depression and anxiety are common in Parkinson's disease.
  – *Sleep disturbances:* Trouble falling asleep or staying asleep.
  – *Autonomic dysfunction:* Symptoms like constipation, urinary problems, and orthostatic hypotension (low blood pressure upon standing).
  – *Loss of smell:* Hyposmia or anosmia, the reduced or complete loss of the sense of smell.
	Management of Parkinson's disease in the elderly involves a combination of medication, therapy, and lifestyle modifications to improve symptoms and enhance the individual's quality of life. Some common approaches to management include:
	• **Medications:** Dopaminergic medications, such as levodopa, are commonly prescribed to replace dopamine in the brain and alleviate motor symptoms. Other medications may be used to manage nonmotor symptoms.
	• **Physical therapy:** Physical therapy and regular exercise can help improve mobility, balance, and overall physical function.
	• **Occupational therapy:** Occupational therapy focuses on helping individuals maintain independence in daily activities.
	• **Speech therapy:** Speech therapy can address speech and swallowing difficulties that may occur in Parkinson's disease.
	• **Supportive care:** A supportive and understanding environment is essential for individuals with Parkinson's disease. Support groups can provide emotional support and helpful tips for coping with the challenges of the disease.
	• **Surgery:** Deep brain stimulation (DBS) is a surgical procedure that may be considered for individuals with advanced Parkinson's disease who are not responding well to medication.
	
	Early detection and early intervention can also help optimize the management of Parkinson's disease in the elderly.

Stroke	
Stroke is a significant health concern, especially among the elderly population. A stroke occurs when there is a sudden interruption or reduction in blood flow to the brain, leading to brain cell damage and potentially long-term disability or even death. Elderly individuals are at a higher risk of stroke due to age-related changes in blood vessels and other health conditions that may increase the risk of stroke. There are two main types of strokes: 1. **Ischemic stroke:** This type of stroke occurs when a blood clot or plaque build-up blocks a blood vessel in the brain, leading to reduced blood flow. Ischemic strokes are more common, accounting for about 85% of all strokes. 2. **Hemorrhagic stroke:** This type of stroke occurs when a blood vessel in the brain ruptures, leading to bleeding and increased pressure on brain tissue. Common risk factors for stroke in the elderly include: • Hypertension • Diabetes • Atrial fibrillation • High cholesterol levels • Smoking • Sedentary lifestyle • Obesity • Previous history of stroke or transient ischemic attack (TIA) Signs and symptoms of a stroke: • Sudden numbness or weakness in the face, arm, or leg, especially on one side of the body • Confusion or trouble understanding speech. • Trouble speaking or slurred speech. • Severe headache with no known cause • Trouble seeing in one or both eyes. • Trouble walking, dizziness, loss of balance, or lack of coordination.	Management and treatment of stroke in the elderly may include: • **Thrombolytic therapy:** For ischemic strokes, clot-busting medications may be administered within a specific time window to dissolve the clot and restore blood flow. • **Mechanical thrombectomy:** For certain types of large vessel occlusions, a procedure called mechanical thrombectomy may be performed to physically remove the clot. • **Blood pressure management:** Controlling blood pressure is essential to prevent further damage to blood vessels. • **Rehabilitation:** After a stroke, elderly patients may require rehabilitation to regain lost function and improve mobility and independence. • **Lifestyle changes:** Encouraging a healthy lifestyle, including a balanced diet, regular exercise, and smoking cessation, can help reduce the risk of recurrent strokes.

Contd...

Contd...

Disorders	Management
Peripheral neuropathy	
Peripheral neuropathy is a common neurological condition that can affect the elderly population. It involves damage to the peripheral nerves, which are the nerves outside of the brain and spinal cord. Peripheral neuropathy can cause a variety of symptoms, depending on which nerves are affected, and it often presents with a combination of sensory, motor, and autonomic symptoms. The elderly are more susceptible to peripheral neuropathy due to age-related changes in nerve function and other health conditions. Common causes of peripheral neuropathy in the elderly include: • **Diabetes:** Diabetes is one of the leading causes of peripheral neuropathy, particularly in older individuals with poorly controlled blood sugar levels. • **Vitamin deficiencies:** Deficiencies in vitamins B1, B6, B12, and E can lead to nerve damage and peripheral neuropathy. • **Alcohol abuse:** Long-term alcohol consumption can damage nerves and cause peripheral neuropathy. • **Medications:** Certain medications, especially chemotherapy drugs and some antibiotics, can cause peripheral neuropathy as a side effect. • **Trauma:** Physical injuries or trauma, such as fractures or compression injuries, can damage peripheral nerves. • **Infections:** Some infections, like shingles (herpes zoster) or Lyme disease, can lead to peripheral neuropathy. • **Autoimmune disorders:** Conditions such as rheumatoid arthritis and lupus can cause nerve inflammation and neuropathy. • **Kidney and liver disease:** Impaired kidney or liver function can lead to a buildup of toxins in the blood, affecting nerves. Common symptoms of peripheral neuropathy in the elderly include: • Numbness or tingling in the hands, feet, or other areas. • Burning or shooting pain in the affected areas. • Weakness and muscle cramps. • Loss of coordination and balance problems. • Sensitivity to touch. • Changes in blood pressure, heart rate, and bowel/bladder function (autonomic symptoms).	Management of peripheral neuropathy in the elderly involves addressing the underlying cause if possible and managing the symptoms. Treatment may include: • **Pain management:** Medications such as over-the-counter pain relievers, topical creams, or prescription medications like gabapentin or pregabalin may be used to manage pain. • **Addressing underlying conditions:** Treating conditions like diabetes, vitamin deficiencies, or infections may help slow or halt the progression of peripheral neuropathy. • **Physical therapy:** Physical therapy can improve strength, balance, and coordination. • **Occupational therapy:** Occupational therapy can help individuals with peripheral neuropathy improve their ability to perform daily activities. • **Foot care:** Proper foot care is essential for individuals with peripheral neuropathy to prevent injuries and complications as patient may not be in a position to feel the pain because of neuropathy and injuries go undetected and unmanaged. • **Lifestyle modifications:** Making healthy lifestyle choices, such as managing blood sugar levels, avoiding alcohol, and quitting smoking, can help improve nerve health. • **Pain management techniques:** Techniques like transcutaneous electrical nerve stimulation (TENS) or acupuncture may help alleviate pain in some cases.
Vertigo and balance disorders	
Vertigo and balance disorders are relatively common in the elderly population and can significantly impact their quality of life. Vertigo is a type of dizziness characterized by a false sense of spinning or movement, while balance disorders refer to difficulties in maintaining equilibrium. These conditions can arise from various causes, and elderly individuals may be more susceptible due to age-related changes in the vestibular system (the part of the inner ear responsible for balance) and other health factors. Common causes of vertigo and balance disorders in the elderly include: • **Benign paroxysmal positional vertigo (BPPV):** BPPV is one of the most common causes of vertigo in the elderly. It occurs when small calcium crystals (otoconia) within the inner ear become dislodged and float into the semicircular canals, leading to a false sensation of spinning with certain head movements. • **Vestibular neuritis:** Vestibular neuritis is inflammation of the vestibular nerve, typically caused by a viral infection. It can lead to severe vertigo, nausea, and imbalance. • **Meniere's disease:** Meniere's disease is a disorder of the inner ear characterized by recurrent episodes of vertigo, hearing loss, tinnitus (ringing in the ears), and a feeling of fullness in the affected ear. • **Age-related changes:** As people age, the structures of the inner ear, including the vestibular system, may undergo degenerative changes, affecting balance. • **Orthostatic hypotension:** A drop in blood pressure upon standing can cause light headedness and imbalance.	Management of vertigo and balance disorders in the elderly involves identifying the underlying cause and providing appropriate treatment. Some management approaches may include: • **Canalith repositioning procedures:** For BPPV, specific maneuvers like the Epley maneuver can reposition the displaced crystals and alleviate symptoms. • **Medications:** Medications may be prescribed to reduce vertigo symptoms or treat underlying conditions. • **Vestibular rehabilitation therapy:** Physical therapy exercises can help improve balance and reduce the sensation of dizziness. • **Lifestyle modifications:** Making changes in daily activities, such as avoiding rapid head movements and using assistive devices for stability, can be helpful. • **Fall prevention:** Implementing fall prevention strategies, such as removing hazards at home and using assistive devices, is essential to reduce the risk of falls.

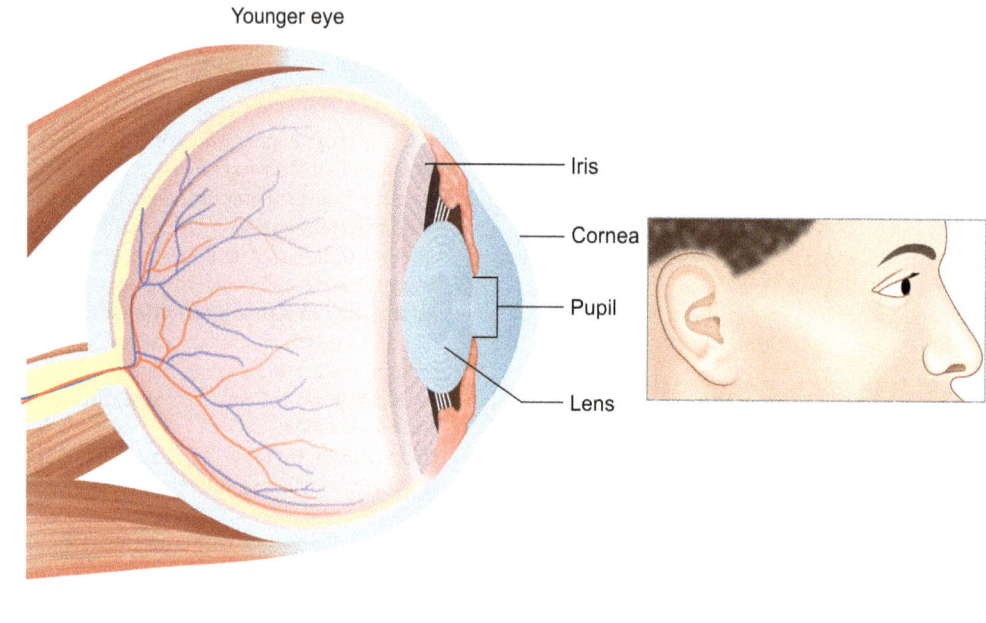

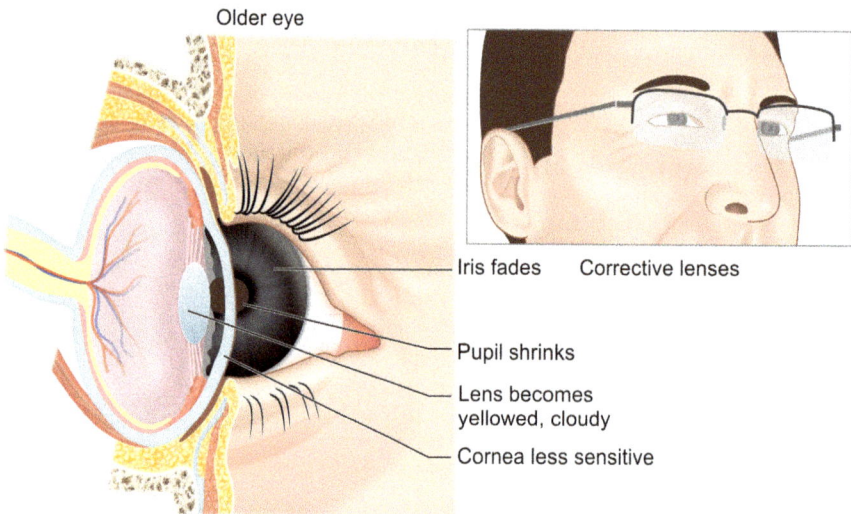

Fig. 47.11: Age-related changes in eye.

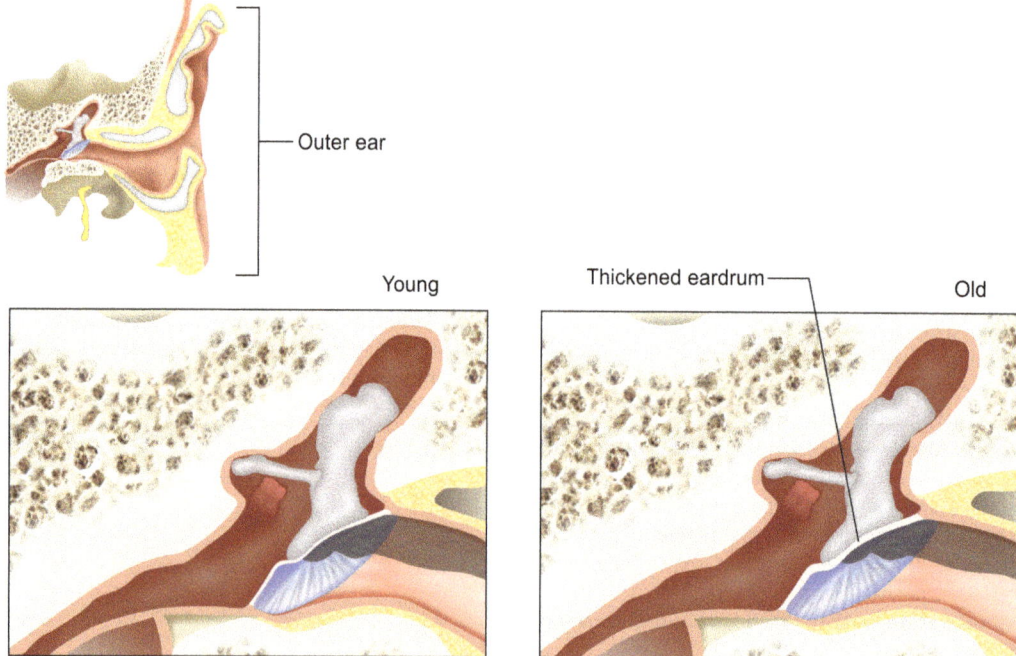

Fig. 47.12: Age-related changes in ear.

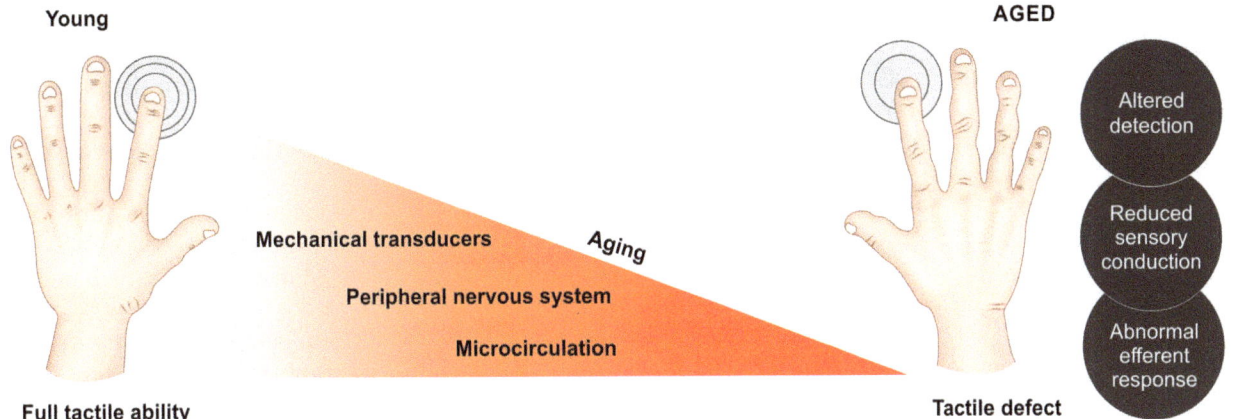

Fig. 47.13: Age-related changes in tactile ability.

- ➢ **Decreased sense of smell:** Ageing can lead to a reduced sense of smell, affecting the ability to detect odors and enjoy food.
- ❖ **Touch (Fig. 47.13):**
  - ➢ *Reduced sensation:* The sensitivity to touch may decrease, making it harder to feel pressure, temperature changes, and pain.
  - ➢ *Slower sensory processing:* Older adults may have slower response times to sensory stimuli.

These sensory changes can impact an elderly individual's quality of life and daily activities. However, it's important to note that sensory changes can vary from person to person and are influenced by factors such as genetics, lifestyle, and overall health.

The following strategies to support older adults with sensory changes:

- ❖ Regular eye and ear check-ups to detect and manage age-related vision and hearing issues.
- ❖ Adequate lighting and reduced glare in the living environment to accommodate visual changes.
- ❖ Using assistive devices such as reading glasses or hearing aids, if necessary.
- ❖ Providing flavorful and aromatic foods to compensate for taste and smell changes.
- ❖ Ensuring safety by adapting the environment to reduce the risk of accidents due to sensory impairments.

Moreover, staying socially active and engaged in stimulating activities can enhance the overall sensory experience and promote cognitive health in elderly individuals.

Table 47.9 depicts the age-related sensory conditions.

INTEGUMENTARY SYSTEM (FIGS. 47.14 AND 47.15)

The skin becomes thinner and less elastic with age, leading to the formation of wrinkles, especially in areas exposed to the

TABLE 47.9: Age-related sensory conditions.

Disorders	Management
Common age-related sensory disorders in the elderly: • **Presbyopia:** Presbyopia is an age-related vision condition in which the eye's lens becomes less flexible, leading to difficulty focusing on close objects. It usually becomes noticeable around age 40 and progressively worsens with age. • **Age-related macular degeneration (AMD):** AMD is a leading cause of vision loss in older adults. It affects the macula, the central part of the retina responsible for detailed vision, leading to a gradual loss of central vision. • **Cataracts:** Cataracts are cloudy areas that form in the eye's lens, causing blurred vision and reduced visual clarity. They are common in the elderly and can be corrected through surgery. • **Glaucoma:** Glaucoma is a group of eye conditions that cause damage to the optic nerve, leading to progressive vision loss and, if left untreated, blindness. It is more common in older adults. • **Hearing loss:** Age-related hearing loss, also known as presbycusis, is a common sensory disorder in the elderly. It involves the gradual loss of hearing sensitivity, especially for high-pitched sounds. • **Tinnitus:** Tinnitus is the perception of ringing, buzzing, or other sounds in the ears when no external sound is present. It can be associated with age-related hearing loss. • **Decreased sense of taste and smell:** Ageing can lead to a decreased sense of taste and smell, which can affect appetite and enjoyment of food. • **Somatosensory changes:** The somatosensory system, responsible for perceiving touch and pressure, may experience changes with age, leading to reduced sensitivity or altered sensations.	Management of age-related sensory disorders in the elderly may involve a combination of medical treatments, assistive devices, and lifestyle adjustments: • Regular vision and hearing screenings are crucial for early detection and intervention. • Prescription glasses or contact lenses can correct refractive errors like presbyopia. • Hearing aids can help individuals with age-related hearing loss. • Surgery is often an effective treatment for cataracts. • Lifestyle changes, such as a healthy diet and exercise, can support overall sensory health. • Fall prevention strategies can be implemented to reduce the risk of injury related to sensory impairment.

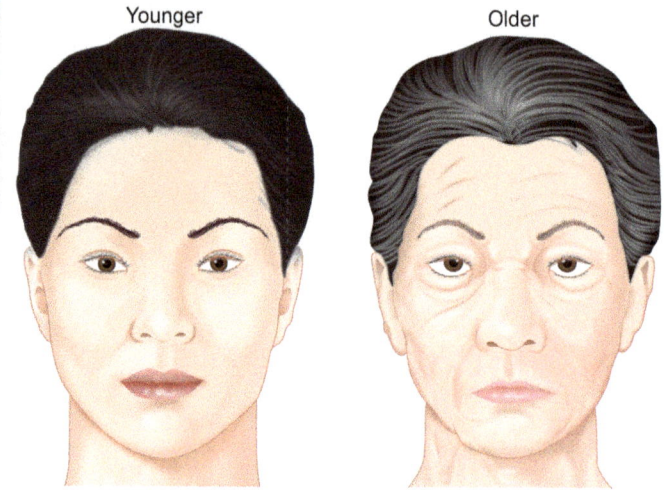

Fig. 47.14: Skin changes in elderly.

sun. Ageing skin tends to produce fewer natural oils, making it more prone to dryness and itching.

Over time, the skin may develop age spots, freckles, or areas of increased pigmentation due to sun exposure and changes in melanin production. Subcutaneous fat, decreases with age, resulting in less padding and potentially contributing to the prominence of veins and bones. Blood vessels become more fragile, and the skin itself becomes thinner, making it more susceptible to bruising and tearing.

Ageing skin has reduced regenerative capacity, leading to slower wound healing and increased susceptibility to skin infections.

Hair may become thinner, drier, and greyer with age, and hair growth may slow down. Nails also may become brittle, thicker, and more prone to ridges and cracks.

The production of sweat decreases with age, affecting the body's ability to regulate temperature. The sebaceous glands produce less oil, affecting the skin's ability to maintain moisture.

Following measures support the integumentary changes:
- Regular use of sunscreen to protect the skin from harmful UV rays and reduce the risk of sun damage and skin cancer.
- Keeping the skin moisturized to prevent dryness and itching.
- Avoiding excessive exposure to hot water during bathing, as it can further dry out the skin.
- Maintaining a balanced diet with adequate nutrients to support skin health.
- Protecting the skin from extreme temperatures, such as wearing appropriate clothing in cold weather and using shade or hats in hot weather.
- Avoiding smoking and limiting alcohol consumption, as they can contribute to skin ageing.

Maintaining good skin hygiene and following a healthy lifestyle can help elderly individuals manage age-related changes in their integumentary system and promote overall skin health.

Various age-related conditions are shown in **Table 47.10**.

IMMUNE SYSTEM (FIG. 47.16)

The immune system plays a crucial role in defending the body against infections and diseases. However, as individuals age, the immune system undergoes certain changes that can impact its effectiveness and responsiveness. Age-related changes in the immune system of elderly individuals include:
- **Immunosenescence:** It refers to the gradual decline in immune function that occurs with ageing. This results in a reduced ability to respond to infections and antigens effectively.
- **Thymus involution:** The thymus, a gland responsible for the maturation of T cells, tends to shrink and become less active with age. This leads to a decrease in the production of new T cells, which are crucial for adaptive immunity.

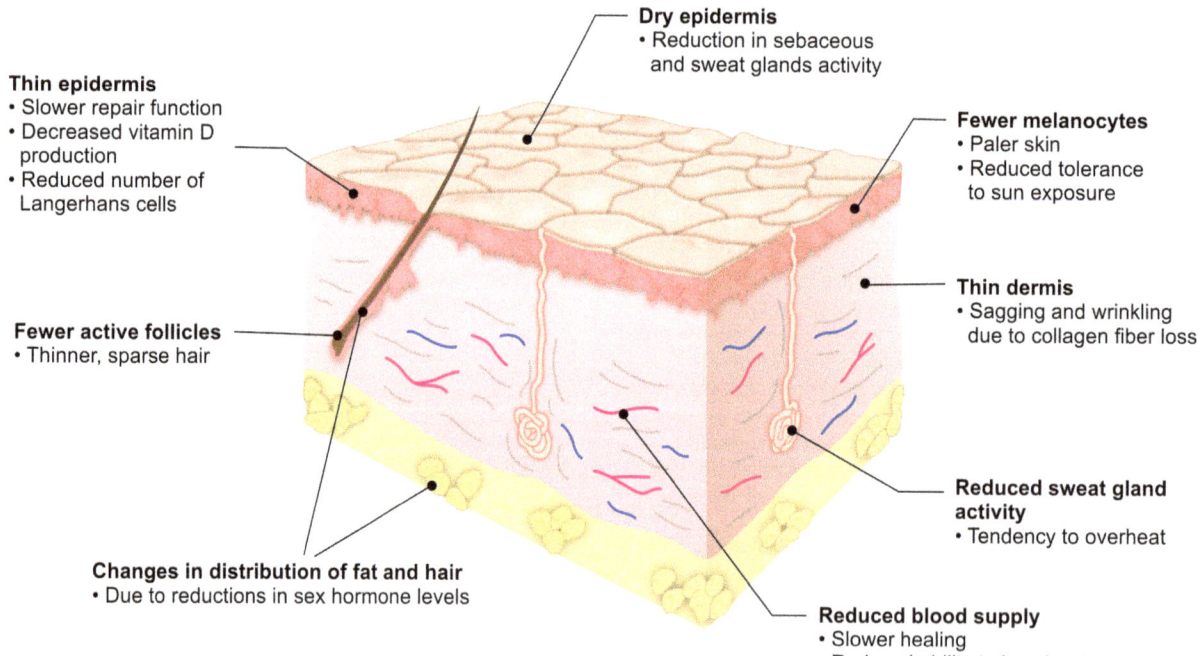

Fig. 47.15: Age-related changes in epidermis and dermis.

TABLE 47.10: Age-related integumentary conditions.

Disorders	Management
Wrinkles and fine lines	
As people age, the skin loses its elasticity and collagen, leading to the formation of wrinkles, fine lines, and sagging skin.	Use moisturizers and creams containing ingredients like retinoids or peptides that may help reduce the appearance of wrinkles. Avoid excessive sun exposure and wear sunscreen daily to protect the skin from further damage.
Dry skin (xerosis)	
The skin tends to become drier as people age due to decreased oil production and reduced ability to retain moisture.	Regularly apply moisturizers to keep the skin hydrated. Avoid hot showers and use mild, fragrance-free soaps to prevent further drying of the skin.
Skin thinning	
The epidermis becomes thinner with age, making the skin more fragile and susceptible to injury.	Prevent skin injuries by wearing protective clothing and using cushioned support surfaces. Keep the skin moisturized to improve its overall health and resilience.
Age spots (solar lentigines)	
These are small, dark spots that appear on the skin due to sun exposure over the years.	Regular use of sunscreen can help prevent new age spots from forming. Topical treatments containing retinoids or hydroquinone may also help fade existing age spots.
Skin tags	
Skin tags are small, benign growths that can appear on the skin, especially in areas where the skin folds or rubs together.	Skin tags can be safely removed by a healthcare professional with methods like cryotherapy, excision, or cauterization if they cause discomfort or become bothersome.
Actinic keratosis	
These are rough, scaly patches on the skin caused by prolonged sun exposure. They may progress to skin cancer if left untreated.	Actinic keratosis should be evaluated and treated by a dermatologist to prevent progression to skin cancer. Treatments may include topical medications, cryotherapy, or other procedures.
Seborrheic keratosis	
These are benign skin growths that can get tan, brown, or black in color and have a waxy, stuck-on appearance.	Seborrheic keratosis is usually harmless and does not require treatment unless it causes irritation. However, if desired, a dermatologist can remove them through cryotherapy or other methods.
Skin cancer	
The risk of skin cancer, including basal cell carcinoma, squamous cell carcinoma, and melanoma, increases with age and with excessive sun exposure.	Early detection and treatment are crucial for skin cancer. Regular skin examinations by a dermatologist and self-checks at home are important for early identification. Treatment may involve surgery, radiation therapy, or other targeted therapies depending on the type and stage of skin cancer.
Pruritus (itchy skin)	
Itchy skin is a common complaint in the elderly, often due to dry skin or underlying medical conditions.	Address the underlying cause of pruritus, such as dry skin or certain medical conditions. Applying moisturizers and using topical or oral antihistamines can help relieve itching.
Nail changes	
The nails may become thicker, more brittle, and develop ridges with age. Fungal nail infections are also common in the elderly.	Proper nail care, regular trimming, and keeping the nails clean can help prevent nail problems. For fungal nail infections, antifungal medications or topical treatments may be prescribed.

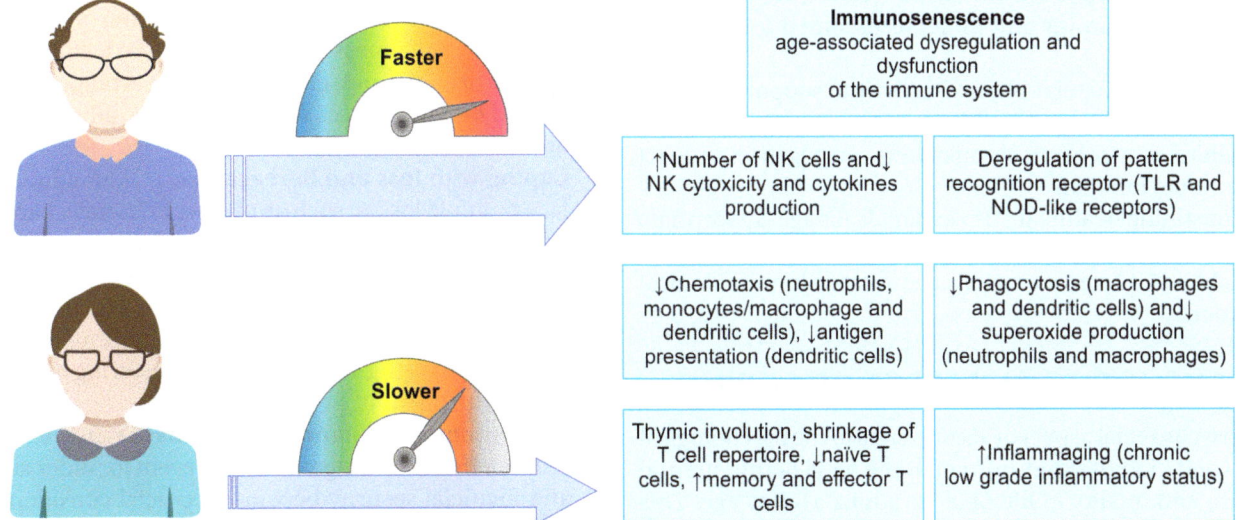

Fig. 47.16: Age-related changes in the immune system.

TABLE 47.11: Common age-related immunological conditions.

Disorders	Management
• **Increased susceptibility to infections:** Age-related changes in the immune system can make the elderly more vulnerable to infections, such as respiratory tract infections and urinary tract infections. • **Autoimmune disorders:** Some autoimmune disorders, such as rheumatoid arthritis and systemic lupus erythematosus, may manifest or worsen in the elderly. • **Immune system dysregulation:** Ageing can lead to immune system dysregulation, which can contribute to chronic inflammation and an increased risk of chronic diseases.	Management of age-related immune system disorders in the elderly involves various strategies to support immune health and reduce the risk of infections and complications. • **Vaccination:** Ensuring that the elderly receive recommended vaccinations, such as the flu vaccine, pneumococcal vaccine, and shingles vaccine, can help protect them from infectious diseases. • **Healthy diet:** A balanced diet rich in fruits, vegetables, whole grains, and lean proteins can provide essential nutrients that support the immune system. • **Regular exercise:** Engaging in regular physical activity can enhance immune function and overall health. • **Proper hygiene:** Encouraging good hygiene practices, such as handwashing, can help prevent the spread of infections. • **Stress management:** Chronic stress can negatively impact the immune system. Implementing stress-reduction techniques, such as meditation or yoga, can be beneficial. • **Adequate sleep:** Ensuring that the elderly get sufficient sleep can help support immune health. • **Avoiding smoking and excessive alcohol:** Smoking and excessive alcohol consumption can weaken the immune system. Encouraging healthy behaviors can benefit overall immune function.

❖ **Decreased T cell function:** T cells, a type of white blood cell, may become less responsive to pathogens and antigens, impacting the immune response.
❖ **Reduced B cell activity:** B cells, responsible for producing antibodies, may also exhibit reduced function and produce fewer antibodies in response to infections.
❖ **Changes in innate immunity:** The innate immune system, which provides the initial defense against infections, may become less efficient with age, leading to a higher susceptibility to certain infections.
❖ **Impaired healing:** The immune system's ability to initiate and regulate wound healing may be compromised in elderly individuals.
❖ **Increased risk of infections:** Due to the changes in the immune system, older adults are more vulnerable to infections.

Strategies that can be beneficial to support the immune system:
❖ Staying physically active and maintaining a healthy lifestyle with a balanced diet to support overall health.
❖ Ensuring adequate nutrition, including sufficient intake of vitamins and minerals essential for immune function.
❖ Engaging in regular physical activity to support immune function and overall well-being.
❖ Minimizing stress, as chronic stress can negatively impact immune function.
❖ Consulting healthcare professionals for age-appropriate health screenings and management of chronic conditions.

Table 47.11 shows various age-related immunological disorders.

PSYCHOSOCIAL ASPECT OF AGEING

The psychosocial aspect of ageing refers to the psychological and social factors that influence the well-being, mental health, and quality of life of older adults as they age. This aspect encompasses a wide range of emotional, cognitive, and social experiences that older individuals encounter during the ageing process. It includes:

❖ **Emotional well-being:** Older adults may experience a mixture of emotions as they age, including feelings of contentment, fulfilment, and satisfaction from a life well-lived, as well as sadness, grief, and anxiety about losses and life changes.
❖ **Mental health:** The prevalence of mental health conditions, such as depression and anxiety, can increase in older adults. However, mental health problems are not a normal part of ageing, and proper diagnosis and treatment are essential for maintaining well-being.
❖ **Self-esteem and identity:** Changes in physical appearance, roles, and status can impact self-esteem and identity in older adults. Adjusting to retirement, loss of independence, or changes in social roles may require adaptation and support.
❖ **Social support:** Social connections and relationships become increasingly important in later life. Maintaining strong social networks can positively impact mental health and overall well-being.
❖ **Loneliness and isolation:** Some older adults may experience loneliness and isolation due to factors such as the loss of loved ones, changes in living arrangements, or limited mobility. These feelings can have adverse effects on mental and physical health.
❖ **Coping with loss and bereavement:** Older adults may face multiple losses, such as the loss of friends, partners, or family members. Coping with grief and bereavement is a significant psychosocial aspect of ageing.
❖ **Positive ageing:** Older adults may embrace the concept of positive ageing, focusing on maintaining an active lifestyle, engaging in hobbies, and fostering a positive outlook on life.
❖ **Retirement and financial concerns:** Transitioning to retirement can be a significant life event for older adults, and financial security becomes a crucial consideration during this phase.

- ❖ **Life satisfaction and meaning:** Finding meaning and purpose in life continues to be essential for older adults, contributing to life satisfaction and overall well-being.
- ❖ **Resilience and adaptation:** Older adults often demonstrate resilience and the ability to adapt to life changes, cope with challenges and find new sources of fulfilment.

Understanding and addressing the psychosocial aspects of ageing are crucial in promoting healthy ageing and improving the quality of life for older individuals. Supportive social networks, access to healthcare and mental health services, engagement in meaningful activities, and fostering a positive and inclusive society are essential components of addressing the psychosocial needs of older adults.

COGNITIVE ASPECT OF AGEING

The cognitive aspect of ageing refers to the changes in cognitive functions, such as memory, attention, problem-solving, and reasoning, that occur as individuals grow older. While some cognitive abilities remain stable or even improve with age, certain cognitive functions tend to decline over time.

Normal ageing is associated with changes in cognitive abilities, such as a decline in processing speed, working memory, and episodic memory (memory for specific events or experiences). These changes are considered a part of the typical ageing process and do not necessarily indicate cognitive impairment or dementia. The cognitive changes that occur with ageing vary widely among individuals. Some older adults may maintain their cognitive abilities relatively well, while others may experience more noticeable declines.

Executive functions, which include abilities like planning, decision-making, and multitasking, can be particularly affected by ageing. Fluid intelligence, which involves the ability to solve new problems and think abstractly, tends to decline with age. In contrast, crystallized intelligence, which is based on accumulated knowledge and experience, may remain relatively stable or even improve over time.

Older adults often possess a wealth of life experience, leading to increased wisdom and expertise in certain domains. Memory, like episodic memory, may decline, semantic memory (general knowledge) and procedural memory (memory for skills and habits) can remain well-preserved in older adults.

Promoting cognitive health in older adults involves engaging in mentally stimulating activities, maintaining social connections, adopting a healthy lifestyle, and managing cardiovascular risk factors. Regular cognitive assessments and early intervention for any cognitive concerns can also be beneficial in ensuring appropriate care and support for older adults.

LATER AGE SEXUALITY

"Later age sexuality" typically refers to the sexual feelings, behaviors, and experiences of individuals who are older in age, often considered to be past their middle age or retirement years. This term is used to recognize that sexuality can remain an important aspect of human life even as people age and that individuals continue to have sexual desires and needs as they grow older.

Important points about later-age sexuality include:
- ❖ **Continued sexual interest:** Contrary to common misconceptions, many older adults maintain a level of sexual interest and desire. While the intensity and frequency of sexual activity may vary, the desire for intimacy and connection can persist throughout life.
- ❖ **Physical changes:** As people age, they may experience physical changes that can impact their sexual functioning. These changes could include menopause in women, erectile changes in men, and other age-related health conditions. However, many of these issues can be addressed with medical help, lifestyle changes, or adjustments in sexual practices.
- ❖ **Emotional and psychological factors:** Emotional and psychological factors can also play a significant role in later age sexuality. Issues such as self-esteem, body image, and relationship dynamics can influence sexual well-being.
- ❖ **Relationships and intimacy:** The importance of emotional intimacy and companionship may become more significant in later age relationships. Non-sexual forms of intimacy, such as cuddling and hugging, can be equally essential in maintaining emotional connection and overall well-being.
- ❖ **Communication and consent:** As with any stage of life, communication and consent are crucial in later age relationships. Discussing desires, boundaries, and expectations with a partner is essential to ensure a mutually satisfying and respectful sexual experience.

NURSING CONSIDERATIONS

Nursing care for older adults involves a holistic approach that addresses the physical, psychosocial, and cognitive aspects of ageing.

- ❖ **Physical aspect:**
  - ➢ *Health assessment:* Regular and thorough health assessments are crucial to identify and address physical health issues promptly. Assessments should include monitoring vital signs, conducting screenings, and assessing mobility and functional abilities.
  - ➢ *Medication management:* Older adults often take multiple medications. Nurses should ensure proper medication administration, educate patients about their medications, and monitor for potential side effects or interactions.
  - ➢ *Fall prevention:* Implement measures to prevent falls, such as ensuring a safe environment, providing assistive devices, and educating both the patient and their caregivers about fall risks.
  - ➢ *Nutrition and hydration:* Older adults may have specific nutritional needs. Nurses should assess dietary intake, offer guidance on balanced nutrition, and monitor hydration status.
  - ➢ *Pain management:* Address and manage pain effectively, as older adults may experience chronic pain. Develop individualized pain management plans, considering nonpharmacological interventions alongside medications.

- ❖ **Psychosocial aspect:**
  - ➢ *Emotional support:* Provide emotional support and create a therapeutic environment that fosters trust and communication. Active listening and empathy can help older adults express their feelings and concerns.
  - ➢ *Social engagement:* Encourage social interactions and maintain connections with family, friends, and support groups to prevent isolation and loneliness.
  - ➢ *Counseling and therapy:* Collaborate with mental health professionals to provide counseling and therapy for older adults dealing with psychosocial challenges, such as grief, depression, or anxiety.
  - ➢ *Life transitions:* Assist in coping with life transitions, such as retirement, loss of loved ones, or changes in living arrangements. Help patients find meaning and purpose in these changes.
- ❖ **Cognitive aspect:**
  - ➢ *Cognitive stimulation:* Engage older adults in cognitive activities that challenge their thinking and memory, such as puzzles, games, or reminiscence therapy.
  - ➢ *Memory aids:* Provide memory aids, such as calendars, reminders, and written instructions, to assist with daily tasks and medication management.
  - ➢ *Communication strategies:* Use clear and simple language, given ample time for responses, and practice patience when communicating with older adults who may experience cognitive changes.
  - ➢ *Family education:* Educate family members and caregivers about cognitive changes, helping them understand how to effectively communicate and provide support.
- ❖ **Holistic care:**
  - ➢ *Individualized care plans:* Develop individualized care plans that address the unique needs and preferences of each older adult, considering their physical, psychosocial, and cognitive aspects.
  - ➢ *Collaboration:* Collaborate with a multidisciplinary team, including physicians, therapists, social workers, and nutritionists, to provide comprehensive care.
  - ➢ *Promote autonomy:* Respect the autonomy and dignity of older adults, involving them in decision-making and care planning as much as possible.

By considering and addressing the physical, psychosocial, and cognitive aspects of ageing, nurses can provide holistic and compassionate care that enhances the quality of life for older adults.

Case Scenario

Case 1
Background: Mrs Kamala Sharma, 72-year-old a retired school teacher, has lived a relatively healthy and active life in New Delhi. She has enjoyed spending time with her family and engaging in community activities. However, as she has aged, she has begun to experience some health challenges.

Presenting health problems:
1. **Hypertension (high blood pressure):** Mrs Sharma has been diagnosed with hypertension, a common health issue among older adults in India. Her blood pressure readings have been consistently elevated, putting her at risk for cardiovascular diseases such as heart attacks and strokes. The nurse assesses her blood pressure regularly and educates her about the importance of medication adherence, maintaining a healthy diet low in salt, and engaging in regular physical activity.
2. **Type 2 diabetes:** During routine health screenings, Mrs Sharma's fasting blood sugar levels were found to be elevated, indicating type 2 diabetes. The nurse provides diabetes education, emphasizing the importance of monitoring blood sugar levels, adhering to prescribed medications, and following a balanced diet. Mrs Sharma is also encouraged to engage in regular exercise to help manage her diabetes.
3. **Osteoarthritis:** Mrs Sharma complains of joint pain and stiffness, particularly in her knees and hips. The nurse assesses her mobility and provides pain management strategies, including gentle exercises, hot and cold therapies, and over-the-counter pain relief. Mrs Sharma is referred to a physical therapist who can design a personalized exercise program to improve her joint function and alleviate discomfort.
4. **Visual impairment:** Mrs Sharma's eyesight has been deteriorating, making it difficult for her to read, watch television, and recognize faces. The nurse arranges for an eye examination and refers her to an ophthalmologist for further evaluation and potential corrective measures, such as glasses or cataract surgery, if necessary.
5. **Social isolation and depression:** As Mrs Sharma's health problems have accumulated, she has become more socially isolated and has started experiencing feelings of sadness and loneliness. The nurse engages in therapeutic conversations, provides emotional support, and encourages her to participate in community events and support groups. Referrals to mental health professionals are also made to address her depression.
6. **Medication management:** Mrs Sharma is taking multiple medications for her health conditions, which can sometimes be confusing to manage. The nurse educates her about the importance of adhering to medication schedules, potential interactions, and possible side effects. A medication organizer is provided to help her keep track of her medications.

Conclusion: This case scenario illustrates some of the common health problems that older adults like Mrs Kamala Sharma may face due to the ageing process. The nursing care provided focuses on addressing these challenges through a holistic approach that encompasses physical health, emotional well-being, and social engagement to improve Mrs Sharma's overall quality of life.

Case 2
Mr Tiwari is a 70-year-old retired school teacher living in a suburban area in India. He has led an active life and maintained a healthy lifestyle, but as he has entered his senior years, he's facing some common health challenges associated with ageing.

Physical aspect: Mr Tiwari has started experiencing joint pain and stiffness, particularly in his knees and back. He finds it difficult to move around as freely as before. His bone density has decreased, making him more susceptible to fractures, and he has been diagnosed with osteoarthritis, which affects his mobility. He is also struggling with weight management, as his metabolism has slowed down, and he's less active due to his joint issues.

Psychosocial aspect: The loss of his spouse a few years ago has left Mr Tiwari feeling lonely and isolated. He misses the social interactions he had with his wife and friends. He finds himself spending most of his time at home, which has led to feelings of sadness and depression. He is concerned about his future and wonders about his purpose in life now that he's retired, and his children have their own families.

Cognitive aspect: Mr Tiwari has noticed that he often forgets where he placed his glasses or keys. He occasionally struggles to recall names of people he has known for years. He's concerned about his memory decline and worries that it might be a sign of a more serious cognitive issue. He's hesitant to participate in social gatherings because of this.

Holistic care approach:
To address Mr Tiwari's health challenges, a holistic care approach is needed:
- **Physical care:** His healthcare provider recommends exercises to improve joint flexibility and strength. Dietary guidance is provided to manage his weight and promote bone health. Medications for pain relief and managing osteoarthritis symptoms are prescribed.

- **Psychosocial support:** Mr Tiwari is encouraged to join local senior citizen groups or hobby classes to meet new people and combat isolation. His family is involved in his care, and they visit him regularly to provide emotional support.
- **Cognitive stimulation:** Cognitive exercises and puzzles are suggested to keep his mind active. His family members engage in memory-boosting activities with him, and he's encouraged to maintain a routine to enhance his cognitive function.

Mr Tiwari's case highlights the interconnected nature of physical, psychosocial, and cognitive aspects of ageing. Through a combination of medical care, emotional support, and cognitive engagement, he can work towards maintaining a higher quality of life as he navigates the challenges that come with ageing.

SUMMARY

- Ageing is a complex and multifaceted process that affects individuals physically, psychosocially, and cognitively.
- Physical aspect of ageing includes the bodily changes like musculoskeletal changes, cardiovascular changes, sensory changes, immune system changes, and metabolic changes.
- The psychosocial aspect of ageing refers to the emotional, social, and psychological changes that occur with age. These changes can include social relationships, potential feelings of loneliness or isolation, coping strategies and emotional resilience through life experiences, identity, and self-esteem changes.
- Cognitive ageing involves changes in cognitive abilities and mental processes. These changes are related to memory, attention, concentration, wisdom, and expertise.
- It's important to note that ageing is a highly individualized process, and not all individuals will experience these changes to the same extent or in the same way. Lifestyle factors, genetics, and overall health play significant roles in shaping how individuals age across these different aspects.

MULTIPLE CHOICE QUESTIONS

1. **Pedal edema is the side effect of which of the following?**
   a. Calcium channel blockers
   b. β-blockers
   c. Angiotensin converting enzyme inhibitors
   d. α-blockers
2. **The most common cancer as per cancer statistics, 2020 is:**
   a. Lung
   b. Prostate
   c. Tongue
   d. Stomach
3. **Steatorrhea is:**
   a. Increase excretion of blood in the stool
   b. Increase excretion of fat in the stool
   c. Increase excretion of pus in the stool
   d. Excessive diarrhea
4. **NUD is manifested as indigestion having no obvious cause. Its full form is:**
   a. Nonulcer dysphasia
   b. Nonulcer dyspepsia
   c. Nonulcer dysphagia
   d. Nonulcer dysplasia
5. **Diagnostic criteria as per WHO for osteoporosis is, when the bone density is:**
   a. < – 2.5
   b. < – 2.0
   c. < –1.5
   d. < – 1.0
6. **Impending pathologic fracture is:**
   a. Complete break of bone
   b. The bone has not broken entirely
   c. Complete crushed bones
   d. The broken ends of the bone line up and are barely out of place.
7. **Loss of urine associated with an abrupt and strong desire to void is called:**
   a. Stress incontinence
   b. Overflow incontinence
   c. Urge incontinence
   d. Functional incontinence
8. **Which of the following does not belong to cognitive aspect of ageing?**
   a. Problem solving
   b. Memory
   c. Attention
   d. Mental health
9. **Emotional well being is the component of which aspect of ageing?**
   a. Physical
   b. Psychosocial
   c. Cognitive
   d. None of the above
10. **Which of the following condition causes due to skin dryness?**
    a. Wrinkles
    b. Xerosis
    c. Seborrheic keratosis
    d. Skin tags

ANSWERS

1. a	2. a	3. b	4. b
5. a	6. b	7. c	8. d
9. b	10. b		

SUGGESTED READING

1. Brunner LS, Suddarth DS, Hinkle JL, Cheever K. Brunner & Suddarth›s textbook of medical-surgical nursing, 13th edition. Philadelphia: Lippincott Williams & Wilkins; 2015. pp. 203-12.
2. Friedman LS, Keeffe EB. Handbook of liver diseases. Elsevier Pub, 2nd edition; 2005.
3. Harrison's Principles of Internal Medicine. Mc Graw Hill Pub, 18th edition; 2008.
4. Lewis SL, Dirksen SR, Heitkemper MM, Bucher L, Harding MM. Medical-Surgical Nursing: Assessment and Management of Clinical Problems. 10th edition. St. Louis: Elsevier; 2017. pp. 65-75.
5. Schaffer DC, Cheskin LJ. Constipation in the Elderly. Am Fam Physician. 1998;58(4):907-14.
6. Singh A, Kaur S, Kishore J. Comprehensive textbook of Elderly Care. Century Publications, New Delhi, 1st edition; 2014. ISBN: 978-81-88132-52-2.
7. Thomas K. Medical Surgical Nursing I & II, 1st edition. New Delhi: Jaypee Brothers Medical Publishers; 2018. pp. 432-42.
8. World Health Organization, Global Surveillance, Prevention and Control of Chronic Respiratory Diseases: A Comprehensive Approach, WHO Press, Geneva, Switzerland; 2007.

CHAPTER 48
Elderly Abuse, Legal and Ethical Issues of the Elderly

Nitasha Sharma, Sunita Sharma

"To care for those who once cared for us is one of the highest honors".

—**Tia Walker**

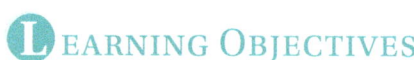 **LEARNING OBJECTIVES**

After going through the chapter, the learner will be able to:
- Define elderly abuse.
- Describe various types of elderly abuse.
- Discuss various risk factors for abuse.
- Describe the role of nurses in the identification and reporting of abuse.
- Discuss the prevention of elderly abuse.
- Discuss ethical principles of elderly care.

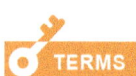 **TERMS**

- **Advance directives:** These are the legal documents that state the person's wishes and preferences about his care and treatment when he/she will lack the capacity for such decisions by virtue of illness/injury or any other cause.
- **Beneficence:** It is promoting the well-being of patients through research and implementation of therapeutic interventions with the highest probability of positive patient outcomes.
- **Elderly abuse:** A lack of appropriate action, occurring within any relationship where there is an expectation of trust, leading to harm or distress to an older person.
- **Euthanasia:** It is the act of deliberately putting an end to a person's life in order to eliminate pain or suffering.
- **Justice:** It implies equitable allocation of healthcare resources.
- **Living will:** A written record of a person's wishes that will help the nominated person(s) to carry out at the appropriate time without any guilt or anguish.
- **Non-maleficence:** Requires the physician to omit any action that would harm the patient.

INTRODUCTION

Elderly abuse is considered a major public health concern. There are pooled estimates from various studies across the world that 1 in 6 people (15.7%) aged 60 years and older have experienced abuse in one or the other form. These rates tend to escalate in institutional settings and other long-stay residential care facilities. Yet, abuse of older people remains a low global priority. Further, the COVID-19 pandemic added to the miseries of the elderly with a sharp rise in the rates of elderly abuse and maltreatment. While the ageing population is increasing in many countries, the rates of elderly abuse are too increasing at an unprecedented pace.

The upcoming section of the chapter describes a basic understanding of elderly abuse, its types, signs, and symptoms followed by the role of healthcare professionals in screening, identification, and reporting of elderly abuse.

DEFINITION OF ELDERLY ABUSE

It is defined as "a single or repeated act, or lack of appropriate action, occurring within any relationship where there is an expectation of trust, which causes harm or distress to an older person." Elderly abuse constitutes of violation of human rights and includes physical, sexual, psychological, and emotional abuse; financial and material abuse; abandonment; neglect; and serious loss of dignity and respect.

TYPES OF ELDERLY ABUSE

There are various types of abuse. While physical abuse is well-known and reported, however abuse in the elderly can be seen in many other forms.

1. **Physical abuse:** The national center on elderly abuse defines physical abuse as "the use of physical force that may result in bodily injury, physical pain, or impairment." It includes other acts of physical harm, such as hitting, kicking, shaking, etc.
2. **Emotional abuse:** Emotional abuse often reported as psychological abuse is defined as "the infliction of anguish, pain, or distress through verbal or nonverbal acts. These acts include the harassment, threats, and intimidation of the elderly.
3. **Sexual abuse:** Sexual abuse occurs when a victim is forced into an unwanted act that is sexual in nature. Such kind of abuse in the elderly encompasses all forms of acts, such as inappropriate physical touch, forced nudity, rape, etc.
4. **Financial abuse:** Acts of directly or indirectly controlling and/or misusing the financial accounts of the victim constitute financial abuse. The acts, such as changing the will by means of fraud or doing financial transactions from the victim's account which are indeed not in the best interest of the elderly also precludes financial abuse.
5. **Neglect:** Neglect refers to situations of non-fulfillment of caretaking responsibilities and duties by caregivers. This includes acts of not providing required medical care and treatment as well as the inability to provide care and support in activities of daily living.

The neglect is very common in institutional settings and is often undetected and unreported. The common forms of neglect in such settings are physically restraining the elderly, lack of dignified nursing care, and non-involvement in decision-making for day-to-day activities and events. The instances of over-medication as well as under-medication are also a form of neglect.

RISK FACTORS FOR ELDERLY ABUSE

Although elderly abuse can occur in a wide array of settings and circumstances, however, there are certain well-known risk factors for elder abuse which need discussion.

- ❖ **Functional dependence/disability/poor physical health:** The probability of abuse likely to be high if the elderly have functional impairment due to an underlying medical condition or disability leading to dependence. Dependence tends to increase the risk of abuse since the ability to escape, seek help, and defend self is reduced. People with a chronic disorder or functional impairment may require more care thus, increasing stress for the caregivers.
- ❖ **Cognitive impairment:** The elderly manifesting cognitive impairment related to dementia and other neurodegenerative processes have more chances of being neglected as well as abused financially. The elderly with dementia have impaired communication, understanding, judgment, and behavior causing dysfunction in day-to-day living and leading to more dependence and frustration in caregivers. It is specifically described in the literature that the disruptive behavior arising out of dementia is a source of stress for the caregivers and thus, a risk factor for elderly abuse.
- ❖ **Gender:** Abuse happens to both older women and older men. While some reports suggest a high prevalence of abuse in women than men, others have contrary findings. Literature also highlights that the severity of abuse, as well as associated physical and emotional impact, is much more grave in women. Though there are cultural and family influences as well.
- ❖ **Living arrangement:** Shared living arrangement has been reported as a major risk factor for elderly abuse while living alone is reported as a protective factor against abuse.
- ❖ **Social isolation:** It is hypothesized that elderly abuse is less likely to happen in families which have strong social ties and networks while families in isolation have high chances of elderly abuse where it is less likely to be detected and reported.

There are also other risk factors in the literature about the perpetrators of elderly abuse:

- ❖ Using or abusing drugs or alcohol
- ❖ High-stress levels
- ❖ Depression
- ❖ Lack of social support
- ❖ Inadequate training in the care of elderly
- ❖ Emotional or financial dependence on the older person

WARNING SIGNS OF ELDERLY ABUSE

Elderly abuse does not always have a uniform presentation as this complex issue has multiple etiologies with varying living arrangements embedded in complex relationships and cultures. Despite such complexities, it is important to know the overt and covert signs of suspected abuse.

- ❖ **Red flags/warning signs for physical elderly abuse:** One must be aware of these overt physical signs of elderly abuse. If there are unexplained bruises, welts, lacerations, or rope marks on the body, one must raise concern for suspected physical abuse. An elderly with bone fractures especially the skull fractures must be assessed for abuse. The presence of wounds and untreated injuries in variable stages of healing indicates potential abuse. It is common to observe sprains and dislocations in the victims of abuse. Other indirect indicators could be the broken spectacles and other physical indicators of being punished, or lacerations around ankles and wrists might reflect signs of physical restraining. Many a time reports of underutilization of prescribed medications or medication overdoses might indicate underlying neglect and abuse.

Other warning signs could be a sudden change in behavior of the elderly. Also, some subtle behaviors, such as the caregiver's disapproval to visitors to meet the elderly alone need to be looked upon.

- ❖ **Warning signs of emotional/psychological abuse:** The warning signs for emotional abuse are very generic, such as an elderly might appear emotionally upset or disconcerted. Certain atypical behaviors, such as sucking, biting, and rocking might be a reflection of emotional abuse. Any change in premorbid behavior in biological functions, such as sleeping and eating and personality changes are warning signs of emotional abuse. One of the most common manifestations of elderly abuse is the presence of depression and anxiety symptoms. An elderly self-report of being verbally or emotionally mistreated should never be disregarded.

- ❖ **Warning signs of financial exploitation:** One must suspect financial exploitation if there are sudden changes in bank accounts or banking practices, such as the withdrawal of huge sums of money by a person escorting the older adult. The inclusion of additional names on an older adult's bank signature card or unlawful drawing of the older adult's funds using their cards are warning signs. If there are any unexpected changes in a will or related documents, one must consider the potential for financial abuse. It is also observed that there is unexplained loss of funds or valuable possessions. If there are unpaid bills in relation to elderly medical care or substandard care being given to the elderly despite having no financial constraints are warning signs of elderly financial abuse. Other covert signs may be the sudden appearance of a relative claiming his right over the property and other possessions who has otherwise never been involved in the care of the elderly. An unforeseen transfer of property to someone who is not an immediate family member must be observed. Many a time the provision of certain costly unnecessary services also indicates financial abuse.

- ❖ **Warning signs of neglect and abandonment:** The warning signs of neglect can be gauzed from the physical condition of the elderly and the elderly's environment. The conditions reflecting neglect could be dehydration and malnutrition. The poor personal hygiene, inadequate clothing, or the presence of unattended pressure sores, and often discounting other physical health problems including pains, aches, or other problems of vision, etc., are possible indicators of neglect. The environmental indicators of neglect include the unsanitary living condition where there is dirt, flies, and lice, soiled and stinking bed linen. The environment can also be hazardous and unsafe with inadequate ventilation, lighting with extremes of temperature with lack of basic amenities, such as water.

- ❖ **Warning signs of sexual abuse:** The warning signs for the sexual abuse of the elderly are overt physical signs, such as bruises around the private parts, the presence of blood on bed sheets, and on their clothing. The victim of sexual abuse would have unexplained venereal disease or genital infections or unexplained vaginal or anal bleeding. Many a time sexual abuse can be suspected if there are sudden changes in an older adult's demeanour, such as appearing withdrawn or fearful in the presence of some specific individual. Self-report of being sexually assaulted or raped is a very important sign.

MANDATORY REPORTING, THE ROLE OF NURSES AND OTHER HEALTHCARE PROVIDERS

The healthcare providers have an ethical and legal responsibility for mandatory reporting of abuse and neglect in the elderly. They must advocate for the victims of all forms of abuse. This is possible if healthcare providers including nurses, doctors, and other paramedical staff have sensitization and the necessary skills to perform screening, identification, and reporting of abuse. It is of paramount importance to educate and equip healthcare professionals with adequate sensitivity and skills to recognize signs of abuse & intervene timely and promptly. Healthcare professionals sometimes may show some resistance and hesitance to report suspected abuse unless they have proof. One of the most common factors of non-reporting is a belief that the suspected abuse was a single incident and it is unlikely to happen again. But mandatory reporting usually protects those who report suspected abuse by maintaining the reporters' anonymity and freeing them from concerns of litigation.

Nursing Care of Elderly Abused Individual

The nurses care for the elderly in a wide array of settings including day care facilities to inpatient settings. Nurses have enough interaction with elderly clients where they are in a position to accurately screen for and assess for any signs of abuse.

- ❖ **Screening for elderly abuse:** Besides looking for overt objective signs of abuse which at times are ignored as these signs are often treated as common signs of ageing, there are objective instruments for screening the elderly for abuse and maltreatment. Elder Assessment Instrument (EAI) is one such tool that has a comprehensive approach for screening suspected elder abuse victims in all clinical settings. The tool reviews signs, symptoms, and subjective complaints of elder abuse and neglect. There are five domains assessed in the instrument viz. general assessment, such as level of hygiene; possible abuse, indicators, such as bruises, fractures, and self-report by elderly; possible neglect indicators, such as dehydration, contractures, etc.; possible exploitation indicators, such as inability to account for money/property; and possible abandonment indicators, such as evidence that the patient is left alone in an unsafe environment for extended periods of time without adequate support. The EAI has no "score," but any positive evidence without clinical explanation, subjective complaints of abuse communicated by an older adult, or a healthcare provider's suspicions of abuse or neglect warrant referral to social services.

- ❖ **Observation and history-taking:** The nurses working with the elderly in outpatient emergency settings can effectively utilize observational skills and history-taking in detecting cases of elderly abuse. Some of the observations that might raise concerns are:

- Older adults and caregivers provide inconsistent explanations of events
- One must observe if there is too much interruption by the caregivers while the elderly are being assessed.
- When the elderly appears hostile, withdrawn, or fearful towards the caregivers.
- If the caregiver is totally unengaged or detached in elderly care, and lacks knowledge about elderly needs and care.
- Caregiver appears burdened which is manifested in the form of frustration, fatigue and anger, and abuse of alcohol and other illicit drugs.

Nurses should try to take the history preferably when the elderly are alone after ensuring confidentiality and privacy. Initiating rapport and trusting relationships are important for such disclosures. Many a time the victims remain silent on these issues owing to perceived guilt, shame, stigma, and fear. There are some subtle indicators from medical history that nurses must be sensitive to acknowledge and report.

❖ **Pointers from the Medical History of Possible Elder Abuse or Neglect:** There are many pointers for elderly abuse in their medical history, e.g., history of unexplained frequent injuries and falls, an obvious and significant delay in medical help-seeking, and very frequent visits to the emergency for similar kinds of injuries. It is noteworthy if there is a history of very frequent changes of physicians and/or treatment settings and there is poor compliance with medications, follow-ups, and other is too an indicator of abuse.

Nursing Interventions in Suspected Abuse

Once a nurse suspects any of her clients to be a victim of abuse, the key nursing interventions must include the following:

1. **Assessment:** The elderly must be assessed for factors that might have provoked abuse. The elderly should be assessed for a history of social isolation, history of mental health-related issues, extreme dependence, and poor family relationships. After making a thorough assessment and considering the present condition of the client, the nursing care must be planned. The various aspects of nursing care include the following:
   - *Treatment of acute medical and traumatic conditions:* Once the abuse is detected, it is important to address the medical needs of the client. Many a time there are wounds related to abuse which might range from mild abrasions to major fractures. These physical injuries can further impair the abilities of daily living, such as walking, bathing, etc. Ensuring timely medical treatment for any physical injuries will help reduce further long-term damage.
   - *Addressing the psychological issues with compassion and dignity:* The elderly often suffer from fear and anxiety related to the re-occurrence of physical aggression. The elderly who are the victims of abuse often have feelings of depression manifesting as sadness of mood, low self-esteem, suicidality, and social isolation. The important element of nursing care is to provide sources of emotional as well as social support to the elderly. Nurses act as advocates for patients to have access to all available services and rights. Nurses can assist in developing new social bonds by educating them about various social groups or organizations working for the cause. Nurses should plan educational interventions to increase awareness and understanding of the elderly about their rights and assist them to make informed choices.
   - *Ensuring patient safety:* Once the abuse is detected, ensuring patient safety is most important to prevent further harm and damage to the patient. The nurses should evaluate the need to refer the elderly to protective services. It must be ensured that the victim does not have any contact with the suspected abuser. If the risk of abuse is high, nurses must ensure patient safety by either offering hospitalization or alternative living arrangements. This may be challenging, particularly when the abuser is either a family member or a nominated representative. In such scenarios, the nurses should not hesitate in involving the hospital administration and legal department to assist with issues including healthcare decision-making and guardianship.

2. **Mandatory reporting:** It is the legal responsibility of nurses to report elderly abuse. This can be done by filing a written complaint to the jurisdictional police.

PREVENTION OF ELDERLY ABUSE

Considering the physical as well as psychological impact of abuse on the elderly and to a large extent on society, prevention of abuse is of paramount importance. Elderly abuse can be prevented with concerted actions and initiatives at various levels. Broadly, this set of actions may be seen in three areas as depicted in **Figure 48.1**.

Preventive Interventions for the Elderly

The most important aspect of elderly-targeted interventions revolves around empowering the elderly to maximize their independence, improve functionality, focus on social support, enhancing their self-efficacy and health locus of control. Social support is well established protective factor against abuse and mistreatment. Elderly people who have someone whom they can count upon for emotional support, somebody for seeking any piece of advice, someone for assistance in daily chores or otherwise trust and may confide in always have a lower risk of mistreatment and abuse. The elderly with strong social networks and bonds often are much more confident and thus have a better sense of self-efficacy

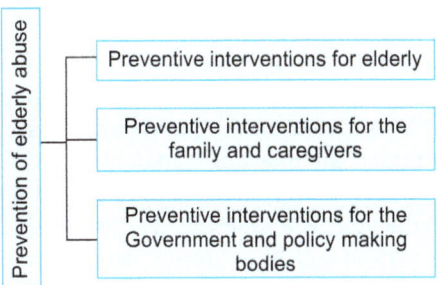

Fig. 48.1: Preventive interventions for elderly abuse.

and even better health. Empowering the elderly is known to be of great importance in the prevention of abuse. Some of the important elements of empowerment of elderly are as follows:

- ❖ Giving information to the elderly about the psychological and physiological changes in advanced age and the required behavioral adaptations that need to be taught for better outcomes. Such adaptive behaviors will assist the elderly to adapt and meet transitional developmental needs in a better way.
- ❖ Education to the elderly about various means to lead an active, productive, and successful life. This can be achieved by joining elderly clubs, engaging in regular physical exercise, such as a morning walk with others of similar age, and keeping on with habits, such as reading, cooking, gardening, etc. The elderly must be in regular touch with their friends outside the family, must possess their own phone, or have access to various means of communication. These small accomplishments would add to their self-esteem and maintain a sense of purpose in them.
- ❖ Imparting education to the elderly about all special benefits and privileges in different policies, etc. These have been detailed in Chapter 49.
- ❖ It is recommended that the elderly should establish a living will or have advanced healthcare planning to ensure that their financial and healthcare decisions are respected.
- ❖ Elderly people must be taught about various means to prevent financial abuse by not giving their banking details to anyone, not lending money without a proper payback schedule, not signing any documents without understanding them, being well informed about all financial affairs, and granting the power of attorney only to a trusted person.

Preventive Interventions for the Family and Caregivers

There are situations when the family members and/or caregivers are perpetrators of the abuse. Some of the risk factors are high caregiver burnout, poor mental health of the caregiver, substance abuse in the caregiver, and lack of training in caregiving. Therefore, the preventive interventions targeting the caregivers are discussed as follows:

- ❖ Provision of training on caregiving can help to minimize abuse in the elderly. The training must focus on essential skills in elderly care with varying levels of dependence. The various components of training include assistance in activities of daily living (bathing, toileting, oral feeding, positioning, mobility assistance, and transfer from bed to wheelchair and vice versa). Well-trained caregivers often have less stress and better mental health.
- ❖ Programs aimed at the promotion of mental health and well-being of caregivers are of great utility in preventing abuse. These include the provision of psychological interventions, such as anger management techniques, cognitive restraining exercises to deal with resentment, stress reduction techniques, etc. The psychosocial support in the form of self-help groups, respite care services, residential respites, and other sitting services can be of great utility.
- ❖ Teaching the caregivers about health promotional behaviors to maintain their own health and seeking help from friends and other social connections is promoted. It is advised not to ignore signs of stress, anxiety, or depression.

Elderly abuse prevention in residential settings can be done by providing formal training to staff, maintaining better communication, keeping a check on caregivers' mental health status and substance use, and screening the elderly for any form of abuse. The family members of such families who often hire paid caregivers must have adequate knowledge about indicators and risk factors for elderly abuse. The verbal report by the elderly about being abused should not be taken, lightly and if possible environmental safety can be ensured by the use of CCTV cameras and other monitoring systems.

Preventive Interventions for the Government and Policy-making Bodies

Government intervention is crucial in enacting and enforcing laws that protect the rights of older adults in India.

- ❖ Governments should continuously review and update existing legislation to ensure its effectiveness in preventing and addressing elder abuse. This includes provisions for increased penalties for offenders and streamlined reporting and investigation procedures. The provision of various laws and national policies for the welfare of the elderly is described in Chapter 49.
- ❖ The government should promote social support networks for senior citizens through community organizations, senior citizen clubs, support groups, and other NGOs. These shall provide avenues to the elderly for socialization, emotional support, and assistance, thereby reducing the vulnerability of older adults to abuse.
- ❖ The implementation of easy and public-friendly reporting systems shall help in the prevention of abuse in the elderly. Establishing accessible and confidential reporting systems in India is essential to encourage individuals to report cases of elder abuse without fear of reprisals. These systems should be supported by clear protocols for reporting, investigation, and follow-up actions.

ETHICAL AND LEGAL ISSUES IN ELDERLY CARE

The ethical principles and code of conduct for medical and paramedical professionals have existed almost for centuries now. The modern ethical principles have their roots in Hippocrates' oath. The four major principles of ethical practice are described as Autonomy, Beneficence, Non-Maleficence, and Justice. The upcoming section shall briefly describe each principle with special reference to elderly care.

Autonomy

This principle basically reflects the obligation of professionals to respect the individual's right to decision-making on their own behalf. It can be better explained as respecting a patient's autonomous choices through self-determination. The healthcare provider can promote autonomy by not standing in the way of what they want to do or by actively supporting their values and goals. Autonomy cannot be equated with the compliance rather it reflects a genuine respect for the patient's autonomous choices. The ground philosophical base for autonomy is that all persons have an intrinsic and unconditional worth, and therefore, should have the power to make rational decisions and moral choices, and each should be allowed to exercise his/her capacity for self-determination. Autonomy requires both "liberty (independence from controlling influences) and agency (capacity for intentional action)" and many a time liberty is destabilized by coercion, persuasion, and manipulation. The principle of autonomy is exercised through the informed consent. Informed consent requires patients to approve or refuse treatment and requires certain other conditions to be met, such as that a patient appreciates:

❖ The nature of the decision or intervention;
❖ Reasonable alternatives to what is proposed; and
❖ Risks and benefits of each alternative.

The incapacity (incompetence) of the person is an important exception to informed consent. The principle of autonomy does not extend to persons who lack the capacity (competence) to act autonomously; examples include infants and children and incompetence due to developmental, mental, or physical disorders.

Personal autonomy runs into particular risk in the clinical setting, owing in large part to the increased dependence and vulnerability that frequently accompany illness. It is important to discuss here that elderly people might lack the capacity for decision-making due to dementia and other age-related cognitive impairments. In such scenarios, the treating team has to rely on a surrogate decision-maker to decide medical decisions on behalf of the patient whose role is to extend the patient's autonomy by representing the patient's wishes. Most of the time this person is selected by the patients themselves by means of a legal instrument, such as a durable power of attorney for healthcare or advanced directives to the physician (living will). As per the landmark case in Supreme Court in 2018, it is recognized that a terminally-ill patient or a person in a persistent vegetative state can execute an "advance medical directive" or a "living will" to refuse medical treatment and gave sanction to passive euthanasia and living will/advance directives.

Justice

The principle of justice implies equitable allocation of healthcare resources. "*Justice* is concerned with the equitable distribution of benefits and burdens to individuals in social institutions, and how the rights of various individuals are realized"

In modern healthcare settings, the principle of justice is usually focused on the distribution of scarce healthcare resources between different individuals and groups in society. Many a time, the age of the person becomes an area of ethical concern especially when distributing the scarce/life-saving resources. One school of thought expresses the idea that an elderly person has already had a fair share of life and thus should step aside to give a chance to the younger groups, especially in a resource-limited scenario. Contrary to this are the arguments that in determining whether or not a person has had a fair share of life, more than the number of years a person has lived is at stake. Another view is that we should choose whatever course of action saves the greatest number of life years or health-related quality of life.

The elderly population accounts for a large share of healthcare expenditure which has led to healthcare rationing based on age. However, the latest evidence substantiates that age should not be taken as the sole criteria for rationing health care especially surgery, chemotherapy, and hemodialysis rather other indicators, such as performance status, comorbid illnesses, etc., must be considered.

Beneficence/Non-maleficence

Beneficence is defined as "the responsibility of healthcare experts to promote the well-being of patients through research and implementation of therapeutic interventions with the highest probability of positive patient outcomes." In addition to these definitions, the principle of beneficence emphasizes the ethical commitment to the benefit, including protecting patients' rights, preventing harm to them, and helping those at risk. It also refers to the course of action that would be in the best interest of the patient and refrain from any such course of action which can have any potential deleterious effect. The principle of non-maleficence requires the physician to omit any action that would harm the patient. Taken together, beneficence and non-maleficence are often understood as maximizing principles, requiring that medical decisions produce the greatest amount of good and the least amount of harm for a particular patient.

The principle is exercised by physicians by performing a risk-benefit analysis for every important treatment decision and avoiding those actions that are inappropriately burdensome and choosing the best course of action for the patient.

Despite well-established principles for ethically sound health care, healthcare providers often encounter various ambiguous scenarios when ethical conflicts arise. Yet irrespective of anything, the healthcare provider's primary commitment must always be the patient's welfare whether the physician is treating the elderly illness or helping the elderly to cope with illness, disability, and even death.

Legal Issues

The most important legal issues in elderly care pertain to end-of-life care. The two worth discussing are advanced directives and living will.

Advance Directives

Advance directives are legal documents that state the person's wishes and preferences about his care and treatment when he/she will lack the capacity for such decisions by virtue of illness/injury or any other cause. The two most common forms of advance directives for health care are the "living will" and the durable "power of attorney for health care".

Living Will

The American lawyer Louis Kutner first proposed the living wills in 1969 as a simple device to allow patients to say no to life-sustaining treatment that they did not want, even if they were too ill to communicate their wishes. The "Living Will" is a written record of a person's wishes that will help the nominated person(s) to carry out the person's wishes at the appropriate time without any guilt or anguish. It is indeed a legal document that tells doctors how the elderly want to be treated at times when they lack the capacity for the same.

It involves aspects, such as their preferred settings of care and even the death (home or hospital), the type of treatment they would, such as to receive, the amount of information about their diseased condition they would, such as to know, and the supports they would, such as to access at end of life. It involves decisions, such as avoidance of any kind of invasive interventions, administration of intravenous fluids, use of antibiotics, administration of blood and blood products, any hospitalization, admission in an intensive care unit, use of dialysis, insertion of feeding tubes and catheters, use of total parenteral nutrition, insertion of the central venous catheter, etc. It also involves confirming a preference not to have invasive medical procedures aimed at resuscitation, mechanical ventilation, use of inotropic drugs, invasive tubes, or artificial machines aimed at keeping a person alive at the end of their life.

There is a provision where the person making the Living Will can alter their preferences and decisions at any moment. They can also modify the name of the Nominated representative at any time.

Euthanasia

"Euthanasia is the act of deliberately putting an end to a person's life in order to eliminate pain or suffering."

Active euthanasia, or assisted suicide, is the act of deliberately and actively doing something, such as injecting a lethal dose of a drug, to end a person's life. Active euthanasia is not permissible in India.

Passive euthanasia is "intentionally letting a patient die by withholding artificial life support, such as a ventilator or a feeding tube." The concept of passive euthanasia entails the desire to hasten death in the patient's best interests. Instances of passive euthanasia can include not giving medication and not performing surgery that would save the patient's life.

There are three conditions that must be met for passive euthanasia to occur:
1. Life-prolonging treatments are being discontinued or withheld.
2. The primary goal of the discontinuation or withholding of the treatment shall be to speed up the death of the patient.
3. The justification for the speed-up death is that the action was taken in the patient's best interests to die, as sooner or later he would die.

The Legalization of Passive Euthanasia in India

Passive euthanasia was legalized in India by the Supreme Court in 2018, subject to the condition that the person is having an advance Directive or a living will. The Supreme Court has given legal recognition to passive euthanasia. According to the ruling, a patient who has competence for a decision on health care as well as a person who lacks competence but has an advance directive shall/may be deemed passive euthanasia. The decision ruled that a patient's living will is a valid legal document in the context of medical decisions, such as withdrawing futile medical treatment. The ruling upholds the right to make an informed decision to decline medical treatment, including withdrawal from life-saving devices.

The Supreme Court has laid down the following guidelines:
- Parents, spouses, or other close relatives are responsible for the decision to discontinue life support, but, in their absence of them, any person or group acting as a friend can make the decision. The patient's doctor can take it as well. Although the decision should be taken in the patient's best interests, it should not be arbitrary.
- Although the decision to withdraw life support can be made by relatives or doctors, the authority for final approval is vested with the high court.
- The procedure laid down upon receipt of such application is depicted in **Figure 48.2**.

A person of sound and healthy mental health can only execute advance directives. It must be voluntary and non-coercive. There shall be a written statement as to when medical treatment may be withdrawn or no medical treatment may be given that would delay the process of death, otherwise causing pain and suffering.
- The document is to be made in the presence of two attesting witnesses when the executor signs the document. The document needs to be countersigned by the Judicial Magistrate of First Class (JMFC) of the concerned jurisdiction. The witness must ensure that the document was signed freely and without any force/coercion.
- The treating physician shall verify the authenticity of the execution from the jurisdictional JMFC if the executor becomes terminally ill with no hope for recovery. The physician must inform the executor or guardian/close relative about the nature of the illness, the available medical care, and the consequences of alternative forms of treatment and remaining untreated if the instructions need to be followed.
- Medical boards shall be formed by the hospital consisting of the head of the treating department and at least three experienced physicians who shall jointly meet with the patient's relatives to decide whether to withdraw medical treatment.

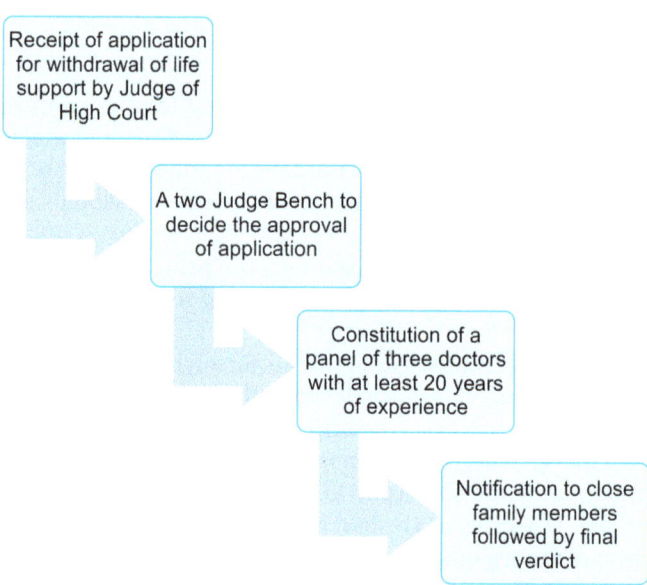

Fig. 48.2: Procedure for passive euthanasia.

❖ The hospital must inform the collector about the proposal if the Medical Board certifies that the instructions should be followed. An additional Medical Board shall be formed by the collector in conjunction with the district's chief medical officer and three expert doctors. If the patient is not able to communicate, the board shall examine the patient and may agree to withdraw the treatment. If the board decides to withdraw the treatment, they should notify JMFC of their decision. After examining all aspects, the JMFC visits the patient and may permit its implementation.

Case Scenario

Mrs SK is an 86-year-old widower staying with her son and daughter-in-law. Her son had major losses in business a few years back after which he increased his alcohol intake to a problematic level. The daughter-in-law works in a private firm and makes some money to run the house. Mrs SK is a known hypertensive and diabetic. She recently had a hypoglycemic shock too as compliance with medications is poor. She has marked cognitive impairment along with wandering behavior recently. What are the probable risk factors, protective factors, and overt indicators of abuse in the case?

SUMMARY

Elderly abuse is a major public health concern with a prevalence rate close to 15%. The abuse can be seen in various forms viz. physical, emotional, sexual, and financial and neglect. It is an ethical as well as a legal responsibility of healthcare providers including nurses to have mandatory reporting of elderly abuse in any form. Nurses working with the elderly population must have adequate training and skills to screen for abuse, make objective assessments for any form of abuse while obtaining history, do basic assessments in routine nursing care, and perform mandatory reporting if abuse is suspected and/or confirmed. The other ethical principles of care include autonomy, justice, and beneficence/maleficence which are equally relevant while providing care to the elderly. The legal aspect of elderly care includes the advance directives/living will. Advance directives are legal documents that state the person's wishes and preferences about his care and treatment when he/she will lack the capacity for such decisions by virtue of illness/injury or any other cause. Passive euthanasia was legalized in India by the Supreme Court in 2018, subject to the condition that the person is having an advance directive or a living will.

MULTIPLE CHOICE QUESTIONS

1. When the abuser is controlling and misusing the victim's financial accounts it is referred as:
   a. Maltreatment
   b. Neglect
   c. Emotional abuse
   d. Financial abuse
2. Which of the following is a sign of sexual abuse:
   a. Dehydration, malnutrition, untreated bedsores, and poor personal hygiene
   b. Unattended or untreated health problems
   c. Bone fractures, broken bones, or skull fractures
   d. Unexplained venereal disease or genital infections
3. An advance directive is a document that does which of the following?
   a. Addresses decisions regarding end-of-life care only
   b. Allows patients to have their wishes honored only in the state in which they live
   c. Becomes effective prior to incapacity in most states
   d. Communicates preferences regarding end-of-life care before incapacitation occurs
4. The concept of justice in ethics is:
   a. An obligation of the patient to the society
   b. That the health resources must be distributed according to the principles of equity
   c. Taken as patients right to choose or refuse treatment
   d. For all medical professionals to do good for all patients under circumstances
5. The four rules of professional–patient relationships set forth and explained by Beauchamp and Childress are:
   a. Autonomy, privacy, respect, and confidentiality
   b. Veracity, privacy, beneficence, and non-maleficence
   c. Respect for autonomy, non-maleficence, beneficence, and justice
   d. Veracity, privacy, confidentiality, and fidelity

ANSWERS

1. d
2. d
3. d
4. b
5. c

SUGGESTED READING

1. Abuse of older people [Internet]. [cited 2023 Apr 9]. Available from: https://www.who.int/news-room/fact-sheets/detail/abuse-of-older-people
2. Advance Care Planning: Advance Directives for Health Care. Available from: https://www.nia.nih.gov/health/advance-care-planning-advance-directives-health-care
3. BBC—Ethics—Euthanasia: Living wills [Internet]. [cited 2023 Jul 14]. Available from: https://www.bbc.co.uk/ethics/euthanasia/overview/livingwills.shtml
4. Chang ES, Levy BR. High Prevalence of Elder Abuse During the COVID-19 Pandemic: Risk and Resilience Factors. Am J Geriatr Psychiatry Off J Am Assoc Geriatr Psychiatry. 2021;29(11):1152-9.
5. Dong X, Simon MA. Is greater social support a protective factor against elder mistreatment? Gerontology. 2008;54(6):381-8. doi: 10.1159/000143228. Epub 2008 Jul 7. PMID: 18600021.
6. EHS—How can institutions prevent and identify Elder Abuse [Internet]. [cited 2023 Jul 23]. Available from: https://www.elderly.gov.hk/english/carers_corner/caring_skills/prevention_of_elder_abuse.html
7. Elder Abuse and Neglect—HelpGuide.org [Internet]. [cited 2023 Jul 23]. Available from: https://www.helpguide.org/articles/abuse/elder-abuse-and-neglect.htm
8. ELICIT-BasicLivingWillAndInstructions-Final.pdf [Internet]. [cited 2023 Jul 14]. Available from: https://palliumindia.org/wp-content/uploads/2020/05/ELICIT-BasicLivingWillAndInstructions-Final.pdf
9. Fulmer T. Elder Abuse and Neglect Assessment. J Gerontol Nurs. 2003;29(6):4–5.
10. Lachs MS, Berkman L, Fulmer T, Horwitz RI. A prospective community-based pilot study of risk factors for the investigation of elder mistreatment. J Am Geriatr Soc. 1994;42(2):169-73.
11. National Research Council (US) Panel to Review Risk and Prevalence of Elder Abuse and Neglect. Elder Mistreatment: Abuse, Neglect, and Exploitation in an Aging America [Internet]. Bonnie RJ, Wallace RB, editors. Washington (DC): National Academies Press (US); 2003 [cited 2023 Apr 9]. (The National Academies Collection: Reports funded by National Institutes of Health). Available from: http://www.ncbi.nlm.nih.gov/books/NBK98802/
12. Patel K, Bunachita S, Chiu H, Suresh P, Patel UK. Elder Abuse: A Comprehensive Overview and Physician-Associated Challenges. Cureus. 13(4):e14375.
13. Podgorica N, Flatscher-Thöni M, Deufert D, Siebert U, Ganner M. A systematic review of ethical and legal issues in elder care. Nurs Ethics. 2021;28(6):895–910.
14. Prevalence of Elder Abuse in India and Steps We Can Take to Address it | TheHealthSite.com [Internet]. [cited 2023 Jul 23]. Available from:

https://www.thehealthsite.com/diseases-conditions/world-elder-abuse-awareness-day-steps-india-can-take-to-combat-elder-abuse-effectively-985229/

15. Prevention F on GV, Health B on G. Medicine I of, Council NR. PREVENTING ELDER ABUSE—HOPE SPRINGS ETERNAL. In: Elder Abuse and Its Prevention: Workshop Summary [Internet]. National Academies Press (US); 2014 [cited 2023 Jul 23]. Available from: https://www.ncbi.nlm.nih.gov/books/NBK208553/

16. Red Flags of Elder Abuse [Internet]. 2019 [cited 2023 Apr 9]. Available from: https://www.justice.gov/elderjustice/red-flags-elder-abuse-0

17. Rosen T, Stern ME, Elman A, Mulcare MR. Identifying and Initiating Intervention for Elder Abuse and Neglect in the Emergency Department. Clin Geriatr Med. 2018;34(3):435-51.

18. Scholarly Articles—Social support system and well being of elderly women—Indian context [Internet]. [cited 2023 Jul 23]. Available from: http://scholararticles.net/social-support-system-and-well-being-of-elderly-women-indian-context/

19. Sedig L. What's the Role of Autonomy in Patient- and Family-Centered Care When Patients and Family Members Don't Agree? AMA Journal of Ethics. 2016;18(1):12-7.

20. Stark S. Elder abuse: Screening, intervention, and prevention. Nursing 2023. 2012;42(10):24.

21. Varkey B. Principles of Clinical Ethics and Their Application to Practice. Medical Principles and Practice. 2020;30(1):17-28.

22. Yon Y, Ramiro-Gonzalez M, Mikton CR, Huber M, Sethi D. The prevalence of elder abuse in institutional settings: a systematic review and meta-analysis. Eur J Public Health. 2019;29(1):58-67.

CHAPTER 49

Provisions and Programs for Elderly

Ruchi Saini, Nitasha Sharma, Sukhpal Kaur

> "A society that does not value its older people denies its roots. Let us strive to enhance their capacity to support themselves when they cannot do so anymore, to care for them".
>
> —**Nelson Mandela**

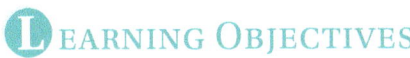

After going through the chapter, the learner will be able to:

- Describe various initiatives taken by the government of India for the welfare of the elderly.
- Enlist various schemes and programs which are running under different ministries for the care of the elderly.
- Appreciate various concessions available for senior citizens.
- Describe various legal frameworks available for the protection of rights, life, and property of older people.

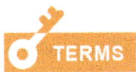

- **Older person/senior citizen:** A person aged more than 60 years.
- **Program:** A set of accessible and affordable services provided for the comprehensive care of the ageing population.
- **Welfare:** Welfare of the elderly pertains to the care of old people in areas of health, medical, housing, social, and financial security.

INTRODUCTION

The population of older people in India has been growing rapidly for the past many years. Though ageing is a natural process of human life, it brings with it numerous problems such as physiological problems, economic problems, social problems, house-related problems, etc. The developed countries have framed many policies and programs to avert the crisis of ageing and promote their economic growth. Similar, initiatives are also taken by the South Asian Countries. The United Nations had taken the initiative as its 1st International Plan of Action on Ageing in Vienna in 1982 and framed Principles for Older Persons in 1991 under the following main themes—Independence, Participation, Care, Self-fulfilment, and Dignity. Based on these themes, India has also made various Constitutional and Legislative Provisions and developed various policies, programs, and schemes for the welfare of the ageing population in the country.

In the upcoming section, we shall provide a synoptic view of provisions and programs available for the welfare of the elderly in India **(Table 49.1)**.

INTEGRATED PROGRAM FOR OLDER PEOPLE

The Integrated Program for Older People (IPOP) is a core divisional program of the Ministry of Social Justice and Empowerment. It came into force in the year 1992.

Objective

To improve the quality of life of the elderly in the country.

Goals

1. Provide the elderly with basic amenities such as housing, food, medical care and entertainment.
2. Support capacity building of various NGOs, Panchayati Raj institutions, and local bodies.

TABLE 49.1: Provisions and programs for the welfare of elderly.

Provision/program	Ministry/organization	Year of implementation
Integrated Program for Older People (IPOP)	Ministry of Social Justice and Empowerment	1992
National Policy on Older Persons (NPOP)	Ministry of Social Justice and Empowerment	1999, updated in 2011
The Maintenance and Welfare of Parents and Senior Citizen	Parliament of India	2007
National Council for Older Persons (NCOP)/ National Council for Senior Citizens (NCSrC)	Ministry of Social Justice and Empowerment	NCOP-1999; NCSrC–2012
Indira Gandhi National Old Age Pension Scheme (IGNOAPS)	Ministry of Rural Development	2007
National Program for the Health Care of the Elderly (NPHCE)	Department of Health and Family Welfare	2010
Health Insurance	Insurance Regulatory Development Authority	2019
Income Tax Rebate	Ministry of Finance	1961
Provisions in Railways	Ministry of Railways	—
Provisions on Airport	Ministry of Civil Aviation	—
Provision in Transport	State Road Transport Undertakings of respective states	—
Protection of Life and Property	Ministry of Home Affairs	Advisories issued in 2008 and 2013
Provisions in Food and Public Distribution	Ministry of Consumer Affairs, Food, and Public Distribution	Antyodaya Anna Yojana – 2000; Annapoorna Scheme – 2000
Rashtriya Vayoshri Yojana	Ministry of Social Justice and Empowerment	2017
Senior Citizen Saving Scheme	Government of India under Government Savings Banks Act, 1873	2004
Rashtriya Swasthya Bima Yojana	Ministry of Labour and Employment	2016
National Pension Scheme	Government of India	2004
Pradhan Mantri Vaya Vandana Yojana (PMVVY)	Government of India	2017

3. Provide financial support to NGOs and organizations for the smooth operation of nursing homes and shelters for the elderly in the country.
4. Support for NGOs and organizations is also provided through the following programs:
   - Programs to meet the basic needs of older people, especially food, housing, and medical care for poorer older people
   - Programs to build and strengthen intergenerational relationships, especially between children/young people and older people
   - Programs that promote active and productive ageing;
   - Programs that provide in-house and out-of-house care/services for older adults
   - Research, advocacy, and awareness programs in the field of ageing
   - All other programs that put the interests of older people first.

On April 1, 2016, the ministry implemented its revised IPOP program. In this program, some elements of the unplanned program are also integrated into the existing planning scheme of the Integrated Programme. These components are: Awareness-raising for the Maintenance and Well-being of Parents and Older Persons (MWPSC) Act, 2007. Establishment of hotlines for senior citizens at the state and district level.

To be eligible for grants under the IPOP program, non-governmental volunteer organizations must be registered under relevant laws. These should also be registered under either the Societies Registration Act of 1860 or the relevant State Societies Registration Act. These must have an adequate management structure and a well-structured governing body with clearly defined powers, duties, and responsibilities set forth in a written charter. An organization should not be aimed at the benefit of any individual or group of individuals and should be founded and managed by its members on democratic principles. Numerous nursing homes have been subsidized to date. Several innovative projects are being implemented under this program, including respite care homes and maintaining homes for continued care. Daycare centers for people with dementia of Alzheimer's type are also cared for under this regulation.

NATIONAL POLICY FOR OLDER PERSONS

In 1999, the Indian government announced a National Policy for the Elderly. This was a positive step towards the passage of UN General Assembly Resolution 47/5, which declared 1999 the International Year of Older Persons and reaffirmed constitutional guarantees for older persons. Article 41 of the Indian Constitution mandates the protection of the rights of the elderly.

A rapidly increasing elderly population and against the backdrop of changing economic and social conditions, medical research, scientific and technological advances, and disadvantaged rural elderly, the Ministry of Social Justice and

Personal Development has formulated the National Policy for Older Persons 2011. The main purposes of this policy are to:
1. Prioritize older people, especially older women, in the implementation of mechanisms established by governments and supported by civil society and older age groups.
2. Promote the concept of ageing in place, or ageing at home, and focus on housing, income security and home care services, old-age pensions, and health insurance plans to promote ageing and maintain dignity. Also, provide access to other programs and services for old age.
3. To achieve this goal, states must provide assistance to older people living below the poverty line both in urban and rural areas, providing social security, health care, housing, and social assistance.
4. Advising countries on the Parent and Elderly Support and Welfare Act.
5. Establish assisted living facilities for abandoned older persons in all districts of the country with adequate financial support.

Activities Carried out Under National Policy for Older Persons, 2011

Here are some of the initiatives that ministries are taking to implement this policy and support older people:
1. Older age benefits and public distribution systems cover all older people living below the poverty line.
2. Tax policy is designed to address the financial problems of the elderly, exacerbated by high medical and long-term care costs, home care, and mobility needs.
3. The health needs of older people are given the utmost attention.
4. The health needs of older people are empowered and prioritized in the development of public health services, health insurance, non-profit health services such as foundations and charities, and private health care.
5. The strategy aims to establish a multilayered system of geriatric care at the national level, with an emphasis on outpatient day care, palliative care, rehabilitation care, and respite care.
6. Rashtriya Swasthya Bima Yojana (RSBY) is promoted in all districts and elderly people are obliged to have health insurance.
7. Web-based services and tools for the safety and welfare of older persons will be promoted and made available in underserved areas.
8. Community awareness and enforcement efforts are being made to address elder abuse and crime against the elderly, especially widows, those living alone, and those with disabilities.
9. Seniors receive 10% of urban and rural low-income housing projects.
10. Reserved public spaces frequently used by the elderly and disabled, such as buses, bus stops, trains, airports, and bus services within airports, banks, hospitals, parks, places of worship, etc., cinemas, and shopping malls.
11. The Government will establish a welfare fund for the elderly, funded by social security contributions.
12. Non-institutional services provided by non-profit organizations are encouraged and supported to improve the ability of older adults and their families to cope with the challenges of ageing.

THE MAINTENANCE AND WELFARE OF PARENTS AND SENIOR CITIZEN ACT, 2007 (MWP ACT, 2007)

The MWP Act, 2007, was enacted in December 2007 by the Parliament of India. It consists of 7 chapters and 32 sections. According to this Act, any Indian citizen with age 60 years or more is called a senior citizen. The issues related to the maintenance of parents and senior citizens which are vital to maintain their dignity and well-being are addressed in this Act. The main provisions under this Act are discussed in brief as under:

Maintenance of Parents and Senior Citizens

In our traditional society, it is expected that the children will support their parents in the old age when it is difficult for them to maintain themselves. Also, the societal changes such as urbanization, industrialization, and migration put a strain on the families and contribute to the neglect of the elderly, if present in the family. Thus, there is a legal provision under this Act where parents can claim for maintenance from their children if the need arises. The children in such cases can be asked to pay a monthly allowance for maintenance if they have sufficient means but refuses to maintain or neglect their father or mother. There is a provision also to secure maintenance from relatives who are eligible for the inheritance of the property if the elderly does not have children.

Establishment of Old-age Homes

There is a provision under this Act for setting up old-age homes for indigent senior citizens and scheme for the management of the old-age homes.

Promoting Medical Care of Senior Citizens

This Act has emphasized the need to provide an adequate number of beds, separate queues, facilities for managing chronic, terminal, and degenerative conditions. It also stresses promoting research and development of dedicated geriatric health facilities. The Ayushman Bharat Pradhan Mantri Jan Arogya Yojana (PM-JAY) improved access to healthcare services for the elderly living below the poverty line.

Protection of Life and Property

The MWP Act of 2007's Section 23 protects the interests of older citizens who sell their property by requiring the transferee to provide ongoing care and protection for them after the transfer. The senior person has the right to reclaim the property by asking the tribunal to declare this transfer null and unlawful if the transferee fails to offer the required support in accordance with this requirement.

Role of Police

Under this Act, each police station is required by this order to keep a list of all senior residents who reside there, with a focus on those who are living alone. In order to facilitate/prompt/aid, when necessary, it has also mandated regular connection with senior persons through social workers or volunteers.

NATIONAL COUNCIL FOR OLDER PERSONS (NCOP)/NATIONAL COUNCIL FOR SENIOR CITIZENS (NCSrC)

Under the leadership of the Minister for Social Justice and Empowerment, the National Council for Older Persons (NCOP) was established in 1999 to oversee the implementation of the National Policy for Older Persons and provide guidance to the government on the creation and execution of age-related policies and programs. In order to promote greater participation from all regions, the NCOP was reorganized in 2012 and given the new name, National Council of Senior Citizens (NCSrC). On June 13, 2018, the Council convened its third meeting. The third meeting of the NCSrC covered topics such as schemes, programs, and acts for the welfare of senior citizens that are handled by several departments and ministries in addition to the Ministry of Social Justice and Empowerment. Significant suggestions made by the council are:

- ❖ The "Maintenance and Welfare of Parents and Senior Citizens (MWPSC) Act, 2007" needs to be strengthened to be more successful.
- ❖ The establishment of more Rashtriya Vayoshri Yojana (RYY) distribution camps throughout the States and UTs.
- ❖ Simplifying the procedures for mandatory empanelment of volunteer organizations and online registration of NGOs.
- ❖ The Senior Citizen's Welfare Fund can be used to provide financial aid to older persons who are cancer sufferers.
- ❖ Revision of the Indira Gandhi National Old Age Pension Schemes' (IGNOAPS') financial assistance policies, including pension amounts and beneficiary identification standards.
- ❖ Suggested that in order to ensure the security and safety of senior citizens in the Union Territories, the Ministry of Home Affairs should play a proactive role.
- ❖ Proposed a discount on airline tickets for seniors and the introduction of 2-tier non-AC trains for the elderly.
- ❖ Proposed making intergenerational bonding counseling sessions a required part of the school curriculum and syllabus.

INDIRA GANDHI NATIONAL OLD AGE PENSION SCHEME (IGNOAPS)

The National Old Age Pension Scheme was renamed "Indira Gandhi National Old Age Pension Scheme (IGNOAPS)" and formally launched on 19th November 2007. IGNOAPS is one of the five sub-schemes of the National Social Assistance Programme (NSAP) under the Ministry of Rural Development.

- ❖ The eligible beneficiaries under IGNOAPS are the Indian citizens living below the poverty line (BPL) and aged 60 years or above.
- ❖ Under this scheme, a monthly pension of ₹ 200/per month is given to an elderly aged 60 years and above.
- ❖ For a senior citizen aged 80 years and above, a monthly pension of ₹ 500/month is given.

Money is distributed by way of the beneficiaries' bank accounts, Post Office Savings Bank accounts, postal money orders, or in open meetings like Gram Sabha meetings in rural regions and neighborhood/Mohalla committee meetings in cities.

NATIONAL PROGRAM FOR THE HEALTH CARE OF THE ELDERLY (NPHCE)

The National Health Care Program for the Elderly (NPHCE) was established in 2010 by the Department of Health and Family Welfare. The main objectives of the program are:

- ❖ Facilitate the provision of promotional, preventive, curative and rehabilitative services to the elderly through a community-based approach to primary health care.
- ❖ Identify health problems in older people and provide appropriate health interventions to the community with strong referral support.
- ❖ Build the capacity of medical professionals, emergency medical professionals, and family caregivers to provide care to older people.
- ❖ Providing referral services for elderly patients through country hospitals and community health facilities.
- ❖ Integration with the National Rural Health Mission, AYUSH, and other specialized departments such as the Ministry of Social Justice and Empowerment.

The main strategies adopted in this program to achieve its goals are:

1. **Preventive and curative care:** Preventive and curative health services such as regular physical activity, healthy diet, vegetarian diet, stress management, smoking cessation, and use of tobacco products through regular home visits by qualified health professionals. Health education about fall prevention, etc., is enhanced by improving access to medical care guaranteed by home visits by qualified healthcare professionals. A weekly clinic will also be set up at the PHC to regularly monitor the elderly and assess them for medical conditions.
2. **Disease control:** Elderly outdoor and indoor specialty medical services to treat chronic and debilitating diseases are provided in PHC, CHC, district hospitals, and community geriatric centers with the support of central and state governments.
3. **Development of health workers for elderly care:** Existing health workers are given in-service training using standardized training modules with the support of medical colleges and local institutions to address the shortage of qualified medical and paramedical staff in geriatric care. Postgraduate courses in geriatric medicine are offered at regional geriatric centers, offering additional educational and support functions.
4. **Medical rehabilitation and therapeutic interventions**: Physiotherapy units in CHCs, district hospitals, and community geriatric centers should have the necessary resources to organize therapeutic exercises, instruction in activities of daily living (ADLs), and therapy. Infrastructure, drugs, and equipment will be provided.

Assessment of pain and inflammation in these identified units will be done.
5. **Information, education, and communication (IEC):** Health education programs are used to disseminate the idea of healthy ageing to target audiences.

HEALTH INSURANCE

Insurance Regulatory Development Authority (IRDA) on 25th May 2019, circulated instructions to all CEOs of General Health Insurance companies regarding health insurance of older persons. These are as follows:
- Entry to health insurance schemes should be allowed up to 65 years of age.
- There should be transparency in the premium charged.
- The reasons for denial of proposals, etc., on health insurance products catering to the needs of older persons should be recorded.
- The insurance companies have no right to refuse renewability without any specific reasons.

INCOME TAX REBATE

According to the Ministry of Finance, the income tax exemption quota for the fiscal year 2022–2023 will be for the elderly (ages 60 and over) and the super-elderly (ages 80 and over). It is:
- For senior citizens (over 60 years old): ₹ 300,000 under the old tax system and ₹ 250,000 under the new tax system.
- Very old (80 years and over): Allowance under the old tax regime is ₹ 5,00,000 and under the new tax regime is ₹ 2,50,000. Electronic filing exemption. Section 194P of the Income Tax Act 1961 exempts persons aged 75 and over from paying income tax. This is in effect from 1 April 2021. Exemption conditions include:
  - Age 75+
  - Seniors must have been "residents" in the previous year.
  - Seniors receive only pension and interest income and accrued/earned interest income from the same designated bank where they receive their annuity.

Exemption from payment of input tax: Under Article 207, resident seniors are exempted from payment of input tax. Under this section 207, resident senior citizens (i.e., persons who were at least 60 years of age in the relevant financial year) who have no commercial or professional income are not required to pay income tax.
- Under Section 80TTB of the Income Tax Act, tax incentives of up to ₹ 50,000 as earned by seniors (people over 60) are available on interest on deposits with banks, post offices, or credit unions. Interest on savings and time deposits is also deductible under this provision.
- Section 194A of the Income Tax Act stipulates that no tax can be deducted from interest payments to senior citizens up to INR 50,000.
- According to Article 80 of the DDB, income tax refunds are available for the treatment of certain diseases in the elderly.
- Older health insurance premiums are also eligible for income tax refund under section 80D.

PROVISIONS IN RAILWAYS

Under the Ministry of Railways, concessions and provisions are available for senior citizens. They are described as under:
- Senior citizens of age 60 years and above can avail concessions on all Mail and Express trains, including Rajdhani, Shatabdi, Jan Shatabdi, and Duronto group of trains. Senior citizens must be at least 58 years old in the case of females and 60 years and above in the case of males to avail the benefits. Concession amounts to 40% for men and 50% for women (11).
- Senior citizens can purchase, book, and cancel tickets at separate counters provided by Indian Railways.
- There is a provision to allot lower berths to senior citizens while booking tickets online.
- Senior citizens have designated sleeping accommodations in all trains. A combined quota of six lower berths per coach in sleeper class and three lower berths per coach in AC-3 tier and AC-2 tier classes has been reserved for senior citizens.
- 'Yatri Mitra Sewa' is a service offered to assist elderly and disabled passengers at the stations who need assistance as well as to improve the current services.
- 'Battery Operated Vehicles for Disabled and Old Aged Passengers' are another complimentary service offered by IRCTC at train stations. Additionally, customers can reserve e-wheel chairs at the IRCTC portal.
- For the convenience of those in need, particularly the elderly, wheelchairs are supplied at all intersections, the district headquarters, and other significant stations.
- At the entrance to major stations, ramps are accessible for wheelchair movement.
- Wheelchair-accessible carriages, handrails, and specially adapted restrooms for people with disabilities have all been implemented.

PROVISIONS ON AIRPORTS

Most airways provide Indian seniors who have reached the age of 60 years, a 50% senior citizen cut price on everyday financial system elegance fares for all home flights, concern to the production of age-proof.

According to the Ministry of Civil Aviation's Annual Report for 2020–21, the subsequent moves were made to enhance the welfare of senior citizens:
- Change the layout of the frisking cubicles withinside the security controls in order that the aged are not always required to climb and descend during the process of security checks.
- Pay special attention to support them, particularly upon getting out of motors at the airports and till the person reaches the check-in counters.
- Give desired reservation and earmarking of seats within side the airways.
- Pay special interest to the aged and people in want of help at the reserving places of airways.

In addition to those moves, the Ministry of Social Justice and Empowerment supplied the Ministry of Civil Aviation with a budgetary guide for senior citizens' welfare from the Senior Citizens Welfare Fund in the fiscal year 2018–19 for 30 electric-powered golfing carts to be operated at certain airports, in addition to price range to the Air Authority of India (AAI) to facilitate senior citizens' movements irrespective of the elegance in their journey and to gain a preferred degree of mobility.

PROVISIONS IN TRANSPORT BY BUSES

- Two seats in the front row of State Road Transport Undertakings buses are reserved for senior citizens.
- Some state governments are creating bus models that are convenient for the elderly.
- State governments are also offering older citizens a concession on bus fares up to 50% while traveling through State Road Transport Undertaking buses.
- Some governments such as Andaman and Nicobar issue free bus passes to senior citizens aged 80 years and above.

PROTECTION OF LIFE AND PROPERTY

The Ministry of Home Affairs, Government of India, has issued advisories to all State Governments in the years 2008 and 2013 to take immediate steps to ensure safety and security and to eliminate all forms of abuse, neglect, and violence against senior citizens. In this regard, the following steps have been taken:

- Identification of senior citizens in the jurisdiction of the police post.
- Sensitization of police personnel for safety and the security of older persons.
- Elimination of all kinds of abandonment, exploitation, and brutality towards senior citizens.
- Regular visits of the police staff to senior citizens.
- Setting up toll-free senior citizens helplines.
- Setting up senior citizen security cell
- Verification of drivers, domestic helpers, etc.

PROVISIONS UNDER THE MINISTRY OF CONSUMER AFFAIRS, FOOD AND PUBLIC DISTRIBUTION

Two schemes for older persons have been run under the Ministry of Consumer Affairs, Food, and Public Distribution. These are:

1. **Antyodaya Anna Yojana:** Under this scheme, families including older persons and living below the poverty line (BPL) are provided with food grains @ 35 kg/family/month. The food grains are issued at ₹ 3/- per kg for rice and at ₹ 2/- per kg for wheat.
2. **Annapoorna Scheme:** Under this scheme, 10 kg food grains per beneficiary per month free of cost are provided to senior citizens not covered under National Old-Age Pension Scheme or under the Targeted Public Distribution System and who have no income of their own.

RASHTRIYA VAYOSHRI YOJANA (RVY)

The Ministry of Social Justice and Empowerment of the Government of India implemented the Rashtriya Vayoshri Yojana in the year 2017. The beneficiaries of the scheme are senior citizens above 60 years of age and living below the poverty line. Benefits under this scheme are the provision of assisted-living devices and aids to senior citizens suffering from disabilities occurred due to age such as impaired hearing, low vision, loss of dentures, and other locomotor disabilities. These aids and assisted-living devices could be wheelchairs, walking sticks, walkers, spectacles, artificial dentures, etc.

SENIOR CITIZENS SAVING SCHEME (SCSS)

This is a government-backed savings scheme for the senior citizens above 60 years of age run by the public or private ban of the Indian Post Office. Under this scheme, a senior citizen can deposit an amount ranging from ₹1000 to ₹15 lacs. The deposit matures in 5 years but can be extended for an additional period of three years just once only. Higher interest rates are fixed and reviewed regularly by the government. The accrued interest is compounded and credited quarterly. The investments made under this scheme are eligible for exemption from tax. A penalty charge of 1.5% of deposit amount will be deducted in case the money is withdrawn prematurely before two years, and 1% after two years.

RASHTRIYA SWASTHYA BIMA YOJANA

It is a centrally sponsored scheme implemented by Ministry of Labour and Employment since 2008 for the families living under poverty line. However, senior citizen health insurance scheme is a top up to existing Rashtriya Swasthya Bima Yojana for the senior citizens aged 60 years and above. It is in effect from 1st April, 2016. Each senior citizen in the eligible family, i.e., below poverty line is given enhanced coverage of ₹30,000. The Senior Citizen Welfare Fund, which is overseen by the Ministry of Social Justice and Empowerment, provides funding for the scheme's premium.

NATIONAL PENSION SCHEME

It is under the purview of the Pension Fund Regulatory and Development Authority (PFRDA) and the Central Government. Any Indian citizen aged between 18–70 years is eligible to subscribe to NPS, including Non-Resident Indians (NRIs). It is mandatory for Central Government employees joining their jobs after 1st January 2004. Monthly income is ensured to the senior citizens for their entire lives. The income is generated from the advantages of market-linked instruments' returns, such as those from stocks, corporate bonds, government bonds, etc.

PRADHAN MANTRI VAYA VANDANA YOJANA (PMVVY)

Seniors who are at least 60 years old are eligible for this program. Any investment between ₹ 1.62 lacs and ₹ 15 lacs can be made here on a monthly, quarterly, half-yearly, or annual basis. The lowest and maximum monthly pensions to which older citizens are entitled are ₹ 1000 and ₹ 9250, respectively. Additionally, he or she benefits from life insurance coverage for the whole policy term. The policy has a ten-year term.

So, from the above discussion, it is observed that the Government of India has provided various welfare services to support the elderly population. But it is also true that the public is not aware of these services. So, the utilization of these services is questionable. A study was carried out to assess the awareness and the extent of utilization of various schemes by senior citizens. Using a systematic random sampling technique, 420 senior citizens visiting the outpatient department of a tertiary care center were enrolled in the study. They were asked about their awareness and utilization of various welfare services. The participants were from the states of Punjab, Haryana, Chandigarh, and Himachal Pradesh. In all four states, the majority of the people were aware of the old age pension scheme. A significant difference was observed in awareness and utilization of most of the schemes. It was concluded that there is a need to generate awareness regarding various schemes for the senior citizens among the general public of India in the Northern region.

Case Scenario

Mr Rahul, 68-year-old, is retired from the government service as a clerk. His spouse had died 5 years ago due to kidney failure. He has his own 10 Marla house and 1-acre agricultural land. He is survived by a son and a daughter. His daughter is married and settled abroad. His son is working in an IT company. He is married and his daughter-in-law is a school teacher. Everything was going well till 6 months before. He decided to transfer his property to his son. But after the transfer of property, his son and daughter-in-law started physically neglecting him. He is given a store room in the house to stay. There is no fan in the store room. Even the toilet is far from the room in the main house. So, it is very difficult for Mr Rahul to reach there when the urge to urination arises. Consequently, sometimes he wet his pants. The clothes are not changed and washed regularly. The same food is served all three times a day. When he used to ask his son to take him to the doctor for follow-up of his diabetes, the son refused to accompany him. This disturbed Mr Rahul. One day, during your home visit as a health worker, he narrated the whole story to you. You identified this as a case of elderly abuse which arises after the transfer of property. Based on your understanding of elderly abuse, The Maintenance of Parents and Senior Citizen's Act, 2007, and the rights to life and property of senior citizens, what action you will take so that Mr Rahul can live with dignity and needed care will be provided to him?

SUMMARY

The elderly population is increasing rapidly and so are the problems due to ageing process. The developed and developing countries have been taking numerous initiatives for the welfare of the elderly. In India, concessions have been provided to the elderly in the fares of buses, railways, and airways. Separate booking counters have been opened and seats are reserved for the senior citizens. Various provisions have been given under various schemes and programs with the target to provide adequate food, housing, shelter, medical care, etc., to older people. The government is also supporting NGOs to come forward and work for the welfare of the elderly. Nowadays, the concept of healthy ageing at home is also promoted through various programs by both the government and nongovernment organizations so that the elderly can live a well-supported and dignified life.

MULTIPLE CHOICE QUESTIONS

1. In which year 'Integrated Program for Older People' is implemented?
    a. 1992
    b. 1999
    c. 2011
    d. 2007
2. Which of the following is NOT part of The Maintenance and Welfare of Parents and Senior Citizen Act, 2007?
    a. Financial support to parents and senior citizens from their children.
    b. Medical care for senior citizens
    c. Right to reclaim property from children or relatives
    d. Exemption from Income Tax
3. Which of the following age group is eligible for an old age pension of ₹ 500/under 'The Indira Gandhi National Old Age Pension Scheme'?
    a. Any person above 60 years
    b. 60 to 70 years
    c. 71 to 80 years
    d. Above 80 years
4. Which of the following ministry run the 'National Program for the Health Care of the Elderly'?
    a. Ministry of Social Justice and Empowerment
    b. Ministry of Health and Family Welfare
    c. Ministry of Rural Development
    d. Ministry of Home Affairs
5. Which of the following step is NOT taken by Ministry of Home Affairs for the protection of life and property of senior citizen in India?
    a. Setting up of old-age homes
    b. Sensitization of police personnel for safety and the security of older persons.
    c. Setting up of toll-free senior citizens helplines
    d. Setting up senior citizen security cell
6. In which year the Maintenance and Welfare of Parents and Senior Citizens Act enacted?
    a. 2001
    b. 2003
    c. 2005
    d. 2007
7. NPOP is one of schemes by Govt of India for the elderly. What is the full form of NPOP?
    a. National program for older people
    b. National policy for older persons
    c. National policy for older people
    d. National program for older persons
8. In which year Indira Gandhi National Old Age Pension Scheme (IGNOPS) was launched?
    a. 2005
    b. 2006
    c. 2007
    d. 2008
9. Under Annapoorna scheme, how much food grain is distributed to the eligible persons above the age of 65 years?
    a. 2 kg
    b. 5 kg
    c. 7 kg
    d. 10 kg
10. IPOP is another scheme for the elderly by Govt of India. Its full form is:
    a. Integrated Program for Older People
    b. Integrated Policy for Older People
    c. Integrated Program for Older Persons
    d. Integrated Policy for Older Persons

ANSWERS

1. a	2. d	3. d	4. b
5. a	6. d	7. b	8. c
9. d	10. a		

SUGGESTED READING

1. Chundawat C. Indian Railways to soon restore senior citizen concession for the sleeper, 3A classes. Business News. 2023 March 14. Available from url: https://www.zeebiz.com/indian-railways/

news-indian-railways-to-soon-restore-senior-citizen-concession-for-sleeper-3a-classes-225800
2. Devi TS, Kaur R, Thakran A, Gudwalia B, Kumari M, Kaur S, et al. Awareness and utilization of various schemes launched by government of India for the welfare of senior citizens Int J Community Med Public Health. 2021;8(4):1809-16.
3. Directorate of Transport. Bus Pass Schemes. [Internet]. Available from url: http://transport.and.nic.in/senior_cit.aspx#:~:text=A%20person%20aged%2080%20years,a%20period%20of%20two%20years
4. Facilities extended to Senior Citizens.[Internet]. Available at url: https://indianrailways.gov.in/railwayboard/uploads/directorate/traffic_comm/FACILITIES%20EXTENDED%20TO%20%20SENIOR%20CITIZENS_170818.pdf
5. Giri M. National Policy for Senior Citizens National Policy on Senior Citizens. 2011;2011:1-10.
6. Government Of India Ministry Of Social Justice And Empowerment An Umbrella Scheme for Senior Citizens. National Action Plan for Welfare of Senior Citizens Scheme of National Action Plan for Welfare of Senior Citizens (NAPSrC). 2020.
7. Health Policy and Health Insurance. Annual Report 2016-17. [Internet]. Available at url: https://main.mohfw.gov.in/sites/default/files/12201617.pdf
8. Issac TG, Ramesh A, Reddy SS, Sivakumar PT, Kumar CN, Math SB. Maintenance and Welfare of Parents and Senior Citizens Act 2007: A Critical Appraisal. Indian J Psychol Med. 2021;43(5_suppl):S107-12.
9. Ministry of Rural Development. NSAP - Indira Gandhi National Old Age Pension Scheme.[Internet]. Available from url: https://www.myscheme.gov.in/schemes/nsap-ignoaps
10. Ministry of Social Justice and Empowerment. Benefits For Old Aged/Differently Abled Persons, 1813733.[Internet]. 2022 April 5. Available from url: https://pib.gov.in/PressReleseDetailm.aspx?PRID=1813733
11. Ministry of Social Justice and Empowerment. National Council of Senior Citizens, 1744553.[Internet].2021 Aug 10. Available from url: https://pib.gov.in/PressReleseIframePage.aspx?PRID=1744553
12. National Health Mission. National Programme for Health Care of Elderly [Internet]. India; updated 2023 June 19. Available from URL: https://nhm.gov.in/index1.php?lang=1&level=2&sublinkid=1046&lid=605
13. National Human Rights Commission. Rights of Senior Citizens. New Delhi: National Human Rights Commission; 2020.
14. Pension Scheme for Senior Citizens.[Internet]. Available at url: https://www.policybazaar.com/life-insurance/pension-plans/articles/monthly-pension-scheme-for-senior-citizens/#:~:text=Features%20of%20the%20National%20Pension%20Scheme%20(NPS)%3A&text=It%20is%20mandatory%20to%20invest,most%20effective%20tax%2Dsaving%20instruments.
15. Programmes and Policies for Promotion of Breast. 2020;(March). Available at url: https://bbau.ac.in/Docs/FoundationCourse/TM/MPDC405/Government%20Schemes%20for%20Senior%20Citizens.pdf
16. Senior Citizen: Problems and Welfare.[Internet]. Available at url: https://loksabhadocs.nic.in/Refinput/New_Reference_Notes/English/SeniorCitizensProblemsandWelfare.pdf
17. Vikaspedia.in. Concessions and Facilities given to Senior Citizens [Internet].India; 2023 Jan 13. Available from URL: https://vikaspedia.in/health/nrhm/national-health-programmes-1/national-programme-for-the-health-care-for-the-elderly-nphce#:~:text=The%20National%20Programme%20for%20the,the%20Government%20of%20India%20in

CHAPTER 50

Care of Elders

Sukhpal Kaur, Alisha Talwar

"Care for your elderly with the same heart as you did for your children in their childhood."
—Sukhpal

LEARNING OBJECTIVES

After going through the chapter, the learner will be able to:
- Differentiate home versus institutional care.
- Enumerate the challenges faced by informal caregivers.
- Discuss the role of nurses in the care of the elderly.
- Discuss the role of family, formal and nonformal caregivers in elderly care.
- Enumerate various aids and prostheses for the elderly.

TERMS

- **Assistive devices:** These are designed to support older adults in various activities to enhance their safety, and improve their overall quality of life.
- **Empty nesters:** The elders staying alone. Either they are not having any children or the children have already left them.
- **Home care:** Care provided in an individual's own home.
- **Institutional care:** Care provided in hospitals, old age homes, nursing homes, daycare centers, etc.

INTRODUCTION

Ageing is a natural process of life. Old age is the last stage of life and is also called the closing period in the life cycle. Even it is named the second childhood. Every individual is likely to come across this process. Old age reduces the immunity level of an individual and makes the elderly more prone to communicable as well as non-communicable diseases leading to more emergency department as well as hospital visits. Consequently, it declines an individual's functioning capacity and makes them dependent on others. They are usually ill-equipped to cope alone with their lives in the face of infirmity and disability.

One of the criteria to judge a prosperous society is how well the elderly are being taken care of. The elderly population needs to be provided with high-quality care either at their own homes by staying with their families, at public institutions, or with the support from private caregivers. India, today is facing a unique challenge in providing care to its elderly. The existing old-age support in the form of family kith and kin is fast eroding. While Western countries have well-organized long-term care facilities for the care of the elderly, however, in India, the growth and development of these kinds of facilities still are inadequate.

The current chapter is all about this. It elaborates on the care of the elderly in homes and institutions, the general measures of caring for the elderly, and also highlights various aids and prostheses which can be used by the elderly for their independence in their daily activities.

HOME CARE OF THE ELDERLY

Being a caregiver can be one of the most fulfilling, however, challenging experiences of one's life. It could be a matter of great joy of helping someone live independently for as long as possible. But it is one of the major decisions a family may have to make to determine how to provide care for elderly parents when they can no longer live independently.

Some of the families provide elders with adequate assistance to remain in their own homes. They personally provide care to their elders. Still, others put them into a formal care facility.

A family is an integral part of everyone's life. The family members should understand and identify the problems an older person is likely to develop. The need for a family increases further once the elderly need more support and help in their later years of life. Families play an important part in informal care provision. Traditionally, only families have been playing the role of primary caregivers. Actually, home is a place where a person finds and expects care, comfort, and security. However, with the ongoing economic development and the consequent changes in family structure, the elderly are often neglected. With the rapid increase in the aging population, the number of empty nesters (the elders either not having any children or the children have already left them) is increasing. So, the care for such kind of elders has emerged as a major social problem. In such a situation, the spouse who himself or herself almost of the same age has been found to assume the role of a primary caregiver and once there is no surviving spouse, the paid caregiver generally assumes caregiver responsibilities. Thus, older people are seen as caring for older people.

Home care, is health care and supportive care provided either by healthcare professionals or nonprofessional caregivers (depending upon the extent or type of care required), in an individual's own home. Nonprofessional caregivers include family members such as a spouse, son, daughter, or friends. The paid informal caregivers are typically home care aides managed by the family or a commercial/government agency in the community. They do not have any formal degree but might be having a certificate of completion of a short-term home healthcare training program. They help and provide care to elderly individuals in their own homes. The professional caregivers include home health visiting nurses, rehabilitation therapists (physiotherapist, speech therapist, occupational therapist, etc.), and healthcare social workers. Home care aims to make it possible for people to remain in their own homes rather than using residential, long-term, or institutional-based nursing care. Home care providers render services in the client's own home. These services may include some combination of professional healthcare services and life assistance services. Professional home health services may include "medical or psychological assessment, wound care, pain management, disease management, physical therapy, speech therapy, or occupational therapy, etc". Life assistance services include "helping the elderly in their daily tasks such as meal preparation, medication reminders, laundry, housekeeping, errands, shopping, transportation, companionship, etc". The elderly people who are dependent for cooking, cleaning, other household work, or getting out and about, home care can be a great help.

Benefits of Home Care

Most elderly people if given the option would choose to remain in their own homes. They will love to avail the opportunity of 'Age in Place'. It can be very difficult for them to go away from their own environment. There are many benefits of home care:

- ❖ Home health care is usually less expensive, more convenient, and may be as effective as institutional care.
- ❖ The elderly enjoy better quality of life (QOL) when they are cared for at home, in surroundings they are familiar with, and amongst the people whom they feel close to.
- ❖ The process of sharing their life of disability with their family members reduces stress among the elderly.
- ❖ The family ties grow stronger.
- ❖ Living at home, elderly people are able to maintain a level of freedom that may not be possible in institutions.
- ❖ They remain to stay physically close to the things they love. There are a lot of sentimental values and memories associated with everything at home. Being able to keep these items readily available gives them a lot of satisfaction and happiness.
- ❖ There is no restriction on the visiting hours at home. So, friends and relatives can visit at their own convenience. This may lead to more frequent visits, which helps the elderly stay connected to their friends and relatives. They feel more secure and happy. This will help in maintaining their well-being and preventing loneliness.
- ❖ Home care can help the elderly maintain better health because they are alone being taken care of by others, there will not be any risk of getting infection from others.
- ❖ With home care, the elderly will not have to adapt to a new routine of a new place, surrounded by new people.
- ❖ The family members can maintain their own schedule and will not disrupt their day-to-day activities.
- ❖ In-home care the number of hours can be tailored as per the requirement of care. Depending upon the need it can be from a few hours to 24 hours.
- ❖ Home care is a good option, especially during a pandemic situation like COVID-19, where it is better to isolate the elderly and receive care in order to prevent the risk of further infection.

Problems/Issues of Home Care

In the nuclear family, the children are more concerned about their career growth and monetary gains. They do not have quality time to spend with their parents and grandparents. And in many cases, they lack the resources to meet their needs (like medical expenses, special food, etc). Thus, in recent times more and more senior citizens hailing even from the Indian middle-class background are seeking accommodation in old age homes. Though there are several benefits of providing care to the elderly in their home care environment, however, there are certain problems associated with such kind of care. There are highlighted as follows:

- ❖ Managing home care for the elderly is a massive challenge specifically once there are financial constraints in the family.
- ❖ There is increased geographical mobility. The family size has been reduced. Even many of young couples either do not want to have any children, or those who want, will go only for one child. So, there is no one to provide home care to the elderly.
- ❖ There is an intergenerational gap. Support or elderly care is no longer considered an absolute obligation by adult children.

- There is a change in the gender role in the care of the elders. In the past females were considered as the primary caregivers in the families. But now after obtaining a higher education, women are becoming more work-oriented women.
- Lack of government involvement and policies.
- Inadequate payment to health workers. The paid/formal caregivers are paid very less. This may affect the quality of care.
- There could be a lack of infrastructure and equipment to care in the home care setting.
- The caregivers might be having irresponsible behaviors especially if it is the paid caregiver and there is no family member to supervise that person.
- This may lead to stress and burnout syndrome among the caregivers if there is a lack of support from others and if they are not trained enough on how to provide care to the elderly, especially in the bedridden stage. They may feel exhausted or depressed.

Requisites for the Caregivers

Managing and providing care to the elderly in the home care settings is a huge challenge. It is a demanding job and may lead to a lot of physical, mental, and emotional stress on the caregivers. Even the caregivers are called "secondary patients or hidden patients". Increased stress among caregivers can result in harmful behaviors in the form of committing errors while administering medicines, elder abuse, neglect, family conflict, etc. They should keep in mind the following points while taking care of elderly people at home.

- The caregivers should reserve time for their own welfare in order to avoid burnout.
- They should continue with social interactions with their friends or significant others even though they are busy providing care to older persons.
- Caring for the elderly is a joint responsibility. They should share responsibility for elderly care with others. They should not try doing everything at their own end.
- All the available resources for such care should be explored.
- They should show thoughtfulness, compassion, and respect for the elderly while providing care.
- There should also be a provision of respite care when the caregivers can take some breaks in between. This will help in rejuvenating their energy.

ELDERLY-FRIENDLY HOME CARE SETTING

With age, there is a lack of physical and mental strength. Elderly people are more prone to slip and fall, or otherwise injure themselves at home. It is important to remember that these injuries of old age are harder to recover. So, we need to follow certain precautions to reduce the risk of injury in the elderly *(please see the following sections on assistive and enabling devices for the use by the elderly).*

- **Living area of the home:**
  - All rugs and loose carpets should be properly taped to the ground. This will prevent the elderly from fall.
  - Electric cables should be secured to the wall or placed under rugs so that no one trips on them.
  - Sharp corners on tables or countertops should be covered to avoid serious injury in the event of a fall.
  - There should be railing on the sides of staircases to support a person's full body weight.
- **Bathrooms:**
  - The toilet seat should be elevated to help elderly individuals to get up and down easily,
  - There should be grab bars on both sides of the toilet for support while sitting/getting up from the toilet seat.
  - The hot water outlet should be labeled or painted red to avoid scalding.
  - Slippery floors can be made safer by adding a non-slip mat in the bathroom.
- **Kitchen:**
  - Make sure that all kitchen appliances are in good working order.
  - All appliances should be placed at waist height so that they do not have to struggle to reach things that are either too high or too low.
  - Ensure that there is adequate lighting. This is especially important in the kitchen, where tools such as knives and shredders are used on a regular basis.

INSTITUTIONAL CARE FOR THE ELDERLY

Institutions are organized establishments, foundations, and societies involved in providing care to the elderly. Institutional care includes old age homes, nursing home care, retirement care home, daycare centers, hospitals, etc. Institutional care is provided in a setting where the functional, medical, personal, social, and housing needs of individuals as a whole are taken care of. Various aspects of care include 24-hour supervision and monitoring, assistance with activities of daily living, skilled nursing care, rehabilitation services, assistive and enabling devices, psychological services, therapies, social activities, etc. The cost of institutional care varies as per the provision of various kinds of facilities and services.

Institutional care includes a trained person in the medical field. This professional may be a nurse who looks after the elderly and support them as per their need including feeding, bathing, exercising or any kind of assistance. Institutional care is quite beneficial to those who find it difficult living at their own, but of course can afford the expenses of that institution. Apart from providing best care, the elderly are helped to achieve their maximum level of independence.

Goals of Care

Various goals of institutional care are to:
- Provide long-term care for elderly patients.
- Promote and maintain the functional status of older adults.
- Motivate the older adults to identify and use their strengths to achieve optimal independence.
- Help the elderly persons to maintain their dignity.
- Maximize autonomy despite the losses pertaining to physical, social, and psychological aspects.
- Use current scientific knowledge to maintain the health of the elderly.
- Collaborate with the interdisciplinary team to provide comprehensive and quality care to the elderly.
- Provide a holistic approach to care.

Benefits of Institutional Care

The elderly people who are living alone, dependent for all of their activities of daily living, at risk of falls, and require frequent medications but often forget, for them staying in the institutions is the best option. Various benefits of providing care to the elderly are:

- In institutional care trained caregivers and medical professionals are available around the clock to provide care to the elderly.
- Personal attention is given to each elderly person as per their requirements, for example, bathing, grooming, dressing, etc.
- The elderly with similar age groups, interests, abilities, and problems get opportunities to interact with one another in institutional care. They get encouragement, satisfaction, and acceptance correlating their own issues with others. They find it nice to have people of their age to talk.
- Staying in the institution decreases loneliness among them because people are always available for companionship.
- There is a lot of recreation and amusements. So, the elderly enjoy celebrating all the occasions in the institution.
- They do have not to worry about household work, shopping, preparing meals, etc.
- The elderly are better secured and safe in nursing homes because of the availability of staff round the clock, which sometimes may not be there in their homes specifically if they are suffering from the problems like dementia or Alzheimer's disease and they tend to wander.
- Many residential care homes allow couples (legally married) to stay together. This can be reassuring for many senior citizens who are afraid of separation.
- Most residential institutions involve the elderly in various activities like gardening, baking, gentle exercises, yoga, laughter therapy, brain exercises, and music, etc., as per their interest and capabilities. They try to engage and make the stay of the elderly enjoyable. They even organize periodical trips for them.

Disadvantages of Institutional Care

Though there are several benefits of institutional care, many still have disadvantages.

- Many elderly people miss their family members and family environment and feel lonely.
- People in institutions often feel depressed watching their peer group passes away.
- The environment of institutional care sometimes becomes uncomfortable because there is no one to spend quality time with them.
- It is quite expensive than living in one's own home because of the fact that services are being provided 24 × 7. So, it may not be accessible for many families who are not able to afford it.
- The food available in the institution may not be appealing and as per the taste and liking of everyone. The choice of food items could be limited there.
- Certain uncongenial and nonadjustable people may spoil the environment of the institution.
- The institutions do not give much independence as is there in their own homes.
- There are generally fixed schedules for all the activities. And not complying with that may lead to problems for the elderly.
- The location of these institutions if away from the market, parks, or other community organizations may further lead to loneliness among the elderly.
- There is also a possibility of poor care including abuse and neglect in many institutions.

ROLE OF NURSES IN THE CARE OF ELDERLY

Caring for the elderly is like caring for a child. They both share many similarities. As a baby is completely dependent on his parents for all his needs, similar is the case especially for very old people. Older adults generally have special needs and nurses are required to provide appropriate care based on their needs. And since each individual is a different entity, nursing care also is to be planned and implemented accordingly. Nurses play a critical role in the care of the elderly, as they are often the primary healthcare providers. Thus, the nurses should be knowledgeable and extremely sympathetic. They should be able to provide respectful and loving care to their patients. He/she needs to have a lot of patience. Nursing care for the elderly may be provided in a variety of settings. This may include home care or institutions such as hospitals, nursing homes, long-term care facilities, old age homes, etc. Some general aspects of elderly care are depicted in **Box 50.1**. Some of the important roles of a nurse in the care of the elderly include:

- Nurses assess the physical, psychological, and social needs of elderly patients and use this information to develop individualized care plans. They also monitor the patient's health status over time, making changes to

---

BOX 50.1: General aspects of care.

- Provide a safe and secure environment for the elderly.
- Keep the activities simple and for a short interval.
- Promote awareness of time, place, and person on a regular basis.
- Always address the elderly person by name with a lot of respect.
- Correct the elderly if he addresses any of the people by the wrong name to maintain the memory intact.
- There should be a clock with big hands and numbers and a calendar with large font size in the room.
- Open the curtains of the room during the day.
- Speak slowly, and clearly, and face the person while talking. Ask clear and simple questions.
- Never rush or hurry in performing any of the activities for the elderly.
- Repeat instructions very patiently. Allow time for them to respond. Avoid arguments.
- Encourage conversations periodically about familiar things or any of the current events to keep them oriented.
- Encourage the use of TV, and radio to watch or listen their favorite programs.
- Make sure they make use of sensory aids.
- Keep familiar objects in view.
- Keep a family photograph adjacent to the elderly person.
- Avoid moving furniture and other belongings in the room. Let everything be in the same place so that the elderly person remains familiar with the immediate environment.
- Encourage independence and self-help whenever possible.

the care plan as needed. Thus he/she should be a good observer of various manifestations related to physical and mental health. These can emerge very quickly in the elderly.

- Nurses provide comprehensive nursing care to the elderly depending on their problems and needs including administering medications, performing wound care, and aiding with activities of daily living, etc.
- Nurses coordinate with the families of the patients while providing care. Many a time the nurses work along with the family caregivers and provide training to family members regarding their health conditions, medications, and self-care strategies in order to maintain the continuity of care after the patients get discharged from the hospital.
- The elderly people require multidisciplinary care. So, the nurses work closely with other healthcare professionals, such as doctors, nutritionists, physiotherapists, social workers, etc., to provide holistic care to elderly patients.
- Working with elderly patients can sometimes be emotionally stressful for the nurses. The elderly people might be victims of neglect and abuse. So, he/she advocates for the rights and needs of elderly patients, working to ensure that they receive the best possible care.

ROLE OF FORMAL AND NONFORMAL CAREGIVERS IN ELDERLY CARE

Formal and nonformal caregivers both play crucial roles in the care of the elderly, each offering unique contributions and support.

Formal Caregivers

Formal caregivers are individuals who provide care and support as part of their professional roles. They may work in various settings, such as hospitals, nursing homes, assisted living facilities, or home care agencies. Some of their roles include:

Medical Care

Formal caregivers, such as doctors, nurses, and medical aides, provide medical attention, administer medications, and monitor the health condition of the elderly.

- It is an essential aspect of ensuring the health and well-being of the elderly. As people grow older, they often face various age-related health challenges that require specialized care. Regular medical health check-ups are crucial for early detection and management of age-related health conditions. These check-ups may include assessments of blood pressure, cholesterol levels, blood sugar, vision, hearing, bone density, and overall physical and cognitive health.
- Many elderly individuals have chronic health conditions such as hypertension, diabetes, arthritis, heart disease, and dementia. Proper management of these conditions is essential to prevent complications and maintain their quality of life. Elderly individuals often take multiple medications, which can lead to potential drug interactions and adverse effects. Healthcare providers should carefully manage and review medications to ensure they are appropriate and safe for the individual.
- Vaccinations, cancer screenings, and other preventive measures are vital to protect the elderly from infections and diseases, as well as to catch potential health issues early.
- A balanced and nutritious diet is also very essential for maintaining health and preventing nutritional deficiencies that can be common in the elderly. It is important to address individual dietary needs and any swallowing or chewing difficulties they may have. Encouraging regular physical activity tailored to an individual's capabilities can help maintain mobility, muscle strength, and overall well-being.
- Addressing mental health concerns like depression, anxiety, and cognitive decline is important for the overall well-being of the elderly. Social engagement, mental stimulation, and emotional support play significant roles in maintaining mental health.
- Elderly individuals are at a higher risk of falls, which can lead to serious injuries. Implementing fall prevention strategies and modifying the living environment can help reduce these risks.
- For elderly individuals with terminal illnesses or those requiring end-of-life care, hospice, and palliative care services can provide comfort and support for both the patient and their family.
- It is important to approach medical care for the elderly with a holistic and person-centered perspective, considering their unique needs and preferences.

Personal Care

- Formal caregivers help with basic activities that the elderly may have difficulty performing independently. This includes tasks such as bathing, dressing, grooming, toileting, and feeding.
- Caregivers also assist elderly individuals with walking, transferring from one place to another (e.g., from the bed to a chair), and using mobility aids such as walkers or wheelchairs. They also ensure that the elderly take their medications as prescribed, and they may also assist with organizing pillboxes and tracking medication schedules.
- Caregivers prepare nutritious meals that meet the dietary needs and preferences of the elderly. They may also consider any special dietary restrictions or conditions. In cases where the elderly have difficulty feeding themselves, caregivers may offer feeding assistance while being mindful of the individual's dignity and comfort. They encourage and monitor the elderly person's fluid intake to prevent dehydration, which can be a common concern among seniors.
- When necessary, caregivers assist with toileting and incontinence care, maintaining the individual's privacy and dignity throughout the process. They also help with skin care, including maintaining skin hygiene, applying lotions or creams, and regularly checking for signs of pressure sores.
- Engaging the elderly in mentally stimulating activities, such as puzzles or reminiscence therapy, can help maintain cognitive function and improve overall well-being. Caregivers provide companionship and emotional support, engaging in conversations and activities to reduce feelings of isolation and loneliness.

- It is essential for formal caregivers to approach their role with empathy, respect, and patience. Building a trusting and compassionate relationship with the elderly individual can significantly enhance the quality of care provided.
- Additionally, formal caregivers should receive adequate training and support to meet the specific needs of the elderly they are caring for.

Skilled Services

Skilled services in elderly care refer to medical and specialized services provided by healthcare professionals to meet the complex and often changing needs of elderly individuals. These services are typically offered by licensed healthcare providers who have received specialized training and have the expertise to address a wide range of medical conditions and age-related challenges.

- Skilled healthcare providers manage and coordinate medical treatments for elderly patients, which may include medication management, wound care, and monitoring of chronic conditions such as diabetes or heart disease.
- For elderly individuals recovering from surgeries, injuries, or strokes, skilled services like physical therapy, occupational therapy, and speech therapy help in restoring mobility, function, and communication abilities.
- Skilled nursing services involve monitoring the health status of the elderly, administering medications, managing medical equipment, and providing wound care. Skilled nurses are trained to assess and address a wide range of medical needs. Healthcare professionals may provide specialized pain management services for elderly individuals dealing with chronic pain or age-related conditions causing discomfort. They also offer advanced wound care techniques to promote healing and prevent infections in elderly patients with wounds or pressure ulcers.
- Specialized care for individuals with dementia or Alzheimer's disease involves cognitive stimulation, behavior management, and creating a safe environment. Skilled services in palliative care focus on providing comfort, pain relief, and emotional support for elderly individuals with serious illnesses, aiming to improve their quality of life.
- Dietitians or nutritionists offer tailored dietary plans to address the specific nutritional needs and challenges faced by elderly patients. Mental health professionals offer assessments and treatment for mood disorders, anxiety, depression, and other mental health issues common in older adults.
- These skilled services are typically delivered in various settings, including hospitals, skilled nursing facilities, home health agencies, and hospice care organizations. The goal of these services is to improve the overall health, well-being, and quality of life of elderly individuals while addressing their unique and changing healthcare needs.

Safety and Supervision

Safety and supervision are critical aspects of elderly care provided by formal caregivers. As the elderly often face physical and cognitive challenges, ensuring their safety and well-being is of utmost importance. Formal caregivers play a crucial role in creating a secure environment and providing the necessary supervision to prevent accidents and address emergencies.

- Falls are a common cause of injuries among the elderly. Caregivers assess the home environment for potential hazards, such as loose rugs or cluttered pathways, and implement measures to reduce the risk of falls. They also assist with mobility and use mobility aids, like walkers or canes, to provide support.
- Caregivers are responsible for administering medications according to the prescribed schedule, ensuring the correct dosages are taken. They may also keep a medication log to track adherence and prevent medication errors. Caregivers regularly monitor the elderly person's physical health, observing for any signs of discomfort, pain, or changes in health conditions. They report any concerning symptoms to healthcare professionals or family members promptly.
- For individuals with cognitive impairments or dementia, caregivers offer close supervision to prevent wandering, ensure safety during daily activities, and provide cognitive stimulation.
- Caregivers conduct regular safety assessments in the home environment, checking for potential hazards and ensuring that safety equipment, like grab bars and handrails, are properly installed and functional.
- Caregivers ensure that the elderly person receives proper nutrition and stays hydrated. They may prepare meals that meet dietary restrictions and encourage regular fluid intake.
- Caregivers are trained to identify potential risks and hazards specific to the individual's health condition or mobility limitations, and they take proactive measures to prevent accidents.
- By focusing on safety and supervision, formal caregivers help elderly individuals maintain their independence and quality of life while minimizing the risks associated with ageing and age-related conditions. Creating a safe and supportive environment is essential for promoting the well-being and comfort of the elderly.

Care Planning

Care planning for the elderly by formal caregivers involves creating a comprehensive and individualized plan to address the specific needs and preferences of each elderly individual under their care. The care plan serves as a roadmap for delivering high-quality care and support, promoting the elderly person's health, safety, and overall well-being. Here are the key steps involved in care planning for the elderly:

- **Assessment:** Formal caregivers start by conducting a thorough assessment of the elderly person's physical health, cognitive function, emotional well-being, and social needs. They also take into account any medical conditions, medications, allergies, and mobility limitations.
- **Goal setting:** Based on the assessment, formal caregivers, along with healthcare professionals and family members, set specific and achievable goals for the elderly person's care. These goals may include improving mobility,

managing chronic conditions, enhancing social engagement, or ensuring safety at home.
- ❖ **Individualized care plan:** Caregivers develop a personalized care plan that outlines the specific actions and interventions required to meet the established goals. The plan should be tailored to the elderly person's unique needs, preferences, and cultural background. The care plan includes details about managing medications, scheduling medical appointments, and coordinating with healthcare providers to ensure proper medical care.

Regularly reviewing and updating the care plan is essential, as the elderly person's needs may change over time. By following a well-structured care plan, formal caregivers can provide effective, person-centered care that enhances the elderly person's quality of life and promotes their overall health and happiness.

Nonformal Caregivers

Nonformal caregivers include family members. The role of the family in the care of the elderly is essential and plays a crucial part in ensuring the well-being and quality of life of older family members. As people age, they may face various physical, emotional, and cognitive challenges that often require additional support and assistance. Family members typically step into provide the care, and their involvement can have a significant impact on the elderly individual's health and happiness. Some key aspects of the family's role in the care of the elderly include:

- ❖ **Emotional support:** Ageing can sometimes be accompanied by feelings of loneliness, isolation, or even depression. Family members can offer emotional support, companionship, and a sense of belonging, which can significantly improve the elderly person's mental well-being.
- ❖ **Physical care:** Family members often help with activities of daily living, such as bathing, dressing, and meal preparation. They may also assist with mobility, transportation to medical appointments, and administering medications.
- ❖ **Household and financial assistance:** Ageing individuals may find it challenging to manage household tasks and finances. Family members can help with chores, bill payments, and managing financial affairs.
- ❖ **Advocacy and healthcare management:** Family members can act as advocates for the elderly person, ensuring they receive appropriate medical care and attention. They can help navigate the healthcare system, communicate with healthcare providers, and monitor the individual's health.
- ❖ **Safety and security:** Families often play a vital role in ensuring the elderly person's living environment is safe and secure. This may involve making necessary home modifications, installing safety devices, or arranging for in-home care services.
- ❖ **Companionship and social engagement:** Regular interaction with family members can prevent feelings of social isolation. Family gatherings, outings, and other social activities can help maintain a sense of belonging and connectedness.
- ❖ **Decision-making:** As individual ages, there may come a time when they are unable to make critical decisions regarding their health and finances. Family members may need to step into make decisions in the best interest of the elderly person, often through legal means like the power of attorney or guardianship.
- ❖ **Memory and cognitive support:** For elderly individuals experiencing cognitive decline or dementia, family members can play a vital role in providing memory cues, engaging in cognitive exercises, and promoting mental stimulation.

ASSISTIVE AND ENABLING DEVICES FOR THE ELDERLY

Aids and prostheses play a significant role in improving the quality of life and mobility for many elderly individuals. As people age, they may experience physical limitations due to age-related conditions or injuries. Assistive devices for the elderly are designed to support older adults in various activities, enhance their safety, and improve their overall quality of life. These devices are intended to compensate for physical limitations, promote independence, and make daily tasks more manageable. Some of the commonly used assistive devices for the elderly are shown in **Table 50.1**.

These assistive devices are often recommended by healthcare professionals or occupational therapists based on the specific needs and abilities of each individual. By incorporating assistive devices into their daily lives, the elderly can maintain their independence, engage in activities they enjoy, and age with greater comfort and dignity.

Special Devices

Special devices for the elderly are designed to address the specific needs and challenges that older adults may face as they age. These devices are created to promote safety, independence, and overall well-being for seniors. Here are some special devices commonly used by the elderly:

- ❖ **Medical alert systems:** These systems include wearable devices or home-based units that enable seniors to call for help in case of emergencies. They can quickly connect the user to a monitoring center or designated contacts.
- ❖ **Smartphones and tablets with senior-friendly features:** These devices may have larger fonts, simplified interfaces, and accessibility options to accommodate the needs of seniors who may have vision or hearing impairments.
- ❖ **Talking pill dispensers:** These devices provide audible reminders to take medications and can dispense the correct doses at scheduled times, helping seniors manage their medications independently.
- ❖ **GPS trackers:** GPS-enabled devices can help caregivers locate seniors with dementia or memory issues in case they wander or become lost.
- ❖ **Easy-to-use remote controls:** Remote controls with simplified buttons and functions are designed to be user-friendly for seniors who may have fine motor skill challenges.
- ❖ **Voice-activated assistants:** Virtual assistants like Amazon Echo or Google Home can be controlled by voice

TABLE 50.1: Commonly used assistive devices for the elderly.

Mobility aids	

Walking canes: Canes provide additional support and stability while walking, assisting those with balance issues or mild mobility impairments. They come in various types, such as single-point canes, quad canes, and folding canes for easy transport. Single-point canes can help with early balance problems. Four-point or "quad" canes add more stability and help even more with balance which is why it is best to use for the elderly.

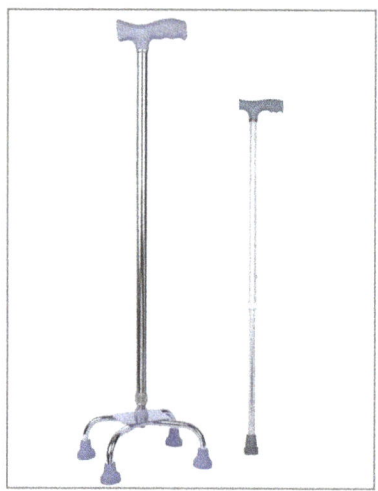
Quad cane   Single point cane

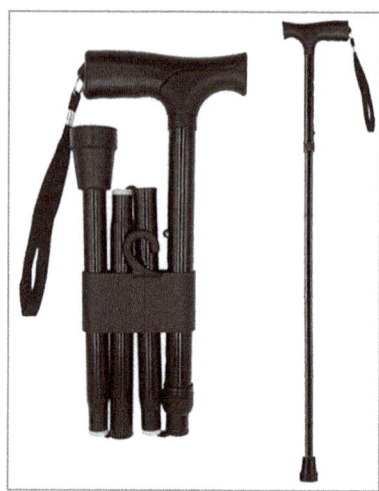
Folding cane

Walkers: Walkers offer more comprehensive support for those with greater mobility challenges. They come in various styles, including standard walkers, rolling walkers, and wheeled walkers.
Standard walkers need to be picked up to move forward. Front-wheeled walkers do not need to be picked up, so they use less energy. Rolling 4-wheeled walkers give support and come with/without seats and brakes.

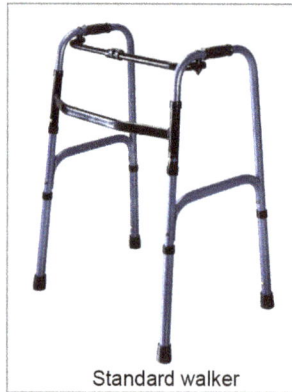
Standard walker

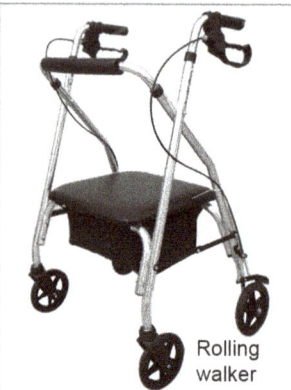
Rolling walker

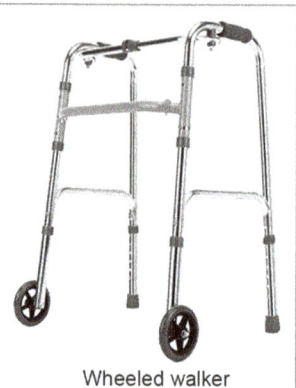
Wheeled walker

Crutches: Crutches are used by individuals who need to keep weight off from one or both legs due to injury and surgery.

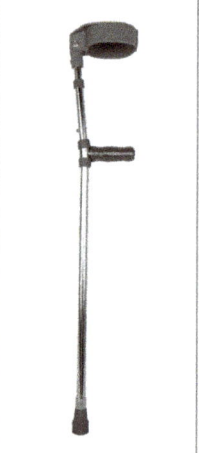

Contd...

Contd...

	Wheelchairs: Wheelchairs are mobility devices for individuals with severe mobility limitations, providing them with independence and mobility. • **Manual wheelchairs:** Self-propelled or pushed by a caregiver, suitable for those with limited mobility. • **Electric wheelchairs:** Powered by batteries, allowing for greater independence in movement. • **Mobility scooters:** Motorized devices designed for outdoor use, providing enhanced mobility. 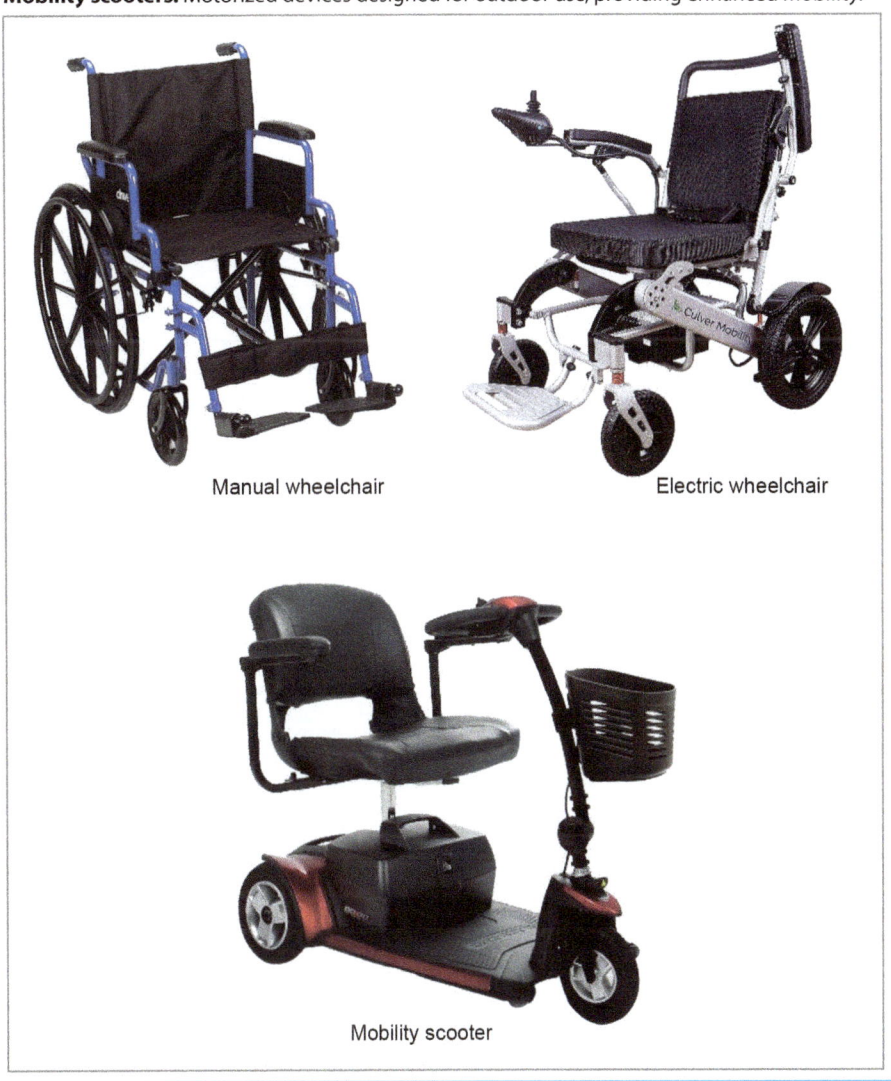 Manual wheelchair Electric wheelchair Mobility scooter
Hearing aids	**Hearing aids:** Amplify sounds and improve hearing for individuals with hearing impairments. • **Behind-the-ear (BTE) hearing aids:** BTE hearing aids sit behind the ear and are connected to a custom earmold that fits inside the ear canal. 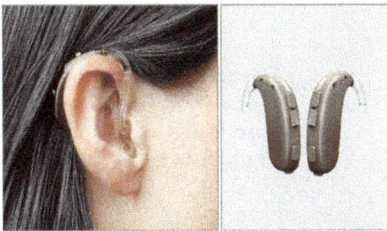 • **In-the-ear (ITE) hearing aids:** ITE hearing aids are custom-made to fit inside the outer ear. 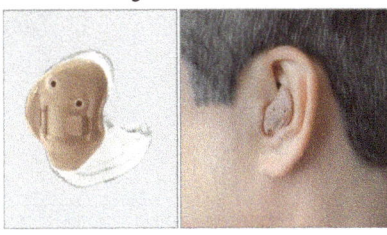

Contd...

Contd...

	- **In-the-canal (ITC) and completely-in-canal (CIC) hearing aids**: These hearing aids are smaller and fit partly or entirely inside the ear canal, making them less visible. 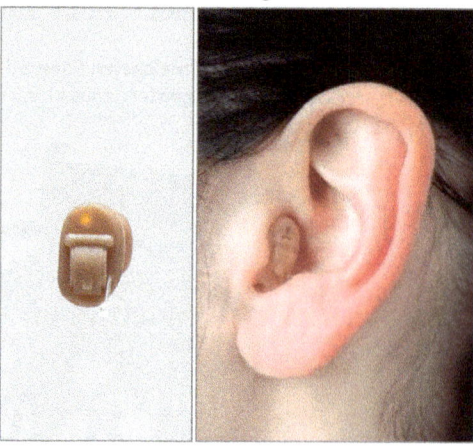
Vision aids	**Reading glasses:** Reading glasses help elderly individuals with presbyopia (age-related difficulty in seeing close objects) to read and perform close-up tasks. 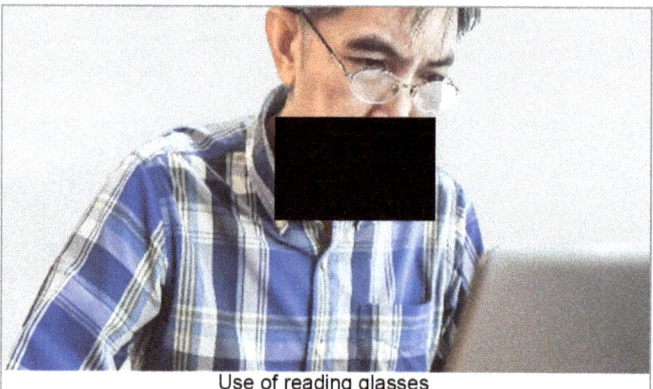 Use of reading glasses 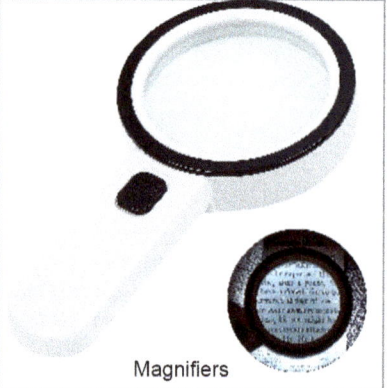 Magnifiers **Magnifiers**: Magnifiers, including handheld magnifiers and magnifying glasses, assist with reading and viewing fine print. **Low vision aids:** Various low vision devices, such as telescopic lenses and electronic magnifiers, help individuals with severe vision loss make the most of their remaining vision. 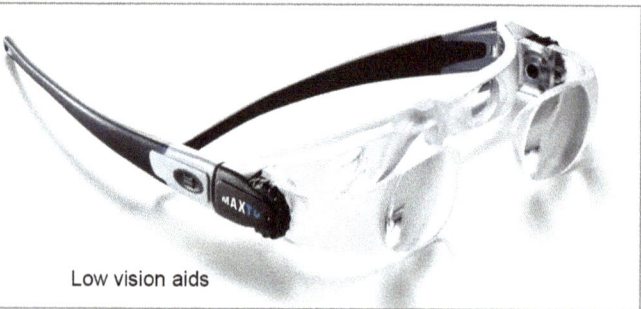 Low vision aids

Contd...

Contd...

Dental prostheses	**Dentures:** Dentures are removable appliances used to replace missing teeth, allowing the elderly to eat, speak, and smile more comfortably. 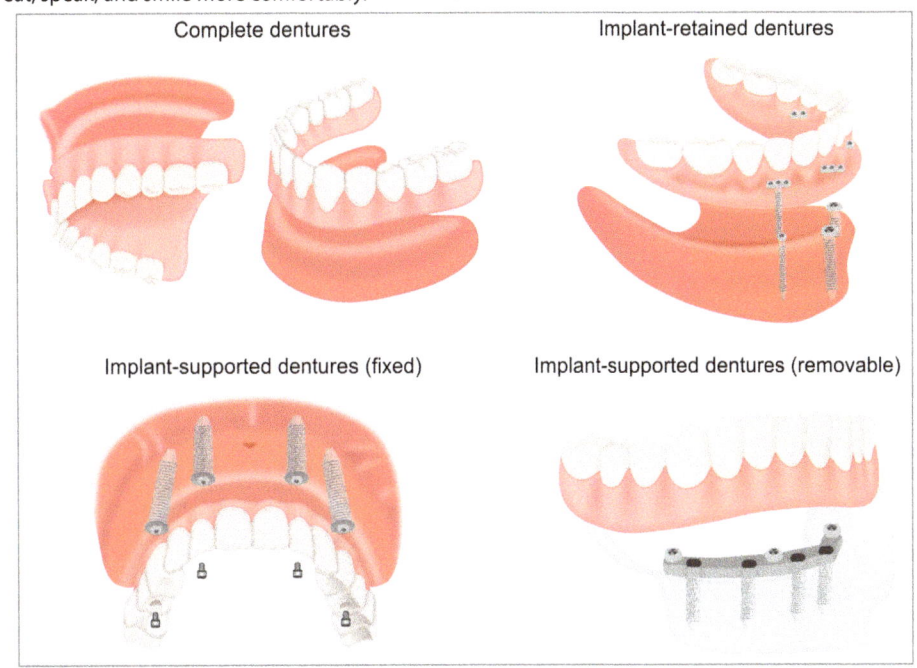
Orthotic devices	**Shoe inserts:** Provide support and alleviate foot pain or conditions like plantar fasciitis. **Ankle braces:** Stabilize and support the ankle joint for individuals with ankle instability or injuries. **Knee braces:** Assist those with knee pain or weakness, offering stability and protection.
Communication aids	**Augmentative and alternative communication (AAC) devices:** These devices help individuals with communication difficulties express themselves through symbols, pictures, or text-to-speech technology. 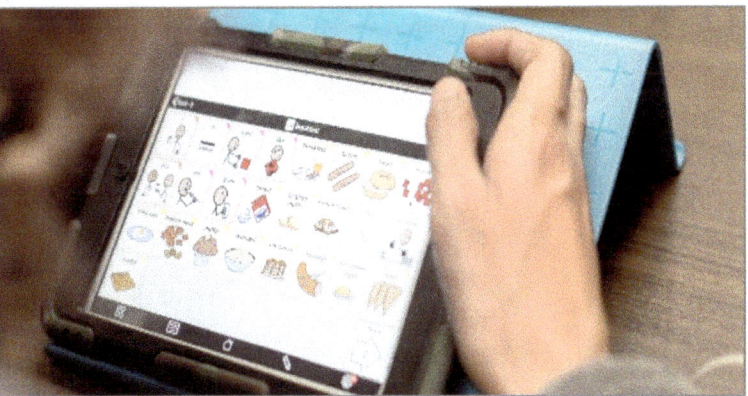
Daily living aids	**Reachers and grabbers:** Reachers and grabbers assist the elderly in reaching objects that are out of their grasp. 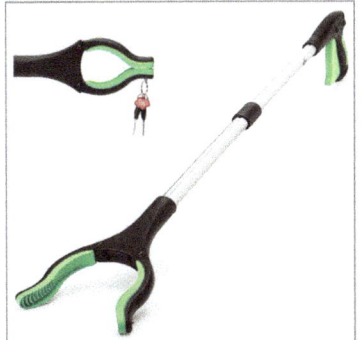 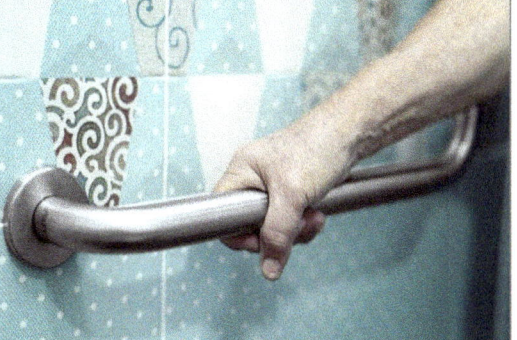

Contd...

Contd...

Adaptive eating utensils: These utensils are designed with modifications, such as larger handles or angled spoons, to make eating easier for individuals with limited dexterity.

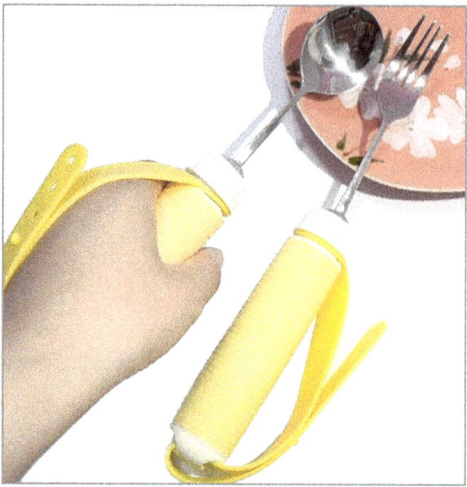

Bed rails: Offer support and prevent falls while getting in and out of bed.

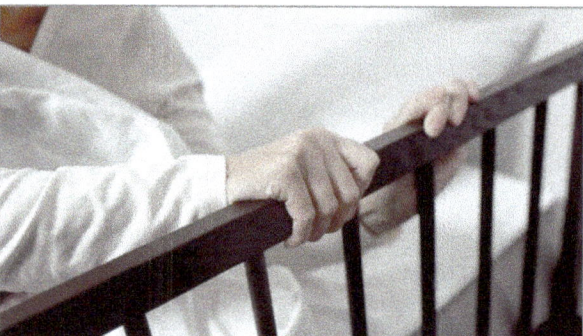

Pill organizers and reminders: Assist in medication management and adherence.

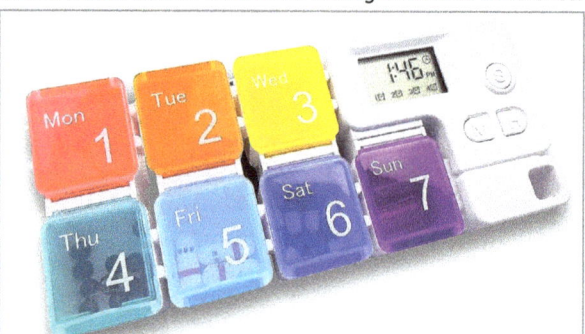

Talking watches and clocks: Provide audible time announcements for individuals with vision impairments.

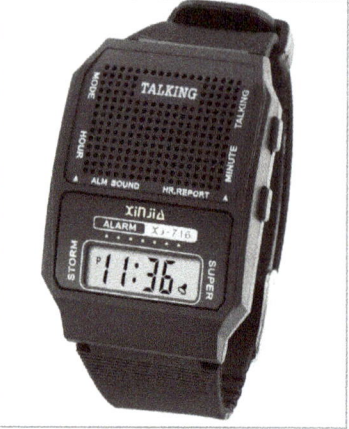

Contd...

Contd...

	Large button phones and cell phones: Easier to use for seniors with visual or fine motor skill challenges. 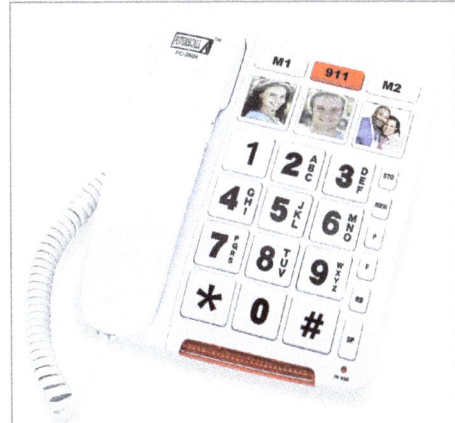 **Electric jar openers:** Help seniors open tight jar lids more easily. 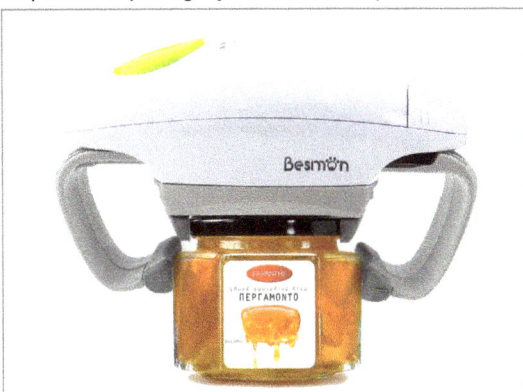
Adaptive dressing aids	**Button hooks:** Assist with buttoning clothes. 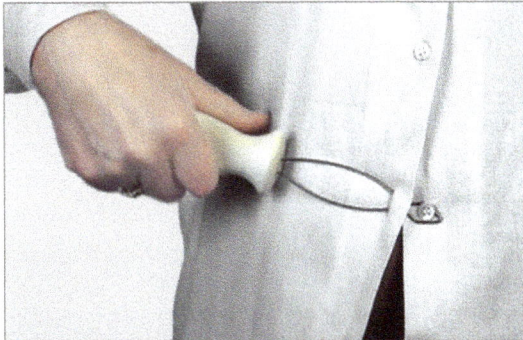 **Zipper pulls:** Make zipping easier for those with limited hand coordination. 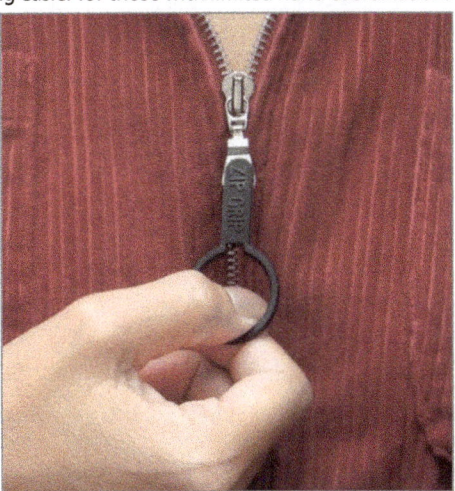

Contd...

Contd...

Bathroom safety aids	**Raised toilet seats:** Increase the height of the toilet for easier use, reducing strain on joints. 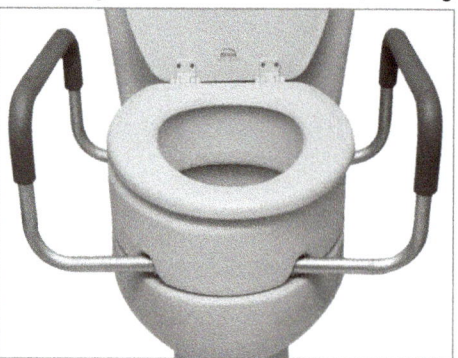 **Grab bars:** Provide support and stability in the bathroom, helping seniors get in and out of the tub or shower safely. 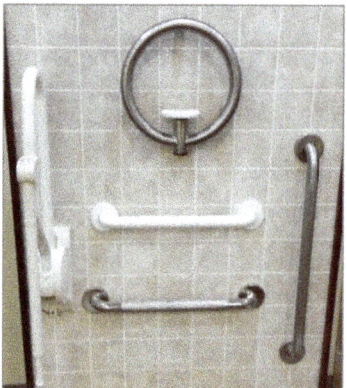 **Bath seats and transfer benches:** Facilitate safe bathing and transferring in and out of the bathtub, reducing the risk of slips and falls. 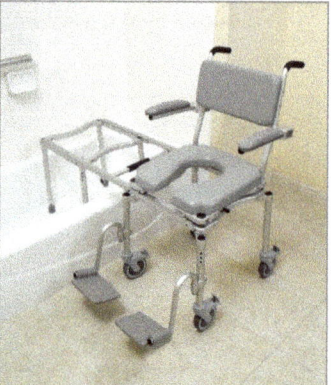
Compression stockings	Improve circulation and reduce swelling in the legs. 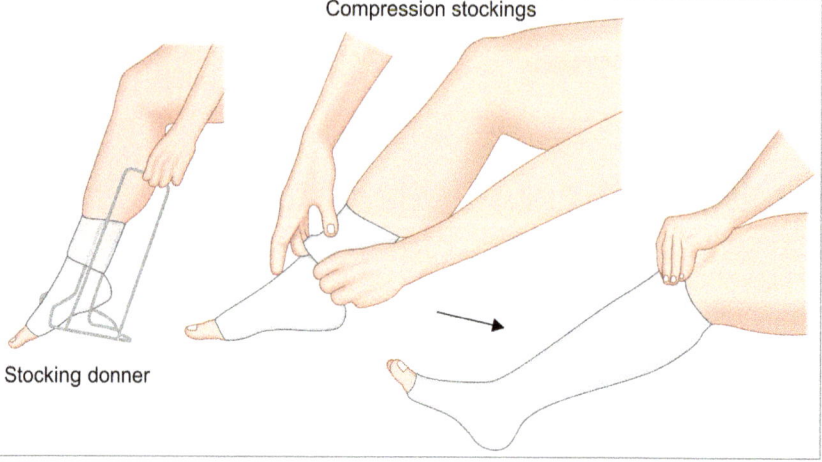

Contd...

Contd...

Emergency alert systems	Personal alarms or wearable devices to call for help in emergencies.
	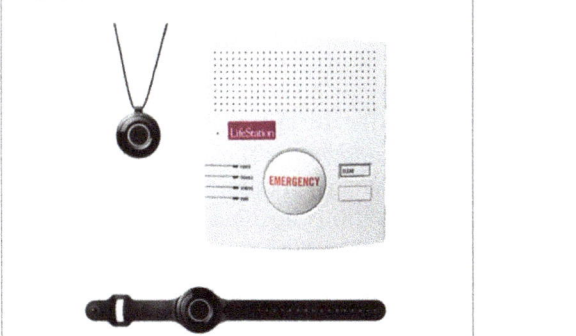

commands, making it easier for seniors to perform tasks like setting reminders, making calls, or getting weather updates.
- **Digital magnifiers:** These devices provide enlarged text and images, helping seniors with low vision read books, newspapers, or other printed materials.
- **Hearing amplifiers:** Similar to hearing aids, hearing amplifiers can boost sound levels for seniors with mild hearing loss.
- **Automatic lights:** Motion-activated or voice-activated lights can improve safety and convenience, especially during night-time trips to the bathroom or kitchen.
- **Video calling devices:** Video calling devices with large screens and simple interfaces enable seniors to stay connected with family and friends, reducing feelings of isolation.
- **Adaptive clothing:** Clothing designed with adaptive features like easy-open closures and magnetic buttons to help seniors dress more independently.
- **One-touch emergency buttons:** These devices can be placed strategically around the home and easily activated to call for help in case of a fall or emergency.
- **Automatic shut-off appliances:** Devices like automatic shut-off coffee makers or stovetop timers can help prevent accidents caused by forgetfulness.
- **Swivel seat cushions:** Assist seniors in getting in and out of chairs or vehicles more easily.
- **Memory aids and reminders:** Devices with voice recording or visual reminders can help seniors remember important tasks or appointments.

These special devices are designed with the unique needs and challenges of seniors in mind, helping them maintain their independence, safety, and comfort as they age. It is essential to choose devices that match the individual's specific requirements and capabilities, and consulting with healthcare professionals or occupational therapists can assist in making appropriate selections.

Smart Technologies for Elderly

Smart technologies for the elderly are designed to enhance the safety, independence, and overall well-being of older adults.
- **Smart home automation:** This technology allows elderly individuals to control various devices in their homes remotely or through voice commands. Smart home systems can adjust lighting, temperature, lock doors, and control appliances, making it easier for seniors to manage their living environment.
- **Smart fall detection systems:** These systems use wearable devices with built-in sensors to detect falls. When a fall is detected, the system automatically sends alerts to caregivers or emergency services, ensuring timely assistance.
- **Medication management devices:** These devices help seniors organize and manage their medications effectively. They can dispense the right dose at the right time and send reminders to take pills, reducing the risk of medication errors.
- **Telehealth and remote monitoring:** Virtual healthcare services allow older adults to consult with doctors or healthcare professionals from the comfort of their homes. Remote monitoring devices can track vital signs and health parameters, enabling healthcare providers to monitor their patients' health proactively.
- **Personal emergency response systems (PERS):** PERS devices are wearable or wall-mounted gadgets that allow seniors to call for help in case of emergencies. They often have a panic button that connects to a monitoring center or designated contacts.
- **GPS tracking devices:** These devices are useful for seniors with dementia or Alzheimer's disease. They can help locate the individual if they wander away from home, providing peace of mind to caregivers.
- **Smart hearing aids:** Advanced hearing aids can be connected to smartphones and other devices via Bluetooth, allowing elderly users to customize settings, stream audio, and adjust the volume more conveniently.
- **Social engagement Apps:** Social networking platforms designed for seniors can help combat loneliness and isolation by connecting them with friends and family, sharing updates, and participating in group activities.
- **Smart pill dispensers:** These devices can sort and dispense medications at scheduled times, and some can even notify family members or caregivers if doses are missed.
- **Voice-activated assistants:** Smart speakers with voice assistants like Amazon Echo (Alexa) or Google Home can provide helpful information, set reminders, answer questions, and even control compatible smart home devices, offering hands-free assistance to seniors.

❖ **Augmentative and alternative communication (AAC) devices:** These are invaluable tools that can greatly benefit elderly individuals who have difficulty with speech or communication. These devices help enhance their ability to express themselves, engage with others, and maintain social connections.

Examples of AAC devices for the elderly:
- *Communication boards and books:* These are low-tech AAC devices that consist of a set of images, symbols, or words representing various needs, emotions, and common phrases. The elderly person can point to the appropriate image or word to communicate their thoughts.
- *Picture exchange communication system (PECS):* PECS involves using picture cards that the elderly individual can exchange with a communication partner to convey their messages or needs effectively.
- *Speech-generating devices (SGDs):* SGDs are electronic devices equipped with pre-recorded or synthesized speech output. They have touchscreens or switches that the user can operate to generate spoken messages.
- *Text-to-speech apps and software:* These applications and programs convert text input into spoken words, allowing the elderly to type out their messages or select pre-written phrases that the app will vocalize.
- *Eye-tracking devices:* Some advanced AAC systems use eye-tracking technology to allow individuals with limited mobility to communicate. The device monitors the movement of their eyes, enabling them to select symbols or words on a screen using their gaze.
- *Head-pointing systems:* These AAC devices use head movements to control a cursor on a screen, enabling the elderly person to select symbols or words and construct messages.
- *Switch-activated devices:* Switches are alternative input methods for individuals with limited motor abilities. They can be activated with various body parts, such as a hand, foot, or even the head, to control AAC devices.
- *Tablet apps with symbol-based communication:* Many tablets and smartphones offer AAC apps with symbol-based communication features. These apps use a grid of symbols that the user can select to create messages.

These smart technologies have the potential to significantly improve the quality of life for elderly individuals, allowing them to age in place more comfortably and safely.

Case Scenario

- Mr Sharma, a 75-year-old retired schoolteacher living in a small town in India. He has three grown-up children and has been a widower for the past five years. Mr Sharma's health has been gradually declining, and he now requires some assistance in his daily activities.
- In Indian culture, it is quite common for elderly parents like Mr Sharma to live with one of their adult children or close relatives. In this case, Mr Sharma lives with his eldest son, Rajesh, and his family. Rajesh's family believes in the traditional Indian value of respecting and caring for their elders. Rajesh's family understands the emotional needs of their father and makes sure to spend quality time with him. They frequently engage in conversations, listen to his stories, and involve him in family gatherings, making him feel loved and valued.
- As Mr Sharma's health declines, his family plays a crucial role in his healthcare. Rajesh's wife, Meera, ensures that he takes his medications on time and schedules regular visits to the doctor. They also accompany him to medical appointments and support him during his treatment.
- As per the Indian scenario, meals are an essential aspect of family bonding. Rajesh's family ensures that Mr Sharma gets nutritious and home-cooked meals that are suitable for his health conditions. They accommodate his dietary preferences and restrictions. With advancing age, Mr Sharma's mobility decreases, and his family assists him with daily activities. They help him with bathing, getting dressed, and other tasks that he may find challenging to do alone. Mr Sharma's children contribute to his financial needs, making sure that he can access the best healthcare and live a comfortable life. Mr Sharma's family encourages him to stay socially active. They take him to community gatherings, religious events, and other social activities that he enjoys. This helps prevent feelings of loneliness and isolation.
- Mr Sharma's family includes him in important decisions, seeking his opinions and valuing his wisdom. They ensure that he feels involved and respected in the family's affairs. Living with his family, Mr Sharma feels safe and secure. They provide him with a warm and nurturing environment, reducing his anxiety and fear related to ageing.
- In this case scenario, Mr Sharma's family plays a significant role in providing him with the care, love, and support he needs during his elderly years. Their collective effort ensures that he can age gracefully and maintain a sense of belonging in a close-knit family structure.

SUMMARY

- The safety and well-being of all the elderly is a matter of concern. The elderly deserve the best care to be provided with a focus on social and mental well-being, economic and social security, and elder abuse to help them to feel as comfortable as possible. Elderly care whether as a home care or institutional care is a decision specific to each family as per the prevailing circumstances. A better old age period can give a real meaning to the remarkable extension of the life span.
- Formal caregivers are individuals who provide care and support as part of their professional roles. They may work in various settings, such as hospitals, nursing homes, assisted living facilities, or home care agencies. They provide medical care, personal care, and skilled services. They also have a role in the safety and supervision and care planning of the elderly. Non-formal caregivers include family. The role of the family in the care of the elderly is essential and plays a crucial part in ensuring the well-being and quality of life of older family members. As people age, they may face various physical, emotional, and cognitive challenges that often require additional support and assistance. Family members typically step in to provide the care, and their involvement can have a significant impact on the elderly individual's health and happiness.
- Assistive devices for the elderly are designed to support older adults in various activities, enhance their safety, and improve their overall quality of life. These devices are intended to compensate for physical limitations, promote independence, and make daily tasks more manageable. Special devices for the elderly are designed to address the specific needs and challenges that older adults may face as they age. These devices are created to promote safety, independence, and overall well-being for seniors.
- It is essential to choose these assistive and special devices that match the individual's specific requirements and capabilities, and consulting with healthcare professionals or occupational therapists can assist in making appropriate selections.

MULTIPLE CHOICE QUESTIONS

1. Formal caregivers provide all the following to the elderly, *except*:
   a. Personal care
   b. Medical care
   c. Safety and supervision
   d. Household and financial assistance
2. For elderly individuals recovering from surgeries, injuries, or strokes which of the following requires the most:
   a. Personal care
   b. Financial assistance
   c. Skilled services
   d. Memory and cognitive support
3. Which of the following assistive device is used for ankle instability?
   a. Walker
   b. Crutch
   c. Cane
   d. Ankle brace
4. Quad canes are better than single-point canes because of:
   a. Stability
   b. Balance
   c. Both a and c
   d. None of these
5. While planning the care of the elderly, healthcare professionals should assess which of the following:
   a. Physical health
   b. Cognitive function
   c. Emotional well-being
   d. All of the above

ANSWERS

1. d   2. c   3. d   4. c
5. d

SUGGESTED READING

1. Bhagoria E, Kaur S, Singh A, et al. Making the Emergency OPD of a Tertiary Care Center Elderly Friendly Through Quality Assurance of Geriatric Syndrome Management Strategies. J Postgrad Med Edu Res. 2021;55(3):114-8.
2. Bhagoria E, Kaur S, Singh A, et al. Pattern of health problems amongst the elderly patients admitted in the emergency department of tertiary care hospital of North India. NMRJ. 2020;16(4):165-72. http://doi.org/10.33698/NRF0324
3. Boland L, Légaré F, Margarita M, et al. Impact of home care versus alternative locations of care on elder health outcomes: an overview of systematic reviews. BMC Geriatrics. 2001;17:20.
4. Kaur S, Gill A, Sharma U, et al. Quality Care Audit of Old Age Homes in a North Indian City. Journal of the Indian Academy of Geriatrics. 2015;11:3-9.
5. Kaur S, Kumar KP A, Kaur B, et al. Knowledge and Attitude Regarding Care of Elderly Among Nursing Students: An Indian Perspective. J Nursing and Care. 2014;3:3: 1000161.
6. Kaur S, Singh A, Gill A, et al. Impact of home-based care package for elderly on prevention of bedsores. J Nursing and Care. 2013;2(3):59.
7. Kaur S, Singh A, Kaur P, Bhalla A, Kumari S, Kaur GP. Assessment of nursing care needs of elderly in Chandigarh, North India: A pilot study. J Nursing and Care. 2013;2(3):83.
8. Kaur S, Singh A, Kumari S, Bhalla A. Assessment of functional status and daily life problems faced by elderly in a North Indian city. Psychogeriatrics; 2019. DOI:10.1111/psyg.12406.
9. Rohilla L, Das K, Kaur S. Assessment of cognitive impairment in the elderly persons admitted in a tertiary care hospital: A pilot study. Journal of Nursing Science and Practice. 2017;7(2):20-4.
10. Saini R, Sharma A, Kaur S, et al. Perceived social support among hospitalized elderly patients in Indian settings. Journal of Geriatric Care and Research. 2020;7(3):133-9.
11. Sharma D, Kaur M, Chaudhary R, Kaur S, et al. Admission of Elderly in Emergency Units: Causes and Problems. Adv Practice Nurs. 2016;2(3), http://dx.doi.org/10.4172/apn.1000119.
12. Sharma S, Thakur M, Kaur S. Assessment of dependency level in the performance of activities of daily living amongst elderly in a suburban population of India. International Journal of Nursing Education. 2012;4(1):94-6.
13. Sharma S, Thakur M, Kaur S. Assessment of dependency level in the performance of activities of daily living amongst elderly in a suburban population of India. International Journal of Nursing Education. 2012;4(1):94-6.
14. Sharma S, Thakur M, Kaur S. Health problems and treatment-seeking behaviour among elderly. HelpAge India-Research and Development Journal. 2012;18(2):21-7.
15. Singh M, Kaur S. Palliative Care in Elderly: A Case Study. Research and Review: A Journal of Health Professions. 2020;10(3):5-9.
16. Vandali V. Role of Nurse in Geriatric Care: A Mini Review. Journal of Nurses Voice and Impact. 2018;1(1):1-3.

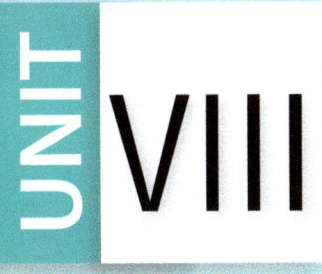

Critical Care Nursing

OUTLINE

51. Critical Care Nursing: General Concepts
Lt Col Lata Mandal

52. Management of Patients in Critical Care Units
Shivani Kalra, Jyoti Sharma

CHAPTER 51

Critical Care Nursing: General Concepts

Lt Col Lata Mandal

"They may forget your name, but they will never forget how you make them feel".
—Maya Angelou

LEARNING OBJECTIVES

After going through the chapter, the learner will be able to:
- Describe the concept of critical care nursing.
- Apply the principles of critical care nursing while caring for critically-ill patients.
- Describe the physical set up, and staffing norms of a critical care unit.
- Identify equipment used in critical care unit and describe their functions.
- Recognize situations in critical care units that have the potential for ethical and legal conflicts.
- Explain the quality indicators in critical care unit.
- Identify cardiac arrest and explain the steps of cardiopulmonary resuscitation.

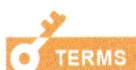

TERMS

- **Adverse patient events:** A preventable or non-preventable event that cause harm to a patient as a result of medical care, for example, patient fall, bedsores, etc.
- **Antibiogram:** A report showing the susceptibility of different strains of pathogens to antibiotics.
- **Burn out:** A syndrome resulting from chronic stress in the workplace.
- **Catheter-associated blood stream infection (CA-BSI):** Blood stream infection caused by intravenous catheter.
- **Critical care nursing:** The specialty of clinical nursing that focus on caring for patients who are critically ill and are hemodynamically unstable.
- **Critical care:** Health care imparted to a person who is facing an actual or potentially life-threatening health condition.
- **Deep vein thrombosis (DVT):** Blood clots in deep veins of the body.
- **ET tube (endotracheal tube):** A flexible plastic tube placed through the mouth into the trachea to maintain airway and help in patient breathing.
- **Hand hygiene:** Act of washing hands with soap and water or using a hand rubbing solution.
- **Healthcare-associated infection:** These are infections that occur in a healthcare setting, such as a hospital.
- Informed consent is the process in which a healthcare provider educates the patient about the risks, benefits, and alternatives of an intervention, so that the patient can make voluntary and informed decision of whether or not to get the procedure done.
- **Pulseless electrical activity (PEA):** Any type of heart rhythm which does not produce detectable pulse.
- **Psychoacoustic therapy:** Branch of psychophysics involving the scientific study of sound perception and audiology.
- **Radial design nursing unit:** Nursing unit designed in a roughly circular form to have maximum visualization of patients.
- **Return of spontaneous circulation (ROSC):** It is the resumption of an uninterrupted heart rhythm required for perfusion. ROSC is detected through return of palpable arterial pulse, measurable blood pressure and breathing.

- **Supraglottic airways:** Devices that can be inserted into the pharynx to allow ventilation, oxygenation, and administration of anesthetic agents.
- **Utility rooms:** An area or room where items required for different functions are kept. These items are useful but may not be used in a daily basis.
- **Ventilator-associated pneumonia (VAP):** An infection in the lung of a patient on ventilatory support.
- **Ventricular fibrillation (VF):** A life-threatening rhythm where the ventricles shiver instead of pumping.
- **Ventricular tachycardia (VT):** A life-threatening rhythm in which the ventricles contract very rapidly but ineffectively.

INTRODUCTION

During the Crimean war in 1850s, Ms Florence Nightingale and her group of nurses set aside an area near the nursing station for caring for the critically ill and injured British soldiers. This can be marked as the healthcare system's first effort in giving focused care to critically-ill patients.

In the early part of the 20th century, efforts of a neurosurgeon named Dr Walter Dandy to create a special area in the John Hopkins Hospital in United States is another landmark in the history of human health that focused in the care of critically-ill patients.

Critical care implies to health care imparted to a person who is facing an actual or potentially life-threatening health condition. **Critical care nursing** is the specialty of clinical nursing that focus on caring for patients who are critically ill and are hemodynamically unstable.

The key characteristics of a critically-ill patient are severe respiratory, cardiovascular or neurological derangement and often these happen in combination. Thus a critically-ill patient often have abnormal physiological observations, such as respiratory distress, hypotension or altered level of consciousness. Critical care nursing is imparted to critically-ill patients in critical care units. **Critical care units** are the specialized areas in the hospitals where skilled personnel and sophisticated equipment are readily available to closely and continuously monitor patients, and impart rapid and intensive therapeutic and nursing interventions. Intensive care units, coronary care unit, neonatal intensive care units are examples of critical care units in the hospital settings.

PRINCIPLES OF CRITICAL CARE NURSING

Nurses working with critically-ill patients need to remember and follow certain basic principles while imparting care. They are as follows:

1. **Principle of anticipation:** A nurse in the critical care unit has to anticipate all types of situations that can arise with patients. This principle helps critical care nurses to keep their units ready at all times, equipment in fully functional condition and keep themselves physically and mentally alert to face any situation.
2. **Principle of holistic nursing:** Most of the time a critically-ill patient is unresponsive and is surrounded and supported by large number of machines. Therefore, it is not uncommon for a nurse to forget the human behind all these gadgets. The principle of holistic care helps in reminding the nurse to meet the patients' overall needs including the physiological, emotional, hygiene, nutrition, and spiritual needs. This principle also demands that a critically-ill patient is cared with dignity and respect as is deserved by a human being.
3. **Principle of collaboration:** The care of a critically-ill patient requires a collaborative team approach with a sense of partnership among nurses, physicians and other healthcare members. A good communication network between the critical care nurse and others helps in getting important inputs from all healthcare members and assist her to make sound and balanced clinical decisions.
4. **Principle of surveillance:** A critical care nurse needs to have very close and consistent surveillance of the patient and the environmental conditions. This principle ensures that a critical care nurse will detect changes in the patients' condition at the earliest and also recognize any errors in the care process and prevent adverse events, such as pressure injuries or patient fall.
5. **Principle of ethical care:** Critically-ill patients are often unresponsive, unconscious, sedated or are too anxious to know whether their ethical rights are violated or not. The nurses caring for these patients may at times forget the human being and the associated ethical rights of the patient, such as his right for autonomy, self-determination, need of justice and fair treatment. This principle ensures that the nursing care rendered to critically-ill patients are abiding to human ethics.

CRITICAL CARE UNITS AND LEVELS

A critical care unit in a hospital should be according to the local needs of the community, and material and human resources available in the hospital. Critical care units can be classified in various levels as per the services they provide.

- **Level 1—critical care unit:** Provides monitoring, observation and short-term ventilation.
- **Level 2—critical care unit:** Provides detailed observation, intervention, including support for a single failed organ system, short-term non-invasive ventilation and post-operative care.
- **Level 3—critical care unit:** Provides comprehensive critical care including complex multi-system life support for an indefinite period. A level 3—critical care unit also should have ongoing research and academic activities.

Critical care units can also be classified based on the management policy of the unit as:

- **Closed critical care** units where the patients' clinical management is done by an Intensivist.
- **Open critical care** unit where the patient management is done by the treating physicians or surgeons.

Physical Setup of a Critical Care Unit

The physical layout of a critical care unit should be in a way that create an environment of caring and make patients and relatives feel calm and reassured. A critical care unit is usually located in an area of the hospital that is close and easily accessible from the emergency department, operation theater, trauma care, blood bank and the laboratory. The lifts, corridors and ramps leading to a critical care unit should be spacious for easy movement of beds and people. There should be a single point of entry for patients and it is mandatory to have an emergency exit point. However, it is desirable to have a separate entry and exit gate, ramp and lifts for healthcare providers, and movement of supplies and wastes. The critical care unit should have uninterrupted power supply with required back up power supply. A critical care unit should be centrally air conditioned and have central supply of oxygen, compressed air and central facility of suctioning. Modern critical care units also have facility for hemodialysis.

Moreover, the physical design of a critical care unit should be such, as to minimize transmission of infection with physical segregation of dirty and clean area, use of air curtains at the entries, adequate spacing between patients, and non-porous easily cleanable walls and surfaces.

The physical layout of a critical care unit can be divided in the following spaces:

- **Patient care area:**
  - Patient care units
  - Nursing station area
  - Work area
- **Clean utility area** for food preparation and eating.
- **Storage area** for drugs, intravenous fluids, equipment, linens.
- **Administrative area** for keeping stationaries, and clerks to sit.
- **Dirty utility area** for collection of soiled linen and storage of bedpans, urinals, etc.
- **Staff and visitors' area** for staff, visitors and relatives of patients
- **Visitor's lounge** for the relatives and friends of the patients.

Patient Care Area

The patient care area should be situated in such a way that patients can see daylight and be aware of the day and night cycle. Lighting in the patient care area should include focused lights in each bed unit and strong central lights for the whole unit. It should also be free from loud or traffic noise and designed in a way to reduce noise. Research study has shown that therapeutic sounds, such as music played in the critical care unit decrease patient's perception of pain. Psychoacoustic therapy, such as sounds of rainfall, waves lapping, mixed with relaxing and soft music, have been shown to calm patients by reducing the pulse rates and blood pressure.

Hand hygiene is the simplest but the most effective method of reducing healthcare-associated infections which are common among critically-ill patients whose immunity is low and have various invasive procedures done on them. Therefore, hand hygiene areas should be conveniently located near the patients' bed space. The hand hygiene areas should have supply of warm water, liquid soap and disposable paper towel or hot air hand drier. A critical care unit should also have sterilizing areas for sterilizing reusable equipment.

Waste disposal in critical care units is very important with segregation of the waste at the point of generation.

- **Patient care units:** The critically-ill patients are generally unable to move and turn their positions themselves and this can lead to various injurious effect to the patients' skin, musculoskeletal, respiratory and the cardiovascular system. Therefore, the beds for critically-ill patients should be adjustable for various positions and the head of the bed should be elevated to 30–45° for preventing respiratory complications. A continuous mattress leads to slipping down of an unconscious or sedated patients. Therefore, split mattresses in the beds help in maintaining body position of patients. Research studies have shown that beds with continuous lateral rotation therapy that rotates the patient at a rate of half a degree per second helps in preventing pressure injuries (bed sores), urinary tract infections, pneumonia and deep vein thrombosis. Even mattresses that have alternate inflation and deflation (commonly known as alternating air mattresses) have also found to be helpful in preventing the above complications. The recommended area for a critical care bed space is 225 square feet per bed. The area around the bed should have hand washing facility, storage space for patients' medications, and intravenous fluids, space for keeping equipment, such as monitors, infusion pumps and chart boards to keep the monitoring records of patients. The bed space should also have electrical outlets of 15 ampere and 5 amperes and outlets for pipeline systems supplying oxygen, compressed air and vacuum from a central supply. Each bed space should have liquid hand sanitizer for quick hand sanitization and color-coded container to receive wastes generated at the bed side. Each bed area should also have a container to receive sharp wastes, such as needles.
- **Nursing station area:** This includes a nursing station with a radial unit design where nurses can have unobstructed view of patients. The nursing station should be in a very short walking distance from each patient care units. This area should have space for storing stationaries, keeping computer terminals, telephones, pagers and space for consultation. Telephones, computers with internet connection and books for referral should be available in this area.
- **Work areas:** The work areas in a critical care unit will include space for preparation of therapy and special procedures. There should be a table top with adequate space and good lighting for nurses to prepare medication. Shelves and refrigerator containing medicines should be in this area. The work area should be within the patient care area. This area should also have a hand hygiene facility.

Clean Utility Area

A critical care unit should have a pantry area with refrigerator and microwave for storing and preparing therapeutic diet for patients.

Storage Area

There should be a large storage area for storing medications, intravenous fluids in bulk and back up equipment. This area should also have cupboards to keep fresh linens.

Administrative Area

This area should be away from the patient care area and should have telephones and computers and space for clerks and managers to sit and work. The area should be fitted with a reception desk where visitors can communicate and address their queries.

Dirty Utility Area

This area is used for storing dirty linens waiting for wash and washing facility for cleaning bedpans, urinals and suction bottles. There should be a large sink for washing the items and also hand washing facility. This area should be physically separate from the clean utility area and the patient care area.

Staff and Visitors' Area

A lounge for staff should be located within the critical care complex where healthcare providers can have comfortable and relaxing environment to rest, eat and change dresses. Lockers to keep personal items and facilities to warm up food, eat, watch TV, read newspapers and books should be available in this area. The area should be in telephonic connection with the nursing station.

Visitors' Lounge

Relatives and friends of critically-ill patients undergo lots of stress and anxiety. Therefore, it is important that they are provided with a comfortable place to seat and relax. Facilities for mobile charging, watching TV, reading, drinking water and eating, etc., should be available in the visitor's lounge.

STAFFING NORMS IN CRITICAL CARE UNIT

The team of healthcare providers who work in the critical care unit should consist of:

- ❖ **Nursing staff:** Nursing staff form the core of the health care team in a critical care unit. Critical patients require continuous and specialized care. Therefore, it is important to maintain an adequate number of nursing staff in a critical care unit. The NABH (National Accreditation Board for hospitals and healthcare providers) India recommends to maintain a nurse—patient ration of 1:1 for beds with ventilation facility and for non-ventilated beds a nurse—patient ratio of 1: 2 (one nurse for two beds). Other than having adequate number of nursing staff, it is important that nurses working in the critical care unit should be especially trained. An adequate nurse patient ratio and the level of training of nurses ensures good quality of care. Research studies have also established that this reduces risks of adverse events, such as patient fall, occurrence of bed sores, DVT, etc.
- ❖ **Medical staff:** A critical care unit should have at least one doctor round the clock who is capable of doing emergency invasive procedures, such as endotracheal intubation, inserting chest drainage or establishing central venous access. In Level III critical care units this responsibility should be with an Intensivist who is a doctor with special training and experience in managing critically-ill patients.
- ❖ **Critical care technical staff:** These members of the team are in-charge of equipment and assist the nursing staff in suctioning and chest physiotherapy of ventilated patients, invasive monitoring, and maintaining the ventilator parameters.
- ❖ **Ancillary and support staff:** This include housekeeping, administrative, pantry and cleaning staff who are permanent members of the critical care team. Other staff, such as radiographers, physiotherapists, clinical pharmacist, dieticians, laboratory technicians who come intermittently for different purposes are also important members of the team. It is essential to remember that these staff should be adequately trained in patient safety and infection control issues of a critical care unit.

EQUIPMENT IN CRITICAL CARE UNITS AND THEIR CARE

The critical care unit is a place in the hospital where one can find various equipment for patient monitoring and treatment. A few important equipment used for critically-ill patients are described below:

- ❖ **Mechanical ventilators:** These are the machines that assist patients to breathe when he is unable to breathe on his own. For example, a patient with severe head injury may not be able to breathe normally. In this case, a ventilator is useful to maintain the patients' respiratory function till the time he recovers his normal breathing function.

  Thus mechanical ventilators help patients to maintain body oxygenation while allowing him to recover from his health condition, and prevents aspiration of gastrointestinal content into the lungs. But patients on mechanical ventilation have high risks of getting respiratory infection. **Ventilator-associated pneumonia (VAP)** has been a significant cause of **healthcare-associated infection (HCAI)** for patients undergoing mechanical ventilation.

  The ventilator is connected to the patient through a closed pipe, known as ventilator circuit which is again connected to an **endotracheal tube**. An endotracheal tube is a flexible plastic pipe that is inserted through the patient's mouth into the trachea. The process of inserting an endotracheal tube in the patient's trachea is called **endotracheal intubation**.

  The Drinker and Shaw tank type ventilator, popularly known as iron lung was one of the first negative-pressure machines introduced in early 20th century. In this machine, the patient was put inside a chamber and a vacuum pump created negative pressure which resulted in expansion of the patient's chest. However, negative pressure ventilators were very uncomfortable for patients and lead to various complications. In the middle of the 20th century, positive pressure ventilation was introduced in the USA. With the development of safe endotracheal tubes, positive pressure ventilators have replaced negative pressure ventilation in the present days.

  In **positive-pressure ventilation**, airway pressure is applied by the ventilator into the patient's airway through an endotracheal tube which causes the compressed air and oxygen to flow into the lungs. As the ventilator stops applying pressure, the airway pressure drops to zero, and the patient's chest recoils and pushes the air out of the chest.

A ventilator has to be kept clean, free from dust and a few inches away from the walls. The ventilator circuits are to be kept sterilized to prevent patient infection. A ventilator requires electric supply for functioning and has battery back up to function for a short duration in case of power failure. This machine is to be taken care by critical care trained nurses or by critical care technicians. The parameters of a ventilator in use for a patient has to be set by an anesthesiologist or by the Intensivist.

❖ **Infusion pumps:** These are the machines that help in infusing medications to patients in minute doses and in a controlled manner. For example a critically-ill patient requires Injection Dopamine at the rate 2 microgram/kg/min. It is difficult for the nurses to accurately deliver this amount through normal infusion sets. Infusion pumps are electric operated with battery backup. They are to be kept clean and free of dust. These pumps are also known as syringe infusion pumps as the medication is loaded in a syringe (usually 50 mL syringe) and set up in the pump. Thereafter the syringe is connected to the patient's venous access through a thin, sterile tube. Generally, syringe pumps have a step motor which pushes the plunger of the syringe which ejects the medication into the patient's blood stream through the tube and venous access. Syringe pumps are just one type of infusion pumps. This machine which came in use in the 1950s have undergone vast changes and presently development of 'smart pumps' have increased accuracy and precision of medication dosages with remote programing.

❖ **Monitoring equipment:** For critically-ill patients sudden and unexpected change in their physiological condition are common. Monitoring equipment are devices that help in detecting and diagnosing these events. Monitoring equipment consist of one or more **sensors** that are either attached to the surface or inside of the patients' body, the **processing components** that converts the signal from the sensor to the display format, and the **display device** that provide information in numerical and waveform formats. Monitoring equipment in critical care unit assess an array of patients' physiological and hemodynamic conditions, such as temperature acquired through probes; blood pressure, acquired both from an **arterial catheter** and external pressure cuff; oxygen saturation of the blood acquired from **pulse oximetry**; heart rate and respiratory rate acquired from external transducers and the electrocardiogram waveform. Critically-ill patients may require additional **hemodynamic monitoring**, such as central venous pressure, right atrial pressure, pulmonary artery pressure, and cardiac output acquired through pulmonary artery catheter. Technological advancement in the monitoring system of critically-ill patients have led to monitors assessing patients' microcirculation, tissue oxygenation, intracranial pressure and respiratory system assessment of ventilated patients. Monitoring equipment in the critical care units come with a number of accessories, such as sensors, probes, transducers, electrical and non-electrical circuits. It is important to keep all these accessories in proper places and in cleaned condition.

❖ **Defibrillator:** A critically-ill patient can have life-threatening arrhythmias and sudden cardiac arrest. Defibrillators are devices that deliver electric current through the heart, thereby depolarizing the heart muscles and restoring normal rhythm of the heart. There are various types of defibrillators, such as external, transvenous, or implanted defibrillators depending on the site where the electric current is delivered. External paddle defibrillators are commonly seen in critical care units. Depending on the direction of current flow, a defibrillator may be biphasic or monophasic. Monophasic defibrillators have been used for a long time since the invention of this machine, however, due to various advantages, the biphasic defibrillators have become more popular. Biphasic machines require lesser energy to defibrillate and they normally do not produce skin burns that can happen with monophasic machines. The invention of defibrillator can be traced back to as early as 1899 and has gone through various technological changes to take its modern form. The defibrillator in the critical care unit should be put on a movable stand, and the battery charged adequately for delivering optimal shock. A bottle of conductive gel that is applied on the external paddles during defibrillation and which helps in decreasing electric resistance thereby preventing burn injury on patient's skin should always be kept near the defibrillator.

POLICIES AND PROTOCOLS OF CRITICAL CARE UNIT

A critical care unit is a place where health care providers are always busy and frequently face uncertain situations where they have to make difficult clinical decisions under time and resource constraints. Therefore it is important to have clear policies and protocols to guide them in these situations. Nurses working in a critical care unit should make themselves acquainted with the policies and protocols of the unit so that they can have standard clinical practice and understand the constraints of other members of the health care team. Every critical care units have certain policies pertaining to the following areas of care, such as:

❖ **Admission policy:** The admission policy of a critical care unit should be based on the belief that the patient should benefit from staying in the unit. Decision for admitting a patient should not be solely based on their medical diagnosis. The critical care unit admission policy can be based on various models, such as **priority model** or **objective parameter model**. However, every critical care unit should have their own admission policy based on the available resource and functioning. The priority model of admission policy classifies patients according to those who will have maximum benefit (priority 1) to those with least benefit from Critical care admission (Priority IV). In this, priority I patients are those with unstable physiological conditions who will require monitoring and intervention that cannot be provided outside the critical care unit. Example, is a patient requiring mechanical ventilation. Priority 2 patients are those who will require intensive monitoring and may require intervention. Example may be of a patient with COPD who has developed acute respiratory problem. Priority 3 are patients who are critically ill but have less likely-hood of recovery. A patient with metastatic malignancy with ARDS is an example of patient in priority 3. Patients with irreversible health condition facing imminent deaths are those under priority 4 and they benefit least from admission to critical care unit. However, numerous research study has shown that admission policy to CCU can be based on objective criteria, such as pulse rate <40 or >150 beats/minute; systolic pressure less by 20 mm Hg from patient's usual SBP; diastolic pressure >120 mm of Hg; mean arterial pressure <60 mm of Hg; and respiratory rate >35 breaths/minute. Similarly laboratory values of serum sodium <110 mEq/L or >170 mEq/L; serum potassium <2.0 mEq/L or >7.0 mEq/L; PaO_2 < 50 mm Hg; pH <7.1 or >7.7; serum glucose >800 mg/dL; serum calcium >15 mg/dL are considered for admission to CCU. In addition physical examination findings of unequal pupils in an unconscious patient; burns covering >10% of body surface area; anuria; airway obstruction; coma; cyanosis; continuous seizures; cardiac tamponade are also used as objective criteria for CCU admission. The admission policy of any CCU should take into consideration the model of admission that is most appropriate for them and make the admitting authority, i.e., physicians in outpatient department, in patient department and emergencies well aware of the policy and the criteria. A proper checklist should be used to receive the patients in ICU.

❖ **Patient management policy:** A critical care unit should have laid out policy regarding the daily management of patient care. It can be a closed management policy with the intensivist being solely responsible for the day-to-day care of patients including admission, discharge and clinical decisions. The management policy of a CCU may also be open type where the admission, discharge and care decisions are taken by the primary attending physician of each patient. In a shared management policy CCU, the attending physician and the intensivist jointly take decisions in combination with the intensivist responsible for the patient's ventilation, oxygenation and resuscitation only and the primary attending physician deciding on medications, antibiotics and discharge.

❖ **Discharge/transfer policy:** The discharge or transfer policy of a critical care unit should be based on the condition of the patient. A patient should be discharged to a lower level of care when the physiological condition of the patient is stable and he does not require constant monitoring. However, to have better resource utilization of critical care beds, patients whose physiological condition has deteriorated but no active interventions are planned may require to be shifted to a lower level of care. Discharge to home or to a lower level of care can lead to gap in communications and continuity of care. Therefore, the discharge policy of a critical care unit should mention the checklist that has to be followed by the healthcare providers while shifting the patient and handing over to a lower level of care or to home. Research studies have shown that the time and day of discharge from a critical care unit are factors that affected mortality and readmission of patients. Therefore, it is important that discharge policy of a critical care unit should stress on avoiding discharge and transfer out in odd hours, night time, weekends and holidays.

❖ **Infection control policy:** Critically-ill patients are vulnerable to infections because of multiple factors. These patients have lower immunity which is additionally compromised by multiple invasive interventions, such as intravenous lines, endotracheal tubes, arterial lines, etc. Moreover these patients are cared by multiple healthcare providers whose hands can be source of transmitting microorganisms. Therefore, a strict infection control policy should exist in a critical care unit with protocols for surveillance and management of healthcare-associated infections. Standard protocols regarding spacing between patients, hand hygiene practices of healthcare providers, assessment of patients at risk for infection, antibiogram surveillance of air, surface, floors of the unit, ventilation and cleaning of surfaces and equipment, movement and segregation of clean and dirty traffic, monitoring and maintaining records of patients' infections and laboratory data, surveillance of medical record of healthcare providers working in the critical care unit are all to be included in the policy.

❖ **Visiting policy in critical care unit:** Patients and their relatives experience high level of anxiety and stress while staying in the critical care units. The presence of relatives near the patients can ease their anxiety and provide emotional support. However, presence of visitors in the critical care unit can cause transmission of infections, interfere with patients' care schedule and intrude into the privacy of other patients. Therefore, a critical care unit should have laid out policy regarding the type of visitation that is permitted; whether unrestricted, partially restricted or restricted visiting policy. While making the visiting policy, the perspective and preferences of the healthcare members should be taken into consideration.

❖ **Communication policy:** Communication of the plan of management, expected course of treatment, positive and negative outcome expected of each intervention, anticipated expenses and any change in the condition of patient should be communicated to the relatives in a timely and periodic manner. Therefore a critical care unit should have clear policy indicating who, when, to whom and what to communicate.

QUALITY INDICATOR OF CRITICAL CARE

Providing care to critical care patients is complex and expensive. A number of errors could occur while working with the critically-ill patients. In addition both the healthcare system and the community expects and demands critical care to be absolutely safe and of the finest quality. This expectation is further escalated by the perpetual challenge of maintaining high quality and safe care in the face of resource constraints. Therefore, it is essential to have objective criteria and measures against which the critical care provided by a unit can be assessed. The quality indicators specific for critical care can be categorized under the following headings:

- Quality indicators related to patients' mortality, such as risk adjusted mortality of the critical care unit. **Risk adjusted mortality ratios** compare the observed mortality rate to the expected mortality rate of the unit. A risk adjusted mortality ratio below 1 (one) suggests good quality and safe care in the unit.
- Quality indicators related to patients' morbidity includes incidences of accidental extubation, procedure related pneumothorax, pressure ulcers, reintubation within 48 hours of extubation, readmission within 48 hours of discharge from critical care, unanticipated cardiac arrest, hypotension and acute renal failure.
- Quality indicators related to patient and staff safety, such as rate of patient fall, medication errors, deep vein thrombosis, nerve injury, dental injury and rate of needle stick injury.
- Quality indicators related to infection control includes rate of ventilator-associated pneumonia (VAP), rate of central line catheter associated blood stream infection (CA-BSI) rate, rate of urinary catheter related infection, etc.
- Quality indicators related to human resource, such as nurse: patient ratio, satisfaction level of healthcare workers in the unit, rate of staff turnover, hours of in-service training for staff.
- Quality indicators related to the care process, such as patients' length of stay in the critical care unit, compliance of healthcare providers to laid protocols, rate of readmission within 48 hours of discharge/transfer from critical care and rate of omission of mouth care, discharge teaching, communication before procedures, etc.

The quality indicators mentioned above can be used effectively in understanding and comparing the quality of critical care of a particular critical care unit. However, it is essential to understand that all these quality indicators can be calculated based on the data provided by the units. Therefore, it is important that the healthcare providers have clear understanding of these indicators, and maintain records of all the data required for the indicators. The staff of the unit should consider these quality indicators as means to improve their performance and should not be used by administrators for punitive purpose.

ETHICAL ISSUES FACED IN CRITICAL CARE NURSING

Nurses working in the critical care frequently face moral distress and ethical conflicts. The responsibility of caring for critically-ill patients in a safe manner, the high intensity work environment, and the use of highly advanced technology in a critical care unit frequently lead to situations where nurses experience moral and ethical distress. In a typical ethically distressing situation, there is always a better option available in front of a person and when it becomes impossible for the person to adopt the best option, the situation leads to moral distress. Some of the common situations in critical care where nurses face ethical dilemma are as follows:

- **Situations of missed care:** Research studies have revealed that while caring for multiple patients a nurse may miss certain aspects of care due to time constraints. The most frequently missed care aspects have been found to be related to mouth care, communication with patients and relatives, doing hand hygiene, etc. A nurse who is well aware of the consequences of missing these activities face ethical distress when the frequency of missing some aspects of care increases.
- **End of life decisions:** Advancement of medical technologies can prolong a person's life. However, technological support, such as a ventilator or parenteral nutrition can prolong life without any promise of recovery and lead to complex situations. These situations lead to loss of dignity for the patient, wasteful healthcare cost and may be against the choice of the patient himself. Therefore, the decision for end-of-life care has to be taken jointly by the patient, relatives, and the healthcare team. The critical care nurse who is in close contact with the patient often find breakdown in communication at this time as many patients are unable to speak, or the relatives are too distraught to discuss and make a proper judgment.
- **Procedures on recently dead patients:** Critical care units in teaching hospitals often have the practice of performing procedures, such as intubation, cannulation on recently deceased patients for educational purposes which is ethically controversial. A recently deceased patient provides a unique clinical opportunity to practice and learn medical procedures for the benefit of future patients in which there is literally no risk to the deceased patient. These situations can lead to ethical distress for nurses.
- **Presence of family members during resuscitation:** Traditionally, family members are not allowed to witness resuscitation attempts on a patient as they may get emotionally traumatized and may interfere with the resuscitation activities. However, research studies have challenged this perspective. The decision of allowing or not allowing the family members during the patient's resuscitation may lead to ethical distress for a critical care nurse.
- **Inadequate pain management:** Critically-ill patients often suffer from great deal of pain. The healthcare team in their singular focus of curing the disease often ignore the pain and suffering of the patient. More importance is given to diagnostic tests, therapeutic interventions and advanced medical technology and less importance to hear the patient's description of pain, prescribing and administering adequate analgesia. Nurses who are in continuous proximity to the patients find these situations morally distressing.

Ethical issues are significantly associated with job dissatisfaction and **burn-out** among nurses in the critical care, and consequently compromise the quality of nursing care. Therefore, it is important that ethical conflicts are recognized and resolved in order to have better quality of care. The ethical principles that can help individual nurses and the administrators to resolve ethical issues are justice, autonomy, beneficence and accountability. Research studies have shown that a good ethical climate in the units help nurses to experience better job satisfaction and render good quality of patient care.

POTENTIAL LEGAL ISSUES FACED IN CRITICAL CARE NURSING

Like any other professionals, a critical care nurse too has the potential for legal liabilities. Some of the potential situations in critical care unit that can lead to legal conflicts are:

- **Malpractice:** This refers to any act of negligence on the part of a professional with license to practice. When a nurse through a negligent act or act of omission causes physical, emotional or financial harm to a patient, malpractice occurs. Malpractice against a nurse can only be proved if it is found that the 4Ds of malpractice are present which are duty, dereliction, damage, and direct cause. For example, a nurse failed to update the surgeon on the change in a postoperative patient's blood pressure level. This was followed by patient requiring inotropic medication and finally the patient went into hypovolemic shock needing ventilation. In this case, it was the duty of the nurse taking care of the patient to update the surgeon about the patient's changing condition but she was derelict in her duty. This also led to physical harm to the patient and loss of time to take corrective measures. In order to avoid legal actions for malpractice, a critical care nurse should be aware of the standard of care in the unit and should always remember that an individual nurse is solely responsible for the activities considered as her duty.
- **Violation of patients' confidentiality:** Nurses working with critically-ill patients are obliged to maintain and respect the confidentiality of the patient's personal and medical history. When health and personal information are improperly disclosed it can harm a person's reputation, social and financial status. Research studies have revealed that patient's medical records are often carelessly kept in open places and disclosed to persons who are not directly involved with care. A nurse working in critical care should be careful of the medical records in her custody. For example, a situation where the nurse leaves the patient's medical folder on the nursing station unattended and open and one of the visitors go through it.
- **Violation of personal space:** While caring for a critically-ill patient a nurse may touch him or expose the person's body often without permission causing embarrassment, shame, discomfort, and nervousness. This is especially true when the patients are conscious and feel threatened to share space with another stranger, such as another patient or the presence of healthcare members in the room.
- **Assault and battery:** While working with critically-ill patients, a nurse may threaten a patient with a nasogastric tube when he refuses to eat. Even if the nurse in this instance has good intention, this can be considered as an assault as the nurses' behavior may be taken as a threat by the patient. Similarly restraining a patient to the bed and administering injection is an example of battery. These situations are potential for legal suits against nurses.
- **Obtaining informed consent from critically-ill patients:** An informed consent for any therapeutic or diagnostic procedures done for the patient is based on the human rights of autonomy and self-determination. Invasive procedures are common in a critical care unit and are often done under emergency condition. Obtaining informed consent from a critically-ill patients can be impossible at times because of altered sensorium, delirium, anxiety or pain. Taking consent from the next of kin is usually practised in most of these situations. The nurse working in the critical care unit should be aware of the standard protocols for informed consent followed in the unit.

BASIC AND ADVANCED CARDIAC LIFE SUPPORT

Introduction

When the brain does not get oxygen supply for 3–4 minutes due to **cardiac or respiratory arrest**, it leads to irreversible cerebral damage and death. Critically-ill patients are highly susceptible for having cardiac or respiratory arrest due to various factors, such as existing cardiovascular diseases, organ failures, use of multiple medications, hypoxemia and so on. Therefore, proficiency in cardiopulmonary resuscitation is considered a core skill for all nurses working in the critical care units.

The causes for cardiac and respiratory arrests are numerous. Cardiac arrest can be caused by almost any known heart conditions. For example, the scarred tissue of an infarcted heart, thickened tissue due to valvular heart diseases, certain medications, abnormalities in the electrical cycle of the heart and abnormalities in the blood vessels are few common causes of cardiac arrest. Similarly **respiratory arrest** is the absence of breathing which can result from respiratory distress caused by severe head injury, pneumonia, obstruction in the respiratory tract, or **asphyxia** due to drowning. Whatever may be the cause, a cardiopulmonary arrest is recognized by two features:

1. **Sudden loss of responsiveness:** The person does not move, speak, blink or respond even when he is tapped hard on his shoulder.
2. **Absence of normal breathing:** The person does not breathe normally or may gasp for breath.

The basic aim of cardiopulmonary resuscitation is to salvage the BRAIN and should have the following goals:
- Improve return of spontaneous circulation (ROSC) in short-term.
- Improve neurological outcome in the long term.

Cardiopulmonary resuscitation is very different in out of hospital cardiac arrest (OHCA) and in hospital cardiac arrest (IHCA). In OHCA, the care of the victim depends solely on the response of the community. It is critical for the community members who are mostly non-healthcare persons to recognize cardiac arrest, ring up emergency ambulance service and perform cardiopulmonary resuscitation (CPR). This process is also called **basic life support (BLS)**. Thus in a situation of OHCA, it is expected that the community members provide BLS following the given steps:

- **Recognition of arrest:** Tap the shoulder of the person hard, call his name, and look for breathing. If the person does not move, speak, blink or respond and there is either no breathing or he is gasping for breath then he is having a cardiac arrest.

- ❖ **Activate response:** The primary responder should immediately call for help. If another person responds he should be directed to activate the emergency response by dialing 102 (ambulance) or 112 (National emergency number) and if possible to get a defibrillator. If no one responds, the rescuer first activates the emergency response system and then begins basic life support.
- ❖ **Start CPR:** Chest compression should be immediately started by giving 30 chest compressions at a rate of 100-120/minute and then opening the airway (lifting the chin and tilting back the forehead) and giving 2 rescue breaths. The cycle of compressions and breaths should be continued without interruption. The technique of doing this is given in details below:
  - ➢ **Compression:** Push down at least two inches in the center of the chest at a rate of 100-120 pushes per minute. We need to push hard and push fast. Allow the chest to completely recoil and come back up to its normal position after each push. A complete recoil of the chest will help in adequate filling of the heart between compressions. Keeping the arms straight, shoulder positioned directly over the hands, fingers interlaced, the compressor should press with the heel of the hands. It is important to remember that the chest compressions should be uninterrupted (interruptions should not be more than 10 seconds). This is because uninterrupted compression will ensure uninterrupted oxygen delivery to the brain (oxygen content in the blood is adequate in the initial stage). Therefore, the compressor should be replaced by another person every 2 minutes. Moreover, if the rescuer is alone and not confident of giving rescue breaths to the victim, it is better to continue with uninterrupted chest compression **(Fig. 51.1)**.
  - ➢ **Maintain airway:** The victim's airway is to be kept open by appropriate positioning of the head and jaw. The **chin lift jaw thrust** method is commonly used and is done by placing the index and middle fingers to push the posterior aspects of the lower **jaw** upwards while their thumbs push down on the **chin** to open the mouth. As the mandible is displaced forward, it pulls the tongue forward and prevents it from obstructing the airway. The chin lift jaw thrust maneuver is done on a supine patient using both hands of the rescuer **(Fig. 51.2)**.
  - ➢ The other method of maintaining airway is the **head tilt chin lift maneuver (Fig. 51.3)** which is used only when cervical spine injury is ruled out for the victim. It is done by tilting the patient's head back by pushing down on the forehead with one hand and placing the tips of the index and middle fingers of the other hand under the chin and pulling up the mandible. This lifts the tongue away from the posterior pharynx and improves airway patency. In both, the maneuver pressure should be applied on the bony parts and not on the soft tissues of the neck which may obstruct the airways and be counterproductive. The airway can be cleaned of any obstruction by sweeping the fingers through the mouth.

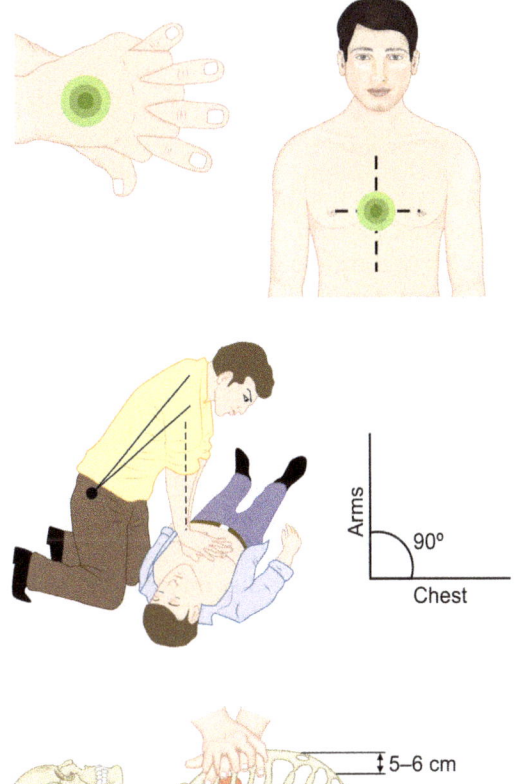

Fig. 51.1: Technique of chest compression.

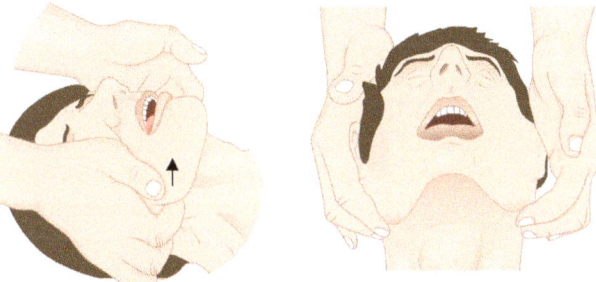

Fig. 51.2: Chin lift jaw thrust technique of opening airway.

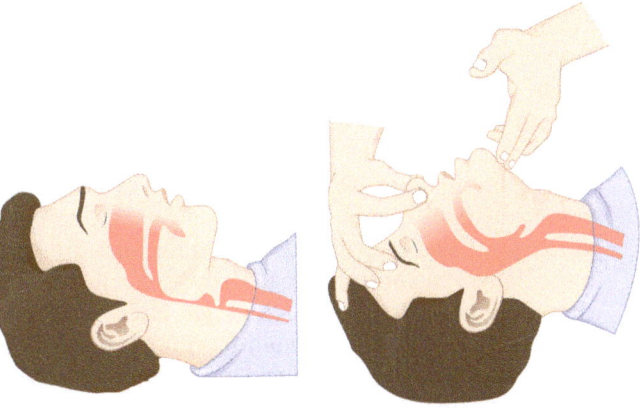

Fig. 51.3: Head tilt/chin lift technique of opening airway.

  - ➢ **Breathing:** It should be clearly understood that less than normal ventilation is adequate during CPR as the cardiac output during this time is only

25–33% of normal cardiac output and therefore a lower ventilation can be optimal. It should also be remembered that breathing is to be started only after initiating chest compressions. Breathing should be given at a rate of 8–10 breathes/minute with the chest of the victim visibly rising with the breath. It is essential to maintain ventilation in a way that cause minimum interruption to chest compression. The ratio of compression: breathing should be 30:2. The breathing can be given either mouth to mouth or given through a self-inflating bag (**AMBU**). If oxygen is available it can be connected to the self-inflating bag and given 10–12 liters/minute. Research studies have shown that **arterial hyperoxia** due to excessive oxygenation during resuscitation is independently associated with increased mortality.

- **Defibrillation:** This refers to electrical shock given to the heart to reset its electrical state. The abnormal rhythms that cause cardiac arrest and also respond to electric shock are **ventricular fibrillation** (VF) and pulseless **ventricular tachycardia**. The recommended energy dose for defibrillation using a biphasic defibrillator is 120 J to 200 J and for monophasic defibrillator is 360 J. It should be remembered that the defibrillator shock delivery should be done immediately after a chest compression and should be immediately followed by a chest compression. Therefore, the person doing compression and the person delivering the shock should have efficient coordination.

Advanced Life Support in Situations of IHCA and OHCA

Once the emergency medical personnel who have the necessary skill and equipment arrives at the scene, they can start with advanced life support which comprises of:

- **Maintenance of airway:** In BLS, the maintenance of airway was done by various maneuvers, such as the jaw thrust chin lift or head tilt chin lift methods depending on the patients' condition. In advanced life support, the airway is maintained by using **oropharyngeal airway** which blocks the epiglottis from covering the airway. An airway can only be used in an unconscious patient without having gag or cough reflexes. The length of the airway should be approximately the length between the patient's tip of nose to tip of earlobe. The oropharyngeal airway in inserted upside down with the tip of the airway facing the roof of the mouth. While inserting, it is gently rotated by 180° till the flange of the airway rests on the patient's lips. Oropharyngeal airways are also known as **Guedel** airway and it not only ensures airway patency but also helps in suctioning through the hole in the flange. **Nasopharyngeal airways** are also useful especially in patients with clenched jaws. However, nasopharyngeal airways are not used for patients with severe craniofacial injury to avoid inadvertent placement of the airway in the intracranial space. Advanced airway adjuncts include **endotracheal tubes** and **supraglottic airways**, such as **laryngeal mask airways (LMA)**. The role of endotracheal intubation during CPR has been studied extensively and research studies have not supported early tracheal intubation for adult in-hospital cardiac arrest.

- **Ventilatory support and oxygenation:** During CPR, bag mask ventilation can ensure oxygenation and ventilation for the patient. But **bag mask ventilation** has the potential to increase the intrathoracic pressure and reduce venous return to the heart. Research studies have concluded that passive oxygenation through face mask, keeping the airway patent have resulted in improved survival.

- **Medications:** The resuscitation team should remember **not to interrupt** chest compression and defibrillation for too long to establish an intravenous access (IV) for administering medications.

  - *Adrenaline:* The American Heart Association guidelines (AHA 2020) **(Table 51.1)** have recommended that the resuscitation team should give injection Adrenaline at 3–5 minutes intervals during the time of resuscitation. If the patient has non-shockable rhythms, such as **pulseless electrical activity (PEA)** or **asystole** then adrenaline can be immediately administered. For shockable rhythms, adrenaline can be administered after the initial attempts to defibrillate fails. The dose of adrenaline is 1 mg IV (intravenous) or IO (Intraosseous). Studies have shown that adrenaline helps in ROCS but has not shown to have any long-term benefit on neurological outcome.

  - *Antiarrhythmic drugs:* Amiodarone is an antiarrhythmic drug that is given intravenous for VF or pulseless VT which are unresponsive to defibrillation. The dose of Amiodarone is 300 mg IV/IO bolus and if the rhythm is not converted then repeat with 150 mg IV/IO bolus. Lignocaine is another antiarrhythmic drug commonly used during CPR for patients with VT/VF not responding to defibrillation. The dosage is 1 to 1.5 mg/kg intravenous initially and the second dose if required is 0.5–0.75 mg/kg.

When to stop CPR: CPR can be stopped in the following conditions:
1. Return of ROSC
2. No return of ROSC by 30 minutes

Post-cardiac Arrest Care of Patient

Once the patient has obtained ROSC, care and support of the patient should continue in the following line and according to his clinical condition:

- Establish intravenous access if not accessed earlier. A central venous access should be established as early as possible.
- Manage the airway with placement of endotracheal tube.
- Manage ventilation with 10 breaths/minute maintaining SpO$_2$ between 92–98%
- Manage hemodynamic parameters by administering crystalloids, and/or vasopressor or inotropes for maintaining systolic blood pressure >90 mm of Hg or Mean arterial pressure >65 mm of Hg.
- Obtain 12 lead ECG (electrocardiogram)

TABLE 51.1: Algorithm for adult cardiac arrest (based on AHA 2020 guidelines).

Recognition of arrest				
1 • Activate response • Start CPR (compression, rescue breaths/bag mask ventilation, maintaining airway) • Attach defibrillator				
Is heart rhythm shockable?				
2 **YES (VF/VT)**			**9** **NO (Asystole/PEA)** • Injection Adrenaline	
3 Defibrillate			**10** • CPR for 2 minutes • IV/IO access • Injection Adrenaline • Look for advanced airway	
4 • CPR for 2 minutes • Look for IV/IO access				
Is heart rhythm shockable?			**Is heart rhythm shockable?**	
YES **5** Defibrillate	**No** (Go to step 12)		**No** **11** • CPR for 2 minutes • Treat reversible cause	**Yes** (Go to 5, 6 or 7, 8)
6 • Continue CPR for 2 minutes • Injection Adrenaline • Look for advanced airway				
Is heart rhythm shockable?			Is heart rhythm shockable?	
Yes **7** Defibrillate	**No** (Go to step 12)		**No** **12** • No ROSC then go to step 10 or 11 • ROSC present then post-cardiac arrest care	**Yes** (Go to step 5, 6 or 7, 8)
8 • Continue CPR for 2 minutes • Antiarrhythmic				
Is rhythm shockable? • If yes follow the loop (step 5, 6, 7, 8) • If No go to step 12				

(IV: intravenous; IO: intra-osseous; VF: ventricular fibrillation; pVT: pulseless ventricular tachycardia)

Reversible causes: Hypovolemia, hypoxia, acidosis, hyperkalemia, hypothermia, tension pneumothorax, cardiac tamponade, toxins, pulmonary thrombosis, cardiac thrombosis.

❖ Obtain glycemic control by maintaining blood sugar between 144–180 mg% and monitoring at regular intervals.
❖ Evaluate and treat any causes that are reversible through expert consultation.
❖ Hyperthermia may compromise post-resuscitation neurologic outcome. However mild-to-moderate hypothermia may improve neurologic outcome and decrease mortality. Monitor the temperature regularly.

Case Scenario

1. A 60-year-old man is admitted in the cardiac critical care unit with complaints of chest pain. His family says that the man has history of high cholesterol and hypertension since last 5 years. As his primary care provider in the unit what are the things that the nurse needs to do initially upon receiving the patient at this time?
   Ans: First of all, it is important for the nurse to do an assessment of the patient and note whether the man is having chest pain at present and have him describe the nature of the pain. Another important assessment task for her is to perform a 12-lead electrocardiogram (ECG) to assess the heart rhythm and observe if there is abnormality in the ECG of the patient. Assessment of the patient will continue with measuring his heart rate, blood pressure and oxygen saturation. The nurse also requires to connect the man to oxygen to help oxygenation of the heart muscle. It is also important to contact the cardiologist at this point for further management.

2. A 48-year-old man who underwent bilateral total knee replacement is transferred from the surgical ward to the critical care unit after he complained of breathlessness on the day following surgery. On entering his cubicle, the nurse finds that the patient is looking anxious, sweating and is on oxygen via venture mask. On asking, the patient answered that he is feeling short of breath and weak. The nurse checked the vitals and checked his chart and observed that there is considerable decrease in BP, increase in HR and decrease in saturation. What should be the nurse's anticipation and action at this point of time?
   Ans: The nurse should stay beside the patient, and reassure him. At the same time keeping in mind the surgical history of the patient the nurse should anticipate that the patient may deteriorate further and faster and get the team alerted to the patient's change in condition.

SUMMARY

- **Critical care** implies to health care imparted to a person who is facing an actual or potentially life-threatening health condition. **Critical care nursing** is the specialty of clinical nursing that focus on caring for patients who are critically ill and are hemodynamically unstable.
- **Critical care units** are specialized areas in the hospitals where skilled personnel and sophisticated equipment are readily available to closely and continuously monitor patients, and impart rapid and intensive therapeutic and nursing interventions. Critical care units can be classified in various levels as per the services they provide. **Level 1 unit** provides monitoring, observation and short-term ventilation; **Level 2 unit** provides detailed observation, intervention, including support for a single failed organ system, short-term non-invasive ventilation and postoperative care; and **Level III unit** provides comprehensive critical care including complex multi-system life support for an indefinite period. A level 3 critical care unit should also have ongoing research and academic activities.
- Nurses working with critically-ill patients need to remember and follow certain basic principles while imparting care. These include principles of anticipation, holistic nursing care, collaboration, surveillance, and ethical care.
- A critical care unit should be located close and easily accessible from the emergency department, OT, trauma care, blood bank and the laboratory. The unit should be centrally air conditioned and have central supply of oxygen, compressed air and central facility of suctioning. The **physical layout** of a critical care unit can be divided in various spaces, such as **patient care area** (patient care units, nursing station area and work area); **clean utility area, storage area, administrative area, dirty utility area, and staff and visitors area**.
- The **staffing in critical care unit** consist of nursing and medical staff in addition to critical care technical personnel and ancillary and support staff.
- The critical care unit is equipped with various **equipment** for patient monitoring and treatment, such as **mechanical ventilators, infusion pumps**, and various **hemodynamic monitoring equipment.** One of the most important equipment in a critical care unit is the **defibrillator**.
- Healthcare providers working in a critical care unit often face uncertain situations where they make difficult clinical decisions under time and resource constraints. Therefore, it is important to have clear policies and protocols to guide them in these situations regarding patient admission, discharge, visitation, management and infection control policy.
- The quality indicators specific for critical care can be categorized under the headings, such as quality indicators related to patients' mortality and morbidity, patient and staff safety, infection control, human resource utilization and the care process.
- Nurses working in the critical care frequently face moral distress and ethical conflicts. Some of the common situations in critical care where nurses face ethical dilemma can be in situations of missed patient care, end of life decision, situations where a newly dead patient's body is used to teach or learn skills, decision of permitting family members during resuscitation and inadequate pain management.
- Like any other professionals, a critical care nurse too has the potential for legal liabilities. Some of the potential situations in critical care unit that can lead to legal conflicts are act of malpractice, assault, battery, violation of patient's confidentiality and personal space, and in situations where consent of a critically-ill patient is required for therapy or procedure.
- Critically-ill patients are highly susceptible for having cardiac or respiratory arrest due to various factors. It is important for the community members to know **basic life support (BLS)** skills when it is an out of hospital cardiac arrest (OHCA). The steps of BLS are: (i) **Recognition of arrest, (ii) Activate response, (iii) Start CPR with** chest compression (30 compressions at a rate of 100–120/minute); opening the airway (lifting the chin and tilting back the forehead) and giving two rescue breaths. The cycle of compressions and breaths should be continued without interruption.
- Once the emergency medical personnel who have the necessary skill and equipment arrives at the scene, they can start with **advanced life support** which comprises of **maintenance of airway, ventilatory support, oxygenation**, and appropriate **medications.** CPR can be stopped at the return of spontaneous circulation (ROSC) or no return of ROSC by 30 minutes. Once the patient has obtained ROSC, care and support of the patient should continue following the laid out protocol of **post-cardiac arrest care**.

MULTIPLE CHOICE QUESTIONS

1. A closed critical care unit means:
   a. No visitors are allowed to meet the patient
   b. Full responsibility of patient management lies with an intensivist
   c. Provides only monitoring and observation facilities
   d. Visitation policy is flexible

2. Head of the bed elevation among ventilated patients improves oxygenation and prevents respiratory complication. The correct angle for HOB is:
   a. Between 20–30°
   b. Between 30–45°
   c. Between 45–60°
   d. 90°

3. The management of pain is an important nursing action for the critical care nurse. When a nurse sees a critically-ill patient to exhibit signs of pain and anxiety, the first action of the nurse is to:
   a. Identify and treat underlying cause
   b. Administer pain medication as ordered
   c. Administer antianxiety medications
   d. Reassess the patient hourly to see whether symptoms resolve on their own.

4. A lady of 75 years who suffered CVA is on ventilatory support in CCU. The nurse wanted to place a feeding tube. However, the spouse and family said that the patient never wanted to be kept alive by tubes. So, the critical care team held a conference along with the family members and decided not to place the feeding tube. This is an example of:
   a. Withdrawal of life support
   b. Withholding life support
   c. Palliative care
   d. DNR

5. The critical care technician in-charge of the equipment of the unit was handling a machine when he noticed that the monitor of a patient is showing irregular and chaotic ECG rhythm. He called the nurse and said that it may be a ventricular tachycardia. What should be the nurse's first action?
   a. Rush the crash cart towards the patient
   b. Check the ECG
   c. Get the defibrillator ready
   d. Raise alarm for CPR

6. Presence of family members during resuscitation and invasive therapies is a debatable issue in a critical care unit. However, many critical care nurses feel numerous benefits of family presence during these times. Please select all that applies:
   a. Families feel that everything possible is done for their relative
   b. Family presence reduces nurses' work of explaining the situation
   c. Staff conversation during resuscitation/therapies is a distressing experience
   d. Family presence encourages litigation

7. The patient in the critical care unit is having ventricular fibrillation. The nurse must have knowledge of what type of defibrillator is available and how many joules to use for defibrillating the patient immediately. Select all that apply:
   a. 200 Joules (biphasic)
   b. 100 Joules (biphasic)
   c. 300 Joules (monophasic)
   d. 360 Joules (monophasic)
8. A patient admitted with head injury in the critical care unit is restless. The nurse restrains him to the bed for administering injection. This is an example of:
   a. Assault
   b. Battery
   c. Malpractice
   d. Negligence
9. CPR in the critical care can be stopped in the following conditions. Select all that apply:
   a. Return of spontaneous circulation
   b. Request from family members
   c. More than half an hour completed after the initiation of CPR
   d. Exhaustion felt by the initial resuscitator
10. A nurse knows that these are signs of ROSC, *except*:
    a. Movement
    b. Palpable pulse
    c. Measurable blood pressure
    d. Occasional gasps

ANSWERS

1. b	2. b	3. a	4. b
5. b	6. a	7. a, d	8. b
9. a, c	10. d		

SUGGESTED READING

1. AHA. Highlights of the 2020 American Heart Association Guidelines for Cpr and Ecc [Internet]. American Heart Association. 2020 [cited 2021 Mar 3]. Available from: https://cpr.heart.org/-/media/cpr-files/cpr-guidelines-files/highlights/hghlghts_2020_ecc_guidelines_english.pdf
2. Almenyan AA, Albuduh A, Al-abbas F. Effect of Nursing Workload in Intensive Care Units. 2021;13(1):1-5.
3. Bala R, Kaur S, Yaddanapudi LN. Exploratory study on nursing manpower required for critically ill patients in intensive care unit. NMRJ. 2010;6(2):71-80.
4. Bala R, Kaur S, Yaddanapudi LN. Nursing Competencies for Caring Critically Ill Patients in Intensive Care Unit. Journal of Nursing Science and Practice. 2013;3(1):10-16.
5. Capuzzo M, Moreno RP AR. Admission and discharge of critically ill patients. Curr Opin Crit Care. 2010;16(5):499-504.
6. Carvalho AS, Martins Pereira S, Jácomo A, Magalhães S, Araújo J, Hernández-Marrero P, et al. Ethical decision making in pain management: a conceptual framework. J Pain Res [Internet]. 2018;11:967-76. Available from: http://www.ncbi.nlm.nih.gov/pubmed/29844699
7. Catalano, Lori A. Werdman E. Avoiding legal risks in critical care nursing. Nurs Crit care. 2017;12(4):30-5.
8. Drews FA. Patient Monitors in Critical Care: Lessons for Improvement. In: Henriksen K, Battles JB, Keyes MA, et al (Eds). Advances in Patient Safety: New Directions and Alternative Approaches (Vol. 3: Performance and Tools). Rockville (MD): Agency for Healthcare Research and Quality (US); 2008 Aug. Available from: https://www.ncbi.nlm.nih.gov/books/NBK43684/
9. George J, Peter JV, Subramani K, Pichamuthu Kishore, Chacko Bimla. Essential of Critical Care. In Hospital Manual. Division of Critical Care, Christian Medical College; 2011.
10. Kaur M, Kaur S, Bhalla A. Knowledge regarding Cardio-Pulmonary Resuscitation among the Nursing Personnel Working in Emergency Department of a Tertiary Care Hospital. Journal of Nursing Science and Practice. 2012:2(2):37-41.
11. Kaur S, Singh A, Dhillon MS, Tewari MK, Sekhon PK. Incidence of bedsore among the admitted patients in a tertiary care hospital. PGMER. 2015;49(1):26-31.
12. Kaushal RK, Kapoor S, Kaur S, Bhagat H. A Methodological study to develop a 'Nursing Checklist' for receiving patients in ICUs. NMRJ. 2015;11(1):1-11.
13. Khaleghparast S, Joolaee S, Ghanbari B, Maleki M, Peyrovi H, Bahrani N. A Review of Visiting Policies in Intensive Care Units. 2016;8(6):267-76.
14. Krishnan N, Kaur S, Yaddanapudi LN. Role of protocol adherence and lack of protocol in the precipitation of nursing care errors amongst the patients admitted in the intensive care units of a tertiary care hospital. Journal of nursing Science and practice. 2014;4(3): 66-71.
15. Krishnan N, Kaur S, Yaddanapudi LN. Role of system based 'latent factors' in the precipitation of nursing errors amongst the patients admitted in intensive care unit of a tertiary care hospital. NMRJ. 2010;6(4):163-171.
16. Lim SH, Wee FC, Chee TS. Basic Cardiac Life Support: 2016; Singapore Guidelines. Singapore Med J [Internet]. 2017;58(7):347-53. Available from: http://www.ncbi.nlm.nih.gov/pubmed/28740995
17. Marshall JC, Bosco L, Adhikari NK, Connolly B, Diaz J V, Dorman T, et al. What is an intensive care unit? A report of the task force of the World Federation of Societies of Intensive and Critical Care Medicine. J Crit Care [Internet]. 2017;37:270-6. Available from: http://www.ncbi.nlm.nih.gov/pubmed/27612678
18. McAndrew NS, Leske J SK. Moral distress in critical care nursing: The state of the science. Nurs Ethics. 25(5):552-70.
19. Rao S. Designing Hospital for better Infection Control: an Experience. Med journal, Armed Forces India [Internet]. 2004;60(1):63-6. Available from: http://www.ncbi.nlm.nih.gov/pubmed/27407581
20. Ray B, Samaddar DP, Todi SK, Ramakrishnan N, John G RS. Quality indicators for ICU: ISCCM guidelines for ICUs in India. Indian J Crit Care Med. 2009;13(4):173-206.
21. Review AN. Ethical Issues Surrounding End-of-Life Care. 2016; 2-7.
22. Rungta N, Zirpe KG, Dixit SB, Mehta Y, Chaudhry D, Deepak Govil D, et al. Indian society of Critical care Medicine experts committee consensus on ICU planning and Designing. Indian J Crit Care Med. 2020;24.
23. Saini R, Kaur S, Das K. Stress, Stress Reactions, Job Stressors and Coping among Nurses Working in Intensive Care Units and General Wards of a Tertiary Care Hospital: A Comparative Study. J Postgrad Med Edu Res. 2016;50(1):9-17.
24. Saini R, Kaur S, Das K. Stress and Burnout among Intensive Care Nurses. Journal of Mental Health and Human Behaviour. 2011;16(1):43-48.
25. Sayed A, Noor M, Al-harthy AM, Aletreby WT. Evaluation of Performance in Intensive Care Unit: Descriptive Study. 2020;10: 35-42.
26. Sharma D, Shruti, Kaur S, Yaddanapudi LN. Problems faced by caregivers of ICU patients and suggestions: A qualitative perspective. NMRJ. 2020;16(4):181-92. http://doi.org/10.33698/NRF0326
27. Society of Critical Care Medicine. Guidelines for intensive care unit admission, discharge, and triage. Task Force of the American College of Critical Care Medicine. Crit Care Med. 1999;27(3):633-8.
28. Suhonen R, Scott PA. Missed care: A need for careful ethical discussion. 2018;25(5):549-51.
29. Wallace DJ, Kahn JM. Florence Nightingale and the Conundrum of Counting ICU Beds. Crit Care Med [Internet]. 2015;43(11):25, 17-8. Available from: http://www.ncbi.nlm.nih.gov/pubmed/26468709

CHAPTER 52

Management of Patients in Critical Care Units

Shivani Kalra, Jyoti Sharma

"It is not how much you do, but how much love you put in while doing."

—Mother Teresa

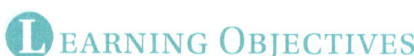 LEARNING OBJECTIVES

After going through the chapter, the learner will be able to:
- Define critical care unit and critically ill patients.
- Describe nursing assessment, monitoring, and management of critically ill patients.
- Elaborate infection control measures including care bundles such as VAP, CAUTI and CLABSI.
- Outline the drugs used in the critical care unit along with their actions, contraindications, side effects, and nursing responsibilities.
- Communicate with patients and family in ICUs.
- Appreciate the importance of maintaining intensive care records.
- Discuss the geriatric considerations related to patients admitted in critical care units.

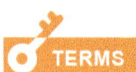

- **Critical care nursing:** It is a specialized field of nursing that focuses on the care of critically ill patients who require comprehensive care and constant monitoring.
- **Critical care unit (CCU) or intensive care unit (ICU):** It is a specialized area of a hospital staffed by highly trained medical professionals and caters to critically ill patients with the use of specialized equipment or devices.
- **Critically ill patient:** The patient with any life-threatening illness who requires continuous monitoring, care, and life support with the use of specialized equipments or devices.
- **End-of-life care:** It refers to care for a person with a disease condition which is progressive, advanced and/or incurable.
- **Hospital acquired infections (HAI):** The infections which are not present or might be incubating at the time of admission and are usually acquired after hospitalization and evident after 48 hours of admission to hospital.
- **Intensive care records:** These are the patient's records, registers and reports that provide information about the patient's condition and also provide data for care studies. Records help medical and nursing students during their clinical experience for case studies.

INTRODUCTION

A critical illness acutely impairs one or more vital organ systems which leads to life-threatening worsening of patient's condition. Critical care nursing focuses on the care of patients who are hemodynamically unstable, require continuous monitoring and advanced care. Critical care nurses have a scope to work in various departments or specialties such as general intensive care units, trauma care units, coronary care units, medical intensive care units, surgical intensive care units, pediatric intensive care units, and neonatal intensive care units. The patients in these units are classified according to the pattern and severity of dysfunction of primarily six organ systems such as cardiovascular, respiratory, neurologic, hematologic, renal, and hepatic. The management and outcome of the patient depend on the severity of organ dysfunction.

NURSING ASSESSMENT OF CRITICALLY ILL PATIENTS

The critically ill patient is a challenge for the ICU team as they require invasive diagnostic tests, advanced procedures, and intensive nursing care. It is always imperative to start with an assessment of the patient to develop a care plan tailored for the individual according to the priorities and concerns. While caring for ICU patients, the assessment and management go hand-in-hand to save time and hence prevent complications or deterioration of patient's condition i.e., *when you identify any life threat during the assessment, begin treatment immediately.* Thus, the two main goals of assessment are: Identifying the life threats and providing immediate treatment.

The assessment includes two steps:
1. **Primary survey/initial assessment:** Evaluates physiology
2. **Secondary survey:** Evaluates anatomy

Primary Survey/Initial Assessment of Critically-ill Patients

The acronym ABCDE is used for quick assessment of the patients **(Table 52.1)**:
- **A:** Airway
- **B:** Breathing
- **C:** Circulation
- **D:** Disability
- **E:** Exposure (environmental)

TABLE 52.1: ABCDE approach of ICU assessment.

Primary survey	Assessment	Signs/symptoms	Management
Airway*	• **Observe the patient for signs and symptoms of airway obstruction:** Such as paradoxical movement of chest and abdominal.** • Is the patient able to talk? Yes? – Inspect for any foreign body – Examine for stridor, hoarseness, gurgling, pooled saliva or blood (indicate partially obstructed airway) – Look for signs of edema, blood vomitus • **Unconsciousness? GCS <8:** Intubate the patient • **Not able to speak:** Probable airway injury	• Breathing difficulty • Bradycardia • Decrease oxygen saturation • Cyanosis • Unconsciousness	• **Opening/maintenance of airway patency:** – The suction of secretions or removal of visible foreign – Chin lift/jaw thrust – Nasopharyngeal or oropharyngeal airway • **Consider definitive airway:** – Endotracheal intubation – Surgical cricothyroidotomy – Tracheostomy • Move the patient in lateral position (secure cervical spine in case of suspected injury)
Breathing	• To detect signs of respiratory distress or inadequate ventilation • Look for bilateral chest movements, tracheal deviation, accessory muscle use, retractions • Check respiratory rate • Diminished or absent breath sounds? • Check spO$_2$ with a pulse oximeter • Auscultate breath sounds for wheezing, crackles, rhonchi, etc. • Observe for S/S of cyanosis: Increasing oxygen requirement • Identify any life-threatening injuries such as rib fractures, massive hemothorax, etc.	• Shortness of breath • Cyanosis • Unconsciousness • Decreased spO$_2$	• Administer 100% or high concentration oxygen and then titrate to maintain spO$_2$ ≥94% • Breathing can be provided by: – Bag-valve mask – Non-rebreather mask • Intubate if the patient is not able to maintain saturation with venturi or NIV. • Obtain Chest X-ray, ECG and ABG once the patient is stabilized. • Tube thoracostomy in case of hemothorax and needle decompression in tension pneumothorax can be performed • Treat appropriately: Oxygen/adrenaline/salbutamol/frusemide/hydrocortisone • The emergent treatment is based on underlying injury
Circulation	• To determine the effectiveness of the cardiac output • Rapid assessment of hemodynamic status • **Look:** Mental status, LOC, skin color • **Feel:** Peripheral pulses • **Check:** BP, HR, urine output and temp	• Tachycardia (HR >100) • Hypotension (SBP <120) • Signs of impaired tissue perfusion • Pale skin color • Cool clammy skin • Delayed capillary refill (>3 sec) • Altered loss of consciousness • Dec. urine output <30 mL/hour • Altered mental status	• Control external hemorrhage • Ensure adequate IV access • IV fluids/blood transfusions • Placement of a Foley catheter to monitor urine output • Placement of a nasogastric tube (to prevent aspiration) • ECG to be taken **Goals** • MAP ≥65 mm Hg • Heart rate should be 60–100 b/m and urine output of 30 mL/h • Prevent hypothermia

Contd...

Primary survey	Assessment	Signs/ symptoms	Management

Disability/ neurologic status	• Level of consciousness (GCS or AVPU)
	• Pupillary size and reactivity
	• Gross neurological examination
	   – Extremity movement
	   – Sensation
	• Check blood glucose level
	• Check external signs of head/neck trauma
		Altered level of consciousness	• Recheck ABC
			• Check for reversible medicine-induced altered level of consciousness

Exposure/ examine	• Remove all clothing's/coverings • Complete head-to-toe examination • Examine axillae and perineum		• Roll to examine back (maintain cervical immobilization) • Avoid hypothermia (hypothermia can cause coagulopathy and increases the risk of hemorrhage)

*Airway and breathing are usually assessed and managed together.
**A state where the chest and abdomen rise and fall vigorously to attempt to remove the obstruction.

Secondary Survey

The secondary survey is started after the completion of the primary survey and when a patient has been adequately resuscitated. It consists of:
- History
- Thorough head-to-toe examination
- Re-evaluation of ABCDE and vital signs
- Diagnostic tests

History

A clinical history includes thorough examination and diagnostic tests. The nurse should collect the complete information from the patient's family or the emergency department nurses while taking charge of a patient in the ICU. The completeness of the history can be summarized using the pneumonic "SAMPLE".
- **S:** Signs and symptoms
- **A:** Allergies
- **M:** Medications
- **P:** Past medical history, pregnancy
- **L:** Last meal taken
- **E:** Events leading to present illness

Head-to-toe Examination

Thorough head-to-examination is required in all patients after primary survey to predict any associated injuries such as deformities, hematomas, discoloration, etc. It includes the examination of:
- Head and skull
- Faciomaxillary injuries
- Neck, chest and spine
- Abdomen
- Perineum/rectum/vagina
- Extremities

Re-evaluation of ABCDE and Vital Signs

Frequent re-evaluation and continuous monitoring are required to find any overlooked findings.

Diagnostic Tests

Various blood tests and radiological evaluations include CBC, serum electrolytes, blood glucose, urea, creatinine, LFT, RFT, toxicology screening, ABG, ABO grouping, and cross-matching, CT scan, X-ray, and MRI.

MONITORING OF CRITICALLY ILL PATIENTS

The goal of continuously monitoring the patient in ICU is to detect problems and manage them as early as possible. This confirms the safety and enhances the quality of care delivered to the patient in the ICU. The enhanced monitoring is done in ICUs with the purpose to measure "real-time" physiologic values that can change rapidly **(Table 52.2)**. After analysis and interpretation of values, certain interventions such as changes in treatment or ventilator settings, etc., can be made on time to prevent serious events.

TABLE 52.2: Monitoring of patient in ICU.

Sr. No.	Types	Monitoring
1.	Vital signs	• Temperature • Blood pressure • Pulse • Respiratory rate • SpO_2
2.	Respiratory	• Gas Exchange: ABG: pH, paO_2, $paCO_2$, HCO_3, estimated base excess or deficit • Oxygenation: paO_2, PaO_2/FiO_2 ratio • Ventilation: $paCO_2$, capnography, capnometry
3.	Cardiovascular	• ECG • Arterial BP monitoring • Central venous pressure • Pulmonary artery pressure
4.	Neurologic	• History • Neurologic examination • Glasgow coma scale • Intracranial pressure monitoring
5.	Renal Function	• Urine output • Urine specific gravity • RFT • Creatinine clearance
6.	Liver Function	• LFT • Hepatic enzymes
7.	Nutritional	• Assessment of nutritional status • Estimating nutritional requirements

Various equipments, instruments, and monitors are used in ICU for monitoring the patients. The monitors can be either placed at the bedside of the patient or can be brought to the bedside (portable equipment). In all of these monitors, alarms are set to detect values that require attention.

Hemodynamic Monitoring

Hemodynamic monitoring is done in ICUs for the assessment of the cardiorespiratory system to assure the adequacy of tissue perfusion. All the patients admitted in ICU require standard basic monitoring **(Table 52.2)** and the patients who are unstable or at risk of instability need a proper assessment of cardiorespiratory function such as central venous pressure, continuous arterial pressure monitoring, and pulmonary artery pressure monitoring **(Table 52.3)**. The patient can be monitored continuously or intermittently using invasive and non-invasive methods of monitoring.

- ❖ **Non-invasive monitoring:**
  - ➢ BP monitoring (using manual BP cuff)
  - ➢ Heart rate
  - ➢ Temperature
  - ➢ Respiratory rate
  - ➢ Pulse oximetry
  - ➢ Urine output
  - ➢ Capnography
  - ➢ Jugular venous pressure
- ❖ **Invasive monitoring:** Classical hemodynamic monitoring is done with the invasive method by inserting arterial, central, or pulmonary catheter for continuous, and accurate monitoring of patient's parameters. Arterial and central line catheters are most commonly used while pulmonary catheters are rarely used in ICUs.
  - ➢ Central venous pressure (CVP)
  - ➢ Mean arterial pressure (MAP)
  - ➢ Pulmonary artery (PA) pressure
  - ➢ Pulmonary capillary wedge pressure (PCWP)
  - ➢ Left arterial pressure

Important Points in Hemodynamic Monitoring

1. Maintaining strict asepsis while caring for the ports.
2. Flush the lines properly to prevent clotting and backflow of blood.
3. Always maintain the closed system to prevent air from going inside the catheter.
4. Zeroing and calibration of equipment every 4–12 hours should be performed to ensure the accuracy of the waveform.
5. The placement of the transducer should be adjusted according to the patient's position keeping in mind the Phlebostatic axis. It is the reference point for zeroing the hemodynamic monitoring device/transducer **(Fig. 52.1)**.

TABLE 52.3: Parameters of hemodynamic monitoring.

Sr. No.	Parameters	Type of catheter used	Normal value	Use in clinical practice
1.	**Mean arterial pressure (MAP)** [Average blood pressure in arteries during a complete cardiac cycle]	Arterial line	70–110 mm Hg	• **MAP >60 mm Hg:** Tissue perfusion is adequate. • **MAP <60 mm Hg:** Indicates impaired tissue perfusion.
2.	**Central venous pressure (CVP)** [Blood pressure in the right atrium of the heart that reflects the circulatory fluid volume and also tells the ability of the heart to pump the blood back into the arterial system]	Central venous catheter (CVC)	2–5 mm Hg or 3–8 cm H_2O	• **CVP>12:** Circulatory (volume) Overload • **CVP<5:** Hypovolemia
3.	**Pulmonary artery (PA) pressure** [Pressure of blood inside the pulmonary arteries]	Swan-Ganz catheter (pulmonary artery catheter)	**Systolic:** 15–30 mm Hg **Diastolic:** 5–12 mm Hg **Mean:** 10–20 mm Hg	• **PA ≥25:** Indicates hypervolemia, pulmonary hypertension, mitral valve dysfunction, tamponade • **PA 21–24:** Abnormal requiring further investigations • **PA <10:** Hypovolemia, excessive vasodilation
4.	**Pulmonary capillary wedge pressure (PCWP)** [Pressure in the left atrium measured by occluding the pulmonary arteriole with an inflated balloon-tipped catheter]	Swan-Ganz catheter	2–14 mm Hg (Mean)	It is used to diagnose the severity of left ventricular failure and mitral stenosis: • **PCWP >14:** Indicates left heart failure with resultant pulmonary congestion, acute mitral insufficiency • **PCWP <2:** Hypovolemia, vasodilation
5.	**Left arterial (LA) pressure** [Pressure created by blood in left atrium when the mitral valve open]	Swan-Ganz catheter	6–12 mm Hg	
6.	**Cardiac output (CO)** The total amount of blood pumped by the heart every minute. It can be calculated by a formula: CO = HR × SV	Doppler echocardiography, Fick's technique	4–6 L/min	• **CO <4 or heart failure:** Transient decrease in systemic perfusion • **CO >6 or high output heart failure:** Due to increased peripheral demands such as anemia, sepsis, etc.

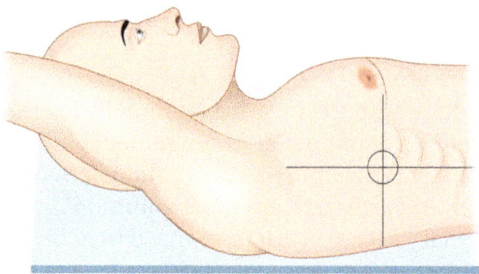

Phlebostatic axis

Fig. 52.1: Phlebostatic axis: It is the anatomical landmark obtained by drawing an imaginary vertical line from the 4th intercostal space at the sternum and finding its intersection with an imaginary horizontal line drawn down the center of the chest below the axillae with patient in supine position.

MANAGEMENT OF CRITICALLY ILL PATIENTS

The critically ill patient requires immediate attention to prevent complications and mortality. The main goal of the management is to identify the problem during assessment and taking quick measures to save a life. Continuous monitoring of vital signs is required, and resuscitation should be initiated using the stepwise approach i.e., airway, breathing, circulation, disability, and exposure (ABCDE) **(Table 52.1)**.

Pain Management in Critically Ill

The International Association for the Study of Pain (IASP) definition of pain is "an unpleasant sensory and emotional experience associated with actual or potential tissue damage or described in terms of such damage". Acute pain is a common problem among patients admitted to ICUs. Most of the patients in ICU are unable to communicate and experience pain due to countless reasons such as mechanical ventilation, sedation, unconsciousness, pulmonary and cardiac dysfunction and hence are at greater risk of inadequate management of pain. Every patient in ICU has the right to be managed for pain regardless of their diagnosis and type of pain (Jarzyna et al., 2011). Pain has multiple negative effects such as delays in healing or recovery, increases the length of stay in ICU, and causes emotional changes in the patient. Pain is multi-dimensional and highly subjective making its assessment challenging at times. Therefore, a compressive pain assessment must be done to keep some points in mind.

Assessment and Management of Pain

Nurses play a central role in the assessment and management of pain. The mnemonic used to assess pain by ICU nurses is *"OLDCART"* **(Table 52.4)**. Patients' self-report about their pain is the most accurate method of assessing the severity of pain.

Various tools are also available to assess the severity of pain in patients such as:

- ❖ Numeric pain rating scale (NRS)
- ❖ Wong-Baker faces a pain rating scale

⎱ Used in sedated patients who are not able to respond

- ❖ Critical care pain observation tool (CPOT)
- ❖ Behavioral pain scale (BPS)

⎱ Used in case of conscious patients who can respond

TABLE 52.4: Pain assessment (OLDCART).		
O	Onset of pain
L	Location of pain
D	Duration of pain
C	Characteristics of pain (burning, stingy, or radiating)
A	Aggravating factors or triggers
R	Relieving factors
T	Treatment that has been tried to reduce pain

There are a majority of factors present that can alter the response of a patient to pain such as anxiety, delirium, sleep deprivation, etc. Light sedation can also be used in conjunction with pain control to reduce anxiety, augmentation of cooperation from the patient, lessening the voluntary motor activity in case of mechanical ventilation. However, in some patients deeper levels of sedation may be required while on mechanical ventilation such as patients with encephalopathy, head injury, etc. Continuous sedation is better as compared to bolus sedation but it prolongs the duration of ventilation and length of stay in the ICU.

Opioids are the most common type of analgesics used in the ICUs as it is a mild sedative and anxiolytic and can be administered through multiple routes. The most commonly used opioids in ICUs are morphine, fentanyl, hydromorphone, and methadone. Patients must be evaluated every hour to consider weaning off opioids as the risk of withdrawal is high with the extended use of opioids.

Nutrition in Critically Ill Patients

Patients in ICU often suffer from critical illness and require adequate nutritional support to meet increased energy requirements. Within few days of admission, the protein breakdown may reach 12–16 g of nitrogen/day and may increase up to 30 g of nitrogen/day in some patients leading to considerable loss of muscle mass.

Indirect calorimetry is a reliable method for assessing appropriate caloric and protein intake in ICUs. The guidelines must focus on the importance of nutritional assessment, detection of malnourished patients, and timely intervention for venerable patients.

Malnutrition is observed in 20–60% of hospitalized patients and is associated with increased morbidity, mortality, and healthcare costs (Correia MI et al., 2003). Most of the patients with a high risk of malnutrition remain undetected during hospitalization due to the lack of standardized nutritional screening tools. The NRS-2002 **(Table 52.5)** is the most commonly used tool in ICUs nowadays and is recommended by the European Society of Clinical Nutrition and Metabolism (ESPEN) as it combines both a measure of current potential undernutrition and a measure of disease severity (Velasco C et al., 2011).

Current guidelines recommend starting enteral feeding early in the course of ICU stay so that caloric energy targets should be reached within 3 days. If caloric goals cannot be reached through enteral feeding, parenteral nutrition can be initiated. Special care should be given to electrolyte status as it may endanger the patient and should be corrected promptly.

TABLE 52.5: Nutritional risk screening (NRS 2002).

Initial screening: 4 criteria
- BMI <20.5 kg/m²
- Weight loss within the last 3 months
- Reduced dietary intake in the last week
- Is the patient severely ill (ICU)?

If no parameter from the above is present, the patient is considered having low risk of malnutrition but if at least one of the above is present, the final screening is applied.

Final screening

Impaired nutritional status			Severity of disease		
Absent	Score 0	Normal nutritional status	Absent	Score 0	Normal nutritional requirements
Mild	Score 1	Weight loss >5% in 3 months or food intake below 50–75% of normal requirement in the preceding week	Mild	Score 1	Hip fracture, chronic patients with acute complications such as cirrhosis, COPD, on hemodialysis, diabetes, etc.
Moderate	Score 2	Weight loss >5% in 2 months or BMI 18.5–20.5 with impaired general condition. Food intake below 25–60% of normal requirement in the preceding week	Moderate	Score 2	Major abdominal surgery, stroke, severe pneumonia, hematological malignancy
Severe	Score 3	Weight loss >5% in 1 month or BMI <18.5 with impaired general condition. Food intake below 0–25% of normal requirement in the preceding week	Severe	Score 3	Head Injury, bone marrow transplantation, Intensive care patients (APACHE >10)
Score	+		Score	=	Total Score

If age is >70 years: Add 1 score to the total score above

Scores for the final screening range from 0 to 7, where the higher the score, the more severe the risk of malnutrition.
Score ≥3: Patient is nutritionally at risk and nutritional care plan should be initiated
Score <3: Weekly rescreening of the patient

Recommended protein intake is 1.3 g/kg/day, although it is dependent on the patient's clinical status. Early nutritional support as per the condition of the patient can improve the metabolic condition, decrease morbidity, and optimize long-term rehabilitation success.

Nursing Diagnosis of Critically Ill Patients (Table 52.6)

- Ineffective airway clearance related to excessive secretions as manifested by increased respiratory rate, crackles heard on auscultation, increased peak pressure in ventilated patients.
- Impaired gas exchange related to altered alveolar-capillary exchange as manifested by hypoxemia, restlessness, cyanosis, hypercapnia.
- Impaired cerebral tissue perfusion related to hemorrhage, interruption of cerebral blood flow, infection, or edema as manifested by changes in consciousness, tachypnea, dyspnea, respiratory rate, and size of the pupil.
- Acute pain related to tissue injury, mechanical ventilation, or cardiac dysfunction as manifested by moaning, grimaces, restlessness, profuse sweating, alterations in BP, HR, and RR.
- Decreased cardiac output related to alteration in heart rate, rhythm, conduction, and impaired contractility as manifested by hypotension, dyspnea, decreased activity tolerance, and dysrhythmias.
- Risk of nosocomial infection related to the presence of invasive lines as manifested by leucocyte count, fever, purulent sputum, cloudy urine, positive cultures.
- Impaired verbal communication related to the presence of alternative airway.
- Risk of fall-related to changes in the level of consciousness and mental status.
- Self-care deficit related to unconsciousness and critical situation.
- Disturbed sensory perception related to sedation and noisy environment of ICU

COMMON INFECTIONS IN CRITICAL CARE UNITS

The prevalence of nosocomial infection/hospital-acquired infection (HAI) is higher in the ICUs as compared to other areas of the hospital. According to WHO, a hospital-acquired infection is an infection acquired by a patient after 48 hours of hospital admission or 3 days of discharge or 30 days of surgery and was not present or incubating at admission. It also includes occupational infections among staff. According to the CDC, 1 in every 25 acute care hospital patients obtains at least one HAI during their inpatient stay. The burden of HAI accounts for 7% in developed and 10% in developing countries. The rate of HAIs varies between 4.36–83.09% in India.

Out of all HAIs, ventilator-associated pneumonia (VAP) is the most common HAI reported followed by central line-associated bloodstream infections (CLABSI), catheter-associated urinary catheter infections (CAUTI), and wound infections **(Table 52.8)**. The most common organisms isolated for HAI are *Acinetobacter baumanii, Pseudomonas aeruginosa, Staphylococcus hemolyticus, E. coli, Klebsiella pneumoniae*, and *Enterobacter cloacae*. HAIs are the major cause of death and increased morbidity among hospitalized patients. Among the patients developing nosocomial infection, the duration of mechanical ventilation, urinary catheterization,

TABLE 52.6: Nursing diagnosis and interventions for a critically ill patient in ICU.

Sl. No.	Nursing assessment	Nursing diagnosis	Nursing interventions	Rationale
1.	**Assess:** • Abnormal breath sounds (crackles, rhonchi, wheezes) • Abnormal respiratory rate, rhythm, and depth • Dyspnea • Excessive secretions • Hypoxemia/cyanosis • Not able to remove airway secretions. • Ineffective or absent cough • Orthopnea	Ineffective airway clearance related to excessive secretions as manifested by increased respiratory rate, crackles heard on auscultation, increased peak pressure in patients on ventilator.	• Provide humidified supplemental oxygen as prescribed. • Tracheal suctioning can be performed. • Consider the need for intubation if secretions cannot be cleared. • Give medications as prescribed such as bronchodilators, antibiotics, mucolytic agents, expectorants, etc.	• Oxygen therapy is recommended to improve spO_2. Humidified air will reduce the thickness of secretions. • Suctioning is required when the patient is unable to cough out secretions properly due to thick mucous plugs, or excessive or tenacious secretions. • Intubation will facilitate the removal of thick and copious secretions and augment oxygenation. • To clear secretions from airways and reduce airway resistance medicines need to be given.
2.	**Assess:** • Respiratory rate, effort, use of accessory muscles. • For the presence of adventitious sounds. • Behavior and mental status such as restlessness, agitation, confusion, etc. • Alteration in BP and HR. • Cyanosis in skin and nails, the color of the tongue, and oral mucous membranes. • Oxygen saturation. • Whether the patient is able to cough out secretions. Take note of the quantity, color, and consistency of the sputum. • Headaches, dizziness, lethargy, response, disorientation, and coma.	Impaired gas exchange related to altered alveolar-capillary exchange as manifested by hypoxemia, restlessness, cyanosis, hypercapnia.	• Position patient with head of the bed elevated (30–45°) as tolerated. • In the case of an obese patient, a reverse Trendelenburg position at 45° can be considered for periods. • Provide humidified supplemental oxygen as prescribed. • Suction out secretions when needed. • Administer prescribed medications. • Monitor the effect of sedation and analgesics on the respiratory pattern of a patient; try sedation vacation daily. • Intubate the patient if needed.	• Upright position allows increased thoracic capacity and increased expansion of lungs preventing aspiration. • Trendelenburg's position helps in increasing tidal volume. • Supplemental oxygen may be required to maintain PaO_2 at an acceptable level (≥90%) • Airway obstruction due to the presence of secretions may block ventilation that impairs gas exchange. • Sedation and analgesics can depress respiration. Continuous use may lead to addiction and late weaning from the ventilator. • Early intubation and mechanical ventilation are recommended to maintain adequate oxygenation and ventilation.
3.	**Assess:** • Signs of decreased tissue perfusion such as pallor, cyanosis, mottling, cool or clammy skin, dec. BP, dec. Urine output, Lactate levels, $ScvO_2$, etc. • Probable contributing factors related to impaired flow of blood. • Respiration pattern or absence of breathing. • Rapid changes in awareness and mental status.	Impaired cerebral tissue perfusion related to hemorrhage, interruption of cerebral blood flow, infection, or edema as manifested by changes in consciousness, tachypnoea, dyspnea, respiratory rate, and pupil size.	• Check the vital signs of the patients. • Record orthostatic changes by recording BP in all positions. • Administer IV fluids as prescribed. • Note urine output to maintain optimal fluid balance. • Maintain oxygen therapy as ordered. • Perform neurological examination. • Avoid measures that may increase ICP such as coughing, vomiting, straining at stool, neck in flexion, supine position, etc. • Maintain patients and environmental temperature. • Position patient in semi-Fowler's to high-Fowler's. • Administer medications as prescribed	• To check the patient's status of tissue perfusion. • Orthostatic hypotension results in decreased cerebral perfusion. • Fluid will maintain adequate filling pressures and improves cardiac output required for tissue perfusion. • Vascular occlusion may lead to reduce renal perfusion. • This enhances myocardial perfusion. • To know about the level of consciousness, mental status, and possibility for increased ICP. • These measures will prevent increased ICP and promote venous outflow. • Fever may reduce cerebral blood flow and ICP can be increased. • Upright position improves alveolar gas exchange. • Medications will facilitate perfusion and improve the condition.
4.	**Assess:** • Expressions of pain such as facial grimaces, moaning, crying, restlessness • Profuse sweating • Alteration in BP, HR, RR • Pain using various tools such as Wong-Baker FACES Rating Scale, NPRS, CPOT to determine pain intensity.	Acute pain related to tissue injury, mechanical ventilation, or cardiac dysfunction as manifested by moaning, grimaces, restlessness, profuse sweating, alterations in BP, HR, and RR.	• Perform a comprehensive assessment of pain (use OLDCART as discussed earlier). • Provide nonpharmacologic pain management such as relaxation, avoiding extra sounds, etc. • Administer analgesics as prescribed and evaluate their effectiveness.	• To know about the type and intensity of pain • In case of mild pain to prevent side-effects of pharmacological therapy. • To relieve the symptoms of patients that may impact outcomes.

Contd...

Contd...

Sl. No.	Nursing assessment	Nursing diagnosis	Nursing interventions	Rationale
5.	**Assess for** • Angina, anxiety, restlessness • Change in level of consciousness. • Dyspnea, orthopnea, tachypnea, crackles • Decreased activity tolerance • Decreased cardiac output • Decreased peripheral pulses; cold, clammy skin/poor capillary refill • Decreased venous and arterial oxygen saturation • Dysrhythmias • Hypotension • Weight gain, edema, decreased urine output • Abnormal heart sounds	Decreased cardiac output related to alteration in heart rate, rhythm, conduction, and impaired contractility as manifested by hypotension, dyspnea, decreased activity tolerance, and dysrhythmias.	• Position patient in semi-Fowler's to high-Fowler's • Administer oxygen therapy as prescribed. • Record hourly urine output and notify decreases in output. • Attach cardiac monitor/defibrillator to monitor for dysrhythmias. • Closely monitor fluid intake and limit fluids and sodium in patients. • Check ABG and electrolytes. • Monitor bowel functions and provide stool softeners as ordered. • Administer medications as prescribed, note any side effects and signs of toxicity.	• Upright position reduces preload and ventricular filling in c/o fluid overload. • Due to an increase in oxygen demands. • Decreased cardiac output reduce renal perfusion. • Atrial fibrillation is common in heart failure. • Poorly functioning ventricles are unable to tolerate increased fluid volumes. The restriction will reduce demands on the heart. • Hypo/hyperkalemia is common in patients with heart problems and may lead to dysrhythmias. • Decreased activity can cause constipation. • Medications will treat the underlying cause and improve the patient's condition.
6.	**Assess for:** • Raised temperature. • Color of respiratory secretions. • Appearance of urine • Signs and symptoms include localized swelling, redness, pain or tenderness, loss of function in the affected area, purulent discharge from incisions or injury, drains, or catheters. • Monitor white blood cell (WBC) count. • Weight, BMI, nutritional status, any history of weight loss, and serum albumin. • Presence of common causes of infection.	Risk of nosocomial infection related to the presence of invasive lines as manifested by leukocyte count, fever, purulent sputum, cloudy urine, positive cultures.	• Maintain strict asepsis in all procedures such as suctioning, tracheostomy care, wound care, intravenous therapy, etc. • Articles should be properly disinfected or sterilized before use. • Use appropriate PPE and infection control measures as discussed in the chapter while caring for the patient. • Place the patient with communicable infection in isolation. • Coughing and deep breathing exercises should be encouraged. • Change position frequently. • Limit visitors.	• This will decrease the chance of infection spread. • Disinfection reduces or eliminates pathogens. • Break the chain of infection and prevent infection. • To prevent transmission of infection to other patients. • Stasis of secretions in the lungs may lead to pneumonia. • By restricting visitors, the transmission of pathogens reduces.

and ICU length of stay was prolonged by 7 days. Infection doubles the ICU mortality rate and the costs associated with infection may be as high as 40% of total ICU expenditures.

Major Contributors of HAIs in ICU

1. Poor set-up of hospitals
2. Inadequate environmental hygienic conditions and waste disposal
3. Understaffing (nurse-to-patient ratio)
4. Overcrowding
5. Length of stay and mechanical ventilation.
6. Usage of invasive devices
7. Type of nutrition
8. Absence of local or national guidelines
9. Improper reporting and surveillance
10. Prolonged and inappropriate use of antibiotics leading to antimicrobial resistance (AMR)

Classification of ICU Infections

According to criterion, ICU-acquired infections are only secondary endogenous and exogenous, whereas primary endogenous are usually imported by the patient during admission.

❖ **Primary endogenous infections:** Infections that occur due to organisms carried at the time of admission to the ICU and are the most frequent infection reported in ICUs i.e., 50–80%.

❖ **Secondary endogenous infections:** Infections that occur by organisms not carried during admission but subsequently acquired usually in 1 week of ICU stay. It accounts for 1/3rd of the ICU infections.

❖ **Exogenous infections:** Infections that may occur at any time during the ICU stay and are typically caused by microorganisms associated with the ICU ecology, e.g., Methicillin-resistant *Staphylococcus aureus* (MRSA) and *Acinetobacter* and *Pseudomonas* species. These account for approximately 15% of all ICU infections.

INFECTION CONTROL PROTOCOLS

It refers to policies, procedures, and standards which are used to reduce the occurrence and spread of infectious diseases in health care settings. It is based on the principle that precautions must be followed for *"all the patients"* in the hospital. The hospital infection control practices advisory committee (HICPAC) and Centre for disease control and prevention (CDC) recommend two tiers of isolation precautions: (A) Standard precautions; (B) Transmission-based precautions. In addition to these two-tier precautions care bundles are also maintained in the hospital to reduce the rate of infection.

Standard Precautions

The standard precautions are to be practiced in all patients in order to prevent the infection. The elements of standard precautions are:
1. Hand hygiene
2. Use of personal protective equipments (PPEs)
3. Prevention of injury from sharps
4. Maintenance of asepsis during procedures
5. Keeping a check on antimicrobial use
6. Following the care bundles regularly
7. Disinfection of surfaces
8. Proper disposal of biomedical waste
9. Changing of lines as per hospital guidelines
10. Respiratory hygiene and cough etiquettes

1. **Hand hygiene:** The most frequent cause of infection in health care settings is by the hands of health care workers. Hand hygiene is the most important element to reduce the transmission of diseases in health care settings. Soap-water or alcohol hand rub can be used to maintain hand hygiene **(Table 52.7)**. Effective handwashing requires at least 20 seconds of vigorous scrubbing and special attention must be given to the area around nail beds and between fingers (high bacterial load). To maintain hand hygiene seven steps **(Fig. 52.2B)** and five moments **(Fig. 52.2A)** are followed.

TABLE 52.7: Alcohol hand rub versus soap-water handwashing.

Alcohol-based hand rub	Soap-water
• When hands are not visibly soiled, i.e., body fluids, excretions, mucous membrane, or wound dressing. • After contact with the patient's intact skin, i.e., checking vital signs or changing the position of the patient. • After contact with inanimate objects in the patient's surroundings. • Before caring for patients with severe immunosuppression. • Before performing any aseptic or clean procedures, i.e., urinary catheter insertion or central venous catheter. • Before donning sterile and after removing gloves.	• When hands are visibly dirty or contaminated with biological material. • Skin allergy to alcohol-based products.

Note: Do not wear artificial nails or nail polish and nails should be kept less than 0.25 inches long.

2. **Use of personal protective equipment's (PPEs):** PPEs such as gloves, mask, face shield or goggles, gown, aprons are used to protect skin and soiling of clothing and to protect nose, mouth, and eyes from splashes of blood, bodily fluids or secretions. Always perform hand hygiene before donning and after doffing the PPEs.

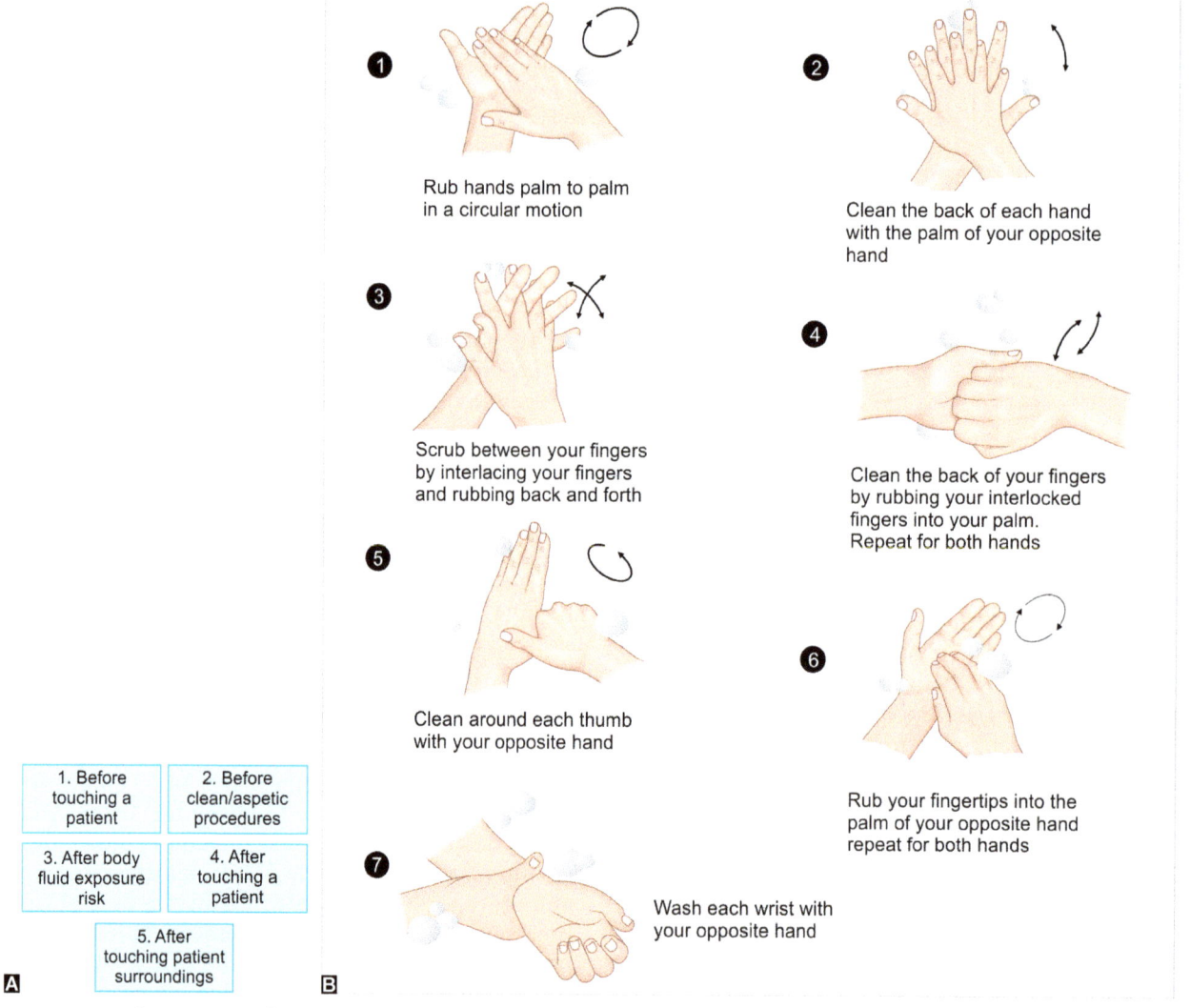

Figs. 52.2A and B: (A) Five moments of handwashing (WHO); (B) Seven steps of handwashing (WHO).

3. **Prevention of injury from sharps:** The most important aspect of preventing blood-borne infections is avoidance of percutaneous injury. Extreme care is essential when using, cleaning, and discarding sharps, i.e., needles or blades. The sharps should never be recapped, instead should be directly placed in the puncture-proof container. If there is a need for recapping, the nurse must use a mechanical device or scoop method to hold the cap or use a one-handed approach. Needlestick injury protocol must be followed if any percutaneous injury occurs **(Box 52.1)**.
4. **Use of aseptic techniques:** All procedures or care such as catheter care, suctioning, oral care, tracheostomy care, or insertion of lines must be done following strict aseptic techniques.
5. **Keeping a check on antimicrobial use:** Antibiotics are used in hospitals to prevent hospital-acquired infections that may lead to resistance towards those drugs. A recent study reported 143 strains of *Acinetobacter* in a tertiary care hospital in India, of which, 126 (88.1%) were extremely drug-resistant (Akula S et al., 2017). With the implementation of proper guidelines, antibiotic resistance can be prevented.
6. **Follow care bundles regularly:** Critical care bundles must be followed for every patient at every single time. A "bundle" is a group of evidence-based interventions when **executed together,** may result in better outcomes than if implemented individually **(Table 52.8)**.

> **BOX 52.1:** What to do in case of needlestick injury?
> - Do not panic.
> - Do not squeeze or apply pressure over the affected area.
> - Wash the area with soap and water until bleeding stops.
> - Do not use alcohol-based hand rub or any chemicals (betadine).
> - Inform to infection control nurse (ICN) immediately.
> - Physician should be consulted.
> - Follow all precautions.

TABLE 52.8: Common hospital-acquired infections in ICU (VAP, CLASBI, CAUTI).

Infection	Definition	Diagnosis	Bundle (evidence-based interventions)
Ventilator-associated pneumonia (VAP)	It is defined as the infection of the pulmonary parenchyma developed after 48 hours of intubation.	Clinical pulmonary infection score (CPIS) developed by Pugin et al. 1991. It includes certain parameters such as tracheal secretions, temperature, leukocytosis, PaO_2/FiO_2 ratio, chest X-ray infiltrates, microbiology report	1. Head of the bed elevated (30–45°) 2. Daily "sedation vacation" and "assessment of readiness to extubate". 3. Daily oral care with chlorhexidine every 4 hourly 4. Peptic ulcer disease (PUD) prophylaxis 5. Deep vein thrombosis (DVT) prophylaxis 6. Subglottic secretion drainage (SSD) every 2 hourly.
Central line-associated bloodstream infection (CLABSI)	It is defined as an infection that develops within 48 hours of central line placement and is not related to an infection at another site.	Paired quantitative blood cultures (one from the central line and the other from the peripheral vein). In case of poor peripheral access, two samples can be drawn from different lumens of the central line catheter.	**Insertion bundle:** 1. Hand hygiene 2. Maximal barrier precautions 3. Optimal catheter site selection (subclavian vein is most preferred while femoral is least preferred) with avoidance of using the femoral vein for central venous access in adult patients. 4. Full body drape 5. Chlorhexidine skin antisepsis **Maintenance bundle:** 1. Hand hygiene 2. Access central line necessity daily 3. Swab ports with chlorhexidine 2% or 70% alcohol swabs (RUB THE HUB) 4. Change dressing as per the hospital protocol (label with date and time) 5. Change of IV bags/tubing every 72 hours 6. Daily review of necessity/early removal (USE IT OR LOSE IT) 7. Screen patients for signs and symptoms of infection (integrated into the daily goal sheet)

Catheter-associated urinary tract infection (CAUTI)	It is a urinary tract infection in a patient that develops after 48 hours of placement of an indwelling urinary catheter.	National Healthcare Safety Network (NHSN) criteria: CAUTI meet the NHSN criteria if positive urine culture with ≥10^5 colony-forming units of 1 or 2 microorganisms per mL of urine is reported along with the following signs and symptoms: No alternative site of infection, fever >100°F or >2°F above baseline, rigors, new hypotension, Leukocytosis, >14000 leukocytes/mm^3, acute mental status, new-onset suprapubic or costovertebral angle pain, purulent discharge around the catheter	**Insertion bundle:**
			1. Insert only for specific reasons
			  – Urinary output in critical ill
			  – Neurogenic bladder or bladder outlet obstruction
			  – Prevent contamination of sacral wounds
			  – Terminal care
			2. Competent healthcare worker should insert the catheter
			3. Aseptic technique to be used during insertion
			4. Closed system with bag below bladder
			Maintenance bundle:
			1. Hand hygiene and PPE before and after any catheter care
			2. Review needs for catheter daily
			3. Maintain unobstructed urinary flow
			4. Keep collection bag below the bladder and off the floor
			5. Check the skin condition around the device daily. Relocate if irritation of the skin is noted.
			6. Use port for urine collection—do no break the catheter system to collect a specimen.

TABLE 52.9: Precaution categories.

Airborne precautions	Contact precautions	Droplet precautions
• The organism that is spread through the air. • Patients must be in a separate room with negative pressure and the door should be closed at all times. • Health care workers must wear an N-95 mask at all times while in the patient's room. • Example: Tuberculosis, smallpox, chickenpox.	• The organism is spread through skin-to-skin contact. • Patients do not require separate rooms and doors do not need to be closed. • Mask is not required. • Example: *Clostridium difficile* infection.	• The organism can be transmitted by close or face-to-face contact. • Patients may be placed in a separate room and doors do not need to be closed. • Health care workers should wear a mask all time. • Example: Influenza, pertussis.

7. **Disinfection of surfaces:** Cleaning, disinfection of environmental surfaces and frequently touched areas should be done regularly. Various disinfectants can be used such as virex, cydex, sodium hypochlorite, etc., with proper instructions for amount, dilution, and contact time as approved by EPA (environmental protective agency). Floors and walls do not need to be disinfected unless visibly soiled with blood or body fluids.
8. **Proper disposal of biomedical waste:** Ensure safe waste disposal according to biomedical waste management. There different color-coding system in biomedical waste management:
   a. *Yellow bin:* Category 1, 2 and 6 (human anatomical or infected waste)
   b. *Red bin:* Category 3 and 7 (gloves or rubber material)
   c. *Blue bin:* Category 4 (sharps – ampules or vials)
   d. *White bin* (puncture proof): Category 4 (sharps: needles, scalpel, etc.)
   e. *Green bin:* General waste (non-infectious)
9. **Changing of lines as per hospital guidelines:** Lines such as a urinary catheter, central line, drains, etc., should be changed regularly as per the hospital guidelines and should be properly mentioned with date and time.
10. **Respiratory hygiene and cough etiquettes:** Health care workers, patients, and visitors should be educated to cover the mouth either by tissue or elbow while coughing sneezing, and wash hands after coming in contact with respiratory secretions. Cough etiquette signs must be displayed where the general public can see them.

Transmission-based Precautions

These precautions are used when standard precautions alone are not sufficient to control and prevent infection. These precautions are used in a patient who is colonized with highly transmissible pathogens or suspected to be infected **(Table 52.9)**.

COMMUNICATION WITH THE PATIENT AND FAMILY IN ICU

Communication with patients in ICU is challenging as patients in the ICU are often deprived of speech and their ability to communicate due to intubation, sedation, and unconsciousness. Severe emotional reactions among ICU patients such as stress or anxiety are directly linked with loss of speech. With effective communication, the patients may be able to convey their basic physiological and psychological needs, decisions, wishes and desires about treatment, and end-of-life decisions that improve clinical outcomes and increase patient satisfaction.

Effective communication with family members is also important as they are frequently involved in decision-making related to treatment and prognosis. Ineffective communication also affects the quality of life of the patients in ICU. Nurses spend more time at the patient's bedside; therefore, they must possess good communication skills to provide complete and comprehensive care. However, various studies have reported that the communication between nurses and mechanically ventilated patients is minimal.

Importance of Communication in ICU

1. Information can be exchanged properly.
2. Establishes an ongoing therapeutic relationship between health care provider and patient.
3. Patients may need to express their final wishes to the family, friends, and providers.
4. Facilitates patient's compliance with therapy and improves clinical outcomes.
5. Increases patient satisfaction.
6. Prevents various physiological effects that occur due to loss of speech.
7. Impact long-term psychological outcomes.

Barriers to Communication in ICU

1. High expectations of patient/family
2. Multiple decision-makers in a family
3. Inadequate prognostication by physicians
4. Not enough time for meeting
5. Cannot assemble an entire team (physicians, intensivists, nurses).
6. Lack of communication skills or training among health care providers.
7. Fear of conflict.

Strategies for Effective Communication

Various strategies are available for improving communication with patients in the ICU that facilitate successful communication with patients receiving mechanical ventilator support:

1. Assess needs of the patient and families.
2. Always start with an open question and make interaction easier for them.
3. Give respect to patient and family during discussions.
4. Speak clearly and slowly.
5. Facilitate lipreading.
6. Give ample time to patient/family to respond or ask questions.
7. Use alternative and augmentative communication devices **(Table 52.10)**

TABLE 52.10: Alternative and augmentative communication devices (communication tool for patients in ICU).

Picture	Communication tool	Description
	Pen and paper	Communication that is made on paper by writing or drawing
	Picture board/charts	These show pictures with descriptive words listed under the picture made according to the needs/desires of the patient. For example, want to sleep, feeling thirsty or hungry, want to meet relatives, etc.
	List of common words or phrases	These include the use of some common words or phrases that may be helpful for the patient to communicate. For example, I have a headache.
	High-tech alternative communication devices	Also known as speech generating devices (SGD). It can be a tablet or iPad with a software program for communication that may have multiple pages and folders. e.g., pressing on "Food" will get to food options, etc.
	Speaking Tracheostomy tube (speaking valves)	These are one-way valves placed onto the tracheostomy tube. The one-way valve allows air in but not out by remaining closed, these redirects exhaled air upwards to vocal cords enabling the patient to vocalize. These are used for the non-ventilator-dependent patient.

Contd...

Contd...

Picture	Communication tool	Description
	Electrolarynx	Also called "throat back", is a device used to produce clear speech in those patients who have lost their voice box, usually due to cancer of the larynx. It is a battery-operated device pressed under the mandible and produces vibrations to allow speech. These are also used in laryngectomy patients for speech recovery.

TABLE 52.11: VALUE.

V	Value and appreciate what the family said
A	Acknowledge the family emotions
L	Listen
U	Understand the patient as a person through asking questions
E	Elicit questions and concerns

8. Listen completely and attentively.
9. Summarize throughout.
10. Keep records and maintain documentation.

The University of Washington End-of-Life Care Research Program at Harborview Medical Center developed a 5-step mnemonic "VALUE" to improve ICU clinician communication with families **(Table 52.11)**.

DRUGS USED IN CRITICAL CARE

Emergency drugs are chemical compounds (natural or synthetic) used during life-threatening conditions to save the life of the patients. These drugs must have short onset of action and be administered in a way to facilitate the rapid onset of action. The purpose of these drugs is used to save the life of a patient, control symptoms, and normalize bodily vital functions. The autonomic nervous system receptors act as on/off buttons that control various sympathetic and parasympathetic effects in the body **(Table 52.12)**.

Classification of Emergency Drugs

- ❖ **Inotropic drugs:** Affects the force of heart contractions.
  - ➢ *Positive inotropes:* Strengthen the force of the heartbeat, e.g., dopamine.

TABLE 52.12: Types of receptors.

Adrenergic receptors		Dopaminergic receptors
α-Adrenergic receptors	β-Adrenergic receptors	
α1 **Site of action:** Smooth muscles of vascular, genitourinary, intestinal, cardiac, and within the liver. **Effects:** Peripheral vasoconstriction, increase peripheral resistance, constriction of smooth muscles of the urinary system, inhibition of renin system, dilation of the pupil (mydriasis).	**β1** **Site of action—heart and kidney** **Effects:** • The force of contraction of the heart. • Increase conduction of AV impulse. • Increase production of renin.	**D1**: Located in substantia nigra pars reticulata, caudate, putamen, nucleus accumbens, olfactory tubercle, and frontal and temporal cortex. **Function:** Memory, attention, impulse control, regulation of renal function, locomotion.
α2 **Site of action:** Platelets, vascular smooth muscle, presynaptic nerve endings, and pancreatic islets. **Effects:** Platelet aggregation, vasoconstriction, inhibit norepinephrine, acetylcholine, and release of insulin.	**β2** Site of action—cardiac muscles, uterine muscles, alveolar type 2, mast cells, mucous glands, epithelial cells, skeletal muscles, vascular endothelium. **Effects:** • Bronchodilation and vasodilation. • Decrease peripheral resistance. • Relaxation of smooth muscles. • Conversion of glycogen to glucose (glycogenesis)	**D2:** Highly expressed in the caudate, putamen (basal ganglia), nucleus accumbens, ventral tegmental area, and the substantia nigra and lower concentrations in the septal region, amygdala, hippocampus, thalamus, cerebellum, and cerebral cortex. Functions: Locomotion, attention, sleep, memory, learning
	β3 **Site of action:** Urinary bladder, gallbladder, and brown adipose tissue. Functions: Smooth muscle relaxation.	**D3:** Ventral striatum including nucleus accumbens, thalamus, hippocampus, and cortex function—cognition, impulse control, attention, sleep **D4:** Cognition, impulse control, attention, sleep **D5:** Decision making, cognition, attention, renin secretion

- ➢ Negative inotropes weaken the force of the heartbeat, e.g., propranolol.
- ❖ **Chronotropic drugs:** Affect the heart rate.
  - ➢ *Positive chronotropic:* Accelerate heart rate, e.g., adrenaline.
  - ➢ *Negative chronotropic:* Slow down heart rate, e.g., digoxin
- ❖ *Dromotropic drugs:* Affect conduction velocity through the conducting tissues of the heart.
  - ➢ *Positive dromotropic:* Increases the electric impulse conduction, e.g., phenytoin.
  - ➢ *Negative dromotropic:* Decreases the electrical impulse conduction, e.g., verapamil.

Common Emergency Drugs Used in ICUs (Table 52.13)

1. Epinephrine and norepinephrine
2. Dopamine and dobutamine
3. Atropine sulfate
4. Digoxin
5. Calcium gluconate
6. Sodium bicarbonate

MAINTAINING INTENSIVE CARE RECORDS

Hospital records are records which includes information related to patients collected during their stay. The records maintained in ICU are more comprehensive and detailed as compared to other units of the hospital. The records are maintained to ensure continuity of care, provide up-to-date status of the patients and justify the hospital policies which furnish the legal aspects of 'duty of care. Various records are maintained for the patients such as vital sign chart, treatment chart, intake-output chart, etc., **(Table 52.14)**. Records are maintained by an on-duty doctor and assigned nurse on daily basis. The nurses working in ICU must be skilled and technologically competent to maintain all the records in ICU.

END OF LIFE CARE

Life and death are two important stages in human life, during which they come across many challenges, diseases, and other problems. End-of-life care refers to the care for a person with a condition which is progressive, advanced and/or incurable. It simply means the support and medical care given during the time surrounding death. A health care provider can have a significant effect on the way patients live, how death occurs, or by creating memories for the families. End-of-life care is called a holistic approach because it deals with a "whole" person, not just illness or symptoms End-of-life care can be provided by healthcare professionals such as consultants, nurses, occupational therapists or physiotherapists trained in palliative care. End-of-life care includes:

- ❖ **Palliative care:** Palliative care is specialized medical care for people living with a serious illness, such as cancer or heart failure. It focuses on symptom management, psychological care, and spiritual support.
- ❖ **Hospice care:** Hospice care focuses on the care, comfort, and quality of life of a person with a serious illness who is approaching the end of life. This compassionate care is provided to a person who is in the last phases (life expectancy of 6 months or less) of incurable illness.

Purposes of End-of-Life Care

- ❖ To enhance the quality of life of patient.
- ❖ To control pain and other distressing symptoms (psychological, social, and spiritual support).
- ❖ To ensure dignified death.

Signs of Approaching Death

The National Cancer Institute (United States) guides the following signs that may indicate that death is approaching:

- ❖ Drowsiness and restlessness, increased sleep, and/or unresponsiveness
- ❖ Disorientation to time, place, and/or identity of loved ones
- ❖ Loss of appetite or decreased interest in food or fluids.
- ❖ Loss of bladder or bowel control along with darkened urine or decreased amount of urine
- ❖ Extremities are cold to touch; skin may become bluish
- ❖ Rattling or gurgling sounds while breathing due to collection of secretions (the sounds may be loud called as death rattle)
- ❖ Shallow and irregular breathing
- ❖ Impaired vision, hearing, and speech
- ❖ Decreased socialization and detachment from the environment
- ❖ Difficulty in controlling pain
- ❖ Involuntary movements (called myoclonus) and loss of reflexes in the legs and arms
- ❖ Report of seeing family or friends who died.

Nursing Care of Terminally Ill Patients

Careful evaluation should be done for physical, psychological, and spiritual problems.

- ❖ **Dealing with psychological issues:** Psychological suffering is a common experience for patients and their families at the end of life related to grief about loss, fear and ambiguity about the future, unsettled issues from the past, and worries about loved ones. The nurse should provide psychological support to patients and their families and also communicate patient's wishes concerning to end of life.
- ❖ **Maintaining communication:** Health care providers must have adequate skills and comfort for assessing patients and their family's response to serious illnesses. After initial discussion or diagnosis of progressive disease, the patient and family will probably have many queries and may need time and support to cope up with changes and the prospect of impending death.
- ❖ **Culturally sensitive care:** During serious illness death, grief, mourning, practices are universally accepted as death approaches and after death. The nurse should share this knowledge with health care providers and facilitate the adaptation of care plans, e.g., nurse may find that a female patient prefers to have her elder son make all of her care decisions. The nurses' role is assessing the preferences, beliefs, values, practices regardless of ethnicity, status, or background regarding end-of-life care includes:

TABLE 52.13: Emergency drugs.

Name of drug	Therapeutic name/ chemical name	Action	Indications	Contraindications	Adverse effects	Nursing responsibilities
Epinephrine hydrochloride *Antidote*— phentolamine *Available form*—1 mg/mL	**Pharmacologic classification:** Adrenergic. **Therapeutic classification:** Bronchodilator, vasopressor, cardiac stimulant, adjunct with a local anesthetic, topical antihemorrhagic	Act on adrenergic receptors • At low dose-β effect • At high dose-α effect β1—positive inotropic, chronotropic and dromotropic effect. β2-bronchial smooth muscle relaxation and dilation of skeletal vasculature. α1—vasoconstriction	• Bronchospasm • Restore cardiac rhythm • Prolong local anesthetic effect • Local superficial bleeding • Anaphylaxis • Antiglaucoma action	• Organic brain damage • Coronary insufficiency • During general anesthesia with halogenated hydrocarbons • In labor • Hypertension • Shock (other than anaphylactic).	**CNS:** Tremors, headache, nervousness, vertigo, disorientation, agitation, drowsiness. **CV:** Hypertension, tachycardia, palpitations, widened pulse pressure, anginal pain, ventricular fibrillation, arrhythmias. **EENT:** Pain, burning, allergic lid reaction. **GI:** Nausea, vomiting.	• Check vital signs (especially B.P). • If given I/M, give it very cautiously, avoid I/M into buttocks. (induced vasoconstriction favors the growth of *Clostridium perfringens*). • Rotate injection sites to prevent tissue necrosis due to vascular constriction. • Maintain mouth hygiene, adequate hydration, and physiotherapy, if used to reduce bronchial spasms. • Intra-cardiac administration requires external cardiac massage (banned by AHA).
Norepinephrine *Drug overdose*—administration of IV fluids and electrolyte replacement. *Available form*—4 mg/4 mL	**Pharmacologic classification:** Catecholamine **Therapeutic classification:** Adrenergic agonist, vasopressor, inotropic agent.	Activation of α adrenergic, β1, and little effects on β2 receptors—stimulation of inotropic effect, vasoconstriction which results increase in BP, increased coronary blood flow, and increased metabolic activity.	• Acute hypotension • Shock • Cardiac arrest	• Known hypersensitivity. • Mesenteric or peripheral vascular thrombosis. • Hypotension	**CNS:** Headache, cerebral hemorrhage **CVS:** Palpitations, bradycardia, hypertension, angina. **GIT:** Nausea, vomiting, anorexia. **Skin:** Necrosis, tissue sloughing with extravasation. **Systemic:** Anaphylaxis.	• Monitor intake/output ratio; notify prescriber if output <30 mL/hr. • Monitor BP, pulse every 3–5 min. • Record or monitor ECG during therapy. • Record CVP or PWP during therapy if possible. • Check for paresthesia and coldness of extremities.
Dopamine *Antidote*—short-acting α-adrenergic blockers and extravasation—phentolamine. *Available form*—200 mg/5 mL	**Pharmacologic classification:** Catecholamine **Therapeutic classification:** Adrenergic agonist, vasopressor, inotropic agent.	Acts through D1, D2 as well as α and β1 receptors. At low dose (0.5 to 3 mic/kg/min)—renal perfusion. At intermediate dose (3–10 mic/kg/min)—stimulates β1 receptors (increase cardiac output). At high dose (>10 mic/kg/min)—α receptors stimulation (pulmonary and systemic vasoconstriction).	• Shock • To increase perfusion • Hypotension • Cardiogenic/septic shock	• Hypersensitivity • Ventricular fibrillation • Tachydysrhythmias • Pheochromocytoma.	**CNS:** Headache **CV:** Palpitations, tachycardia, hypertension, angina, wide QRS complex, peripheral vasoconstriction. **GI:** Nausea, vomiting, diarrhea. **Skin:** Necrosis, tissue sloughing with extravasation.	• Monitor ECG for dysrhythmias. • Assess for heart failure—dyspnea, crackles, neck vein distension. • Regularly monitor saturation. • Stop infusion and notify the physician, if BP drops 30 mm Hg. • Monitor extravasation.
Dobutamine hydrochloride Side effects—metoprolol (1–5 mg) or esmolol. Chest pain or arrhythmias -do not resolve after the termination of dobutamine infusion then Nitroglycerine can be used. *Available form*- 250 mg/5 mL	• Vasopressor • Sympathomimetic	• Act on both α and β1, β2 adrenergic receptors- more inotropic effect • Increase the force of cardiac contraction and output- At a dose of 2.5–10 µg/kg/min IV	• Cardiogenic shock • Severe heart failure • Cardiac stress test • Open heart surgery • Myocardial infarction.	• Hypersensitivity. • Pheochromocytoma. • Recent myocardial infarction. • Unstable angina pectoris. • Heart failure. • Stenosis of LCA.	**CVS:** Hypertension, angina, arrhythmia, and tachycardia. Used with caution in atrial fibrillation increasing the atrioventricular (AV) conduction. **Metabolism:** Hypokalemia **CNS:** Headache, tremor, restlessness, anxiety **Renal:** Urinary urgency **GIT:** Nausea, vomiting	• Monitor vital signs and ECG. • Monitor urinary output and maintain intake/output chart. • Protect from sunlight and do not store above 25 degree Celsius. • Regularly monitor serum potassium levels. • Check blood glucose levels if the patient is diabetic. • Instruct patient to report if chest (anginal) pain occurs.

Contd...

Contd...

Name of drug	Therapeutic name/chemical name	Action	Indications	Contraindications	Adverse effects	Nursing responsibilities
Atropine sulfate *Antidote*—physostigmine. *Available form*—0.6 mg/mL	**Pharmacologic classification:** Anticholinergic **Therapeutic classification:** Antiarrhythmic, vagolytic **Antidote:** Antimuscarinic	**CNS:** <ul><li>Stimulates medullary center.</li><li>Blocking cholinergic property.</li></ul> **CVS:** Blockade of M2 receptors on SA node. <ul><li>Vasodilation action at high doses.</li><li>Act as α1 adrenergic agonist and antagonist.</li><li>Decreases secretions by blockade of M3 receptors, i.e., saliva, sweat, lacrimal</li></ul>	<ul><li>Preanesthetic medication.</li><li>Symptomatic bradycardia</li><li>Reduce salivation and bronchial secretions</li><li>Blocks cardiac vagal reflexes</li><li>Antidote for cholinesterase poisoning.</li></ul>	<ul><li>Hypersensitivity</li><li>Obstructive uropathy</li><li>Toxic megacolon</li><li>Asthma</li><li>Bowel disease (ulcerative colitis)</li><li>Enlarged prostate</li><li>Thyrotoxicosis</li><li>Severe heart disease</li><li>Heartburn (reflux esophagitis)</li><li>Acute closed-angle glaucoma</li></ul>	**CNS:** Headache, dizziness, excitement, restlessness, agitation, confusion ataxia, disorientation, hallucinations, delirium, insomnia. **CV:** Palpitations, bradycardia (from lower dose), tachycardia (from higher dose) **EENT:** Photophobia, blurred vision, eye dryness, eye irritation **GI:** Dry mouth, thirst, constipation, nausea, vomiting **GU:** Urine retention, impotence **SKIN:** Dryness, decreased sweating, dermatitis, rashes, pruritis	<ul><li>Check vital signs very carefully.</li><li>Check pupil size.</li><li>To prevent constipation, provide plenty of fluids and a high-fiber diet.</li><li>Report to the physician, if signs of toxicity are observed.</li><li>Discontinue drug if platelet count decreases to below 1,00,000/mm³</li><li>Continue drug if mild diarrhea but notify the physician if the blood in the stool occurs.</li><li>Assess skin for rashes</li><li>Monitor stomatitis and metallic taste in mouth.</li></ul>
Digoxin *Antidote*—digoxin immune Fab (Digibind) *Available form*—inj-250 mcg/mL Tab 0.25 mg	**Pharmacological classification:** Digitalis preparation **Therapeutic classification:** Cardiac glycoside, positive inotropic effect, negative chronotropic effect.	<ul><li>It inhibits the Na-K pump thus increasing calcium leading to more contraction of heart muscles.</li><li>Positive inotropic, negative chronotropic, and negative dromotropic effect.</li></ul>	<ul><li>Congestive heart failure</li><li>Atrial fibrillation</li><li>Atrial flutter</li><li>Supraventricular tachycardia</li></ul>	<ul><li>Hypersensitivity to digitalis</li><li>Ventricular fibrillation</li><li>Carotid sinus syndrome</li><li>2nd and 3rd-degree heart block</li></ul>	**CNS:** Headache, confusion drowsiness and disorientation. **EYE:** Visual disturbance such as diplopia, blurred vision, yellow-green halos. **GI:** Anorexia, diarrhea, Nausea and vomiting. **CV:** Bradycardia **Toxicity:** <ul><li>Shock</li><li>Cardiac arrest</li><li>Severe ventricular dysrhythmias</li><li>Bradycardia</li><li>Hypokalemia</li></ul>	<ul><li>Monitor for toxicity</li><li>Monitor serum levels (therapeutic range is 0.5 to 2 mg/mL)</li><li>Administer with caution in elderly clients.</li><li>IV medicine should be given slowly.</li><li>An increased risk of toxicity exists in clients with hypercalcemia, hypokalemia, hypomagnesemia, hypothyroidism, renal disease.</li><li>Monitor potassium levels and notify the physician.</li></ul>
Calcium gluconate *Antidote*—Sodium thiosulfate and hyaluronidase *Available form*—950 mg/10 mL	**Pharmacologic classification:** A calcium supplement **Therapeutic classification:** Therapeutic agent for electrolyte balance	<ul><li>Stabilizing the membranes of cardiac cells.</li><li>(Counteract the toxicity of hyperkalemia and reducing fibrillation).</li></ul>	<ul><li>Hypocalcemia</li><li>Hyperkalemia</li><li>Hypermagnesemia</li><li>Cardiac resuscitations</li><li>After open-heart surgery</li><li>Beta-blocker and calcium channel blocker overdose.</li></ul>	<ul><li>Hypercalcemia</li><li>Renal calculi</li><li>Renal and cardiac diseases</li><li>Respiratory acidosis</li><li>Respiratory failure</li></ul>	**CNS:** Tingling sensation, headache, irritability, weakness, syncope. **CV:** Fall in BP, bradycardia, vasodilation, arrhythmias, cardiac arrest. **GI:** Nausea, abdominal pain, constipation, chalky taste, hemorrhage, rebound hyperacidity, thirst. **GU:** Renal calculi, hypercalcemia, polyurea	<ul><li>Monitor vital signs and ECG.</li><li>To prevent extravasation and necrosis, IV should be administered through a large bore cannula.</li><li>Monitor frequent calcium levels.</li><li>Should be administered slowly.</li><li>Monitor toxicity in patients.</li><li>If tetany develops, protect the patient from injury.</li><li>Oxalic acid (spinach), phytic acid (bran and whole-sale cereals), and phosphorus (milk and its products) may interfere with absorption.</li></ul>
Sodium bicarbonate *Available form*—1 mL/1 meql	**Pharmacologic classification:** Trace material **Therapeutic classification:** Alkalinizing agent, systemic hydrogen ion buffer, oral antacid	<ul><li>Buffers excess hydrogen ion concentration to form water and carbon dioxide.</li><li>Neutralizing excess stomach acid.</li><li>IV administration increases plasma bicarbonate, Raises blood pH.</li></ul>	<ul><li>Stomach upsets related to hyperacidity</li><li>Adjunct to advanced cardiac life support</li><li>Metabolic acidosis</li><li>Urinary alkalinization</li></ul>	<ul><li>Hypocalcemia (alkalosis may produce tetany)</li><li>Metabolic or respiratory alkalosis.</li><li>Hypokalemia.</li><li>Vomiting or prolonged GI suction</li><li>Use with extreme caution in heart failure, renal insufficiency, edema.</li></ul>	**GI:** Gastric distention **CNS:** Headache, weakness **Others:** Hypersensitivity **Metabolic:** Metabolic alkalosis, hypernatremia	<ul><li>Monitor urine pH and vital signs carefully.</li><li>Prevent extravasation.</li><li>Always flush line before and after administration.</li><li>If using from long term, assess the patients for Milk-Alkali-Syndrome.</li><li>Oral preparations should be used 1 hr or 2 hrs. prior or after enteric coated tablets</li></ul>

TABLE 52.14: Types of records maintained in ICU.

Sl. No.	Records	Components
1.	Initial assessment	Time of receiving, chief complaints, present/history, vital signs, the signature of doctor and nurse, etc.
2.	Vital sign monitoring	Temperature, pulse, respiration, blood pressure, signature of the nurse with time, date, etc.
3.	Treatment chart	Patient identification, drug allergies, date of starting medication, Inj/tab form, name of the medicine (dose, frequency, route), the signature of doctor, etc.
4.	Doctor order sheet	Prescriptions, medical investigations, diet, etc.
5.	Intake/output chart	Patient identification, day/date/time, diagnosis, input (enteral, IV fluids/injections), output (urine, stool, vomitus/NG aspirate, drains), balance 24 hourly, and signature of the nurse.
6.	Patient transfer form	Patient identification, admitting unit, consultant in charge, diagnosis, transferred from, receiving unit, the status of the patient at transfer and receiving status with the signature of doctor and nurse, etc.
7.	Pain assessment form	Patient identification, date/time, pain score, treatment given, treatment response or side effects and signature of doctor and nurse, etc.
8.	Investigation sheet	Patient identification, date, and lab reports (LFT, RFT, CBC, X-ray, CT, MRI), etc.
9.	ICU daily monitoring sheet	Patient identification, vital signs, peripheral pulses, CVP, pupil status, GCS, suction/secretions, eye/mouth care, skin care, position with date/time and signature of the nurse, etc.
10.	Patient and family counseling form	Patient identification, date/time, the purpose of the meeting, condition of the patient, name of the doctor, signature of patient relatives/relation and signature of doctor and nurse, etc.
11.	Nursing shift handover record	Patient identification, Date/time/shift, vital signs, intake output and condition of the patient, etc.
12.	Blood sugar chart	Patient identification, date/time, RBS, ketones, insulin administered and signature with code, etc.
13.	Nursing care process	Patient identification, date/time/shift, nursing process (assessment, diagnosis, planning, implementation, evaluation), the signature of the nurse, etc.
14.	Consent forms (diagnostic/therapeutic procedures, i.e., mechanical ventilation, central line, restraining, any surgery.	Patient identification, explanation about the procedure with benefits and risk, the signature of doctor and patient or relatives with relation/date/time/place, etc.
15.	Ventilator chart	Patient identification, vital signs, ventilator mode, settings and signature of the nurse, etc.
16.	Critical care bundles, i.e., CAUTI, CLABSI, SSI, VAP	Patient identification measures to prevent infection, the signature of the nurse, etc.
17.	Registers	Statistics (admission/discharge), daily census, round register, attendance register for doctors, nurses and other personnel's working in ICU etc.

- ➢ Truth-telling to the patients or their family, i.e., the person responsible for disclosure.
- ➢ The person is responsible for decision-making in their family.
- ➢ Any advance directives (discussed below).
- ➢ Location of dying, i.e., home or any other location.
- ➢ Care of body after death and funeral or burial practices.
- ➢ Any special spiritual practices or rituals followed in their family.
- ➢ Expression of grief and mourning practices in their family.

❖ **Setting the goals of care:** It is the responsibility of the nurse to help patients and their family members to clarify goals, expected outcomes, and treatment options. In addition, nurses should coordinate with colleagues to ensure that the family and patient are referred for psychological support, symptom management or hospice care, referral for financial support.

❖ **Spiritual assessment:** Spiritual assessment is a key component of assessment in nursing for terminally ill patients as well as their families, i.e., religious faith, religious affiliation or preference, rituals, etc. Many studies have suggested that spiritual wellbeing affects suffering at the end of life.

❖ **Hopefulness:** Hope is a multidimensional construct that provides comfort as a person endures life threats and personal challenges. The hope can be nurtured or delayed due to various factors such as love of family and friends, faith, dreams, positive relationships, etc. Nurses can support hope for patients and their family by listening, encourage to share feelings, accurate information, encouraging realistic goals, effective communication, psychological and spiritual counseling.

Management of Physiologic Responses at End-of-Life

A patient who is approaching to end of life may experience many physical symptoms which may be directly caused by disease condition or indirectly by the treatment **(Table 52.15)**.

Legal and Ethical Issues in End-of-Life Care

During terminal stages of illness, patients and their family members struggle with many decisions. It is the responsibility of health care providers to assist patients with their decisions.

❖ **Organ donation:** The decision of organ donation may be made by a person before death or their family members after death. At the time of donation decisions from

TABLE 52.15: Management of physical symptoms at the end of life.

Physiological symptoms	Management
1. Pain	
Pain is a common symptom in the final stages of illness i.e., cancer, heart disease, and renal disease which affect the psychological, emotional, social, and financial wellbeing of patients. Pain can be: • Acute • Chronic	• Assess pain (use VAS, numeric rating scale). Determine the location, nature, quality, pattern, and contributing factors of pain. • If the patient is unable to communicate, it should not be equated with the absence of pain. (McGuire et. al., 2011). • Administer around-the-clock medications that are prescribed by physician, e.g., opioid or non-opioid analgesics, i.e., morphine. • Also provide non-pharmacological measures, i.e., massage, guided imagery, and various relaxation techniques.
2. Dyspnea	
Dyspnea is the most challenging and prevalent subjective symptom to manage. The underlying cause of dyspnea should be identified and treated.	• Assessment of severity of dyspnea can be assessed by using the dyspnea scale. • Elevate or assist the patient in fowlers position to improve chest expansion. • Provide an adequate environment to facilitate air movement. • At bedside or in-room there should be a call bell or light source near the patient. • Administer oxygen therapy via nasal cannula or mask if tolerated. • Suctioning to remove secretions if any and cautiously in the terminal phase. • Administer bronchodilators, corticosteroids, diuretics, and fluid balance (based on underlying pathology) as prescribed by a physician.
3. Nutrition and Hydration	
Depending upon underlying disease condition, level of disability, or stage of illness anorexia, dysphagia and cachexia are most common in patients at end of life. Cachexia refers to severe lean muscle loss with or without a fat loss that cannot reverse (Fearon, Strasser, Anker et.al., 2011).	• Assess the patient frequently for dryness in the mucous membrane that can lead to discomfort. • At the end of life, nutritional demands or needs change. The ability to use, eliminate or store nutrients, fluids, or desire for food or fluids is diminished. • Offer small portions of their favorite foods (High calorie and high protein diet). • Give cold foods as compared to hot (maybe better tolerated). • Give more fluids or liquid supplements with a straw i.e. milkshakes, fruit juices. • Do not force feed the patient. • Schedule meals when family members are present. • If not able to swallow then enteral or parenteral feeding considered. • Apply lubricant to lips and mucous membrane as needed. • Administer antiemetics as prescribed by the physician if needed.
4. Delirium	
The state in which disturbances in the level of consciousness, attention, awareness, and cognitive capability develop over a short period. (Wright et al. 2014).	• Assess the patient for causes of delirium. • Identify the underlying cause of delirium and educate family members about how to interact, safety for the patient, and what is normal. • Spiritual intervention, music therapy, gentle massage, and therapeutic touch may provide relief. • Reduce environmental stimuli, presence of familiar faces, and regularly reorientation and reassurance could be helpful. • Pharmacologic interventions are required. • Neuroleptic drugs, i.e., haloperidol, olanzapine, quetiapine and risperidone, and benzodiazepines are administered as prescribed by a physician.
5. Skin Integrity	
Impaired skin integrity at end of life may be due to immobility, bowel pattern and urinary incontinence, anemia, decreased circulation.	• Assess the skin for signs of breakdown. • Follow protocol for the management of wounds, drainage, odor, and keep it dry.
6. Bowel Movement and Bladder control	
Constipation or diarrhea can occur due to immobility, use of drugs, or lack of hydration and high fiber diet.	• Assess pattern and remove fecal impactions. • Give a high fiber diet and fluids. • Administer laxatives, enemas, or antidiarrheal if needed as directed by a physician. • Assess urine output and use of absorbent pads. • Make use of indwelling or external catheters if needed.

family members are taken. It is the responsibility of the physician to notify immediately organ donation agencies after the death of the patient e.g., donation of the eye, tissues, etc. Nurses have got an important role to play in counseling the patients regarding organ donation. So, they should be knowledgeable enough regarding the process of organ donation. They should also be skillful in providing quality care to the brain-dead patients.

❖ **Advance directives:** These are the written documents based on the principle of autonomy that provide information about the decision of medical treatment or patient desires and who is his/her surrogate decision-maker.

Types of advance directives:

a. *A living will:* A legal document that gives instructions about future medical care treatment that patient wants or not to keep him alive and measures should be taken when the patient is unable to communicate.

b. *Power of attorney:* A legal document that describes the legal authority to a particular person to make medical treatment decisions on the behalf of a patient when he/she will lose the ability to communicate.

- **Do not attempt resuscitate (DNAR):** It is a legal document of patient desires, the decision of surrogate decision-maker or the patient who is terminal ill/incurable illness that CPR should not be initiated when it is required. This document is counter-signed by the treating physician. DNAR is practiced in most of the ICUs or hospitals between patient's relatives and doctors but it is not yet a legal practice in India.
- **Euthanasia:** It is a deliberate act of hastening death by removing the life support system. Euthanasia is of two types: Active and Passive. In march 2018 passive euthanasia became legal in India under certain legislations like a person who is deliberately ill or in a permanent vegetative state.

GERIATRICS CONSIDERATIONS IN ICU

Elderly care is paramount due to its distinctive requirements. Advanced age brings physiological changes that demand specialized attention. Comorbidities frequently accompany elderly patients, intensifying the complexity of ICU care. Managing multiple conditions necessitates a holistic approach, where medical interventions are intricately tailored to individual needs. Age-related alterations in basal metabolism and organ functioning can influence the efficacy and dosing of medications. This mandates vigilant monitoring and adjustments to ensure optimal treatment outcomes. Moreover, elderly individuals often face financial dependence, impacting decisions regarding interventions, post-ICU care, and potential complications. Clear communication with patients and their families is vital to ensure shared decision-making aligned with the patient's preferences and circumstances. In conclusion, geriatric ICU care demands a nuanced understanding of age-related changes, comorbidities, financial limitations, and emotional factors. By integrating medical expertise with empathy and interdisciplinary collaboration, healthcare providers can offer optimal care for geriatric patients in the ICU.

Case Scenario

1. You are the infection control nurse in a 20 bedded Medical ICU. One of your staff nurses has returned after a week vacation and has fever and cough. You suspect that this staff nurse may have contracted a respiratory infection that has just recently been seen in the community. How would you identify and manage ill staff nurses? What extra precautions would need to be taken for other staff nurses? What training would staff need?
   You can prepare a self-reporting questionnaire for all those who are new or joining after vacations to identify potential carriers of infection. Those who have symptoms or at risk should be sent to physician for diagnosis and investigations. Make sure that other staff nurses should take proper contact precautions while working with ill staff nurses such as using PPE and proper handwashing. The staff should be trained about understanding importance of reporting symptoms, taking precautions, using adequate PPE, using infection control measures while caring the patient, taking regular vaccinations as per hospital protocols.
2. Mr Rakesh 65-year-old male was admitted in oncology ward. Rakesh arrived to hospital with dyspnea, chest pain, cough with purulent sputum, fatigue and weight loss. Two years ago, he diagnosed with small cell lung cancer. He was on chemotherapy treatment. He has a history of alcoholism since 25 years, hypertensive, still suffering from reflux, reformed smoker. Quit 2 years ago (30 cigarettes/day for the past 20 years). Recent (3 weeks ago) repair of bleeding gastric ulcer and 1 month ago diagnosed with COPD. As per the social history, he used to work in spin mill, long hours. Married with two children and has grandchild.
   On examination, he is alert and oriented, airway is patent, breathing—RR 32 breaths per minute, SpO$_2$ 84/minute on R/A, not talking in full sentences, circulation—BP 170/90 mm Hg, HR 102 (regular), temperature 36.8°C. On physical examination dullness on percussion, decreased breath sounds. X-ray shows right hilar mass and right upper lobe mass. PET scan shows metastasis in brain. In ED he managed with oxygen administration, bronchodilators, analgesics, corticosteroids and to manage nutritional status NG tube inserted. Family counselled about the condition. The family informed health care providers about his desire of DNR (do not resuscitate).

SUMMARY

A critical illness acutely impairs one or more vital organ systems which leads to life-threatening condition. The critically ill patient is a challenge for the ICU team as they require invasive diagnostic tests, advanced procedures, and intensive nursing care. The management and outcome of the patient depend on the severity of organ dysfunction. Critical care nursing focuses on the care of patients who are hemodynamically unstable, require continuous monitoring, advanced care and infection control protocols must be followed in collaboration with various other departments. The communication with critically ill patients is important to meet their physical, psychological needs, their wishes or desires as well as to their family members for decision making process. In life-threatening conditions in order to save the life of the patient, control symptoms, and normalize bodily vital functions emergency drugs are used and these drugs must have short onset of action and be administered in a way to facilitate the rapid onset of action. A patient who is approaching to end of life may experience many physiological symptoms. So, compassionate, symptomatic and quality care must be provided in collaboration with other departments. To ensure continuity of care, provide up-to-date status of the patient and justify the hospital policies which furnish the legal aspects of care, the records are maintained which include the detailed information related to the patient during their stay. The records maintained in ICU are more comprehensive and detailed as compared to other units of the hospital.

MULTIPLE-CHOICE QUESTIONS

1. **The single most important way to control the spread of infection is by:**
   a. Covering the mouth and nose when sneezing and coughing
   b. Disinfecting equipment and surfaces
   c. Thorough handwashing
   d. Wearing gloves, gowns, and mask
2. **What is the color-coding of the bag used in hospitals to dispose of human anatomical wastes such as body parts?**
   a. Yellow   b. Black
   c. Red   d. Blue
3. **Antidote for digoxin toxicity:**
   a. Diltiazem   b. Digibind
   c. Dicyclomine   d. Doxepin
4. **Which of the following is considered as the priority element of the primary survey?**
   a. Brief neurological examination
   b. Diagnostic tests
   c. Assessment of vital signs
   d. Head-to-toe examination
5. **Mr X arrives at the emergency department and suffered from multiple injuries after a road-side accident. Which of the following should be assessed as the highest priority?**
   a. Unequal pupils
   b. Irregular pulse
   c. Ecchymosis on flank area
   d. Deviated trachea

6. When attending a client with a head and neck trauma following a roadside accident, the nurse's initial action is to?
    a. Provide oxygen therapy   b. Start I/V fluids
    c. Immobilize cervical area   d. Perform suctioning
7. Effective treatment of VAP can be ensured by diagnosis based on findings from which of the following?
    a. Chest radiographs   b. Pathological studies
    c. Bronchial alveolar lavage d. Blood Glucose level
8. What test is needed to determine the cause of a central line-associated bloodstream infection?
    a. Blood cultures   b. Complete blood count
    c. Chemistry   d. Glucose
9. Which of the following statement is TRUE for end-of-life care?
    a. It is synonymous with palliative care
    b. It is defined by a specified period
    c. It does not include a focus on the family
    d. It is one aspect of palliative care
10. When documenting in patients' notes what must always be there?
    a. Date, time, signature, name, designation, ward
    b. Date, time, ward, signature
    c. Date, time, signature, name, designation with a code number
    d. Date, time, signature, name

ANSWERS

1. c	2. a	3. b	4. a
5. d	6. c	7. a	8. a
9. d	10. c		

SUGGESTED READING

1. Adams A, Mannix T, Harrington A. Nurses' communication with families in the intensive care unit - a literature review. Nursing in Critical Care. 2015;22(2):70-80.
2. Akula S., Manderwad G, Reddy RS, Rajkumar HRV. Emergence of Extensively drug-resistant Acinetobacter spp in a tertiary care centre of Hyderabad, Telangana state. Indian J Microbiol Res. 2017;4(4):448-52.
3. Al Barraj M, Fawaz M, Badr L. Needs of family members of critically ill patients: A comparison of nurses and family perceptions. Journal of Nursing Education and Practice. 2019;9(9):81.
4. ALBERT R. End-of-Life Care: Managing Common Symptoms. American Family Physician. 2017;95(6):356-361.
5. Arora B, Bhardwaj U, Rajlaxmi R, Bansal P, Girdhar K. Visual Communication Board for Communication Compromised Patients. IOSR Journal of Nursing and Health Science. 2017;06(03):01-07.
6. Babbar P, Biswal M, Behera D, Gupta A. Healthcare-associated infections in intensive care units: A pilot study in a tertiary care public hospital in India. Journal of Prevention & Infection Control. 2019; 5(1):1-5.
7. Bheemavarapu H, Arief M, Ahmad A, Patel I. Nosocomial infections in India: The unaddressed lacunae! Journal of Pharmacy Practice and Community Medicine. 2018;4(2):43-43.
8. Boscart VM. A communication intervention for nursing staff in chronic care. J Adv Nurs. 2009;65:1823-32.
9. Choudhuri A, Chakravarty M, Uppal R. Epidemiology and characteristics of nosocomial infections in critically ill patients in a tertiary care intensive care unit of Northern India. Saudi Journal of Anaesthesia. 2017;11(4):402.
10. Correia MI, Waitzberg DL. The impact of malnutrition on morbidity, mortality, length of hospital stay and costs evaluated through a multivariate model analysis. Clin Nutr. 2003 Jun;22(3):235-9. doi: 10.1016/s0261-5614(02)00215-7. PMID: 12765661.
11. Dithole K, Thupayagale-Tshweneagae G, Akpor O, Moleki M. Communication skills intervention: promoting effective communication between nurses and mechanically ventilated patients. BMC Nursing. 2017;16(1).
12. Drews FA. Patient Monitors in Critical Care: Lessons for Improvement. Advances in Patient Safety: New Directions and Alternative Approaches (Vol. 3: Performance and Tools). Rockville (MD): Agency for Healthcare Research and Quality (US); 2008 Aug. Available from: https://www.ncbi.nlm.nih.gov/books/NBK43684/
13. Ducel G, Fabry J, Nicolle L. Prevention of hospital-acquired infections: A practical guide [Internet]. 2nd ed. Geneva: World Health Organization; 2021 [cited 5 September 2021]. Available from: https://www.who.int/csr/resources/publications/whocdscsreph200212.pdf
14. Edwardson S, Cairns C. Nosocomial infections in the ICU. Anaesthesia & Intensive Care Medicine. 2019;20(1):14-18.
15. Finke E, Light J, Kitko L. A systematic review of the effectiveness of nurse communication with patients with complex communication needs with a focus on the use of augmentative and alternative communication. Journal of Clinical Nursing. 2008;17(16):2102-15.
16. Fox M. Improving Communication with Patients and Families in the Intensive Care Unit. Journal of Hospice & Palliative Nursing. 2014;16(2):93-98.
17. Giordano J, Abramson K, Boswell MV. Pain assessment: subjectivity, objectivity, and the use of neurotechnology. Pain Physician. 2010;13(4):305-15. PMID: 20648198.
18. Happ M, Seaman J, Nilsen M, Sciulli A, Tate J, Saul M et al. The number of mechanically ventilated ICU patients meeting communication criteria. Heart & Lung. 2015;44(1):45-49.
19. Hariharan U, Garg R. Sedation and analgesia in critical care. Journal of Anesthesia & Critical Care: Open Access. 2017;7(3). 00262.
20. Haskey E. Nursing critically ill patients in the intensive care unit. In Practice. 2016;38(S4):25-29.
21. Hazra A, Dasgupta S, Das S, Chawan N. Nosocomial infections in the intensive care unit: Incidence, risk factors, outcome and associated pathogens in a public tertiary teaching hospital of Eastern India. Indian Journal of Critical Care Medicine. 2015;19(1):14-20.
22. Huygh J, Peeters Y, Bernards J, Malbrain MLNG. Hemodynamic monitoring in the critically ill: an overview of current cardiac output monitoring methods [version 1; referees: 3 approved] F1000Research 2016, 5(F1000 Faculty Rev):2855 (doi: 10.12688/f1000research.8991.1)
23. Jain R, Agarwal R, Agarwal N, Prabhat N. Nosocomial Infections in ICU-Review article. Flora and Fauna. 2015;21(2):283-92.
24. Jarzyna D, Jungquist C, Pasero C, Willens J, Nisbet A, Oakes L, et al. American Society for Pain Management Nursing Guidelines on Monitoring for Opioid-Induced Sedation and Respiratory Depression. Pain Management Nursing. 2011;12(3):118-45.e10.
25. Kaplan S, Greenfield S, Ware J. Assessing the Effects of Physician-Patient Interactions on the Outcomes of Chronic Disease. Medical Care. 1989;27(Supplement):110-27.
26. Kaur S, Bhagat H. Nursing management of brain dead organ donors. In Kaur S, Singh M. Clinical Neurosciences and Critical Care Nursing. Jaypee Medical Publishers, New Delhi, 1st Edition; 2014 ISBN 978-93-5152-200-3.
27. Kaur S, Ghai S, Krishnan N, Rana D, Kathania D, Kaur G, et al. Knowledge, attitude and perception regarding organ donation among the Nursing students. J Postgrad Med Edu Res. 2015;49(3):105-10.
28. Khan H, Baig F, Mehboob R. Nosocomial infections: Epidemiology, prevention, control and surveillance. Asian Pacific Journal of Tropical Biomedicine. 2017;7(5):478-82.
29. KONDRUP J. Nutritional risk screening (NRS 2002): a new method based on an analysis of controlled clinical trials. Clinical Nutrition. 2003;22(3):321-36.
30. Kozier. Fundamentals of Nursing: Concepts, Process, and Practice. 5th edition. Addison-Wesley; 163-183.673-701.
31. Kumari S, Kaur S, Singh A, Mukherjee KK. Reliability of a 'Communication Chart' for Conscious Patients on Mechanical

Ventilator or Tracheostomy Admitted in Intensive Care Unit of a Tertiary Care Referral Center, India. Journal of Nursing Science and Practice Volume. 2011;1(3):28-3.
32. Kumar S, Sen P, Gaind R, Verma P, Gupta P, Suri P, et al. Prospective surveillance of device-associated health care–associated infection in an intensive care unit of a tertiary care hospital in New Delhi, India. American Journal of Infection Control. 2018;46(2):202-6.
33. Kynoch K, Chang A, Coyer F, McArdle A. The effectiveness of interventions to meet family needs of critically ill patients in an adult intensive care unit. JBI Database of Systematic Reviews and Implementation Reports. 2016;14(3):181-234.
34. Lewis's. Medical-Surgical Nursing. Assessment and Management of problems. 2nd south Asian Edition. Vol.1. Elsevier; 138-51.
35. Magill SS, Edwards JR, Bamberg W, et al. Multistate point-prevalence survey of healthcare–associated infections. N Engl J Med. 2014;370:1198-208 (CDC HAI Prevalence Survey).
36. Martin S J, Yost RJ. Infectious Diseases in the Critically Ill Patients. J Pharm Pract. 2011;24(1):35-43. doi:10.1177/0897190010388906
37. McGuire D, Reifsnyder J, Soeken K, Kaiser K, Yeager K. Assessing pain in nonresponsive hospice patients: Development and preliminary testing of the multidimensional objective pain assessment tool (MOPAT). Journal of Palliative Medicine. 2011;14(3):287-92.
38. Muhasin Gowda N. Nosocomial infections: A review article. International Journal of Science and Research (IJSR). 2020;9(9):431-34.
39. Murray A, Chambers J, Van Saene. Infections in patients requiring ventilation in intensive care: application of a new classification. Clinical Microbiology and Infection. 1998;4(2):94-99.
40. Müller M, Dahdal S, Saffarini M, Uehlinger D, Arampatzis S. Evaluation of Nutrition Risk Screening Score 2002 (NRS) assessment in hospitalized chronic kidney disease patient. PLOS ONE. 2019;14(1):1-11.
41. Nursing: Record of Intensive Care Unit (rajnursing.blogspot.com). 2017.
42. Olsen H, Strom T, Lars M, Oxlund J, Wian K, Kroken B, et al. Non-sedation or light sedation in critically ill, mechanically ventilated patients. New England Journal of Medicine. 2020;382(26):1103-11.
43. Pandharipande P, Hughes, McGrane. Sedation in the intensive care setting. Clin Pharmacol: Advances and Applications. 2012;4:53-63
44. Patak L, Wilson-Stronks A, Costello J, Kleinpell RM, Henneman EA, Person C, et al. Improving Patient-Provider Communication A Call to Action. Journal of Nursing Administration 2009;39(9):372-6.
45. Patel F, Vegad M. Prevalence of nosocomial infections by multidrug-resistant organisms in patients admitted to the critical care area of the regional cancer center, Gujarat, India. Sri Lankan Journal of Infectious Diseases. 2019;9(2):129.
46. Petosic A, Viravong M, Martin A, Nilsen C, Olafsen K, Berntzen H. Above cuff vocalization (ACV): A scoping review. Acta Anesthesiologic Scandinavica. 2020;65(1):15-25.
47. Puntillo K. Pain assessment and management for intensive care unit patients: Seeking best practices. ICU Management & Practice. 2016;16(4):233-6.
48. Raja SN, Carr DB, Cohen M, Finnerup NB, Flor H, Gibson S, et al. The revised International Association for the Study of Pain definition of pain: concepts, challenges, and compromises. Pain. 2020;161(9):1976-82.
49. Ramasubramanian V, Iyer V, Sewlikar S, Desai A. Epidemiology of healthcare acquired infection: An Indian perspective on surgical site infection and catheter related blood stream infection. Indian Journal of Basic and Applied Medical Research. 2014;3(4):46-63.
50. Ratna H. The importance of effective communication in healthcare practice. Harvard Public Health Review. 2019;23:1-6.
51. Sharma KS. Textbook of Pharmacology, Pathology, and Genetics for Nurses, 1st edition. Jaypee brothers; 2016;1:326-43.
52. Singer P, Blaser A, Berger M, Alhazzani W, Calder P, Casaer M, et al. ESPEN guideline on clinical nutrition in the intensive care unit. Clinical Nutrition. 2019;38(1):48-79.
53. Singer P. Preserving the quality of life: nutrition in the ICU. Critical Care. 2019;23(S1):139.
54. Suddarth's and Brunner. Textbook of Medical-Surgical Nursing. South Asian Edition. Vol II. Wolters Kluwer; 2029-2050.
55. Taj A, Shamin A, Khanday S, Ommid M. Prevalence of common nosocomial organisms in Surgical Intensive Care Unit in North India: A hospital-based study. International Journal of Critical Illness and Injury Science. 2018; 8(2):78-82.
56. Ten Hoorn S, Elbers P, Girbes A, Tuinman P. Communicating with conscious and mechanically ventilated critically ill patients: a systematic review. Critical Care. 2016;20(1).
57. Tripathi K. Essential of Pharmacology for Dentistry, 3rd edition. New Delhi, India: Jaypee Brothers Medical Publishers(P) Ltd; 2005. pp. 94-107.
58. Velasco C, Garcia E, Rodriguez V, Frias L, Garriga R, Alvarez J, et al. Comparison of four nutritional screening tools to detect nutritional risk in hospitalized Patients: a multicentre study. European journal of clinical nutrition. 2011;65(2):269-74. Epub 2010/11/18. pmid:21081958.
59. Wright D, Brajtman S, Cragg B, Macdonald M. Delirium as letting go: An ethnographic analysis of hospice care and family moral experience. Palliative Medicine. 2015;29(10):959-66.
60. Wright J, Williams R, Wilkinson J. Health needs assessment: Development and importance of health needs assessment. BMJ. 1998;316(7140):1310-3.
61. Yoo H, Lim O, Shim J. Critical care nurses' communication experiences with patients and families in an intensive care unit: A qualitative study. PLOS ONE. 2020;15(7):e0235694.

UNIT IX

Occupational and Industrial Disorders

OUTLINE

53. Occupational and Industrial Disorders (Occupational Hazards Among Nurses)
Khaiwal Ravindra, Pooja Parihar, Suman Mor

Occupational and Industrial Disorders (Occupational Hazards Among Nurses)

CHAPTER 53

Ravindra Khaiwal, Pooja Parihar, Suman Mor

"I believe in protecting people and not killing people through easily preventable occupational diseases."
—Steven Magee

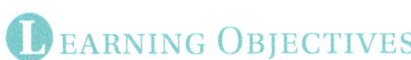

After going through the chapter, the learner will be able to:
- Define occupational hazards among nurses.
- Describe the related diagnostic modalities.
- Elaborate the efforts to solve the problems of nurses suffering from occupational disorders.

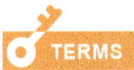

- **Hazard:** Something which is dangerous and, such asly to cause damage.
- **Occupational diseases:** A disorder caused by the work environment.
- **Occupational hazards:** A hazard experienced at the workplace.

INTRODUCTION

Occupational health is defined as the highest degree of physical, mental, and social well-being of workers in all occupations. It is the branch of healthcare which deals with all aspects of health and safety at the workplace.

A workplace incident or exposure that triggers or leads to a disease or worsens a pre-existing condition is referred to as an occupational illness. There are a number of factors that are related to the workplace environment and other risk factors which may lead to the occurrence of occupation-related illnesses. Various categories of occupational diseases include ergonomics-related factors leading to occupational injuries; the chemical occupational factors involving exposure to dust, gases, acid, alkali, metals, etc.; physical factors including exposure to noise, heat, radiation, etc. The major occupational diseases are silicosis, musculoskeletal injuries, coal workers' pneumoconiosis, chronic obstructive lung diseases, asbestosis, byssinosis, anthracosis, pesticide poisoning, noise-induced hearing loss, contact dermatitis, and occupational cancer, etc. All these disorders are already discussed in various other chapters under related systems. The current chapter specifically focuses on the occupational hazards among nurses.

One of the most common occupational diseases among hospital employees is musculoskeletal disorders (MSDs) and occupational stress is also found to be very common. Among hospital employees, nurses are the most vulnerable to MSDs and occupational stress. Musculoskeletal disorders (MSDs), such as low back, shoulder, and arm pain, are pervasive worldwide and are associated with high costs for people, employers, and society.

Musculoskeletal disorders are a serious issue in terms of absenteeism and workability. Adult patients with acute and chronic diseases, as well as a wide range of medical and surgical complications, are cared for by registered nurses, who work mainly in hospitals. Nurses play a vital role in healthcare institutions, and the healthcare system's performance will be jeopardized without a practical and resourceful nursing staff. Physical and mental health issues among nurses and increased work-related stressors are undeniably essential factors in lowering the quantity and quality of their work, particularly when caring for patients. Working three shifts in challenging areas, such as cancer or emergency rooms and caring for ill patients puts nurses under many mental, emotional, and physical strains.

Due to a combination of increased risk and fewer safety procedures, nurses in underdeveloped nations have a higher risk of contracting blood-borne infections through occupational contact. Nurses are subjected to a combination of work environment and personal factors that cause occupational stress. Nurses must have advanced critical thinking skills, a broad understanding of disease states and body systems, strong management abilities, and the ability to remain calm under pressure. Developing countries confront numerous challenges in reducing the danger of occupational exposure among nurses. On the international and national levels, efforts have been undertaken to solve the issues of nurses suffering from occupational diseases and are vulnerable to get suffering.

CONCEPT AND DEFINITION

Occupational disease is defined as any disease contracted mainly as a result of exposure to risk factors resulting from job activity.

An occupational/industrial worker may be exposed to five types of hazards, depending upon his occupation **(Table 53.1)**.

TABLE 53.1: Types of occupational hazards.

Physical hazards	**Heat and cold**	• Heat is a very common physical hazard. The direct exposure to heat causes the heat exhaustion, burns, heat cramps, and heat stroke. Heat also affects indirectly which in turn causes decreased efficiency, increased fatigue and enhanced accident rates • Radiant heat is the main problem in foundry, glass and steel industries, while heat stagnation is the principal problem in the jute and cotton textile industry • Physical work under such conditions is very stressful and impairs the health and efficiency of the workers • According to the study by Rao (1952, 1953) and Mookerjee et al. (1953) indicates that a corrected effective temperature of 69–80°F (20–27°C) is the comfort zone in this country and temperatures above 80°F (27°C) cause discomfort • Important hazards associated with cold work are erythrocyanosis, frostbite and immersion foot as a result of cutaneous vasoconstriction
	Noise	• **Auditory effects:** Temporary or permanent hearing loss • **Non-auditory effects:** Nervousness, fatigue, interference with communication by speech, decreased efficiency and annoyance
	Light	• Exposure to poor illumination causes headache, eye strain, eye pain, lachrymation and congestion around the cornea its chronic effect includes "miner's nystagmus" • Exposure to excessive brightness or "glare" is associated with discomfort, annoyance and visual fatigue. Intense direct glare may also result in blurring of vision and lead to accidents • Therefore, sufficient and suitable lighting which can be natural or artificial should be there wherever persons are working
	Ionizing radiation	• **Ionizing radiation:** X-rays and radioactive isotopes • Radiation hazards includes genetic changes, malformation, cancer, leukemia, depilation, ulceration, sterility and in extreme cases death • The International Commission of Radiological Protection has set the maximum permissible level of occupational exposure at 5 rem per year to the whole body
	UV radiation	• Exposure occurs mainly in arc welding • These radiations affect the eyes, causing intense conjunctivitis and keratitis (Welder's flash)
	Vibration	• Vibration especially in the frequency range 10 to 500 Hz, may be encountered in work with pneumatic tools, such as drills and hammers • Exposure to vibration may also produce injuries to the joints of the hands, elbows and shoulders
Chemical hazards	**Local action**	Causes dermatitis, eczema, ulcers and even cancer by primary irritant action
	Inhalation	**Dust** • Produced in a number of industries mines, foundry, quarry, pottery, textile, wood or stone working industries • Particles smaller than 5 microns are directly inhaled into the lungs arid are retained there. This fraction of the dust is called "respirable dust", and is mainly responsible for pneumoconiosis • **Inorganic dusts:** Silica, mica, coal, asbestos dust • **Organic dusts:** Cotton and jute • The most common dust diseases in this country are silicosis and anthracosis **Gases** • **Simple gases:** Oxygen and hydrogen • **Asphyxiating gases:** Carbon monoxide, cyanide gas, sulfur dioxide and chlorine • **Anesthetic gases:** Chloroform, ether and trichlorethylene • Carbon monoxide hazard is frequently reported in coal-gas manufacturing plants and steel industry
Biological hazards		• Workers may be exposed to infective and parasitic agents at the place of work • Brucellosis, leptospirosis, anthrax, hydatidosis, psittacosis, tetanus, encephalitis, fungal infections and schistosomiasis are occupational disorders under this category

Contd...

Contd...

Mechanical hazards		About 10% of accidents in the industry are due to mechanical causes
Psychosocial hazards		Frustration, lack of job satisfaction, insecurity, poor human relationships, emotional tension are some of the psychosocial factors that may undermine both physical and mental health of the workers
		The effects can be classified in two categories: 1. **Psychological and behavioral changes:** Including aggressiveness, anxiety, depression, alcoholism, drug abuse and sickness 2. **Psychosomatic ill health:** Including fatigue, headache; pain in the shoulders, neck and back; peptic ulcer, hypertension, heart disease and rapid ageing

Occupational disease in nurses varies from physical to mental disorders. Nurses are highly vulnerable to musculoskeletal disorders that may be confined to muscles, joints, tendons, ligaments, and nerves that may lead to lower back pain, neck, knee and shoulder discomfort, and discomfort in the wrist and elbow.

CLASSIFICATION OF OCCUPATIONAL DISORDERS

Occupational disorders can be classified into several categories based on their nature and causative factors. Here are some of the common classifications of occupational disorders:

1. **Musculoskeletal disorders (MSDs):** These are disorders that affect the muscles, joints, and bones due to repetitive strain, awkward posture, or other physical factors associated with work. Some examples of MSDs include back pain, carpal tunnel syndrome, and tennis elbow.
2. **Respiratory disorders:** These disorders are caused by exposure to dust, chemicals, fumes, or other harmful substances that can damage the lungs and respiratory system. Examples of respiratory disorders include asthma, pneumoconiosis, and chronic obstructive pulmonary disease (COPD).
3. **Skin disorders:** These disorders are caused by exposure to chemicals, radiation, or other substances that can irritate or damage the skin. Examples of skin disorders include dermatitis, eczema, and skin cancer.
4. **Psychological disorders:** These disorders are caused by stress, pressure, and other psychological factors associated with work. Examples of psychological disorders include anxiety, depression, and post-traumatic stress disorder (PTSD).
5. **Cardiovascular disorders:** These disorders are caused by exposure to physical and emotional stress associated with work. Examples of cardiovascular disorders include hypertension, heart disease

EPIDEMIOLOGY

The highest level of physical, mental, and social well-being of workers in all industries is described as occupational health. Occupational disorders, such as musculoskeletal disorders, mental stress, etc., lead to absenteeism among nursing practitioners. Approximately 180.8 per 100,000 capita injuries are globally attributable to occupations and in low middle-income countries of South-East Asia, occupational injuries accounted for 97.5 per 100,000 capita in 2004. Out of these injuries, 2.51 per 100,000 deaths were attributable to occupations in low-middle-income countries in South-East Asia in 2004. Globally, 5.48 per 100,000 capita deaths were attributable to occupations in 2004.

Ergonomic-related stress globally had affected approximately 13.99 per 100,000 capita and in lower-middle-income countries in the South-East Asia region were affected 15.65 per 100,000 capita in the same year. Specific work-related hazards, such as injuries, noise, oncogenic agents, air pollutants, and ergonomic hazards, make for a significant portion of the chronic illness burden—back pain accounts for 37% of all cases, hearing loss for 16%, the chronic obstructive pulmonary disease for 13%, asthma for 11%, injuries for 8%, lung cancer for 9%, leukemia for 2%, and depression for 8% of all cases.

Global Scenario

A comprehensive review of the literature was conducted, which included the majority of publications published in peer-reviewed journals on the topic of 'Occupational and Industrial Disorders'. On a global scale, a wide range of workplace threats were observed in the nursing profession as reported in **Table 53.2**.

A study conducted in New Zealand reported that among the musculoskeletal disorders, low back pain and wrist pain had the highest proportion (76% each). Another study reported that the prevalence of musculoskeletal disorders among nurses was 79.52% and the waist (64.83%), neck (61.83%), and shoulder (52.36%) were the most affected. However, in another study, 58.1% of the nurses reported low back pain. The factors associated with low back pain were high BMI, poor physical condition, working in awkward postures, etc.

In another study, mild-to-severe depression (50.5%), anxiety (51.8%) and stress (41.7%) were reported among nurses and 61.9% of the nurses reported psychological effects of COVID-19. Another study reported that the incidence rate of occupational skin diseases among nurses and assistant nurses were 3.3 and 2.7/10000 per year. The most common cause of skin diseases among healthcare workers was the use of rubber chemicals and preservatives.

A study conducted in Ghana reported that nurses are aware of the risk of occupational hepatitis B infection; however, 94.4% of the nurses perceived that they were at high risk of HBV infection and post-exposure management could be managed by only 23.4% of the subjects. Another study conducted in Mexico City reported that communicable diseases and musculoskeletal injuries are the most common problems in the nursing profession. Musculoskeletal

TABLE 53.2: Studies highlighting the occupational disorders among nurses.

Authors	Major observation
Harcombe et al., 2014	Among the musculoskeletal disorders, low back pain and wrist pain had the highest prevalence (76% each)
Yan et al., 2018	The prevalence of musculoskeletal disorders among nurses was 79.52% and it affected mainly the waist (64.83%), neck (61.83%), and shoulder (52.36%)
Boughattas et al., 2017	A major proportion (58.1%) of nurses reported low back pain
Chowdhury et al., 2021	Mild-to-severe depression (50.5%), anxiety (51.8%) and stress (41.7%) were reported among nurses and 61.9% of the nurses reported psychological effects of COVID-19
Aalto-Korte et al., 2021	The incidence rate of occupational skin diseases among nurses and assistant nurses were 3.3 and 2.7/10000 per year
Konlan et al., 2017	94.4% of the nurses perceived that they were at high risk of getting HBV infection
Silva et al., 2018	Musculoskeletal disorders were reported among a maximum of 86.24% of workers and almost 43% of nurses showed signs of drowsiness
Kshetrimayum et al., 2019	Occupational stress among 49.8% of nurses. Perceived level of stress among 55.4% of the nurses
Chaudhari et al., 2018	Mild stress was reported in 51.5% of nurses, moderate stress in 34% of nurses and severe stress in 2.10% of nurses
Bhatia et al., 2010	Occupational stress was found to be in 87.4% of nurses
Jain et al., 2010	Dermatitis was reported in 64% of nurses
Nair RS, 2020	Low back pain was reported in 73.8% of nurses. Reasons for low back pain were lifting patients (61.9%), moving trolly (47.6%) and long duration of file works (45.2%), etc.

disorders were reported among a maximum of 86.24% of workers and almost 43% of nurses showed signs of drowsiness.

Indian Scenario

A study conducted in Mysuru (Mysore) city in India reported that 49.8% of the nurses suffered from occupational stress and the perceived level of stress was in 55.4% of the respondents. A similar study conducted in Maharashtra reported that mild stress was reported in 51.5% of nurses, moderate in 34% of nurses and severe stress in 2.10% of nurses. However, in another study, occupational stress was found in 87.4% of nurses and they perceived that time pressure is one of the causes of stressful life as they have to handle simultaneous work, such as along with occupation household work, caring for children and parents, etc. According to a study conducted in Northern India very high incidence of contact dermatitis was seen in nurses. According to 64% of nurses, dermatitis is caused by repeated exposure to allergens or irritants in the workplace.

A study conducted in South India reported that approximately 73.8% of the nurses reported low back pain. A maximum of the nurses (66.7%) reported that low back pain was caused by standing for a long duration of time. Other reasons for low back pain were lifting patients (61.9%), moving trolly (47.6%) and long duration of file works (45.2%), etc.

RISK FACTORS AND ETIOLOGY

Risk factors of occupational health disorders include physical, biological, ergonomic, chemical, and psychological factors.

- ❖ Musculoskeletal pains or physical hazards and accidents are caused due to:
  - ➢ Physically lifting and moving patients
  - ➢ Handling sharp objects
  - ➢ Uncomfortable working conditions
  - ➢ Standing and walking for long periods of time
- ❖ Working in three shifts in stressful environments, such as in emergency rooms, as well as caring for sick patients, puts nurses under a lot of mental and physical strain.
- ❖ Communicable and contagious diseases can threaten the health of the nurses because of exposure to injections, suturing and blood and other body fluids.
- ❖ Chemical hazardous material includes disinfectants and sterility materials, such as glutaraldehyde and ethylene oxide, chemotherapy drugs, and latex contact, etc.

PATHOPHYSIOLOGY

Occupational hazards among nurses result from performing long duration or repetitive tasks, such as lifting patients, moving trollies, etc. These repeated tasks lead to an inflammatory response that leads to tissue injury or breakdown of tissues that causes fibrosis resulting in pain and loss of motor function. Long duration of forceful tasks results in chronic inflammation of the tissues that lead to sickness, depression, and anxiety-like conditions, as shown in **Flowchart 53.1**.

CLINICAL MANIFESTATIONS

- ❖ Work overload causes stress and fatigue.
- ❖ Sleep deprivation due to night shifts.
- ❖ Working in awkward positions, lifting, or moving of obese patients, etc., may lead to back injuries or back pain, or temporary and permanent disabilities.
- ❖ Exposure to ionizing radiation results in an increased risk of miscarriage, stillbirth, cancers, such as leukemia, bone and skin cancer.
- ❖ Nurses working in mental health services have long been targets of patient abuse.
- ❖ Exposure to blood-borne pathogens leads to infectious diseases, such as hepatitis B, tuberculosis, HIV, etc.

DIAGNOSTIC MODALITIES

To diagnose an occupational disease, various variables must be investigated that are typically overlooked while taking only the patient's medical history. Questions could be used to enhance the clinical history. Some of the questions for a causal relationship of occupational diseases are:

1. How long does it take from the initial exposure to the onset of symptoms?

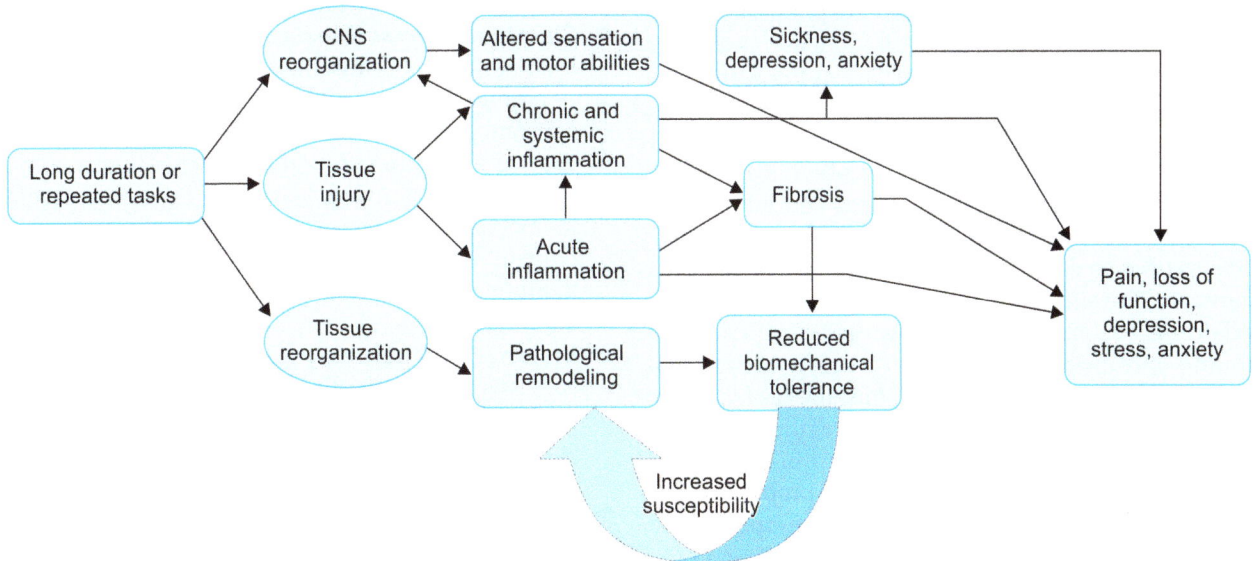

Flowchart 53.1: Occupational hazards among nurses resulting from performing long duration or repetitive tasks.

2. If you are not exposed anymore, have the symptoms been improved?
3. If you are still exposed while doing the same work, have the symptoms got worsened or increased?
4. Are your coworkers experiencing the same symptoms as you as a result of the same exposure?

   Examining for the presence of an occupational ailment frequently necessitates the assessment of:
   - Evidence from epidemiological research demonstrates that the same environmental agents caused the specific ailment or disease.
   - Chemical components found in each product describe the kind of symptoms that the material could induce also include information, such as "risk phrases".
   - Enlist occupational diseases associated with that chemical, activity, or practice.
   - Notify the public health authorities about the incidence of the occupational illness case.

Needle stick injury (NSIs)
- Needle stick injuries refer to injuries that occur when needles or other sharp medical instruments pierce the skin of healthcare workers or other individuals. These types of injuries are common in healthcare settings and can occur in any clinical environment where sharp objects are used.
- The consequences of needle stick injuries can be serious, and can include infection with diseases, such as HIV, hepatitis B, and hepatitis C. These infections can have long-term consequences for healthcare workers, and can even result in death.
- In addition to the physical consequences of needle stick injuries, there are also psychological consequences. Healthcare workers who experience needle stick injuries may become anxious or fearful about future exposure to needles or other sharp objects. This can lead to a decrease in productivity and quality of care, as well as an increased risk of turnover.
- To prevent needle stick injuries, healthcare workers should take precautions, such as wearing protective clothing and gloves, disposing of used needles appropriately, and avoiding unnecessary handling of sharp objects. Healthcare facilities should also have policies and procedures in place to minimize the risk of needle stick injuries, and should provide education and training to healthcare workers on how to prevent and manage these injuries.

- In conclusion, needle stick injuries are a serious risk to healthcare workers and others who come into contact with sharp objects in clinical settings. Preventative measures should be taken to minimize the risk of these injuries, and healthcare workers should be provided with education and training to protect themselves from this occupational hazard.

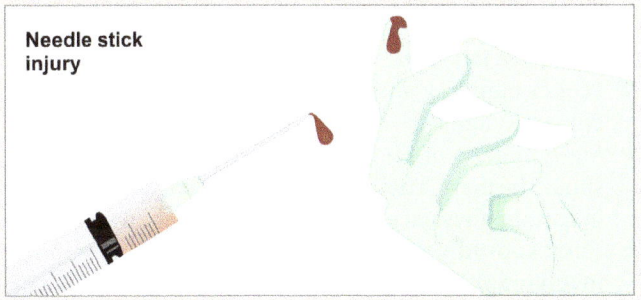

Needle stick injury

OCCUPATIONAL HEALTH MANAGEMENT

Avoid occupational diseases or illnesses through continuous workplace monitoring, early detection, evaluation, and control of work-related health hazards. For this, there should be:
- ❖ Periodic medical examination
- ❖ Availability of special medical examinations for specific health hazards
- ❖ Training and understanding of occupational health hazards and how to avoid them, ergonomic training, and so on.

To prevent occupational diseases, a system must be established, implemented, and continued to encourage safe and healthy working habits and provide a healthy work environment. Healthy working policies must be established to prevent the occupational diseases. Hygienic eating place at healthcare facilities should be there. Such areas should have sufficient rest place and should be away from hazardous areas. Workers should remove their PPE (personal protective equipment) kit and relax away from potentially dangerous work locations.

Prevention of Occupational Hazards Among Nurses

Occupational health is the highest degree of physical, mental, and social well-being of workers in all occupations. It deals with all the aspects of health and safety at the workplace with special emphasis on primary prevention of hazards. The safe, healthy, and positive work environment will have a positive impact on productivity and economic and social development. So, prevention of hazards should form an essential part of economic activities.

Nurses have an essential role in providing patients care. As shown in **Flowchart 53.2**, the management of patients includes initial estimate and tracking, care of patients with acute and chronic symptoms, treatment of critically-ill patients, and care of the deceased. Thus, the protection of nurses' health at healthcare facilities requires the prevention of occupational dangers also. To prevent occupational hazards among nurses, there is a need to prepare action protocols and training and information campaigns on preventive matters.

- ❖ Nurses must follow good hand hygiene practices, such as washing hands properly before and after caring for a patient.
- ❖ Preventative measures for infectious accidents include wearing personal safety gear, such as masks, face shields, eye protectors, etc.
- ❖ Safer injection techniques such as needlestick injuries might put nurses' health at risk. So, safe injection practices should be followed.
- ❖ Proper handling and disposal of material that could be contaminated.
- ❖ Maintenance of both physical and mental well-being should be there. They should regularly engage themselves in certain physical exercises to build up their stamina.
- ❖ They should practice principles of body mechanics involving proper moving and lifting techniques while caring for their patients.
- ❖ Everyone should try to create a positive work environment.

GERIATRIC CONSIDERATIONS

When it comes to occupational hazards, nurses who are caring for elderly patients must take special geriatric factors into mind. Elderly patients sometimes have several long-term medical conditions, necessitating a more all-encompassing strategy for nursing care. When caring for old patients, nurses should consider the following geriatric factors and occupational hazards:

- ❖ **Management of drugs:** Elderly patients frequently take several medications, which raises the risk of negative drug responses and interactions. Nurses must make sure that patients are properly taking their prescriptions and monitoring for any negative side effects.
- ❖ **Emotional stress:** Nursing staff must take care of their mental health because handling geriatric patients can be emotionally taxing. They ought to take breaks, look for assistance, and take care of themselves.
- ❖ **Prevention of infection:** Older patients' immune systems may be compromised, leaving them more susceptible to infections. Nurses are required to adhere to infection control standards, which include maintaining good hand hygiene, donning the proper PPE, and sanitizing equipment.
- ❖ **Violence and aggressive behavior:** Elderly patients suffering from dementia or delirium may exhibit violent or aggressive behavior, endangering nursing. To stop violence, nurses should be able to spot the warning signals of hostility and take the necessary precautions
- ❖ **Cognitive impairment:** Elderly persons who suffer from cognitive impairment, such as dementia or delirium, may find it challenging to comprehend instructions or express their demands. To support patients with intellectual disabilities, nurses must utilize tactics for effective communication.
- ❖ **Falls:** Nurses must take the necessary precautions to prevent falls in elderly patients because they are more vulnerable. However, when helping patients, nurses also run the risk of suffering injuries from falls. Nurses must employ the proper tools, such as bed supports, transfer belts, and gait belts, to prevent falls. Additionally, they must determine the patients' fall risk and create a fall prevention strategy.

When it comes to occupational or industrial dangers, nurses who care for elderly patients must take special geriatric factors into mind. They must be aware of the dangers involved in taking care of and take the necessary precautions to protect patients' safety and prevent harm. In addition to providing safe and effective care for older patients, nurses can safeguard their own health and well-being by being aware of these hazards and taking the appropriate safeguards.

> **Case Scenario**
>
> 1. A 15-year-old boy was diagnosed with acute myelocytic leukemia. He was in severe agony, enraged, terrified, and completely reliant on others to supply his bodily requirements. The boy realized he was dying as his health worsened. The boy's physical and emotional requirements grew as his condition deteriorated. The nurses vowed that he would not be left alone and that he would not be permitted to suffer. He was assigned a primary care nurse, by the staff, who would coordinate and organize the increasing amount of care he would require. Boy was unable to walk within a few days due to the discomfort he was experiencing as a result of his sickness. He was frequently feverish, with nausea, vomiting, and diarrhea. For the boy and his nurses, nighttime was especially challenging. One evening, he requested his nurse to stay with him, even though that she had already worked all day. Also, she suffered from severe back and arm pain (musculoskeletal disorder) due to long working hours. She remained in the ward to take care of her patients. Unfortunately, another member of the staff nurse fell ill and there was a shortage of staff nurses to take care of patients. One of the nurses was with the boy for the most part. If the patient has not recovered, the nurses would undoubtedly experience guilt, irritation, and resentment, etc.

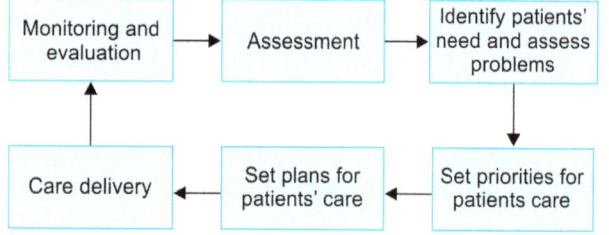

Flowchart 53.2: Nursing management of patients.

This seems that work overload and stress are two major variables that endanger nurses' health and can lead to burnout and weariness. Working three shifts, in challenging areas, such as emergency rooms, and caring for incurable patients puts nurses under a lot of mental, emotional, and physical strain.

2. Maggie is a licensed nurse that works in a hospital's emergency room. Her right shoulder and lower back have both been giving her pain and discomfort for a while now. After each shift, she experiences physical and emotional exhaustion. Maggie decides to see a doctor since she believes her problems are caused by her work as a nurse. Maggie is diagnosed with a musculoskeletal issue that was brought on by the repetitive lifting and shifting of patients throughout her shifts. Her employer has recommended her take some time off work so she may relax and get physical rehabilitation. Maggie's situation is common. The risks that nurse experience on the job can result in infections, injuries, and psychological discomfort. The physical strain of lifting and carrying people has resulted in a musculoskeletal injury in Maggie's case, which necessitates medical attention.

In conclusion, workplace risks for nurses are a serious issue that calls for attention from healthcare providers and employers. By giving nurses the right training, tools, and support, they may work in a secure setting that enhances their well-being and quality of life.

3. Sam is a licensed nurse who works at a busy hospital in a significant urban area. She has been employed in the healthcare sector for more than 10 years and enjoys her profession, but she has recently been exposed to a number of workplace dangers that are negatively affecting her health and well-being.

Physical strain: Sam suffers from severe back discomfort and heel pain as a result of spending most of her shift standing up. Along with helping a patient who had fallen out of bed, she also suffered a shoulder injury.

Sam is continuously at risk for contracting infectious diseases, such as COVID-19 and TB. She must put on personal protective equipment (PPE), such as gloves, a mask, and a dressing gown to shield herself from these infections.

Sam works in a hospital that employs a variety of chemicals, including chemotherapeutic drugs, cleaning products, and disinfectants. Her exposure to these substances led to skin inflammation and breathing issues.

Violence: Patients and even coworkers have abused Sam verbally and physically. A patient who was agitated and disoriented attacked her.

Conclusion: Numerous workplaces risks that Sam is exposed to have an impact on her health and well-being. These risks are frequent among nurses, so it is essential for healthcare companies to offer the right training, tools, and assistance to reduce the dangers of the profession. In order to protect herself from these risks, Sam should take the appropriate measures, such as using PPE, reporting any instances of abuse or violence, and taking regular breaks to reduce both physical and mental stress.

SUMMARY

Medical-surgical nursing is subjected to various occupational hazards. Among occupational diseases, musculoskeletal disorders and mental disorders are the most common. Some of the infections, such as hepatitis B virus, HIV, COVID-19 and many others are serious health problems that can be transmitted from patients to healthcare workers. During COVID-19 time, the occupational stress was higher among nurses. Also, nurses are highly exposed to the risk of infection transmission. The physical and psychological tear (tiredness and drowsiness) has negative effects on attentiveness and observation. It could be a risk factor for nursing personnel losing their capacity to work. Creating a secure and supportive work environment at healthcare facilities could be regarded as an institutional strategy for preventing chronic fatigue as well as physical and psychological tear.

MULTIPLE CHOICE QUESTIONS

1. Why nursing diagnosis is different from medical diagnosis?
   a. For the direction of suitable actions, nursing diagnosis is based on medical diagnoses
   b. Nursing is focused on caring, while medical diagnosis is primarily focused on curing
   c. Nursing diagnosis focuses on human response, whereas medical diagnosis is mostly focused on pathology
   d. Nursing focused on psychological characteristics, whereas medical diagnosis focuses on physiologic characters

2. The assessment feedback process for it to be effective, medical surgical nurse who is also a manager:
   a. Organize a weekly meeting with the staff
   b. When delegating work, takes into account the interests and abilities of the employees
   c. Inform employees frequently about how well they are doing their duties
   d. Establishes objectives for employees to achieve

3. In ICUs, the most often employed model of care is:
   a. Functional nursing   b. Total patient care
   c. Team nursing   d. Primary nursing

4. The nurse realizes at the end of the shift that she missed documenting a dressing change she did for a patient. Which of the following actions should the nurse take?
   a. Before departing, fill out an incident report
   b. Nothing needs to be done; the next nurse will take care of it
   c. Make a note of the dressing change in a previous note
   d. As an addendum to the narrative notes, add a late entry

5. When working as a nurse and a conflict arises between your client's demands and what the family and/or physician desires, and/or hospital norms, according to the nursing code of ethics, your first commitment is to the:
   a. Hospital   b. Family
   c. Client   d. Physician

6. An occupational health nurse observes the different types of injuries and diseases that people can get from their jobs. Which of the following recommendations about workplace safety would the nurse most, such asly make?
   a. To get the physical activity done, find another job, such as physical labor
   b. The safest option for employment is a professional position
   c. Choose white-collar jobs that have the lowest risk of harm
   d. There is no such thing as a risk-free job or career

7. Several nurses from one unit have missed work after catching a communicable disease from a patient, according to a nurse who works in a hospital. Which of the following statement most accurately characterizes the host factor?
   a. The hospital   b. The communicable disease
   c. Each sick nurse   d. The patient

8. Which of the following is the most important reason to wash your hands?
   a. To improve the circulation of the hands
   b. To avoid the spread of microorganisms
   c. To stay away from the client with a dirty hand
   d. To provide cleanliness

9. Before administering medication, the nurse must confirm the client's identity. Which method is the safest for identifying the client?
   a. Inquire about the client's name
   b. Examine the client's identification bracelet
   c. Inquire about the room number
   d. Mention the client's name aloud and have the client repeat it

10. When examining a client's ability to get up in a chair, which of the following actions should the nurse take?
    a. Lift the client's arms by bending at the waist and placing arms under the client's arms
    b. Ask the client to spread their feet apart
    c. Face the client, bend your knees and lay your hands on the forearm of the client
    d. Ask the client to tighten their pelvic muscles
11. Primary role of occupational health nurse:
    a. Providing tertiary prevention
    b. Providing secondary prevention
    c. Providing health promotion and emergency care
    d. Primary prevention
12. In terms of education and follow-up evaluation, to which of the following groups should the occupational health nurse devote the most time?
    a. To newly recruited workers of less than 1 years
    b. To chronically unwell elder workers
    c. To women in their reproductive years
    d. Older workers with diminished hearing
13. The best strategy for preventing hearing loss at work or healthcare facility is to:
    a. Always wear ear protection to protect your ear
    b. A routing hearing test can be used to track your hearing loss over time.
    c. Monitor noise level using administrative and engineering controls to reduce over exposure
    d. None of the above
14. Which of these should be the initial action in a risk assessment?
    a. Assessing the risk
    b. Hazard identification
    c. Review what you found
    d. Update risk assessment
15. Which of the following can be caused on by exposure to loud noise?
    a. Hypertension
    b. Gastrointestinal problem
    c. Chronic fatigue
    d. All of the above

ANSWERS

1. c	2. c	3. b	4. d
5. c	6. d	7. c	8. b
9. a	10. c	11. c	12. a
13. c	14. b	15. d	

SUGGESTED READING

1. Aalto-Korte K, Koskela K, Pesonen M. Allergic contact dermatitis and other occupational skin diseases in health care workers in the Finnish Register of Occupational Diseases in 2005–2016. Contact dermatitis. 2021;84(4):217-23.
2. Alefi M, Sadeghi Yarandi M, Karimi A. Modeling of occupational risk factors in the development of musculoskeletal disorders in nurses. Archives of Occupational Health. 2020;4(1):474-9.
3. Association AN. Nursing administration: Scope and standards of practice: Nursesbooks. Org; 2009.
4. Azma K, Hosseini A, Safarian MH, Abedi M. Evaluation of the relationship between musculoskeletal discomforts and occupational stressors among nurses. North American journal of medical sciences. 2015;7(7):322.
5. Barbe MF, Barr AE. Inflammation and the pathophysiology of work-related musculoskeletal disorders. Brain Behav Immun. 2006;20(5):423-9.
6. Bergen G, Stevens MR, Burns ER. Falls and Fall Injuries Among Adults Aged ≥65 Years—United States, 2014. Morbidity and Mortality Weekly Report [Internet]. 2016;65(37):993-8. Available from: https://www.jstor.org/stable/24858985 Accessed on 20 May 2021.
7. Bhatia N, Kishore J, Anand T, Jiloha RC. Occupational stress amongst nurses from two tertiary care hospitals in Delhi. Australasian Medical Journal (Online). 2010;3(11):731.
8. Boughattas W, El Maalel O, Maoua M, Bougmiza I, Kalboussi H, Brahem A, et al. Low back pain among nurses: prevalence, and occupational risk factors. Occupational Diseases and Environmental Medicine. 2017;5(1):26-37.
9. Cegolon L, Lange JH, Mastrangelo G. The Primary Care Practitioner and the diagnosis of occupational diseases. BMC public health. 2010;10(1):1-4.
10. Chaudhari AP, Mazumdar K, Motwani YM, Ramadas D. A profile of occupational stress in nurses. Annals of Indian Psychiatry. 2018;2(2):109.
11. Chowdhury SR, Sunna TC, Das DC, Kabir H, Hossain A, Mahmud S, et al. Mental health symptoms among the nurses of Bangladesh during the COVID-19 pandemic. Middle East Current Psychiatry. 2021;28(1):1-8.
12. Harcombe H, Herbison G, McBride D, Derrett S. Musculoskeletal disorders among nurses compared with two other occupational groups. Occupational Medicine. 2014;64(8):601-7.
13. Jain A, Chander R, Mendiratta V. Contact dermatitis in nurses and paramedicals in a tertiary care hospital of northern India; 2010.
14. Konlan KD, Aarah-Bapuah M, Kombat JM, Wuffele GM. The level of nurses' knowledge on occupational post exposure to hepatitis B infection in the Tamale metropolis, Ghana. BMC health services research. 2017;17(1):1-7.
15. Kshetrimayum N, Bennadi D, Siluvai S. Stress among staff nurses: A hospital-based study. Journal of Nature and Science of Medicine. 2019;2(2):95.
16. Masoudi Alavi N. Occupational hazards in nursing. Nursing and midwifery studies [Internet]. 2014;3(3):e22357. Available from: https://www.ncbi.nlm.nih.gov/pmc/articles/PMC4332998/ Accessed on 23 May 2021
17. Nair RS. Prevalence and risk factors associated with low back pain among nurses in a tertiary care hospital in south India. International Journal of Orthopaedics. 2020;6(1):301-6.
18. Rao MN, Lundgren NPV. A Review of Occupational Health Research in India, ICMR, New Delhi; 1955.
19. Rice R. Home care nursing practice: concepts and application: Elsevier Health Sciences; 2006.
20. Saha RK. Occupational Health in India. Ann Glob Health. 2018;84(3):330-3.
21. Silva T, Araújo W, Stival MM, Toledo A, Burke TN, Carregaro RL. Musculoskeletal discomfort, work ability and fatigue in nursing professionals working in a hospital environment. Rev esc enferm USP. 2018;52(e03332):1-8.
22. World Health Organisation 2013 [Available from: https://www.who.int/data/gho/data/indicators/indicator-details/GHO/occupational-ergonomic-stressors-attributable-dalys-per-100000-capita#.
23. World Health Organization. Occupational Health [Internet]. Who. int. World Health Organization: WHO; 2019. Available from: https://www.who.int/health-topics/occupational-health accessed on 25 May, 2021
24. Yan P, Yang Y, Zhang L, Li F, Huang A, Wang Y, et al. Correlation analysis between work-related musculoskeletal disorders and the nursing practice environment, quality of life, and social support in the nursing professionals. Medicine. 2018;97(9).

UNIT X

Special Topics

OUTLINE

54. **Patient Safety**
    Arti Saini, Neha Pundir, Pankaj Arora

55. **Organ Donation and Transplantation**
    Navdeep Bansal, Sukhpal Kaur

56. **Importance of Yoga for Nursing Professionals**
    Tanmya Deswal, Pooja Nadholta, Sadhana Verma

54

Patient Safety

Arti Saini, Neha Pundir, Pankaj Arora

"If I'm doing whatever is best for my patients, then I'm doing what's best for me and for our system."
—Kelly Tayler

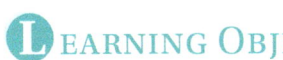

Learning Objectives

After going through the chapter, the learner will be able to:
- Define patient safety.
- Understand various components of patient safety.
- Enumerate various types of harms and healthcare-associated errors.
- Discuss in detail the types of errors, their incidence, risk factors, and potential solutions.
- Discuss patient safety with regard to elderly patients.

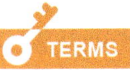

- **Adverse events:** Undesirable outcome of care.
- **Adverse reaction:** It is the unanticipated and undesirable harm occurring following a justified and correct process.
- **Near misses:** An undesirable incident that did not reach the patient.
- **Patient safety:** It is the protection of patients from unnecessary potential healthcare-associated harm.

INTRODUCTION

Patient safety is a matter of life and death. It is as important as health is. It is one of the important dimensions of quality of care. Protecting the safety of the patients is a basic principle of health care. Patient safety includes various components critical to the delivery of quality healthcare services including surgical safety, safe childbirth, injection safety, blood and medication safety, medical device safety, and safe organ, tissue, and cell transportation and donation. Other important aspects of patient safety are biomedical waste management and the prevention of healthcare-associated infections. Patient safety is not only limited to these aspects of care, but it also involves care of each and every component of the journey of the patient starting from his entry into the hospital to discharge and further to his/her rehabilitation.

In 2015, the 68th WHO Regional Committee for Southeast Asia endorsed the "Regional Strategy for patient safety in the WHO South-East Asian Region (2016–2025)." This initiative aims to support the development of national quality of care and patient safety strategies, policies, and plans to ensure patient safety. The Institute of Medicine report "To Err is Human" in 1999 shook the world wherein it stated that up to 98,000 patients die every year in the US healthcare system due to medical errors. Acting on its report on patient safety, World Health Assembly in its 55th Session adopted a resolution "Quality of care: Patient Safety" urging the Member States to:
- "Pay the closest possible attention to the problem of patient safety;"
- "Establish and strengthen science-based systems, necessary for improving patients' safety and the quality of health care, including the monitoring of drugs, medical equipment, and technology."

Patient safety can be defined as a framework of an organized set of activities that lead to lesser risks, reduced incidence of avoidable harm, and reduced chances and impact of error if it occurs. This is accomplished by creating sustainably and consistently safe and conducive cultures, processes, technologies, behaviors, and environments in the healthcare system.

In other words, patient safety is 'freedom from unintended harm during healthcare'.

It is the protection of patients from unnecessary potential healthcare-associated harm.

According to WHO, one in 10 patients is estimated to have experienced an adverse event while receiving care in a hospital in the developed world. Though the data is not robust for developing countries, estimates suggest that in the hospitals of low and middle-income countries, about 134 million adverse events occur annually due to unsafe care. This contributes to a mortality of around 2.6 million yearly. Besides the tremendous financial burden of adverse events (1 trillion to 2 trillion US$ a year), intangible costs are equally distressing for patients/families and healthcare workers. These include, but are not limited to, mistrust in the healthcare system, reduced quality of life, and loss of confidence amongst HCWs. Adverse events are just the tip of the iceberg. The number of near-miss events far outnumbers the adverse events. Therefore, it is all the more important to identify and rectify near-miss events to reduce adverse events.

Globally, many countries and organizations have instituted steps to address various aspects of safe healthcare. WHO has identified three Global Patient Safety Challenges to focus the world's attention on these three key areas. These are:
1. "Clean Care is Safe Care"
2. "Safe Surgery Saves Lives"
3. "Medication Without Harm"

PATIENT SAFETY INDICATORS

Patient safety indicators (PSI) refer to the methods used to ascertain whether a patient has experienced any adverse event because of exposure to the health care system. Patients can be protected from these potentially preventable adverse events by making certain modifications in the health care organization, which can be at the system or provider level. Patient safety indicators can be defined on two levels, which are:

Provider Level

Provider level PSIs are utilized to measure the avoidable complications for the patient who experienced this complication in the same period of hospitalization in which they received their initial care. Examples include accidental puncture or laceration, a complication of anesthesia, pressure sores, inadvertently retained foreign objects, transfusion reaction, sepsis in the postoperative period, etc.

Area Level

Area-level PSIs are used to estimate all cases of avoidable complications that occur in each geographical area, during hospitalization, or leading to subsequent hospitalization of the patients. Examples are—dehiscence of the surgical wound, certain nosocomial infections, foreign body left during the procedure, etc.

PATIENT SAFETY IN INDIAN SCENARIO

Many strategies have been adopted by the Government of India and the health care institutions to ensure patient safety and prevention of healthcare-induced harm. To strengthen the patient safety initiatives, the Ministry of Health and Family Welfare developed an overarching framework for patient safety in India known as the "National patient safety implementation framework (2018–2025)" to promote patient safety at all levels of healthcare. Some other significant examples are:

1. **Surgical safety:** There is no formal nationwide policy or plan to regulate surgical services at different levels of healthcare. However, many healthcare institutions have adopted and implemented the WHO surgical safety checklist.
2. **Injection safety:** Many agencies like the Indian Academy of Paediatrics and the National Center for Disease Control have published various guidelines to promote safe injection practices. WHO (2015) also issued "New policy guidance on safe injections."
Excellent surveillance of needle stick injuries is being conducted in all accredited hospitals.
3. **Infection prevention:** National health policy recommends vaccination of health care workers against hepatitis B. Biomedical waste management rules mandate vaccination of waste handlers against hepatitis B and Tetanus. There is variable implementation of infection prevention/control guidelines in the healthcare sector but accreditation and programs like Kayakalp have squarely brought heightened sensitivity to the topic. A major area for potential improvement is the availability of post-exposure prophylaxis in areas like emergency and operation theaters.
4. **Blood safety:** The Drugs and Cosmetics Act categorizes blood as a drug, thus, blood banks are considered manufacturing units that can only function under a license issued by the FDA with the approval of DCGI. All collected blood units undergo mandatory screening for HIV, HBV, HCV, malaria, and syphilis.

DOMAINS OF PATIENT SAFETY/TYPES OF HARM

Certain important domains of healthcare practices which can affect the safety of the patients are depicted in **Box 54.1**.

MEDICATION ERROR

Definition

The "United States National Coordinating Council for Medication Error Reporting and Prevention" defines a medication error as: *"any preventable event that may cause or lead to inappropriate medication use or patient harm while*

BOX 54.1: Domains of healthcare practices.

- Medication errors
- Health care-associated infection
- Unsafe surgical care practices
- Unsafe injection practices
- Diagnostic errors
- Unsafe transfusion practices
- Radiation errors
- Venous thromboembolism

the medication is in the control of the health care professional, patient, or consumer. Such events may be related to professional practice, health care products, procedures, and systems, including prescribing, order communication, product labeling, packaging, and nomenclature, compounding, dispensing, distribution, administration, education, monitoring, and use". The definition emphasizes that medication errors can be avoided at different levels. Another definition of medication error is a reduced probability of timely and effective treatment or an increased risk of medication-related harm compared with the generally accepted practice.

Classification of Medication Errors

- ❖ Classification is based on the point at which the error occurs in the process of medication use. The error can occur while prescribing, transcribing, dispensing the medication, during administration, or during the monitoring stage.
- ❖ Another way of classifying is based on the type of error occurring for example—wrong medication, dose, frequency, administration route, or patient etc.
- ❖ Errors can also be classified as:
  - ➢ *Knowledge-based or rule-based mistakes/errors*—these are the errors that occur from mistakes made when planning actions.
  - ➢ *Action-based errors (slips, lapses, or memory-based errors)*—these are the errors in the execution of appropriately planned actions.
- ❖ Another way to classify the errors is according to the level of severity which is mild, moderate, and severe.

No strong evidence exists that supports a particular method of classification of errors thus the selection of classification approach is guided by the setting and the purpose for which the classification is being done.

Prevalence of Medication Errors

The prevalence of medication errors is difficult to estimate because of various reasons like; varying definitions, different classification systems, and the type of denominator used (patient prescription or medication). The prevalence rates reported from various parts of the world are highly variable. A study was conducted in the United Kingdom which highlighted that around 12% of the patients receiving primary care may have been subjected to a medication error whereas another study conducted in Saudi Arabia stated that errors were found in as many as 1/5th of the prescriptions at the primary care level.

Causes of Medication Errors

Various causes of medication errors are depicted in **Table 54.1**.

POTENTIAL SOLUTIONS TO MEDICATION ERRORS

The following are the possible solutions to prevent medication errors:
- ❖ **Training of healthcare professionals and patients:**
  - ➢ Providing education to primary caregivers about the common reasons for medication errors.

TABLE 54.1: Causes of medication errors.

Factor	Types of errors
Heath professional associated factors	• Insufficient knowledge related to drugs • Inadequate clinical experience • Inability to estimate risks • Overworked or fatigued staff • Ineffective communication between patients and health professionals • Inadequate therapeutic training • Inadequate knowledge related to patient
Patient-related factors	• Characteristics of the patients—literacy, language barriers, personality • The complexity of the case—polypharmacy, high-risk medications, multiple co-morbidities.
Work environment-related factors	• Time pressures and heavy workload • Distractions and interruptions from other staff and patients • Non-availability of standard policies and protocols • Problems related to the physical environment, for example—lighting, ventilation, and temperature. • Inadequate resources
Medication-related factors	• Ambiguous naming, labeling, or packaging of medication
Task-related factors	• Repetitive system of ordering, processing, and authorization • Patient monitoring
Factors related to computerized information systems	• Complicated processes for generating first prescriptions • The cumbersome process of generating repeat prescriptions correctly • Inaccurate patients' records • Complicated design that allows for human errors

  - ➢ Providing simple tools to primary care providers to assist them in error-free prescription and usage procedures. Provide tools for patient involvement to combat non-adherence.
- ❖ **Reconciliation and implementation of medication reviews:**
  - ➢ Making sure pharmacists actively evaluate prescriptions.
  - ➢ Supporting and encouraging physicians' use of medication reconciliation.
- ❖ **Encourage electronic tool usage:** The electronic systems need to be strengthened to improve safety features irrespective of the status of the patient. Examples include improving the accuracy and comprehensiveness of records using 'electronic health records', supporting the diagnosis, surveillance, and treatment of various disease conditions, reduction of health risk and effective behavior change, sharing reliable health data, and enhancing patient and caregiver participation in care. Electronic usage also reduces errors and improves coordination between healthcare professionals.
- ❖ **Prioritizing areas for immediate gains:**
  - ➢ Target interventions for the treatment of children and the elderly.

- Target interventions linked to injection use as a major source of mistakes.
- Implement multicomponent interventions that include education, health informatics, medication reviews, and the participation of community chemists.

KEY ISSUES ASSOCIATED WITH PRIMARY CARE-RELATED MEDICATION ERRORS

1. **Use of injection:** Injection is associated with the risk of transmission of infectious diseases. According to the findings of a study, 1.67 million HBV infections, 3,15,120 cases of HCV infections and 33, 877 HIV infections are associated with unsafe injections (Pèpin J et al).
2. **Pediatrics:** Children who utilize medications have some unique difficulties. Widespread off-label and unlicensed use of medications raises the possibility of unnecessary medication-related damage. Compared to the adult population, there is a higher risk of injury from a slight medicine dosage mistake in children. Additionally, weight-related dosage adjustments and other dosing computations are needed for pediatric prescriptions, which are less frequent in adults.
3. **Home care setting:** The elder people may experience particular problems with medication errors. For instance, residents at care facilities are frequently weak, have several medical issues, and require various prescriptions. The administration of medicine in this setting frequently differs from that in patients' homes since it is done by nursing staff or other professionals, which leads to issues related to medication dispensing, administration, monitoring and surveillance, and staff training.

HEALTHCARE-ASSOCIATED INFECTIONS

Definition

"Healthcare-associated infections (HAIs), commonly referred to as nosocomial infections, that individuals contract while undergoing treatment for a medical or surgical problem."

HAIs can develop in various settings including hospitals, ambulatory clinics, surgical centers, and long-term facilities like nursing homes and rehabilitation centers. HAIs may present themselves during hospitalization or post-discharge.

Risk Factors of HAIs

All the patients in the hospital are at risk of developing a nosocomial infection especially at extremes of age, and immunocompromised patients are more susceptible to contract infection from other hospitalized patients. Many common factors responsible for healthcare-associated infections include prolonged hospitalizations, use of invasive devices and indwelling catheters, improper hand hygiene practices, and inappropriate use of antibiotics.

Prevalence of HAI

The Centres for Disease Control (CDC) reports that around 1.7 million infections and 99,000 deaths occur annually in American hospitals alone due to healthcare-associated infections. Among these infections:

- ❖ Urinary tract infections account for 32% of all healthcare-associated infections.
- ❖ Surgical site infections constitute 22% of all HAIs.
- ❖ Lung infections make up 15% of cases of pneumonia.
- ❖ Infections in the bloodstream account for 14%.

Most Important Types of HAIs

1. Central line-associated bloodstream infection (CLABSI)
2. Catheter-associated urinary tract infections (CAUTI)
3. Surgical site infection (SSI)
4. Ventilator associated pneumonia (VAP)

Potential Solutions to Reduce HAIs

Recent research evidence strongly recommends careful adherence to evidence-based best practices to avoid many hospital-acquired infections. Some recommendations are:

- ❖ Healthcare professionals should perform hand washing with soap and water or use an alcohol-based hand rub before and after treating any patient **(Figs. 54.1 and 54.2)**.
- ❖ Catheters must be used judiciously and only when necessary and frequent assessments should be done to remove them as soon as possible. The skin around the surgical site or the catheter insertion site should also be cleaned and assessed frequently. When necessary, healthcare professionals should use gloves, masks, gowns, and hair coverings when cleaning the surgical site or the area where the catheter is being implanted.

For more information related to various care bundles for HAI prevention refer to the further reading section.

UNSAFE SURGICAL CARE PROCEDURES

The World Health Assembly (2002) adopted a resolution urging the countries to strengthen their healthcare safety and monitoring systems. This came as the consequence of growing worldwide evidence of substantial public health harm secondary to inadequate patient safety.

Millions of individuals have surgery every year, data suggests that around 13% of all disability-adjusted life years are related to surgical procedures worldwide.

Surgeries are a lifesaving treatment modality however poor surgical care can lead to serious mortality and morbidity. The various important implications related to the prevalence of surgery are:

- ❖ 0.5–5% reported crude mortality rate following major surgery and nearly 25% of patients undergoing inpatient procedures also experience problems.
- ❖ About half of the adverse outcomes experienced by hospitalized patients in industrialized nations are related to surgical treatment with half of these problems being avoidable.
- ❖ It is reported that in some parts of sub-Saharan Africa, the death rate due to general anesthesia alone is quite high.

Potential Solutions to Overcome the Burden of Unsafe Surgical Care Procedures

WHO has launched various national and international initiatives to promote surgical safety. WHO second global

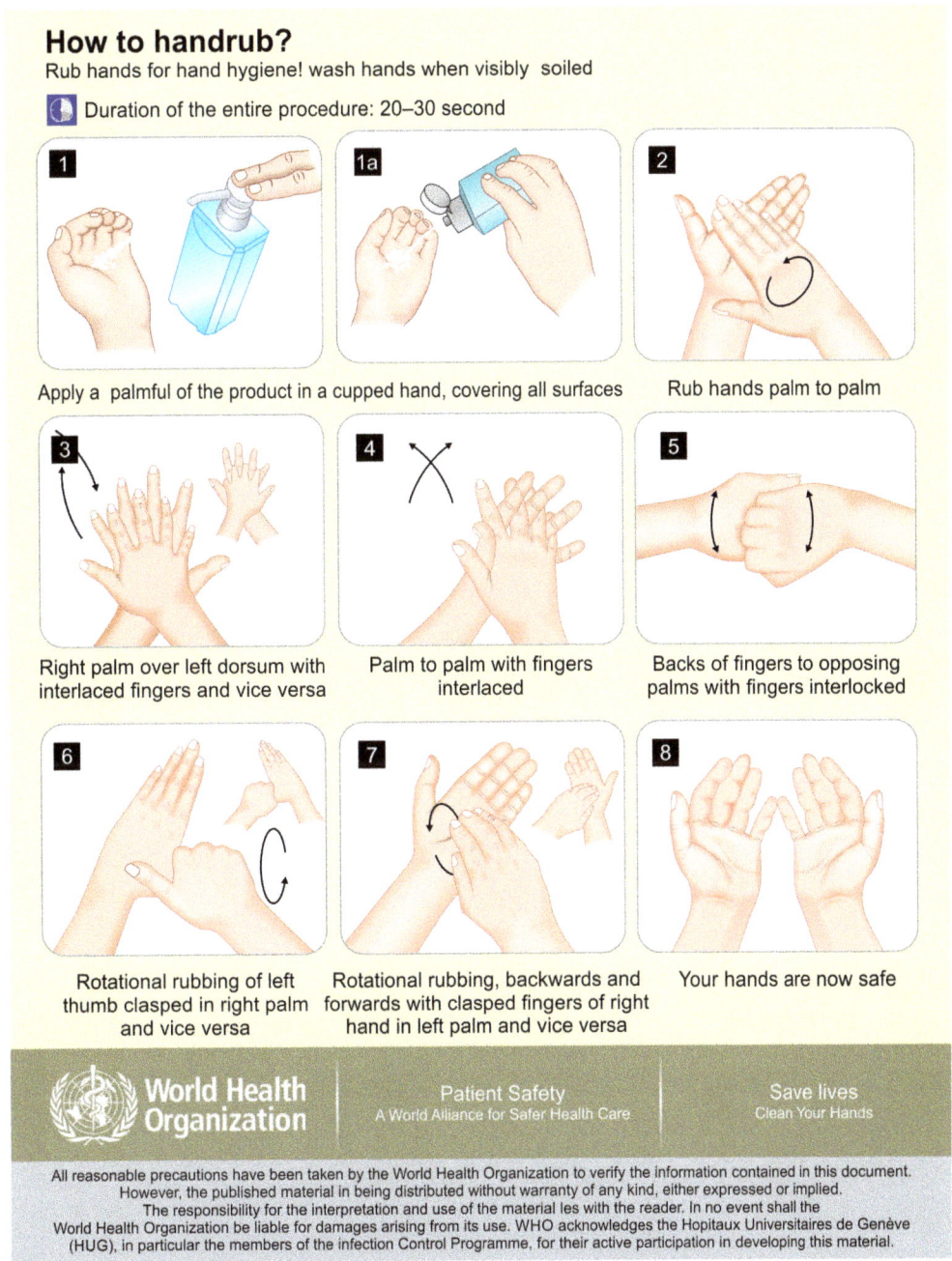

Fig. 54.1: Hand hygiene (using handrubs).

patient safety challenge "Safe surgery saves lives" was an inspiration for a large portion of this effort. "Safe surgery saves lives" helped to increase surgical safety globally by providing a fundamental set of safety requirements that could be implemented in all the WHO member states. It seeks to improve surgical safety and reduce the mortality and morbidity related to surgeries:

- ❖ By providing clinicians, hospital administrators, and public health officials with information on the role and patterns of surgical safety in public health.
- ❖ By defining a minimal set of uniform measures, or "surgical vital statistics," for national and international surveillance of surgical care.
- ❖ By testing the checklist and surveillance tools at pilot sites in all WHO regions and then distributing the checklist to hospitals worldwide.
- ❖ By identifying a straightforward set of surgical safety standards that can be used in all countries and settings and are compiled in a "surgical safety checklist" for use in operating rooms.

Highlights of "Safe Surgery Saves Lives Program"

The established framework for safe intraoperative care in hospitals entails a regular series of events, each with specific risks that can be mitigated: Preoperative patient evaluation, surgical intervention, and preparation for appropriate postoperative care.

1. **Preoperative patient evaluation:** This includes obtaining informed consent, ensuring the right identity, procedure site, the integrity of the anesthesia machine, the availability of emergency medications, and adequate preparation for any intraoperative events.

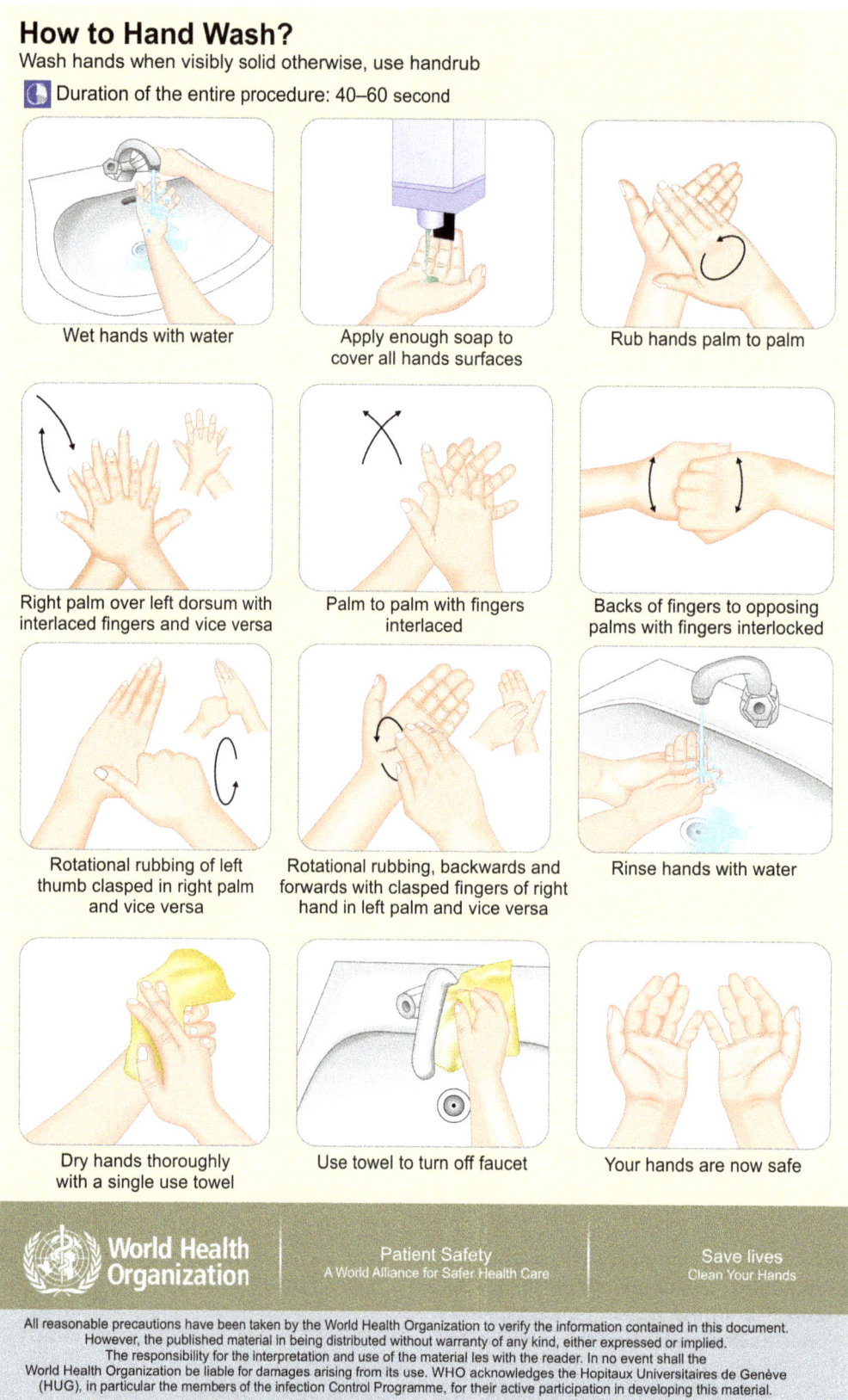

Fig. 54.2: Steps of handwashing.

2. **Surgical intervention:** Positive surgical outcome can be achieved by ensuring the following points:
   - The right antibiotic should be used
   - All the vital imaging should be available
   - The patient should be appropriately monitored
   - Effective teamwork should be there
   - The anesthetic and surgical judgments are made
   - Meticulous surgical technique is used
   - There is good communication between the surgeons, anesthetists, and nurses.

3. **Preparation of appropriate post-operative care:** Following surgery, a clear care plan, knowledge of potential and anticipated intraoperative events, and adherence to adequate monitoring have the potential

to strengthen the surgical system, enhancing patient safety and enhancing results. Additionally, there is a recognized requirement for qualified workers and functional resources, like sterilization tools and suitable illumination. Last but not the least, constant quality control and supervision are necessary for safe surgery.

Three Main Aspects of "Safe Surgery Saves Lives"

- **Safe surgical teams:**
  - Improvement in communication
  - Ensuring correct patient, site, and procedure.
  - Informed consent
  - Ensuring the availability of all team members
  - Adequate preparation of the team
  - Adequate planning for the procedure
  - Confirmation of any patient allergies before the procedure
- **Safe anesthesia:**
  - Availability of trained anesthetist
  - Anesthesia machine and medication safety check
  - Monitoring of pulse oximetry, heart rate, blood pressure and temperature
- **Prevention of surgical site infection:**
  - Proper hand washing
  - Judicious use of appropriate antibiotics
  - Antiseptic skin preparation
  - Atraumatic wound care
  - Maintenance of sterility and adequate decontamination of instruments

The 10 essential objectives for safe surgery, as given by WHO, are:

The team will:
1. Operate on the correct patient at the correct site.
2. Use methods proven to prevent harm due to the use of anesthetics while protecting the patient from pain.
3. Recognize and prepare for life-threatening procedures (airway/respiratory function).
4. Recognize and prepare for high-risk blood loss.
5. Avoid inducing allergies or adverse drug reactions.
6. Use methods to reduce the risk of surgical site infection.
7. Prevent unintended retention of surgical items in the wound.
8. Secure and correctly identify all surgical specimens.
9. Effectively communicate and exchange critical information for the safe conduct of surgery
10. The health systems will establish routine surveillance of surgical capacity volume and results.

Surgical Safety Checklist

It includes a simple set of surgical safety standards which can be applied to all countries and settings and have been compiled in the form of a checklist for use in operating rooms. The checklist divides the surgery into three phases, each one corresponding to a specific time in the normal flow of the procedure that is, before induction of anesthesia, before the incision, and during or immediately after wound closure but before the patient is shifted out of the operating room. A single person is made responsible for performing the safety checks on the list, usually the circulatory nurse. During each phase, the checklist coordinator should confirm that the surgical team has completed the respective tasks of that phase before proceeding to further steps. All the steps of the checklist must be verbally verified with the appropriate team member to ensure compliance **(Fig. 54.3)**.

UNSAFE INJECTION PRACTICES

Unsafe injections are responsible for around 9.2 million years of life lost due to mortality or morbidity worldwide (Disability Adjusted Life Years or DALYs). With respect to the health care settings, unsafe injections can transmit infections like HIV, hepatitis B, and C and are a direct threat to healthcare workers. To prevent unsafe injection-related harm, WHO has developed guidelines to promote the use of safety-engineered syringes for subcutaneous, intradermal, and intramuscular injections in healthcare settings. Another set of guidelines is the WHO best practices for injections and related procedures tool kit.

DIAGNOSTIC ERRORS

Accurate and timely diagnosis depends on a variety of variables, including the resources that primary caregivers have access to as well as their knowledge, experience, and expertise. Diagnosis is a high-risk area for errors especially in primary care. Primary care professionals often see a large number of patients, and because of this sometimes their diseases are frequently challenging to diagnose. Primary care doctors could be familiar with rare diseases and have variable levels of access to diagnostic testing. When a diagnosis is overlooked, improperly postponed, or incorrect, a diagnostic error occurs.

Prevalence of Diagnostic Errors

- According to research done in a developed country, every year, about 5% of individuals have diagnostic mistakes in the OPDs. The potential for serious injury existed in more than half of these mistakes. The researchers hypothesized that this was probably an underestimate and that diagnostic error rates in low-income nations may be far higher.
- Due to restricted access to diagnostic testing resources, a lack of experienced primary care providers or specialists, and constrained record-keeping systems, there may be even larger issues in low- and middle-income nations. These elements could make diagnostic mistakes more common in primary care.

Causes of Diagnostic Errors

- The diagnostic method is susceptible to committing an error in every step. Studies on diagnostic errors frequently identify many underlying explanations for each instance. Cognitive mistakes, such as incorrectly summing up the available evidence or improperly using data from physical examinations or tests, may be the root of the problem.
- There is proof that more than half of diagnostic mistake instances may be attributed to cognitive errors. As a result of issues with communication or care coordination, issues with the accessibility of medical record data, and limited access to experts, system defects may potentially cause diagnostic mistakes.

SURGICAL SAFETY CHECKLIST (FIRST EDITION)
World Health Organization

Before induction of anesthesia ▶▶▶▶▶▶▶ **Before skin incision** ▶▶▶▶▶▶▶ **Before patient leaves operating room**

Sign in
- ☐ Patient has confirmed
  - Identity
  - Site
  - Procedure
  - Consent
- ☐ Site marked/not applicable
- ☐ Anaesthesia safety check completed
- ☐ Pulse oximeter on patient and functioning

Does patient have A:
Known allergy?
- ☐ No
- ☐ Yes

Difficult airway/aspiration risk?
- ☐ No
- ☐ Yes, and equipment/assistance available

Risk of >500 mL blood loss (7 mL/kg in children)?
- ☐ No
- ☐ Yes, and adequate intravenous access and fluids planned

Time out
- ☐ Confirm all team members have Introduced themselves by name and Role
- ☐ Surgeon, anesthesia professional and nurse verbally confirm
  - Patient
  - Site
  - Procedure

Anticipated critical events
- ☐ Surgeon reviews: what are the Critical or unexpected steps, Operative duration, anticipated Blood loss?
- ☐ Anesthesia team reviews—are there any patient-specific concerns?
- ☐ Nursing team reviews—has sterility (including indicator results) been confirmed? Are there equipment issues or any concerns?

Has antibiotic prophylaxis been given within the last 60 minutes?
- ☐ Yes
- ☐ Not applicable

Is essential imaging displayed?
- ☐ Yes
- ☐ Not applicable

Sign out
Nurse verbally confirms with the Team:
- ☐ The name of the procedure recorded
- ☐ That instrument, sponge and needle Counts are correct (or not Applicable)
- ☐ How the specimen is labelled (including patient name)
- ☐ Whether there are any equipment problems to be addressed
- ☐ Surgeon, anesthesia professional and nurse review the key concerns for recovery and management of this patient

Fig. 54.3: WHO surgical safety checklist.

- The patient-practitioner clinical encounter (79%), referral issues (20%), patient-related factors (16%), follow-up and tracking of diagnostic information (15%), and the execution and interpretation of diagnostic tests (14%), were found to be the process breakdowns that occurred most frequently in one developed country.

Common Conditions Involved in Diagnostic Errors

The disease conditions identified as diagnostic difficulties and errors in primary care are heart attack, cancer, dementia, meningitis, asthma, anemia due to iron deficiency, HIV, and tremors in the elderly population. In patients with pneumonia (7%), decompensated congestive heart failure (7%), acute renal failure (5%), malignancy (5%), and urinary tract infection (5%) mistakes were widespread, according to a study of 190 cases of diagnostic errors (Singh H et al).

Overall, it seems that the commonest forms of hazardous diagnostic errors encountered in primary care include missed diagnoses of cancer, infections, and cardiovascular disease.

Potential Solutions to Reduce Diagnostic Errors

1. **Provide assistance to the workforce:**
   - Ensuring that patient safety education is provided to the primary care workers. Ensuring that the health professionals in the primary care setup have enough time to adequately assess the patient. Education related to delayed and missed diagnosis must be a part of mandatory training and continuing education programs.
   - Incorporating, thinking and cognitive psychology into the curricula can help the healthcare providers to understand the root causes and significance of various system-level approaches.
   - In order to appropriately assess and examine the patients make sure that primary health care providers have sufficient time.
   - Encouraging a conducive work culture that makes providers comfortable about recognizing and sharing errors.
   - Encouraging and assisting service providers to collaborate in multidisciplinary teams.
2. **Making patients a member of the care team:**
   - Encouraging patients to voluntarily ask questions and follow up.
   - To make patients a genuine partner in the diagnostic process, healthcare professionals must be taught to collaborate with patients and promote these queries.
3. **Adopting supporting tools:**
   - Creating error-reporting systems to promote learning from mistakes.
   - Ensuring closed-loop systems through clinical process redesigning.
   - Implementing electronic records with decision support and using mnemonics, checklists, and

web-based assistance to generate an appropriate differential diagnosis.
- Utilizing health technologies, such as remote consultations, so that healthcare providers can quickly access specialists and senior colleagues and ensure that information is accurate and up to date.

4. **Developing diagnostic facilities:**
   - Enhancing system design by taking human factors into consideration.
   - Increasing access to diagnostic tests in primary care, including point-of-care testing.
5. **Setting improvement priorities:**
   - Investing in research into the causes and treatments of diagnostic errors so that interventions may be customized to the local environment.
   - Focusing interventions for improvement on diseases with high rates of diagnostic errors, such as cancer, cardiovascular diseases, and infections.

UNSAFE TRANSFUSION PRACTICES

Blood products have been designated as an essential medicine by WHO. Blood and blood products can save lives and patients around the world. Along with the need for an adequate supply of blood, there is also a need to ensure the safety of the harvested blood because the blood products carry inherent biological hazards, and process-related hazards can result in serious or fatal consequences. With unsafe transfusion practices, there is a possibility of adverse transfusion reactions and the transmission of infections. An average incidence from a group of 21 countries shows 8.7 serious transfusion reactions per 10,000 distributed blood components.

To avoid transfusion-related harm:
- Blood must be used only when needed, clinically appropriate
- When the patients' condition can be improved only by transfusion
- When no alternative therapy is available
- When the administration of transfusion can be properly monitored

Reasons for inappropriate use of blood:
- Lack of education and training in the appropriate use of blood
- Weak system to safely manage the series of processes starting from education and recruitment of volunteer donors to the donation, testing, processing, and distribution, through transfusion and follow-up of patients.

Safety measures during collection, testing, and storage of blood products:
- Blood must be collected from healthy donors who are at low risk of infections transmissible by blood.
- Donated blood must be tested carefully against well-recognized standards, to protect the safety of the recipient as well as the donor.
- Each product must be tested and labeled showing its product type, storage requirements, expiry dates, and any modifications as well as other relevant information like ABO grouping and RhD group.
- Plasma can transmit most of the infectious agents present in whole blood and can cause other reactions also therefore the indications for its transfusion are limited and must be carefully weighed.
- Plasma derivatives produced by pharmaceutical manufacturing processes from large volumes of plasma collected from many individual blood donations. They must be tested to minimize the risk of transmitting infections and must undergo pathogen inactivation to ensure safety.
- Whole blood has a higher volume than the red cell concentrates due to the presence of an entire unit of plasma therefore it must be carefully used in patients with the risk of circulatory overload.
- For the recipients of multiple non-ABO identical whole blood units, low titer O whole blood is preferred.
- Completion of the transfusion within four hours of commencement should be ensured.
- Never add any medication to a unit of blood.
- Plasma must normally be ABO compatible to avoid the risk of hemolysis in the patient. However, in trauma patients with an unknown ABO group, Group A plasma has been demonstrated to be safe and effective.
- Before use, plasma must be thawed between 30°C and 37°C. High temperatures must be avoided as they can inactivate clotting factors and other proteins. Appropriate equipment like water baths or any other recommended equipment according to manufacturers' instructions must be used.
- After thawing, plasma must be infused within four to six hours or stored in a refrigerator at a temperature between 2 to 6°C.
- For transfusing plasma, a standard blood transfusion set must be used (**Fig. 54.4**).
- Transfusion-related acute lung injury can occur if donors are not screened for HLA antibodies.
- When using cryoprecipitate, use an ABO-compatible product preferably, after thawing infuse as soon as possible through a blood transfusion set. Preferably cryoprecipitate must be infused within six hours of thawing and four hours of pooling.
- Platelet concentrate should be slowly infused over at least two hours in a nonbleeding patient, this helps to prevent administering a large bolus of cytokines quickly which can lead to a febrile reaction.
- Platelets must not be refrigerated before infusion as this can impair platelet function.
- One standard blood transfusion set can be used for four to six units of platelet concentrates.

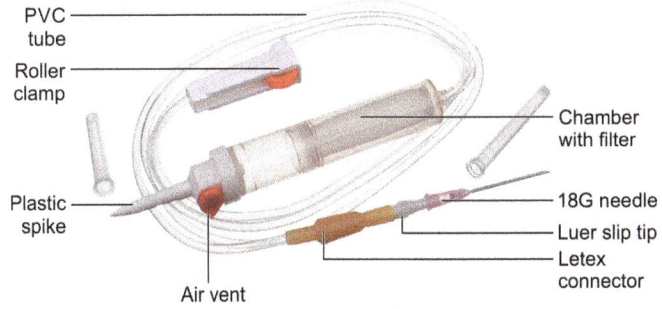

Fig. 54.4: Blood transfusion set.

- Rh compatibility should be considered while administering platelets.
- Every unit of donated blood must be screened for the following infections:
  - HIV-1 and HIV-2 antibody
  - Hepatitis B surface antigen
  - Hepatitis C antibodies
  - Treponema pallidum antibodies
  - Chagas disease (for donors living in countries where Chagas disease is prevalent).
  - Malaria where the donors are exposed to the infection risk.
- Screening for other infectious agents can be done according to national policies.
- No blood and blood product can be released for transfusion until all the required tests have been completed and shown to be non-reactive.
- Providing right blood component to right patient at right time must be ensured.
- Clear communication strategies, written standardized protocols and establish policies for the training of staff are essential for safe transfusion practices.

RADIATION ERRORS

It includes patients who are overexposed to radiation, and also involve cases with wrong patient and wrong site identification while conducting radiation procedure. The overall incidence of radiation errors estimates at around 15 per 10,000 treatment courses, according to the analysis of 30 years of data published on safety in radiotherapy.

VENOUS THROMBOEMBOLISM

It is one of the common and preventable causes of patient harm accounting for one-third of hospitalization-related complications. According to the estimates, 6 million cases in low- and middle-income countries and 3.9 million cases in high-income nations are reported annually. Venous thromboembolism can be prevented by early ambulation, active and passive limb exercises, and prescribing DVT prophylaxis (unfractionated heparin or low molecular weight heparin) unless contraindicated, in all bedridden patients. Frequent assessments of limbs for signs of deep vein thrombosis are also necessary for early detection and treatment, and prevention of life-threatening pulmonary embolism.

GERIATRIC CONSIDERATIONS

Geriatric patients are particularly at risk of medical errors. Data suggest that the rate of adverse events tends to increase with age, leading to a two-fold higher risk of adverse events in individuals ≥65 years of age, as compared to younger patients. Predominant adverse events frequently encountered in the elderly are adverse drug reactions, procedure-related events, and falls. The potential reasons for their increased vulnerability can be multiple comorbidities resulting in increased hospital stay, and frailty. Various geriatric syndromes like falls, delirium, pressure ulcers, and underfeeding can also be counted as medical errors, which significantly increase mortality and morbidity. These syndromes are usually preventable by proper assessment and timely intervention. Example of prevention strategies for underfeeding using a clinical guide that may assist in preventing malnutrition during long-term care. Use of agents like megestrol acetate help to prevent unintended weight loss, and improve calorie intake, appetite, and weight gain in nursing home residents. Staff education and multidimensional interventions are also important to prevent geriatric syndromes.

Acute care for the elderly (ACE) units provide an optimal physical environment to geriatric patients to prevent functional decline and promote functionality and independence. Some structural features of ACE units are-handrails, carpeting, large clocks and calendars, uncluttered hallways, elevated toilet seats, and door levers so that the elderly can perform Activities of daily living with minimal assistance.

Intervention programs for staff including education, training in gait and transfer skills, strengthening exercises, changes in environmental hazards, fall-risk education, nutrition counseling, etc. can improve safety in geriatric patients.

Case Scenario

A nurse was instructed by the physician to administer 140 mg of calcium chloride to an 8-month-old patient. The nurse thought that there was 10 mg per mL instead of 100 mg per mL of calcium chloride in the ampoule. She made the calculation in her mind and administered 14 mL of calcium to the baby, a dose that was 10 times higher than the prescribed. By the time she discovered her mistake, the patient had already died.
What type of medication error she committed and how can you prevent this type of error? Incorrect dose calculation error.
What to do to prevent: Calculations must be double or triple-checked before administering the medication. It may be tempting to rely on the brain to calculate dosages but it must be remembered that there is always a chance of human error especially if the staff is busy or tired. The dosage calculator app can be downloaded to check the accuracy of the calculation. The colleagues or supervisor may be asked to cross-check the calculation before administering.

SUMMARY

Patient safety is regarded as one of the care quality characteristics for people, along with adequacy, efficacy, accessibility, and capability. Errors can happen in any setting of the hospital i.e. general wards and intensive care units. Standardized protocols of various practices may help in preventing errors. Patient safety includes various features pivotal to the delivery of standard healthcare including surgical safety, medicine and blood safety, medical equipment safety, safe use of injectables, safety during the birth of a child, and safe transportation and donation of tissue, cell, and organ. Other important aspects of patient safety are biomedical waste management and the prevention of healthcare-associated infections. Patient safety measures are a collection of procedures that aid in identifying potential adverse events that a patient could suffer after being exposed to the medical system. In contrast to commonly recognized practice, a medication error is described as a decreased likelihood of timely and effective treatment or an increased risk of medication-related injury. Such incidents could have something to do with clinical practice, medical tools, protocols, and systems, such as prescription writing, order communication, product labeling, packaging, nomenclature, compounding, dispensing, distribution, administration, education, and monitoring.

Every admitted patient is susceptible to developing a hospital-acquired infection due to prolonged hospitalization, the use of invasive devices, a lack of handwashing by medical staff, and the improper administration of antibiotics. Also, venous thromboembolism is one of the frequent and avoidable causes of harm in patients accounting for one-third of hospitalization-related complications. Therefore, before treating each patient, healthcare professionals strictly follow proper hand hygiene steps using hand rub or soap and when necessary, medical professionals should use a personal protective equipment kit for safety. To address surgical safety, the WHO has started several global and regional projects. The WHO "Second Global Patient Safety Challenge"- "Safe Surgery Saves Lives" act as the framework for surgical safety standards which can be applied to all operating room settings in the form of a checklist. In hospital settings, unsafe injection practices can spread infections, along with hepatitis B and C, and HIV, and provide an immediate threat to patients as well as medical professionals. To prevent this WHO has presented recommendations for using safety-engineered syringes for injecting drugs to the patient in the hospital. Healthcare professionals often see a large number of patients, and because of this sometimes their diseases are frequently challenging to diagnose. Ensuring that healthcare providers have sufficient time for patient investigation and evaluation. Additionally, mandatory training and ongoing professional development should include concerning any delayed and missed diagnoses. Implementing electronic records, utilizing health technologies, such as remote consultations, so that medical professionals can quickly approach experts and senior faculty and ensure that details are accurate and up to date. In unsafe transfusion practices, there is a possibility of detrimental transfusion reactions and the transmission of infections. Along with the need for an adequate supply of blood, there is also a need to ensure the safety of the harvested blood because the blood products carry inherent biological hazards, and process-related hazards can result in serious or fatal consequences. Radiation errors occur when the patients are overexposed to radiation and also involve cases with the wrong patient and wrong site identification while conducting radiation procedures. Over 5 million people die from sepsis every year as they get resistant to antibiotics frequently, impacting an estimated 31 million people globally. It can be concluded that most patient safety issues can be mitigated by Effective education and training, proper communication, robust documentation, and adherence to protocols and guidelines.

MULTIPLE CHOICE QUESTIONS

1. Which of the following blood products must be kept at room temperature:
    a. Packed RBCs
    b. Cryoprecipitate
    c. Plasma
    d. Platelet concentrate
2. 'Safe Surgery Saves Lives' is associated with:
    a. World Health Organization
    b. World Health Assembly
    c. Joint Commission
    d. Royal College of Surgeons
3. Which of the following steps is the part of 'time out' of WHO surgical safety checklist?
    a. Ensuring site marking
    b. Anesthesia safety check
    c. Introduction of team members
    d. Proper collection and labelling of specimen
4. Blood transfusion must be finished within _____ hours of commencement:
    a. 2 hours
    b. 4 hours
    c. 3 hours
    d. 6 hours
5. Select the example of health professional-associated factors related to health care-associated errors:
    a. Time pressures and heavy workload
    b. Distractions and interruptions from other staff and patients
    c. Lack of standardized protocols and procedures
    d. Inability to estimate risk
6. Which of the term defines, "An incident that did not reach the patient"?
    a. Adverse event
    b. Patient event
    c. Near misses
    d. Adverse reaction
7. Which of the following is not a component in "Global Patient Safety Challenges"?
    a. Clean Care is Safe Care
    b. Safe Surgery Saves Lives
    c. Medication without harm
    d. Diagnosis without error
8. Which is the most common type of medication error in pediatric patients?
    a. Administering the wrong drug
    b. Administering drugs through the wrong route
    c. Administering an improper dose
    d. Administering drugs to the wrong patient
9. The temperature range in which plasma must be thawed before use?
    a. 30–37°
    b. 20–27°
    c. 27–30°
    d. 37–39°
10. Select the correct statement:
    a. Rh compatibility is not important while administering platelets.
    b. For the recipients of multiple non-ABO identical whole blood units, high titer O whole blood should be preferred
    c. Blood must be collected from healthy donors who are at low risk of infections.
    d. Transfusion-related acute liver injury can occur if donors are not screened for HLA antibodies

ANSWERS			
1. d	2. a	3. c	4. b
5. d	6. c	7. d	8. c
9. a	10. c		

SUGGESTED READING

1. Agency for healthcare research and quality-quality indicators [Internet]. [cited 2023 Jul 4].Available from: https://qualityindicators.ahrq.gov/Downloads/Modules/PSI/V30/2006-Feb-PatientSafetyIndicators.pdf.
2. Brennan TA, Leape LL, Laird N, et al. The nature of adverse events in hospitalized patients: Results of the Harvard Medical Practice Study I. N Engl J Med. 1991;324:370-6.
3. Diagnostic errors- Technical series on safer primary care[Internet]. [cited 2023 Jul 9]. Available from: https://apps.who.int/iris/bitstream/handle/10665/252410/9789241511636-eng.pdf
4. Guidelines and principles for Safe Blood Transfusion Practice - Introduction [Internet]. World Health Organization; [cited 2023 Jul 9]. Available from: https://www.who.int/publications/m/item/guidelines-and-principles-for-safe-blood-transfusion-practice
5. Kohn KT, Corrigan JM, Donaldson MS. To err is human: Building a safer health system [Internet]. US National Library of Medicine; [cited 2023 Jul 9]. Available from: https://pubmed.ncbi.nlm.nih.gov/25077248/

6. Krishnan N, Kaur S, Yaddanapudi LN. Role of protocol adherence and lack of protocol in the precipitation of nursing care errors amongst the patients admitted in the intensive care units of a tertiary care hospital. Journal of Nursing Science and Practice. 2014;4(3):66-71.
7. Krishnan N, Kaur S, Yaddanapudi LN. Role of system-based 'latent factors' in the precipitation of nursing errors amongst the patients admitted in intensive care unit of a tertiary care hospital. NMRJ. 2010;6(4):163-71.
8. Medication errors- Technical series on safer primary care[Internet]. [cited 2023 Jul 9]. Available from: https://apps.who.int/iris/rest/bitstreams/1070139/retrieve
9. National patient safety implementation framework (2018-2025) [Internet]. [cited 2023 Jul 4].Available from: https://main.mohfw.gov.in/sites/default/files/national%20patient%20safety%20implimentation_for%20web.pdf
10. Patient safety [Internet]. World Health Organization; [cited 2023 Jul 9]. Available from: https://www.who.int/teams/integrated-health-services/patient-safety
11. Pèpin J, Chakra CN, Pèpin E, Nault V, Valiquette L. Evolution of the global burden of viral infections from unsafe medical injections, 2000-2010. PLoS One. 2014;9(6):e99677.
12. Safe surgery saves lives [Internet]. [cited 2023 Jul 9]. Available from: https://apps.who.int/iris/bitstream/handle/10665/70080/WHO_IER_PSP_2008.07_eng.pdf?sequence=1
13. Singh H, Giardina TD, Meyer AN, et al. Types and origins of diagnostic errors in primary care settings. JAMA Intern Med. 2013;173:418-25. 10.1001/jamainternmed.2013.2777
14. The clinical use of blood: Handbook [Internet]. World Health Organization; 1970 [cited 2023 Jul 9]. Available from: https://apps.who.int/iris/handle/10665/42396
15. The clinical use of blood: Handbook [Internet]. World Health Organization; 1970 [cited 2023 Jul 9]. Available from: https://apps.who.int/iris/handle/10665/42396

CHAPTER 55

Organ Donation and Transplantation

Navdeep Bansal, Sukhpal Kaur

"You are a piece of the puzzle of someone else's life. You may never know where you fit, but others will fill the holes in their lives with pieces of you."

—Bonnie Arbon

LEARNING OBJECTIVES

After going through the chapter, the learner will be able to:
- Define organ donation.
- Define brain death.
- Enumerate various types of organ transplantation.
- Identify the organ failure patient potential for organ donation.
- Discuss pathophysiology of brain death.
- Describe various legal frameworks and policies to promote and regulate various activities related to organ donation in India.
- Discuss nursing management of a brain-dead patient potential for organ donation.

TERMS

- **Brain death:** As per Section 2(d) of the THOTA brain death is "the stage at which all functions of the brain stem have permanently and irreversibly ceased" and is so certified under Section 3(6) of the act. It was legalized in India in 1994.
- **Deceased organ/tissue donation:** It is the process of taking out an organ or tissue at the time of death of a donor for the purpose of transplantation to another person.
- **Donation after circulatory death (DCD):** It is the process of organ donation happening after the heart stops beating.
- **Potential donor:** An individual whose clinical condition is suspected to fulfill brain death criteria, but is not, yet recognized as a donor.
- **The Transplantation of Human Organs and Tissues Act, 1994 (THOTA):** It has the provisions for regulation of removal, storage, and transplantation of human organs and tissues for therapeutic purposes and for the prevention of commercial dealings in human organs and tissues.

INTRODUCTION

Organ transplantation is the last hope to save the lives of patients who are having end-stage failure of an organ. However, many people lose their lives due to the non-availability of organs. But, because of the awareness of people, an increase in the number of organ transplants in the last two decades has been observed. It has provided excellent results in children and young adults. The result of Organ Transplantation continues to improve, due to innovations and the improvements in peri-operative management. The organs donated by one single cadaver donor can save up to eight lives.

- **Organ donation can be defined as** "giving an organ or part of an organ to be transplanted into another person having terminal organ failure".
- **Organ transplantation can be defined** as a "surgical procedure to replace a diseased organ with a healthier donor organ such as liver, kidneys, heart or lung".

CURRENT SCENARIO OF ORGAN DONATION

There is an acute shortage of organs globally. India is quite behind in the process of organ donation. In India, every year nearly 6 lac people die because of organ failure and due to scarcity of organs for transplant. A disproportionate and huge gap is there between the demand and supply of organs. It is not that in India, there are not enough organs to transplant. Nearly every person who dies naturally or in an accident can be a potential donor for any organ or tissue donation. India is a hub of accidents. During the calendar year 2021, a total number of 4,12,432 road accidents have been reported by the Police Departments of States and Union Territories (UTs) in the country, claiming 1,53,972 lives and causing injuries to 3,84,448 persons (Road Accidents in India, 2021). Although there are strong laws and regulations, even then, India has been unable to prevent the growing number of accidents on its roads. Having 1,53,972 deaths annually because of accidents is a huge number. The lack of awareness and misconceptions about organ donation among the public are the major factors for the shortage of organs. The other causes of organ shortage include refusal by the family to donate; not recognizing a potential organ donor by the medical fraternity; cultural considerations among people influencing the willingness to donate; and even the knowledge and attitudes of health professionals regarding organ donation.

Currently, India has a 0.4 per million population deceased organ donation rate, whereas countries such as Spain and the United States have 38 deceased donors per million population followed by Portugal which has about 25 donors per million population. These countries have an opt-out system of transplant whereas India has to opt-in system for transplant.

Opt-out System

It is a donation policy, wherein it is presumed that all the individuals residing in a country/state are willing deceased organ donors unless they specifically opt out of doing so, also known as presumed consent. Opting out requires individuals to state their preference against deceased organ donation during their lifetime. Usually, such a preference is recorded in a national opt-out register.

Opt-in System

This system is opposite to the opt-out system of donation. It is a donation policy, wherein the individuals express their own willingness for being a deceased organ donor. So, in this system, no one is presumed to be a willing donor unless they make a statement regarding their preference for a deceased donation. It is also known as an express consent policy.

TYPES OF TRANSPLANTATION (FIG. 55.1)

- ❖ **Autograft or autotransplantation:** It is the transplantation of an individual's own tissue to another side of his own body. For example, retrieval of skin from the legs and transplantation of it on damaged skin of the face or another part of the body.
- ❖ **Allograft or allotransplantation:** It is the transplantation of an organ or tissue between two genetically non-identical individuals of the same species. Mostly all human tissues and organs transplant are examples of allograft or allotransplantation.
- ❖ **Iso-transplantation or iso-graft:** It is the transplantation of organs or tissues between two genetically identical

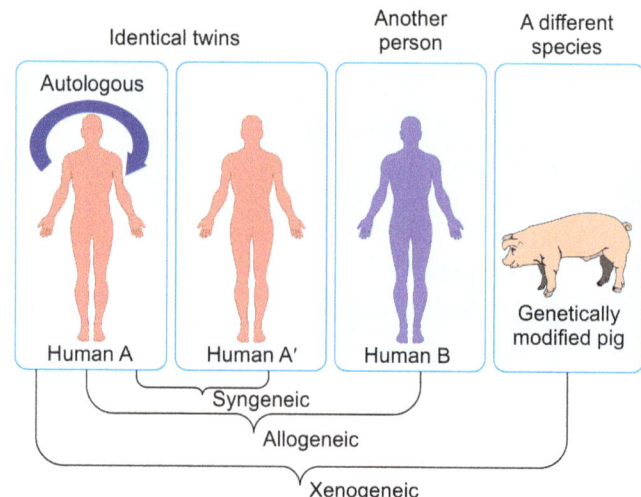

Fig. 55.1: Different types of transplants.

individuals, i.e., monozygotic twins. There will be no immune response, so there will be no transplant rejection.
- ❖ **Xenotransplantation or xenograft:** The transplantation of tissues or organs from one species to another species is called xenotransplantation. For example, the tissues and organs from pigs are tried to transplant into human beings, but still, this is in the infancy phase and requires more innovations.
- ❖ **Split transplant:** The transplantation when an organ is divided into two parts and given to more than one recipient, it is called split transplantation. For example, the liver from a deceased donor can be divided into two recipients usually an adult and a child.
- ❖ **Domino transplant:** It is also called sequential transplant. It happens rarely. It is the transplantation in which the recipient also acts as a donor at the same time. For example, if a patient needs lungs, but the best management is to give that patient a combination of heart and lung, and as his heart was in good condition, it can be transplanted in another patient who requires only a heart.
- ❖ **ABO-incompatible transplants:** With the advancement in medical science, it is now also possible to transplant organs between ABO incompatible individuals, it permits more efficient use of available organs regardless of ABO blood type, but this type of transplant involves the use of expensive procedures like plasma pheresis and use of powerful monoclonal antibodies to prevent rejection.
- ❖ **Swap transplants:** This method of transplantation is used to overcome the shortage of organs and to avoid ABO incompatible transplants. In this transplant, in legal ways, the blood group incompatible donor and recipient couples are matched with couples having the same problems.

TYPES OF DONORS

Organ donors can be living or deceased organ donors. Deceased donors can be further classified based on manner of death, i.e., they can be donated after circulatory death or donation after brain death. Some of the renewable tissues and organs like blood, skin, kidney, and liver can be taken from living donors. But the maximum number of organs

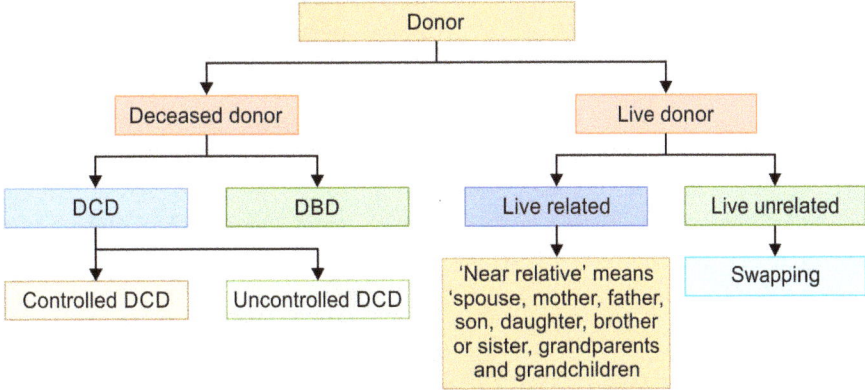

Flowchart 55.1: Different types of transplants.

(DBD: donation after brain death; DCD: donation after circulatory death)

and tissues can be taken from deceased organ donors only **(Flowchart 55.1)**.

Live Donor

The prerequisites for a living donor are that the person is above 18 years of age, and should be mentally and physically healthy. The person can donate one of a paired organ, part of an organ, or a tissue. The different types of organs that can be transplanted from living donors are the kidney, a segment of the liver, the lobe of one lung, a portion of the pancreas, and the intestine. The most common organs that are taken from living donors are the kidneys and the liver.

The live donor can be further classified as live-related donors and live unrelated donors. Live-related donor means donation between family members or near relatives. As per THOTA rules 2014, near relative means spouse, son, daughter, father, mother, brother, sister, grandmother, grandson, and granddaughter. Live unrelated cases include two cases of swapping and cases based on altruistic donations.

Deceased Donors

Deceased donation is the donation of organs after death. Deceased donors are the maximum source of organs currently. Deceased donors can be further classified on the basis of/manner of death, i.e., donation after circulatory death (DCD) and donation after brain death (DBD).

The patients after brain stem death are the donors who are at a stage where all the brain functions are permanently and irreversibly ceased. In this case, it is important to establish the cause of irreversible coma. Pre-conditions should be met. The confounding factors are to be ruled out.

Donation after Circulatory Death (DCD)

Donation after circulatory death means that organ donation happens after the heart stops beating, in contrast to donation after brain death where the heart is still beating, it is also referred to as donation after cardiac death.

Currently, donation after circulatory death is low in India but it is gaining more and more prominence with time. As in these donors, circulatory arrest has occurred and there is no circulation of blood to the organs so organ retrieval must start as soon as possible after death has been determined. Donations after circulatory death can be further classified into two types based on the circumstances of cardiac arrest.

TABLE 55.1: Difference between natural death and brain death.

Natural death	Brain death
No spontaneous respiratory activity	No spontaneous respiratory activity
No consciousness (coma+)	No consciousness (coma+)
No cardiac activity	Cardiac activity present
All organ systems shut down	Organ systems other than brain preserved
The irreversible state has completed all organ system shutdowns.	Irreversible neurological state—could slowly progress to another organ dysfunction.

Uncontrolled DCD

In this, there is sudden and unexpected cardiac arrest, which makes it very difficult to retrieve organs, and warm ischemia time is also increased.

Controlled DCD

In this, the elective withdrawal of ventilation in an end-of-life situation leads to cardiac arrest. So, this donation is comparatively easy than uncontrolled circulatory death, also warm ischemia time is less which makes it more suitable for organ donation.

Table 55.1 depicts the difference between natural death and brain death.

NATIONAL ORGAN TRANSPLANT PROGRAMME

As there is a huge gap between the demand and supply of organs, so to promote organ donation, the Director General of Health Services of Government of India implemented the National Organ Transplant Programme to carry out the activities as per the amendment act, for the training of manpower and promotion of Organ Donation from deceased donors.

Objectives

1. To organize a system of organ and tissue procurement and distribution for transplantation
2. To promote deceased organ and tissue donation.
3. To train the required manpower
4. To protect vulnerable poor from organ trafficking.
5. To monitor organ and tissue transplant services and bring about policy and program corrections wherever required.

Flowchart 55.2: Transplant organizations at various levels.

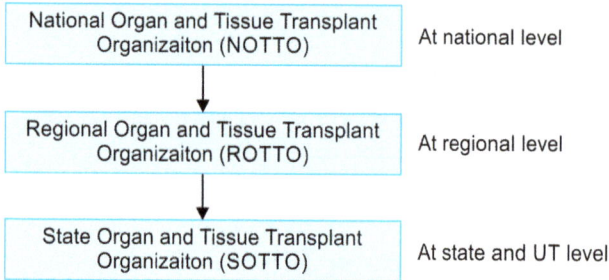

Under this program, an apex-level National Organ and Tissue Transplant Organization (NOTTO) at New Delhi, five Regional Organ and Tissue Transplant Organizations (ROTTOs), and sixteen State Organ and Tissue Transplant Organizations (SOTTOs) have been established **(Flowchart 55.2)**. The main role of these organizations is to control and regulate all the activities related to organ donation at the National, Regional, and State levels respectively, and is to publicize appropriate information about organ donations to the general public.

Legal Framework in India

In India Transplantation of Human Organ Act (THOA) was passed in 1994. It provides a system to regulate the removal, storage, and transplantation of Human Organs for therapeutic purposes. Further, it also regulates a system for the prevention of commercial dealing in human organs. This act was amended in 2011 following which, transplantation of human organ and tissues rules 2014 were notified in March 2014. Some of the points defined in this act are:

- ❖ Regulation of human organ retrieval and transplant centers.
- ❖ Next of kin who can give consent in case of cadaver organ donation.
- ❖ Regulations regarding live donation between near relatives, unrelated, and foreigners.
- ❖ Various tests, members, and procedures of brain death.
- ❖ Punishments if someone is involved in commercial dealings of organs.

PATHOPHYSIOLOGY OF BRAIN DEATH

Severe trauma, hemorrhage, tumors, etc., cause damage to neuronal tissue. This may lead to edema and an increase in intracranial pressure and thereby compromising cerebral perfusion. A vicious cycle is initiated in which decreasing cerebral perfusion and increasing ICP interact with each other until no further blood flows in the cranial cavity and herniation of the brain occurs. A continuous uncontrolled rise in the intracranial pressure gradually decreases the venous return from the brain initially and a further rise in intracranial pressure chokes the brain of its arterial blood supply eventually resulting in neural death.

ROLE OF NURSES IN ORGAN DONATION

The success of organ retrieval of a brain-dead patient is highly dependent on organ preservation. Nursing professionals play an imperative role in every successful organ donation

---

BOX 55.1: Role of nurses in organ donation.

- Educating the public with accurate and objective information concerning donations.
- Participating in activities to identify possible donors
- Working closely with the healthcare facility, the organ procurement organization (OPO) and/or tissue bank, and members of the health team to seek consideration for such donations
- Proving emotional support and objective and accurate information to families considering organ and tissue donation.
- Advocating patients and families in the informed choice process
- Recognizing and respecting their cultural and religious beliefs
- Demonstrating clinical expertise while providing care to the brain-dead patients potential for organ donation (discussed later)

---

program **(Box 55.1)**. They can also choose their carrier in the field of organ donation by becoming transplant coordinators, by taking training from NOTTO, and from other organizations which provide training courses for transplant coordinators. As per the THOTA Act, it is mandatory for every hospital to keep transplant coordinators if any hospital wants to start transplant-related activities. Nurses can resume various responsibilities by becoming cadaver donor coordinators, recipient coordinators, and live donation coordinators.

It is estimated that about 1–4% of people who die in hospitals and from 10 to 15% of those who die in intensive care units are potential donors. Among all the healthcare professionals nurses are the ones who are with the patients for most of the time. So, it is imperative that they should be knowledgeable enough regarding the early identification of potential donors and the care of brain-dead patients. The gift of life can be given to needy persons by making the organ available to that particular person. Organs and tissues of a brain-dead body must be meticulously maintained, and remain hemodynamically and thermodynamically stable to avoid damage and to maintain optimum function for procurement. It is the nurse who maintains hemodynamic stability so that the organs of the donor remain viable by the time the other related formalities are completed. The nurses need to know various physiologic changes that occur at the time of brain death and the essential nursing interventions.

BRAIN DEATH

Brain death is the irreversible end of brain activity that occurs because of total necrosis of the cerebral neurons following the loss of oxygenation to the brain. Patients classified as brain dead can be eligible candidates for the removal of their organs surgically for organ donation. Brain death is a legal death, but still with the heart beating, and with mechanical ventilation all other vital organs may be kept completely alive, viable, and functional for organ transplantation. Clinical evaluation of the patient is carried out to determine brain death. A neurological examination is done to document the irreversible loss of total brain functions. The criteria for determining brain death include assessment for coma or unresponsiveness, absence of brainstem reflexes, and apnea **(Fig. 55.2)**.

- ❖ **Coma or unresponsiveness:** The brain-dead person cannot be awakened by any stimulus. He does not respond to pain or speech. Pressure is applied at the supraorbital

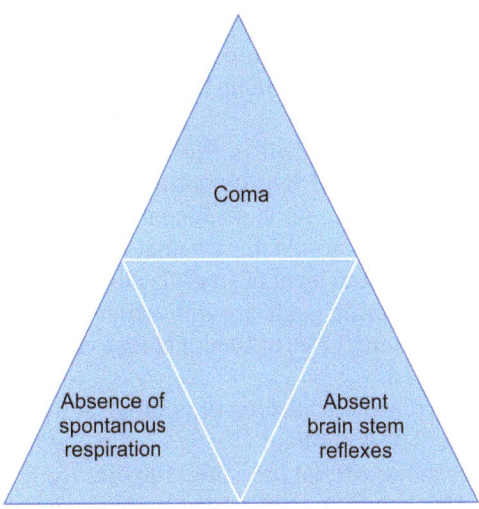

Fig. 55.2: Brain death triad.

area to test the response to painful stimuli. A GCS score of 3 indicates profound unresponsiveness.

❖ **Absence of brainstem reflexes:** These include checking the pupillary reflex, corneal reflex, cough and gag reflexes, and jaw reflex. The following tests are performed to confirm the absence of brainstem reflexes **(Fig. 55.3)**:
  ➤ *Pupillary reflex*: This is checked by throwing a light beam with a torch into the patient's eyes. Normally the pupils constrict. In brain-dead patients, the pupils do not react to light. The fixed and dilated pupils of size greater than 4 mm are suggestive of brain death.
  ➤ *Oculocephalic reflex or Doll's eyes reflex*: This is also known as the "doll's eyes" test. This involves turning the patient's head rapidly at 90° to both sides. In a normal doll's eye reflex, the eyes move in the direction of movement of the head. A brain-dead patient's eyes will stay fixed at the midline. A negative doll's eye reflex signifies severe brain damage or brain death. So, when this reflex is absent, the eyes remain fixed at midline irrespective of the head-turning in either direction. This test should not be performed in unstable cervical spine injuries.
  ➤ *Vestibulo-ocular reflex*: This is also called the caloric test. It involves instilling about 50 mL of cold water or saline into the ear canal. Normally, the patient's eyes will turn toward the stimulated ear. The eyes are to be observed for a minute after the completion of irrigation. After five minutes repeat the test on the other side. No eye movement occurs in a brain-dead person. Before testing this reflex, it is important to inspect both ears using an auroscope in order to confirm that the tympanic membrane is intact and there is no obstruction in the external auditory canal with wax or any other material.
  ➤ *Corneal reflex*: The tip of a sterile cotton swab is gently touched to the patient's cornea from the side. Normally there will be blinking of the eyelids and/or eye movement. In brain dead person, neither there will blinking nor eye movement.
  ➤ *Cough reflex*: To check the cough reflex, deep bronchial suctioning is performed through the patient's endotracheal tube. There will be no cough response in case of brain death.
  ➤ *Gag reflex:* It can be assessed either by manually manipulating the endotracheal tube or by touching a cotton-tipped applicator to the posterior pharynx. There will be no gag reflex in a brain-dead person.
  ➤ *Apnea test*: In order to perform this test, the patient is taken off mechanical ventilation and is administered 100% oxygen at the rate of 6 L/min for eight minutes. The patient is observed for signs of attempted breathing. An arterial blood gas (ABG) is performed to ensure adequate $PaCO_2$ to stimulate respiration. With $PaCO_2$ level greater than 60 mm Hg and no attempt of breathing confirms brain death.

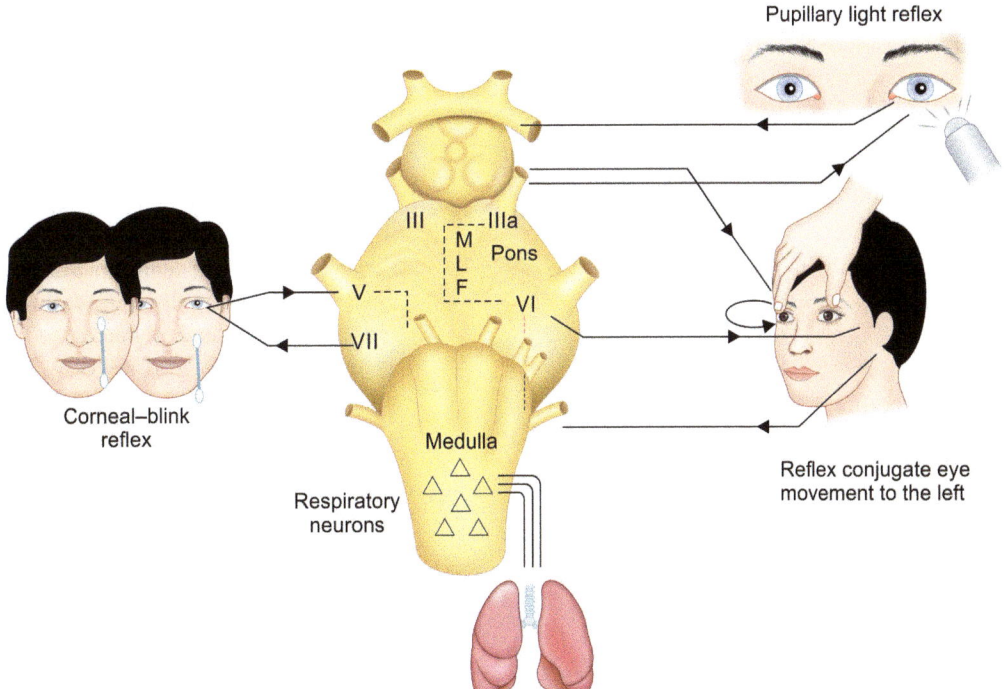

Fig. 55.3: Brainstem reflexes.

Management of Brain Death Patients: Nurses' Role

Once the brain death is confirmed, the focus of care shifts from treating the patient with a brain injury to preserving the organs. It is important to remember that the care of potential brain-dead organ donors is **"caring for multiple recipients"**. A multidisciplinary team approach is required for successful organ donation. Maintenance of the physiology of all the available organs in the donor is extremely imperative till the time of organ retrieval.

Management of deceased donors is discussed under three aspects as depicted in **Figure 55.4**.

1. **Physiological care**: Maintenance of deceased donors requires high standards of nursing care, invasive monitoring, and prompt treatment to preserve organ function. Brain death alters the physiology and the cellular biochemistry of all organic systems drastically. Various physiologic changes that occur with brain death include:
   - Hemodynamic instability
   - Endocrine abnormalities
   - Hypothermia
   - Coagulopathy
   - Respiratory dysfunction
   - Cardiovascular system changes
   - Impairment in renal function
   - Electrolyte imbalances
   - Corticosteroid deficiency
   - *Maintenance of hemodynamic instability:* Hemodynamically instability is observed even prior to the diagnosis of brain death in a patient. The functioning of all the vital parameters is altered. With the progression of cerebral ischemia and as it reaches the brainstem, a severe increase in systemic vascular resistance (SVR) and blood pressure occurs because of the release of endogenous catecholamines, commonly referred to as a "catecholamine storm." These reflect the body's attempt to maintain cerebral circulation and reverse brain ischemia. However, at the peak of increased SVR, cardiac output decreases, and intense vasoconstriction leads to decreased perfusion to abdominal organs. As ischemia continues, the catecholamine storm subsides with a decline in SVR. Blood pressure then drops further leading to hypoperfusion of vital organ systems unless treated. Hypotension is the most common hemodynamic instability observed in up to 91% of brain-dead organ donors.

Fluid resuscitation is the main therapy for the management of hypotension. The choice of fluid depends on the patient's hematocrit and electrolyte status. It is suggested that a hematocrit level of 25–30%, or hemoglobin level of 10 g/dL should be targeted. If hemodynamic goals are not achieved with volume replacement (CVP: 6–10 mm of Hg), vasoactive drugs are added.

"To achieve the various physiological parameters, a rule of 100 is applied:
- Systolic arterial pressure >100 mm Hg
- Urine output >**100 mL/h**
- PaO_2 >**100 mm Hg**
- Hemoglobin concentration >100 g/L (10 g/dL)
- Blood sugar 100 mg/dL

- *Maintenance of endocrine abnormalities:* Brain death affects the hypothalamus-pituitary axis. In most of the cases, vasopressin release is decreased which results in diabetes insipidus (DI). It occurs in about 80% of these patients. The various features of DI include:
  - Urine output >4 mL/kg/hour
  - Increasing serum sodium >145 mmol/L
  - Increasing serum osmolarity >300 mOsm/L
  - Urine osmolarity <300 mOsm/L, urine specific gravity (<1.005).

Management of DI involves the replacement of fluid to maintain hourly urine output and vasopressin (Pitressin) infusion. Observe urine output of at least 0.5 mL/kg/h to determine the need for fluid resuscitation and vasopressin infusion. Replace the fluid deficit and ongoing fluid losses with hyponatremic fluid. 0.45% saline is an appropriate first choice of fluid administration.

The patients following brain death are also at risk of developing hyperglycemia. Various factors like stress response to injury, reduced insulin levels due to catecholamine release or inotropic infusion, and resuscitation with glucose-containing fluids lead to hyperglycemia. The main consequences of hyperglycemia are a hyperosmolar state leading to dehydration and a shift in electrolytes from intracellular to extracellular fluids, osmotic diuresis with a subsequent loss of water and electrolytes, metabolic acidosis, and ketosis.

Hyperglycemia is managed by IV administration of insulin by infusion at least 1 unit/hour and may be titrated to a serum glucose level of 120 to 180 mg/dL. This prevents additional fluid loss due to osmotic diuresis. Hyperglycemia can lead to osmotic diuresis and cellular dehydration, resulting in hypovolemia. Regular blood-glucose monitoring with corrective interventions is very important. Finger-stick measurement is usually adequate.

- *Hypothermia: body temperature maintenance:* Body temperature is regulated by the hypothalamus through a homeostatic feedback mechanism. In a healthy

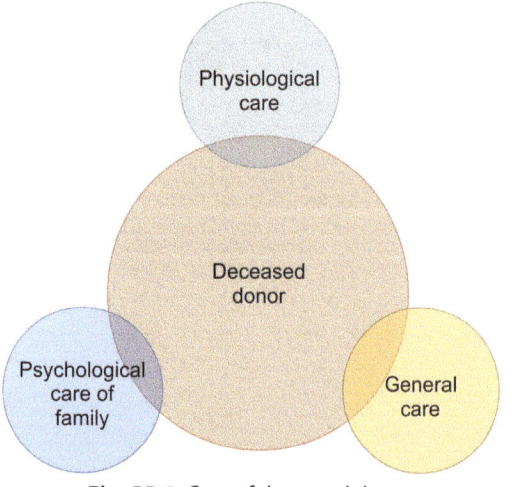

Fig. 55.4: Care of deceased donor.

person, if the body becomes too hot, the hypothalamus prompts vasodilation, resulting in sweating. If the body becomes too cool, the hypothalamus prompts vasoconstriction in the skin, shivering, and piloerection, resulting in heat retention. After brain death, because of the loss of thalamic and hypothalamic central temperature control mechanisms, the body becomes poikilothermic. Hypothermia contributes to hemodynamic instability. Various harmful effects of hypothermia include myocardial depression leading to decreased cardiac output; reduced tissue oxygen delivery; impaired ability of the kidneys to maintain tubular concentration gradients, and coagulopathy. Management of hypothermia is accomplished ideally by prevention and frequent monitoring of body temperature. The various measures to maintain body temperature could be aggressive surface warming with heat lamps at a distance of 0.5–1 m from the donor, the use of warm blankets, warmed IV fluids, and heated humidified ventilator systems. The donor's body temperature should be maintained at 36.5–37.5°C (97.7–99.5°F).

> *Maintenance of coagulation function:* Release of a large amount of tissue thromboplastin and plasminogen from ischemic or necrotic brain tissue results in coagulopathy. Hypothermia and the release of catecholamines contribute to coagulation disorders. Fluid resuscitation to manage hypovolemia causes dilution of coagulation factors in circulation.

Bleeding from any site like gingival bleeding, hematuria, GI, or skin should alert the nurses to suspect coagulation disorders. It is also important to confirm and match blood groups and various blood components to avoid mismatch reactions that can initiate or aggravate clotting disorders.

> *Maintenance of respiratory functions:* Central control of breathing which occurs from pons and medulla oblongata is lost after brain death. Coexisting problems like pneumonia, gastric aspiration, ARDS, etc., lead to further respiratory compromise. Pneumothorax, lung trauma caused by the initiating event will aggravate the respiratory compromise. Sterile and frequent suction of respiratory secretions is very important after brain death. Ventilation-perfusion mismatch, atelectasis, and increased body oxygen demand will further aggravate respiratory problems. Standard management is aimed at maintaining PaO_2 between 70–100 mm Hg, using tidal volumes of 8–12 mL/kg, FiO_2 <0.6, and PEEP <5 cm H_2O, keeping $PaCO_2$ within the normal range. If PaO_2 is <70 mm Hg, FiO_2 is increased to maintain SaO_2 >95%, and PEEP is increased carefully, monitoring its effect on cardiac output and plateau pressure (<30 cm H_2O), to reduce the risk of barotrauma.

> *Cardiovascular system changes and maintenance of cardiovascular functions:* Hypovolemia is the most common cause of hypotension in organ donors whereas the contributory factors include dieresis with osmotic solutions and drugs to reduce cerebral edema, inadequate replacement of fluid losses, polyuria due to diabetes insipidus, and diuretics. Arrhythmias may be caused by metabolic, cardiac, or hormonal consequences and will further add to hypotension. On the contrary, hypertension may occur in these patients due to the release of catecholamines and thus increase systemic vascular resistance which ultimately culminates into hypotension due to loss of vasomotor tone and left ventricular dysfunction. Half of brain-dead persons develop hypotension due to brain herniation.

As the ultimate aim of care is to maintain adequate organ perfusion, it is of paramount importance to stabilize the donor's hemodynamic status irrespective of the underlying cause of the hypotension. In most of the situations, liberal fluid therapy to maintain intravascular volume should help maintain the hemodynamic equilibrium as hypovolemia is invariably the underlying factor although central venous pressure monitoring can better guide the management. Complete loss of organs and/or impaired quality of the donor organs can be the result of under or over-fluid resuscitation. Low levels of hemoglobin or hypoproteinemic states need to be tackled with appropriate transfusions. Depending upon fluid losses and electrolyte status, crystalloids or colloids will do the job in the rest of the donors. Even with appropriate fluid infusion, donors will invariably require inotropic support to achieve adequate organ perfusion. Dopamine in low doses will usually be the first choice while other vasopressors can be used as per need-based circumstances with regular monitoring and titration. Nursing care is required while maintaining vasopressin infusion, vitals monitoring, and urine output status assessment.

> *Maintenance of renal function:* Good renal function involves maintaining adequate systemic perfusion pressure and urine output (>1–2 mL/kg/hr), while minimizing the use of vasopressors. If urine output is less (<1 mL/kg/hr) after adequate volume loading, loop diuretics (furosemide), or osmotic diuretics (mannitol) should be used. The use of nephrotoxic drugs (aminoglycosides) and agents that adversely affect renal perfusion (e.g., NSAIDs), should be avoided. Nursing interventions include closely monitoring fluid intake and urine output and the patient's overall state of hydration as well. Frequently measure the urine output, heart rate, and blood pressure, or invasively by using a central line to monitor central venous pressure.

> *Maintenance of electrolytes:* All the body electrolytes get deranged in brain-dead patients. Hypernatremia is common in these patients because of dehydration, sodium administration, and diabetes insipidus. Hyponatremia is uncommon in these patients that may occur secondary to hyperglycemia. Hyperkalemia, though rare, may result from impaired renal elimination of potassium (i.e., kidney failure) or the causes leading to the movement of potassium into the extracellular fluid (i.e., metabolic acidosis). A majority (90%) of brain-dead patients develop hypokalemia because of various causes like the use of diuretics, polyuria from any cause, and alkalosis.

Hypocalcemia, hypophosphatemia, and hypomagnesemia are most often related to the polyuria associated with osmotic diuresis, the use of diuretics, and diabetes insipidus. Hypocalcemia is often present when the brain-dead patient has been aggressively transfused with blood. Hypercalcemia, hyperphosphatemia, and hypermagnesemia because of brain death are rare.

> *Corticosteroid deficiency:*
> - The presumed reason for corticosteroid deficiency is firstly hypothalamic-pituitary-adrenal (HPA) axis failure which could mediate hemodynamic instability.
> - Secondly, hemodynamic instability and hormonal imbalances in brain-dead donors lead to the release of pro-inflammatory and immunological mediators. This has been associated with reduced graft function.
> - High doses of corticosteroids may reduce brainstem death-induced inflammation and help to modulate immune function. This may improve the donor organ quality and post-transplant graft functioning. This has also been shown to improve donor lung quality.

2. **General care:** It is important to remember that the brain-dead patient should be provided care as that of a normal patient. So, along with prompt care to achieve various physiological parameters, these brain-dead donors require general care also.
   > Practice all the general measures of infection control as per standard care. The presence of infection may complicate the donor organs and further the recipient. Bacteremia or sepsis are not contraindications to donation, provided pathogen-specific antibiotics have been administered for at least 48 hours before procurement.
   > Frequent turning of patients and meticulous skin care for the prevention of bedsores.
   > Provide oral care and back care at least once in 6 hours and sponge bath once a day.
   > Change the dressing, and provide urinary and intravascular catheter care as per the guidelines to minimize the risk of infection. Ideally, it should be done daily or early, if these get soiled.
   > Maintain bronchial hygiene to improve the elimination of secretions.
   > Provide eye care to ensure that there are no corneal abrasions or ulcers. This will improve the chance of corneal donation. So,
   > - Cover the eye with a sterile gauze or sterile surgical pad
   > - Clean eyes with normal saline every three hourly
   > - Apply lubricant or eye drops (as prescribed) every three hours to maintain the area clean and moist.
   > A nasogastric tube must be inserted for gastric decompression and prevention of aspiration.
   > The patient should be administered feed as prescribed. It can be total parenteral nutrition (TPN) or any other as per prescription. These can be high protein and high-calorie feed --(A-1 (Milk based), A-2 (soya based); Lactulose and gluten-free (A-3 (100% Whey protein), and Khichdi feed.
   > Arterial and central venous lines should be inserted preferably into the upper extremities because femoral line readings can become inaccurate during surgical procedures for organ procurement.

3. **Psychological care:** There is never anything easy or routine in Organ Donation. It is a huge challenge and emotionally draining dealing with any and every case. On one hand, it is difficult to handle the grieving family's emotional and psychological issues, which is quite understandable in view of the unbearable loss of a family member. But more challenging is sorting the difficulties related to brain death declaration administrative issues, building a consensus among decision-makers of family, and police permission in MLC cases.

So, along with the maintenance of the deceased donor, there will be lots of psychological needs of the family of brain-dead patients as soon as the patient is declared brain-dead. The family needs to be assured that every effort has been made to save the life of their loved one. It is extremely important that the team attends to the family of the potential donor in the most cordial and friendly way. The family should be answered any questions they ask. They should be provided with the necessary information. They may be allowed to visit their potential donor if they wish.

MEASURES TO PROMOTE ORGAN DONATION

As the organ donation rate is very low in India due to various myths and misconceptions related to organ donation among the general population, some of the measures that can be taken to promote organ donation are:

❖ **In curriculum:** As the concept of organ donation is added in the syllabus of medical and nursing students, similarly it should be added in the syllabus of children at the school level so that they should become aware of this at their early phase of life.

❖ **Large-scale awareness:** By organizing large-scale awareness programs, deceased organ donation can be promoted. These should aim to educate people about the benefits of organ donation, and clear all prevalent myths and misconceptions. The concept of brain death needs to be adequately dealt with so that a maximum number of families with brain-dead patients should opt for organ donation. Positive messaging on organ donation can be done using the following media:
> TV, Radio, In-cinema halls
> Social Media
> Celebrity endorsements
> Theater and Street Plays
> Organizing events such as marathons, concerts, etc. to promote organ donation
> On-ground awareness drives at Schools, Colleges, Corporate offices, Clubs, etc.

❖ Option on driving license and ID cards as has been started by some of the states like Tamil Nadu and Chandigarh

❖ Option for pledging of organs should be asked from the person when he or she is going to apply for a driving license

- It should also be the policy of every organization or company to ask for pledging of organs when a new employee is going to apply for ID card.
- **Declaration of brain death should be mandatory**—declaration of brain death should be made mandatory in every intensive care unit because that patient can be a potential donor and can save the lives of many needy people.

Case Scenario

1. A 16-year-old male from Haryana was diagnosed with spontaneous ICH on 12-01-2019. He was referred by a local hospital to PGIMER on 14-1-2019 and was immediately shifted to OT, but due to increased intracranial pressure could not be operated upon. His GCS was 3. He was kept in the intensive care unit. On 17-01-19, he was suspected of potential brain dead. A brain death declaration committee was constituted and the patient was declared brain dead at 9.04 pm on the 17th itself. The family gave verbal consent for organ donation. The second committee was planned in the morning of 18-01-19. This committee deferred brain death due to the presence of some flickering movements. It was planned by committee members for re-evaluation after 12 hours. Even after 12 hours, it was observed that some movements were still present and were even increased somewhat. The benefit of the doubt was given to the patient and the patient was not declared brain dead and was kept under observation. Opinions were taken from various experts from different fields regarding those movements, some were saying these as spinal reflexes but some were not convinced. Even video was sent to experts in this field outside India. All other mandatory tests like the apnea test was positive, the doll's eye was absent, cold calorie test was negative. The patient was in the same condition for more than one week. It was a tragic situation for the family, and even for the health care professionals that what to explain to the family? After 10 days it was decided to go for a confirmatory test. So, a four vessels angiography was planned for the patient. The scan was showing no blood supply to the brain. The committee was again constituted on 28-1-19 and the patient was declared brain dead on 29-01-19 after the second committee as no movements were present. The family gave written consent for organ donation. Liver, both kidneys, and cornea were retrieved successfully.

   This case has shown that the situations where a complete and accurate clinical evaluation is impossible, clinicians must use additional tests, called ancillary tests, to confirm the neurological death of the patient. Brain blood flow imaging, such as four-vessel angiography, and functional tests, such as radionuclide imaging, have traditionally been used as the gold standard ancillary tests for the neurological determination of death (NDD). And secondly, the patient was brain-dead for more than one week, even then four organs were retrieved successfully. This shows that the patient was provided meticulous nursing care to maintain the viability of the organs.

2. A 21-year-old male from Punjab, unmarried, was admitted at PGIMER on 1/03/2019 after a roadside accident (RSA) with a severe head injury. He was kept in the Intensive care unit. But declared brain dead on 9/03/2019. Male members of the family usually accompany patients in the hospital, so the same was in this case. All male Family members (father, brother, uncle) were available in the hospital and were counseled for organ donation. They gave consent for organ donation.

   Being medicolegal case (MLC), information was sent to investigating officer for NOC. He was not aware of organ donation and refused to give NOC for organ donation. So higher officials like SHO, DSP, and SP were contacted for help. Even though they were not aware, they said investigating officer (IO) will take the decision. Even after efforts of one day, he did not give NOC. Father was still willing to donate but IO was not ready to listen to him or to come to the hospital. Forensic team clearance was already taken, when asked for their opinion in this case, they said to proceed without NOC as they are going to ascertain the cause of death. When more pressure was put on investigating officer, he sent some police personnel to the house of the patient and they bought the mother and sister of the patient to the police station. They took in writing from the mother of the patient that she does not want to donate the organs of her son. Instead of sending NOC to us, they sent a statement of the mother. Later, the father said it will cause a dispute in their family, and due to fear of the police, they took patient LAMA. So, we lost one healthy potential donor to convert into an actual donor.

   This case reflects that instead of making the family more comfortable with their decision, the police generate unnecessary concerns. Not surprisingly, requests for donations are more likely to be honored if the police and the health care personnel work together as a team. This case also highlights the importance of awareness generation regarding organ donation among the public.

SUMMARY

Organ donation is one of the best gifts which a person can give to another. Due to various myths and misconceptions in the general public as well as a lack of clarity regarding various issues of organ donation and brain death among healthcare professionals as well, the rate of deceased organ donation is very low in India. There is a need to spread lots of awareness among the general public as well as among healthcare professionals to improve organ donation rates and to save various crucial lives. Nurses being important members of the health care team as well as their interaction with family members of patients and the community can play a crucial role in improving the rate of organ donation.

MULTIPLE CHOICE QUESTIONS

1. Which of the following conditions is an absolute contraindication to organ donation?
   a. Bacteremia
   b. Squamous cell carcinoma of the skin
   c. HIV infection
   d. Hospital-acquired infection

2. How many potential solid organ transplant recipients can receive organs from a single deceased donor:
   a. 2
   b. 4
   c. 6
   d. 8

3. The process of removal and replacement of damaged tissues or organs with healthy ones from a donor is called:
   a. Organ retrieval
   b. Organ transplantation
   c. Replacement therapy
   d. All of the above

4. The transfer of an individual's own tissue to another part of the body is called:
   a. Autograft
   b. Xenograft
   c. Allograft
   d. Syngeneic graft

5. The transfer of tissue/organs between genetically identical individuals/twins is called:
   a. Autograft
   b. Syngenic graft
   c. Xenograft
   d. Allograft

6. Which of the following organs survive shortest outside the body:
   a. Kidneys
   b. Heart
   c. Liver
   d. Pancreas

7. Major sources of organs in India are:
   a. Living donors
   b. Cadaver donors
   c. Organ from other species
   d. Artificially created organs

8. Which of the following is not consistent with brain death:
   a. Diabetes insipidus
   b. Hyperglycemia
   c. Pinpoint pupils
   d. Hypothermia
9. Which of the following does not need to be ruled out before assessing for brain death:
   a. Fractures
   b. Electrolyte imbalances
   c. Hypothermia
   d. Drug intoxication
10. Which of the following conditions would not fulfill the criteria for brain death?
    a. Absence of brain stem reflexes
    b. No response to painful stimuli in all four extremities
    c. Absence of EEG activity in a sedated patient
    d. Absence of blood flow to the brain on the brain scan
11. All the following are pre-requisites for brain death certification, *except*:
    a. Hypothermia excluded and spontaneous respiration has ceased
    b. Severe metabolic and endocrine disturbances excluded
    c. Reversible causes of coma due to sedatives, neuromuscular blocking agents, or anesthetic drugs excluded
    d. The patient should not be on inotropic support

ANSWERS

1. c	2. d	3. b	4. a
5. b	6. b	7. a	8. c
9. a	10. c	11. d	

SUGGESTED READING

1. Gordon JK, McKinlay J. Physiological changes after brainstem death and management of the heart-beating donor. Contin Educ Anaesth Crit Care Pain 2012. First published online: May 24, 2012.
2. http://www.anaesthesia.ie/archive/ICSI/ICSI%20Guidelines%20MAY10.pdf. Diagnosis of brain death and medical management of organ donors. Guidelines for adult patients 2010.
3. https://dghs.gov.in/content/1353_3_NationalOrganTransplantProgramme.aspx
4. https://dghs.gov.in/WriteReadData/userfiles/file/RTI/THOA_NOTP_NOTTO_ROTT O_SOTTO_16-7-2020.pdf
5. https://notto.gov.in/WriteReadData/Final_sop/ICU/Intensive_Care_Unit.pdf
6. Kaur S, Bhagat H. Nursing management of brain-dead organ donors, In: Kaur S, Singh M (Eds). Clinical Neuroscience and Critical Care Nursing, 1st edition. Jaypee Brothers Medical Publishers, New Delhi. 2014:364.
7. Kaur S, Ghai S, Krishnan N, Rana D, Kathania D, Kaur G, et al. Knowledge, attitude, and perception regarding organ donation among Nursing students. J Postgrad Med Edu Res. 2015;49(3):105-10.
8. Liberato SMD, Mendonça AED, Freire ILSF, Dantas RAND4, Torres GV. Nursing care of the potential donor of organs after brain death: Integrative review. J Nurs UFPE online. 2012;6(10):2521-6.
9. Ministry of Road Transport and Highways https://morth.nic.in › files › RA_2021_Compressed
10. Swarnalatha G, Sahay M. Manual for Transplant Coordinators, 1st edition.

CHAPTER 56

Importance of Yoga for Nursing Professionals

Tanmya Deswal, Pooja Nadholta, Sadhana Verma

"Yoga means addition—addition of energy, strength, and beauty to body, mind, and soul."

—Amit Ray

LEARNING OBJECTIVES

After going through the chapter, the learner will be able to:
- Enlist the causative factors of stress and burnout among nurses.
- Explore the scientific evidence supporting the beneficial impact of yoga on nursing students and professionals.
- Appreciate the role of yoga in managing psychosocial stress and enhancing the overall quality of life of an individual.
- Understand various yoga asanas for the beginners.

TERMS

- **Allostatic load:** It is "the wear and tear on the body" which gets accumulated as a result of repeated exposure to stress.
- **Burnout:** A state of physical, emotional, and mental exhaustion caused by prolonged stress and overwork, commonly experienced by healthcare professionals.
- **Compassion fatigue:** A form of secondary trauma experienced by healthcare professionals due to prolonged exposure to patients' suffering, leading to emotional exhaustion and reduced empathy.
- **Holistic approach:** An integrated and comprehensive approach that considers physical, emotional, and mental well-being, emphasizing the importance of addressing all aspects of a person's health.
- **Mindfulness:** A practice of being present in the moment, which can help manage stress, improve focus, and enhance the overall mental health of an individual.
- **Resilience:** The ability to bounce back and cope with challenging situations, a crucial trait for healthcare workers to maintain their well-being and continue providing quality care.

INTRODUCTION

The healthcare field is tough due to various associated challenges and environmental pressures, which may make it hard to work proficiently, especially nurses who work tirelessly to care for patients day and night. Because of the nature of the job, burnout is quite common in the medical field. There is a need to find ways to help healthcare workers stay healthy and keep giving good care. Yoga, a type of exercise and relaxation, could help them prevent burnout and stress.

Healthcare is a challenging and demanding field, requiring hours of work and unwavering commitment from those who choose to serve in it. The entire healthcare system is undergoing a rapid transformation in response to the environmental pressures owing to pandemics, climate change, shortage of manpower, financial constraints, and other such problems. Healthcare workers, such as nurses, stand at the frontline of this realm, braving the challenges that come with a strong dedication to saving lives and serving the sick and afflicted. There is no question that nursing is a physically and emotionally demanding profession, which makes nursing staff prone to stress, burnout, and other stress-related disorders.

In the 21st century, the nursing profession has undergone a remarkable transformation, expanding its horizons far beyond the traditional hospital setting. Today, nurses play an important role in different environments, such as community health departments, corporate sectors, home healthcare, teaching, and laboratories. Despite the specific responsibilities in different settings, the role of a professional nurse is to provide the best care to their patients, guided by research-based evidence. Healthcare is evolving rapidly and nurses have emerged as dynamic and adaptable healthcare professionals who are providing their services beyond hospitals, and engaging with individuals from all walks of life, addressing unique health needs, and empowering communities with knowledge and resources to lead healthier lives.

However, despite the challenging nature of their work, which puts them at a higher risk of burnout and stress-related illnesses, there is limited research on this topic. The need for a solution-directed approach towards the issues is essential to maintain the quality of life of the medical professionals and the high standard of healthcare for the patients.

It is also important to not just exclusively focus on the current medical practitioners but also give adequate attention to the future of healthcare, medical students, or in this case specifically, nursing students. There is a need to address their concerns and provide them with tools to help manage the heavy workload and stress levels fostered by the competitive nature of medical education and practice.

To address the current challenges in our medical workforce, it is crucial to consider Complementary and Alternative Medicine (CAM) alongside mainstream and traditional solutions. By adopting a comprehensive and holistic approach, we can better support the well-being of healthcare professionals. The exploration of Yoga as a potential tool to tackle these issues has shown promise, but further in-depth research is necessary in this area. Embracing CAM, including Yoga, can open new avenues for enhancing the overall health and resilience of our medical workforce.

NURSES IN DIVERSE SETTINGS

In educational settings, nurses act as catalysts, providing health literacy and essential clinical skills to future generations, ensuring a healthier and more productive society. Community health departments provide nurses with a platform to reach out to underserved populations and address pressing public health issues. Through proactive interventions and health promotion campaigns, nurses create positive impacts that transcend individual care, benefiting entire communities and driving transformative changes in healthcare outcomes. The corporate sector is recognizing the value of nurses in promoting employee wellness and optimizing workplace productivity. By implementing health programs, and mental health support, nurses contribute to a healthier workforce and foster a positive work environment, ultimately benefiting both employees and employers. Home healthcare has become an increasingly vital aspect of modern healthcare delivery. Nurses provide compassionate care within the comfort of patients' homes, ensuring continuity of care and enhancing the overall patient experience. This personalized approach fosters stronger patient-nurse relationships, leading to better treatment adherence and improved health outcomes. In laboratories and research settings, nurses actively participate in groundbreaking studies and evidence-based research, contributing to advancements in healthcare practices and patient-centered interventions. Amidst the vast array of diverse roles they undertake and the unwavering support they provide to others, it is crucial to prioritize the well-being of nurses themselves. In the pursuit of delivering compassionate care, nurses often find themselves facing challenges, such as heavy workloads, job dissatisfaction, traumatic incidents, and undervalued compensation, which can lead to significant mental and physical stress. To ensure a resilient and thriving nursing workforce, it becomes quite important to address these issues through holistic approaches that prioritize their overall health and wellness. Overwhelming workloads can lead to burnout and emotional exhaustion, hindering their ability to provide the best care to their patients. Furthermore, encounters with traumatic incidents can take a toll on their mental health, necessitating specialized support and interventions to cope with the emotional impact. Considering these facts there needs to be a holistic approach to proactively manage both physical and emotional stress among nurses. Beyond conventional approaches, incorporating holistic practices, such as yoga, mindfulness, and meditation can significantly contribute to alleviating stress and enhancing overall well-being. These mind-body practices can help nurses to cultivate resilience, manage stress more effectively, and develop inner balance amidst the demanding nature of their profession. Additionally, promoting a supportive work culture and fostering open communication channels can create an environment where nurses feel comfortable seeking assistance when needed. Establishing peer support programs, counseling services, and debriefing sessions after traumatic events can be instrumental in helping nurses process their emotions and cope with the challenges they encounter. Recognizing the pivotal role nurses play in healthcare, organizations and policymakers must address issues related to workload and compensation to ensure that nurses receive the recognition and remuneration they rightfully deserve. Investing in nursing staff not only enhances patient care but also elevates the overall healthcare system. Addressing the mental and physical stress experienced by nurses requires a comprehensive and holistic approach, encompassing mind-body practices, supportive work environments, and recognition of their invaluable contributions. By fostering a culture of well-being and investing in the holistic health of nurses, we can build a resilient nursing workforce that continues to excel in delivering compassionate and exceptional care to those they serve.

CHALLENGES AMONG NURSES IN HEALTHCARE

Stress, anxiety, and burnout are pervasive challenges in the lives of nurses and other healthcare professionals. The demanding nature of the healthcare industry, with its long hours, high-stakes decision-making, and emotionally charged environments, often affects the mental and emotional well-being of those dedicated to caring for others. Nurses, in particular, face unique stressors as frontline workers, responsible for providing compassionate care and support to patients during times of vulnerability and distress.

The constant pressure to deliver optimal care amidst limited resources and an ever-increasing workload can lead to chronic stress and feelings of anxiety. Over time, this chronic stress can lead to burnout, "characterized by emotional exhaustion, depersonalization, and a diminished sense of personal accomplishment". Recognizing and addressing these mental health challenges is crucial to preserving the well-being of healthcare professionals, ensuring their ability to continue providing high-quality care while also safeguarding their own mental health. Supportive workplace environments, access to mental health resources, and self-care practices, such as Yoga, mindfulness, and exercise are essential components in mitigating stress, anxiety, and burnout among nurses and healthcare professionals.

STRESS, BURNOUT, AND PTSD AMONG NURSES

When the body experiences any physical or psychological stimuli that disturb its internal balance (homeostasis), it triggers a stress response. These stimuli, known as stressors, lead to physiological and behavioral changes as a reaction. The stress response involves a complex interplay of the nervous, endocrine, and immune systems, which activate the sympathetic-adreno-medullar (SAM) axis, the hypothalamus-pituitary-adrenal (HPA) axis, and the immune system. The acute stress response is an adaptive mechanism that enables an organism to react to environmental or physiological shifts and restore equilibrium. However, chronic stress, in contrast, can be maladaptive and is associated with various harmful conditions, such as depression, anxiety, cognitive decline, and heart disease. One outcome of prolonged and intense stress is burnout.

Burnout refers to a prolonged reaction to ongoing emotional and interpersonal stressors in the workplace, encompassing exhaustion, cynicism, and a sense of inefficacy. Extensive research over the past 25 years has revealed the intricacies of this phenomenon, highlighting that burnout is not solely an individual experience but also influenced by the larger organizational context and how people relate to their work.

In recent years, there has been growing concern surrounding physician well-being, especially owing to the increasing evidence of burnout and stress among medical professionals. Physicians and nurses experiencing burnout not only face challenges, such as substance abuse, strained relationships, and thoughts of suicide, but they also perceive a decline in the quality of care they provide. Patients, in turn, appear to be less satisfied with healthcare professionals experiencing burnout, impacting patient outcomes, including patient experiences, quality of care, and the occurrence of medical errors. Burnout is a work-related stress syndrome, and so is found to exist in all professional fields. However, the risk of burnout amongst nurses has been found to be significantly higher owing to the demanding and challenging nature of their profession. With the increasing workloads on healthcare systems and clinicians, the demands on nurses have also risen, leading to a negative impact on the nursing work environment. Nurses work in a variety of settings within the healthcare framework, including intensive care units (ICUs). The ICU is a common setting for cardiopulmonary resuscitation, end-of-life issues, and medical malpractice disputes, subjecting ICU nurses to prolonged exposure to stressors and significant mental strain. Furthermore, ICU nurses face substantial challenges in their daily work due to the high morbidity and mortality rates of their patients and must exhibit both care and patience towards their patients while working tirelessly during day and night shifts. ICU nurses operate in a challenging setting characterized by repetitive exposure to traumatic situations and stressful events putting them at an increased risk of post-traumatic stress disorder (PTSD).

IMPACT OF THE COVID-19 PANDEMIC

COVID-19 shook the world and had a profound impact on healthcare professionals like nurses, who were at the forefront of the crisis. It subjected them to immense physical and emotional strain owing to the overwhelming patient influx, prolonged working hours, and increased exposure to the virus.

They faced issues like inefficient infection control, inadequate protective equipment, and patient assaults/verbal abuse, further impacting their safety and well-being. As a result, during the COVID-19 pandemic, healthcare workers, particularly nurses, were highly susceptible to experiencing post-traumatic stress disorder (PTSD), leading to a negative impact on their overall quality of life. Studies on past SARS and Ebola epidemics indicate that the abrupt emergence of highly life-threatening illnesses can create tremendous pressure on healthcare workers. Healthcare workers faced added challenges to their resilience during the pandemic period, such as isolation, reduced social support, infection risks to loved ones, and significant changes in their work environment, making them particularly susceptible to mental health issues, such as fear, anxiety, depression, PTSD, and insomnia. In a systematic literature search conducted until April 17th, 2020, which included thirteen studies with a total of 33,062 participants, findings revealed that the pooled prevalence rates were 23.2% for anxiety and 22.8% for depression, while the prevalence of insomnia was estimated as 38.9% across five studies. Subgroup analyses indicated higher rates of affective symptoms among female healthcare providers and nurses compared to male and medical staff, respectively.

This highlights how crises, such as the pandemic can take a severe toll on the mental health of healthcare workers, and brings attention to the critical need for robust and ongoing support systems to safeguard their mental health, not only during emergencies but also as a fundamental aspect of their overall welfare.

DEPRESSION, ANXIETY, AND INSOMNIA IN NURSING STUDENTS

While recognizing the demanding and stressful nature of the medical profession, it is essential to consider the well-being not only of those presently practicing but also of those aspiring to join the field.

Universally, there is growing concern about the prevalence of poor mental health among university students.

Depression and anxiety symptoms are frequently observed among students across various global regions, significantly affecting their quality of life and academic performance. Apart from the challenges faced by students in general, nursing students encounter additional unique issues specific to their healthcare training, and as a result, stress, depression, and anxiety are commonly observed among nursing students in different countries around the world. In a 2018 meta-analysis conducted by Tung et al., comprising of 27 cross-sectional studies and 8,918 nursing students with a mean age ranging from 17.4 to 28.4 years, the prevalence of global depression was reported as 34.0%. This indicates a significantly higher prevalence of depression among nursing students compared to the general population, which was only 4.7%. The included studies showed a proportion of female students ranging from 79.0% to 100.0%.

Nursing students encounter novel challenges both in the academic setting and clinical education, including adapting to new teaching methods and providing care to real patients during their initial clinical practice. They must navigate the higher education system, often necessitating living away from their families, while also contending with the pressure to excel academically and confronting peer-related hurdles. All these factors put them at a higher risk of mental distress and related issues such as anxiety, insomnia, etc.

Studies have indicated that medical students with elevated stress levels and subclinical depression are more susceptible to experiencing sleep disorders. Engaging in late-night study routines and participating in internships can lead to sleep deprivation and disrupt their regular sleep habits. Additionally, research has found a link between shift work and an increased prevalence of sleep disorders, such as insomnia.

Stress and anxiety is also a widely prevalent problem in the nursing student population.

A cross-sectional correlational descriptive study by Onieva-Zafra et al. included a sample of 190 nursing students from Ciudad Real University in Spain, with a mean age of 20.71 ± 3.89 years (range 18–46 years). Approximately, 47.92% of the students reported a moderate level of stress, with a mean Perceived Stress Scale score of 22.78 (± 8.54). Senior nursing students perceived higher stress levels compared to novice students. The findings indicated significant correlations between perceived stress and state anxiety ($r = 0.463$, $p < .000$) as well as trait anxiety ($r = 0.718$, $p < .000$).

Assessing the mental health of nursing students and implementing appropriate mental health interventions is of utmost importance to support this vulnerable group. Given the nature of nursing as a profession that relies on empathetic human interaction, depression, and anxiety can negatively impact cognitive processes and communication skills, potentially leading to suboptimal clinical decision-making and an increased risk of medical errors during practice. (Prioritizing the mental well-being of future healthcare providers is a fundamental aspect of nursing education.

YOGA FOR MANAGEMENT OF STRESS AND PTSD

The demands and challenges of today's fast-paced world have created a fertile breeding ground for stress and mental health problems to foster. Post-Traumatic Stress Disorder is a psychological condition characterized by unwanted memories, trauma flashbacks, negative thoughts and feelings, active avoidance of triggers, and hyperarousal. While a few validated treatment approaches are available, most PTSD patients retain their diagnosis and some symptoms despite the intervention of modern psychiatric techniques. A significant number of people exhibit a sense of distrust and skepticism towards modern psychiatric medicine due to its limited efficacy and numerous side effects.

Complementary and Alternative Medicine (CAM) has the potential to cater to that segment of the population that is not adequately assisted by the conventional approaches. Flourishing research in the realm of CAM has prompted individuals to integrate alternative therapy, such as yoga in the treatment of excessive stress and mental health disorders, such as PTSD. Hatha yoga includes physical postures (asanas), breathing techniques (pranayama), and meditation as integral components of its practice, and has become increasingly popular as a form of exercise as well as relaxation across the globe. The growing recognition of yoga's ability to alleviate stress and promote mental well-being has contributed to its popularity in recent times. It is believed that stress causes disruption of balance within the autonomic nervous system (ANS), with decreased parasympathetic nervous system (PNS) activity and an increase in sympathetic nervous system (SNS) activity, while at the same time leading to reduced activity of the inhibitory neurotransmitter, gamma amino-butyric acid (GABA) and an elevated allostatic load. Yogic practices address the under activity of the parasympathetic nervous system (PNS) and the GABA system, partly by stimulating the vagal nerves. Furthermore, it is believed that yoga can decrease allostatic load, leading to a reduction in stress and other symptoms of anxiety.

Post-traumatic stress disorder is a condition that is bolstered by stress, characterized by low PNS and GABA system activity, and hence also shows improvement in response to yoga-based interventions. Yoga and yogic practices have also been reported by researchers to influence the functioning of the hypothalamus and stress response, which play a vital role in regulating blood pressure, blood sugar, heart rate, and respiration. By promoting relaxation responses, these practices are believed to have an impact on the anterior cingulate cortex and hippocampus, regions of the brain associated with empathy, decision-making, emotion, and memory.

In recent times, a growing body of research has emerged exploring the potential of yoga as a therapeutic intervention for post-traumatic stress disorder, along with speculations regarding the physiological mechanisms that may be involved. The use of yoga in individuals with PTSD has shown promising outcomes in several cases.

A study by Bessel A. van der Kolk et al involved 64 women with chronic, treatment-resistant PTSD, who were randomly assigned to either attend a trauma-informed yoga class or a supportive women's health education class, both consisting of weekly 1 hour sessions for a total of 10 weeks. The results demonstrated that 52% of the participants in the yoga group did not meet the criteria for having PTSD anymore, compared to 21% in the control group. While both groups experienced notable reductions in PTSD symptoms during the initial phase of treatment, only the yoga group sustained those improvements whereas the control group relapsed after the initial progress. Yoga significantly helps individuals dealing with PTSD navigate the complexities of their trauma and manage their symptoms better, especially those dealing with hyperarousal symptoms by helping calm the nervous system down.

People with PTSD and C-PTSD often experience alexithymia, which is characterized by challenges in recognizing, articulating, and/or conveying emotions, accompanied by a cognitive style that tends to focus more on external factors. Yoga is a practice that can assist these individuals in reestablishing a mind-body connection, allowing them to regain a sense of self within the world. Breathing exercises help individuals center themselves within their body and significantly improves their relationship and control over their own bodies.

In his book, "The Body Keeps the Score" Dr Bessel A Van Der Kolk writes that those with PTSD and C-PTSD frequently encounter difficulties in managing emotions and impulses, which is often attributed to the relationship between the regulating systems of the amygdala and the medial prefrontal cortex, which are usually at an imbalance in a traumatized body. However, that too can be assisted significantly by yoga, which can better equip individuals with the capacity to self-regulate and gain bodily control, by strengthening the capacity of the medial prefrontal cortex to motor bodily sensations.

While there is a surge of interest in yoga as a complementary approach to managing PTSD, the scope of research still remains limited and challenging due to the myriad of styles and practices within yoga. Further investigation into the question of optimal frequency and duration of treatment is necessary in order to gain a deeper understanding of yoga as a therapeutic intervention for PTSD.

The efficacy of yoga in reducing stress and its potential to assist with PTSD, depression, anxiety, and other mental disorders is widely recognized and constantly researched. However, it is important to acknowledge that there is still significant scope for further investigation. Continued research efforts will help us better our understanding, refine therapeutic applications, and uncover new insights into the profound benefits that yoga can offer in promoting mental well-being.

YOGA FOR THE MANAGEMENT OF INSOMNIA AND ANXIETY

Insomnia is a term that finds varied usage in both the medical literature and popular media, but its most common definition revolves around an individual's self-reported difficulty with sleep. It is the most common clinical sleep disorder, with its prevalence ranging from 3% to 22%, depending on the classification system used. While the general understanding of insomnia is well-established, its classification has been ever-changing, following the guidelines of ICSD-3, ICD-10, and DSM-V. Currently, insomnia is defined as difficulty initiating or maintaining sleep, leading to daytime disturbances, despite adequate time for sleep and it often co-occurs with medical and psychiatric comorbidities and may be linked to substance use as well. Insomnia's high prevalence contributes to a significant annual loss of quality-adjusted life-years, surpassing other medical and psychiatric conditions. Moreover, it is associated with higher healthcare utilization and costs, especially in individuals with concurrent medical or psychiatric disorders, making it a crucial issue for managed care. Cognitive behavioral therapy (CBTI) is considered the first line of treatment for insomnia but its extensive cost and insufficient availability of trained providers have hindered its widespread adoption. Anxiety is a fear response that arises when confronted with stressful or threatening situations. While it is a normal reaction to danger, persistent or overwhelming feelings of anxiety may indicate an anxiety disorder. According to the Royal College of Psychiatrists, anxiety disorders, which encompass conditions, such as panic disorder, post-traumatic stress disorder, and social anxiety disorder, affect approximately one in ten individuals. Anxiety is commonly associated with insomnia, with each condition often amplifying the other. Anxiety can disrupt sleep, leading to difficulty falling or staying asleep, which contributes to insomnia. Likewise, chronic insomnia can increase feelings of anxiety, as sleep deprivation affects mood and cognitive functioning. This creates a cyclic pattern that can significantly impact a person's mental and physical health. Addressing both insomnia and anxiety through appropriate interventions is crucial in breaking this cycle and promoting better sleep and overall well-being. Exploring alternative approaches to address these issues is essential in order to complement existing treatment methods and achieve a more comprehensive and holistic approach to managing them. As one turns to CAM, Yoga emerges as a prominent choice. Yoga's three main components—postures, breathing, and meditation, have been found to offer numerous benefits in addressing sleep, anxiety, and insomnia-related issues by helping calm the nervous system, reduce stress, and promote relaxation. Regular yoga practice has been associated with increased muscle strength, flexibility, range of motion, and balance, promoting a sense of relaxation and overall well-being. The deep relaxation induced by yoga can help reduce sympathetic arousal and anxiety, contributing to improved sleep quality. Additionally, the practice of controlled breathing and mindfulness in yoga can aid in better pain and stress management, positively impacting sleep patterns.

To evaluate the effectiveness of mindfulness-based interventions (MBIs), Lomas et al., conducted a meta-analysis of 35 randomized controlled trials, encompassing various occupations, MBIs, and wellbeing-related outcomes. The findings indicated that mindfulness had moderate effects on reducing deficit-based outcomes, including stress, anxiety, distress, depression, and burnout. Additionally, mindfulness had moderate to small effects on enhancing asset-based outcomes, such as health, job performance, compassion, and empathy, as well as promoting mindfulness and positive well-being. These results emphasize the beneficial impact of mindfulness on both reducing negative mental health aspects and fostering positive well-being-related outcomes.

Yoga offers a holistic and natural approach to addressing anxiety and insomnia, providing individuals with practical tools to cultivate mental and emotional well-being. Yoga has demonstrated its potential as a valuable complementary approach to managing conditions, such as anxiety, depression, and insomnia when used alongside standard treatment methods, such as medication and therapy. Utilizing yoga as an adjunctive therapy may offer individuals a more comprehensive approach to addressing these challenging mental health conditions. It is important to consult with a healthcare professional or qualified yoga instructor to tailor a yoga practice that suits individual needs and health conditions.

SELF-CARE AND YOGA FOR NURSES

The nursing profession demands the provision of compassionate, empathetic, culturally sensitive, skilled, and ethical care, often within settings with limited resources and growing responsibilities. This disparity between delivering high-quality care and managing stressful work environments can result in burnout, compromised productivity, performance, and the quality of patient care.

Self-care, a fundamental aspect of holistic nursing, goes beyond caring for the patient and encompasses the well-being of the nurse themselves. Nurses are an integral component of the healing environment for their patients and a holistic approach underscores the importance of practicing self-care as a responsibility rather than simply a personal choice. It is one of the philosophical principles that serve as the foundation of holistic nursing practice. The inclusion of mind-body (MB) yoga techniques in nurses' self-care routines can enhance their knowledge and understanding, enabling them to better interpret regimens of care and serve their patients more effectively in the healing environment. Prioritizing self-care is vital for the nursing profession as it empowers nurses to maintain their physical and emotional health, leading to improved patient care and overall job satisfaction.

Numerous mindfulness and spirituality-based programs have reported a reduction in perceived stress levels among nurses and healthcare professionals (HCPs). MB yoga, encompassing mind-body awareness through postures, breathing techniques, and mindful practices, is accessible to nearly everyone. Herrick and Ainsworth (2000) highlight the physiological, psycho-emotional, and spiritual benefits of MB yoga practices, including stress reduction, increased energy, and significant improvements in the overall sense of well-being among nurses. The incorporation of MB yoga practices can play a crucial role in mitigating stress and promoting the well-being of nurses in their demanding profession.

Kabat-Zinn (2003) suggests that MB interventions not only contribute to stress reduction in nurses and healthcare professionals during challenging times but also foster an increased awareness of their capacity to respond with unattached observance rather than reacting impulsively to stressful situations. This cultivation of "moment-to-moment" awareness empowers them to remain composed and grounded, even in high-stress work environments, effectively reducing instances of feeling overwhelmed and promoting a more balanced and mindful approach to their work and daily experiences. By practicing MB interventions, nurses and other healthcare practitioners can enhance their ability to navigate stressful situations with greater resilience and self-awareness.

In Fang and Li's clinical trial, 120 nurses were randomly assigned to two groups—one group participated in a six-month yoga program, while the other group had no intervention. The follow-up analysis revealed that the yoga group reported significant reductions in stress levels ($\chi2 = 16.449$; $p = 0.001$). Similarly, Alexander et al.'s study involving nurses who participated in an eight-week yoga program demonstrated higher levels of self-care compared to a non-participating group.

In another trial by Bond et al. focusing on medical students, an 11-week mind-body course resulted in statistically significant improvements in self-regulation values (increasing from 3.49 to 3.58; $p = 0.003$) and self-compassion values (increasing from 2.88 to 3.25; $p = 0.04$). While perceived stress scores decreased from 1.55 to 1.48 and empathy levels increased from 5.64 to 5.80, these changes were not statistically significant ($p = 0.70$ and $p = 0.30$, respectively)

These findings suggest that incorporating yoga programs into the lives of nurses can lead to meaningful improvements in stress management and self-care. They underscore the importance of considering MB practices as potential strategies to enhance the overall mental and emotional health of healthcare workers, thereby contributing to a more sustainable and fulfilling healthcare profession (**Fig. 56.1**).

YOGA FOR THE DEVELOPMENT OF COMPASSION AND SATISFACTION IN NURSING PROFESSIONALS

Compassion is a fundamental virtue for all healthcare professionals, particularly nurses, and doctors. Its presence is crucial for providing effective clinical care. However, the demanding workload in healthcare settings can lead to compassion fatigue or barriers to compassion, adversely affecting both patient care and the professional efficiency of healthcare providers. As front-line workers directly interact with patients, nurses carry a significant responsibility to be compassionate towards their patients. Nevertheless, due to various professional and personal reasons, some nurses may find it challenging to maintain this level of compassion consistently. Addressing these challenges and fostering compassion in healthcare remains imperative to ensure the well-being of both patients and healthcare professionals.

Yoga, as a transformative practice, holds immense potential for fostering compassion and satisfaction among nurses. The demands of the nursing profession can often lead to emotional exhaustion and stress, making it essential for nurses to prioritize their mental well-being. Engaging in yoga offers nurses a pathway to develop self-compassion and cultivate empathy for themselves and their patients.

Mindfulness, as described by Kabat-Zinn, involves paying deliberate attention in the present moment, without judgment. Different theories have been proposed to understand the underlying mechanisms of mindfulness practice. Davidson et al. utilized electroencephalography to suggest that meditation activates the relative left frontal lobe,

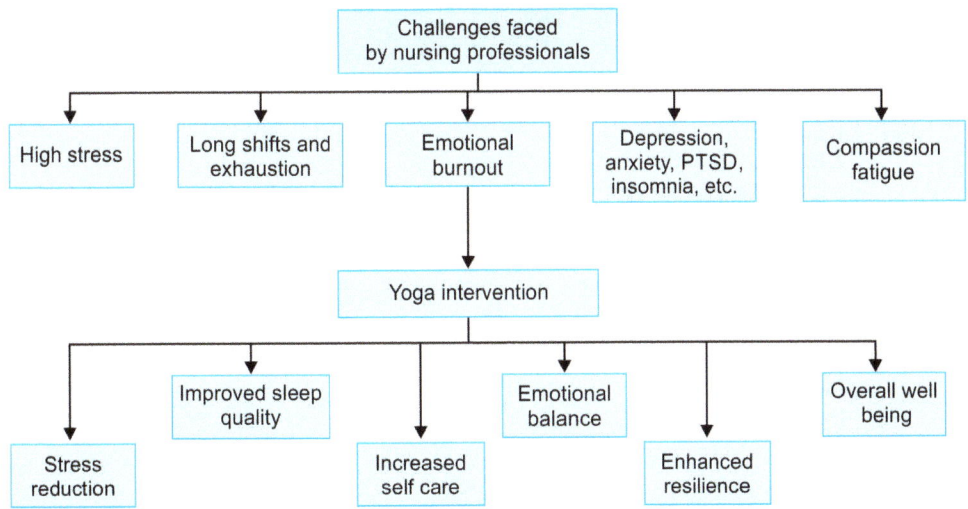

Fig. 56.1: Schematic indicating the challenges faced by nurses and benefits of yoga intervention for management of the challenges.

which is linked to reduced anxiety and negative emotions while increasing positive emotions. Additionally, Fox et al. reported that meditation is associated with changes in brain anatomical structures, including the frontal lobes. These neurobiological changes may play a role in fostering compassion through mindfulness practice.

By cultivating mindfulness, individuals become more attuned to their thoughts and emotions without judging them. This heightened self-awareness enables individuals to recognize and understand their own suffering and that of others with compassion and empathy. Mindfulness practice encourages individuals to respond to difficult emotions and challenging situations with a kind and nonjudgmental attitude, fostering compassion towards themselves and others. As individuals develop their capacity for mindfulness, they become more sensitive to the needs and feelings of those around them, enhancing their ability to respond to others with empathy and care. Ultimately, mindfulness plays a crucial role in fostering compassion and promoting a deeper connection with oneself and others. Not only in the healthcare profession but among nursing students also, compassion and empathy need to be inculcated and practiced. Moreover, the physical aspects of yoga, such as postures and breath work, promote relaxation and reduce stress, contributing to an overall sense of satisfaction and well-being. Numerous research studies have shown that yoga interventions positively impact compassion, satisfaction, and overall mental health among the nursing professionals.

YOGA PRACTICE AND ASANAS

A suggested structured yoga program for stress management and improving workplace quality of life has been proposed and validated by *Suprakash Mandal et al.* which includes warm-up practices, a few postures (Asana), breathing practices (pranayama), and relaxation techniques **(Table 56.1)**.

YOGA NURSING STUDIES

The extensive research on yoga and its benefits, spanning beyond nursing professionals to a wide array of domains, serves as a testament to the profound impact this ancient practice has on holistic well-being. These studies provide us with empirical evidence, demonstrating how yoga weaves into the fabric of comprehensive healthcare strategies. As the body of research expands, it provides a solid foundation for refining yoga protocols tailored to specific populations and conditions. This targeted approach resonates deeply with the principles of integrative health, where interventions are customized to meet individual needs and preferences.

The diverse applications of yoga underscore its significance and call for extensive research to fully explore its benefits. As we look for more holistic approaches to healthcare, rigorous research will help harness yoga's potential and empower individuals to lead healthier lives **(Tables 56.2 and 56.3)**.

FORMALIZING CURRICULUM

There are certain educational institutes in India dedicated to Yogic studies, such as SVYASA (Swami Vivekananda Yoga Anusandhana Samsthana), which provide a comprehensive range of undergraduate (UG), postgraduate (PG), and PhD academic programs focused on yoga. Similarly, there exist other institutions, such as the Bihar School of Yoga, the University of Patanjali, the Indian Institute of Yogic Science and Research, and many more, which offer comprehensive courses as well as Teacher Training Programs in the field of yoga.

While yoga courses abound in India's traditional and alternative education landscape, their integration into schools, colleges and formal medical curricula, such as Nursing, MBBS, MD, DM, and PhD programs remains limited. This highlights a significant gap in healthcare education, one that could potentially hinder the holistic well-being and comprehensive care of patients. One reason for this can be the separation of modern medicine and traditional practices, such as yoga, which has been ingrained for decades, leading to a lack of integration in formal medical education. Moreover, the existing medical curricula are often packed with essential subjects, leaving little room for additional courses, such as yoga. The lack of resources, infrastructure, and faculty becomes another contributing factor.

TABLE 56.1: Suggested yoga protocol adapted from Suprakash Mandal et al. phase II trial among nursing staff for the management of stress among nurses.

Preparatory practices			*Duration (minutes)*
Sukshma Vyayama	1. Jogging 2. Twisting 3. Forward and backward bending		05
Preparatory movements with breathing	1. Hand stretch breathing 2. Ankle stretch breathing 3. Straight leg raise breathing 4. Pawanmuktasana breathing		05
Suryanamaskar	Six rounds		10
	Asanas		
Standing	1. Ardha-kati chakrasana		05
	2. Trikonashana		
	3. Veerabhadrasana		
	4. Vrikshasana		

Contd...

Contd...

Preparatory practices			Duration (minutes)
Sitting	1. Vakrasana/Ardhmatseyndrasana	Or	05
	2. Ustrasana		
	3. Paschimauttanasana		
Prone	1. Bhujangansana		05
	2. Shalabhasana—ardha or full		
	3. Dhanurasana		

Contd...

Contd...

Preparatory practices			Duration (minutes)
Supine	1. Setubandhasanas		05
	2. Ardhahalasana		
	3. Naukasana		
Pranayama	1. Nadishudhi 2. Kapalbhati 3. Bhramhari		05
Relaxation technique	Deep relaxation technique		05
Total duration in minutes			**50**

TABLE 56.2: Summary of key research studies exploring the diverse benefits of yoga practices for nurses.

Sl. No.	Name of study	Conclusion	References
1.	**Holistic nursing in practice:** Mindfulness-based yoga as an intervention to manage stress and burnout	The MB yoga intervention demonstrated a statistically noteworthy impact on the health and well-being of nurses and healthcare professionals, particularly in relation to stress-related indicators	Hilcove K, Marceau C, Thekdi P, Larkey L, Brewer MA, Jones K. Holistic nursing in practice: Mindfulness-Based yoga as an intervention to manage stress and burnout. Journal of Holistic Nursing. 2020 May 27;39(1):29–42.
2.	The effect of laughter yoga on perceived stress, burnout, and life satisfaction in nurses during the pandemic: A randomized controlled trial	Laughter yoga proves to be an efficacious approach for decreasing perceived stress and burnout, simultaneously enhancing overall life satisfaction	Sis Çelik A, Kılınç T. The effect of laughter yoga on perceived stress, burnout, and life satisfaction in nurses during the pandemic: A randomized controlled trial. Complementary Therapies in Clinical Practice. 2022 Nov;49:101637.
3.	Effect of Yoga on the quality of life of nurses working in intensive care units. Randomized controlled clinical trial	The implementation of yoga exercises proved to be successful in enhancing the quality of life among ICU nurses	Rostami K, Ghodsbin F. Effect of Yoga on the Quality of Life of Nurses Working in Intensive Care Units. Randomized Controlled Clinical Trial. Investigación y Educación en Enfermería. 2019 Oct 23;37(3).
4.	A randomized trial comparing effect of Yoga and exercises on quality of life in among nursing population with chronic low back pain	Integrated yoga demonstrated greater enhancements in quality of life when compared to physical exercises in nursing professionals with chronic low back pain	Patil N, Nagaratna R, Tekur P, Manohar P, Bhargav H, Patil D. A randomized trial comparing the effect of yoga and exercises on quality of life in among nursing population with chronic low back pain. International Journal of Yoga. 2018;11(3):208.
5.	A regular yoga intervention for staff nurse sleep quality and work stress: A randomized controlled trial	Regular yoga can lead to better sleep quality and reduced work stress for staff nurses	Fang R, Li X. A regular yoga intervention for staff nurse sleep quality and work stress: a randomized controlled trial. Journal of Clinical Nursing. 2015 Oct 19;24(23–24):3374–9.

Contd...

Contd...

Sl. No.	Name of study	Conclusion	References
6.	Restorative yoga for occupational stress among Japanese female nurses working night shift: A randomized crossover trial	Restorative yoga could be beneficial in reducing occupational stress for female nurses on night shifts.	Miyoshi Y. Restorative yoga for occupational stress among Japanese female nurses working night shift: Randomized crossover trial. Journal of Occupational Health. 2019 Jul 31;61(6):508–16.
7.	Determining the effect of yoga on job satisfaction and burnout of nurse academicians	Engaging in yoga practice effectively reduces burnout and enhances job satisfaction among nursing academicians	Kavurmaci M, Tan M, Bahcecioglu Turan G. Determining the effect of yoga on job satisfaction and burnout of nurse academicians. Perspectives in Psychiatric Care. 2021 Apr 30;58(1):404–10.
8.	Using Yoga Nidra to improve stress in psychiatric nurses in a pilot study	Derived from a limited sample of nurses, the outcomes exhibited favorable results concerning perceived stress levels and muscle fatigue	Anderson R, Mammen K, Paul P, Pletch A, Pulia K. Using Yoga Nidra to Improve Stress in Psychiatric Nurses in a Pilot Study. The Journal of Alternative and Complementary Medicine. 2017 Jun;23(6):494–5.
9.	The effectiveness of a stress coping program based on mindfulness meditation on the stress, anxiety, and depression experienced by nursing students in Korea	The mindfulness-based stress program effectively reduced stress and anxiety in nursing students and could be used for managing stress in student nurses	Kang YS, Choi SY, Ryu E. The effectiveness of a stress coping program based on mindfulness meditation on the stress, anxiety, and depression experienced by nursing students in Korea. Nurse Education Today. 2009 Jul;29(5):538–43.
10.	Effect of mindfulness-based stress reduction therapy on work stress and mental health of psychiatric nurses	MBSR therapy reduces work stress, anxiety, and depression, and improves the mental well-being of psychiatric nurses	Yang J, Tang S, Zhou W. Effect of Mindfulness-Based Stress Reduction Therapy on Work Stress and Mental Health of Psychiatric Nurses. Psychiatria Danubina. 2018 Jun 19;30(2):189–96.

TABLE 56.3: Overview of research studies investigating the positive effects of yoga across various populations.

1.	Effectiveness of yoga lifestyle on lipid metabolism in a vulnerable population—A community-based multicenter randomized controlled trial	Yoga lifestyle regulates blood lipid levels in prediabetic and diabetic individuals, adjusting them as needed in both rural and urban Indian communities	Nagarathna R, Kumar S, Anand A, Acharya IN, Singh AK, Patil SS, et al. Effectiveness of Yoga Lifestyle on Lipid Metabolism in a Vulnerable Population—A Community-based Multicenter Randomized Controlled Trial. Medicines. 2021 Jul 13;8(7):37.
2.	War-related mental health issues and need for Yoga intervention studies: A scoping review	Incorporating Yoga and Mindfulness into daily routines for military personnel and war-affected populations can help prevent and manage mental health disorders related to conflict	Anand A, Ghani A, Sharma K, Kaur G, Khosla R, Devi C, et al. War-related mental health issues and need for yoga intervention studies: A scoping review. International Journal of Yoga. 2021;14(3):175.
3.	Potential benefits of Yoga in pregnancy-related complications during the COVID-19 Pandemic and implications for working women	Yoga proves effective in reducing stress, and anxiety, and enhancing immunity for pregnant working women facing the COVID-19 pandemic	Nadholta P, Bali P, Singh A, Anand A. Potential benefits of Yoga in pregnancy-related complications during the COVID-19 pandemic and implications for working women. Work. 2020 Nov 9;67(2):269–79.
4.	Ayurveda body-mind constitutional types and role of Yoga intervention among type 2 diabetes mellitus population of Chandigarh and Panchkula regions	Yoga was found to have significant positive results on individuals with diabetes	Sivapuram MS, Srivastava V, Kaur N, Anand A, Nagarathna R, Patil S, et al. Ayurveda Body–Mind Constitutional Types and Role of Yoga Intervention Among Type 2 Diabetes Mellitus Population of Chandigarh and Panchkula Regions. Annals of Neurosciences. 2020 Jul;27(3–4):214–23.
5.	Yoga practice is beneficial for maintaining healthy lifestyle and endurance under restrictions and stress imposed by Lockdown during COVID-19 Pandemic	Yoga has the potential to mitigate COVID-19 risks by reducing stress and bolstering immunity if specific yoga protocols are enacted through a global public health initiative	Nagarathna R, Anand A, Rain M, Srivastava V, Sivapuram MS, Kulkarni R, et al. Yoga Practice Is Beneficial for Maintaining Healthy Lifestyle and Endurance Under Restrictions and Stress Imposed by Lockdown During COVID-19 Pandemic. Frontiers in Psychiatry. 2021 Jun 22;12.
6.	Common Yoga Protocol Increases Peripheral Blood CD^{34+} cells: An Open-Label Single-Arm Exploratory Trial	Common Yoga Protocol practice led to a rise in CD^{34+} cells in the bloodstream and resulted in a notable alteration in BDNF levels following the intervention. Additionally, an enhancement in the overall well-being and psychological state of the participants was evident	Sharma K, Maity K, Goel S, Kanwar S, Anand A. Common Yoga Protocol Increases Peripheral Blood CD^{34+} Cells: An Open-Label Single-Arm Exploratory Trial. Journal of Multidisciplinary Healthcare. 2023 Jun;Volume 16:1721–36.

Contd...

Contd...

7.	Effects of one month of Common Yoga Protocol practice appear to be mediated by the angiogenic and neurogenic pathway: A pilot study	The practice of CYP might impact cell survival pathways through the interaction of angiogenic and neurogenic signals. Therefore, CYP could serve as a preventive approach for conditions linked to compromised angiogenic and neurogenic mechanisms	Sharma K, Pannu V, Sayal N, Bhalla A, Anand A. Effects of one month of Common Yoga Protocol practice appear to be mediated by the angiogenic and neurogenic pathway: A pilot study. EXPLORE. 2021 Sep;17(5):451–7.
8.	Prevalence of prediabetes, and diabetes in Chandigarh and Panchkula region based on glycated hemoglobin and Indian diabetes risk score	A significantly higher occurrence of diabetes was observed in the sampled group compared to the national average	Kumar S, Anand A, Nagarathna R, Kaur N, Sivapuram MS, Pannu V, et al. Prevalence of prediabetes, and diabetes in Chandigarh and Panchkula region based on glycated haemoglobin and Indian diabetes risk score. Endocrinology, Diabetes & Metabolism. 2020 Nov 11;4(1).
9.	Yoga as a Preventive Intervention for Cardiovascular Diseases and Associated Comorbidities: Open-Label Single Arm Study	The findings emphasize the importance of additional research to gain a deeper understanding of how yoga impacts the primary prevention of cardiovascular diseases	Sharma K, Basu-Ray I, Sayal N, Vora A, Bammidi S, Tyagi R, et al. Yoga as a Preventive Intervention for Cardiovascular Diseases and Associated Comorbidities: Open-Label Single Arm Study. Frontiers in Public Health. 2022 Jun 13;10.

KNOWLEDGE, ATTITUDE, AND PRACTICE GAP

The realm of Yoga witnesses a complex interplay between knowledge, attitude, and practice, revealing a multifaceted gap that not only influences the individual's engagement with Yoga but also influences the decision of healthcare workers specifically consultants to advise Yoga to the patients. Being the most trustworthy professionals for patients, healthcare workers should be exposed to Yoga so that they can experience the benefits of Yoga and then advise patients to incorporate it into their life. While the popularity of Yoga has surged, a notable knowledge gap persists. Many individuals hold a limited understanding of Yoga's comprehensive philosophy, historical roots, and diverse practices beyond the physical postures (asanas). This gap in knowledge can hinder practitioners from fully appreciating the holistic benefits of yoga and embracing its profound teachings. Yoga is a holistic practice that encompasses physical, mental, and spiritual well-being. The knowledge gap often pertains to the interconnectedness of these dimensions. Many might not realize that yoga is not just about flexibility or stress reduction, but it offers a path toward self-awareness, mindfulness, and inner transformation. Misconceptions, such as yoga is only for certain age groups, body types, or belief systems, or assuming that it requires a specific level of physical fitness are also contributing factors.

The attitude gap in yoga refers to the diversity of perspectives and beliefs that individuals hold toward the practice. This gap encompasses a wide range of attitudes, from deep reverence and dedication to skepticism or misconceptions about yoga's purpose and benefits. This diversity in attitudes often reflects societal, cultural, and personal influences. Bridging the knowledge and attitude gap entails fostering an open-minded and inclusive perspective that recognizes the multifaceted nature of yoga. Emphasizing the holistic nature of yoga and its ability to address physical, mental, and spiritual well-being can help individuals appreciate its multifaceted benefits. Providing comprehensive education about the different aspects of yoga, its history, philosophy, and benefits is also extremely crucial to bridging the gap. Engaging in consistent and authentic yoga practice is where a significant gap frequently emerges. Despite possessing knowledge about yoga's potential benefits and holding positive attitudes, individuals may struggle to translate this into sustained practice. Factors, such as time constraints, lifestyle demands, and lack of motivation contribute to the practice gap. Establishing clear and achievable goals for yoga practice can provide individuals with a sense of purpose and direction, making it more likely for them to commit to consistent practice. Starting with small, manageable steps and gradually building up their practice can also help prevent overwhelm and sustain long-term engagement. Partaking in structured yoga programs, classes, or routines can also help individuals overcome the practice gap.

LIMITATIONS AND WAY FORWARD

After the comprehensive exploration of the impact of yoga on the various challenges faced by nursing professionals, certain limitations of the discussion need to be considered and discussed. We have extensively focused on the impact of yoga; however, nursing professionals' well-being is influenced by a multitude of factors, such as personal life circumstances, job demands, social support, and access to healthcare services. These external factors can potentially confound the observed effects of yoga interventions. Additionally, it is important to conduct further investigations into the sustainability of the observed benefits over an extended period of time. While initial results may highlight positive outcomes, it is important to understand whether these effects continue to positively impact nursing professionals' well-being in the long run. It is also essential to give due consideration to the influence of cultural factors. The cultural diversity within the nursing community can significantly impact the receptiveness and effectiveness of yoga interventions. Studying how culture affects intervention adoption and outcomes in nursing can help customize approaches for diverse nursing groups. Moreover, many of the case studies and research papers discussed in this chapter may have focused on specific populations of nursing professionals, which could limit the generalization of the findings of those studies.

The field of yoga's impact on nurses remains underexplored, highlighting the necessity for more extensive studies. Further comprehensive research is essential to grasp and effectively harness the benefits of yoga interventions. Upcoming studies should aim to broaden their participant pools to encompass various contexts, while also emphasizing the importance of cultural diversity. Tailoring interventions to different cultures can enhance their effectiveness and relevance. Future research needs to build on what we already know and further help explore the effectiveness of yoga intervention.

Case Scenario

Rekha, is a hardworking and caring nurse who never fails in her responsibility of taking care of patients and always prioritized her patients. She used to be busy looking after others that she hardly had time for herself. The stress from work and family responsibilities was piling up, and she was feeling worn out. As a result, she was not able to perform her duties well. One day, Rekha heard about how yoga could help manage stress and emotional burnout and increase the quality of life and work. Rekha decided to try it out. At first, it was a bit hard to fit yoga classes into her schedule, but she was determined and kept going. Even on days when she could not make it to class, Rekha practiced yoga at home using online videos. Over time, she noticed that her mood improved, and she felt less tired and more energized, and more mindful at work. The yoga poses, breathing practices, relaxation techniques, meditation, and mindfulness she learned became a regular part of her day. After a busy day at work, she would look forward to her yoga session. She found that she was more relaxed and better able to connect with her patients, understanding their feelings. Rekha's newly explored strength and calmness helped her handle both her professional and personal life calmly. She kept doing yoga and encouraged her coworkers to take care of themselves too. Her journey with yoga made her a healthier and happier nurse.

SUMMARY

In the current situation, nurses and nursing students in the healthcare system face various challenges that significantly impact their well-being and performance. Stress, burnout, anxiety, PTSD, insomnia, and other mental health challenges have become prevalent issues, leading to potential adverse effects on their quality of life and the quality of care provided, and the overall functioning of healthcare professionals. Looking into alternative approaches, such as yoga can offer significant potential in alleviating these burdens and supporting the overall well-being of nursing professionals and other healthcare practitioners. Yoga's holistic benefits make it a promising tool to help mitigate stress, burnout, and other mental health challenges. As evident FROM the above literature, Yoga has shown promising results in addressing the mental and emotional struggles faced by nurses. A combination of physical postures, breathing techniques, and mindfulness practices offers an effective tool to manage stress and combat burnout. By regularly engaging in Yoga, nurses can enhance their ability to cope with the emotionally and physically demanding healthcare environment. Yoga's versatility in addressing various mental health challenges, including anxiety, PTSD, burnout, and insomnia, makes it a valuable complement to traditional and mainstream treatment methods. Incorporating yoga into healthcare practices would make it easier to tackle the challenges encountered by nurses and nursing students in the healthcare field. Its advantages extend beyond managing stress, burnout, and other mental health issues, encompassing compassion development and self-care. Continued research and acknowledgment of yoga's potential in healthcare are essential to harness its full potential and benefit, and to incorporate it into our healthcare professionals' lives, helping enhance their quality of life as well as the quality of patient care.

MULTIPLE CHOICE QUESTIONS

1. What is the primary objective of a professional nurse in diverse healthcare settings?
    a. Conduct groundbreaking research
    b. Manage financial constraints in healthcare
    c. Deliver the highest quality of patient care backed by evidence-based research
    d. Promote wellness programs for employees in corporate sectors

2. What is the term used to describe a state of physical, emotional, and mental exhaustion caused by prolonged stress and overwork?
    a. Compassion fatigue
    b. Burnout
    c. Resilience
    d. Mindfulness

3. How can nurses benefit from practicing yoga?
    a. Improve laboratory research skills
    b. Enhance patient-nurse relationships in home healthcare
    c. Manage stress, build resilience, and find inner balance
    d. Provide health literacy to future generations in educational settings

4. Which term refers to an integrated and comprehensive approach that considers physical, emotional, and mental well-being?
    a. Holistic approach
    b. Psychosocial stress
    c. Sympathetic-adreno-medullar (SAM) axis
    d. Hypothalamus-pituitary-adrenal (HPA)

5. What is the role of nurses in corporate sectors?
    a. Provide health literacy and clinical skills to employees
    b. Conduct transformative community health campaigns
    c. Administer compassionate care to patients at home
    d. Participate in groundbreaking research in laboratories

6. Which practice helps nurses be present in the moment, manage stress, and improve focus?
    a. Yoga
    b. Mindfulness
    c. Meditation
    d. Holistic medicine

7. What is the term used to describe a form of secondary trauma experienced by healthcare professionals due to prolonged exposure to patients' suffering?
    a. PTSD
    b. Resilience
    c. Compassion fatigue
    d. Burnout

8. What can organizations and policymakers do to support nurses' well-being?
    a. Implement peer support programs
    b. Ignore issues related to workload and compensation
    c. Avoid counselling services for nurses
    d. Discourage the practice of yoga in healthcare settings

9. What is the primary purpose of embracing complementary and alternative medicine (CAM) in healthcare?
    a. To ignore evidence-based research
    b. To focus solely on traditional solutions
    c. To support the overall health and resilience of healthcare professionals
    d. To increase healthcare costs

10. What can nurses do in community health departments to address pressing public health issues?
    a. Conduct groundbreaking research
    b. Provide health literacy to employees
    c. Engage in health promotion campaigns and proactive interventions
    d. Practice yoga for personal well-being

ANSWERS

1. c	2. b	3. c	4. a
5. a	6. b	7. c	8. a
9. c	10. c		

SUGGESTED READING

1. Alexander GK, Rollins K, Walker D, Wong L, Pennings J. Yoga for Self-Care and Burnout Prevention Among Nurses. Workplace Health and Amp; Safety. 2015;63(10):462-70.
2. Aryuwat P, Asp M, Lövenmark A, Radabutr M, Holmgren J. An integrative review of resilience among nursing students in the context of nursing education. Nursing open. 2023;10(5):2793-818.
3. Bond AR, Mason HF, Lemaster CM, Shaw SE, Mullin CS, Holick EA, et al. Embodied health: the effects of a mind-body course for medical students. Medical Education Online. 2013;18(1):20699.
4. Buckner JD, Bernert RA, Cromer KR, Joiner TE, Schmidt NB. Social anxiety and insomnia: the mediating role of depressive symptoms. Depression and Anxiety. 25(2):124-30.
5. Chu B, Marwaha K, Sanvictores T, Ayers D. Physiology, Stress Reaction. NCBI Bookshelf. 2022. Available from: https://www.ncbi.nlm.nih.gov/books/NBK541120/
6. Cocchiara RA, Peruzzo M, Mannocci A, Ottolenghi L, Villari P, Polimeni A, et al. The Use of Yoga to Manage Stress and Burnout in Healthcare Workers: A Systematic Review. Journal of clinical medicine. 2019;8(3):284.
7. Cocker F, Joss N. Compassion Fatigue among Healthcare, Emergency and Community Service Workers: A Systematic Review. International Journal of Environmental Research and Public Health. 2016;13(6).
8. Davidson RJ, Kabat-Zinn J, Schumacher J, Rosenkranz M, Muller D, Santorelli SF, et al. Alterations in Brain and Immune Function Produced by Mindfulness Meditation. Psychosomatic Medicine. 2003;65(4):564-70.
9. Dean E. Anxiety. Nursing Standard. 2016;30(46):15-15.
10. Does Mindfulness Decrease Stress and Foster Empathy Among Nursing Students? [Internet]. Journal of Nursing Education. Available from: https://journals.healio.com/doi/abs/10.3928/01484834-20040701-07
11. Dopheide JA. Insomnia Overview: Epidemiology, Pathophysiology, Diagnosis and Monitoring, and Nonpharmacologic Therapy. AJMC. 2020 Apr 13; Available from: https://www.ajmc.com/view/insomnia-overview-epidemiology-pathophysiology-diagnosis-and-monitoring-and-nonpharmacologic-therapy
12. Fang R, Li X. A regular yoga intervention for staff nurse sleep quality and work stress: a randomised controlled trial. Journal of Clinical Nursing. 2015;24(23-24):3374-9.
13. Flo E, Pallesen S, Magerøy N, Moen BE, Grønli J, Hilde Nordhus I, et al. Shift work disorder in nurses --assessment, prevalence and related health problems. PloS one. 2012;7(4):e33981.
14. Fox KCR, Nijeboer S, Dixon ML, Floman JL, Ellamil M, Rumak SP, et al. Is meditation associated with altered brain structure? A systematic review and meta-analysis of morphometric neuroimaging in meditation practitioners. Neuroscience & Biobehavioral Reviews. 2014;43:48-73.
15. Guarda The impact of COVID-19 pandemic on mental health of Nurses. La Clinica Terapeutica. Available from: https://clinicaterapeutica.it/ojs/index.php/1/article/view/246/206.
16. Guixia L, Hui Z. A Study on Burnout of Nurses in the Period of COVID-19. Psychology and Behavioral Sciences. 2020;9(3):31.
17. Haldorsen H, Bak NH, Dissing A, Petersson B. Stress and symptoms of depression among medical students at the University of Copenhagen. Scandinavian Journal of Public Health. 2013;42(1):89-95.
18. Herrick CM, Ainsworth AD. Invest in Yourself: Yoga as a Self-Care Strategy. Nursing Forum. 2000;35(2):32-6.
19. Hilcove K, Marceau C, Thekdi P, Larkey L, Brewer MA, Jones K. Holistic Nursing in Practice: Mindfulness-Based Yoga as an Intervention to Manage Stress and Burnout. Journal of Holistic Nursing. 2020;39(1):29-42.
20. How yoga can help ease PTSD symptoms --PTSD UK. Available from: https://www.ptsduk.org/how-yoga-can-help-ease-ptsd-symptoms/
21. Interventions to reduce burnout of physicians and nurses: Medicine. LWW. 2020. Available from: https://journals.lww.com/md-journal/ Fulltext/2020/06260/Interventions_to_reduce_burnout_of_ physicians_and.89.aspx
22. January J, Madhombiro M, Chipamaunga S, Ray S, Chingono A, Abas M. Prevalence of depression and anxiety among undergraduate university students in low- and middle-income countries: a systematic review protocol. Systematic Reviews. 2018;7(1):1-5.
23. Kabat-Zinn J. Mindfulness-based interventions in context: Past, present, and future. Clinical Psychology: Science and Practice. 2003;10(2):144-56.
24. Kamaraj M. The Impact of Yoga on Mental Health. Indonesian Journal of Community and Special Needs Education. 2023;3(2):141-6.
25. Kelly UA, Evans DD, Baker H, Noggle Taylor J. Determining Psychoneuroimmunologic Markers of Yoga as an Intervention for Persons Diagnosed with PTSD: A Systematic Review. Biological Research for Nursing. 2017;20(3):343-51.
26. Ketchesin KD, Stinnett GS, Seasholtz AF. Corticotropin-releasing hormone-binding protein and stress: from invertebrates to humans. Stress. 2017;20(5):449-64.
27. Khamisa N, Oldenburg B, Peltzer K, Ilic D. Work related stress, burnout, job satisfaction and general health of nurses. International journal of environmental research and public health. 2015;12(1):652-66.
28. Kiecolt-Glaser JK, Christian L, Preston H, Houts CR, Malarkey WB, Emery CF, et al. Stress, Inflammation, and Yoga Practice. Psychosomatic Medicine. 2010;72(2):113-21.
29. Kinchen E, Loerzel V, Portoghese T. Yoga and perceived stress, self-compassion, and quality of life in undergraduate nursing students. Journal of education and health promotion. 2020;9:292.
30. Kolk B van der. The Body Keeps the Score: Mind, Brain and Body in the Transformation of Trauma. Penguin UK; 2014.
31. Lin CC, Yeh CB. Factors associated with PTSD symptoms and quality of life among nurses during the COVID-19 pandemic: A cross-sectional study. PloS One. 2023;18(3):e0283500.
32. Li P, Kuang H, Tan H. The occurrence of post-traumatic stress disorder (PTSD), job burnout and its influencing factors among ICU nurses. American journal of translational research. 2021;13(7):8302-8.
33. Liu CY, Yang YZ, Zhang XM, Xu X, Dou QL, Zhang WW, et al. The prevalence and influencing factors in anxiety in medical workers fighting COVID-19 in China: a cross-sectional survey. Epidemiology and infection. 2020;148:e98.
34. Lomas T, Medina JC, Ivtzan I, Rupprecht S, Eiroa-Orosa FJ. Mindfulness-based interventions in the workplace: An inclusive systematic review and meta-analysis of their impact upon wellbeing. The Journal of Positive Psychology. 2018;14(5):625-40.
35. Magtibay DL, Chesak SS, Coughlin K, Sood A. Efficacy of Blended Learning with Stress Management and Resilience Training Program. The Journal of Nursing Administration. 2017;47(7/8):391-5.
36. Mandal S, Misra P, Sharma G, Sagar R, Kant S, Dwivedi S, et al. Effect of Structured Yoga Program on Stress and Professional Quality of Life Among Nursing Staff in a Tertiary Care Hospital of Delhi --A Small Scale Phase-II Trial. Journal of Evidence-Based Integrative Medicine. 2021;26:2515690X2199199.
37. Maslach C, Schaufeli WB, Leiter MP. Job Burnout. Annual Review of Psychology. 2001;52(1):397-422.

38. Mealer ML, Shelton A, Berg B, Rothbaum B, Moss M. Increased Prevalence of Post-traumatic Stress Disorder Symptoms in Critical Care Nurses. American Journal of Respiratory and Critical Care Medicine. 2007;175(7):693-7.
39. Miyoshi T, Ida H, Nishimura Y, Ako S, Otsuka F. Effects of Yoga and Mindfulness Programs on Self-Compassion in Medical Professionals during the COVID-19 Pandemic: An Intervention Study. International Journal of Environmental Research and Public Health. 2022;19(19).
40. Onieva-Zafra MD, Fernández-Muñoz JJ, Fernández-Martínez E, García-Sánchez FJ, Abreu-Sánchez A, Parra-Fernández ML. Anxiety, perceived stress and coping strategies in nursing students: a cross-sectional, correlational, descriptive study. BMC Medical Education. 2020;20(1):1-9.
41. Pappa S, Ntella V, Giannakas T, Giannakoulis VG, Papoutsi E, Katsaounou P. Prevalence of depression, anxiety, and insomnia among healthcare workers during the COVID-19 pandemic: A systematic review and meta-analysis. Brain, behavior, and immunity. 2020;88:901-7.
42. Park J, Jun JY, Lee YJ, Kim S, Lee SH, Yoo SY, et al. The association between alexithymia and posttraumatic stress symptoms following multiple exposures to traumatic events in North Korean refugees. Journal of Psychosomatic Research. 2015;78(1):77-81.
43. Qualities, teaching, and measurement of compassion in nursing: A systematic review. Nurse Education Today. 63:50-8.
44. Roth T. Insomnia: definition, prevalence, etiology, and consequences. Journal of clinical sleep medicine: JCSM: official publication of the American Academy of Sleep Medicine. 2007;3(5 Suppl):S7-10.
45. Saoji AA. Yoga: A Strategy to Cope up Stress and Enhance Wellbeing Among Medical Students. North American Journal of Medical Sciences. 2016;8(4):200-2.
46. Shah MK, Gandrakota N, Cimiotti JP, Ghose N, Moore M, Ali MK. Prevalence of and Factors Associated with Nurse Burnout in the US. JAMA Network Open. 2021;4(2):e2036469.
47. Sonmez Y, Akdemir M, Meydanlioglu A, Aktekin MR. Psychological Distress, Depression, and Anxiety in Nursing Students: A Longitudinal Study. Healthcare. 2023;11(5).
48. Streeter CC, Gerbarg PL, Saper RB, Ciraulo DA, Brown RP. Effects of yoga on the autonomic nervous system, gamma-aminobutyric-acid, and allostasis in epilepsy, depression, and post-traumatic stress disorder. Medical Hypotheses. 2012;78(5):571-9.
49. Tiwari GK. Yoga and Mental Health: An Underexplored Relationship. The International Journal of Indian Psychology. 2016;4(1):19-31.
50. Tung YJ, Lo KKH, Ho RCM, Tam WSW. Prevalence of depression among nursing students: A systematic review and meta-analysis. Nurse Education Today. 2018;63:119-29.
51. van der Kolk BA, Stone L, West J, Rhodes A, Emerson D, Suvak M, et al. Yoga as an Adjunctive Treatment for Posttraumatic Stress Disorder. The Journal of Clinical Psychiatry. 2014;75(06):e559-65.
52. Watts BV, Schnurr PP, Mayo L, Young-Xu Y, Weeks WB, Friedman MJ. Meta-Analysis of the Efficacy of Treatments for Posttraumatic Stress Disorder. The Journal of Clinical Psychiatry. 2013;74(06):e541-50.
53. Weber P, Peltonen LM, Junger A. The Essence and Role of Nurses in the Future of Biomedical and Health Informatics. In: Studies in Health Technology and Informatics. IOS Press; 2022. Available from: http://dx.doi.org/10.3233/shti220948
54. West CP. Physician Well-Being: Expanding the Triple Aim. Journal of General Internal Medicine. 2016;31(5):458-9.
55. Wilson A, Attarian HP. Defining Insomnia [Internet]. Springer International Publishing. 2017. Available from: https://link.springer.com/chapter/10.1007/978-3-319-41400-3_1
56. Wynn GH. Complementary and Alternative Medicine Approaches in the Treatment of PTSD. Current Psychiatry Reports. 2015;17(8).
57. Zeichner SB, Zeichner RL, Gogineni K, Shatil S, Ioachimescu O. Cognitive Behavioral Therapy for Insomnia, Mindfulness, and Yoga in Patients with Breast Cancer with Sleep Disturbance: A Literature Review. Breast Cancer: Basic and Clinical Research. 2017;11:117822341774556.

Annexures

ANNEXURE 1: IMPORTANT CLINICAL SIGNS

Sign	Description
Battle's sign	Bruising behind the ears (mastoid ecchymosis) due to a skull fracture, often associated with basilar skull fractures.
Brudzinski's sign	Involuntary flexion of the hip and knee when the neck is passively flexed. Like Kernig's sign, it suggests meningeal irritation and is associated with meningitis.
Cullen's sign	Periumbilical ecchymosis (bruising) due to bleeding in the abdominal wall, often associated with pancreatitis or intra-abdominal bleeding.
Chvostek's sign	Facial muscle contraction (twitching) induced by tapping the facial nerve just anterior to the ear. Like Trousseau's sign, it is associated with hypocalcemia and tetany.
Grey Turner's sign	Bruising of the flanks, usually indicative of retroperitoneal bleeding, often associated with conditions like pancreatitis or ruptured abdominal aortic aneurysm.
Homans' sign	Pain in the calf or posterior knee when the foot is dorsiflexed, indicating deep vein thrombosis (DVT).
Kernig's sign	Resistance or pain when attempting to straighten the knee with the hip flexed at a right angle. It is indicative of meningeal irritation and is often seen in cases of meningitis.
Murphy's sign	Pain or cessation of deep inspiration during palpation of the right upper quadrant of the abdomen, often associated with cholecystitis
Trousseau's sign	Carpal spasm induced by inflating a blood pressure cuff above the systolic pressure for a few minutes. It is associated with hypocalcemia and is seen in conditions like tetany.
Psoas sign	Pain in the right lower quadrant of the abdomen when the patient lifts his right thigh against resistance, indicating irritation of the psoas muscle often due to appendicitis.
Mcburney's point	A point located one-third of the distance from the anterior superior iliac spine to the umbilicus. Tenderness at this point is indicative of appendicitis.
Rovsing's sign	Pain felt in the right lower quadrant of the abdomen when pressure is applied to the left lower quadrant, indicative of appendicitis.
Three C's of measles	Cough, coryza, conjunctivitis

ANNEXURE 2: CLINICAL TRIADS

Beck's triad (cardiac tamponade)	A triad of symptoms—hypotension, distended neck veins, and muffled heart sounds—often seen in cardiac tamponade, a condition where fluid accumulates in the pericardial sac and compresses the heart
Cauda equina syndrome	Low back pain + Bowel/bladder dysfunction + Saddle anesthesia
Charcot's triad	Ascending cholangitis, fever with rigors + Right upper quadrant pain + Jaundice
Congestive heart failure triad	Tachycardia, tachypnea, tender hepatomegaly
Cushing's triad	A combination of three signs—hypertension (elevated blood pressure), bradycardia (slow heart rate), and irregular respirations—indicative of increased intracranial pressure
Danny's triad	Painful urination, testicular pain, diarrhea. Seen in *Chlamydia*
Fanconi syndrome triad	Aminoaciduria, proteinuria, phosphaturia. Seen in Fanconi syndrome.
Graves disease triad	Goiter, exophthalmos, pretibial myxedema. Seen in Grave's disease
Hakims triad	Gait disturbance + Dementia + Urinary incontinence
Horner's syndrome triad	Ptosis + Miosis + Anydrosis
Leriche syndrome	Buttock claudication + Impotence + Symmetrical atrophy of bilateral lower extremities
Lethal triad also known as the trauma triad of death	Hypothermia + Coagulopathy + Metabolic acidosis
Mackler's triad—esophageal perforation (Boerhaave syndrome)	Vomiting + Lower thoracic pain + Subcutaneous emphysema
Meniere's disease	Tinnitus + Vertigo + Hearing loss
Meningitis triad	A triad of symptoms often associated with bacterial meningitis—involving fever, headache, and neck stiffness (nuchal rigidity).
Neurogenic shock	Bradycardia + Hypotension + Hypothermia
Opioid overdose	Pinpoint pupils + Respiratory depression + CNS depression
Pheochromocytoma	Palpitations + Headache + Perspiration (diaphoresis)
Reactive arthritis	Can't See (conjunctivitis) + Can't Pee (urethritis) + climb a tree (arthritis). Arthritis, urethritis and, conjunctivitis.
Rigler's triad – gallstone ileus	Gallstones + Pneumobilia + Small bowel obstruction
Ruptured abdominal aortic aneurysm	Severe abdominal/back pain + hypotension + pulsatile abdominal mass
Saint's triad	Gallstones, diverticulosis, hiatus hernia
Sjögren's triad	A combination of dry eyes (keratoconjunctivitis sicca), dry mouth (xerostomia), and arthritis, is often seen in Sjögren's syndrome.
Tetany in children—triad	Stridor, carpopedal spasm, convulsions
Triad of kwashiorkor	Growth retardation, mental changes, edema
Triad of renal cell carcinoma	Hematuria, palpable abdominal mass, flank pain
Virchow's triad	A triad of factors that contribute to the formation of blood clots (thrombosis) in veins—endothelial injury, stasis of blood flow, and hypercoagulability.
Wernicke's encephalopathy—thiamine deficiency	Confusion + Ophthalmoplegia + Ataxia
Whipple's triad	A triad of symptoms used to diagnose insulinoma—a rare tumor of the pancreas that causes excessive insulin secretion. The triad consists of symptoms of hypoglycemia, a low blood glucose level during symptoms, and symptom relief after glucose administration.
Wolf parkinson white syndrome	Delta waves + Short PR interval + Wide QRS complex
Reiter's syndrome triad (reactive arthritis)	A triad of symptoms—arthritis, urethritis (inflammation of the urethra), and conjunctivitis (eye inflammation)—often seen in reactive arthritis, which can follow certain infections.

Appendix

URINE CHEMISTRY—NORMAL VALUES

Sl. No.	Test	Specimen	Conventional units	Possible etiology	
				Higher	*Lower*
1.	Acetone	Random	Negative	Diabetes mellitus, high fat and low carbohydrate diets, starvation states	
2.	Bence Jones protein	Random	Negative	Multiple myeloma, biliary duct obstruction	
3.	Bilirubin	Random	Negative	Hepatitis.	
4.	Calcium	24 hours	100–250 mg/day	Bone tumor, hyperparathyroidism	Hypoparathyroidism, malabsorption of Ca and vitamin D
5.	Chloride	24 hours	110–250 mEq/day	Addison's disease	Burns, excessive perspiration, vomiting, diarrhea, menstruation
6.	Creatine	24 hours	<100 mg/day	Carcinoma of liver, hyperthyroidism, diabetes, infections, burns	Hypothyroidism.
7.	Creatinine	24 hours	0.8–2.0 g/day	Anemia, leukemia, muscular atrophy	Renal disease.
8.	Creatinine clearance	24 hours	85–132 mL/min		Renal disease.
9.	Glucose	Random	Negative	Diabetes mellitus, low renal threshold for glucose resorption, pituitary disorders	
10.	Hemoglobin (Hb)	Random	Negative	Extensive burns, hemolytic transfusion reaction, glomerulonephritis, hemolytic anemia	
11.	Ketone bodies	24 hours	20–50 mg/day	Marked ketonuria	
12.	Myoglobin	Random	Negative	Crushing injuries, electric injuries, extreme physical exertion	
13.	pH	Random	4.0–8.0	Chronic renal failure, compensatory phase of alkalosis, vegetarian diet	Compensatory phase of acidosis, dehydration, emphysema
14.	Phenyl pyruvic acid	Random	Negative	Phenylketonuria	
15.	Protein	24 hours	<150 mg/day	Cardiac failure, inflammatory processes of urinary tract, nephritis, nephrosis, toxemia of pregnancy	
16.	Sodium	24 hours	40–250 mEq/day	Acute tubular necrosis	Hyponatremia
17.	Specific gravity	Random	1.003–1.030	Albuminuria, dehydration glycosuria.	Diabetes insipidus
18.	Uric acid	24 hours	250–750 mg/day	Gout, leukemia	Nephritis.
19.	Urobilinogen	24 hours	0.5–4.0 EU/day	Hemolytic disease, hepatic parenchymal cell damage, liver disease	Complete obstruction of bile duct

HEMATOLOGY—NORMAL VALUES

Sl. No.	Test	Conventional units	Possible etiology	
			Higher	Lower
1.	Bleeding time	3.0–9.5 min	Defective platelet function, thrombocytopenia	
2.	Activated partial thromboplastin time (APTT)	24–36 sec	Deficiency of factors I, II, V, VIII, IX and X, XI, XII, hemophilia, liver disease, heparin therapy	
3.	Prothrombin time	10–14 sec	Warfarin therapy, deficiency of factors I, II, V, VII and X, vitamin K deficiency Liver disease	
4.	Fibrinogen	200–400 mg/dL	Burns (after first 36 hours) inflammatory disease	Burns (during first 36 hours) DIC, severe liver disease
5.	Erythrocyte count Male Female	$4.5–6.0 \times 10^6/\mu L$ $4.0–5.0 \times 10^6/\mu L$		
6.	Mean corpuscular volume (MCV)	82–98 fL	Macrocytic anemia	Microcytic anemia
7.	Mean corpuscular hemoglobin (MCH)	27–33 pg	Macrocytic anemia	Microcytic anemia.
8.	Mean corpuscular hemoglobin Concentration (MCHC)	32–36%	Spherocytosis	Hypochromic anemia
9.	Erythrocyte sedimentation rate (ESR) Male <50 years	<15 mm/h	Moderate increase: Acute hepatitis, myocardial infarction, rheumatoid arthritis.	Malaria, severe liver disease, sickle cell anemia
	>50 years	<20 mm/h		
	Female <50 years >50 years	<20 mm/h <30 mm/h	Marked increase: Acute and severe bacterial infections, malignancies – Pelvic inflammatory disease – Dehydration, high altitudes, polycythemia	Anemia, hemorrhage, overhydration
10.	Hematocrit Male Female	40–54% 38–47%	COPD, high altitudes, Polycythemia	Anemia, hemorrhage.
11.	Hemoglobin Male Female	13.5–18.0 g/dL 12.0–16.0 g/dL		
12.	Glycosylated hemoglobin	4.0–6.0 %	Poorly controlled diabetes mellitus	Sickle cell anemia, chronic renal failure, pregnancy.
13.	Platelet count (thrombocytes)	$150–400 \times 10^3/\mu L$	Acute infections, chronic granulocytic leukemia, chronic pancreatitis, cirrhosis, collagen disorders, polycythemia, postsplenectomy	Acute leukemia, DIC, thrombocytopenic purpura
14.	White blood cell count (WBC)	$4.0–11.0 \times 10^3/\mu L$	Inflammatory and infectious processes, leukemia	Aplastic anemia, side effects of chemotherapy and irradiation
15.	Lymphocytes	20–40%	Chronic infections, lymphocytic leukemia, mononucleosis, viral infections.	Corticosteroid therapy, whole body irradiation
16.	Monocytes	4–8%	Chronic inflammatory disorders, malaria, monocytic leukemia, acute infections, Hodgkin's disease.	
17.	Eosinophils	0–4%	Allergic reactions, eosinophilic and chronic granulocytic leukemia, parasitic disorders, Hodgkin's disease	Corticosteroid therapy
18.	Basophils	0–2%	Hypothyroidism, ulcerative colitis, myeloproliferative diseases	Hyperthyroidism stress

SERUM, PLASMA AND WHOLE BLOOD CHEMISTRY

Sl. No.	Test	Conventional units	Possible etiology	
			Higher	*Lower*
1.	Acetone	0.3–2.0 mg/dL	Diabetic ketoacidosis, high fat diet, low carbohydrate diet, starvation	
2.	Albumin	3.5–5.00 g/dL	Dehydration	Chronic liver disease, malabsorption, malnutrition, nephrotic syndrome, pregnancy
3.	α-fetoprotein	<15 ng/mL	Cancer of testes and ovaries, carcinoma of liver	
4.	Ammonia	30–70 µg/dL	Severe liver disease	
5.	Amylase	0–130 U/L (method dependent)	Acute and chronic pancreatitis, mumps, perforated ulcers	Acute alcoholism, cirrhosis of liver, extensive destruction of pancreas
6.	Bicarbonate	20–30 mEq/L	Compensated respiratory acidosis, metabolic alkalosis	Compensated respiratory alkalosis, metabolic acidosis
7.	Bilirubin Total Indirect (unconjugated) Direct (conjugated)	0.2–1.3 mg/dL 0.1–1.0 mg/dL 0.1–0.3 mg/dL	Biliary obstruction, impaired liver function, hemolytic anemia, pernicious anemia, prolonged fasting	
8.	Blood gases Arterial pH Venous pH Arterial pCO_2 Venous pCO_2 Arterial pO_2 Venous pO_2	7.35–7.45 7.35–7.45 35–45 mm Hg 45–52 mm Hg 75–100 mm Hg 30–50 mm Hg	Alkalosis. • Compensated metabolic alkalosis. • Respiratory acidosis. • Administration of high concentration of oxygen	Acidosis • Compensated metabolic acidosis • Respiratory alkalosis • Chronic lung disease • Decreased cardiac output
9.	Calcium	9–11 mg/dL (4.5–5.5 mEq/L)	Acute osteoporosis, hyperparathyroidism, vitamin-D intoxication, multiple myeloma	Acute pancreatitis, hypoparathyroidism, liver disease, malabsorption syndrome, renal failure, vitamin D deficiency
10.	Chloride	95–105 mEq/L	Metabolic acidosis, respiratory alkalosis, corticosteroid therapy, uremia	Addison's disease, diarrhea, metabolic alkalosis, respiratory acidosis, vomiting
11.	Cholesterol HDL (high density lipoproteins) Male Female LDL (low density lipoproteins)	140–200 mg/dL (Age dependent) >45 mg/dL >55 mg/dL <130 mg/dL	Biliary obstruction, hypothyroidism, idiopathic hypercholesterolemia, renal disease, uncontrolled diabetes	Extensive liver disease, hyperthyroidism, malnutrition, corticosteroid therapy
12.	Cortisol	8 am: 5–25 µg/dL 8 pm: <10 µg/dL	Cushing syndrome, pancreatitis, stress	Adrenal insufficiency, panhypopituitary states.
13.	Creatine	0.2–1.0 mg/dL	Active rheumatoid arthritis, biliary obstruction, hyperthyroidism, renal disorders, severe muscle disease	Diabetes mellitus.
14.	Creatine kinase (CK) Male Female	15–105 U/L 10–80 U/L	Musculoskeletal injury or disease, myocardial infarction, severe myocarditis, exercises, myocarditis numerous intramuscular injections, brain damage	
15.	CK-MB (CK–2)	0–9 U/L	Acute myocardial infarction	
16.	Creatinine	0.5–1.5 mg/dL	Severe renal disease	
17.	Glucose fasting	70–120 mg/dL	Acute stress, cerebral lesions, Cushing's disease, diabetes mellitus, hyperthyroidism, pancreatic insufficiency	Addison's disease, hepatic disease, hypothyroidism, insulin overdosage, pancreatic tumor, pituitary hypofunction

Contd...

Contd...

Sl. No.	Test	Conventional units	Possible etiology	
18.	Lactic acid	5–20 µg/dL	Acidosis, congestive heart failure, shock	
19.	Lactic dehydrogenase (LDH)	50–150 U/L	Congestive heart failure, hemolytic disorders, hepatitis, metastatic cancer of liver, myocardial infarction, pernicious anemia, pulmonary embolus, skeletal muscle damage	
20.	Lipase	0–160 U/L	Acute pancreatitis, hepatic disorders, perforated peptic ulcer	
21.	Magnesium	1.5–2.5 mEq/L	Addison's disease, hypothyroidism, renal failure	Chronic alcoholism, hyperparathyroidism, hypoparathyroidism, severe malabsorption, hyperthyroidism
22.	Phosphatase acid	0–0.6 U/L	Advanced Paget's disease, cancer of prostate, hyperparathyroidism	
23.	Phosphatase alkaline	30–120 U/L	Bone diseases marked hyper-parathyroidism, obstruction of biliary system, rickets	Excessive vitamin D ingestion, hypothyroidism, milk alkali syndrome
24.	Potassium	3.5–5.5 mEq/L	Addison's disease, diabetic ketosis, massive tissue destruction, renal failure	Cushing syndrome, diarrhea (severe), diuretic therapy, gastrointestinal fistula, pyloric obstruction, starvation, vomiting
25.	Sodium	135–145 mEq/L	Dehydration, impaired renal function, primary aldosteronism, corticosteroid therapy	Addison's disease, diabetic ketoacidosis, diuretic therapy, excessive loss from gastrointestinal tract, excessive perspiration, water intoxication
26.	Proteins total Albumin Globulin Albumin-globulin ratio	6.0–8.0 g/dL 3.5–5.0 g/dL 2.0–3.5 g/dL 1.5:1–2.5:1	Burns, cirrhosis, dehydration. Multiple myeloma (globulin fraction) shock and vomiting.	Congenital agammaglobulinemia, liver disease, malabsorption Malnutrition, nephrotic syndrome, proteinuria, renal disease, severe burns
27.	T4 (thyroxine) total T4 (thyroxine) free T3 uptake T3 (triiodothyronine) TSH (thyroid stimulating hormone)	5–12 µg/dL 0.8–2.3 ng/dL 25–35% 110–230 ng/dL 0.3–5.4 µU/mL	Hyperthyroidism, thyroiditis Hyperthyroidism, metastatic neoplasms. Myxedema, primary hypothyroidism, Graves' disease	Cretinism, hypothyroidism, myxedema Hypothyroidism, pregnancy Secondary hypothyroidism
28.	Serum glutamic oxaloacetic (SGOT) or aspartate aminotransferase (AST). Serum glutamate pyruvate SGPT or alanine aminotransferase (ALT)	7–40 U/L 5–36 U/L	Liver disease, myocardial infarction, pulmonary infarction, acute hepatitis Liver disease, shock	
29.	Triglycerides	40–150 mg/dL	Diabetes mellitus, hyperlipidemia, hypothyroidism, liver disease	Malnutrition
30.	Blood urea nitrogen (BUN)	10–30 mg/dL	Increase in protein catabolism, renal disease, urinary tract infection	Malnutrition, severe liver damage
31.	Uric acid Male Female	 4.5–6.5 mg/dL 2.5-5.5 mg/dL	Gout, gross tissue destruction, high protein weight reduction diet, leukemia, renal failure, eclampsia.	Administration of uricosuric drugs

CEREBROSPINAL FLUID ANALYSIS

Sl. No.	Test	Conventional units	Possible etiology	
			Higher	Lower
1.	Pressure	60–150 mm H_2O	Hemorrhage, intracranial tumor, meningitis	Head injury, spinal tumor, subdural hematoma
2.	Blood	Negative	Intracranial hemorrhage	
3.	Cell count WBC RBC	 0–5 cells/µL 0	Inflammations or infections of CNS	
4.	Chloride	100–130 mEq /L	Uremia.	Bacterial infections of CNS
5.	Glucose	40–75 mg/dL	Diabetes mellitus, viral infections of CNS	Bacterial infections and TB of CNS
6.	Protein Lumbar Cisternal Ventricular	 15–45 mg/dL 15–25 mg/dL 5–15 mg/dL	• Guillain–Barré syndrome, poliomyelitis, traumatic tap • Syphilis of CNS • Acute meningitis, brain tumor, chronic CNS infections, multiple sclerosis	

FECAL ANALYSIS—NORMAL VALUES

Sl. No.	Test	Conventional units	Possible etiology	
			Higher	Lower
1.	Urobilinogen	30–220 mg/100 g of stool	Hemolytic anemia.	Complete biliary obstruction.
2.	Mucus	Negative	Mucous colitis, spastic constipation.	—
3.	Pus	Negative	Chronic bacillary dysentery, chronic ulcerative colitis, localized abscesses.	—
4.	Blood	Negative	Anal fissures, hemorrhoids, malignant tumor, peptic ulcer, inflammatory bowel disease.	—

5.	Color
	  Brown
	  Clay
	  Tarry
	  Red
	  Black
		—	• Various color depending on diet.
			• Biliary obstruction or presence of barium sulfate.
			• More than 100 mL of blood in GI tract.
			• Blood in large intestine.
			• Blood in upper GI tract or iron medication.
				—

Tumor marker	Normal range	Units
Alpha-fetoprotein (AFP)	Less than 10	ng/mL
Carcinoembryonic Antigen (CEA)	Less than 5 (nonsmokers) Up to 10 (smokers)	ng/mL
CA 15-3	Less than 30	U/mL
CA 19-9	Less than 37	U/mL
CA 125	Less than 35	U/mL
Prostate-specific antigen (PSA)	0–2.5: Normal for a man 40–50 years 2.5–3.5: Normal for a man 50–60 years 3.5–4.5: Normal for a man 60–70 years 4.5–5.5: Normal for a man 70–80 years	ng/mL
Beta-2 microglobulin (B_2M)	0.8 - 2.2	mg/L
Chromogranin A	Less than 100	ng/mL
Human chorionic gonadotropin (hCG)	In non-pregnant adults: Less than 5 In pregnant women (depending on gestational age): Varies	mIU/mL
Neuron-specific enolase (NSE)	Less than 16	ng/mL

Contd...

Contd...

Tumor marker	Normal range	Units
Progastrin-releasing peptide (ProGRP)	Less than 65	pg/mL
Thyroglobulin (Tg)	Less than 2.0	ng/mL
Calcitonin	Less than 10 (non-smokers) Up to 100 (smokers)	pg/mL
Alpha-methylacyl-CoA racemase (AMACR)	Less than 1.0	ng/mL
Cancer antigen 27.29 (CA 27.29)	Less than 38	U/mL
Cancer antigen 125 (CA 125 II)	Less than 35	U/mL
Cancer antigen 72-4 (CA 72-4)	Less than 6.9	U/mL
Squamous cell carcinoma antigen (SCCA)	Less than 1.5	ng/mL

Index

Page numbers followed by *b* refer to box, *f* refer to figure, *fc* refer to flowchart, and *t* refer to table.

A

Abdomen 480
    radiotherapy involving 480*t*
Abdominal aortic aneurysm, ruptured 716
Abducens nerve 262
Abducent nerve palsy 216
Abductor pollicis brevis muscle 390*f*
ABO-incompatible transplants 690
Abscess 279
    abrupt rupture of 383
    formation 122*f*
    parapharyngeal 43
    peritonsillar 33, 43, 44
    postauricular 26
    zygomatic 26
Absolute bone conduction test 13
Accessory ganglion 90*f*
Accredited social health activist 235, 237
Acetaminophen 364
Acetylcholine 197, 245
    inhibitors 197
Acetylcholinesterase
    enzyme 197
    inhibitors 426
Achilles reflex 268
Acid-fast bacteria 278
Acinetobacter baumanii 649
Acoustic evoked potentials 419
Acoustic neuroma 29
Acquired monocular elevation deficiency, causes of 217
Acquired palsy, causes of 215
Acquired voice disorders 64
    etiology of 64
Actinic keratosis 589
Acute otitis media 19, 23
    suppurative phase of 23*f*
Acyclovir 109, 378, 409
Adalimumab 578
Adaptation 591
Adaptive clothing 625
Adaptive dressing aids 623
Adaptive eating utensils 622
Adenoid facies 44
Adenoid hypertrophy 44
Adenoiditis 44
Adequate fluid status 293
Adequate hydration and rest 43
Adequate nutrition 457
Adequate sleep 590
Adequate tissue oxygenation, maintenance of 453
Adie's tonic pupil 184
Adjuvant chemotherapy 473

Administer pain medications 367
Admission policy 635
Adopting supporting tools 684
Adrenal insufficiency, monitor signs of 379
Adrenaline 640
Adrenergic receptors 656
Advance care planning 506
Advance directives 594, 599, 661
Advanced bionics 81
Advanced cardiac life support 638
Advanced diabetic retinopathy 153*f*
Advanced life support 640, 642
Agitation 428
Agnosia 256
Airborne precautions 654
Air-conduction 72
Airway 289, 290, 298, 315, 639
    and breathing 646
    breathing, circulation, disability, and exposure 524, 648
    compromises 315
    disease, chronic obstructive 571
    maintenance of 640, 642
    management 451
    obstruction 454
        malignant 494
    protection 392
    supraglottic 632, 640
Akinesia 423
Alanine aminotransferase 276
Alcohol
    abuse 585
    avoidance of 574
    based hand rub 652
    hand rub 652*t*
    intoxication 286
    use of 528
    withdrawal syndrome 286
Alemtuzumab 441
Alexithymia 703
Alkaline phosphatase 276
Alkylating agents 483
Allergen, avoidance of 37
Allergic conditions 24
Allergic rhinitis 35
    classification of 37*f*
    management of 37
Allergy
    biochemical mechanism of 36*f*
    mechanism of 36
Alloderm 455
Allogeneic bone marrow transplantation 486*f*
Allogeneic stem cell transplantation 486
Allograft 690

Allotransplantation 690
Alopecia 484
Alpha-adrenergic receptors 656
Alzheimer's disease 423, 424, 427, 560, 583
    pathophysiology of 424, 425*f*
    risk factors for 424
    stages of 425
    types of 424
Alzheimer's illnesses 424
Amantadine 437
Amaurosis fugax 193
Amblyopia 200, 210, 217
    mixed 211
    treatment of 211, 216
    types of 210
Ametropia 111
Aminoglycoside 132, 695
Aminophylline 409
Amiodarone 193, 409, 640
Amitriptyline 409
Ammetropic amblyopia 211
Amnesia 256
Amoxicillin 109
Amphetamines 286
Amphotericin 409
    B 109, 132, 378
Amygdala 423
Amyloid beta protein 423
Amyotrophic lateral sclerosis 280, 433, 434*f*
Anakinra 578
Anal sphincter, loss of control of 492
Analgesia 298, 299
Analgesic
    anticipatory 456
    ladder 511*f*
    rebound 364
Anaplasia 463, 464
Anasarca 450
Ancillary 634
    tests 189
Androgen receptor blockers 482
Andropause 577, 581
Anemia 454, 484
    nursing implications for 484
Anesthesia, safe 683
Aneurysm 285
    classification of 336, 337*t*
    clipping of 339*f*
    complications of 340
    formation 337
    pathophysiology of 337*f*
    ruptured 337, 338
    unruptured 337, 338
Angiogenesis 466
Angiography 314

Angiotensin 1-converting enzyme 424
Angular conjunctivitis 146
Anhidrosis 184
Animal bites 532
    management of 533
Anisocoria 184f
Anisometropic amblyopia 211
Ankle
    braces 621
    fractures 579
    jerk 252
Ankyloglossia 62
Ann Arbor system 466
Annulus of Zinn 180
Anorexia 485, 512
Antecubital vein 167
Anterior chamber angle 137, 139
Anterior cord syndrome 311, 319, 321
Anthracosis 667
Antibiogram 631
Antibiotic 109
    therapy, role of 168
Anticholinergic drug toxicity 286
Anticonvulsant therapy 384
Antidepressants, tricyclic 286
Antifungal therapy 379
Antiglaucoma
    medications 136
    therapy 132
Antihistamine 37, 418
Anti-infective agents 109
Anti-inflammatory agent 109
Antimetabolites 483
Antimicrobial therapy 454
Antimicrobial use 653
Antioxidants 555
Anti-parkinsonism medications 432
Anti-platelets 333
Anti-progression medications 441
Antipsychotic medications 437
Anti-seizure
    medications 338
    therapy 299
Anti-snake venom 533
Antitumor antibiotics 483
Antiviral medications 574
Antrochoanal polyp 55
Anxiety 58, 509, 512, 700, 701, 703
    assess level of 430
    disorders 703
Apert-Crouzon syndrome 201
Aphakia 91
Aphasia 256
Apheresis 486, 487
Apnea test 693
Apnea-hypopnea index 59
Apocrine hydrocystoma 121, 123
Appetite, loss of 340
Apraxia 256
Aqueous humor drainage 137
Aqueous outflow
    pathways 137fc
    system 137
Archimedean spiral drawn 409f
Arcus 134
    senilis 134
Ardhahalasana 708
Ardha-Kati chakrasana 706
Ardhmatseyndrasana 707
Areflexia 389
Argyll-Robertson pupil 184
Argyrosis 150
Aripiprazole 437
Arnold-Chiari malformation 189

Arrhythmia 285
Arterial blood gas 693
Arterial catheter 635
Arterial hyperoxia 640
Arterial pressure, left 647
Arterial thrombosis 499
Arteriovenous malformations 276, 281
Arthritis, reactive 716
Arthropod-borne viral encephalitis 380
Articulation disorders 62
Articulation treatment procedure 63
Asanas 706
Asbestosis 667
Ascites 574
Aseptic techniques, use of 653
Asparaginase therapy 499
Aspartate aminotransferase 276
Aspergillus 131
    fumigatus 379
Asphyxia 638
Aspiration 399
Aspirin 364, 419
    intolerance 55
Assistive devices 611
Asthma 55
    acute 571, 572
    bronchial 571
    chronic phases of 572
Astrocytoma 345
Asystole 420
Ataxia 177, 256, 370, 423
Athetosis 411
Atonic seizures 368
Atrial fibrillation 333
Atrioventricular block, types of 534
Atrioventricular system 566
Atrophic rhinitis 35
Atrophy 423
Atropine 132
    sulcate 169
    sulfate 168, 657, 659
Atypical parkinsonian syndromes 274
Audiogram 71, 75f, 418
Audiological examination 12
Audiometric examination 419
Audiometric test 419
Audiometry 71
Auditory brainstem response 71, 78
    test 78f
Auditory canal, external 11f, 14, 20f
Auditory discrimination 582
Auditory effects 668
Aura 362, 363f
    phase 361
    presence of 362
Aural fullness 418
Aural methods 83
Aural syringing 20
Aural toileting 20, 22, 24
Auricle 4
Auscultation 469
Autograft 690
Autoimmune disorders 585, 590
Autologous bone marrow transplantation 486f
Autologous peripheral blood stem cells 485
Autonomic dysfunction 392, 584
Autonomic nervous system 243, 254, 702
Autonomic symptoms 418
Autorefractometry 96
Autotopagnosia 259
Autotransplantation 690
Awareness, loss of 368
Axonal injury 313
Azithromycin 147

B

Babinski's reflex 265, 267f
Babinski's signs 252
Baclofen 322, 410
Bacteria 465
Bacterial growth, caries-producing 512
Bag and mask 522
    ventilation 640
Bagolini striated glass 205f
    test 205, 206f
Balance disorders 585
Barbiturate 286, 316, 370
    coma therapy 299
Baroreceptor sensitivity 567
Barotrauma 24
Bartonella henselae 191
Basal cell carcinoma 121
Basal ganglia 409, 423
Basic life support 642
Basic vital signs 258
Basilar artery occlusion 286
Bath seats 624
Bathroom 613
    safety aids 624
Battle's sign 715
Beck's triad 716
Bed rails 622
Behavioral changes 583
Behavioral observation audiometry test 76f
Behavioral pain scale 648
Behavioral tests 76
Behcet's disease 176
Bell's palsy 414, 416
    risk factors for 416
Bell's phenomenon 414
Benign prostatic
    hyperplasia 581, 582
    hypertrophy 576
Benzodiazepine 285, 286, 370, 410, 412, 418, 419, 661
Bereavement support 506
Beta-adrenergic receptors 656
Beta-blockers 365
Betamethasone 109
Bezold's abscess 25
Bhopal Gas Tragedy 539
Bhramhari 708
Bhujangansana 707
Bielschowsky type 213
Bile duct disorders 574
Billroth surgery 475
Binocular double vision 185
Binocular eye movements 201
Binocular vision 98, 220
    physiology of 202
Binocularity, grades of 204f
Biological grafts 455
Biological hazards 538, 668
Biomedical waste
    management 654, 677
    proper disposal of 654
Biopsy 281, 306, 347
Bipolar cells 170
Bisacodyl 510
Bitemporal hemianopia 174f
Bladder
    capacity 575
    control 661
    dysfunction 440
    elimination 350
    function, loss of 492
    management 392
    training 576

Blastomyces dermatitidis 379
Bleeding 470, 476
Blepharitis 121, 122
Blepharoptosis 121
Blindness 111
Blood
    glucose level, check 288
    loss 454
    mechanism 466
    products 685
    proteins 467
    safety 678
    sugar, control of 580
    tests 276, 277*t*, 427, 467
    transfusion set 685*f*
    type 451
    vessels, narrowed 340
Blood flow
    and vascular spasm, blockage of 530
    insufficient 338
Blood pressure 258, 298, 522, 567
    abnormalities 320
    control 340
    high 340, 592
    lowering medications 365
    management 584
Blood serum
    creatine-kinase 451
    infection, catheter-associated 631
Blood-borne infections, contracting 668
Blood-brain barrier 249, 376
Bloodstream infection, central line with 649, 653, 680
Blood-sucking parasitic insects 533
Blunt trauma 49, 139*f*, 222, 224
Body
    electrolytes get 695
    hearing aid 79, 79*f*
    image, loss of 471
    physiological functions of 560
    temperature maintenance 694
    weight, changes in 470
Boerhaave syndrome 716
Bone
    conduction 71
    health 581
    nerve compression 510
Bone marrow
    aspiration needle 487*f*
    depression 483
    donating 487, 487*b*
    stem cells, sources of 485
    suppression 479
    transplantation 485
        procedure of 487
Bony labyrinth 4*f*, 5*f*
Bony spur 52*f*
Borrelia 191
Botox injections 365
Botulinum
    injection 412*f*
    neurotoxin 410
    toxin 214, 411
Bowel changes 470
Bowel dysfunction 440
Bowel elimination 350
Bowel function 292
    loss of 492
Bowel management 392
Bowel movement 661
Bowman layer 135
    dystrophies 133
Bowman membrane 89, 130
Brachial plexus 254

Brachioradialis reflex 268
Brachytherapy 344, 473, 477
Bradycardia 420, 450
Bradykinesia 431
Bradypnea 450
Brain 245, 340
    aneurysm, ruptured 339
    blood vessels of 328*f*
    computed tomography 347
    edema, diffuse 294
    function tests 437
    functional areas of 247*f*
    herniation 285
    imaging tests 437
    inferior aspect of 250*f*
    inferior surface of 253*f*
    iron accumulation 411
    lobes of 246*f*
    magnetic resonance imaging 347
    parts of 245, 245*t*, 380
    poles of 246*f*
    right side of 332*f*
    sagittal section of 246*f*
    scans 427
    stimulation, deep 306, 371, 371*f*, 409, 432
    venous drainage of 250
    ventricles of 248
    vessel 334*f*
    waves, types of 275, 275*t*
Brain abscess 376, 382
    causes of 382
    pathophysiology of 382*fc*
Brain death 689, 691*t*, 692
    donation after 691
    management of 694
    pathophysiology of 692
    patient's eyes 693
    triad 693
Brain injury
    closed 311
    non-penetrating 312
    primary 312
    secondary 312
    traumatic 294, 312, 318*f*
Brain tissue
    compared to 314
    death of 327
Brain tumor 280, 297, 344
    grading of 345
    pathophysiology of 346*fc*
    treatment of 348
    types of 345, 345*t*
Brainstem 380
    nuclei 175
    reflexes 693*f*
        absence of 693
    tumor 286
Branch retinal artery occlusion 155
Branch retinal vein occlusion 155
BRCA-1 469
BRCA-2 469
Breast
    changes in 470, 581
    conserving surgery 474, 474*f*
Breast cancer 464, 467, 477, 479, 479*t*
    hormone therapy for 482
    surgery for 474
    treat 482
Breathing 289, 315, 639
    absence of normal 638
    difficulty 479
    techniques 702
Brimonidine 109
Bronchospasm 167

Brooke army formula 452
Brown-Séquard syndrome 311, 319, 321, 492
Bruch's membrane 90
Brudzinski's sign 377, 378*f*, 715
Bruising 470
B-scan 100*f*
Buccal mucosa 16
Bulbar muscles 395
Buphthalmos 141*f*
Burn 447
    accidental
        corneal 110
        retinal 110
    care at hospital 451
    care, rehabilitation phase of 457
    chemical 527
    classification of 448, 448*t*
    degree of 448
    estimating extent of 449*f*
    first aid for 451
    fourth degree 448*f*
    injury 447, 448
    out 631, 699
    partial thickness 448*f*
    pathophysiology of 449, 450*fc*
    second degree of 448*f*
    severity of 451
    surface area 447, 449
Burn wound
    cleaning procedure 454
    dressing procedure 454
    grafting 455
    healing, disorders of 456*f*
Burr holes 303*f*
Busulfan 483
Butyrophenone 430
Byssinosis 667

C

Cachexia 513
Caffeine 364
Calcium
    channel blockers 338, 365
    gluconate 657, 659
Caloric diet, high 465
Caloric test 418
Campylobacter jejuni 388
Canalith repositioning procedures 585
Cancer 463, 510*t*
    awareness about 470
    causes of bleeding in 499
    cell 464, 464*f*
        genetic material of 467
    diagnosis of 467, 467*t*
    early detection of 469, 469*t*
    epidemiology of 464
    etiopathogenesis of 465
    high-grade 467
    low-grade 467
    pathophysiology of 465*fc*
    prevention of 469
    psychosocial aspects of 470
    screening of 469
    signs of 470*t*
    staging of 466
    surgery, principles of 474
    symptoms of 470*t*
    treatment 470, 473
    warning signs of 469, 470
Candida 131, 379
    albicans 454, 500
Cane stick 232
Canine distemper 439

Capsulotomy 285
   posterior 110
Carbamazepine 370, 437
Carbon
   dioxide levels, high 570
   monoxide 526
      poisoning 286, 451
Carboxyhemoglobin 519
Carboxymethylcellulose 109
Carcinoma larynx 55
Cardiac arrest 638, 641t
Cardiac changes 340
Cardiac effects 450
Cardiac impulse generation 566
Cardiac monitors 522
Cardiac muscle 567
Cardiac output 567, 647
Cardiac rehabilitation 568
Cardiac symptoms 420
Cardiac tamponade 493, 716
Cardiotoxicity 479
Cardiovascular conditions, age-related 568t
Cardiovascular disorders 669
Cardiovascular emergencies 493
Cardiovascular functions, maintenance of 695
Cardiovascular management 324
Cardiovascular reflexes 566
Cardiovascular system 566, 567f, 695
Care
   cultural aspects of 507
   ethical aspects of 507
   extreme 523
   general aspects of 614b
   goals of 613
   high-quality 701
   legal aspects of 507
   physical aspects of 506
   planning 616
   psychological aspects of 506
   regarding safety 419
   social aspects of 506
   supportive 430, 512
Care-related information, documentation of 523
Carpel tunnel syndrome 280
Castroviejo's conjunctival scissors 106f
Cat scratch disease 191
Cat's paw 103
Cataract 114, 115f, 116, 116f, 220, 231, 587
   acquired 117
   anterior polar 116
   blue dot 116, 117f
   classification of 116
   complicated 166
   congenital 114, 116
   cortical 114, 117
   geriatric considerations for 119
   incipient 118
   lamellar 114, 116f
   nursing management of 119
   pathophysiology of 115fc
   polar 114, 116
   posterior
      polar 116, 118f
      subcapsular 117f
   subcapsular 114, 117
   surgical rate 236
   sutural 116
   traumatic 223f
   type of 116
Cataract formation
   risk factors for 115
   stages of 118
Cataract surgery
   complications of 118
   endothelium during 134
   extracapsular 118
   laser-assisted 110
Catarrhal pharyngitis, chronic 38
Catarrhal tonsillitis, acute 42
Catastrophe theory, error 561
Catecholamine 245
   storm 694
Catheter, types of 647
Cauda equina
   lesions 319, 321
   syndrome 311, 716
Cavernous sinus 180, 182f
   syndrome 181
Cell
   body 244
   membrane, selective permeability of 244
   normal 464
   number of 464
   phones 623
   type 467
Central chiasmal lesion 173
Central cord syndrome 311, 319, 321
Central gas pipelines 522
Central nervous system 243, 245, 345
Central retinal
   artery 156f
      occlusion 155
   vein occlusion 154
Central serous chorioretinopathy 159
Central trans herniation 295
Central venous
   catheter 647
   pressure 647
Cephalalgia 360
Cerebellar dysfunction 440
Cerebellar function 265
   testing 266t
Cerebellar nuclei 409
Cerebellothalamic circuit 409
Cerebellum 248
Cerebral aneurysm 336
   repair 306
Cerebral angiography 281
Cerebral artery 336
   of brain, right middle 332f
Cerebral autoregulation, effect of 295f
Cerebral blood
   circulation 250
   flow 276, 294, 296, 349, 362
Cerebral circulation 249
Cerebral circulatory system, arrest in 276
Cerebral cortex 246
Cerebral emboli 276
Cerebral functions 259
Cerebral hemisphere, left 246f, 247f
Cerebral hypertension, prevalence of 294
Cerebral irritation 341
Cerebral ischemia 338
Cerebral palsy 201
Cerebral perfusion pressure 294, 311
Cerebral tissue perfusion 307
Cerebral tumor 364
Cerebral venous drainage, facilitation of 298
Cerebral volume 295f
Cerebrospinal fluid 278, 294, 389
   absorption of 249
   analysis 276, 278t, 348, 390, 721
   drainage 341
   examination 378
   functions of 249
   test 338, 427
Cerebrovascular accident 327
Cerebrovascular disease, ischemic 276
Cerebrovascular disorders 327
Cerebrum 245
Certolizumab 578
Cerumen 19, 71
   impaction 19, 20f
Cervical
   collar 522
   compression 492
   dystonia 412, 412f
   injuries 320
   plexus 254
   vascular disease 361
Cervix, cancer of 470
Cetirizine 419
Chaddock's reflex 265
Chalazion clamp, closed 106f
Chalcosis 226
Charcot's triad 716
Chemical agents 465
Chemical burn, symptoms of 527
Chemical disinfectants 105
Chemical injury 222, 448
Chemical occupational factors 667
Chemical spills 541
Chemosis 127f
Chemotherapeutic agents 409
   safe handling of 485
Chemotherapy 348, 356, 463, 482, 500
   extravasation of 500
   side effects of 483
Chest
   and abdomen rise 646
   compression 642
      technique of 639f
   infections 480
   pain 658
   X-ray 289
Chevallet fracture 54
Cheyne-Stokes respirations 256
Chiasm 172
   lesion, lateral 173
Chilblain 519, 528
Chin lift jaw thrust technique 639, 639f
Chlamydia trachomatis 147
Chloroquine 193
Chlorpromazine 409
Cholinergic crisis 397
Cholinesterase inhibitors 427
Chorea 405, 406
   causes of 406t
Chorioretinal degeneration, diffuse 162
Choroid 90, 225
Choroidal melanoma 201
Choroidal neovascular membrane 151, 164
Choroidal vessels 157f
Chronic obstructive pulmonary disease, treatment of 572
Chronic otitis media 19, 24
   mucosal 25
   squamous 25
Chronological age 558
Chvostek's sign 715
Ciliary body 89, 90, 137, 224
   anatomy of 137f
   suspends 90
Ciliary ganglion 90f
Ciliary motility, disorders of 55
Ciliary muscle 137
Ciliary spasm 169
Cingulate herniation 295
Cingulotomy 285, 305
Cinnarizine 409
Ciprofloxacin 109, 168
Circle of Willis 184, 250, 250f
Circulatory anticoagulants 499

Circulatory death 691
  donation after 689, 691
Cisplatin 409, 483
Citelli's abscess 26
Citrus fruits 469
Claustrophobia 272
Clean utility area 633
Cleft lip 61
Clinical phenotype 167*fc*
Clinically isolated syndrome 440
Clonazepam 410, 437
Clonidine 286
Clonus 368
Close off aneurysm 339
Clot-busting medications 333
Clotrimax 512
Clotting, disruption of 476
Coagulation function, maintenance of 695
Coagulopathy 316
Coal workers' pneumoconiosis 667
Cobalamin 193
Cocaine 286
Coccidioides immitis 379
Cochlea 4
Cochlear canal, divisions of 4*f*
Cochlear corporation 81
Cochlear implant 71, 81, 81*f*
  candidacy 81, 82
  surgery, assessment for 82
Cogan microcystic epithelial dystrophy 133
Cognitive behavioral therapy 69, 703
Cognitive changes 566, 584
Cognitive development 560
Cognitive dysfunction 60, 440
Cognitive impairment 595, 672
Cognitive rehabilitation 442
Cognitive test 427
Cogwheel rigidity 423
Cold injury 448
Cold spatula test 15, 15*f*, 53
Collagen fibrils 130
Colles' fractures 578
Colloids 317, 452
Colon cancer 467
Color vision 98, 110
  testing 186
Color-coding system, different 654
Coma 285, 311, 692
Comatose 288
Common cold 33
Communication 61, 259, 544, 657
  aids 621
  and consent 591
  devices 621, 626
  impaired 257
  policy 636
  system 626
  tool 655
  with team 543
Community health centers 545
Community ophthalmology 234
Compartment syndrome 447, 454
Compassion fatigue 699
Complementary medicine 700, 702
Complete blood count 289, 378, 467
  analysis 415
Compound muscle action potential 390*f*
Compression stockings 624
Concha bullosa 15
Concussion 311
Cone dystrophy 152, 160
Cone-rod dystrophy 152
Confrontation test 187, 187*f*

Congenital motor nystagmus 188
Congenital nasolacrimal duct obstruction 121, 124
Congestive heart failure triad 716
Conjunctiva 88*f*, 89, 105, 149*f*
  degenerative changes in 149
  disorders of 145
  tumor of 149
  wounds of 225
Conjunctival disorders 145, 146
Conjunctival sac 89
Conjunctivitis 145, 146
  allergic 145, 147
  chemical 148
  chronic 147
  hemorrhagic 146
  infective 130, 145
Conjunctivochalasis 150
Consciousness
  altered level of 285, 286, 286*t*-288*t*
  clouding of 287
  level of 260, 340
  loss of 368
Consecutive exotropia 213
Consensual pupillary reaction, loss of 172
Constipation 292, 480, 510, 512, 574
  laxatives in 512
Contact lenses 112, 231
Continuity theory 562
Contrast sensitivity test 186
Control anxiety 533
Contusion 311, 313
Conus medullaris 311
  syndrome 319, 321
Conventional adenoidectomy, steps of 44
Convergence-retraction nystagmus 177, 189
Cooking equipment 527
Copper 193, 426
Cor pulmonale 43
Cord concussion 311
Cord injury, incomplete 321
Cornea 89, 105, 139, 149*f*, 224
  diseases of 130
  disorders of 130
  hazy 141*f*
  layers of 89*t*
  wounds of 225
Corneal cross-linking 134
Corneal curvature, abnormal 111
Corneal diseases 131
Corneal dystrophies 133
Corneal edema 131, 132*f*
Corneal integrity, preserving 291
Corneal laceration 223*f*, 225
Corneal opacity 131
Corneal penetrating injury 127*f*
Corneal perforation 132
Corneal reflex 693
Corneal thickness, peripheral 139*f*
Corneal tissue storage 230*f*
Corneal topography 112
Corneal transplantation 134, 135, 232
Corneal ulcer 130, 131
  complications of 132
Corneoscleral coat 89
Coronary artery disease 568
Coronavirus disease-2019 (COVID-19) 612
  pandemic 594, 701
  psychological effects of 669
Corpectomy 324
Corpus callosotomy 305, 370
Corrosive chemicals 519
Cortical gray matter 380

Corticospinal tract mediates, lateral 251
Corticosteroid 37, 109, 322, 349, 384, 396, 418
  deficiency 696
Cortisol regulation 577
Corynebacterium diphtheriae 51
Coryza 33
Co-trimoxazole 409
Cottle's test 53
Cotton wool test 15
Cough 470, 480
  etiquettes 654
  reflex 693
Cover test 208
  alternate 205, 209
Cover-uncover test 205
Cranial cavity 4
Cranial dura 249*t*
  mater 249
Cranial nerve 177, 253, 253*f*, 260, 260*t*
  assessment of 270
  disorders 414
  dysfunction of 440
  examination 189
  functions of 253*t*, 260
  palsy
    multiple 180
    treatment of 179
  third 177
  types of 253*t*
Cranial surgical approaches 303*t*
Craniectomy 285, 305, 311
  decompressive 299
Craniopharyngioma 345
Craniotomy 302, 311
  procedure of 304
  types of 303
Cranium, disorder of 361
C-reactive protein 278
Critical care 631, 632, 642
  nursing 631, 632, 638, 644
  quality indicator of 636
  technical staff 634
Critical care unit 632, 642, 644
  equipment in 634
  physical layout of 633
  physical setup of 632
  policies of 635
  protocols of 635
  waste disposal in 633
Critical facilities 538
Critically-ill patient 644, 645, 650
Cromolyn sodium 109, 147
Crutch glass 217*f*
Crutchfield tongs 323*f*
Cryoprecipitates 499
Cryptococcal
  disease 192
  meningitis 378
  neoformans 192, 377, 379
Cryptococcus 191
Cullen's sign 715
Cultivating mindfulness 705
Cupric oxide 157
Curative treatment 491
Curriculum 696
Cushing's triad 295, 716
Cushing's ulcers 318
Cutaneous areas, distribution of 252
Cyber security breaches 541
Cyclic esotropia 212, 213
Cyclitic membrane 166
Cyclizine 418
Cyclopentolate eyedrops 168

Cyclophosphamide 483
Cycloplegic drugs, role of 168
Cycloplegics agents 109
Cyclosporine 109, 409
Cyst
  laryngeal 50
  of Moll 121, 123
  sebaceous 121, 123
  tonsillar 43, 43f
  vocal 65f
Cystic fibrosis 55
Cystic swelling 11
Cystitis, hemorrhagic 495
Cystoid macular edema 151, 164
Cystoid retinal degeneration, peripheral 162
Cytomegalovirus 191, 388, 499
Cytotoxic T-lymphocyte associated antigen inhibitor abatacept 578

D

Dacryoadenitis 123, 120, 124
Dacryocystorhinostomy 124
Danny's triad 716
Daratumumab 481
Dawson's fingers 191
De Wecker's scissors 105
Deaf, educational approaches for 82
Deafness 72
  grading 13f
Death
  fear of 471
  manner of 691
  natural 691t
  trauma triad of 716
Debridement 447
Debulking 474
Deceased donor 691
  care of 694f
Deceased organ donation 689
Deceased tissue donation 689
Decompression sickness 519, 530, 531f
Deep vein thrombosis 341, 631
  prophylaxis 391, 392
Degenerative diseases 134
Dehydration 115, 512
  test 418
Delirious 288
Delirium 428, 509, 661, 686
  types of 429
Dementia 426, 560
  frontotemporal 427
  mixed 427
  prevention of 428
  symptoms, cause of 426
  types of 427
  vascular 427
Demyelinating disease 286
Demyelinating type 388
Denial, phase of 534
Denosumab 481
Dental prostheses 621
Dentate nucleus 409
Dentate-olivary circuits 409
Denture 621
Depression 180f, 428, 559, 592, 701
  cortical spreading 361
  mild-to-severe 669
Dermal substitutes 455
Dermatitis, contact 667
Dermatome 254, 254t, 455
Dermis, age-related changes in 588f
Descartes-Sherrington's law 202
Descemet's membrane 89, 130, 135

Desensitization 68
Desmetocele 132
Deviated nasal septum, types of 52
Deviation
  causing suppression 217
  primary 208f
  secondary 208f
Dexamethasone 109, 298, 378
  loading dose of 492
Dexmedetomidine infusion 316
Dhanurasana 707
Diabetes 115, 585
  management of 580
  mellitus 153f, 580, 592
Diabetic macular edema 152, 153
Diabetic retinopathy 109, 151, 152, 153f, 231, 238
Diarrhea 485
Diencephalon 245, 246
Dietary factors 465
Dietary management 419
Dietetics 34, 37, 45, 49, 51, 56, 334, 372
Diethylstilbestrol 465
Diffuse axonal injury 311
Digital rectal examination 470
Digitalis 193
Digoxin 657, 659
Dihydroergotamine 364
Dilation, effects of 99f
Diphtheria 146
Diplopia 185, 200, 203, 205f, 214-217, 370
  test 206
Disability 315
Disability-adjusted life-years, causes of 448
Disaster 539
  characteristics of 539
  classification of 540, 540t
  environmental 540
  epidemiology of 540
  future 542
  hospital management 545
  human-made 540
  natural 540
  preparedness 541, 545
  response, control 542
  risk management cycle 543f
  technological 540, 541
  types of 550
Disaster management 538, 543, 546, 546b
  cycle 542
  principles of 542
  structure 546f
Disc
  edema sectoral, inferior 192f
  edema, stages of 195f
  neovascularization of 152
Discharge planning 58
Disengagement theory 562
Disinfection 103
Diskectomy 323
Disseminated disease 466
Disseminated intravascular coagulopathy 499
Diuretics 299, 418
Divalproex 437
Diver's disease 519
Divergence excess 207f
Dizziness 28, 370
Dobutamine 657
  hydrochloride 658
Doll's eyes reflex 693
Domino transplant 690
Donepezil 426, 427
Donor
  site 447
    care of 456
  types of 690

Dopamine 657, 658
  receptor agonists 432
Dopaminergic receptors 656
Dorsal kyphosis 492
Dorsal midbrain syndrome 176
Dorzolamide 109
Down's syndrome 115, 201, 424
Drop attack 418
Droplet precautions 654
Drugs
  administration 318, 485
  anthelmintic 384
  antiallergic 109
  antiarrhythmic 640
  anticancer 193
  anticholinesterase 396
  antiepileptic 369, 371f
  antifungal 378
  antiglaucoma 109
  anti-inflammatory 384
  antimitotic 109
  anti-nausea 364
  anti-seizure 365
  antitubercular 193
  antiviral 378
  atorvastatin 333
  body cells killing 491
  chronotropic 657
  classes of cytotoxic 483
  classification 409
    of emergency 656
  concentration 108
  critical care 656
  cycloplegic 169
  cytotoxic 483, 491
  dromotropic 657
  emergency 658t
  group of 397
  immunomodulatory 480t
  immunosuppressive 109
  inotropic 656
  preparation 485
  rosuvastatin 333
  sedative 528
  side effects of 399
  topical cycloplegic 169
  vasoconstrictor 109
Dry eye disease 149
Dua's layer 89, 130
Duane's retraction syndrome 200, 217, 218f
Duane's syndrome 216
Duchenne muscular dystrophy 387, 400
Dysarthria 423
Dysautonomia 389
Dyskinesia 423
Dyslipidemia 154
Dyspepsia 479
Dyspeptic symptoms 573
Dysphagia 16, 399, 479, 480
Dysplasia 463, 464
Dyspnea 509, 511, 661
Dystonia 405, 410, 410t
  severity action plan 410, 410t
Dystonic storm 410

E

Ear 3, 10, 80
  age-related changes in 586f
  behind 80
  deformity 456
  disorders of 19
  drops 20
  examination of 10

external 3f, 4, 11
hearing aid
behind 80f, 619
receiver in 80f
inner 3f
level hearing aids 80
ossicles 4
Ear, nose and throat
anatomy and physiology of 3
diagnostic evaluation of 10
disorders of 1
Eardrum 4
Early stage symptoms 436
Earmold 79
Earthquakes 539, 540
Eating and nutrition 438
Eating disorder 470
Ectatic conditions 134
Ectodermal layer 243
Ectropion 120, 121
bilateral severe 120f
Edema 340, 450
Edinger-Westphal nucleus 90f
Edrophonium 197
chloride test 395
Efferent pupillary defect 183f
Efferent visual system 175
Elastic cartilage 4
Elderly abuse 594, 595
preventive interventions for 597f
risk factors for 595
screening for 596
types of 595
warning signs of 595
Electric jar openers 623
Electric wheelchairs 619
Electrical injury 448
Electrical stimulation 370
Electrocardiogram 451
Electrocochleography 418
Electrode 275f
array 81
Electroencephalogram 272, 274, 275f
Electrolyte 452
disturbance 287, 309
imbalance 341
maintenance of 695
Electromyography 280
Electronystagmography 272, 275
Electrophysiological tests 395
Elschnig spots 151
Elsper therapy 499
Embryonic subdivisions 245, 245t
Emergency
alert systems 625
care, medicolegal aspects of 522
department, palliative care for 508f
management 315, 542
principles of 519, 520
nurse, role of 520
nursing 517
ethics of 523
principles of 520, 520b
response 544
room management 317
services, organization of 521
Emmetropia 111
Emotional abuse 595
warning signs of 596
Emotional status 198
Emotional stress 672
Emotional support 617
Emotional well-being 566, 590

Employment, loss of 555
Encephalitis 286, 287, 376, 380
Encourage electronic tool usage 679
End of life, symptoms at 509b
Endocrine
abnormalities 426
system 576
conditions, age-related 579f, 580t
therapy 481, 482
End-of-life
care 402, 644, 657, 660
decisions 637
issues 701
Endogenous
endophthalmitis 168
infections, secondary 651
Endolymph 19, 414
Endolymphatic sac 19
decompression 418
Endophthalmitis 165, 168
Endothelial corneal dystrophy 133
Endothelial surface 166f
Endotheliitis 132
Endothelium 89
Endotracheal intubation 634
Endotracheal tube 631, 634, 640
Endovascular coiling 340f
Endovascular treatment 339
Enterobacter cloacae 649
Enterococcus faecalis 500
Entropion 120, 121
Envenomation 286, 519
Environmental aspects 439
Environmental temperature 528
Enzyme reactions, series of 482
Ependymomas 345
Ephedrine 24
Epidermis, age-related changes in 588f
Epidural hematoma 313, 315f
Epiglottitis 33, 41, 41f
Epilepsy 360, 368
pathophysiology of 369f
Epileptic seizures 370
Epinephrine 409, 657, 658
Epipodophyllotoxins 483
Epiretinal membrane 158
Episcleritis 165
Episodic cluster 365
Epistaxis 14, 47, 53
artery of 48
cause of posterior 48
types of 47
Epithalamus 247
Epithelial defect 130, 131, 131f
Epithelial dystrophy 133
Epithelium 89
Epstein-Barr virus 388, 416, 439
Equilibrium, anatomy and physiology of 5
Equipment 257, 278, 522
Erectile dysfunction 581, 582
Ergot derivatives 432
Errors theory 561
Erythema chronicum migrans 534
Erythrocyte sedimentation rate 193
Erythromycin 147
Eschar 447
Escherichia coli 131, 454
Esophageal perforation 716
Esotropia 200, 205f, 211
acute concomitant 213
concomitant 212
infantile 212, 212f

non-accommodative 212
nonrefractive
hyperaccommodative 212
hypoaccommodative 212
types of 211
Esotropic Duane retraction syndrome 219
Estrogen
levels, lower 482
receptor 482
block 482
Etanercept 578
Ethambutol 193
Ethanol 286
Ethical care, principles of 632
Ethmoid, posterior 15
Ethmoidal polyps 55
Ethylene oxide 105
Eustachian tube opening 12
Euthanasia 594, 600, 662
legalization of passive 600
procedure for passive 600f
Evisceration 126, 128, 164, 169
Excedrin migraine 364
Excessive stress, treatment of 702
Excimer 109
Exercise 340
tolerance 567
Exogenous endophthalmitis 168
Exogenous infections 651
Exostoses 21
Exotropia 200, 205f, 213
congenital 213
right 198f
types of 213
Exotropic Duane retraction syndrome 218
External auditory canal, examination of 11
External beam
radiation 478
radiotherapy 476
Extranodal extension 57t
Extraocular movements 201, 127f
Extraocular muscles 88, 88f, 88t, 201, 201f, 202t
Eye 226
affected 215
age-related changes in 586f
anatomy and physiology of 87
artificial 230f
astigmatism 111, 112f
blood 109
conditions, increased risk of 582
contralateral 183
deformity 456f
diagnostic evaluation of 93
dilation 99
disease study, age-related 158t
disorder of 85, 361
donation 228-230
down and out 177
emmetropic 112f
examination 93-96
grades of 229f
hypermetropic 112f
ipsilateral 183
myopic 112f
response 260
strain 364
structure of 87f
tracking devices 626
Eye bank 228, 229f, 230f
basic infrastructure of 229
functions of 228
staff 229
system 229, 229f

Eye care 417
    cadre distribution 236*t*
    comprehensive primary 234, 236*f*
    delivering comprehensive 237
    human resources 236
    primary 234
Eye movements 188
    physiology of 200
    types of 175
Eyeball 87
    abnormal size of 112
    coats of 89
    fluids in 91
    interior of 91
Eyelash, malposition of 121
Eyelid 88, 88*f*, 97
    benign lesion of 121, 123
    disorders of 120, 121*b*
    inflammatory disease of 121, 122
    malignancies 120
    malignant lesion of 121, 123, 123*t*
    malposition of 120, 121
    margin 88*f*
    speculum 106*f*

F

Facial expression 259
Facial muscles 417
Facial nerve 262, 414, 416
Facial pain 53
Facial structural anomalies 61
Falx cerebelli 249
Falx cerebri 249
Family eye history 95
Fanconi syndrome triad 716
Fasciculus 177
    medial longitudinal 176
Fasciotomy 447
Fatigue 382, 397, 470, 479, 511
Fatty liver disease, nonalcoholic 574
Febrile transfusion reactions 499
Fecal analysis 721
Felbamate 370
Fertility decline 581
Fever 382
    control 298
Fexofenadine 24
Fibrosis 479
Fibrotic tonsillitis, chronic 42
Fibrovascular proliferation 152
Filamentary keratopathy 131
Financial abuse 595
Fine finger movements 266
Finger to nose 266
First aid 48
First-tier treatment 298
Fit, first aid management of 372
Flaccid paralysis 389
Fleischer ring 134
Fletcher suit applicator 477*f*
Floor of mouth 16
Fluconazole 378, 512
Fluency disorders 61, 67, 67*f*
Fluent aphasia 259
Fluid
    balance 291
    disturbances 309
    imbalance 341
    therapy 316, 317*b*, 318
Fluorescein angiography 166, 189
Fluoroquinolone 132, 168
Fluphenazine 409

Focal brain edema 294
Focal injuries 313
    types of 313*f*
Focal neurological deficit 347
Foerster's sponge-holding forceps 106*f*
Folate 193
Follicular tonsillitis 42
Food and drug association 81
Food poisoning 526
Foraminotomy 324
Forced expiratory volume 572
Forearm fractures 579
Foreign body 20, 20*f*, 223, 226
    injuries 224
    intraocular 226
Fornix, inferior 88*f*
Foscarnet 109
Fourth nerve 177, 215
    anatomy 179*f*
Fovea 90*f*
    centralis 90
Franceschetti type 213
Free radical 561, 561*f*
    break cells down 561
    scavengers 561
    theory 561
Fresh frozen plasma 499
Frostbite 448, 528
Frostnip 528
Fuch's endothelial dystrophy 134
Functional endoscopic sinus surgery 55
Fundus
    autofluorescence 151, 164, 168
    camera 100*f*
    evaluation 188
    fluorescein angiography 93, 100, 151, 164
        procedure 167
    photograph 161*f*
        left eye 154*f*, 155*f*, 158*f*
        right eye 157*f*
Fungal meningitis 377-379
Fungal sinusitis, allergic 55
Fungal ulcer with hypopyon 132*f*
Fungus 377
Furosemide 695
Fusarium 131
Fusional amplitude 215

G

Gabapentin 370, 409
Gag reflex 43, 693
Gaits, abnormal 265*t*
Galantamine 426, 427
Gallstone ileus 716
Gamma aminobutyric acid 245, 702
Gamma knife radiosurgery 415
Gamma-glutamyl transferase 276
Gancyclovir 109
Ganglion cell 91, 170
    analysis 190*f*
Gardner-wells tongs 322, 323*f*
Gas
    bubbles 530
    exchange, improving 308
    lasers 109
Gasserian ganglion 132
Gastric acid secretion 572
Gastric dysmotility 389
Gastritis 480
Gastroesophageal reflux disease 572, 573
Gastrointestinal bleeding 495
Gastrointestinal cancer, surgery for 475

Gastrointestinal emergency 495
Gastrointestinal system 570
    age-related changes in 573*f*
Gastrointestinal tract, cancer of 573
Gaze and yoke muscles, cardinal positions of 203*f*
Gaze control 175
Gaze disorders 176
Gaze stabilization 175
General public health system 235*f*
Genetic predisposition 465
Genetic test 427
    and counselling 437
Geniculate body, lateral 90*f*
Geniculate nucleus, lateral 172*f*
Genitourinary emergencies 495
Genitourinary management 324
Gentamycin 109, 418, 419
Geographic atrophy 157*f*
Geriatric nursing 553
Geriatric syndromes 686
Gerotransdence theory 563
Giant cell arteritis 181, 198, 366
Glasgow coma scale 260*t*, 289, 313, 317
    assessment, frequency of 258*f*
Glatiramer acetate 441
Glaucoma 91, 105, 136, 140, 142*t*, 231, 587
    childhood 136
    classification of 140, 141*fc*
    closed angle 136
    hemifield test 140*f*
    laser
        iridotomy in 110
        procedures in 141
    open angle 136
    primary angle closure 136
    risk factors of 138
    secondary 136, 166
    terminology of 140
    treatment of 140
Gliomas 345
Glomerular filtration rate 575
Glomerulonephritis 43
Glossopharyngeal nerve 414
Glossopharyngeal neuralgia 419
Glottic anomalies 63
Glottic tumor 56
Glottic web 50
Glucocorticoids 298
Glucose management 318
Glutamate 245, 368
Gluten-free 696
Glycerol dehydration test 418
Glycine 245
Golimumab 578
Gonioscopy 136
Gonorrheal conjunctivitis 146
Gordon's sign 265
GPS
    trackers 617
    tracking devices 625
Grab bars 624
Grady coma scale 289
Grafts
    care of 455
    types of 455
Graft-*vs*-host disease 488, 489
Gram-negative
    bacilli 181
    organisms 454
Gram-positive cocci 500
Granulomatous polyangiitis 165*f*
Graphesthesia 269

Grave's disease 580, 716
Grey turner's sign 715
Growth hormone deficiency 577
Guedel airway 640
Guillain-Barré syndrome 278, 387, 388f
Gums and teeth 16
Gynecologic cancer, surgery for 474
Gynecological cancers 477, 582

H

H1 and H3 antagonists 418
Habenular nuclei 247
Haemophilus influenzae 23-25, 76, 377, 388
Hakims triad 716
Halitosis 512
Haller cells 15
Hallucinations 428
Halo device 322, 323f
Haloperidol 286, 409, 430, 661
Hamper communication abilities 62
Hand
    held magnifier 232f
    hygiene 484, 631, 652, 681f
    magnifiers 232
Handwashing
    five moments of 652f
    soap-water 652t
    steps of 652f, 682f
    technique, good 476
Hard palate 16
Harms trabeculotome 105
Hazard 538, 667
    chemical 668
    environmental 538
    geological 538
    geophysical 538
    mechanical 669
    occupational 667, 671fc
    prevention of 672
    psychosocial 669
Head
    of bed, elevation of 298
    posture 205, 206
    trauma 424
Head and neck 479, 484
    cancer, surgery for 474
Head injury
    open 312
    types of 311
Head tilt
    chin lift maneuver 639
    right 215f
Headache 53, 341, 349, 360, 364, 370, 379
    acute single 362
    chronic daily 364
    classification of 361
    cluster 365
    disorder, active 361
    epidemiology 360
    medication overuse 366
    nursing management of 366
    phase 361
    potential precipitating factors of 361
    primary 361
    secondary 360, 361, 366
    subacute 363
    tension 364, 365
Head-impulse test, positive 418
Head-pointing systems 626
Head-to-toe examination 646
Health
    assessment 591
    emergencies 540

financing 237
history 468
insurance 604, 607
management information system 236
system framework 235
Health care
    basic principle of 677
    management 617
    power of attorney for 599
    practices, domains of 678b
    primary 234
    products 679
    professionals 377, 701, 704
Healthcare-associated infection 631, 634, 680
Healthy diet 590
Healthy lifestyle 583
Hearing
    amplifiers 625
    anatomy and physiology of 4
    assessment for 76
    devices, implantable 81
    impairment 72
    problems 428
    process of 4
Hearing aid 26, 79, 80, 619, 620
    bone-anchored 82, 82f
    digital 80
    in-the-ear 619
    selection and fitting 81
    smart 625
    types of 79, 80f
Hearing loss 10, 26, 28, 72, 418, 587
    age-related 582
    bilateral
        conductive 73f
        mixed 75f
        sensorineural 74f
    causes of 75
    classification of 72
    conductive 71, 73, 75
    configuration of 75
    congenital causes of
        conductive 75
        sensorineural 76
    degree of 73, 74, 74f
    epidemiology of 72
    mixed 73, 76
    noise-induced 667
    prevention of 78
    sensorineural 73, 76
    types of 72
Heart
    failure 568
    rate 258
        and rhythm, changes in 567
        rhythm shockable 641
    size 567
Heartbeat, irregular 333
Heat exhaustion 528
Heat stroke 528
Heavy metals 193
Heel to toe walk 267
Heel walk 267
Helicobacter pylori 572
Hematemesis 484
Hematologic emergencies 498
Hematoma 311
    intracerebral 313
    intracranial 315f
Hematopoietic stem cell transplantation
    complications of 488
    types of 485
Hemiparesis 256
Hemispherectomy 305

Hemispherotomy 370
Hemodynamic monitoring 635, 647, 647t
    equipment 642
Hemorrhage 157f, 177
    cerebellar 286
    intracranial 278
    intraocular 110
    intraventricular 313
    pontine 286
    primary 43
    reactionary 43
    secondary 43
    splinter 192f
    subarachnoid 276, 278, 313, 336, 338f
    subconjunctival 145
Hemorrhagic stroke, types of 328
Hemostatic emergencies 499
Hepatic encephalopathy 287, 574
Hepatobiliary disease 574
Heredity 116
Hering's law 202
Herniation, sites of 296f
Herpes simplex
    encephalitis 381
    virus 416
Herpes zoster 181
    ophthalmicus 132
Herpetic keratoconjunctivitis 147
Heterochromia 184
Heterophoria 200
    control of 208
    detect 208
    method 212
Heterotropia 208
Hiatal hernia 573
Hip fracture 578, 579
Hippocampus 423
Hirschberg's test 205, 206, 207f, 208f
Histamine 245
Histopathology tests 467
Histoplasma capsulatum 379
Hoarse voice 479
Holistic approach 699
Holistic care 505, 592
Holistic nursing, principles of 632
Homans' sign 715
Homatropine 168, 169
Home care 324, 611, 612
    setting 680
        elderly-friendly 613
Home remedies 438
Homeostasis 701
    disorder of 361
Homocysteinemia 154
Homonymous hemianopia, right 173, 174f
Homonymous quadrantanopia, left upper 173
Hopkin's endoscopic picture 56f
Hormonal agents 465
Hormonal changes 581
Hormone
    production 576
    therapy 481, 482
Horner's pupil 184
Horner's syndrome 184
    triad 716
Hospice care 503, 509, 657
Hospital cardiac arrest, out of 638
Host disease 488
Hot air oven 105
House fire 527
Hughes-Roper-Hall classification 223t
Human bites 532
    management of 533
Human herpes virus-6 439

Human papillomavirus 464
  vaccine 470
Humidified air 51
Humphrey single field 140f
Humphrey visual field analyzer 98f
Huntingtin gene 406f
Huntington's disease 408, 435
  nursing care plan for 408t
  pathophysiology of 436
  staging of 407t
Hydrated nucleus pulposus extrusion 279
Hydration 66, 401, 591, 661
Hydrocephalus 189, 285, 340
Hydrochloride 658
Hydrochlorothiazide 418, 419
Hydrogen peroxide 105
Hydrometeorological factors 538
Hydroxychloroquine 193
Hydroxyethylcellulose 109
Hymenopteran stings 532
Hyoid bone 51
Hyperactive delirium 429
Hyperacusis, presence of 416
Hyperbaric oxygen therapy 527
Hypercarbia 570
Hyperemia 190f
Hyperemic zone 449
Hyperglycemia
  management of 290
  relieve symptoms of 580
Hyperkinetic movement disorders 406fc
Hyperleukocytosis syndrome 498
Hypermature senile cataract 118
Hypermetropia 111
Hyperplasia 40, 463, 464
Hyperplastic laryngitis, chronic 40
Hypertension 154, 329, 568, 592
  portal 574
  systemic 153
Hypertensive retinopathy 151, 153
Hyperthermia management 379
Hyperthyroidism 580
Hypertonic saline 316, 317
Hypertrophic laryngitis, chronic 40
Hypertrophic pharyngitis, chronic 38
Hypertrophic rhinitis 35
Hypertrophic scarring 456f
Hypertropia 200, 215
Hyperventilation 299, 318
Hyperviscosity syndrome 498
Hypoglossal nerve 264
Hypoglycemia, management of 290
Hyponatremia 341
Hypoproteinemia 454
Hypotension 450
Hypothalamic nuclei 248
Hypothalamospinal tract 252
Hypothalamus 247
  functions of 247
  nuclei of 248t
  pituitary-adrenal axis 701
Hypothermia 450, 529, 529t, 694
Hypothetical care plan 393t
Hypothyroidism 580
Hypotropia 200
Hypoxic ischemic injury 313
Hysterectomy 474

I

Ibuprofen 384
Idiopathic headache, diagnosis of 364
Idiopathic intracranial hypertension 195
Idiopathic macular hole 158
Ifosfamide 409
Imipramine 409
Imminently dying, care of 507
Immobilization 322
Immune disorders 426
Immune system 588, 701
  age-related changes in 589f
  dysregulation 590
  failure 465
  vital components of 562
Immunity 555
  theory 562
Immunization programs 78
Immunologically mediated diseases 133
Immunomodulating therapies, long-term 396
Immunosuppression 454
Immunosuppressive agent 109
Immunotherapy
  adverse effects of 481f
  side effects of 481
Impedance audiometry test 13, 77, 77f
Implantable devices 79
Impulse generation, artificial 566
Income tax rebate 604, 607
Incongruous hemianopia 174f
Incus 4
Indira Gandhi National Old Age Pension Scheme 604, 606
Indocyanine green angiography 164, 168
Indomethacin 109
Industrial accidents 527, 541
Industrial disorder 665, 667
Infection 50, 309, 341, 426, 476, 488, 585, 653
  control policy 636
  control protocols 651
  deep neck space 51
  hospital-acquired 644, 653t
  increased risk of 590
  increased susceptibility to 590
  induced cancers, case of 464
  prevention of 454, 484, 672, 678
  signs of 450
  symptoms of 450
  systemic 450
Infectious agents 439
Infectious causes 181
Infectious orbital inflammatory disease 126, 127t
Inflammatory airway obstruction, progressive 572
Inflammatory bowel disease 572
Inflammatory conditions 50
Inflammatory demyelinating polyneuropathy 388, 391
Infliximab 578
Influenza A virus 388
Infusion pumps 635, 642
Ingested poisoning 526
Inhaled anticholinergic bronchodilators 572
Inhaled poisoning 526
Inhibit calcium channels 370
Inhibitory neurotransmitter, activity of 702
Injection
  practices, unsafe 683
  safety 678
  tenecteplase 334
  use of 680
Injury
  acceleration 312
  depth of 448
  mechanism of 448
  mild 315
  prevention of 653
  primary 312
  secondary 312
  severe 316
Innate immunity, changes in 590
Inner ear
  disorders of 26
  internal 4
Inorganic dusts 668
Insomnia 701, 703
  management of 703
Institutional care 614
Instrument 104, 219
  classification of 104
  faster drying of 104
  sterilization, cycle of 104
Insulin sensitivity 577
Integumentary system 324, 484, 587
Intense inflammatory reaction 226
Intensity 71
  pain scale, self-reporting 510
Intensive care records 644
Intensive care unit 644, 701
  assessment, ABCDE approach of 645t
  infections, classification of 651
Interferon 441, 465
Intermittent exotropia 213, 213f
Internuclear ophthalmoplegia 176, 176f
Internuncial fibers 90f
Interstitial implant 477f
Intervertebral disc 251
Intra-arterial thrombolysis 334
Intracranial hypertension 296, 297
Intracranial pressure 278, 294t, 295, 295f, 312
  elevation 294
  increased 294, 340, 341, 492
  manifestation of 297b
  monitoring 297
    indications for 297t
  pathophysiology of increased 296f
  values, normal 294t
Intracranial surgery 302, 306
  types of 302
Intracranial tumors 344
  distribution of 345f
  grading of 345t
Intramedullary intervertebral disc extrusion 279
Intraocular injections 108
Intraocular lens
  implantation 112
  replacement surgery 112
Intraocular pressure 93, 96, 136, 138, 151, 164
Intra-orbital part 178, 179
Intraparenchymal hematoma, frontal 338f
Intraparenchymal hemorrhage, right 315f
Intraretinal microvascular abnormalities 152
Intrathecal baclofen 441
Intravenous fluids 316
Intravenous immunoglobulin
  G therapy 391
  therapy 396
Intravenous thrombolytic therapy 334b
Intraventricular pressure, monitor 300
Intravitreal antibiotics 168
Intravitreal injection, site of 91
Invasive neurodiagnostic tests 276
Invasive neurological procedures 273
Ionizing radiation 448, 668
Ipratropium 572
Ipsilateral anopia 172
Iridodialysis 222, 224, 224f
Iris 89, 105, 224, 226
  forceps 105
  tear of 224
Irwin Moore sign 42

Ischemia 312
Ischemic heart disease 568
Ischemic injury 340
Ischemic optic neuropathy, posterior 192
Ischemic stroke treatment, acute 333, 333f
Ishihara chart 99f
Ishihara plates 186, 186f
Isoniazid 193
Isotonic glucose 317
Isotonic saline 317
Itchy skin 589
Itraconazole 378

J

Jaeger's chart 185f
Jameson's muscle hook 106f
Japanese encephalitis 380
Jarjaway fracture 54
Jaw claudication 193
Joint
    pain 534
    positioning, sensation of 269
Junctional scotomas 172, 174f
Juvenile Huntington's disease symptoms 436

K

Kapalbhati 708
Kelly Descemet membrane punch 105
Kendrick extrication device 522, 522f
Keratic precipitates, large 166f
Keratitis 130
    acanthamoeba 133, 133f
    bacterial 131, 132
    disciform 132f
    epithelial 132
    fungal 131, 132
    herpetic 132
    infectious 131
    marginal 133
    neurotrophic 134
    phlyctenular 133
    punctate 145
    stromal 132
    treatment of infectious 132
    viral 132
Keratoconjunctivitis
    atopic 148
    epidemic 146
    sicca 149
    vernal 147, 148f
Keratoconus 134
Keratoglobus 134
Keratomileusis 112
Keratopathy
    band-shaped 134, 164, 166
    exposure 134
Keratoplasty 130, 132, 135, 135f
Kernig's sign 378f, 715
Ketoconazole 512
Kidney 585
    failure 695
Killian's incision 53
Kinetic tremors 409
Klebsiella 454
    pneumoniae 649
    species 500
Knapp procedure 217
Knee 252
    braces 621
    reflex 268

Krimsky test 209, 209f
Kwashiorkor, triad of 716

L

Labyrinth 4
    dense bone of 14
Labyrinthectomy 418
Labyrinthitis 28
Lacrimal drainage system, disorders of 121, 123
Lacrimal gland 88
    tumor 128, 128f
Lacrimal punctum, displaced 120f
Lacrimal sac
    acute inflammation of 124
    chronic inflammation of 124
    external landmark for 88f
Lacrimal system 123
    disorders of 120, 121b
Lactated ringer's solution 452
Lactobacillus acidophilus 452
Lactulose 696
Ladder method 510
Lamellar separation 118
Laminectomy 312, 323, 356
Lamotrigine 370, 437
Language 61
    problems 583
Lantern test 186
Large-scale awareness 696
Laryngeal cartilages 7f
Laryngeal cavity 8
Laryngeal cleft 64
Laryngeal diphtheria 51
Laryngeal edema 167
Laryngeal mask airways 640
Laryngeal nerve injury, bilateral recurrent 50
Laryngeal obstruction 49, 51
    causes of 49b
Laryngeal webs 63
Laryngitis 33, 40
Laryngomalacia 49
Laryngopharynx 6
Laryngoscopy, indirect 16, 16f
Laryngospasm 49
Laryngotracheobronchitis, acute 50
Larynx 6, 7f
Laser 108
    complications of 110
    interstitial thermal treatment 370
    tissue interactions 109
    treatment 156t
    types of 109
Laser-assisted in situ keratomileusis 112, 135
Lashes, malposition of 120
Lasmiditan 364
Lattice degeneration 162
LE SO palsy 216f
Lead 193
Leber's hereditary optic neuropathy 194
Left eye 123f, 140f, 161f, 178f, 184f
    esotropia 207f
    hypertropia of 216f
    miotic pupil in 184f
    ptosis, severe 178f
    suppression 205f
Lemniscus pathway, medial 251
Lenalidomide 480
Lennox-Gastaut syndrome 370
Lens 91, 105, 224, 226
    crystalline 89
    fogging 215
    injury, management of 226

    localized opacification of 110
    perforation of 115
    subluxation of 225f
    transparency, loss of 115
Leptomeningeal disease 493
Leriche syndrome 716
Lesion, site of 173f
Lethal triad 716
Leukemia 128
Leukotriene receptor antagonists 37
Levator palpebrae superioris 177
Levetiracetam 370, 437
Levocetirizine 24
Levodopa 432
Levothyroxine 409
Lewy body 423
    dementia 427
Lhermitte's sign 423
Lid
    inferior 184f
    retraction 121, 122
        bilateral 177
Life assistance services 612
Life limiting disease 503
Life satisfaction 591
Lifestyle 438
    changes 340, 584
    modifications 568, 574, 585
    patterns 468
Life-threatening complications 167
Ligaments 7f
Light reflex 177, 182
    indirect 183f
    pathway 90f, 182f, 283f
Light sedation 648
Lighthouse effect 26
Light-near dissociation 185, 187
Lim's forceps 105, 106f
Limb muscles 395
Limbic system 250, 251
Limbus 89, 91
Linac machine 477f
Line diagram depicting refraction 112f
Lipid
    dysfunction 123f
    solubility 108
Lips 16
Liquids, gastric emptying of 572
Lithium 409
Live donor 691
Liver
    disease 574, 585
        end-stage 574
    failure 574
    function 276, 646
        tests 289
    segment of 691
    transplantation 574
Living arrangement 595
Living will 594, 599, 661
Lobectomy 370, 474
Lobotomy 305
Loop diuretics 695
Lotepredonol 109
Louder voices 8
Low mood 399
Low vision
    aids 231, 232, 620
    distance systems 231
    near systems 231
    telescope 231f
Lower eyelid chalazion 122f

Lower lid 124f
    malignant tumor 123f
Lower motor neuron 252
    lesions 252t
Lubricating agent 109
Luc's abscess 26
Lumbar puncture 191, 272, 276, 297, 348, 382, 440
    contraindications of 277
    indications for 277
    set 279
Lumbar sacral injuries 321
Lumbosacral plexus 254
Lumen, contents of 11
Lumpectomy 473
Lumps 470
Lumpy bumpy appearance 197f
Lund-Browder
    diagram 449f
    method 449
Lung
    cancer 467, 572
    diseases, chronic obstructive 667
    fibrosis 480
Lutein 157
Lyme disease 519, 534
Lymphatic mechanism 466
Lymphoma 124, 128
Lymphoproliferative disorders 128

M

Mackler's triad 716
Macular corneal dystrophy 134f
Macular degeneration, age-related 151, 152, 157, 231, 587
Macular disorders 152, 157
Macular dystrophy 152, 161
Macular edema, clinically significant 153f
Macular hole 158
Maddox rod 200, 206, 209, 210f
    test 210f
Maddox tangent scale 206, 209, 211f
Magnifying glasses 231
Maintenance and Welfare of Parents and Senior Citizen Act 604, 605
Malignant cells, characteristics of 465, 465t
Malignant neoplasm, surgical management of 473
Malleus 4
Malocclusions 61
Mammogram 463
Mandibular branch 262
Manifest nystagmus, face turn in 207f
Mannitol 316, 317
Manual laryngeal musculoskeletal tension reduction technique 67
Maslow's hierarchy of needs 564f
Mass casualty management 544
Mass lesions, resection of 299
Massive hemoptysis 495
Mast cell stabilizers 37
Mastectomy 473
    simple 474
    types of 474
Mastoid air cells 14
Mastoiditis 25
    pathology 25
Maxillary sinus 15
Maximal tremor amplitude 409
McBurney's point 715
McDonald criteria 440

McGill questionnaire 510
Measles 439
    three C's of 715
Mechanical injuries 223
    classification of 223fc
Mechanical thrombectomy 334, 584
Mechanical ventilators 634, 642
Meclizine 418, 419
Medical alert systems 617
Medical care 615
Medication
    administration of 529
    management devices 625
Medication errors
    causes of 679
    classification of 679
    primary care-related 680
Medicine, alternative 700, 702
Medroxyprogesterone 409
Medulla oblongata 248
Medulloblastoma 345
Meibomian glands, opening of 88f
Melanocytic nevus 121, 123
Melatonin production 577
Memantine 428
Membranous labyrinth 5f
Membranous tonsillitis, acute 42
Memory 259
    disorders 560
    immediate 259
    impaired 257
    loss 583
Meniere's disease 28, 417, 418, 585, 716
Meniere's syndrome 28
Meningeal infection 276
Meningeal irritation 340
    signs of 378f
Meninges 249, 376
Meningioma 345
Meningitis 286, 287, 376, 377b
    bacterial 378
    hospital-acquired 377
    pathophysiology of 377fc
    triad 716
Meningococcal meningitis 379
Meningoencephalitis 379
Menopause 577, 581
Mental health 428, 590
    disorders 702
    resources 701
Mental status, altered 382
Mental stimulation, lack of 424
Mentally stimulating activities 615
Mercury 193
Mesenchymal tumors 128
Metabolic emergencies 495
Metabolic problems 426
Metaplasia 463, 464
Metastasis 128, 463, 465
Metastatic pathways 465
Metastatic spinal tumors 356
Metastatic tumor 128, 345
Methicillin-resistant *Staphylococcus aureus* 651
Methotrexate 109, 193
Methylprednisolone 193
Metoclopramide 409, 418
Metoprolol tartrate 365
Microbial organisms 454
Microphone 79
Microtropia 212, 213
Microvascular decompression 415
Midazolam 316
Midbrain 248

Middle ear 3f, 4
    disorders of 22
    examination of 12
    implant 82
    mucosa 12
    routes of infection of 23
Midfacial hypoplasia, left sided 215f
Migraine 360-362, 363f, 364
    classification of 362
    diagnostic criteria 362
    phase of 361, 361f
    triggers of 361
Migratory thrombophlebitis 499
Miller-Fischer syndrome 389
Mind-body
    practices 700
    yoga techniques, inclusion of 704
Mindfulness 699, 701
    practice 705
Mindfulness-based interventions, effectiveness of 703
Minimally invasive endonasal endoscopic surgery 306
Minimally invasive neuroendoscopy 306
Mini-stroke, significance of 328
Miosis 184
Mirror prism glasses 198
Misconceptions 690
Mitigation 538, 542
    activities 542
Mobilization 473, 485, 487
Modiolus 4f
Monoamine oxidized inhibitors 432
Monoclonal antibodies 480
    types of 480f
Monocular elevation deficiency 217
Monofixation syndrome 205
Mono-ocular blindness 172
Monosodium glutamate 364
Monozygotic twins 690
Monro-Kellie concept 295
Montelukast 37
Mood 259
    disorders 584
Mooren ulcer 133
Moraxella catarrhalis 23, 24
Morgagnian hypermature cataract 118
Morphine 510
Mosquito forceps 103
Motion sickness 27
Motivation 68
Motor cortex 409
Motor deficits 340
Motor dysfunction 440
Motor nerve conduction 390f
Motor neuron disorder 280
Motor neuronopathy 280
Motor symptoms 584
Motor system functions 264
Mouth
    breathing 39, 512
    care 291
    method 510
Movement disorder 405, 411, 412
    emergency in 411
    treatments for 437
Moxifloxacin 168
Mucositis 479, 489
Multi-hazard early warning systems 538
Multiorgan
    failure 450
    infection 534

Multiple dot contusions 313
Multiple sclerosis
   pathophysiology of 439*f*
   symptoms of 440*t*
Murine 480
Murphy's sign 715
Muscle
   actions, laws of 202
   clonus 252
   disorders of 280, 387
   hook 105, 219*f*
   spasm 510
   strength 264
      assessment of 265*t*
      procedure 219
   structure 567
   tone 252
   wasting 252
Muscle-specific tyrosine kinase, antibody against 394
Muscular dystrophy 280, 387, 400, 400*t*
Muscular mass, minor tension of 265
Musculoskeletal disorders 115, 667, 669
Musculoskeletal health 576
Musculoskeletal injuries 667
Musculoskeletal management 324
Musculoskeletal system 576
   age-related changes in 577*f*
   conditions, age-related 578
Myasthenia
   crisis 387, 397
   generalized 394
   gravis 197, 216, 217, 387, 393, 395*f*, 395*fc*, 395*t*, 397*t*, 398*t*
   types of 394
   seronegative 394
Mycobacterium tuberculosis 148, 571
Mycoplasma pneumoniae 388
Mycostatin lozenges 512
Mydriatics 109
Myelography 279
Myocardial function 450
Myocardial muscle cells 566
Myoclonic seizures 368
Myoclonus 368, 411
Myopia 96, 111
   high 216
Myopic shift 115
Myringoplasty 23
Myringotomy 24

N

Nadishudhi 708
Nagel's anomaloscope 186
Nail 588
   artificial 652
   changes 589
   polish 652
Naphazoline 109, 147
Narcotics 286
Nasal bleeding 14
Nasal blockage 46
Nasal bone 15
   fracture of 54*ff*
Nasal cavity 5
   medial wall of 6*f*
Nasal disc margin, blurring of 190*f*
Nasal discharge 14
Nasal floor 14
Nasal obstruction 14
Nasal packing 47, 49, 49*f*, 54
Nasal patency, tests for 53
Nasal polyps 54

Nasal septum 5
   cartilage forming 6*f*
   deviated 52, 53*f*
Nasal trauma 53
Nasopharyngeal airways 640
Nasopharynx 6
   X-ray 44
Natalizumab 441
Natamycin 109
   topical 132
National Cancer Control Programme 504
National Council for Older Persons 604, 606
National Disaster Management Authority 546
National Disaster Response Force 546
National Elderly Policy 558
National Health Mission 235
National List of Essential Medicines 237
National Organ Transplant Programme 691
National Pension Scheme 604, 608
National Policy for Older Persons 604
National Program for Control of Blindness and Visual Impairment 235
National Program for Health Care of Elderly 604, 606
National Tuberculosis Elimination Programme 571
Naukasana 708
Nausea 483, 510, 512
Near drowning 529
Near sightedness 96
Nebulizers 522
Neck
   disorder of 361
   dissection 474
   injuries 320
Necrotizing scleritis 165
Needle stick injury 671
   case of 653
Neisseria 147
   gonorrhoeae 131, 147
   meningitis 377
Neoadjuvant chemotherapy 473
Neoplasia 463, 465
Neoplasms 49, 51
Neostigmine reduce breakdown 197
Neovascular membrane, greenish yellow 157*f*
Nephrotoxic drugs, use of 695
Nerve
   accessory 264
   conduction velocity 280
   damage, peripheral 280
   disorders of 280, 387
   fibers 265
   infiltration 510
   palsy, signs of 177-179
   roots 253
   variant 260
Nervous system 243
   age-related changes in 583*f*
   anatomy and physiology of 243
   cells of 243
   disorders of 241
   functional unit of 243
   health of 193
   subdivisions of 243*fc*
Neural tumors 128
Neuritic plaques 423
Neuroanatomy 177
Neurocysticercosis 376, 383
   pathophysiology of 384*fc*
Neurodegenerative diseases 423
Neuroectoderm 243
Neuroendocrine theory 562
Neurofibrillary tangles 423

Neuroglial cells 243
Neuroimaging, indications for 179
Neuroleptic malignant syndrome 286
Neurologic deficits, severe onset of 341
Neurologic dysfunction 315
Neurologic emergencies 491
Neurologic evaluation, comprehensive 440
Neurological assessment, components of 258*f*
Neurological category 320
Neurological classification 320
Neurological conditions, age-related 583*t*
Neurological diagnostic tests 273*t*
Neurological disorders 256, 258*t*, 276, 360
   diagnostic evaluation in 272
   group of 405
   spectrum of 405
Neurological examination 256
Neurological infections 376
   geriatric considerations for 385
Neurological problems 470
   chronic 360
Neurological status, monitor 300
Neurological system 581
   neoplasms of 344
Neurological test 427
Neuromuscular blockade 299
Neuromuscular blocking agents 300
Neuromuscular diseases, geriatric considerations for 402
Neuromuscular disorders 61
Neuromuscular junction 394*f*
   disorders 201
   normal 394*f*
Neuron 243
   damage 393
   first order 184
   geniculocalcarine 170
   parts of 244*fc*
   second order 184
   structure of 244*f*
   third order 184
   typical 243
Neuro-ophthalmic field defects 189
Neuro-ophthalmology 170
   diagnostic evaluation for 185
Neuropathy 280
   demyelinating 280
   peripheral 585
Neuropsychiatric disorders 280
Neuropsychological testing 437
Neuroretinitis 190, 190*f*
Neuroscience critical care unit 341
Neurosyphilis 191
Neurotransmitter 244, 245
   deficit 424
Neutropenia 483
Neutropenic enterocolitis 495
Neutropenic fever 500
Neutrophil count 483
   absolute 500
Night sweat 470
Nitric oxide 245
Nitrosoureas 483
N-methyl D-aspartate receptor antagonist 426
Nodes of Ranvier 244
Nodular episcleritis 165
Nodular scleritis 165*f*
Noise 668
Non-acceleration injuries 312
Non-auditory effects 668
Noncontact tonometer 97*f*, 139*f*
Noninvasive neurological procedures 272
Non-opioids 511
Non-optical devices 232

Non-ostial obstruction 38
Non-polio enteroviruses 377
Nonsteroidal anti-inflammatory drugs 109, 356
Nonsteroidal immunosuppressive agents 396
Non-toothed Bonaccolto's forceps 106f
Nonulcer dyspepsia 573
Nonvascular intracranial disorder 361
Norepinephrine 409, 657, 658
Nose 5, 14, 15
    bleeding from 47
    disorder of 361
    examination of 14
    external 5, 14f
    parts of 14
Nosocomial infection, risk of 649
Nostrils 5
Nuchal rigidity 376, 377
Nuclear
    accidents 541
    complex 177
    sclerosis 117f
Nucleus 177, 178
Numbness 257
Numeric pain scale 510
Nurse
    role of 471, 543, 544, 614, 692
    strikes 265
Nurse Led Disaster Management Program 545
Nursing responsibilities 52
Nutrition 318, 401, 476, 591, 661
    imbalanced 417
Nutritional care 512
Nutritional deficiencies 426
Nutritional management 317
Nutritional risk screening 649t
Nutritional status 350, 649
Nystagmus 188, 256, 370
    acquired 189
    congenital 188
    downbeat 189
    end-point 188
    infantile 188
    latent 189
    optokinetic 188
    periodic alternating 189
    physiological 188
    upbeat 189
    vestibular 188
Nystatin 512

O

Obesity 439
Obstructive sleep apnea 43, 58
Occipital cortex 90f
Occupational cancer 667
Occupational diseases 667, 668
Occupational disorder 665, 667, 670t
    classification of 669
Occupational health 667
    disorders 670
        risk factors of 670
    management 671
Occupational injuries 667
Occupational therapy 435, 438, 442
Ocrelizumab 441
Ocular deviation 214
Ocular drugs, modes of administration of 109f
Ocular examination 95, 117
Ocular injuries 222, 227
Ocular malignancies 201
Ocular movements 188, 209
Ocular muscles 395
Ocular myasthenia 394
Ocular myopathies 197
Ocular pain, severe 169
Ocular pharmacology 108
Ocular prosthesis 228, 230
    insertion of 129
    removal of 129
Ocular prosthetic devices 232
Oculocephalic reflex 693
Oculomotor evaluation 188
Oculomotor nerve 89, 90f, 217, 261
    palsy 214
Oculosympathetic palsy 184
Odisha cyclone 539
Ofatumumab 441
Olanzapine 437, 661
Old-age homes, establishment of 605
Olfactory nerve 260
Oligodendrogliomas 345
Olivary nucleus, inferior 409
Olopatadine 109, 147
Omentectomy 474
Omissions 62
Oncological disorders 461, 467
Oncological emergencies 491, 492f
Onodi cell 15
Open globe injury 222, 223
Open Lambert's chalazion clamp 106f
Ophthalmia neonatorum 147
Ophthalmic branch 262
Ophthalmic surgeries, routine 105, 105t
Ophthalmic surgical instruments 103
Ophthalmoplegia 491
Ophthalmoscope
    direct 97, 98f
    indirect 98, 98f
Opioid 511
    medications 364
    overdose 286, 716
    weak 511
Oppenheim's sign 265
Optic
    atrophy, bilateral 194f
    canal 180
    foramen 180
    pathway 170, 171f
    tract 90f, 171
Optic chiasma 90f
    anatomy 172f
    flattened 91
    Willebrand knee of 174f
Optic disc 90, 136, 170
    cup 140f
    drusen 197f
    edema 190f
    waxy pallor of 161f
Optic nerve 90, 170, 171, 225, 261
    anterior, lesions of 172
    head 139, 197f
    parts of 90t
    pathway 90f
    sheath diameter 297
Optic neuritis 189, 191
    atypical 191
    infective 191
    typical 191
Optic neuropathy
    anterior ischemic 192
    arteritic ischemic 193
    ischemic 192
    nonarteritic ischemic 192, 198
Optic radiation 90f, 172, 174f
    lesion of 173
Optical coherence tomography 93, 99, 100f, 151, 164, 168, 189
    angiography 151, 164, 168
Opt-in system 690
Optokinetic system 175
Opt-out system 690
Oral antifungal agents 132
Oral candidiasis 512
Oral cavity 16f
    changes in 470
    examination of 16
Orbit 128
Orbital anatomy 181f
Orbital apex syndrome 181
Orbital cellulitis 126
Orbital disorders 126
Orbital fissure, inferior 180
Orbital floor fractures 217
Orbital implant 228, 230, 231f
    types of 231
Orbital inflammatory
    disease 126, 127t
    pseudotumor 181
Orbital myositis 216
Orbital pathology 128
Orbital tumors 126
    differential diagnosis of 128f
    types of 128t
Orbital wall blowout fracture, medial 216
Organ donation 660, 689, 692
    concept of 696
    role of nurses in 692
Organ transplantation 689
Organic dusts 668
Orofacial structures, examination of 63
Oropharyngeal airway 640
Oropharynx 6
    examination of 16
Orthopnea 491
Orthoptic therapy 214
Orthostatic hypotension 585
Orthotic devices 621
Osmotic diuretics 695
Ossicles 12
Osteoarthritis 578, 592
Osteoporosis 578
    diagnosis of 578
    prevalence of 560
Ostial obstruction 38
Otalgia 19, 20
Otitis
    externa 19, 21
        bacteriology of 21t
    media 24
Otoacoustic emissions 78
Otorrhea 10
Otosclerosis 26, 71
Otoscopic examination 12f
Ototoxicity 26
Ovarian cancer 467
Oxcarbazepine 370
Oxygen therapy 512
Oxygenation 640, 642
Oxymetazoline 24

P

Pachychoroid neovasculopathy 159
Pachychoroid pigment epitheliopathy 159
Pachychoroid spectrum 159
Pain 127, 341, 379, 476, 509, 661
    acute 393
    and suffering, fear of 471
    assessment of 509, 510t, 648t
        principles of 510
    causes of 510t
    contralateral loss of 492

control 430
level of 510
management 391, 452, 510, 591, 648
relievers 338
sensation of 269
Palliative care 463, 503, 504, 504b, 505, 512, 657
communication in 506
community-based 508
continuum of 504f
domains of 506
home-based 508
hospital-based 507
models of 507
principles of 505
processes of 506
setting of 506
structure of 506
team 505, 505f
units, acute 507
Palsy, double elevator 217
Pancreas, portion of 691
Panic disorder 703
Panitumumab 481
Panophthalmitis 165, 169
Panum's fusional area 205
Panuveitis 165, 166
Papanicolaou test 463, 470
Papillae 146f
Papilledema 195, 196f, 256
Papillitis 190, 190f
Papillomacular bundle 194f
loss 171f
Paralysis 257
divergence 216
extended 252
lead to 492
superior rectus 217
Paralytic strabismus 214t
Paranasal sinus 6, 15
examination of 15
Paraophthalmic aneurysm, large 339f
Paraplegia 312
Parapontine reticular formation 176
Parasympathetic innervation pathway 182
Parasympathetic nervous system 254, 702
Parathyroid function 577
Parenchymatous tonsillitis 42
Parenteral nutrition, total 696
Parinaud syndrome 176
Parkinson's disease 431, 584
management of 432
pathophysiology of 431f
staging of 280, 431
tremor 409, 432
Parkinson's illnesses 424
Parks-Bielchowsky three-step test 215
Paroxysmal symptoms 414
Pars plana vitrectomy 151, 164, 169
Pars plicata 90
Paschimauttanasana 707
Patch test 209
Patellar reflex 268
Patient safety, domains of 678
Pelli Robson chart 98f, 186, 186f
Pellucid marginal degeneration 134
Pelvic
fractures 579
organ prolapse 582
Penetrating injury, management of 225
Peptic ulcer 572, 573
Perceptual sign 64-66
Perceptual symptoms 65-66
Percutaneous balloon microcompression 415
Pericardial effusion 491

Perimetry 136, 139, 189
Perinatal care, improved 78
Periocular injections 108
Peritonitis 287
Peritonsillar space 44f
Periwinkle plant 483
Persistent fetal vasculature 117
Personal emergency response systems 625
Personal protective equipment 671
use of 652
Personality development
Erikson' stages of 564f
theory, stages of 564
Person-environment-fit theory 563
Pesticide poisoning 667
Petit mal seizure 368
Phacoemulsification 114, 118
procedure 118f
Pharyngeal wall, posterior 16
Pharyngitis 33, 38, 39
Pharynx 6
sagittal section of 5f
Phenothiazines 286, 430
Pheochromocytoma 716
Phlebostatic axis 648f
Phlyctenular conjunctivitis 148f
Phlyctenular keratoconjunctivitis 148
Photoablation 108
Photodisruption 108
Photoreceptor dystrophy, diffuse 152, 160
Phthisis bulbi 166
Physical abuse 595
Physical care 592, 617
Physical fitness, level of 710
Physical hazards 668
Physical strain 673
Physical therapy 401, 434, 437, 442
Physiologic voice therapy 67
Physiotherapy 432
Pineal gland 247
Pinguecula 149
Pinna 4, 11
landmarks of 11f
Pituitary apoplexy 181
Pituitary tumors 345
Plantar reflex 265
Plantar responses 270
Plasma 105, 719
derivatives 685
exchange 442
therapy 391
Plica seminularis 88f
Pneumoencephalus tension 299
Pneumonia, ventilator-associated 632, 634, 649, 653, 680
Pneumonitis 480
Podophyllum pellatum 483
Poisoning 525
Police, role of 605
Polydipsia 450
Polyp, unilateral 64f
Polypharmacy 409
Polypoidal choroidal vasculopathy 159
Polytrauma 519, 523
Pomalidomide 480
Pork tapeworm infestation 376
Post-bone marrow transplant management 488
Post-cardiac arrest care 640, 642
Post-dural puncture headache 279
Posterior cord syndrome 312
Postnatal care, improved 78
Post-traumatic stress disorder, increased risk of 701
Postural changes, age-related 577f

Postural tremor 409
Potential brain-dead organ donors, care of 694
Pradhan Mantri Jan Arogya Yojna 237
Pradhan Mantri Vaya Vandana Yojana 604, 608
Pranayama 702, 708
Praziquantel 384
Preauricular region 11
Pre-cachexia 513
Prednisolone 109, 419
Pregabalin 370
Pre-hospital field care 545f
Prenatal care, improved 78
Presbycusis 71, 582
Presbyopia 112, 582, 587
Preseptal cellulitis 121, 122, 122f, 126
Pressure, sensation of 265
Pretectal nucleus 90f
Pre-thrombolysis nursing management 334
Primary health centers 234, 545
Prism bar cover test 209, 209f
Prochlorperazine 409, 418
Prodromal phases 361, 362
Promethazine 409, 410
Propranolol 365
Proptosis 126, 127, 127f
Prostate
changes 581
malignancy of 582
Prostate cancer 467
cell androgen production 482
hormone therapy for 482
treat 482
Prothrombin complex concentrate 316
Pruritus 589
Pseudo disc edema 197, 197f
Pseudoenophthalmos 184
Pseudoesotropia 200
Pseudoexotropia 200
Pseudomonas 25, 76, 131, 454, 651
aeruginosa 454, 500, 649
Pseudophakia 91
Pseudophakic bullous keratopathy 134
Pseudotumor cerebri 195, 364
Psoas sign 715
Psychiatric
disorders 361
problems 437
signs 437
symptoms 437
Psychoacoustic therapy 631
Psychogenic tremors 410
Psychological abuse, warning signs of 596
Psychological care 696
Psychological disorders 669
Psychological support 544
Psychological testing 437
Psychosocial intervention 426
Psychosocial support 593
Psychotherapy 437
Pterygium 149, 149f
Ptosis 120, 121, 179f, 214, 395f
bilateral 198f
mild 184, 184f
Public health system 235
Pulmonary airway, chronic obstructive 572
Pulmonary artery
catheter 647
pressure 647
Pulmonary capillary wedge pressure 647
Pulmonary catheters 647
Pulmonary disease, chronic obstructive 571, 572
Pulmonary embolism 341, 499
Pulsation 127
Pulse oximetry 635

Pulseless electrical activity 631, 640
Punctum, lower 88f
Pupil 97, 214
    examination 186
    size, assessment of 186
    tonic contraction of 184
Pupillary abnormalities 184
Pupillary defect, afferent 183f
Pupillary fibers 178f
Pupillary light reflex
    consensual 187
    direct 186
    pathway 182
    test 206
Pupillary reaction 170
    loss of direct 172
Pupillary reflex 182, 186, 693
Pupillomotor fibers 177
Pupils, assess 288
Pure tone audiometry 13, 77
    test 77f
Pursuit system 175
Pyridostigmine 197
Pyridoxine 193

Q

Quadriplegia 492
Quetiapine 661
Quinine 193

R

Radial ciliary muscle 137
Radial design nursing unit 631
Radial keratotomy 112
Radiation 478
    controlling external 478f
    errors 686
    pneumonitis 479
    safety 478
Radiation therapy 348, 356
    internal 477
    principles of 476
    types of 356
Radical hysterectomy 474
Radical neck dissection 475f
Radioablation 580
Radiofrequency thermal rhizotomy 415
Radiotherapy 476
    treatment, effects of 479t
Raised intracranial pressure 510
    management of 297
Raised jugular venous pressure 572
Rapid eye movement sleep 581
Rapid immune-modulating therapies 396
Rashtriya Swasthya Bima Yojana 604, 605, 608
Rashtriya Vayoshri Yojana 604, 608
Raynaud's diseases 528
Reactive oxygen species 561
Rectal bleeding 484
Rectus, medial 88, 177
Rectus-oblique intrigue 202, 202f
Recurrent laryngeal papillomatosis 51
Reflex 256, 265
    accommodation 182
    acoustic 71
    direct light 183f
    hammer 257
    type 268
Reflexometry test 78
Refraction 96
    abnormal index of 112

Refractive accommodative esotropia 212, 212f
Refractive errors 111, 212
    spectacle correction of 213
    types of 111
Refractive power 111
Refractive procedures 135
Refractive surgery 105, 110, 112
Refractory cachexia 513
Regular exercise 435, 590
Regular sleep patterns 364
Rehabilitation 228, 230, 232, 324, 351, 358, 442, 473, 476, 539, 584
Reinke's edema 65, 65f
Reiter's syndrome 716
Relaxation technique 708
Remote controls, easy-to-use 617
Remote memory 259
Renal cell carcinoma, triad of 716
Renal disorders 115
Renal failure, acute 454
Renal function 646
    maintenance of 695
Reoxygenation 476
Repetitive nerve stimulation test 395
Reproductive hormones 577
Reproductive steroid hormones 482
Reproductive system 579
    conditions, age-related 582t
    female 581f
    male 581f
Reservoir sign 25
Resonant voice therapy 67
Respiration, examine 288
Respiratory arrest 638
Respiratory care 434
Respiratory conditions, age-related 571t
Respiratory disorders 669
Respiratory distress 43
Respiratory disturbance index 59
Respiratory emergencies 494
Respiratory failure, acute 453
Respiratory functions, maintenance of 695
Respiratory hygiene 654
Respiratory infections 571
Respiratory management 324
Respiratory muscles 395
Respiratory rate 258
Respiratory status, monitoring 391
Respiratory system 567
    age-related changes in 570f
Respiratory therapy 322
Respiratory tract infections 388
Restless leg syndrome 360, 374
    diagnosis of 375f
Reticular activating system 250, 285
Reticular formation 250
Reticular system, descending 250
Retina 90, 91, 170, 225, 226
    disorders of 151
    vascular disorders of 152
Retinal artery occlusion 155
Retinal break 110
    large 159f
    sealing of 159
Retinal complications 166
Retinal correspondence 203, 204
Retinal degeneration 162
    types of 162
Retinal detachment 152, 159
    exudative 160
    rhegmatogenous 159, 159f
    surgery, basic principles 159
    tractional 153f, 159
Retinal dystrophy 152, 160, 161f

Retinal nerve fiber layer
    loss of 194f
    scans 190f
Retinal points 203f
Retinal vein occlusion 154
    classification of 154
Retinitis pigmentosa 152, 160, 161f
Retinoblastoma 201
Retinopathy of prematurity 155
Retinoschisis, acquired 162
Retinoscopy 112
Retrobulbar neuritis 189
Retrocolumellar vein 48f
Retromolar trigone 16
Reye's syndrome 297
Rheumatic heart disease 43
Rheumatoid arthritis 578
Rhinitis 33, 34
    acute 34
    caseosa 35
    chronic 35
    medicamentosa 35
    sicca 35
Rhinoscopy
    anterior 14, 14f, 37, 38, 53, 54, 55
    posterior 15, 15f, 55
Rhinosinusitis 37, 55
Rhythm shockable 641
Rib fractures 579
Ribbon retractors 103
Riboflavin 193
Richter scale earthquakes 549
Right eye 153f, 161f
    adduction deficit 176f
    congenital severe ptosis 121f
    esotropia 212f
    exotropia 207f
    hypertropia 207f
    hypotropia 207f
    lower eyelid entropion 121f
    suppression 205f
Rigler's triad 716
Ring ulcer 133f
Ringer's lactate 317
Rinne's test 12, 13f
Risperidone 661
Rituximab 441, 578
Rivastigmine 426, 427
Rods and cones 170
Romberg's test 267
Rovsing's sign 715
Rufinamide 370
Rule of Nine 449, 449f
Ruptured aneurysm, bleeding from 276

S

Sabouraud dextrose agar 131
Saccades 175, 188
Saccadic system 175
Safe care 678
Safe surgery saves lives 678, 687
    program 681
Safe surgical teams 683
Saint's triad 716
Salbutamol 409
Salicylate 286
    toxicity, chronic 286
Saline, normal 317
Saliva, artificial 512
Salmeterol 409
Salpingo-oophorectomy 474
Sarcoidosis 124, 181
Scala media, endolymph of 4

Scald injury 448
Schiotz tonometer 97f
Schuller's view 14
Schwalbe's line 139
Schwannoma 345
Sclera 89, 224
 disorders of 164, 165
 inflammations of 165
Scleral spur 139
Scleral wounds, management of 225
Scleritis 165
 anterior 165
 diffuse anterior 165f
 non-necrotizing 165
Sclerosis, multiple 438
Sclerotic hypermature cataract 118
Scotoma, large 205
Screamer's node 64
Sebaceous cell carcinoma 121
Seborrheic keratosis 589
Sedation 298, 299, 316
Sedative 418
See-saw nystagmus 189
Seizures 257, 286, 341, 360, 368, 378, 493
 absence 368
 activity 309
 classification of 368
 clonic 368
 focal 368
 generalized 368
 post-traumatic 316
 prophylaxis 316
 types of 368, 369
Self-care 704
 difficulty with 584
 practices 701
Self-inflating bag 640
Senescent bone loss 566
Senile cataract 118
Senile retinoschisis 162
Senior Citizen Saving Scheme 604, 608
Sensation 587
 loss of 492
Sense of smell 15
 decreased 587
Sense of taste, decreased 587
Sense organs 582
Sensors 203, 635
Sensory conditions, age-related 587t
Sensory deficit nystagmus 188
Sensory deprivation 308
 amblyopia 210
Sensory disturbances 389
Sensory dysfunction 440
Sensory esotropia 212, 213
Sensory evaluation 202, 270
 tests for 205
Sensory evoked responses 440
Sensory exotropia 213
Sensory functions 265
 assessment of 269t
Sensory ganglionopathy 280
Sensory incomplete 320
Sensory perception 246
 disturbed 417
Sensory perceptual factors 62
Sensory problems 437
Sensory stimulation 292
Sepsis 287, 450
Septal correction, steps of 53
Septoplasty 53
Septum 14
Serologic testing 396

Serotonin 245
 syndrome 286
Serous otitis media 24
Serum 719
 lactate 451
 procalcitonin 277
Setubandhasanas 708
Sexual abuse 595
 warning signs of 596
Sexual assault 534, 535
 nurse examiner 534
Sexual dysfunction 440
Sexual habits 468
Sexual interest, continued 591
Shalabhasana 707
Shiotz indentation tonometer 139f
Shock 378, 450
 circulatory 167
 distributive 454
 hypovolemic 476
 neurogenic 312, 716
 septic 454
Shoulder fractures 579
Siderosis 226
Siegerts streaks 151
Silent cough 66
Silicone sponge 159
Silicosis 667
Sinemet 432
Singer's node 64
Single cadaver donor 689
Single-fiber electromyography 396
Single-word testing 63
Sinus
 disorder of 361
 plate 14
Sinusitis 33, 37, 53
Sinusoidal gratings 186
Sixth nerve 178
 anatomy 180f
Sjögren's syndrome 149
Sjögren's triad 716
Skeletal fracture reduction 322
Skilled activities, execution of 259
Skin 478
 artificial 455
 barrier loss 449
 cancer 589
 changes 470, 588f
 contamination 527
 disorders 669
 dry 589
 integrity 661
 prick test 37
 reactions, minimize radiation 479b
 sparing mastectomy 474
 tags 589
 thinning 589
Skull fractures 313
Sleep
 disordered breathing, development of 58
 disturbances 428, 584
 hygiene 428
Sleepiness 370
Slight reverse ptosis 184f
Slit-lamp 99f, 139f
 biomicroscopy 99
 examination 112, 116
Small incision
 cataract surgery 118
 lenticule extraction 135
Small intestine 574
Smart home automation 625

Smart pill dispensers 625
Smell 582
 loss of 14, 584
Smoker, chronic 127f
Smoking, avoiding 590
Snail tract degeneration 162
Snakebite 533
Snellen visual acuity chart 95f
Snellen's chart 185f
Social anxiety disorder 703
Social isolation 592, 595
Sociological theories 562
Sodium
 bicarbonate 657, 659
 channel inactivation 370
 fluorescein 167
 level, change in 340
 potassium pump 244
 valproate 370
Soft palate 16
 infiltration 510
Soiled linen, collection of 633
Solar lentigines 589
Solid silicone band 159
Sonata systems 81
Sound pressure waves 4
Spaeth Richman contrast sensitivity test 186
Spasmus nutans 189
Spaulding's classification 104, 104t
Spectacle correction, prescription of 112
Speculum, examination 11
Speech 61, 259, 324, 399, 442
 audiometry 77
 defect 61, 62
 difficulties 399f
 disorder 61, 62
 geriatric considerations in 69
 generating devices 626
 motor processes 62
 reading 71, 83
 sound disorder 62f, 63
 therapy 61, 63, 435, 437
Sperm quality 581
Sphenoid 15
Spinal column 354f
Spinal cord 251, 252, 323, 354f
 compression 491
 lesions 279
 thoracic level of 492
 transverse section of 252f
 tumor, pathophysiology of 354f
Spinal cord injury 318
 complete 311, 320
 incomplete 312
 pathophysiology of 320fc
 types of 311, 319f
Spinal disorders, degenerative 280
Spinal dura 249, 249t
 mater 249
Spinal injuries 320f
Spinal nerve 254
 number of 254t
 root compression 280
Spinal reflexes 252
Spinal shock 312
Spinal tumor 353
 primary 356
 symptoms of 355
 treatment of 355
 types of 353, 353t, 354f
Spine
 board 522f
 fractures 579

magnetic resonance imaging of 440
stabilization 356
X-rays 355
Spinothalamic pathway, lateral 251
Spiral ganglia 4*f*
Spirochetes 181
Split thickness skin graft 447, 455*f*
Split transplant 690
Squamous cell carcinoma 121
Squamous papilloma 121, 123
Squint 200, 203, 205*f*, 206
    accommodative 207*f*
    causes of 201
    comitancy of 208*f*
    latent 200
    measurement of 209
    surgery, caliper for 219*f*
Stapedectomy 71
Staphylococci aureus 382
Staphylococcus 34, 131, 133, 181, 454
    aureus 24, 25, 377, 454, 500
    hemolyticus 649
    proteins 133
Stargardt disease 152, 161, 161*f*
Status dystonicus 410
Status epilepticus 286, 372
Status migrainosus 360
Steatohepatitis, nonalcoholic 574
Steele-Richardson-Olszewski syndrome 176
Stenosis 276
Stereo-butterfly test 206*f*
Stereognosis 269
Stereopsis testing 205
Stereotactic radiosurgery 306, 356
Sterilization 103, 104
    types of 104
Steroid 54, 168, 298, 492
    therapy, role of 168
Stethoscope 522
Stevens-Johnson syndrome 148, 149
Stomatitis 512
Strabismic amblyopia 211
Strabismus 99, 200
    incomitant 214
    measurement of 209
    restrictive 214*t*
    surgery 219
Strauss syndrome 55
Streptococci 382
    viridans 500
Streptococcus 34, 131, 181
    aureus 23
    group B 377
    pneumoniae 23, 76, 377, 500
    pyogenes 500
Streptomycin 193
Stress 700, 701
    disorder, post-traumatic 703
    ergonomic-related 669
    fractures 280
    management of 590, 702
    occupational 667
    related illnesses 700
    ulcers, prophylaxis for 318
Stretch reflex 252
Stridor 43, 51
Stroke 198, 281, 327, 338, 584
    acute 335
    diagnostic evaluation of 332*f*
    epidemiology of 328
    hemorrhagic 328, 328*f*, 332*f*, 335, 584
    ischemic 177, 328, 328*f*, 332*f*, 584
    pathophysiology of 330*fc*

risk factors of 329*f*
signs of 584
site 330*f*
symptoms of 584
types of 328
unit 330
Stroma 89, 130
Stromal dystrophies 133
Subarachnoid hemorrhage, diffuse 339*f*
Subdural hematoma 313, 314, 315*f*
Subepithelial dystrophy 133
Subglottic anomalies 63
Subglottic hemangioma 50, 63
Subglottic stenosis 50
Subpial transection, multiple 305, 370
Sulcus vocalis 66, 66*f*
Superior oblique paralysis, left 179*f*
Superior orbital fissure syndrome 180, 181, 181*f*
Superior vena cava syndrome 494
Supportive therapy 169
Suppression 200, 204
Supraglottic anomalies 63
Supranuclear gaze palsy 176
Supranuclear palsy, progressive 198
Surgery
    choice of 219
    indications for 217, 218
    psychological effects of 476
    timing of 117
Surgical care procedures, unsafe 680
Surgical instruments 103
    cleaning of 104
Surgical oncology focuses 473
Surgical procedure 118, 128
Surgical safety 678
Surgical site infection 680
    prevention of 683
Swallowing therapy 442
Swan-Ganz catheter 647
Swap transplants 690
Swelling 470
Swinging flashlight test 187, 187*f*
Switch-activated devices 626
Symblepharon 150, 222
Sympathetic adrenomedullar axis 701
Sympathetic nervous system 254
    activity 702
    function of 254*b*
Sympathetic visual system 184, 184*f*
Synapses, types of 244
Syncope 569
    management of 289
Syndrome of inappropriate antidiuretic hormone secretion 496
Synechiae 164
Synoptophore 210, 211*f*
Synthesis 370
Syphilis 124, 191
Systemic skeletal disease 578
Systemic vascular resistance 694

T

T cell function, decreased 590
Tachyphylaxis 491
Tacrolimus 109, 409
Tactile ability, age-related changes in 587*f*
Tactile agnosia 259
Tamoxifen 193, 409
Tamsulosin 119
Tandem gait 256
Tardive dyskinesia 411
Tarry stools 484

Taste 582
    and smell, changes in 479
    sensitivity 582
Tau proteins 423
Taxanes 483
Tear
    artificial 109
    film 145
Technological hazards originate 538
Teeth, malocclusions of 62
Telangiectasia 479
Telescopes 231
Teletherapy 473
Temperature 258, 269
    control 317
    monitoring equipments 522
    senses 492
Temporal bone 14*f*
Temporomandibular joint 14
Tendon reflex 252
    deep 268*t*, 270
Tenon's capsule 89
Tenonplasty 222
Tensilon test 197, 395
Tentorium cerebelli 249
Testicular androgen production, lower 482
Testosterone deficiency 582
Tetraplegia 312
Text-to-speech apps and software 626
Thalamotomy 432
Thalamus 246, 380
    functions of 246
Thalidomide 409, 480
Thallium 193
Theophylline 409
Therapeutic hypothermia 299
Therapeutic recreation specialists 324
Thermal ablation 370
Thermal emergencies 528
Thermal injury 222, 448
Thermoregulation 291
Thiamine 193
    deficiency 716
Thioridazine 409
Third nerve
    anatomy 177*f*
    palsy 214, 217
    paresis 217
Thoracic injuries 320
Thoracic nerves 254
Thorax 479, 480*t*
Throat 16
    pain 16
Thrombectomy 306
Thrombocytopenia 484, 489
Thrombolysis 333, 335
    complications of 335
Thrombolytic therapy 584
Thrombosis 499
Thumb sign 41*f*
Thymus
    gland, removal of 197
    involution 588
Thyroid
    function 576
    hormones, overproduction of 580
    orbitopathy 181, 217
Thyroidectomy 474
Thyrotropin-releasing hormone 322
Tiagabine 370
Tic 411
    douloureux 414
Tick bite 533

Timolol 109
Tingling 257
Tinnitus 19, 26-28, 418, 587
Tiotropium 572
Tissue destruction 465
T-lymphocytes 465
TNO test 206f
Tocilizumab 578
Toe
    tapping 266
    walk 267
Tolosa Hunt syndrome 181
Tongue 16
    base of 16
    blade 257
    tie 62
Tonic clonus 368
Tonic seizures 368
Tonic-clonic seizures 368
Tonometers 139f
Tonometry 136, 138
Tonsil 16, 42
Tonsilitis 33
Tonsillar herniation 295
Tonsillar pillar, anterior 42
Tonsillectomy 43
    complications of 43
Tonsillitis 42
    acute 42, 42f, 43
    chronic 42, 43, 43f
Tonsilloliths 43
Topical bacteriostatic agents 456
Topiramate 370
Torchlight eye examination 97
Tortuous optic nerve sheath 196f
Tourette syndrome 410
Toxic
    alcohol ingestion 286
    optic neuropathy 193
Toxins 286
Toxoplasmosis 192
Trabeculectomy 136
Tracheostomy 51
Trachoma 147, 231
Transcalvarial herniation 295
Transcranial Doppler flow tests 285
Transfer policy 636
Transfusion practices, unsafe 685
Transient ischemic attack 328
Transplantation of Human Organ Act 692
Transplantation of Human Organs and Tissues Act 689
Transplants, types of 690f, 691fc
Trauma 585
Traumatic brain injury
    mild 314t
    moderate to severe 314t
    pathophysiology of 314fc
Traumatic mydriasis 224
Tremor 257, 405, 409
    drug-induced 409
    essential 409
    supportive management of 410
Treponema 181
    pallidum hemagglutination 191
Triamterene 418
Triazoles 378
Trichiasis 121
Trichloroacetic acid 48
Trigeminal nerve 414
Trigeminal neuralgia 414
Trikonashana 706
Triptans 364
Trochlear nerve 262
    palsy 215

Tropicamide 167
Trotter's method 48, 48f
Trousseau's sign 715
Trunk 178
    stability of 266
Tsunami 539
Tubercular meningitis 377
Tuberculosis 124, 191
Tumbling e-chart 95
Tumor 149f, 279, 344, 466
    axial 344
    category 466
    cells, survival of 466
    extra-axial 344, 345
    grading 467
    histological type of 347
    infratentorial 345
    location of 467
    lysis syndrome 495
    malignant 345
    marker 467, 721
    necrosis factor-alpha inhibitors 578
    primary 345
    resection 356
    staging 57t
    supraglottic 56
    supratentorial 345
    types of 128
Tuning fork 257
    tests 12, 12t
Tympanic cavity 14
Tympanic membrane 4, 12f
    examination of 11
    perforation 22, 22
    right 12f
Tympanograms, types of 78f
Tympanometry 77
Tympanoplasty 23
Typoscope 232

U

Ulcers, pressure 686
Uncover test 208
Universal Eye Health Plan 235
Unruptured cerebral aneurysms, prevalence of 341
Up-gaze palsy 177
Upper airway
    infections 33
    obstruction 47
Upper extremity, swinging 265
Upper lid, left 122f
Upper motor neuron 252
    lesions 252t
Upper respiratory airway, trauma of 47
Uremic encephalopathy 287
Urge incontinence 576
Urinary bladder changes 470
Urinary catheter infections, catheter-associated 649
Urinary incontinence 576
Urinary retention 285, 292
Urinary system 574
    age-related changes in 575f
    conditions, age-related 575tt
Urinary tract infection 287, 291, 575
    catheter-associated 653, 680
    risk of 575
Urine
    chemistry, normal values 717
    output, decreased 450
Ursodeoxycholic acid 574
Ustrasana 707

Uvea
    disorders of 164, 165
    inflammation of 165
Uveal tissue, disorders of 165
Uveitic cystoid macular edema 168
Uveitis 165, 166
    acute anterior 167fc
    anatomical classification of 166
    anterior 165, 166
    complications of 166
    granulomatous anterior 166f
    intermediate 165, 166
    posterior 165, 166, 167f
    sequelae of 166
    surgical management of 168

V

Vaccination 590, 615
Vaginal atrophy 582
Vagus nerve 264, 371, 414
Vakrasana 707
Valproic acid 370, 409
van Herick method 139f
Van Riper's approach 68
Varicella zoster virus 132, 416
Vascular abnormalities 279
Vascular defects 499
Vascular disorders 151
Vascular endothelial growth factor 152
Vascular malformations 128
Vasomotor control, loss of 389
Vasomotor rhinitis 35
Vasopressors, use of 695
Veerabhadrasana 706
Veno-occlusive disease 488, 489
Venous thromboembolism 686
Venous thrombosis, deep 499
Ventilation 298
    positive pressure 634
Ventral spinocerebellar tracts 251
Ventricular fibrillation 632, 640
Ventricular tachycardia 632, 640
Ventriculoperitoneal shunt 384
    malfunction 286
Ventrolateral thalamus 409
Verapamil 365
Vergence 188, 200, 202
    system 175
Vertebra
    characteristics of typical 251
    parts of typical 251f
Vertebral column 251
Vertebral compression fractures 579
Vertebral decompression 323
Vertical diplopia 215
Vertical gaze palsy 176
Vertigo 418, 585
    attack, acute phase of 418
    benign paroxysmal positional 585
Vessels, rupture of 48
Vestibular nerve section 418
Vestibular neurectomy 418
Vestibular neuritis 585
Vestibular rehabilitation therapy 585
Vestibular suppressant 418
Vestibular system 175
Vestibule 14
Vestibulocochlear nerve 262
Vestibulo-ocular reflex 693
Vibratory senses, loss of 492
Victim's airway 639
Video calling devices 625
Vinca alkaloids 483

Vinca rosea 483
Vincristine 193
Vinke tongs 323f
Violence 534, 672, 673
Viral conjunctivitis 146
Viral hepatitis 574
Viral meningitis 378
Virchow's triad 716
Virus 181, 192, 465
Viscosity 108
Vision 582
 aids 620
 assessment 94
 blurred 116f, 297
 blurriness of 257
 double 297
 impairment, causes of 231
 loss of 172, 185
 physiology of 91
Visual acuity 93, 95, 297, 582
 decrease in 110
 testing 185
Visual agnosia 259
Visual cells, external layer of 90
Visual cortex 170, 175f
 causes of lesions of 174
 lesions of 174
 primary 172, 173f
Visual disturbances 297
Visual field 136
 defect 171f, 174f, 175f, 185
  types of 173f
 loss 297
 test 98
Visual fixation 175, 188
Visual impairment 592
Visual pathway 91
 afferent 170, 173t
 lesions of 172
Visual reinforcement audiometry 77
Visual system, immature 203
Visual-evoked
 potential 189, 191
 slow 440
Vital organ systems, hypoperfusion of 694
Vital signs 469, 525, 646
 monitor 366
Vitamin
 B_1 193
 B_{12} 193, 426
  deficiency 439
 B_2 193
 B_6 193
 B_9 193
 C 157

 consume adequate 428
 D 439
 deficiencies 585
 E 157
  deficiency 426
Vitelliform
 dystrophy 161
 lesions, adult-onset 152
Vitrectomy, role of 169
Vitreomacular adhesion 158
Vitreomacular traction syndrome 158
Vitreoretinopathy, familial exudative 159
Vitreous 226
 disorders of 151
 tap, diagnostic 168
Vocal cord
 cyst 65
 immobility 63
 paralysis 50, 63
 swelling 341
Vocal fold 8
 length of 65f
 nodule 64f
 polyps 64
 right 64f
Vocal function exercises 67
Vocal hygiene program 66
Vocal nodule 64
Vocational rehabilitation 442
Vogt's striae 134
Voice 61
 disorder 63
 rest 66
Voice therapy 66
 accent method of 67
 hygienic 66
 symptomatic 67
Volcanic eruptions 541
Vomiting 483, 510, 512
von Willebrand's disease, acquired 499
Voriconazole 109, 132
Vossius ring 224
Vrikshasana 706

W

Waterhouse-Friderichsen syndrome 378
Wave
 alpha 275
 beta 275
 obliteration of 275
 theta 275
Weakness 257
Wear-and-tear theory 561
Weber's test 13, 13f

Wegener's granulomatosis 181
Weight loss 513
Weisenberg syndrome 419
Wernicke's encephalopathy 189, 287, 716
West Nile encephalitis 380
Whipple's surgery 475, 475f
Whipple's triad 716
Whisper test 262
White blood
 cell 278
 chemistry 719
Widespread disease 466
Withdrawal reflex 252
Wolf Parkinson white syndrome 716
Wong Beker pain scale 510
Word recognition score 77
Worsening dystonia, monitor 410
Worsening muscle weakness 197
Worth four dot test 205, 205f
Wound
 appearance of 448
 care, surgical management of 452
Wrist fractures 579

X

Xanthelasma 121, 122, 123f
Xenograft 690
Xenotransplantation 690
Xerophthalmia 149
Xerosis 149, 589
Xerostomia 463, 479, 512
X-linked recessive disorder 400
Xylometazoline 24

Y

Yoga 699, 701-704, 710
 diverse applications of 705
 exploration of 700
 instructor, qualified 704
 interventions, benefits of 711
 nursing studies 705
 practice 705
Young's procedure 35

Z

Zafirlukast 37
Zeaxanthin 157
Zinc oxide 157
Zipper pulls 623
Zonisamide 370

EU GSPR Authorised Reprsentative
Logos Europe, 9 rue Nicolas Poussin
1700, La Rochelle, France
Phone: +33 (0) 6 67 93 73 78
E-mail: contact@logoseurope.eu

www.ingramcontent.com/pod-product-compliance
Ingram Content Group UK Ltd.
Pitfield, Milton Keynes, MK11 3LW, UK
UKHW051847210426
5322IPUK00019B/287